THE JOURNAL
OF
PEDIATRICS

A MONTHLY JOURNAL DEVOTED TO THE PROBLEMS AND DISEASES OF INFANCY AND CHILDHOOD

Official Organ for The American Academy of Pediatrics

VOLUME 13
JULY—DECEMBER, 1938

ST. LOUIS
THE C. V. MOSBY COMPANY
1938

1954

Printed in the
United States of America

Press of
The C. V. Mosby Company
St. Louis

The Journal of Pediatrics

Vol. 13 JULY, 1938 No. 1

Original Communications

PRESIDENTIAL ADDRESS

Philip Van Ingen, M.D.
New York, N. Y.

IT IS my privilege to open this general session of the Eighth Annual Meeting of the American Academy of Pediatrics. Those who are here represent 1,229 recognized pediatrists from forty-seven states of the Union, the District of Columbia, Hawaii, and five Provinces of Canada. To have been elected president of such an organization is an honor of honors, and I thank you most humbly for having placed on my unworthy shoulders the mantle worn by my distinguished predecessors.

Since our last meeting, two of our most valued fellows have passed from our circle. It is just and fitting that a word of appreciation should be recorded here.

In the death of Dr. Barnet E. Bonar, the Academy has lost one of its early and most assiduous workers.

Dr. Bonar was a member of the first regional committee of Region IV. He took a great deal of interest in the Academy and was especially active in the work in Utah and Idaho.

Dr. Bonar did not confine his work to pediatrics but did a large amount of obstetrics and as a consequence would not, under present conditions, be eligible for membership in the Academy, but his chief interest was always pediatrics and his investigative work was confined to pediatric subjects, especially concerning the newborn infant.

In a region where very little investigative work has ever been done, Dr. Bonar, by his industry and persistence, succeeded in turning out several very good pieces of work. He became nationally known as a result of this work and several years before he died was elected to membership in the American Pediatric Society. His was a genial, placid character, of rare good humor and the friendliest of spirits. He was an excellent clinician, and his patients loved him. His colleagues trusted him as is indicated by his various positions in the local com-

---

Presented at the Eighth Annual Meeting of the American Academy of Pediatrics, Del Monte, Calif., June 11, 1938.

munity where he was on the Utah State Board of Health and had been secretary of the Salt Lake County Medical Society.

The Academy and the members of the Academy have lost a friend in the tragic death of Dr. Bonar, and we cannot but feel his loss when we gather together, especially in this western country.

Dr. Louis Schroeder's life was one of ceaseless, unfaltering effort to make the most of his opportunities and to do his bit. With no backing but his own indomitable courage, he passed from high school to a job in a carriage factory. By hard work he saved enough money and studied enough at night to obtain admission to the College of Physicians and Surgeons in New York, from which he graduated in 1911. His ability won immediate recognition, and after serving in medicine as intern at Bellevue Hospital and in pediatrics as intern and resident, he was picked by such men as John Howland and Oscar Schloss for important administrative and teaching positions. He was intensely practical, and it was that characteristic which attracted students and patients. Always abreast of the times, he applied knowledge where it would do the most good.

Louis Schroeder gave freely of all he had, too freely for his own health. Utterly fearless, he fought every wrong or reactionary force he met. He gave his best to this Academy as a regional chairman, to his hospital, to the American Child Health Association, to the Boy Scouts, in the reorganization of whose health work he was actively engaged up to the time of his death, and to many other activities. He loved children, understood them, and served them well.

Besides all of this work he was an omnivorous reader on many subjects, an ardent student of Shakespeare, an eager and appreciative listener to music, and a sculptor of merit. He was a founder and an active booster of the Physicians' Art Exhibition held every year at the New York Academy of Medicine.

Never afraid, he always took a strong stand for what he thought right, but withal he was tolerant and fair. With a fine sense of humor, a knack for telling stories, and a cheerful disposition, he will be missed by a host of friends. It may be truly said of him that the world was a little better for his having lived.

This general meeting is held to hear the reports of the regional chairmen and those of special committees, to evaluate the work done, and, looking ahead, to consider what we shall do next to carry out our specific purposes: (a) to establish and maintain the highest possible standards for pediatric education in medical schools and hospitals, pediatric practice, and research; (b) to perpetuate the history and best traditions of pediatric practice and ethics; (c) to maintain the dignity and efficiency of pediatric practice in its relationship to public welfare; (d) to promote publications and encourage contributions to medical and scientific literature pertaining to pediatrics.

These reports have all been distributed to you, and I hope you will read them through from start to finish; they are well worth it. And what is more to the point, these reports are presented to *you,* not to the Executive Board. This is your Academy, not the Executive Board's. The fellowship as a whole is strangely and often discouragingly silent concerning what has been done and what might well be undertaken. The Executive Board exists to carry out your wishes as far as it is practicable to do so. It would like more suggestions from you. Dr. Morse warned you in his presidential address that what you get out of the Academy will be according to what you put in.

This is the first and last time that I shall address you as president and, before I return to a peaceful fellowship in the Academy, I want to call your attention to certain parts of some of those reports, and to make a suggestion or two.

Committee on Immunization Procedures.—I feel that Dr. Toomey's committee has done a great service to the fellows of the Academy and to the profession at large by its frank, brief report. None of us are more familiar with the evidence concerning the results of immunization than the members of that committee. They have presented a statement of our actual proved knowledge on these various procedures and, while some of us may be more optimistic concerning certain methods than they are, they have helped us to make our own decisions or to keep our minds open.

Many of us are pestered by conscientious but overenthusiastic parents to carry out all kinds of preventive procedures, some of which we do not approve. One friend of mine tells me he carries this report about with him in his bag to show to parents when overpressed.

I hope the committee will be continued and will be asked, as occasion demands, to submit any changes which should be made. The Academy should make this a "loose-leaf" or "living" document for the guidance and help of its fellows.

It has been suggested, and may be well, that we should prepare and distribute similar reports on methods concerning which such all-embracing claims are made, about certain vitamins, for instance. This is an activity which should be developed.

Committee on Contact Infections.—This committee was appointed by the Executive Board at its December meeting, on the initiative of Dr. Fairfax Hall. He called the attention of the Board to the need for our action. It is a complicated problem, but that it can be met is shown by the success in Westchester County, N. Y.; Knoxville, Tenn.; Newark, N. J.; and other places.

We are all of us only too familiar with the tragic results of exposure of children to infection from their nurses, relatives, and household servants. Dr. Hall has traveled across the continent to present this report, and it is worthy of your careful consideration, discussion, and action. I can think of no more valuable contribution to preventive medicine which this Academy could make than to initiate a campaign such as he outlines. We should not need more evidence than the Knoxville experience, of which he will tell you.

School Health and School Health Education.—Last year Dr. Mitchell's committee presented a report of deep interest which caused much comment. The report this year is of equal importance. The problem of the health of the school child is a very difficult and complicated one. It is one that vitally interests us as an Academy and individually. Over forty-five years ago we began to realize it was a problem. In 1892, New York City appointed one public medical school officer. I am afraid there was more gesture or politics in that than real effort. Two years later Boston appointed fifty physicians, one for each school district, to inspect children for the detection of contagious disease. Chicago became enthusiastic in 1895 and divided the city into nine districts, appointing one inspector for each district, for the same purpose. As each district covered approximately twenty square miles, the effectiveness of the plan may be imagined. In 1897, five years after the appearance of its lone medical school officer, New York City appointed 134 medical inspectors to visit each school daily, again to exclude infectious diseases. Vermont was the first state to officially go further when, in 1903, it passed a law requiring an annual examination of the eyes, ears, and throats of all school children. And so it has gone on—ever increasing in personnel involved and in the millions spent each year throughout the country in discovering physical defects. That is fairly easy; but there the progress has broken down, for the correction of those defects, which should be the object, is a difficult problem. It requires the cooperation of school principal, schoolteacher, school physician, school nurse, *and* parent, *and* private physician. It involves a clash of authority—a division of responsibility.

Ten years or more ago the American Child Health Association carried on a series of investigations on the health of school children, and as a result a continuation study was made by it with funds provided by the Metropolitan Life Insurance Company. The report, entitled "Physical Defects, the Pathway to Correction," was published in 1934 and aroused much interest. Professor Rogers, Dean of Student Health and Physical Education of Boston University, said: "The very least consequence of its publication should be a complete overhauling of medical examination and follow-up services in practically every school in the land."

But the trouble is, how are you going to improve it? It is an intensely practical problem and one that can be solved in its details only by careful trial and retrial. Fortunately, it is being tried out by practical and analytical experts in a limited district in New York City from funds provided from three sources. The interest, cooperation, yes, enthusiasm of the various groups concerned has been secured; each individual step in procedure is studied, new methods tried out in the experimental schools, improved, and then, owing to the interest and splendid cooperation of the Departments of Health and Education, which share the responsibility in New York City, is or will be gradually extended to the whole school system. I mention these New York activities chiefly because Dr. Mitchell participated in all the original studies mentioned and now is district health officer where this tryout is being carried on. He can speak with authority in the report he has presented. The most interesting address I could have made to you, were it permissible, would have been to read you the "Progress Report" of this demonstration, presented to the directing committee by Dr. Dorothy Nyswander, the executive director, two weeks ago.

Until we have a system which has been tried out and proved practicable, we shall blunder on, in the hit or miss method, doing as much effective work as possible. The formation of the American School Health Association is a recognition of the complexity of the problem and the necessity for team work. Succeeding reports from Dr. Mitchell's committee will be awaited with much interest.

Committee on Mental Hygiene.—This whole subject has been one which has baffled us for years. In the White House Conference on Child Health and Protection there was a committee on psychology and psychiatry, of which Dr. Bronson Crothers was chairman. He worked very hard to produce a report which would be constructive, but as far as he and his committee could get was to present "The Problem."

Dr. Beverly's committee has presented a program, and it is to be hoped that a formal course in mental growth and development may be given in our medical schools, but it must be a course given in medical words of one syllable. Dr. Beverly will present this report. It is a very valuable one because it has a definite program to offer, and I believe the Academy should get behind it and push it hard. It is at least an attempt to improve an intolerable situation.

Medical Education.—One of the outstanding contributions of the Academy has been its work for the improvement of the character and scope of pediatric education. Dr. Veeder was chairman of the committee on that subject of the White House Conference, which made a most valuable report, and he, as chairman, and the members of our committee on medical education have rendered invaluable service. In medicine, as in everything else, with a change in ideas the pendulum tends to swing from one extreme to the other and only comes back to a reasonable position after a time.

Thirty-five years ago medical education consisted largely of didactic lectures, recitations, or quizzes, clinics on ambulatory patients, and a smattering of bedside instruction. We "walked the wards," as it was called long ago, a few times; we saw a few operations in a crowded amphitheatre if we could see. That was practically our medical education, apart from simple laboratory work of various kinds, and anatomy. Clinical clerkships were practically nonexistent. Bedside experience we obtained as interns. We went out with our heads very full of book knowledge and learned to apply it in the hospital. Today clinical clerkships are practically universal. That is as it should be. Laboratory work and research have been taking more and more of the time of the undergraduate student. So-called "book learning" has become less and less emphasized. The pendulum has swung a long way. Has it swung too far? I think it has. From my experience of a good many years in examining candidates for internship in a general hospital, I have been increasingly impressed and depressed by the often pathetic lack of knowledge of the principles of medicine and the symptomatology of disease.

Only this past spring a young man came up for examination for internship, concerning whom letters had been received which were very laudatory, and several were personal letters ending, "I really mean this." That man was asked, in oral examination, to give the symptoms of typhus fever. He paused a moment and very calmly replied, "I'm sorry, I am afraid I can't. I never saw a case of typhus fever." And another, equally well recommended, gave as three of the most suggestive early symptoms of scarlet fever, "malaise, anorexia, and a rash."

And in our examinations for the American Board of Pediatrics I have been impressed by the woeful ignorance shown of the "art" of medicine. And I think many other examiners have also.

Several of my precedessors have called attention to this. Dr. Morse said: "The only danger I see is that in some of our Class A schools, in which many or most of the instructors have had no experience in practice, the student may be taught too much laboratory and too little bedside pediatrics. . . . Young men and women, entirely unsuited for research work, are urged to undertake *Arbeits* when they ought to be learning how to keep children well, how to find out what is the matter with them when they are sick, what to do about it, and finally, how to practice medicine. Some men have the scientific mind and are natural investigators. They cannot be kept away from investigation any more than a duck from water. They should be encouraged in every way. Puddles, ponds, and lakes should be provided for them according to their size and ability. Chickens and young turkeys do not like the water and are not intended to go in the water. Water is bad for them. They should therefore be kept on dry land and not forced into it."

Dr. John Ruhräh said, "In our devotion to the science of pediatrics we are liable to forget that it is also an art. The earlier pediatrists were all art and no science, and our present day graduates are likely to be all science and no art." He also said, "There should be two professors of pediatrics in every medical school, one to teach the science, and one to teach the art."

And let me finally quote a professor of applied physiology in one of our full-time universities. At a stated meeting of the New York Academy of Medicine last February he said: "One may occasionally wish that the premedical education of today might have more science, and the medical education less science and more art."

In the 1937 educational number of the *Journal of the American Medical Association* there are listed fifteen medical schools that require an internship before the degree is granted. During the years 1936 to 1937, 5,484 of the 5,836 graduates of the previous year were interning (nearly 95 per cent).

My experience may be different from that of others. I may be old-fashioned, but I feel that a very valuable contribution of the section on undergraduate education of our committee on medical education would be to investigate how much attention is paid to—for want of a better term—"book-learning." I believe that the medical graduate of my day knew more of the symptomatology of disease when he graduated than the present generation, and I think in that respect he was better equipped.

The American Board of Pediatrics.—The report of the three Academy members of the American Board of Pediatrics is a brief and formal one. It gives you a few facts but tells you little of its activity. I have been a member of that Board since its organization and, while I am accredited as a member of the American Pediatric Society, I would remind you that all nine members are fellows of the Academy.

In his address as our first president, Dr. Abt stated, "In the future deliberations of our organization it will become necessary to define the qualifications of a pediatric specialist."

The Academy accepted this responsibility and was the prime mover in the organization of the American Board of Pediatrics. That Board has done a prodigious amount of work, much of it extremely disagreeable. It has investigated carefully every person applying for certification. It has planned its examinations with care and given them in utter fairness. No candidate is examined by an examiner from his own immediate locality or by one whom he personally knows. The certification of 1,226 pediatrists has involved more hard work than you can fully appreciate, and the bulk of that work has fallen upon the Secretary, Dr. Aldrich.

I have mentioned the work of only a few of the committees. All have had important questions to deal with and all have done yeoman service.

What has the Academy done for us individually? Eight years ago there was no country-wide organization open to all qualified pediatrists and to them only. There was the pediatric section of the American Medical Association which was bringing scientific pediatric knowledge to the rank and file of the profession. Good work it has done and long may it continue to do so. There was the American Pediatric Society, a small group, which from the very nature of its organization could not possibly take in all qualified pediatrists, and then there were local groups, large and small, also doing excellent work, many of them, in developing better pediatrics in their own areas.

There were no standards for judging who should be considered as qualified to practice pediatrics as a specialty. I have mentioned our part in the founding of the American Board of Pediatrics. I believe its establishment of standards has been of real value to each one of us, and that it will become of greater importance in the years to come.

The annual meeting of the Academy has provided an opportunity for pediatrists from all over the country to meet together as pediatrists to discuss problems in an informal way at round tables and to present present knowledge, or our lack of it, on important subjects by panel discussions. Its regional meetings have taken up problems of special local interest or importance. All the facts brought out have been made available to the fellows, and to many others, through our Journal.

Besides giving all this information in permanent form, the Journal has provided a much needed addition to American pediatric literature. It does not conflict with other journals because not only is it primarily devoted to practical pediatrics, but the *American Journal of the Diseases of Children* cannot possibly publish all worth-while contributions.

The Academy has made a start in other services to our Fellowship. It has presented an authoritative statement on immunization procedures and will probably render other services along such lines.

It has attempted to help in the development of pediatric research, a field which has been exploited in the name of science to a serious degree, and has resulted in a great waste of money which could have been better used. The Council on Pediatric Research has had a difficult job but it has worked carefully, and we feel it is at a point where definite results may be expected.

In these and in other ways, trivial perhaps individually, but bulking large the Academy has given pediatrics a dignity and a unity which it never had before.

I have taken up enough of your time, perhaps too much. There are many other things I would like to have touched upon. You will hear the report of the executive board from Dr. Helmholz. May I be permitted to say that I entered that board two years ago a novice. It has been a liberal education. Many of its members have served you long, all have served you faithfully, and I have been deeply impressed by their loyalty, their devotion, and their hard work. One has to work on that board, for it has a stern taskmaster in Dr. Grulee; but its members don't mind his driving, for each and every one of us knows that he drives himself ten times harder than he drives us. He has mercy on us, occasionally, but he never has any mercy on himself.

And finally, may I repeat to you, Fellows of the Academy, this is your Academy. Your board and officers have tried to carry out what they think are your wishes. It is greatly to be hoped that your interest and participation will continue and that you will increasingly express your ideas and offer your suggestions. The older Fellows are getting older, so are the younger. We are well launched. It is time the younger men take more initiative.

THE EARLY LESIONS OF POLIOMYELITIS AFTER INTRANASAL INOCULATION

With Comments on Their Relationship to the Early Clinical Manifestations and to the Nonparalytic Cases

Harold K. Faber, M.D.
San Francisco, Calif.

At THE onset of human poliomyelitis certain signs and symptoms appear, almost, if not quite invariably, which are not referable to the spinal cord. Among these may be mentioned fever, vomiting, headache, drowsiness, irritability, affective disturbances, general hyperesthesia, and malaise. It is noteworthy that one or more of these manifestations occur in all recognizable cases of the disease irrespective of whether paralysis eventually develops or not. At this stage abnormalities of the spinal fluid are usually, though not always, present. The appearance of signs and symptoms of involvement of the spinal cord, when they occur, is separated from the manifestations of the onset by a definite interval which may be short or extend over a period of several days.

The origin of the early manifestations has been the subject of much debate. Until recently the theory has been widely popular that they are due to "systemic" or "general" infection without involvement of the central nervous system; that following the "systemic" infection the virus penetrates the choroid plexus and meninges and thus infects the central nervous system.[1] Serious and probably conclusive objections to the "systemic" theory, which have been reviewed elsewhere[2] and which are based on anatomic, pathologic, experimental, and clinical considerations, have led to its virtual abandonment by critical students of poliomyelitis. There remains, however, some disagreement as to the actual channels followed by the infecting virus in entering the body and reaching the spinal cord. It seems fair to state that at the present time the nasal-olfactory-nerve portal of entry is in better harmony with the available evidence and is open to fewer critical objections than others. There is general agreement that the virus is highly, if not exclusively, neurotropic and that preceding trauma (insect bites, lacerations, abrasions, etc.) is not a factor of etiological importance. If these considerations are correct, it is necessary to postulate an all-nerve route from the body surfaces into the central nervous system, and only one such route exists: the olfactory nerve ends in the nasal mucosa, which are actually exposed on the

From the Department of Pediatrics, Stanford University Medical School.

Presented April 30, 1937, at the meeting of the American Pediatric Society, Hot Springs, Va.

This study was supported by a grant from the Rockefeller Fluid Research Fund.

surface and connect directly with the central nervous system. It is extremely important in applying the results of experimental work in poliomyelitis to the interpretation of the human disease to remember that no experimental method of inoculation that is dependent on trauma for success is reasonably comparable with the human infection. Certain rare exceptions, such as poliomyelitis following tonsillectomy[3] or prophylactic injections of imperfectly sterilized virus, definitely prove the rule. By such a criterion, the nasal route is the only one supported by adequate experimental evidence; and the others fail conspicuously. Animals can be infected regularly by nontraumatic methods by the nasal route[4] but not by other routes.

The probability that poliomyelitic virus enters the body by the olfactory route raises various interesting and practical questions: particularly, the neural routes by which virus eventually reaches the spinal cord, the lesions or reactions which may be set up along those pathways, and their relationship to the clinical manifestations of the onset and other early nonparalytic stages of poliomyelitis. A continuous route of invasion along nervous pathways alone, extending from the olfactory bulb through the brain stem and thence to the spinal cord, was demonstrated in a previous experimental study,[5] which also showed that a period of about three days elapsed between the appearance of virus in the olfactory bulb and its appearance in the spinal cord. During this interval, virus in large amounts was found in the brain stem. It was therefore suggested that the chief source of the early manifestations of poliomyelitis was the brain stem, particularly the diencephalon (thalamus, etc.).

Attention has been generally focused on the pathologic lesions of the spinal cord, and these have been held to be alone characteristic of poliomyelitis (the term itself denotes an inflammatory disease limited to the cord), so that the occurrence and importance of cerebral lesions are customarily forgotten or overlooked. The observations of Harbitz and Scheel[6] which, with those of E. Müller,[7] remain the most thorough histologic studies of the entire central nervous system in poliomyelitis available in medical literature, bear witness to the fact that inflammatory changes in human patients dying during the acute stage of the disease are constantly present in the central nervous system *above* the cord level, with marked intensity throughout the brain stem, which is involved to a relatively greater degree than the forebrain. These changes, to be sure, are largely perivascular and meningeal (small cell infiltrations and hyperemia) except in the medulla where gross nerve cell changes are not infrequent. Hurst[8] has shown, however, that such changes are in all probability secondary to primary neural invasion by the virus, as are the alterations in the cerebrospinal fluid.

Therefore, while it is probable that during the earliest period of clinical manifestations pathologic lesions are present in the brain stem, and during this period the disease is really an encephalitis which becomes during the ensuing stages an encephalomyelitis, actual proof that this is true cannot be obtained from human material because patients do not die during the initial stage. We have therefore attempted to obtain information on the point from animal experiment.

Since it is highly probable that under natural conditions poliomyelitis infection enters the body through the olfactory mucosa, the experiments have been designed on that basis.

PROCEDURE

Macacus rhesus monkeys were inoculated intranasally with MV virus by the method of Schultz and Gebhardt[4] and killed at various intervals after inoculation and after receiving injections of trypan blue according to the method, slightly modified, of McClellan and Goodpasture.[9] The average interval after intranasal inoculation and before paralysis in the monkey is a little more than eight days but there is considerable individual variation. Paralysis, while rare before the seventh day and usually present by the tenth, occasionally occurs as early as the fourth and as late as the twentieth day. Infection fails sometimes, but in less than 5 per cent of cases by the method used. Trypan blue stains most of the extranervous tissues but not the intrinsic nervous tissues in the normal animal. According to McClellan and Goodpasture,[9] who worked with herpetic encephalitis in rabbits, damaged nerve cells are stained by the dye given intravitally and hence areas of nerve cell damage become grossly visible. Our own observations which will be presented in detail in the protocols show that areas of capillary hyperemia, even without demonstrable damage to the nerve cells, also become grossly visible mainly from blue stain in the plasma of the distended loops. The time of appearance and distribution of macroscopically visible areas of blue staining in relation to the interval after inoculation, together with histologic changes in various parts of the central nervous system, have been investigated in the present study as a means of observing the evolution of the inflammatory process in the central nervous system during the preparalytic period of poliomyelitis.

One day before the time selected for killing the animal, 25 c.c. of a 1 per cent solution of trypan blue made up in sterile distilled water was given intramuscularly. This was usually done in the afternoon, and the next morning the skin and mucous membranes were found to be stained deep blue.

About two hours before killing, the monkey was given 25 c.c. of the same dye solution intravenously, or sometimes intraperitoneally, as in monkey 9. Some of the samples of dye proved to be toxic, and a number of specimens became useless, for in such cases, presumably because of toxic injury to nerve cells, all the gray matter in the central nervous system became intensely and uniformly stained blue. That this had nothing to do with the poliomyelitic infection itself was shown by the occurrence of the same phenomenon in an uninoculated animal intended for a control.

When toxic phenomena did not occur or were slight, the animal was killed under ether anesthesia about two hours later. The jugular veins were cut, and as much blood as would flow with the animal suspended head down was permitted to run out. The carotid arteries were then injected with as much 10 per cent neutral formalin solution as would run in easily by gravity, usually 50 to 75 c.c. This procedure gave an immediate fixation of the central nervous system and prevented post-mortem diffusion of the dye. The brain was then cut sagittally with a long knife into slices of about 2 mm. thickness. Portions of the cord from the cervical, thoracic, and lumbar regions were cut transversely, and other portions from the same regions, longitudinally, into sections of about the same thickness. The cut sections were then run through graded alcohols into absolute alcohol, then into benzene, and finally into a mixture of benzyl benzoate and artificial oil of wintergreen, in which they became transparent and were mounted; the procedure followed, with slight modifications, the Spalteholz technique.

In the control animal, uninoculated with virus, the central nervous tissues proper are unstained or merely show a trace of greenish color in the gray matter. In the inoculated animals a positive reaction is shown by the appearance of areas of definite blue color in the nerve substance, largely confined to the gray matter. For the sake of brevity in description, the intensity of blue staining (as viewed by the unaided eye by transmitted light) has been designated as follows: Grade 1, faint blue; Grade 2, moderate blue; Grade 3, marked blue; Grade 4, very intense blue.

Nearly all the extranervous tissues are stained by trypan blue. Thus, the dura mater was very deep blue; the leptomeninges, a faint blue; the choroid plexus and velum interpositum, a deep blue; the walls of the larger vessels, moderate blue; and the infundibulum of the hypophysis, a moderate blue. These changes occurred, of course, in the control as well as in the test animals.

Microscopic examination was made of several specimens from the control animal (No. 5), No. 6 (three days), No. 24 (four days), No. 9 (five days), and No. 3 (six days); and of a few from No. 4 (seven days), No. 13 (seven days), and No. 2 (nine days). Specimens were taken and examined from various parts of the brain and spinal cord. Stains used were hematoxylin and eosin, cresyl violet, Giemsa, and methylene blue and phloxin. A careful search was made for intranuclear inclusions, which were found only in No. 3 (6 days), and then mainly in the medulla.

The present report is based on the results obtained in eight animals, of which one, the control, was not inoculated with virus; one killed three days; one, four days; one, five days; one, six days; two, seven days; and one, nine days after inoculation. It is a matter of regret that, owing to various technical difficulties, the work could not be extended to afford duplicate studies of any except the seventh day, permitting a fuller sampling of variability, and that some of the specimens intended for microscopic examination were lost.

PROTOCOLS

CONTROL.—Monkey 5, not inoculated with virus, was given 25 c.c. of 1 per cent trypan blue solution intramuscularly on Nov. 24, 1935. On November 25, 25 c.c. of 1 per cent trypan blue solution were given intravenously at 5:30 P.M. The animal was killed two hours later under ether anesthesia by exsanguination, followed by injection of 75 c.c. of 10 per cent neutral formalin solution into the internal carotid arteries.

Gross inspection showed there is no bluish staining of the nervous tissue in brain or spinal cord. The dura mater is intensely blue and so are the choroid plexuses and velum interpositum. The infundibulum of the pituitary is likewise stained deep blue. Similar changes are seen in all the inoculated animals.

Microscopic Examination, Olfactory Bulb.—For purposes of comparison, the microscopic appearance of the normal animal after trypan blue injection is of interest. The pial meshes show no leucocytes or lymphocytes. In the substance, microglial cells are of rare occurrence. Most conspicuous is the large number of small glial nuclei, most of which appear to be oligodendroglia rather than astrocytes, in the mitral and other nerve cell layers. With heavy staining with hematoxylin and eosin, the characteristic chromatin dotting of these nuclei is obscured, and the cells may easily be mistaken for lymphocytes. In thick sections they may cover the nerve cells so that the latter are difficult to find. Visible capillaries are rather widely spaced.

Tissues from other portions of the central nervous system appear quite normal.

THREE DAYS' INCUBATION.—Monkey 6 was inoculated intranasally Jan. 17, 1936, and received intramuscular dye on January 19. Intravenous dye was given January 20, and the animal was killed about two hours later. No temperatures were taken. No paralysis was apparent.

Macroscopic Appearance.—One small spot (1 by 2 mm.) of Grade 2 staining is seen at about the position of the subthalamic nucleus, and faint to doubtful staining just above the roof of the descending cornu of the lateral ventricle. No other areas in brain and spinal cord show any trace of the dye.

Microscopic Examination.—The spinal cord only was examined and found to be normal.

Summary.—Early or doubtful localized reaction in inferior portion of interbrain, and amygdaloid nucleus.

FOUR DAYS' INCUBATION.—Monkey 24 was inoculated Sept. 23, 1936. On September 25 behavior was normal, and temperature 103.6° F. On September 26, behavior was normal, temperature, 104.1° F. Cisternal puncture revealed clear fluid, 108 cells per cubic millimeter. Trypan blue solution was given intramuscularly.

On September 27, behavior was normal; temperature, 104.7° F. At 2:30 P.M. trypan blue solution was given intravenously. At 4:00 P.M. under ether anesthesia, the carotid arteries were cut, exsanguination performed, and 10 per cent neutral formalin solution injected in the carotid.

Macroscopic Appearance.—The staining as a whole is heavy, and the gray matter throughout the central nervous system shows a faint greenish cast.

Olfactory bulbs are stained blue with more intense staining in a small spot in the anterior pole and more diffusely (Grade 2-3) in the posterior third up to the stalk.

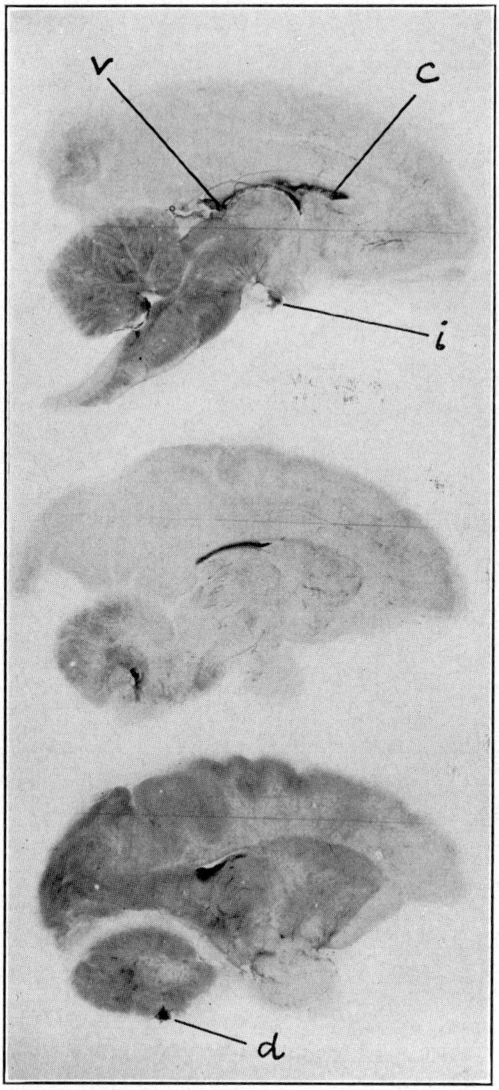

Fig. 1.—Uninoculated control, monkey 5. Blue staining is confined to the choroid plexus (*c*), velum interpositum (*v*), infundibulum (*i*) and a small bit of dura mater (*d*) adhering to the cerebellum. The darker areas in the top and bottom specimens are at places where the sections are thicker because of uneven cutting, and are not blue in the original.

In this and succeeding photographs, the top specimen is nearest the midline, the next below is the next laterally, and so on.

Forebrain: Grade 2 staining is limited to the mesial portions of the second and third temporal convolutions and, slightly more intense, to the uncinate gyrus. Just anterior and lateral to the exit of the optic nerve and below the anterior commissure an area of intense blue, about 1 by 2 mm., is probably the parolfactory area.

Corpus striatum is unstained except in one area about 6 by 2 mm. of very intense blue just above the descending cornu of the ventricle which occupies the position of the tail of the caudate nucleus and the amygdaloid nucleus.

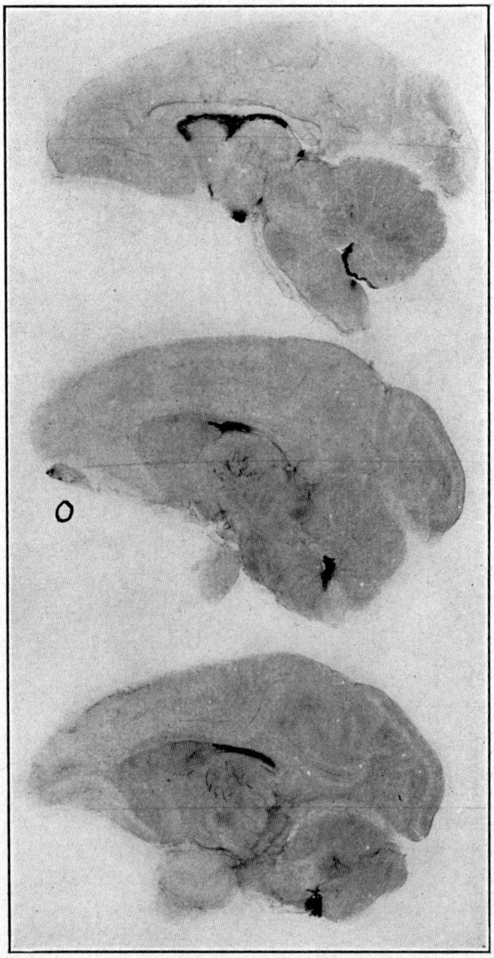

Fig. 2.—Five days' incubation, monkey 9, first stage. This animal had a slower rate of invasion than the four-day monkey (No. 24). That the first stage of reaction is represented here is shown by the fact that the olfactory bulb (*o*) is stained, and the remainder of the central nervous tissues is unstained.

Interbrain: The thalamus shows Grades 2 and 3 staining of the mesial, anterior, and lateral nuclei. Grade 1 staining is seen in the hypothalamic area (corpora mammillaria). The pulvinar is unstained.

Midbrain: The red nucleus is unstained. The corpora quadrigemina show Grade 1 staining. A narrow band of Grade 2 staining is seen just above the pons in the region of the substantia nigra.

Pons Varolii: Grade 4 staining, the most intense in the entire specimen, is seen in the ventral gray matter of the pons (nuclei pontis) over an area measuring 3 by 7 mm. extending from the midbrain level nearly to the medulla, and from a plane slightly lateral to the midline to or almost to the lateral boundaries of the pons. Dorsally, a narrow band of Grade 2 staining extends through the tegmental

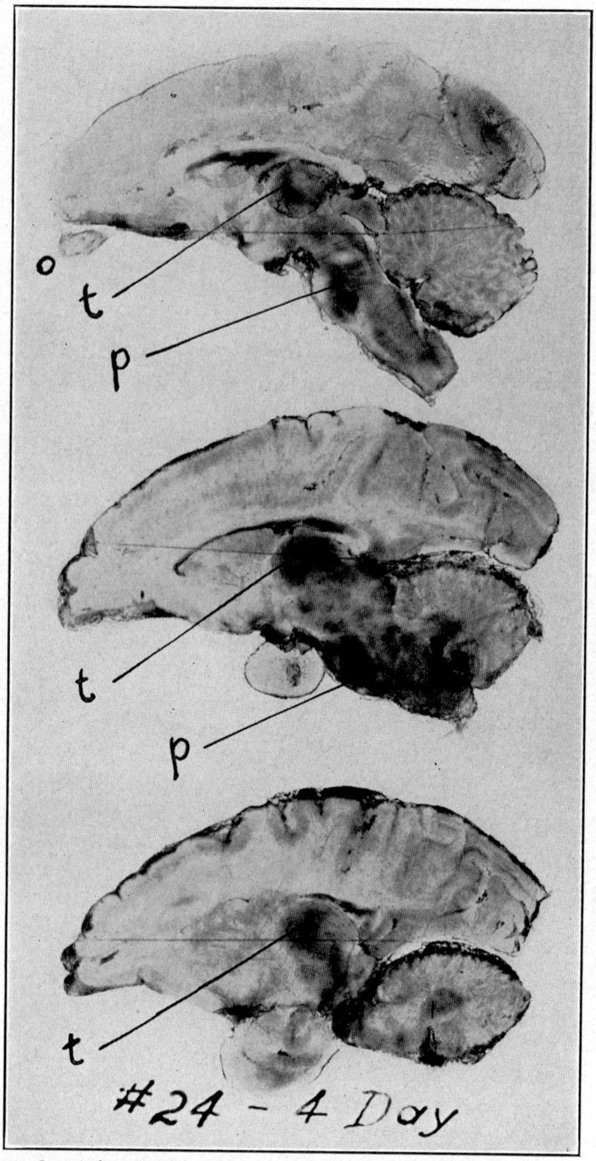

Fig. 3.—Four days' incubation, monkey 24. The dark areas are very deep blue. The olfactory bulb (*o*) in the original is bluer than the photograph shows. Note the particularly dense staining in the thalamus (*t*) and ventral region of the pons (*p*). The cerebral and cerebellar cortex is unstained.

region from the midbrain (continuous with the band of the substantia nigra) down to, and including, the floor of the fourth ventricle, and this is probably the formatio reticularis.

Medulla: Staining is less intense than in the pons. Besides the stained formatio reticularis just mentioned, there is an area of grade 1-2 staining about 1 by 5 mm. long and about 1 mm. inside the ventral margin in the region of the olivary body. The rest of the medulla is unstained.

Cerebellum: No blue staining.

Spinal Cord: No blue staining is visible anywhere in the gray or white matter of the cord. The dural covering of the roots and dorsal ganglia is intensely stained.

Microscopic Examination.—Olfactory Bulb: Throughout the substance and particularly in the glomerular and next two subjacent layers there is an enormous increase in the microglial (rod) cells. In the mitral cell layer these are clumped in places, suggesting neuronophagia, but a careful search failed to reveal degenerating nerve cells within the clumps. No nerve cells could, however, be found in any of the sections: whether they had entirely disappeared or were merely overlaid by the heavy infiltration of microglia could not be determined. In the pial meshes there is a heavy infiltration with lymphocytes and polymorphonuclear leucocytes, and some lymphocytes were also found scattered in the substance of the bulb.

Thalamus: There is marked capillary dilatation throughout. No perivascular infiltrations, no increase in microglia, no degenerated nerve cells are seen.

Cerebral Cortex: Some capillary dilatation but no other changes in the substance, meninges, or vessels are noted.

Pons (Ventral Region): There is conspicuous increase in the rod cells throughout the gray matter, also very marked dilatation of the capillary bed. The nerve cells appear normal. There are no perivascular or meningeal infiltrations.

Medulla: No changes are apparent other than a slight or doubtful increase in the rod cells.

Spinal Cord: No abnormalities are noted.

Summary.—Selective localizations of trypan blue staining were in the olfactory bulbs, olfactory areas of the forebrain, thalamus, pons and (slight) in the medulla. There were no localizations in the remainder of the cerebral cortex, in the cerebellum, or in the spinal cord. Microscopic changes were seen in the olfactory bulb, in which they are more advanced than elsewhere, in the thalamus, and in the ventral region of the pons. Invasion by rod cells (microglia) is notable.

FIVE DAYS' INCUBATION.—Monkey 9, inoculated intranasally on July 17, 1936, behaved normally throughout experiment. Temperatures were as follows: July 18, 101.0° F.; July 21, 101.7° F.; July 22, 103.4° F. On July 21, trypan blue solution was given intramuscularly; July 22, 9 A.M., 25 c.c. trypan blue was given intraperitoneally, and at 1 P.M., 10 c.c., intravenously. At 4 P.M. the monkey was killed by exsanguination under ether anesthesia; 10 per cent neutral formalin solution was injected in the carotids.

Macroscopic Appearance.—The dura, choroid plexuses, velum interpositum, and infundibulum show the usual deep blue staining. Both olfactory bulbs in their rostral halves show streaks of Grade 2-3 of blue staining. None of the other portions of the brain or spinal cord substance shows any staining at all, with the possible exception of the amygdaloid nucleus in which a very faint bluish tinge is barely visible. The specimen is unusually good in that it shows none of the greenish tint seen in several of the other specimens in unaffected areas, which is probably due to toxic effects of the dye itself.

Microscopic Examination.—Olfactory Bulb: Moderate capillary dilatation is seen in several places. There are a few areas in and near the glomerular layer which show a distinct increase of microglial cells. Meningeal infiltration is absent. The nerve cells appear normal.

The tissues from other portions of the central nervous system appear entirely normal.

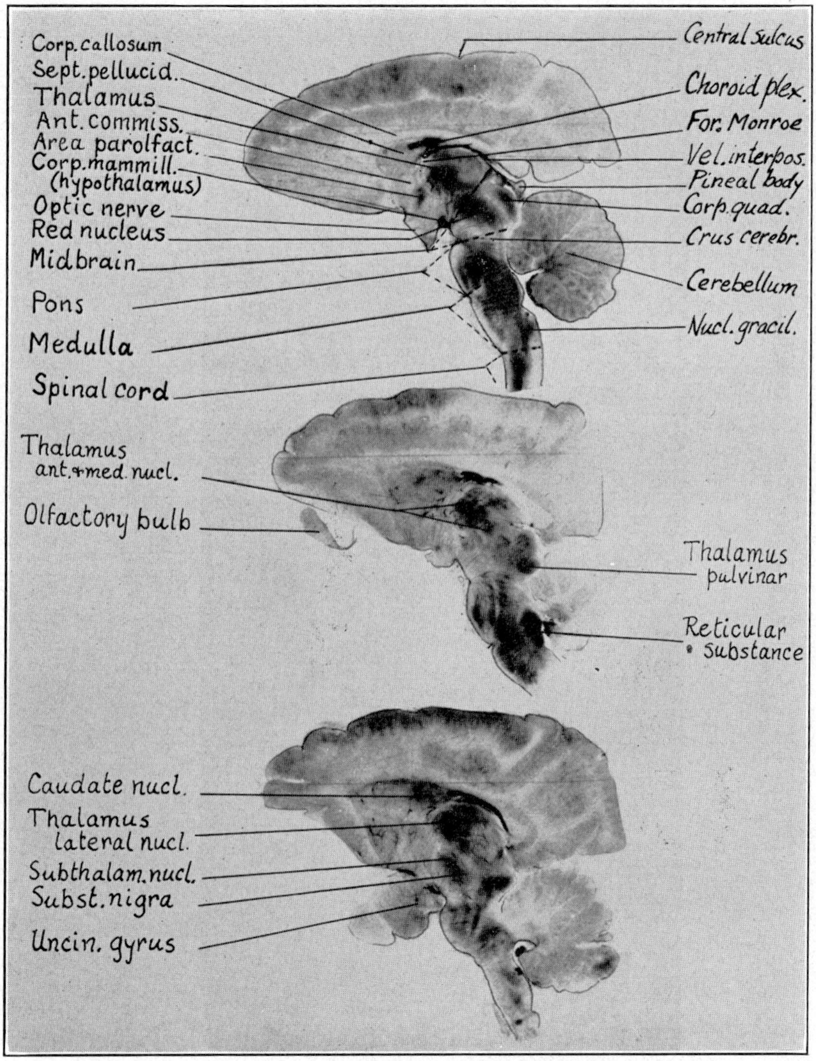

Fig. 4.—Six days' incubation, monkey 3, third stage. Intense staining in the brain stem and cervical cord. The legend on this and the succeeding specimen may be used as an anatomic guide to the other specimens as well. The contrast between the stained and unstained areas is particularly sharp.

Summary.—Lesions are limited to the olfactory bulbs, where they are slight, in an animal with a slower than average rate of invasion.

Six Days' Incubation.—Monkey 3 was inoculated intranasally Nov. 13, 1935. Temperatures were not taken. No paralysis had occurred up to time of death.

On November 18, trypan blue solution was given intramuscularly and on November 19, trypan blue was given intravenously at 4:30 P.M. At 6:30 P.M. the animal was killed.

Macroscopic Appearance.—The staining is somewhat lighter than in No. 24; the gray matter outside the areas of positive reaction showing only a very faint greenish color.

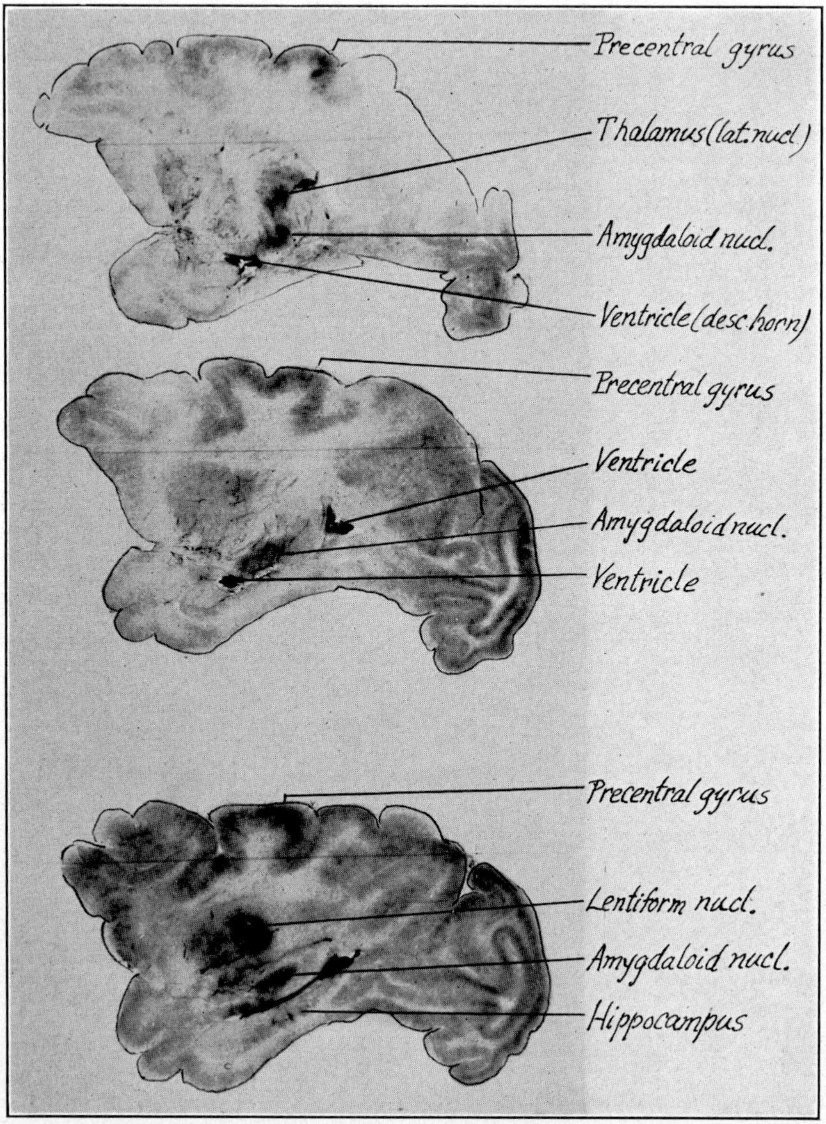

Fig. 5.—Six days' incubation, monkey 3. These sections are just lateral to those of Fig. 4. The amygdaloid nucleus (perhaps including the tail of the caudate nucleus) is deep blue. The lentiform nucleus, though appearing dark in the photograph, is not stained blue in the original. Marked staining is seen in two areas of the cerebral cortex, the precentral gyrus and the hippocampus (uncinate gyrus). This is the only specimen in which any considerable staining was found in the cerebral cortex outside of the uncinate gyrus.

Olfactory Bulbs: No staining.

Forebrain: No bluish staining excepting in the precentral gyrus on the convexity which shows Grade 2 staining and the uncinate gyrus (Grade 2).

Corpus Striatum: Unstained excepting an area about 2 by 6 mm. just above the descending horn of the lateral ventricle, in the position of the tail of the caudate nucleus and the amygdaloid nucleus (Grade 2-3). The same area was stained in No. 24.

Interbrain: The mesial, anterior, and lateral nuclei and also the pulvinar of the thalamus show Grade 3 staining. The corpora mammillaria show Grade 1 staining.

Midbrain: The red nucleus and corpora quadrigemina show Grade 2-3. No staining is seen in the region of the substantia nigra.

Pons Varolii: The ventral gray matter shows Grade 2-3 staining, and Grade 1-2 also shows in the dorsal portions in continuity with a rather diffuse area in the mesial portions of the medulla. The staining in the pons thus is somewhat more extensive than in No. 24.

Medulla: In the mesial portion the gray matter is rather diffusely stained (Grade 2-3). In the more lateral portions the stain is more localized in the portions below the floor of the fourth ventricle, but scattered small areas of blue (Grade 1-2) are seen throughout the substance. The staining in the medulla is more extensive than in No. 24.

Cerebellum: No staining.

Spinal Cord: In the cervical region the gray matter is intensely stained, with a distinct difference between the two lateral halves, one being Grade 3 and the other Grade 4. The posterior horns, the intermediate portions, and the anterior horns are almost equally blue. The white substance shows no visible staining. The thoracic portion is also well stained, and the lumbar region, while blue (Grade 2), is much less intensely stained than the cervical and thoracic segments. In longitudinal sections the dye is seen to be unevenly distributed at different levels.

Microscopic Examination.—Olfactory Bulbs: Throughout the nerve substance and in the pial meshes there is a notable infiltration with lymphocytes and a few polymorphonuclear leucocytes; and one perivascular cuff is seen. There is also a marked increase in the microglial (rod) cells with several small focal accumulations. No neuronophagia was found after careful search. The mitral cells show clear outlines in protoplasm and nucleus, and the nucleoli are centrally placed. The capillary bed is not conspicuously dilated, which may explain why macroscopic staining is not present.

Cerebral Cortex (frontal): No changes are seen except slight hyperemia.

Amygdaloid Nucleus: Slight capillary hyperemia and a slight or doubtful increase in the microglial cells are the only changes found.

Uncinate Gyrus: Moderate capillary dilatation is present, and also a few lymphocytes and polymorphonuclear cells are found in the pial meshes.

Choroid plexus and *ependyma* are entirely normal.

Thalamus: Marked capillary dilatation is present, the plasma appearing bluish in sections without counterstain and many of the capillary endothelial nuclei showing a deep blue color. In several places there are foci of rod cells. Cuffing, which is slight, is seen around one small vessel.

Medulla: The changes here are marked and relatively advanced in the gray matter, though slight or negligible in the meninges. Several degenerated nerve cells are surrounded and overlaid with rod cells; lymphocytes and a few polynuclear leucocytes are seen. Many clumps of microglial cells are seen. Several small vessels with moderate, but not deep, perivascular infiltrations are present. Several nerve cells with intranuclear inclusions are found, the only instance in the series of experiments. A few nerve cells are stained by trypan blue. Marked capillary dilatation is present.

Cerebellum: No notable abnormalities are found.

Spinal Cord: In striking contrast to other portions of the central nervous system, the ganglion cells contain considerable amounts of trypan blue, especially in the nuclei which are quite densely stained. This is much more marked in the cervical and upper thoracic than in the lumbar levels. The majority of stained

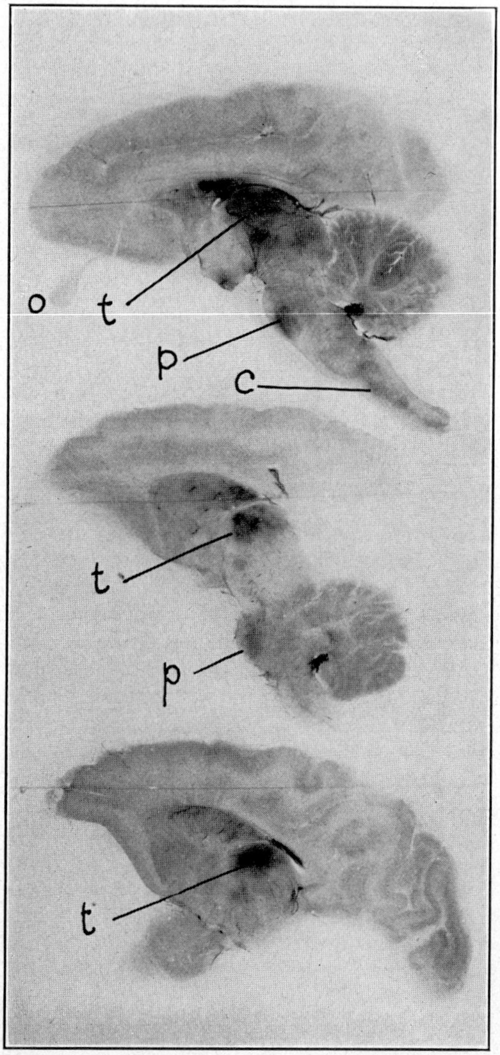

Fig. 6.—Seven days' incubation, monkey 4. The thalamus (*t*) is deeply stained, and lighter staining is seen in the ventral area of the pons (*p*) and in the cervical cord (*c*). The olfactory bulb (*o*) is unstained. The cerebral cortex is unstained.

cells are in the anterior half of the gray matter, but scattered stained cells are seen also in the mid-portion and a few in the posterior horns. In the cervical level the nerve cells stain very poorly, and the Nissl substance has disappeared; there are dense patches of microglial infiltration, some of which may represent neurophagia, although nerve cells were not found within them; there are slight infiltration of lymphocytes and a few polymorphonuclear leucocytes in the anterior fissure and slight cuffing of one small vessel. In the thoracic cord the nerve cells stain poorly; there is heavy rod cell infiltration in the gray matter but no meningeal or perivascular infiltration. In the midlumbar level the contrast with the upper levels is sharp; the nerve cells stain excellently and show normal appearance, with well-stained and normally distributed Nissl substance; no rod cell aggregations or increase and no meningeal or perivascular infiltrations are seen. Apart from a fairly marked dilatation of the capillary bed, the changes in the supporting tissues,

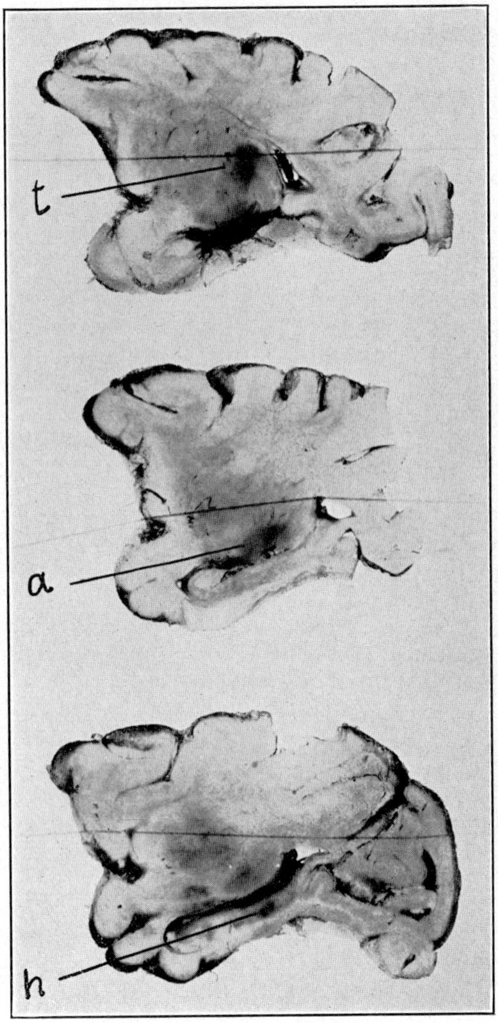

Fig. 7.—Seven days' incubation, monkey 4. Sections lateral to those of preceding photograph (Fig. 6). Localizations of dye in the thalamus (lateral nucleus) (*t*), amygdaloid nucleus (*a*), and uncinate gyrus (*h*) are conspicuous.

white matter, larger vessels, and meninges are very slight. No intranuclear inclusions are found. The picture as a whole is of a primary insult in the nerve cells, which permits dye to pass through the membranes both of the outer protoplasm and of the nucleus.

Summary.—The olfactory bulbs show microscopic abnormalities but no gross staining. Selective localizations of trypan blue are present and marked in the uncinate gyrus, amygdaloid nucleus, thalamus, midbrain, pons, medulla, and spinal cord. Evidences of nerve degeneration are advanced in the medulla and in the gray matter of the cord, especially in its upper portions. It is evident that this animal had a heavier than average infection and would have become paralyzed very shortly.

SEVEN DAYS' INCUBATION (TWO SPECIMENS).—Monkey 4 was inoculated Nov. 13, 1935. No temperatures were taken. Paralysis did not occur up to time of death. Dye was injected intramuscularly on November 19, and intravenously on November 20. The animal was killed on November 20, about two hours after the last dye injection.

Macroscopic Appearance.—Olfactory Bulbs: No staining.

Forebrain: No stain is found anywhere except in the uncinate gyrus, where it is quite intense (Grade 3-4).

Corpus Striatum: A small area of Grade 3 staining is seen in caudate nucleus just above the thalamus, and again in the tail of this nucleus and the amygdaloid nucleus above the descending cornu of the lateral ventricle in the same area which was found stained in previous specimens.

Interbrain: The mesial, anterior, and lateral nuclei of the thalamus are blue (Grade 3), but the pulvinar is not. The mammillary bodies (hypothalamus) are not stained.

Midbrain: A small area of blue, Grade 2, is seen in the region of the red nucleus.

Pons: The ventral region shows staining, Grade 2, in the same area noted in previous specimens.

Medulla: Very little stain is visible between the pons and the level of the cuneate tubercle, where in the central portions and in continuity with the gray matter of the cervical cord Grade 2 staining is seen.

Cerebellum: No staining.

Cervical Cord: In the uppermost portion, one side of the gray matter shows Grade 2 stain, most marked in the anterior horn. No stain is seen in the remainder of the cervical cord, nor in the thoracic and lumbar regions.

Microscopic Appearance.—Left Olfactory Bulb: There is a diffuse, and in places very marked, microglial infiltration especially marked in the glomerular, subglomerular, and central layers. There is also a fairly marked capillary dilatation. One pial vein shows a moderate perivascular infiltration with lymphocytes and a few polymorphonuclears. In the substance cuffing of a small vessel is seen. The pial infiltration is only slight. The nerve cells are fairly numerous and probably normal, although the fixation of the specimen as a whole is imperfect.

No other portions of the central nervous system were examined microscopically.

Summary.—There are localizations in the upper brain stem and olfactory cortex and in the upper part of the spinal cord. The specimens give the impression of a relatively mild infection with beginning invasion of the cord.

MONKEY 13 was inoculated Aug. 4, 1936. On August 6, the animal appeared "nervous"; August 7, nervous and irritable with temperature of 104.4° F.; and on August 8, nervous and irritable with temperature of 105.2° F. Same condition continued on August 9; temperature, 105.0° F. August 10, dye was injected intramuscularly. On August 11 symptoms were nervousness, fine tremors, weakness of legs; temperature, 104.4° F. Dye was given intravenously at 1:15 P.M., and the specimen was killed at 4:15 P.M.

Macroscopic Appearance.—Olfactory Bulb: Heavy staining, about Grade 4.

Forebrain: No staining is found, except very faint (Grade 1) in uncinate gyrus, especially at the tip (uncus).

Corpus Striatum: No staining except in same area as in previous specimens in roof of descending horn of ventricle (tail of caudate and amygdaloid nucleus) where it is Grade 2.

Interbrain: The staining is rather faint (Grade 1-2) and is seen in the anterior and lateral nuclei. The mammillary bodies are unstained.

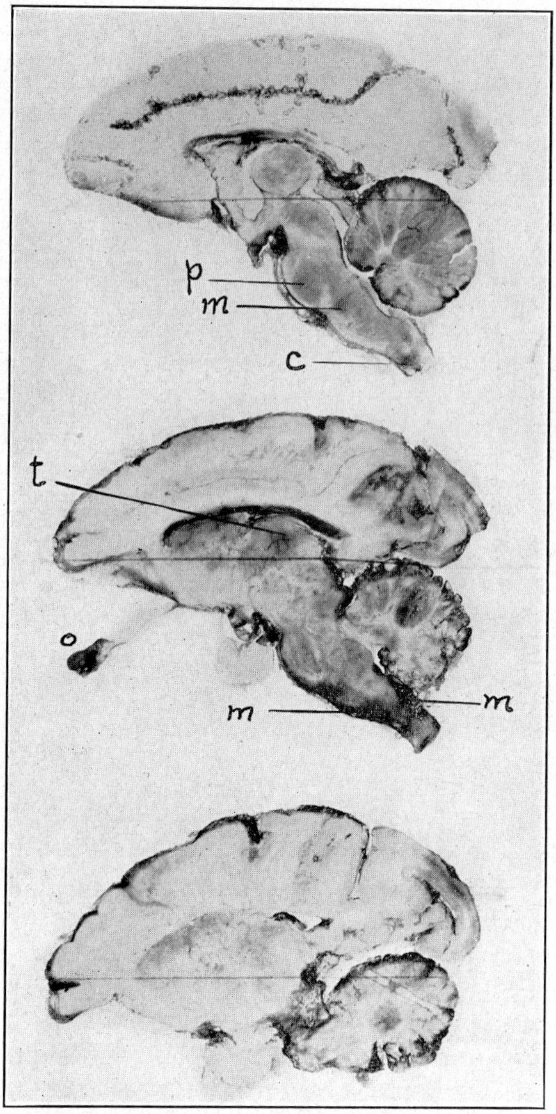

Fig. 8.—Seven days' incubation, monkey 13. The olfactory bulb (*o*) is rather deeply stained. There is faint staining in the thalamus (*t*). The chief involvement appears to be in the pons (*p*) and medulla (*m*) and in the cervical cord (*c*). The cerebral cortex and cerebellum are unstained. The cervical cord below the section is quite heavily stained.

Midbrain: Grade 1 staining appears in the region of the red nucleus.

Pons: The ventral area shows streaks of Grade 2 staining, and there are also a few spots in the dorsal region.

Medulla: Small spots of intense stain are seen in the ventral region at about the level of the pyramid. In the central region just below the pons an area of somewhat more diffuse stain, Grade 2, is seen.

Cerebellum: No staining.

Spinal Cord: By contrast with the brain, the staining in the cord is intense, especially in the cervical region where the gray matter, both anterior and posterior, is Grade 4. The gray matter of the thoracic cord is also deeply stained. In the lumbar cord, in one section, one of the anterior horns is deep blue (Grade 4), while the other is lightly stained (Grade 2). In longitudinal sections, some unevenness of staining is apparent at different levels, but the stain in the cervical region throughout is very much more intense than in the thoracic and lumbar levels.

Microscopic Examination.—Right Olfactory Bulb: The sections are thick, making it difficult to find mitral cells. There is an enormous infiltration with microglia in the glomerular and subjacent layer, extending into the granular layer. In the pia a fairly heavy infiltration with lymphocytes and some polymorphonuclears is found in places. Some cuffing of veins in the substance of the bulb is also found. The nerve cells are difficult to locate, being covered by heavy layers of oligodendroglia; the few that were found appear normal. It is impossible to determine whether or not neuronophagia is present.

No other sections from this animal were examined.

Summary.—There is selective staining in the brain stem, olfactory bulb, and spinal cord. The relative intensities of stain give the impression of a subsiding reaction in the brain stem and a much more active and severe reaction in the cord. The reaction in the olfactory bulb appears to be still very active.

NINE DAYS' INCUBATION.—Monkey 2 was inoculated Oct. 22, 1935. No temperature record was taken. Dye was injected intramuscularly on October 30, and intravenously on October 31, at 2 P.M. The specimen was killed at 5 P.M. No paralysis occurred.

Macroscopic Appearance.—Olfactory Bulbs: The right bulb is unstained; the left shows Grade 2 staining.

Forebrain: There is no staining anywhere, even in the uncinate gyrus.

Corpus Striatum: No staining appears except in the gray matter in the roof of the descending horn (tail of caudate nucleus and amygdaloid nucleus), where it is Grade 1-2.

Interbrain: The stain is rather faint (Grade 1-2) and diffuse, being seen mainly in lateral and posterior nuclei.

Midbrain: Grade 1-2 staining appears in the region of the red nucleus and substantia nigra.

Pons: There is Grade 2 staining in the dorsal portions, but none in the ventral area which was so well stained in the earlier specimens. The stained area in the pons is continuous with that in the medulla.

Medulla: Rather diffuse Grade 2-3 staining appears, especially conspicuous in the floor of the fourth ventricle and extending through the central portions to about 1 mm. from the ventral surface and from the level of the pons to the lower level of the pyramid. The region of the cuneate nucleus is unstained.

Spinal Cord: In the uppermost portion and again in the middle portion of the cervical cord, a deep blue area, rather sharply limited, of staining (Grade 3-4) is seen in the gray matter, involving both horns. The thoracic and lumbar regions are unstained.

Microscopic Appearance.—Left Olfactory Bulb: There is a notable increase in microglial cells, especially in the glomerular and subglomerular layers. Several moderate perivascular infiltrations are seen, and the pial meshes show a moderate infiltration with small round cells and polymorphonuclears. The nerve cells are numerous and apparently normal. In a few places the rod cells occur in clumps, which may represent neuronophagia, but no degenerating nerve cells are seen among them.

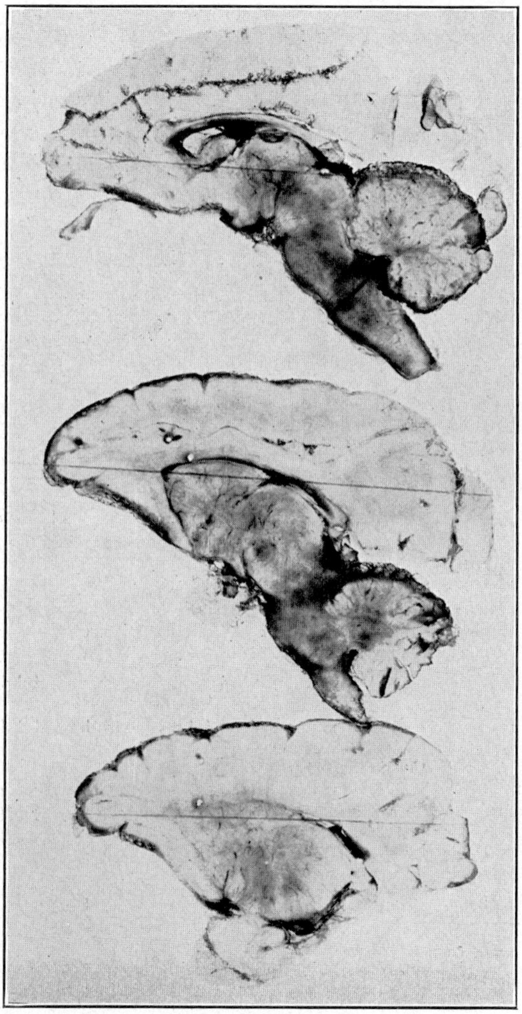

Fig. 9.—Nine days' incubation, monkey 2. Staining here is entirely limited to the brain stem and is deepest in the pons and medulla.

Thalamus: There is moderate capillary dilatation. There are several patches of microglial infiltration, one quite large, but no definite neuronophagia. Moderate cuffing of a few veins is seen. The ependyma appears normal.

Medulla: The veins are distended and some of them show slight cuffing. There are several areas of marked rod cell infiltration, with a few small clumps suggestive of neuronophagia. The rod cells are also increased throughout the substance.

Cervical Cord: There is slight perivascular cuffing in one place but no meningeal infiltration. In the anterior horn one large and one small collection of rod cells are seen; in the latter a degenerating nerve cell is visible. Several nerve cells look normal, but the majority stain poorly, without Nissl substance.

Thoracic Cord: The sections are small and unsatisfactory, but in one a small perivascular infiltration and a few small aggregations of rod cells are seen.

Lumbar Cord: In striking contrast with the cervical cord, the nerve cells stain well with normal Nissl substance. No perivascular or meningeal infiltrations nor aggregations of microglial cells are found.

Summary.—There is rather diffuse and light staining in the brain stem with less marked involvement of its uppermost portions than in previous specimens, and marked staining, rather sharply localized, in the midcervical cord. One olfactory bulb is stained; the other, unstained. The impression is that of a subsiding reaction in the brain stem, with discrete localized reaction in the cord, in an animal that might perhaps have survived the infection.

SUMMARY OF LOCALIZATIONS

These are shown in Table I. The control animal, No. 5, shows no visible staining with trypan blue. The small spot of blue in the subthalamic nucleus of the three-day animal, No. 6, is of doubtful and

TABLE I

	INCUBATION							
	CONTROL	3 DAYS	5 DAYS	4 DAYS	6 DAYS	7 DAYS		9 DAYS
	NO. 5	NO. 6	NO. 9	NO. 24	NO. 3	NO. 4	NO. 13	NO. 2
Olfactory bulb	0	0	++	+++	++*	0*	++++	0 right ++ left
Forebrain								
Precentral	0	0	0	0	++	0	0	0
Temporal	0	0	0	++	0	0	0	0
Uncinate	0	0	0	+++	++	+++	+	0
Corpus striatum								
Amygdaloid nucleus	0	±	±	+++	++	+++	++	++
Interbrain								
Thalamus								
Medial nuclei	0	0	0	++	+++	+++	+	0
Anterior nuclei	0	0	0	++	+++	+++	+	+
Lateral nuclei	0	0	0	++	+++	+++	+	+
Pulvinar	0	0	0		++	0	0	
Hypothalamus								
Corpora mammillaria	0	0	0	+	+	0	0	0
Subthalamic nucleus	0	+	0	0	0	0	0	±
Midbrain								
Red nucleus	0	0	0	0	++	++	+	+
Corpora quadrigemina	0	0	0	+	++	0	0	0
Substantia nigra	0	0	0	++	0	0	0	+
Cerebellum	0	0	0	0	0	0	0	0
Pons varolii								
Ventral region	0	0	0	++++	+++	++	+	0
Dorsal region	0	0	0	++	++	0	+	++
Medulla								
Ventral region	0	0	0	+	++	0	++	++
Dorsal region	0	0	0	+	++	0	++	++
Central	0	0	0	0	++	++	++	++
Cord								
Cervical	0	0	0	0	++++	++	++++	+++
Thoracic	0	0	0	0	+++	0	++++	0
Lumbar	0	0	0	0	++	0	+++	0

*No macroscopic staining, but marked histologic abnormalities.

perhaps negligible significance. The earliest stage of definite reaction in the central nervous system is shown in No. 9, killed on the fifth day after inoculation and a few hours after fever had begun, in which trypan blue staining is limited to the olfactory bulbs. Infection and invasion in this animal were a day or so slower in appearing than average, an example of the considerable variability so characteristic of poliomyelitis, both experimental and human.

The second stage is illustrated by No. 24, killed four days after inoculation, in which infection and invasion were rapid and severe. Here, the staining is extensive and intense but still limited to the areas of the central nervous system above the spinal cord, and is particularly marked in the olfactory bulbs and the brain stem above the medulla.

The third stage is illustrated by No. 3, killed six days after inoculation, in which the distribution in the brain stem is much like that in No. 24 (though more marked in the medulla), but the inflammatory change has now extended to the spinal cord where the upper (cervical) portions are more heavily stained than the lower. In this specimen for the first time definite degeneration of nerve cells is found, as shown by the normal microscopic signs and also by deposition of trypan blue in the cytoplasm and nucleus.

Specimens 4, 13, and 2, representing the seventh and ninth days, illustrate some of the later, preparalytic developments and variations, such as increasing involvement of the lower spinal segments, irregularities of distribution of lesions within the cord, and suggestions of subsidence of the inflammatory reaction in the olfactory bulbs and brain stem.

The experimental observations may be summarized as showing the progress of reaction to poliomyelitic infection during the incubation or preparalytic period as follows: (1) a primary stage of rhinencephalitis (olfactory bulbs only), succeeded by (2) a secondary stage of basal encephalitis, rather explosive in nature, consisting largely of hyperemia and microglial infiltration, succeeded by (3) a stage of myelitis with beginning nerve cell destruction, followed by (4) a stage of advancing and localizing myelitis simultaneous with beginning subsidence of the encephalitis.

The early and consistent involvement of the secondary olfactory centers (amygdaloid nucleus, uncinate gyrus) is of interest in relation to the olfactory route of invasion. The experiments as a whole give convincing evidence of the descending or caudad direction of poliomyelitic invasion into and through the central nervous system, after intranasal inoculation.

The nature of the inflammatory reactions in the early stages of infection is of considerable interest. That the localized areas of trypan blue staining are due to the presence of virus in those areas seems reasonably assured by comparison with the previous series of experiments in which the localizations of virus were determined and by comparison with the absence of stained areas in the central nervous system in the uninoculated control. The correspondence between the localizations of dye and of abnormalities in the microscopic appearance is also reasonably good; although in a few places (for example, the olfactory bulbs in No. 6) histologic changes were present where trypan blue was not visible, and in some of the trypan blue stained areas, histologic changes were slight or doubtful. Under the microscope the trypan blue becomes difficult to see except in the spinal cord and occasionally in the medulla where it has invaded the nerve cells. In most other places its macroscopic visibility seems to depend upon dilatation of the capillary bed, in which a faint bluish tint of the plasma and occasionally a more marked staining of the endothelial nuclei can be detected. Hyperemia is familiar as one of the most constant and marked features of the central nervous tissues in poliomyelitis, and the present observations suggest that it is probably the first tissue response to the virus. In addition, the present observations corroborate the studies of Hurst[8] that invasion by the microglial (rod) cells is an early and characteristic feature of the pathologic histology of poliomyelitis. These cells, the ''leucocytes of the central nervous system,'' not only constitute the principal element in areas of neuronophagia, but also are increased rather diffusely in infected areas before changes in nerve cells are manifest and can be found in the perivascular infiltrations.*

They are readily identified by the shape of their nuclei, which are pleomorphic and irregular in outline, usually with reentrant angles or curves such as are not seen in other glial cells. The cytoplasm is not seen except with special stains.

The present observations further confirm the contentions of Fairbrother and Hurst[11] that the perivascular and meningeal reactions are secondary phenomena; in most of the sections the meningeal infiltrations were either absent or slight in degree, even at times and in places when the parenchymal lesions were well advanced. Perivascular infiltrations (cuffing) were commoner than meningeal but were relatively slight.

In contrast with the report of Sabin and Olitsky,[13] neuronophagia in the olfactory bulbs was not identified with certainty in any of the specimens. This is not to say that it may not have been present. The mitral cells are bedded in a dense mass of small round glial cells

*I suspect that, if looked for, they would often be found in the cerebrospinal fluid in poliomyelitis and perhaps other virus diseases of the central nervous system. Fraser's description[10] seems quite characteristic of the microglial cell. Speaking of the cerebrospinal fluid in poliomyelitis he says: "In the more acute stages, larger cells with very irregular nuclei and a faintly basophilic and vacuolated cytoplasm were present in considerable numbers."

which conceal them in thick or heavily stained sections, and early degenerative changes are easily overlooked. In a few of the present specimens, clumps of microglial cells in or near the mitral cell layer may have concealed degenerated nerve cells within, but in no case were the latter seen. On the other hand, definite neuronophagia was found in the medulla and cord in some of the specimens, and manifest degeneration without neuronophagia was found in the cord in a few.

It seems correct to state that with the exception of necrosis of the nerve cells, the various tissue alterations described are of a reversible (recoverable) nature and that above the level of the medulla, nearly all the lesions noted in the present series were of that kind.

Finally, attention is directed to certain interesting features of the localizations of the spinal lesions in the seven- and nine-day animals. Thus, in No. 4 (seven-day incubation), dye was limited not only to a single level of the cord but to one lateral half of the anterior horn. In No. 13 (seven-day incubation), in which the distribution of trypan blue was much more extensive and intense in most places than in No. 4, there was a marked difference in the two lateral halves of the lumbar cord. In No. 2 (nine-day incubation) two separate areas in the cervical cord were stained while the rest of the cord was unstained. Differences in staining between the two lateral halves of the cord were also noted in No. 3. These observations may well be of importance as analogues of the varying and restricted sites of paralysis, so often one-sided, in man, thus illustrating the possibilities of variation in spinal localization after infection by the olfactory route.

DISCUSSION

The results of the present experiments on visualization of the evolution of poliomyelitic lesions during the period of invasion conform reasonably well, if not in all details, with the earlier series in which the localizations of the virus itself during the same period were determined. Both series bring out the following facts: (1) that both virus and lesions are first detected in, and limited to, the olfactory bulbs; (2) that both spread next to the basal regions of the central nervous system above the spinal cord; (3) that both are next found (sixth or seventh day after inoculation) in the spinal cord. Variations and discrepancies in time of localization amount to not more than one day, and the exact localizations differ only in minor details. The cerebral cortex, excepting the olfactory areas, contains no virus and shows only infrequent and mild lesions.

Both series of experiments also harmonize, I believe, with the pathologic process which probably occurs in human poliomyelitis during its early stages, consisting of a progressive, descending infection, with accompanying inflammatory reactions, of the central nervous system successively involving the olfactory bulb,* the brain stem and, in paralytic cases, the spinal cord. Indeed, it is difficult to account for the character and order of appearance of the clinical manifestations of acute poliomyelitis and even more difficult to explain the failure of paralysis to appear in the nonparalytic cases, in which the clinical manifestations (usually including abnormalities in the cerebrospinal fluid) are identical with the preparalytic manifestations in cases going on to paralysis, on any other basis than a descending infection which shows a strong tendency to halt at one point or another in its anatomic progress through the central nervous system. It is hard to conceive of a blood-borne infection acting in this way and, in particular, permitting the anterior horns of the cord, the most highly susceptible parts of the central nervous system to poliomyelitic virus, ever to escape. The fact that the cerebrospinal fluid does not contain virus does not harmonize with transport by the blood stream. Moreover, the fact that the meningeal and perivascular lesions of the disease are secondary to a primary infection of the nerve cells and, in severe cases, may even fail to appear in areas where nerve cells are already dead, has long been apparent from human material studied post mortem and has more recently been proved by the experiments of Fairbrother and Hurst.[11] There can be little, if any, question that the virus of poliomyelitis exerts its primary and characteristic effects exclusively on the nerve cells. The recent experiments on dermal infection[14] do not contradict this since no dermal lesions have been described, nor do they, in my opinion, disprove the theory of axonal transmission.

The considerable difficulty encountered in infecting monkeys by the blood stream has to be taken into consideration. Very large amounts of virus suspension injected directly into the blood stream

*The observations of L. W. Smith[12] on 56 human olfactory bulbs from fatal cases of poliomyelitis have repeatedly been cited as showing no or only minor and presumably insignificant abnormalities and hence as evidence against the nasal route of infection. Indeed, such is the conclusion drawn by Smith himself. His description, however, not only shows pathologic changes to be present but is in agreement with my own contention that the changes in the olfactory bulb are probably like those in other portions of the central nervous system above the level of the medulla (e.g., the thalamus), that is, of a mild and recoverable nature. Smith's statement is as follows: "Examination of fifty-six olfactory bulbs microscopically has shown a surprisingly small amount of pathologic change. *There has frequently been edema and congestion, harbingers of more extensive damage, but in less than a fourth of them do the characteristic cellular infiltrative changes, as seen in the ganglia and nerve roots, appear.* Either any inflammatory reaction in these organs is extremely short-lived, unlike the lesions of poliomyelitis elsewhere in the central nervous system, or the virus passes along these structures without leaving its identifying signature." [Italics added.]

The fact therefore seems established that abnormalities do occur frequently in the human olfactory bulbs, that even infiltrative changes occur not uncommonly (20 per cent?). The assumption that the mildness of the lesions points to another than the nasal route of entry seems to be quite gratuitous. Certainly the clinical evidence, as well as some pathologic evidence (see Harbitz and Scheel's observations[6] on two patients dying during the stage of repair) points very clearly to the existence of lesions, often widespread, in the central nervous system that subside without leaving residual effects. How else can the nonparalytic cases with nervous symptoms and characteristic changes in the cerebrospinal fluid be explained; or the recovery, partial or complete, that is so frequent in the paralytic cases?

Indeed, the changes noted by Smith in the olfactory bulbs are exactly what I have expected would be found.

are required and do not always succeed in breaking down the effective normal blood-brain barrier.[15] The human analogue to such experimental conditions is difficult to envisage. One would have to assume the existence of some extranervous tissue or organ in which the virus multiplied, and virus has been conspicuously absent when searched for in the extranervous tissues of man save in the nasopharynx and its regional lymph nodes. On the other hand, it has been recovered several times from the nasopharyngeal washings.[16, 17]

There seems to be no valid reason to assume that in "abortive" poliomyelitis, infection has not yet entered the central nervous system, simply because the cerebrospinal fluid shows no abnormalities.* Such abnormalities have been shown by Fairbrother and Hurst[11] to be secondary and subsequent to primary nerve tissue infection and to arise from drainage through the perivascular channels into the subarachnoid space of the products of inflammation, protein and cells, in the nervous parenchyma. The symptoms in the cases reported by Paul, Salinger, and Trask,[17] fever, vomiting, and headache, are the ordinary onset symptoms of poliomyelitis in general, such as are not uncommonly accompanied by abnormalities in the cerebrospinal fluid in nonparalytic and paralytic cases.

Objections to the gastrointestinal route are, to my mind, convincing. Experimentally, it has been clearly shown[19, 20] that when trauma to the tract and contact with the nasopharynx are avoided, virus, even in very large amounts, passes through it without causing infection and can even be recovered from the stools. The only successful experiments have depended either upon access to the nasopharynx or upon trauma to the tract. Since preceding trauma or infection or mechanical disorders of the bowel (such as volvulus, ulceration, etc.) are certainly of rare occurrence in man, the gastrointestinal portal can probably be dismissed as of little significance. The nasal portal remains the only one for which preceding trauma is not essential. The following comments are based on the thesis that it is the actual route of entry in man.

When poliomyelitic infection does enter the human body through the olfactory mucosa, it seems highly probable that it sets up in the central nervous system, as it has been shown to do in the monkey, a succession of inflammatory reactions which constitute the anatomic basis and source of the various clinical manifestations of the disease.

This concept is particularly illuminating in the interpretation of character and course of the onset and other early symptoms of poliomyelitis; of the so-called abortive and nonparalytic cases which form about 80 per cent of all recognizable poliomyelitic infections; and of

*Levinson[18] has shown from five cases of paralytic poliomyelitis that in the preparalytic stage with weakness already apparent the cerebrospinal fluid may show no increase of cells and only a slight increase of globulin. His review of the literature reveals the fact that the fluid in such cases is not infrequently entirely negative at a time when the central nervous system is unquestionably infected.

the usual absence of symptoms referable to the cerebral cortex (neopallium). We may envision the disease as one due to progressive invasion of nervous tissue by a virus which is not only neurotropic but, even within the nervous tissues themselves, exercises a rather striking degree of selectivity, being capable of producing only transient and recoverable lesions (hyperemia, cell infiltrations) in certain parts of the central nervous system (upper brain stem); destructive lesions (cell degeneration) in only a few (anterior horn cells, motor cells of the medulla); and slight lesions or none at all in others (cerebral cortex, cerebellum).

Furthermore, the conclusion is inescapable that in many instances the virus implants itself for a brief time only and, after invading the olfactory bulb and sometimes the brain stem, dies out without reaching the vulnerable lower motor neurons. Such appears to be the process in abortive and nonparalytic cases. The possibility that infected nerve cells in poliomyelitis frequently recover is one to which too little attention has been paid. Indeed, clinical experience indicates that in a certain proportion of cases even the vulnerable lower motor neurons recover from infection, since in nonfatal cases patients quite regularly regain part and sometimes all of the muscular strength lost during the acute stages of the disease.

The symptomatology of the disease shows an order of progression corresponding with the advancing distribution of lesions, and may, I believe, be properly divided into three main phases. The first phase is manifested by fever alone, and the lesions are confined to the olfactory bulb. The second consists of a symptom-complex in which more or less generalized affective, sensory, and autonomic phenomena are conspicuous, and the lesions consist mainly of a basal encephalitis without involvement of the spinal cord. During the third phase, in which lesions are now present in the spinal cord, there occur, usually in rapid succession, two kinds of symptoms: (a) localized autonomic and sensory phenomena arising in the lateral and posterior horns and dorsal root ganglia and (b) localized motor phenomena arising in the anterior horns. *The advance of infection may cease at any of the phases short of flaccid paralysis and place the case in the subclinical, abortive, or nonparalytic category.* The classification is given in greater detail in Table II.

The relationship of the various symptoms to their probable anatomic sources in the central nervous system has been discussed in considerable detail in another paper and need not be repeated here. With regard to fever, however, it now appears likely from the data in experiment 9 of the present series and from the recent experiments of Howe and Ecke[21] that this symptom, which is the earliest and most constant in poliomyelitis, may have its origin in infection of the

TABLE II

PHASE	SITE OF VIRUS AND LESION	SYMPTOMS	CEREBRO-SPINAL FLUID	CLASSIFICATION WHEN PROCESS FAILS TO ADVANCE BEYOND GIVEN PHASE
1	Olfactory bulb	Fever only	?	Subclinical
2	Brain stem	Fever, vomiting, headache, general hyperesthesia, drowsiness alternating with irritability, malaise, apprehensiveness	a) 0 b) +*	Abortive Nonparalytic
3a	Posterior and lateral horns and dorsal ganglia of spinal cord	Localized pains and tenderness, localized sweating, spine sign, painful Kernig	+	Preparalytic
3b	Anterior horns	Tremor,† weakness, flaccid paralysis	+	Paralytic

*Pleocytosis, increased protein. Negative fluid does not indicate that infection has not yet reached the central nervous system.

†Tremor may in some instances be due to involvement of the red nucleus.

olfactory bulbs alone and not primarily, as was previously suggested, in involvement of the hypothalamic centers. The affective and sensory disturbances of the second phase are reasonably referable to the diencephalon; and the autonomic disturbances to the base of the diencephalon, where, as Bard[22] states, there is a "dominant mechanism . . . capable of causing a simultaneous discharge over the entire series of preganglionic neurones." The functional disturbances of the bladder (retention) and of the gastrointestinal tract (constipation, occasional diarrhea) may also be due to disturbances in the higher autonomic centers. The preganglionic neurones have their origin in the lateral horns of the thoracic and lumbar segments. The origin of the localized autonomic disturbances of the third phase would seem to be here, just as that of the localized sensory and motor phenomena must be in the posterior horns and dorsal ganglia, and the anterior horns, respectively.

The speed of evolution, as well as the order of evolution of symptoms in man may quite reasonably be analogous to the speed and order of evolution of lesions in the experiments. The order seems to be quite regularly from above downwards, but the speed varies greatly. Thus in No. 9 only the olfactory bulbs showed lesions, and these mild, on the fifth day, while in No. 24 both the extent and severity of the lesions were vastly greater on the fourth. The extent and severity of the spinal lesions were more marked in No. 3 on the sixth day than in No. 2 on the ninth. The marked variations in the experiments obviously have their counterpart in the human disease which is so characteristically variable in the extent and severity of symptoms, and also in the period of time over which they develop. A survey of any well documented series of cases of some size will bear this out. For example, in Draper's series[1] the majority of paralytic cases showed weakness or paralysis within two or three days of the onset, some within a few hours and some within several days. In one case paralysis occurred eleven days after the onset. In a considerable number (dromedary cases) there was an interval, in one case of eight days, of symptomatic silence between the initial stage and the paralytic stage. Finally, as is true in all epidemics, a large proportion showed only the initial stages and developed no paralysis at all. Thus, the disease may run a slow course, a mild course, or a fulminant and explosive course. In practically all cases, however, the symptoms and signs of the onset are similar and do not point to implication of the cord.

SUMMARY

1. Intravital staining with trypan blue of monkeys intranasally inoculated with poliomyelitis virus gives selective staining in the central nervous system of areas of gray matter corresponding with those in which virus has previously been found to be present—particularly in the olfactory bulb and olfactory areas of the cortex and of the corpus striatum, in the brain stem, and spinal cord.

The localizations of the dye are due largely to capillary dilatation of the capillary bed and partly to staining of tissue cells (endothelium of capillaries) and, in the medulla and cord, to staining of the nerve cells themselves. It is assumed that the capillary hyperemia is the first response to invasion of nerve cells with virus after the latter has reached the critical concentration necessary to affect the cellular metabolism.

2. By sacrificing animals, intravitally stained, on various days of the preparalytic period, the order of appearance and the descending progress of the lesions can be followed.

3. The first stage consists of lesions limited to the olfactory bulb and is accompanied by fever.

4. The second stage consists of a marked and extensive reaction in the brain stem down to the medulla, with implication of the secondary olfactory centers (amygdaloid nucleus, uncinate gyrus).

5. The third stage consists of an increased involvement of the medulla and beginning implication of the spinal cord.

6. Later stages show localization in restricted areas in the cord itself, sometimes unilateral, with beginning subsidence of the reactions in the brain stem.

7. No significant variations were found in the *order* of development of the lesions, but conspicuous variations occurred in their *speed of evolution,* their extent, and severity and in their localizations in the cord.

8. The present experiments suggest that, since the host cells for poliomyelitis virus are in all probability nerve cells, and since nerve cell degeneration in most of the areas manifestly invaded above the level of the medulla was conspicuously slight or absent, these cells must in many instances be invaded by virus without undergoing destruction and are therefore capable of full recovery. This principle is probably true even in the highly susceptible anterior horns of the cord and may account not only for the nonparalytic cases but also for the recovery, partial or complete, of the many patients with paralysis.

9. Reasons are discussed for believing that the present experiments can fairly be applied to human poliomyelitis; that inflammatory reactions in the brain stem occur in the brain stem in nonparalytic cases and in the preparalytic stage of paralytic cases, and that they are responsible for the initial and other early symptoms which are constant in recognizable cases of the disease.

10. It is not necessary or correct to postulate a preliminary period of ''systemic,'' ''general,'' or extranervous infection. The concept of poliomyelitis as a primary disease of the central nervous system is reaffirmed.

Technical assistance in the experiments was given by Mr. Edward K. Blasdel and by Dr. Albert W. Snoke and Dr. William J. Newman.

REFERENCES

1. Draper, G.: Philadelphia, 1917, P. Blakiston's Son & Co.
2. Faber, H. K.: Medicine **12**: 83, 1933.
3. Aycock, W. L., and Luther, E. H.: New England J. Med. **200**: 164, 1929.
4. Schultz, E. W., and Gebhardt, L. P.: Proc. Soc. Exper. Biol. & Med. **30**: 1010, 1933.
5. Faber, H. K., and Gebhardt, L. P.: J. Exper. Med. **57**: 933, 1933.
6. Harbitz, F., and Scheel, O.: Pathologisch-anatomische Untersuchungen über akute poliomyelitis und verwandte Krankheiten von den Epidemien in Norwegen 1903-1906, Christiania, 1907, Jacob Dybwad.
7. Müller, Eduard: Die spinale Kinderlähmung. Eine klinische und epidemiologische Studie, Berlin, 1910, Julius Springer.
8. Hurst, E. W.: J. Path. & Bact. **32**: 457, 1929.
9. McClellan, R. H., and Goodpasture, E. W.: J. M. Research **44**: 201, 1924.
10. Fraser, F. R.: J. Exper. Med. **18**: 242, 1913.
11. Fairbrother, R. W., and Hurst, E. W.: J. Path. & Bact. **33**: 17, 1930.
12. Landon, J. F., and Smith, L. W.: Poliomyelitis: A Handbook for Physicians and Medical Students, p. 50, New York, 1934, The Macmillan Company.
13. Sabin, A. B., and Olitsky, P. K.: J. A. M. A. **108**: 21, 1937.
14. Trask, J. D., and Paul, J. R.: Science **87**: 44, 1938.
15. Flexner, S., and Amoss, H. L.: J. Exper. Med. **25**: 525, 1917.
16. Taylor, E., and Amoss, H. L.: J. Exper. Med. **26**: 745, 1917.
17. Paul, J. R., Salinger, R., and Trask, J. D.: J. A. M. A. **98**: 2262, 1932.
18. Levinson, S. O.: J. Pediat. **1**: 337, 1932.
19. Clark, P. F., Roberts, D. J., and Preston, W. S., Jr.: J Prev. Med. **6**: 47, 1932.
20. Flexner, S.: J. Exper. Med. **63**: 157, 1936.
21. Howe, H. A., and Ecke, R. S.: Proc. Soc. Exper. Biol. & Med. **37**: 125, 1937.
22. Bard, P.: In ''The Vegetative Nervous System,'' pp. 67-91, Baltimore, 1930, Williams and Wilkins Company.

FUTURE OF CHEMOPROPHYLAXIS AS A MEASURE FOR THE PRACTICAL CONTROL OF POLIOMYELITIS

E. W. Schultz, M.D.
Stanford University, Calif.

THE thought that certain chemical agents might serve to prevent the implantation of poliomyelitis virus at the portal of entry is not new. Soon after it was discovered that this disease could be transmitted to monkeys by the intranasal application of virus, Levaditi and Danulesco (1912)[1] attempted to prevent infection by first treating the nasal mucosa with chemical agents. However, the agents employed by them were chosen for their virucidal action rather than for their power to modify the permeability of the portal of entry and included such substances as potassium permanganate, hydrogen peroxide, phenol, menthol, iodine, and immune serum. Among those which were tested, potassium permanganate (1:500) protected two out of three monkeys, and one of five monkeys escaped infection in the iodine-treated group. Eight years later Flexner and Amoss (1920)[2] carried out similar experiments with chloramine T and dichloramine T, in both instances with negative results.

Present interest in chemoprophylaxis may be said to date from the observations by Olitsky and Cox[3] in 1934, who found that tannic acid instilled intranasally in mice protected a large percentage of animals against the virus of equine encephalomyelitis instilled intranasally four days later. In 1935 Armstrong[4] reported that a 3 per cent solution of alum protected mice against the virus of St. Louis encephalitis instilled intranasally several days later.

We are indebted to Armstrong and Harrison[5] for reviving interest in the possibilities of chemical prophylaxis in poliomyelitis. In May, 1935, they reported that a 4 per cent solution of alum applied intranasally conferred on monkeys a temporary resistance to virus instilled intranasally. Later, similar results were obtained with picric acid and with a combination of picric acid and alum.[6] These observations naturally suggested the practical possibilities of a chemical approach in the control of this disease; this became more apparent following the observations by Sabin, Olitsky and Cox (1936),[7] and by ourselves (1936),[8] which indicated that the protection afforded by chemical treatment may in some instances persist for months. It was this rather lasting effect which encouraged us to make a fairly comprehensive inquiry into the practical possibilities afforded by chemical prophylaxis.

Read before the Portland Academy of Medicine, Portland, Ore., Mar. 10, 1938.

Our attention was directed to the possible use of chemical agents in the control of this disease early in 1935 after we had been engaged in an extensive search for evidence that immune serum and vaccines really afford significant protection against this disease.[9] This shift was prompted largely by a realization that its practical control would not be possible by such orthodox measures.

After preliminary tests with tannic acid, which yielded equivocal results, it occurred to us that such substances as picric acid and mercurochrome, because of their staining action, might modify the permeability of the olfactory mucosa, including the olfactory cells and hairs. Our first report dealt with the protective action of these two substances. This report appeared almost simultaneously with that of Armstrong and Harrison on picric acid. The observations presented in these two papers were in harmony so far as the results could be compared. Those obtained by the Eastern workers applied to the protection afforded a few days following the period of treatment, while our observations extended over periods of more than a month. What came as a real surprise in this early work was the duration of the protection afforded—a point which still remains unexplained.

With this as a background, we set out on an extensive study to determine the range of substances which are able to produce more lasting protection. Many chemical substances have been tested under more and more exacting conditions in an effort to elicit those possessing more outstanding protective powers. Instead of testing monkeys for resistance to infection several days to several weeks after treatment, we now follow the practice of waiting at least a full month before subjecting treated monkeys to virus instillations. The number of treatments have been reduced from three to five to one; and in carrying out the resistance tests, the intranasal instillations of virus are repeated until 100 per cent of an equal number of controls have succumbed.

Up to the present we have investigated more than fifty chemical agents. While most of these have been tested only in a limited way, others have been subjected to an extensive study. It is not my purpose to present the observations in detail. I have only time enough to say that a number of agents, some of them quite unrelated to each other, are protective and that among those which have been tested more fully, zinc sulfate solution seems to be the most effective. A 1 per cent solution of this agent thoroughly applied to the olfactory mucosa will protect about 90 per cent of monkeys a month later against virus instillations sufficiently heavy to infect 90 to 100 per cent of an approximately equal number of controls.

MODE OF ACTION

While we are not yet ready to express an opinion as to how chemicals may act to produce this protection, a few general remarks on this aspect of the subject may be of interest. My remarks, however, must be regarded as purely tentative since we are still quite unenlightened as to the precise mechanism underlying chemical protection. Besides, there is a possibility that different chemicals may confer protection by actions which differ from each other, and a given agent may act in more than one way. While this may be true, we feel certain that in no case does the type of resistance under discussion depend on a virus-destroying action, but rather on some effect on the portal modifying its permeability to the virus. How this permeability is influenced is not clear. While most of the protective agents are fairly acid and strong protein precipitants, there is no absolute correlation either between the power to precipitate egg white in solution and protective power, or between acidity and protecting power. For example, 1 per cent zinc sulfate, C. P., in distilled water (pH 5.9), is more protective than either 1 per cent tannic acid (pH 3.6), 1 per cent picric acid (pH 1.72), or 1 per cent uranium nitrate (pH 2.9), despite the fact that all three of the latter are more acid and are at least as good protein precipitants as zinc sulfate. While certain agents such as nickel sulfate (pH 3.2) and barium chloride (pH 8.0), possessing low protein-precipitating powers, also display low protective powers, it is possible to point to some agents which are highly protective and yet incapable of marked protein precipitation. For example, 1 per cent mercurochrome, which is alkaline in reaction (pH 8.8) and precipitates proteins only very slightly, if at all, is quite highly protective. Among the zinc compounds, 1 per cent solutions of zinc sulfate (pH 5.9), zinc chloride (pH 6.2), zinc bromide (pH 5.5), zinc acetate (pH 6.6), and zinc sulfocarbolate (pH 5.4) are all more or less protective; while 1 per cent zinc permanganate, which is very acid (pH 3.5) and a very strong protein precipitant, seemingly possesses little if any protecting powers.

In the case of zinc compounds, we feel that the protection may possibly depend on some union of the zinc ion with the protoplasm of the olfactory endings, a zinc proteinate being formed which is less permeable to the virus than the unmodified protoplasm. It is also possible that the protection may result from an actual destruction of the olfactory dendrites, possibly even of the olfactory cells themselves, and that the susceptibility returns only after these have been regenerated. Later in this paper I shall mention certain difficulties attending a satisfactory study of the anatomic effects produced by such chemical treatment.

PORTAL OF ENTRY

Any attempt to control poliomyelitis by devoting attention to the olfactory area should naturally be supported with good evidence that this is actually the region through which the virus gains admission to the body. It therefore seems proper that I should introduce this discussion with a review of the evidence concerning the olfactory area as the natural portal of entry. You may wonder why I stop to consider this question in the face of the quite general recognition of the olfactory area as the sole natural portal. This widely held view, however, cannot yet be said to rest on unequivocal evidence. There are a few investigators who believe that in man the gastrointestinal tract is a more likely route of entrance, and recently it has been inferred that under natural conditions the virus may even enter through the skin.

Soon after the first successful transmission of the disease to monkeys by Landsteiner and Popper[10] in 1908, several investigators succeeded in infecting these animals by applying virus to the nasal mucosa. However, up to a few years ago the incidence of infection by this route was low, and little use was made of the intranasal method in experimental work. Recently, with a better technique and more virulent strains of virus, it has been possible to infect a high percentage of monkeys by this route. Establishment of the fact that infection can be easily induced in monkeys by the intranasal route further localized the problem as to through which portion of the nasal mucosa entrance is actually effected. Is it possible for the virus to pass through any portion, or does it pass through a restricted portion? As early as 1912, Flexner and Clark[11] made observations indicating that invasion may occur through the olfactory area. This was suggested by the fact that forty-eight hours after intranasal inoculation, virus was demonstrable in the olfactory bulbs, but not in the medulla and cord. This naturally raised the question, just how did the virus reach the bulbs? In 1917, Flexner and Amoss[12] made the following pertinent statement: "Having reached the upper respiratory mucosa, the virus may take either of two routes in invading the central nervous organs. It may penetrate first into the local blood vessels and be carried into the circulation and thence to the nervous tissue, or it may pass into the lymphatic vessels surrounding the olfactory nerves and ascend more directly to the brain, medulla, and spinal cord." The possibility that the virus may actually penetrate the nerve cell and be disseminated axonally, a view now widely held, was not considered, at least not seriously, at this time.

Before I go on with this discussion, I should like for the sake of clarity to review briefly the anatomy of the olfactory apparatus. In man the olfactory portion of the nasal mucous membrane occupies the upper third of the nasal septum, nearly the whole of the superior concha, and a small portion of the middle concha (Schaeffer, 1920, 1928).[13] In the healthy and fresh state, this area is demarcated from the adjacent mucosa by its yellowish or brownish tint and slightly greater thickness. Histologically, three kinds of cells may be recognized: (1) olfactory nerve cells, (2) supporting or sustentacular cells, and (3) small stellate basal cells. These cells rest directly on the tunica propria, without an intervening basement membrane. The supporting or sustentacular cells are tall, columnar cells, with oval nuclei. The superficial end of the cell extends a considerable distance peripheral to the nucleus and gives rise to a superficial zone in the olfactory membrane which is practically devoid of nuclei. The deep-lying part of the cell is frequently forked, the processes ramifying with those of neighboring cells to form a sort of network. The small stellate basal cells lie within this network. These are pyramidal, cuboid, or round cells, which like the sustentacular cells present ovoid nuclei. They are regarded by some as additional and younger forms of supporting cells.

The olfactory nerve cells lie between the deep processes of the sustentacular cells. They are fusiform and bipolar cells with large spherical nuclei surrounded by a small zone of finely granular protoplasm. The nuclei of these cells are quite round and also larger than the nuclei of the sustentacular cells and are found for the most part below the zone of oval nuclei of the sustentacular cells. This cell has two processes: (1) The superficial process, or dendrite, is short and relatively thick, its actual length depending on the level of the cell within the mucosa. It courses through the nonnuclear zone of the epithelium and terminates slightly beyond the free surface of the epithelium in a small hemispherical or bulbous enlargement. This enlargement is surmounted by six to eight short cilia-like olfactory hairs, which project, often spinelike, from different parts of the rounded end. Occasionally the dendrite does not present this bulbous enlargement but itself projects spinelike and terminates in one or more hairs. (2) The deep process of the cell is threadlike from the beginning and is continued centrally as an axone. The axones from neighboring cells run together to form eventually about twenty nerve filaments which pass through as many openings in the cribriform plate to end finally in the glomeruli of the olfactory bulb. Each of the main filaments or branches of the nerve receives a tubular sheath from the dura and piarachnoid, the former being continued into the periosteum, the latter into the neurolemma of the nerve. Years ago Key and Retzius[14] concluded from experimental observations that the olfactory nerve filaments in the nasal mucosa are surrounded by a loose connective tissue with spaces continuous with those in the piarachnoid. More recently similar observations have been reported by other investigators, including W. E. LeGros Clark,[15] who has emphasized the role which these spaces play in the spread of septic processes from the nose to the meninges and brain. It was these spaces, which in reality are not "lymph spaces," which Flexner, no doubt, had in mind as the route by which the virus might pass to the central nervous system. But while there is evidence that bacteria and certain neurotropic viruses, such as that of equine encephalomyelitis (Rake,[16] 1937), may take this route, it seems quite unlikely from available evidence that this is the route actually taken by the virus of poliomyelitis.

In the olfactory bulb the deep processes or axones of the olfactory cells form a feltwork of interlacing fibers over the surface of the bulb lying in contact with the cribriform plate. Here they come in contact with the bushlike dendritic processes of the large mitral cells, which constitute a part of the relatively superficial and circumferential zone of gray matter in the bulb. Peripheral to these cells in the gray matter are the smaller, less conspicuous tufted nerve cells, sharing in this relay. These two groups of nerve terminals—those coming from the olfactory cells on the one hand and those coming from the two kinds of nerve cells in the bulb on the other—give rise grossly to a circumscribed, more or less spherical thickening on the lower surface of the bulb, known as the olfactory glomerulus. Microscopically, this region presents a large number of small glomerular bodies containing the terminal arborizations of the respective processes. The axonal processes of the mitral cells go into the formation of the olfactory tracts, while those of the tufted cells pass through the anterior commissure to the opposite bulb.

In the gross the olfactory tracts are flat or triangular white bands which pass posteriorly on each side on the orbital surface of the frontal lobe to the so-called olfactory peduncle, located approximately at the level of the optic chiasma. Here the fibers diverge to form the lateral and medium striae and pass into substance of the cerebrum. It is unnecessary for our purpose to carry this anatomic description any farther.

In 1934 Brodie and Elvidge[17] and Gebhardt and myself[18] simultaneously reported the important observation that after the olfactory tracts have been cut, monkeys can no longer be infected by the intranasal route. This observation demonstrated for the first time the important fact that infection by the intranasal route under otherwise normal conditions can occur only through the olfactory portion of the nasal mucosa. This has been confirmed by Lennette and Hudson[19] (1935), who made the additional observation that the incidence of infection following the intravenous injection of virus is reduced some by a previous section of the olfactory tracts, suggesting that even when virus is introduced into the circulation, invasion of the central nervous system occurs more easily if the virus can enter from the olfactory mucosa. Armstrong[20] (1936) has reported that infection by the intravenous route occurs less easily in animals previously given intranasal treatments with picric acid. As further evidence, Sabin and Olitsky[21] (1937) have reported that monkeys infected by the intranasal route always show lesions in one or both bulbs, while those inoculated by other routes do not show these changes. A cellular infiltration was always observed in the outer layer of the bulb, which consists largely of olfactory nerve fibers, and also in the adjacent layer of glomeruli and in the underlying lamina granulosa externa and the lamina gelatinosa. We have been able to confirm these observations and have extended them some by tracing the infiltrative reactions from the olfactory mucosa to the olfactory bulbs. With a little experience it is possible in the monkey to remove the olfactory mucosa, nerve filaments, and bulbs of both sides, all in one piece. A study of such material shows that the inflammatory reaction is also present in the smaller nerve bundles in the tunica propria and that these changes become more marked in the larger filaments approaching the bulbs.

While such observations as these exclude the probability that the virus passes readily through any portion of the nasal mucosa and definitely fixes the portal as the olfactory area, they do not wholly exclude the possibility that the virus may pass centrally by the way of the perineural spaces. But while this is true, I think that the perineural spaces as an important route can be almost entirely excluded on the basis of supplementary evidence pointing to the olfactory neurons themselves. A part of this evidence is presented by the fact that the virus has only on very rare occasions been demonstrated in the spinal fluid where we would expect to find it if transmission occurs by the way of these spaces. Another line of evidence is supplied by the fact that the virus is so strictly neurotropic that it probably becomes intimately associated with neurons immediately, in other words, with neurons of the olfactory nerve, which are easily accessible to it.

During recent years much light has been thrown on the pathogenesis of virus diseases in general. A fact which is clearly recognized in viruses is their dependence on tissue cells of one type or another. This is often such a highly specialized dependence that only certain cells may be attacked to the exclusion of all others. From this we must conclude that the requirements for multiplication are met only by very intimate association with the particular cells suited to their propagation, an association such as would result from an actual invasion of the cells which are attacked. That this type of relationship exists is evidenced by the rather distinctive pathology of the virus diseases and by the exacting growth requirements of the viruses when they are cultivated outside of the body. The pathologic effects produced on cells by different viruses range from a rapid degeneration as in poliomyelitis to a stimulation of growth and division as in certain virus induced tumors in animals. In addition to these changes one may observe the presence of characteristic inclusion bodies in the affected cells in many virus diseases. These are generally eosinophilic reaction products which in some infections occur in the cytoplasm, in others in the nucleus. While similar cytologic reaction may be induced by some nonvirus agents and not all virus infections are associated with the formation of inclusions, the presence of such reaction products in a virus disease may, I believe, be regarded as reasonably good evidence that the causal agent is acting from inside the cell.

To what I have just said, I might add that no filter-passing virus has as yet been propagated outside the body in the absence of living tissue cells. While many viruses have now been cultivated outside of the natural host in cultures of embryonic tissues and in the chorioallantoic membrane of the developing chick, they differ in their capacity to multiply in cells other than those parasitized under natural conditions. The virus of poliomyelitis, for example, has resisted cultivation in various kinds of tissue cultures, and, as Sabin and Olitsky[22] (1936) have recently shown, yields to cultivation in such media only in the presence of nervous tissue from the human embryo. Tissues other than the nervous tissue from the same human embryos failed to provide the conditions necessary for growth, and nervous tissue from the adult monkey also failed to meet the growth requirements of this virus. While we have not had an opportunity to repeat this work with human embryonic tissue, we have spent more than a year in unfruitful efforts to grow the virus in cultures of various other tissues. All of this testifies to the very high selectivity of this virus, a fact which should be remembered in considering the possible routes by which the virus may gain entrance to the body.

Support of the view that the virus probably invades the olfactory nerve directly and reaches the central nervous system through the fibers of this nerve is also to be found in what we know of the pathogenesis of this disease. At one time it was believed that the destruction of the anterior horn cells in the medulla and cord was the indirect result of pressure by inflammatory exudate, a view which was predicated on the presence of an interstitial action. We know now, largely from the work of Hurst and others, that the nerve cell degeneration is a primary phenomenon and that the inflammatory response seen represents a purely secondary reaction. Hurst[23] (1929) came to this conclusion from direct observations of the changes found in different stages of the experimental disease. Later, in collaboration with Fairbrother,[24] he found by sampling different regions of the nervous system during the preparalytic period that the infection spreads along neural pathways. This work was extended by Faber and Gebhardt[25] (1933), who found that by the fourth day following intranasal inoculation the virus becomes established in the olfactory bulbs. By the fifth or sixth day it reaches the hypothalamus, and from here it spreads explosively to the medulla, thalamus, and midbrain, and finally to the cord. Certain portions of the central nervous system, including the frontal and parietal lobes and the cerebellum never contained demonstrable amounts of virus. From this work and a critical review of the literature, Faber[26] (1933) came to the conclusion that throughout its entire course this disease is primarily an infection of the central nervous system, that the virus is transmitted axonally and in intimate association with the neurons from the portal of entry onward.

Recently, Gebhardt and I[27] have extended these studies and not only tested different parts of the central nervous system for the presence of virus but have titrated the concentration of the virus in different parts of the nervous system as the infection advanced during the preparalytic period. These studies were carried out not so much to satisfy ourselves of the correctness of the earlier mentioned observations, as to check the validity of an hypothesis we have entertained regarding one aspect of the pathogenesis of this disease. This is to the effect that degeneration of susceptible nerve cells does not occur until a certain rather high concentration of virus has been reached—that in the presence of lower concentrations all but very susceptible cells escape damage. We believe that while the virus is transmitted neuronally, injury to the neurons is not necessarily a consequence of an intraneural infection. We believe that nerve cell damage is determined both by the concentration of the virus and the level of resistance of the individual neurons. I cannot discuss this view any further here. I can say, however, that our observations not only lend additional support to the view that the transmission of this virus is primarily axonal, but show also that virus may be present in fairly high concentrations, even in the cord, before any paralysis makes its appearance. It is commonly recognized by experimental workers that in monkeys paralysis of the legs usually precedes paralysis of the arms. This rather frequent observation has suggested to some observers that there must be a fallacy in the theory of axonal transmission, since, if the virus progresses downward from the medulla through the cervical cord, the upper extremities should become involved before the lower. The fact that in man also the legs are commonly involved first has been evoked in favor of the view that the virus enters the central nervous system by the way of autonomic nerves supplying the digestive tract. Our investigations, however, show that the cervical cord may contain a high concentration of virus in advance of its appearance in the lumbar cord. This suggests that the motor nerve cells in the lumbar cord are for some reason more susceptible to this virus than are those in the cervical cord. It seems altogether possible that less usual distributions of paralysis in man may rest on a somewhat greater susceptibility of corresponding groups of nerve cells, rather than that the virus is restricted to the regions showing involvement. At any rate, it may prove helpful in understanding some of these distributions if we bear in mind the possibility that there may be not only an inherent difference in the susceptibility of motor nerve cells in individuals taken as a whole, but that some groups in a given individual may be more susceptible than others.

Also in harmony with an intraneural infection is the presence of inclusion bodies in the nuclei. While not numerous, they have been conclusively demonstrated by Covell[28] (1930), Hurst[29] (1931), and by ourselves (Schultz,[30] 1932) and may be regarded as bearing witness to the location of the virus.

If the evidence I have reviewed concerning the axonal transmission of the virus appeals to you, I should like to put before you this question: How is this virus, which measures only about 10 millimicrons[31] and is among the smallest of the known viruses, actually propagated along the nerve processes? Are autonomously dividing virus particles pushed, carried, or moved along by streaming protoplasm, or, is the virus propagated along the nerve as the result of some catalytic type of action in which one activator particle activates a precursor next to it in series along the axone? Whatever the actual mechanism may be, it is known that the concentration of the virus tends to decrease from above downward after the infection has advanced to the cord[24] and that the concentration in the cord decreases during the days which follow the onset of paralysis. How this inactivation is effected is not known.

It seems clear that once the virus has reached the central nervous system, its propagation is definitely associated with neurons. If we accept this view, it then is not a long step to the concept that the initial infection, under natural as well as under experimental conditions, occurs as a direct invasion of the olfactory neurons in the olfactory mucosa, the only region in the body where nerve cells are exposed to the exterior. We should remember that not only the hairlike endings are exposed at the surface of the olfactory mucosa but also the bulbous enlargements bearing these hairs. This accessibility of neurons to a highly neurotropic virus should explain satisfactorily enough why section of the olfactory tracts prevents the passage of virus to the central nervous system and makes it apparent why the olfactory perineural spaces and the spinal fluid need not be expected to play important roles in carrying it to the central nervous system.

A few investigators do not share this view and believe that in man the olfactory nerve is probably not a frequent portal of entry. On the basis of epidemiologic observations, Kling,[32] of Sweden, in 1929 published the view that the disease may be spread through the medium of water and that the digestive tract may be the most important portal. Experimental observations in collaboration with Levaditi and Lépine[33] (1929) seemed to support this view. However, later work carried out with Levaditi and Hornus[34] (1934) showed quite definitely that it is easier to infect monkeys by the intranasal route than by the alimentary route.

In this country Toomey[35] (1932-1936) has enthusiastically supported the gastrointestinal hypothesis and has offered arguments drawn from both clinical and experimental observations in support of it. I have time only to say that those who do not share his view would point out that the clinical observations to which he has given weight are not necessarily at variance with the more generally accepted view, also, that his experimental procedures have been rather too artificial and drastic to be convincing. It is generally well understood by investigators that any method in which virus is forcibly introduced into the tissues may result in infection. Virus inoculated into the sciatic nerve finds its way to the cord (Hurst,[36] 1930); it does so also following intradermal injection. It should not be surprising then to find that infection follows the injection of virus subserosally into the wall of the gut; that infection results following the introduction of virus into the lumen of the gut under a ballooning pressure; or, that infection follows when virus is introduced there along with toxic substances which help to provide artificial access to nerve terminals in the wall of the gut.

Clark, Roberts, and Preston[37] (1932), Flexner[38] (1936), and especially Lennette and Hudson[38] (1936) have reported observations which demonstrate that when injury to the intestinal mucosa is avoided and something approaching a natural exposure is imitated, it is exceedingly difficult to infect monkeys by this route. While it does not necessarily follow that in man infection by this route would be equally difficult, it is, nevertheless, not yet evident why the intestinal mucosa in man should be any more accessible to this virus than that in the monkey.

Recently Harmon[40] (1937, 1938) has reported that the injection of monkeys with rectal and nasal washings from twenty convalescent patients produced "takes" in only four animals, all resulting from rectal washings. At first glance such an observation seems to afford a strong argument in favor of the intestinal tract as the portal of entry. Let us, however, analyze the possible significance of this observation. In the first place, it seems unlikely that an amount of virus sufficient to be demonstrable in the feces would be ingested with food or water. It is much less likely that virus ingested in any amount multiplies in the gut. We can be certain about this from our knowledge of its exacting growth requirements. How else then can such an amount of virus come to be present in the feces? There is, as I see it, only one satisfactory explanation possible, namely, that it comes to be there as the result of repeatedly swallowing virus-contaminated secretions from the nasopharynx; being highly resistant, the virus is eventually concentrated sufficiently in the gut to be demonstrable. A less likely possibility is that it may be eliminated into the gut from infected autonomic nerves. While it is difficult to demonstrate virus in oral and nasal washings, it has been demonstrated in such washings in patients, in human convalescents, and in infected monkeys (Flexner,[38] 1936; and Kramer, Sobel, Grossman and Hoskwith,[41] 1936). The difficulty of demonstrating virus in such washings probably rests in a large measure on the fact that it is moved downward and outward very rapidly and is not readily detected unless it is present in fairly large amounts. Its low concentration in the nasal washings may indeed mean that higher and more easily demonstrable concentrations are to be found in tissues and organs which lie below the olfactory area and in a position to receive virus from above. One would, therefore, expect to be able to recover virus from tonsils and adenoids. Indeed, this has been done in convalescents and contacts. Kramer[42] (1935) recovered virus from the tonsils and adenoids of a child who had no known contact with the disease. If it can be demonstrated in the adenoid tissue of the upper respiratory passages, there is then no reason to doubt its reaching the digestive tract from the same general source. Until recently, however, little success has attended attempts to recover virus from the stools of human beings or of monkeys dying of the disease, even with the aid of methods for concentrating any virus that might happen to be present (Clark, Roberts and Preston, 1932[37]; and Flexner, 1936[38]).

Important arguments against the theory that the olfactory nerve in man is the common pathway for this virus are the observations made by Landon and Smith[43] (1934) on some fifty-six olfactory bulbs from fatal human cases. They found surprisingly little pathologic change in most of the bulbs which they examined. While edema and congestion were rather frequently observed, fewer than one-fourth showed cellular infiltrations. They conclude that either the inflammatory reaction is short lived, or the virus passes along these structures without leaving traces. A third possibility seemed more logical, namely, that in human beings the olfactory bulb is not necessarily a frequent pathway and that nerve roots elsewhere may be of equal importance as portals of entry, possibly indirectly by the way of the blood stream to their ganglia. Harmon and Levine[40] (1938) have reported that only two of nine fatal cases disclosed lesions in the olfactory bulbs. Such negative observations as these are, of course, of great important, especially in the light of the recent observations of Sabin and Olitsky[44] (1937), who have found that the olfactory bulbs of intranasally infected monkeys show definite lesions, which are absent when the invasion of the nervous system has been by other pathways. They found, however, that the type and extent of the lesions varied considerably and that one of the olfactory bulbs frequently showed more extensive lesions than the other. In almost a third of the animals receiving instillation of virus in both nares, only unilateral involvement of the bulbs was observed. Such observations suggest that in man minor lesions may be altogether missed unless both bulbs are carefully examined by the serial section method. After all, should one necessarily expect to always find lesions in the olfactory bulbs in man? I, personally, do not feel certain that the virus always leaves an easily recognizable trail to mark the route it has taken. In any case a more extensive study of the olfactory bulbs from fatal cases in man is certainly needed now to help clear up this important question. Sabin and Olitsky, at the Rockefeller Institute, are at present engaged in such a study and will, I know, greatly appreciate the cooperation of pathologists who send them such material for study.

Before I leave the question of the portal of entry, I should refer briefly to recent observations (Trask and Paul,[45] 1936, 1938; and Howitt,[46] 1937) which indicate that freshly isolated, so-called human strains exhibit a greater capacity to infect monkeys by intradermal inoculation than do monkey passage strains, the practical inference being that natural infection in man may possibly result from cutaneous contact with virus. What the actual practical significance of these observations really may be is yet too early to say. This much, however, may be said. All the facts to date seem to indicate clearly that the virus of this disease is highly neurotropic and is capable of multiplying only in nervous tissue. Since this is true, it would be indeed surprising to find that it can spontaneously establish itself in the nervous tissue of a new host by penetrating a barrier so unfavorable as squamous epithelium. This would prove especially surprising in view of the fact that even an intact mucous membrane affords a considerable barrier for this virus. I have already mentioned that in monkeys infection by the gastrointestinal tract is difficult if we take care not to traumatize the mucosa. I have also mentioned that after cutting the olfactory tracts, one may instill virus freely and repeatedly into the nasal passages without inducing infection. It appears then that infection through intact mucous surfaces does not occur. It would seem, therefore, that to have infection through the skin, one would have to presuppose an abrasion or injury sufficient to allow a skin containing virus to come in contact with cutaneous nerves. That such a combination of circumstances may play an important part in the epidemiology of this disease seems unlikely from the information we have at the present time.

I have dwelt at some length on the portal of entry because any prediction as to the value of chemoprophylaxis in the control of this disease must depend in the first place on how valid the evidence is that the olfactory nerve is the usual portal of entry. If it is not the usual portal in man, then my story ends here. If it is the usual portal, then I can go on and say that the future of chemoprophylaxis as a practical measure depends on the eventual answers to at least three important questions: (1) Are the results which have been obtained in monkeys transferable to man? (2) Are the practical difficulties of applying such a prophylactic measure in man sufficiently surmountable to make it a reasonably attractive public health measure? And (3) are there any serious contraindications to the general use of such a prophylactic measure?

ARE THE RESULTS OBTAINED IN MONKEYS TRANSFERABLE TO MAN?

Whether or not the results which have been obtained in monkeys are in any measure transferable to man is still too early to say. Observations with the picric acid-alum spray in Alabama in 1936 were inconclusive, but, as Armstrong[47] has pointed out in his analysis of this field test, the results in this test could not have been anything more than inconclusive in the absence of a dependable method of applying the prophylactic treatments. We now know that solutions cannot be applied to the olfactory area with an ordinary atomizer. It follows as a corollary that there can be no evaluation of this type of prophylaxis in the absence of a method which can be depended upon to bring the solution in contact with all of the olfactory surface. I want to emphasize this, for I have heard the Alabama experience mentioned as evidence that chemoprophylaxis has nothing to offer. I grant that eventually the application of chemical solutions may be proved worthless in preventing the disease in man, but we should be sure to view such an experience in the proper light—as a failure in the technique of its application and not necessarily as evidence against the protective value of the agent used.

Unfortunately, the Alabama field test is not the only field test which has failed to contribute an answer to our first question. From another report it appears that a second field test, carried out during the past summer in Toronto, in which zinc sulfate solution was used, also failed to yield information on this point. The report to which I refer appeared in the November (1937) issue of the *Canadian Public Health Journal* under the authorship of Tisdall and others.[48] It presents the results obtained on a group of about 5,000 children treated with zinc sulfate solution. These treatments were carried out according to a technique recommended by Peet, Echols, and Richter[49] (1937), which I shall describe later. Here, too, the results were such as to suggest, on superficial examination of the data, that the measure is not of value in man, for in a group of 4,713 children sprayed twice at intervals of ten to twelve days there were 11 cases of poliomyelitis, with only 18 cases in a control group of 6,300. In the period from seven days after the first spraying to thirty days after the second spraying the attack rate was 2.1 in the sprayed group and 2.9 in the control group. Statistically, there was no significant difference between the two groups. In writing their conclusions, they stated that their study furnishes no evidence of the protective value of the "spray." While this statement is basically correct, it is a little misleading without some qualification to indicate that the success of the measure might have depended somewhat on how thoroughly the solution was applied to the portal of entry. The following statement in the body of the report helps to convey the impression that this particular field test was in a sense crucial. It reads: "In the opinion, however, of the attending otolaryngologists, the olfactory area was satisfactorily sprayed in the majority of children." Since this is an important statement let us examine the data presented for evidence that this was true. Probably the only dependable criterion at present available of complete coverage of the olfactory area is the development of anosmia. Their figures show that of a total of 5,233 children sprayed, less than 20 per cent were tested for the presence of anosmia and that of the total number tested a grand average of only 14 per cent showed impairment of the sense of smell. The degree of the impairment and its duration are not discussed. At any rate, we must conclude from the figures they themselves have given us that in about 85 per cent of those sprayed the solution was not applied thoroughly enough to cover all of the olfactory area. Naturally, any failure to cover this area tends to invalidate conclusions drawn as to the prophylactic value of the solution used. The only conclusion which seems justifiable from the results of this field test is that the method of applying the solution failed.

But while this field test also failed to give us information as to the effectiveness of chemical prophylaxis in man, some information has been gathered which should prove helpful in conducting future field tests. Foremost is the probable importance of using the presence of anosmia as a criterion of adequate treatment. There can be no assurance that the olfactory area has been completely covered unless anosmia is produced in all individuals treated. Furthermore, functional tests repeatedly applied to determine the continued presence of anosmia should be, I believe, the basis for deciding the interval of time which may elapse between treatments, rather than results obtained in monkeys. We now know that anosmia invariably follows a thorough application of zinc sulfate solution, and, since this is the case, there can be no better guide as to when another treatment is due. The method employed for testing the anosmia should be entirely dependable, one in which the results are not influenced by natural anatomic conditions in the nose. Such a method, I understand, is that devised by Esbach. I can appreciate what all this testing would mean from the standpoint of time and skill, but I see no easier road to the information we now need. It seems certain that a sufficient number of functional tests will have to be carried out in the beginning to determine whether the method employed for applying the solution can be depended on to cover the olfactory area completely. As to the interval of the treatments, experience will have to be our guide if the duration of the anosmia is to serve as a criterion.

ARE THE PRACTICAL DIFFICULTIES OF APPLYING SUCH A PROPHYLACTIC MEASURE IN MAN SUFFICIENTLY SURMOUNTABLE TO MAKE IT A REASONABLY ATTRACTIVE PUBLIC HEALTH MEASURE?

Unfortunately, the olfactory area in man is rather inaccessible. Because the middle turbinate tends to encroach on the septum, the chances of adequately covering this area with an ordinary atomizer are small. To surmount this obstacle Peet, Echols, and Richter[49] (1937) suggested the use of a special atomizer tip, which can be introduced along the septum past the middle turbinate. This special tip overcomes some of the difficulties, but to use it requires the service of a nose and throat specialist. It is hazardous in the hands of unskilled operators and cannot be applied to young children and others who do not cooperate fully. The fact that in the Toronto outbreak of poliomyelitis the use of this method resulted in producing an anosmia in less than 15 per cent of those treated suggests that it is not trustworthy, even in the hands of nose and throat specialists.

Measures are often discovered when a need becomes urgent. The need for a simple and effective method for covering the olfactory area has not existed before. To most of us this area is new territory. Therefore, it is not surprising that a simple way to inundate this surface with a medicinal solution had to be discovered.

During recent months it has become evident that this can be accomplished without the aid of an atomizer and with little or no instrumentation. It has been established that when the head is completely inverted, a fluid properly introduced into the nares will flow freely into and fill the superior meatal space.

Before I enlarge on this observation, I want to refer briefly to a method introduced by Pentecost[50] (1937) during the recent epidemic in Toronto. Anticipating that he might be called upon to apply zinc sulfate, Pentecost began experiments in July to ascertain the best method for applying the solution. He settled on a technique which consisted of introducing the solution with the aid of a flexible olive-tipped ureteral catheter. This he inserted between the nasal septum and the middle turbinate; then, with a Luer syringe attached to the free end, 0.5 c.c. of the solution was forced through the catheter, the patient being recumbent with the head in the Proetz position ("head inverted so that the chin and external auditory meatuses are in the same vertical plane"). This procedure seemed the easiest to carry out, the least hazardous, and the least discomforting to the patient. Especially noteworthy is the fact that by this method immediate anosmia was produced in 100 per cent of those treated. Approximately 100 children, 8 years of age and older, were treated in this way with no serious effects. The method, unfortunately, was developed too late to receive more extensive application in this outbreak. There were no cases of poliomyelitis among those treated by the method, but, of course, the group was too small for this to be of any significance.

Early during the past summer Shahinian, Bacher, McNaught and Newell[51] at Stanford undertook studies to determine the best way of applying solutions to the olfactory area. Soon after they began this work they showed me a method which was similar to that described a short time later by Pentecost. However, they abandoned this method when they discovered that correct posture alone suffices to overcome much of the difficulty. The Proetz position, a position commonly used in filling the sphenoidal sinuses with solution, was recognized as not an optimum position for obtaining good coverage of the olfactory area. From radiologic and other observations it became evident that when the head is completely inverted, that is, when the line between the infra-orbital ridge and the external auditory meatus is in the horizontal plane, limited quantities of the fluid, if introduced slowly into the olfactory sulcus at the limen nasi, will flow along the nasal groove and fill the inverted common nasal meatus in a highly selective manner and to a height usually sufficient to immerse most of the estimated olfactory area. This method was found fully as efficient as direct placement of fluid by means of a delicate ureteral catheter introduced between the middle turbinate and septum.

To apply the solution by this procedure, the patient is put on a table with the head in the fully inverted position. A maximum of 0.5 c.c. of fluid is then introduced slowly and steadily, drop by drop, with a medicine dropper into each nasal space. After the required amount has been introduced, the patient is kept in the inverted position for one minute. He is then turned over to the prone position and instructed to lift his head and sniff outwardly to help discharge any excess fluid. Previous shrinkage of the mucous membranes is believed unnecessary and probably undesirable.

Information from other groups of nose and throat specialists investigating this question indicates that this purely postural method is finding favor. It is much more easily carried out than the spray method and can be applied by any physician or public health worker after a little instruction.

ARE THERE ANY CONTRAINDICATIONS TO THE GENERAL USE OF ZINC SULFATE AS A PROPHYLACTIC MEASURE?

This question deserves careful consideration. In addition to temporary discomfort, such as local irritation and headache lasting for several hours, which is more severe in adults than in children, there is possibly some risk of inducing a lasting anosmia. I have emphasized the importance of applying the treatments thoroughly enough to induce anosmia, but no one wants such an effect to be permanent. While the information I have obtained to date from various sources indicates that the anosmia induced by zinc sulfate solution in the vast majority of cases disappears in less than two weeks, I have also been informed of cases in whom the sense of smell did not return until after periods of two to four months. While I have no knowledge at this time of permanent anosmia having been produced in any one, nevertheless, I feel that there is this risk, one which may be greater if the treatments are carried out with temporary anosmia as an objective. Dr. Pentecost has recently informed me that all of his group have now regained the sense of smell, "although in a few it is still not 100 per cent." So far as my information goes, all of the cases of more lasting anosmias have been in adults, in whom the immediate local reaction following treatment is likely to be much more severe than in children. This posttreatment reaction is associated with a more or less severe headache, which generally begins about twenty minutes following the application of the solutions and lasts from three to six hours. The headache is usually frontal, localized between the eyes and referred to the occiput. I am told that it ends suddenly, as though a hot iron had suddenly been removed. This difference between adults and children, both in the severity of the immediate reaction and in the duration of the anosmia may possibly be explained on an anatomic basis. In adults the superior meatus is narrower than in children;[51] it may indeed be narrow and deep enough to hold considerable solution by capillary action. This would naturally result in a solution being held in contact with the olfactory mucosa for a longer period of time than would be likely in children, who have a wider superior meatus. Such longer contact would of course intensify and prolong the immediate discomfort and no doubt add to the local injury, whatever the character of this injury may be. One may well ask, is there a relationship between the degree of this immediate reaction and the duration of the anosmia? Is an immediate edema as well as more intense drug action responsible for the pain? Is the more lasting anosmia in adults due in part, at least, to a persisting inflammatory reaction, or, does it rest wholly on a more profound injury to the olfactory apparatus, the result of prolonged and uncontrolled drug action? If the latter is the case, how may we account for the return of function months after treatment? I wish that I could answer these questions. The answers would, no doubt, be more apparent if we knew more about the way zinc sulfate acts in producing protection in monkeys. I recall that during the early part of our studies, I experienced at one time considerable uneasiness when it occurred to me that the protection we had observed might have resulted from an edema of the olfactory mucosa, closing off mechanically the very narrow olfactory cleft. However, careful dissections of the area in untreated and recently treated monkeys ruled out this possibility. It was ruled out also by the fact that the protection in monkeys often lasts for several months.

I would not have you believe that we are unmindful of the possibility that the protection observed may be the result of an actual destruction of the olfactory receptors. In this case susceptibility or the sense of smell would not be expected to return unless structural regeneration can and does take place. This brings up the question, to what extent can the olfactory nerve regenerate? We, of course, all know that ordinary nerve cells are not restored and that only the dendrites and axones of otherwise normal neurons can be regenerated, but so far as I know there is no information available bearing on the regenerative powers of the olfactory nerve. To me it does not seem entirely improbable that these rather primitive receptors, whose cell bodies are no doubt exposed to naturally induced injuries, may possess powers of regeneration beyond those we see in ordinary nerve cells. As I have already pointed out, there are certain reasons for keeping open minded on this question; among these are the restoration of susceptibility in monkeys and the restoration of the sense of smell in man after a prolonged anosmia.

During recent months we have been engaged in studies designed to determine how the resistant state in monkeys is produced, especially with a view to determining whether the protection is associated with recognizable anatomic changes in the olfactory cells or their peripheral processes. This investigation has proved more difficult than we anticipated. An important difficulty lies in the lack of altogether practical staining methods for demonstrating olfactory cells and their processes. In describing the structure of the normal olfactory mucosa, I spoke with some assurance on the differences between three types of cells found in the membrane. However, when one is confronted with the immediate problem of identifying olfactory cells with certainty, he begins to appreciate some of the difficulty which attends such a study. With regard to the more obvious histologic changes, we can say that varying grades of exudative inflammation may be present in the olfactory mucosa even a week or more after treatment, but this is frequently no more than one may observe in untreated monkeys. One may also see some desquamation of the olfactory epithelium, but this also is sometimes observed in sections from normal monkeys. There may be some disorder in the arrangement of the epithelial cells. This, too, has been observed in the olfactory mucosae of some untreated monkeys.

Recently we have examined membranes removed one to five days after treatment. These examinations were prompted by evidences of epithelial regeneration in several membranes which were removed two days after treatment, also, by the fact that the membranes from some of the monkeys treated a week or so previously presented certain signs of having been repaired. What is important is that several membranes removed a day after treatment with 1 per cent zinc sulfate have presented a marked exudative inflammation associated with some desquamation and necrosis of epithelial cells. This inflammation, however, seems to subside rapidly and to be followed very promptly by regeneration of the epithelium. To what extent the olfactory nerve cells themselves figure in this regeneration, if at all, is now being investigated. At present we can only say that if the protection described is wholly the result of a destruction of the peripheral processes of the olfactory cells, or of the cell bodies themselves, it must then follow that there is regeneration of these processes, possibly even of olfactory cells. This only would explain why practically all monkeys become susceptible again to intranasal instillation of virus several months after the treatments. A regeneration of the peripheral processes only would not be novel, but evidence that destroyed neurons are replaced in some way would indeed be new.

I wish to repeat, however, what I said earlier, that it is quite possible that the protection may result, in part at least, from a more or less lasting chemical union of the zinc ion with the dendrite of the olfactory cell, altering its permeability but not necessarily associated with visible anatomic change, or the dendrite alone may be destroyed and subsequently regenerated.

In closing, I should like to make a few more general remarks regarding this type of prophylaxis. Should further field tests show that chemical agents can be used effectively in preventing this disease in man, and should there prove to be no serious contraindications to the widespread use of such a measure, regarding which we may well be uncertain, this would still leave us with a measure which would be far from ideal. It would not be ideal for the reason that such protection as may be afforded would be at best of short duration, thus making it necessary to repeat the treatments several times during the "polio" season. Furthermore, it would not be practical to use it widely enough to protect against the more sporadic occurrence of the disease. Its usefulness would be limited to checking an incipient epidemic, after enough "sentries" give the signal that an epidemic is approaching. An ideal prophylactic measure would be one that would be sufficiently effective to help stamp out the disease entirely. Because of the relatively short duration of the protection and the unlikelihood that a chemical measure ever will be applied to a large part of the population, it is not likely to afford an effective means for the eventual conquest of this disease. But while all this is true, such a measure seems to possess certain virtues not likely to be found in methods which may leave a more lasting immunity. A chemical solution is simple to prepare and inexpensive. It carries nothing which may induce infection and probably will prove simple enough to apply. I am aware there are many who cherish the hope that a method will be found by which a permanent resistance to this disease may be artificially induced, possibly by the application of a specific antigen to the olfactory area. While I would be unwilling to say that there is no prospect of such a solution of the problem, such a measure would have to be not only proof against accidental infections, but financially within reach of the public purse to have wide application. Any measure which requires material from infected monkeys is likely to prove prohibitive from the cost angle alone. This cost, of course, would prove considerably less if we had a simple test to identify those in need of artificial help, but from the results of extensive studies in our laboratory and elsewhere I can say that such a test is not in prospect.

Because of these facts, it is my opinion that the possibilities of chemical prophylaxis should be explored further, for at the present moment such a measure seems to offer the only promise of a practical solution. Investigations should be continued to elicit the most effective, the least irritating, and least harmful agent for trial in man; there should be an agreement on what constitutes a thorough application and how frequently a solution should be applied to insure a continued effect. Above all, we need a satisfactory field test to tell us whether this type of prophylaxis, so effective in monkeys, is in any measure applicable to man.

REFERENCES

1. Levaditi, C., and Danulesco, V.: Compt. rend. Soc. de biol. **73**: 252, 1912.
2. Flexner, S., and Amoss, H. L.: J. Exper. Med. **31**: 123, 1920.
3. Olitsky, P. K., and Cox, H. R.: Science **79**: 566, 1934.
4. Armstrong, C.: Pub. Health Rep. **50**: 43, 1935.
5. Armstrong, C., and Harrison, W. T.: Pub. Health Rep. **50**: 725, 1935.
6. Armstrong, C., and Harrison, W. T.: Pub. Health Rep. **51**: 203, 1936.
7. Sabin, A. B., Olitsky, P. K., and Cox, H. R.: J. Bact. **31**: 35, 1936; J. Exper. Med. **63**: 877, 1936.
8. Schultz, E. W., and Gebhardt, L. P.: Proc. Soc. Exper. Biol. & Med. **34**: 133, 1936; California & West. Med. **45**: 138, 1936.
9. Schultz, E. W., and Gebhardt, L. P.: California & West. Med. **43**: 111, 1935; J. Pediat. **7**: 332, 1935.
10. Landsteiner, K., and Popper, E.: Wien. klin Wchnschr. **21**: 1830, 1908.
11. Flexner, S., and Clark, P. F.: Proc. Soc. Exper. Biol. & Med. **10**: 1, 1912-1913.
12. Flexner, S., and Amoss, H. L.: J. Exper. Med. **25**: 525, 1917.
13. Schaeffer, J. P.: The Nose and Olfactory Organ, pp. 370, Philadelphia, 1920. P. Blakiston's Son & Co.; Special Cytology, Edit. by E. V. Cowdry, Vol. 1, p. 47, New York, 1928, Paul B. Hoeber, Inc.
14. Key and Retzius: Anatomie des Nervensystems und des Bindesgewebe, Stockholm, 1876.
15. Clark, W. E. LeG.: Great Britain Reports on Public Health and Medical Subjects, Ministry of Health, No. 54, 1929.
16. Rake, G.: J. Exper. Med. **65**: 303, 1937.
17. Brodie, M., and Elvidge, A. R.: Science **79**: 235, 1934.
18. Schultz, E. W., and Gebhardt, L. P.: Proc. Soc. Exper. Biol. & Med. **31**: 728, 1934.
19. Lennette, E. H., and Hudson, N. P.: Proc. Soc. Exper. Biol. & Med. **32**: 1444, 1935.
20. Armstrong, C.: Pub. Health Rep. **51**: 241, 1936.
21. Sabin, A. B., and Olitsky, P. K.: J. A. M. A. **108**: 21, 1937.
22. Sabin, A. B., and Olitsky, P. K.: Proc. Soc. Exper. Biol. & Med. **34**: 357, 1936.
23. Hurst, E. W.: J. Path. & Bact. **32**: 457, 1929.
24. Fairbrother, R. W., and Hurst, E. W.: J. Path. & Bact. **33**: 17, 1930.
25. Faber, H. K., and Gebhardt, L. P.: J. Exper. Med. **57**: 933, 1933.
26. Faber, H. K.: Medicine **12**: 83, 1933.
27. Schultz, E. W., and Gebhardt, L. P.: Studies on the Pathogenesis of Poliomyelitis. I. Relationship Between the Concentration of Virus and Nerve Injury. Unpublished Observations.
28. Covell, W. P.: Proc. Soc. Exper. Biol. & Med. **28**: 927, 1930.
29. Hurst, E. W.: J. Path. & Bact. **34**: 331, 1931.
30. Schultz, E. W.: J. Pediat. **1**: 358, 1932.
31. Clifton, C., Schultz, E. W., and Gebhardt, L. P.: J. Bact. **22**: 7, 1931; Theiler, M., and Bauer, J. H.: J. Exper. Med. **60**: 767, 1934; Elford, W. J., Galloway, I. A., and Perdrau, J. R.: J. Path. & Bact. **40**: 135, 1935.
32. Kling, C.: Acta psychiat. et neurol. **6**: 337, 1931 (a review).

33. Kling, C., Levaditi, C., and Lépine, P.: Bull. Acad. de méd. **102**: 158, 1929.
34. Kling, C., Levaditi, C., and Hornus, G.: Bull. Acad. de méd. **111**: 709, 1934.
35. Toomey, J. A.: J. Pediat. **8**: 664, 1936 (a review).
36. Hurst, E. W.: J. Path. & Bact. **33**: 1133, 1930.
37. Clark, P. F., Roberts, D. J., and Preston, W. S.: J. Prev. Med. **6**: 47, 1932.
38. Flexner, S.: J. Exper. Med. **63**: 209, 1936.
39. Lennette, E. H., and Hudson, N. P.: J. Infect. Dis. **58**: 10, 1936.
40. Harmon, P. H.: J. A. M. A. **109**: 1061, 1937; Harmon, P. H., and Levine, V.: Ibid. **110**: 602, 1938.
41. Kramer, S. D., Sobel, H. E., Grossman, L. H., and Hoskwith, B.: J. Exper. Med. **64**: 173, 1936.
42. Kramer, S. D.: Proc. Soc. Exper. Biol. & Med. **32**: 1165, 1935.
43. Landon, J. F., and Smith, L. W.: Poliomyelitis, pp. 275, New York, 1934, The Macmillan Company.
44. Sabin, A. B., and Olitsky, P. K.: J. A. M. A. **108**: 21, 1937.
45. Trask, J. D., and Paul, J. R.: J. Bact. **31**: 527, 1936; Science **87**: 44, 1938.
46. Howitt, B. F.: Science **85**: 268, 1937.
47. Armstrong, C.: Am. J. Pub. Health **27**: 103, 1937.
48. Tisdall, F. F., Brown, A., DeFries, R. D., Ross, M. A., and Sellars, A. H.: Canad. Pub. Health J. **28**: 523, 1937.
49. Peet, M. M., Echols, D. H., and Richter, H. J.: J. A. M. A. **108**: 2184, 1937.
50. Pentecost, R. S.: Canad. Pub. Health J. **28**: 493, 1937.
51. Shahinian, L., Bacher, J. A., McNaught, R. C., and Newell, R. R.: J. A. M. A. **110**: 1254, 1938.

PERSISTENT ANOSMIA FOLLOWING ZINC SULFATE NASAL SPRAYING

F. F. TISDALL, M.D., ALAN BROWN, M.D., AND R. D. DEFRIES, M.D.
TORONTO, ONT.

DURING the outbreak of poliomyelitis which occurred in Toronto during the months of August, September, and October, 1937, a study[1] was conducted to furnish information concerning the possible prophylactic value of the zinc sulfate nasal spray, the use of which was suggested by the findings of Schultz and Gebhardt,[2] and Peet, Echols, and Richter.[3] Observations were made on a group of 4,713 children, aged 3 to 10 years, who received two sprayings with an interval between the sprayings of ten to twelve days, and 520 additional children who received only one spraying. The spraying was conducted in special clinics by otolaryngologists. Schultz and Gebhardt, and Peet and his collaborators expressed their belief that the satisfactory covering of the olfactory area was indicated by the loss of the sense of smell. From the observations made in the Toronto study, it would appear that not more than 25 per cent of the children sprayed developed anosmia (temporary). Inquiries have indicated that very few, if any, of the children who were sprayed in the special clinics reported subsequently to the various hospital clinics complaining of persisting anosmia. It is to be remembered that this age group consisted of children of from 3 to 10 years of age.

Through the cooperation of the otolaryngologists of the various city hospitals, reports were supplied concerning the persons sprayed by them in their private practice. Data were kindly furnished regarding age and the number of sprayings. Information was also supplied concerning the presence of anosmia at the end of two months, with or without disturbance of the sense of taste, and similar information at the end of six months. Reports were received from thirty-two otolaryngologists. Statements were not made in their reports concerning the method of determining the loss of the sense of smell or the disturbance of the sense of taste. The number recorded having anosmia with or without disturbance of the sense of taste at the end of two months was thirty-six, and the number at the end of six months was fifty-two, indicating that a number of patients did not consult their otolaryngologist until several months had elapsed. These data, arranged in age groups, are presented in Table I; in Table II, data are presented, arranged according to the number of sprayings.

From the Hospital for Sick Children and the School of Hygiene and Connaught Laboratories, University of Toronto.

TABLE I

PATIENTS REPORTING DISTURBANCE OF SENSE OF SMELL WITH OR WITHOUT DISTURBANCE OF SENSE OF TASTE

(Toronto, 1937)

AGE (YR.)	AFTER 2 MONTHS				AFTER 6 MONTHS			
	SMELL ONLY	TASTE ONLY	SMELL AND TASTE	TOTAL	SMELL ONLY	TASTE ONLY	SMELL AND TASTE	TOTAL
Less than 10	2	3	–	5	–	–	1	1
10 to 14	4	–	4	8	1	4	5	10
15 to 19	7	4	5	16	5	3	13	21
20 to 24	2	2	–	4	1	1	13	15
More than 25	–	–	3	3	–	–	5	5
Total	15	9	12	36	7	8	37	52

TABLE II

DISTURBANCE OF SMELL AND TASTE IN RELATION TO THE NUMBER OF SPRAYINGS

(Toronto, 1937)

NO. OF SPRAYS	AFTER 2 MONTHS				AFTER 6 MONTHS			
	SMELL ONLY	TASTE ONLY	SMELL AND TASTE	TOTAL	SMELL ONLY	TASTE ONLY	SMELL AND TASTE	TOTAL
1	–	1	3	4	1	–	10	11
2	11	8	9	28	6	7	26	39
3	4	–	–	4	–	1	1	2
Total	15	9	12	36	7	8	37	52

Although data were not available regarding the total number of persons sprayed by the various otolaryngologists, the total number probably did not exceed 5,000. That this is not too conservative an estimate is indicated by the fact that records of only 741 children receiving two sprayings in private practice were received from the otolaryngologists of the city for inclusion in the report of the original study. The findings as presented in Table I indicate that the complaint of persistent anosmia occurred more frequently in the older age groups. Although it is not possible to state the methods of testing the sense of smell used by the various otolaryngologists, there can be little doubt that these patients at the end of six months had definite complaints of disturbance of the sense of smell and, in many instances, of taste. It will be noted from Table I that only five children less than 10 years of age were reported by the group of otolaryngologists, in their private practice, as having anosmia at the end of two months and only one at the end of six months. These findings are in accord with the opinion of the attending otolaryngologists that few, if any, of the children who received the nasal spraying in the special clinics subsequently suffered from a continuing disturbance of the sense of smell. Persisting disturbance of taste and smell was noted in eleven cases (Table II), in which the patients received only one spraying, and in thirty-nine who received two sprayings. The clinical reports relating to the fifty-two patients, who at the end of six months had disturbances of the sense of smell and taste, include patients with marked loss of the sense of smell as well as others in whom the sense of smell is returning. Some complained of unpleasant odors and others of a distorted sense of smell. Disturbances of taste were frequently associated with disturbances of smell (Table I).

DISCUSSION

Schultz and Gebhardt based their belief that the application of 1 per cent zinc sulfate with 0.5 per cent pontocaine, in the small amounts required to cover the olfactory area, would not produce any undesirable or harmful effects on the finding that no noteworthy gross or microscopic changes were found in the nasal mucous membranes of monkeys treated repeatedly with zinc sulfate, other than a mild grade of inflammation. Peet and his collaborators recorded anosmia following the application of the spray in a group of medical students but found that the sense of smell returned within one or two weeks. Dr. Peet[4] reported that all children sprayed by him and by his associates in Michigan last summer had been re-examined, and in every one the sense of smell had returned. In some adults, however, the sense of smell did not return to normal for three months or even longer.

The persisting disturbance of sense of smell and taste in certain individuals, after a period of six months, is difficult to explain on the basis of a persisting inflammation of the olfactory mucous membrane, causing a mechanical blocking of the olfactory area. A study of the changes in the olfactory mucous membrane following the instillation of zinc sulfate in rats,[5] and similar observations made in ferrets[6] suggest that the effect of a one per cent solution of zinc sulfate on the mucous membrane of human beings should be carefully studied to determine if the persisting disturbance of smell and taste may be due to injury to the olfactory area.

REFERENCES

1. Tisdall, F. F., Brown, Alan, Defries, R. D., Ross, M. A., and Sellers, A. H.: Canad. Pub. Health J. **28**: 523, 1937.
2. Schultz, E. W., and Gebhardt, L. P.: J. A. M. A. **108**: 2182, 1937.
3. Peet, M. M., Echols, D. H., and Richter, H. J.: J. A. M. A. **108**: 2184, 1937.
4. Peet, M. M.: Personal communication, University of Michigan, Ann Arbor, Mich.
5. Smith, C. G.: Personal communication, Department of Anatomy, University of Toronto.
6. Stuart-Harris, C. H.: Personal communication, Rockefeller Institute for Medical Research, New York.

ACUTE ANTERIOR POLIOMYELITIS FOLLOWING TONSILLECTOMY AND ADENOIDECTOMY

With Special Reference to the Bulbar Form

R. Cannon Eley, M.D., and Carlyle G. Flake, M.D.
Boston, Mass.

THE portal of entry of the virus of poliomyelitis into the central nervous system has always received a great deal of attention and even today warrants further clinical and experimental study. The fact that the bulbar form of acute anterior poliomyelitis has been reported[1, 2] following recent tonsillectomy and adenoidectomy has suggested that this procedure might, in some manner, influence the entrance of the virus. A study of 418 consecutive patients with acute poliomyelitis admitted to the medical wards of the Infants' and the Children's Hospitals of Boston adds further evidence as to this possibility and strongly suggests that in those instances in which the operation is of an elective nature, it may be advisable to postpone it during that period when poliomyelitis is prevalent. The following information is offered in support of this statement.

Table I

Total Number of Admissions of Patients With Acute Poliomyelitis

Number of cases of spinal poliomyelitis	287
Number of cases of bulbar poliomyelitis	131
Total number of admissions	418

The large percentage of bulbar poliomyelitis cases included in the total number of admissions in Table I is striking. This is probably explained by the fact that this form of the disease causes deeper concern than the spinal form, with the result that the patient suffering from bulbar poliomyelitis is more frequently referred to the hospital.

CASES OF ACUTE ANTERIOR POLIOMYELITIS

Record No. 154106.—J. R., female, 4¼ years of age, had a tonsillectomy and adenoidectomy on Oct. 14, 1931, and on Oct. 24, 1931, complained of headache and malaise. Two days later she developed a stiff back, resisted anterior flexion of her head, and complained of headache. On October 28 she was admitted to the hospital with temperature 101° F., pulse rate 120 per minute, and respiration rate 28 per minute. The physical examination and the examination of the cerebrospinal fluid were sufficient to warrant a diagnosis of acute anterior poliomyelitis. A few days after her entry the patient developed weakness of her abdominal muscles.

Record No. 182418.—J. I., male, 5 years and 11 months old, had a tonsillectomy and adenoidectomy on Aug. 13, 1934, and on Sept. 7, 1934, he complained of head-

From the Infants' and the Children's Hospitals, the Department of Pediatrics of the Harvard Medical School, and the Department of Communicable Diseases of the Harvard School of Public Health, Boston, Mass.

ache, malaise, abdominal pain, and developed a temperature of 102° F. During the following thirty-six hours these symptoms persisted, but for the next twelve hours he felt well so was allowed out of bed. When he began to walk he complained of weakness in his legs. On admission to the hospital his temperature was 102.6° F., pulse rate, 115 per minute, and respiration rate, 25 per minute. Examination revealed definite signs of meningeal irritation and weakness of the extensor muscles of the lower extremities. The changes in the cerebrospinal fluid were consistent with those noted in acute poliomyelitis.

RECORD NO. 214299.—B. P., female, 4½ years of age, had a tonsillectomy and adenoidectomy performed on July 1, 1937. On July 26, 1937, she complained of headache and pains in her muscles. On July 29 these hyperesthesias of her muscles became more pronounced, her neck resisted anterior flexion, and her back was stiff. On August 2 she was admitted to the hospital with a temperature of 98.6° F., pulse 120 per minute, and respiration 28 per minute; there was weakness of the right shoulder girdle. Examination of the cerebrospinal fluid showed clinic and cytologic changes consistent with a diagnosis of acute anterior poliomyelitis.

RECORD NO. 214691.—G. J., male, 5 years and 9 months of age, had a tonsillectomy and adenoidectomy performed on July 22, 1937. On Aug. 18, 1937, he developed a temperature, headache, and became irritable. At the time of examination, August 22, his temperature was 101.4° F., pulse 130 per minute, and respiration 40 per minute. The neck resisted anterior flexion, the back was stiff, and there was weakness of the right lower extremity. Examination of the cerebrospinal fluid presented changes consistent with acute anterior poliomyelitis.

RECORD NO. 138479.—H. P., male, 3 years and 10 months of age, had a tonsillectomy and adenoidectomy on July 27, 1930. On August 26 he became restless, complained of headache and abdominal pain. The following day the same symptoms were present and there was temperature, resistance to anterior flexion of the neck, and stiffness of the back. On admission the temperature was 99.8° F., pulse 140 per minute, and respiration 40 per minute. The physical examination as well as the examination of the cerebrospinal fluid supported a diagnosis of acute anterior poliomyelitis.

RECORD NO. 142785.—C. K., male, 9 years of age, had a tonsillectomy and adenoidectomy on Aug. 29, 1930, and on Oct. 1, 1930, complained of headache, abdominal pain, and nausea. On the following day the patient vomited, continued to complain of headache, and developed a temperature, stiff neck, and stiff back. On admission his temperature was 100.4° F., pulse 90 per minute, and respiration 25 per minute. The physical examination and the examination of the cerebrospinal fluid warranted a diagnosis of acute anterior poliomyelitis.

PATIENTS WITH BULBAR POLIOMYELITIS

RECORD NO. 108099.—J. S., female, 7⅓ years of age, had her tonsils and adenoids removed on Aug. 11, 1927, and on Aug. 21, 1927, she became nauseated, complained of a headache, and regurgitated fluid through her nose. At the time of admission to the hospital on August 22 her temperature was 100.4° F., pulse 110 per minute, and respiration 20 per minute. Physical examination and examination of the cerebrospinal fluid supported the diagnosis of acute anterior poliomyelitis with pharyngeal paralysis.

RECORD NO. 62593.—D. V., male, 4 years and 11 months of age, had a tonsillectomy and adenoidectomy performed on Aug. 5, 1927. On August 15 he complained of malaise, headache, and vomited. On August 18 he developed a nasal voice, became unable to swallow, and regurgitated fluids through his nose. At the time of admission to the hospital his temperature was 100.4° F., pulse 120 per minute, and respiration 24 per minute. The physical examination and the examination of the cerebrospinal fluid confirmed the diagnosis of acute anterior poliomyelitis with pharyngeal paralysis.

RECORD NO. 108514.—M. D., female, 8 years of age, had her tonsils and adenoids removed on Aug. 14, 1927, and on Aug. 24, 1927, she became drowsy, irritable, and complained of a headache. On August 28 her speech became indistinct and some difficulty was encountered on swallowing. At the time of her admission, August 30, her temperature was 104° F., pulse 120 per minute, and respiration 30 per minute. Physical examination and examination of the cerebrospinal fluid confirmed the diagnosis of acute anterior poliomyelitis with pharyngeal paralysis.

RECORD NO. 162714.—W. E., male, 6 years of age, had a tonsillectomy and adenoidectomy performed on July 22, 1933, and on Aug. 6, 1933, complained of headache and malaise; he refused food and developed a temperature. On August 8 he complained of stiff neck and back, and on August 9 he became unable to swallow fluids. At the time of admission his temperature was 101° F., pulse 130 per minute, and respiration 30 per minute. Physical examination and examination of the cerebrospinal fluid warranted a diagnosis of acute anterior poliomyelitis with right facial paralysis and partial paralysis of both shoulders and left hip.

RECORD NO. 162675.—M. McG., female, 4 years and 2 months of age, had a tonsillectomy and adenoidectomy on Aug. 16, 1932, and on Aug. 28, 1932, she developed a temperature and vomited. Twenty-four hours later she complained of a stiff neck and back. On August 30 her voice assumed a nasal tone and she began to regurgitate fluids through her nose. Physical examination and examination of the cerebrospinal fluid established a diagnosis of acute anterior poliomyelitis with pharyngeal paralysis.

RECORD NO. 153356.—A. T., female, 6¾ years of age, had her tonsils and adenoids removed on Sept. 11, 1931. On Sept. 21, 1931, the school teacher observed that the child had a nasal voice and seemed to swallow with difficulty. The child was sent home from school and on the following day admitted to a hospital where the diagnosis of acute anterior poliomyelitis with pharyngeal paralysis was made. On September 26 she was transferred to the Children's Hospital where the same diagnosis was made, as the physical examination and examination of the cerebrospinal fluid were consistent with this infection.

RECORD NO. 195745.—E. B., male, 9 years of age, had a tonsillectomy and adenoidectomy performed on Sept. 1, 1935. On Sept. 14, 1935, he developed a temperature, vomited, and complained of difficulty in swallowing. He was admitted to the hospital on September 15, at which time his temperature was 102.4° F., pulse 106 per minute, and respiration 24 per minute. Physical examination and examination of the cerebrospinal fluid established the diagnosis of acute anterior poliomyelitis with pharyngeal paralysis.

RECORD NO. 191189.—J. D., male, 4¾ years of age had his tonsils and adenoids removed on July 31, 1935, and on August 14 complained of malaise, headache, and developed a nasal voice. He was admitted to the hospital on August 17, at which time his temperature was 101.6° F., pulse 152 per minute, and respiration 32 per minute. Physical examination as well as examination of the cerebrospinal fluid established the diagnosis of acute poliomyelitis with pharyngeal paralysis.

RECORD NO. 153131.—M. T., female, 6 years of age, had a tonsillectomy and adenoidectomy performed on Sept. 2, 1931. On Sept. 16, 1931, she became listless and complained of being tired. The following day she became unable to swallow fluids. At the time of admission her temperature was 102.4° F., pulse 140 per minute, and respiration 24 per minute. Physical examination as well as the examination of the cerebrospinal fluid confirmed the diagnosis of acute anterior poliomyelitis with pharyngeal paralysis.

Record No. 142337.—G. B., female, 6 years and 2 months of age, had her tonsils and adenoids removed on Sept. 4, 1930. On Sept. 18, 1930, she complained of headache and developed a temperature of 101.6° F. Forty-eight hours later she began to regurgitate fluids, and her voice became nasal in character. On admission, her temperature was 102.4° F., pulse 90 per minute, and respiration 30 per minute. Physical examination and examination of the cerebrospinal fluid confirmed the diagnosis of acute anterior poliomyelitis with pharyngeal paralysis.

Record No. 124487.—T. K., male, 2¾ years of age, had his tonsils and adenoids removed on Aug. 3, 1931. On Aug. 17, 1931, he became irritable and fussy, developed a nasal voice, and began to regurgitate fluids. At the time of admission his temperature was 103° F., pulse 130 per minute, and respiration 30 per minute. Physical examination and examination of the cerebrospinal fluid confirmed the diagnosis of acute anterior poliomyelitis with pharyngeal paralysis.

Record No. 172937.—M. N., female, 6 years and 2 months of age, had her tonsils and adenoids removed on Aug. 7, 1933, and on Aug. 22, 1933, became sick with temperature, nausea, malaise, and headache. The following day, August 23, her neck became stiff, and her voice developed a nasal quality. She was admitted to the hospital on August 24 with temperature 99.8° F., pulse 92 per minute, and respiration 24 per minute. Physical examination disclosed paralysis of the pharynx and stiff neck. The changes in the cerebrospinal fluid were consistent with those noted in acute anterior poliomyelitis.

Record No. 188272.—N. M., female, 5 years and 5 months of age, had a tonsillectomy and adenoidectomy performed on Aug. 28, 1935. On September 13, after a day or two of not feeling very well, the child developed a nasal voice and began to regurgitate fluids through her nose. She was admitted to the hospital on September 15, at which time her temperature was 102.8° F., pulse 128 per minute, and respiration 28 per minute. The physical examination and the cytochemical changes within the cerebrospinal fluid confirmed the diagnosis of acute anterior poliomyelitis with pharyngeal involvement.

Record No. 109687.—P. L., male, 6½ years of age, had his tonsils and adenoids removed on Sept. 27, 1927. On Oct. 13, 1927, he complained of headache, muscle pains, and fever. At the time of admission, Oct. 17, 1927, his temperature was 99.8° F., pulse 110 per minute, and respiration 20 per minute. Physical examination and examination of the cerebrospinal fluid supported a diagnosis of acute anterior poliomyelitis with right facial paralysis.

Record No. 153511.—R. P., male, 5 years and 1 month of age, had a tonsillectomy and adenoidectomy on Aug. 21, 1935, and on Sept. 8, 1935, he developed a temperature, headache, stiff neck, and began to talk with a nasal voice. On September 10 he was admitted to the hospital, at which time his temperature was 102.2° F., pulse 120 per minute, and respiration 24 per minute. Physical examination and the examination of the cerebrospinal fluid warranted a diagnosis of acute anterior poliomyelitis with pharyngeal paralysis.

Record No. 152204.—E. B., male, 9 years of age, had a tonsillectomy and adenoidectomy performed on July 28, 1931, and on Aug. 16, 1931, he developed a temperature and complained of a stiff neck. The following day his speech became nasal in quality, and there was difficulty in swallowing. At that time he was admitted to the hospital with a temperature of 101° F., pulse 146 per minute, and respiration 26 per minute. Physical examination and examination of the cerebrospinal fluid justified a diagnosis of acute anterior poliomyelitis with pharyngeal paralysis.

Record No. 196760.—R. L., male, 3 years of age, had a tonsillectomy and adenoidectomy on Nov. 13, 1935, and on Dec. 4, 1935, he became irritable, feverish, and vomited several times. On the following day his condition remained unchanged with the exception of the fact that he developed a stiff neck and stiff back. He was admitted to the hospital on December 9, at which time his temperature was 102° F., pulse 140 per minute, and respiration 40 per minute. Physical examination and cytoclinical examination of the cerebrospinal fluid established the diagnosis of acute anterior poliomyelitis. A few hours after entry the patient developed palatal paralysis, paralysis of both arms and the diaphragm. Death occurred on December 9.

PATIENTS WITH SPINAL POLIOMYELITIS

Record No. 205037.—E. F., male, 11 years of age, had his tonsils and adenoids removed on July 24, 1936, and on July 21, 1937, he complained of headache and developed a temperature of 103° F. On August 1 he was admitted to the hospital, at which time his temperature was 105° F., pulse 136 per minute, and respiration 32 per minute. His neck resisted anterior flexion, the back was stiff, the muscles were tender, the reflexes were hyperactive, and there was a positive Kernig sign. Examination of the cerebrospinal fluid showed chemical and cytologic changes consistent with those found in acute anterior poliomyelitis.

Record No. 142311.—A. G., male, 5¾ years of age, had his tonsils and adenoids removed on Aug. 25, 1930, and on Sept. 2, 1930, he became ill with headache, vomiting, stiff neck, stiff back, and hyperesthesia of his muscles. At the time of admission to the hospital, his temperature was 99.8° F., pulse 100 per minute, and respiration 24 per minute. Physical examination and examination of the cerebrospinal fluid supported a diagnosis of acute anterior poliomyelitis. At the time of discharge from the hospital the patient presented weakness of the left intercostal muscles as well as weakness of the right leg.

Table II

Spinal Poliomyelitis in Relation to Tonsillectomy and Adenoidectomy

Number of patients with spinal poliomyelitis with tonsils and adenoids present	184
Number of patients with spinal poliomyelitis with tonsils and adenoids previously excised	95
Number of patients with spinal poliomyelitis with tonsils and adenoids excised within 30 days prior to illness	8

Table III

Bulbar Poliomyelitis in Relation to Tonsillectomy and Adenoidectomy

Number of patients with bulbar poliomyelitis with tonsils and adenoids present	40
Number of patients with bulbar poliomyelitis with tonsils and adenoids previously excised	74
Number of patients with bulbar poliomyelitis with tonsils and adenoids excised within 30 days prior to illness	17

Tables II and III indicate the number of cases of spinal and bulbar poliomyelitis in relation to the presence or absence of the tonsils and adenoids. The occurrence of eight cases of the former type and of seventeen cases of the latter type within a short period of time following the removal of the tonsils and adenoids is demonstrated in the following tables.

Table IV presents a tabulation of the number of cases of spinal poliomyelitis occurring within thirty days following the excision of the tonsils and adenoids. Although 287 patients with this form of the disease were admitted to the hospital, yet there were only eight patients with a history of a recent tonsillectomy and adenoidectomy, a percentage of 2.78. It will be further noted that of the eight pa-

TABLE IV

ACUTE ANTERIOR POLIOMYELITIS, SPINAL FORM, DEVELOPING WITHIN 30 DAYS FOLLOWING OPERATION

Total No. cases of spinal form = 287
No. cases following operation = 8
Percentage = 2.78

RECORD NO.	DATE OF OPERATION	DATE OF ONSET OF ILLNESS	DAYS BETWEEN OPERATION AND ONSET	CELL COUNT OF CEREBROSPINAL FLUID	PARALYSIS
205037	7/24/36	7/31/36	7	350	0
142311	8/25/30	9/ 2/30	8	17	+
154106	10/14/31	10/24/31	10	270	+
182418	8/13/34	9/ 7/34	24	210	0
214299	7/ 1/37	7/26/37	25	12	+
214691	7/22/37	8/18/37	26	62	+
138479	7/28/30	10/ 1/30	29	60	0
142785	8/29/30	10/ 1/30	30	90	0

TABLE V

ACUTE ANTERIOR POLIOMYELITIS, BULBAR FORM, DEVELOPING WITHIN 30 DAYS FOLLOWING OPERATION

Total No. cases of bulbar form = 131
No. cases following operation = 17
Percentage = 12.98

RECORD NO.	DATE OF OPERATION	DATE OF ONSET OF ILLNESS	DAYS BETWEEN OPERATION AND ONSET	CELL COUNT OF CEREBROSPINAL FLUID	PARALYSIS
108099*	8/11/27	8/21/27	10	63	+
62593	8/ 5/27	8/15/27	10	22	+
108514	8/14/27	8/25/27	11	180	+
162714	7/26/33	8/ 6/33	11	80	+
162675	8/16/32	8/28/32	11	101	+
153356	9/11/31	9/21/31	10	110	+
195745	9/ 1/35	9/14/35	13	39	+
191189	7/31/35	8/14/35	14	96	+
153131	9/ 2/31	9/16/31	14	180	+
142337	9/ 4/30	9/18/30	14	23	+
124487	8/ 3/31	8/17/31	14	120	+
172937	8/ 7/33	8/22/33	15	130	+
188272	8/28/35	9/13/35	16	95	+
109687	9/27/27	10/13/27	16	105	+
153511	8/21/35	9/ 8/35	18	49	+
152204	7/28/31	8/16/31	19	60	+
196760	11/13/35	12/ 4/35	20	166	Died

*This case had an adenoidectomy without tonsillectomy.

tients with the disease, only three developed it between the seventh and eighteenth day (the commonly accepted incubation period of poliomyelitis) following the operative procedure.

From Table V it can be seen that the number of cases of bulbar poliomyelitis occurring within thirty days following the removal of the tonsils and adenoids is in marked contrast to the number of cases of the spinal form following the same procedure. Of 131 patients with bulbar poliomyelitis admitted to the wards, seventeen or 12.98 per cent had had this operation performed within twenty days prior to the onset of their illness. Furthermore, fifteen of the seventeen patients developed the disease within the usual incubation period. Statistical computations demonstrate that the occurrence of this number of cases within the given period of time cannot be attributed to chance, nor can it be attributed to the usual frequency of poliomyelitis. The interval between the operation and the onset of both forms of the disease is indicated in Fig. 1.

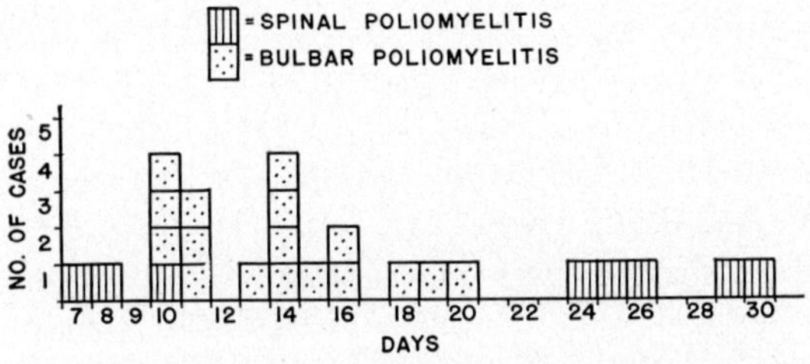

Fig. 1.—Interval between operation and onset of disease, in days.

Table VI, which demonstrates what might be called "scatter cases" (i.e., cases developing after a sufficient period of time has elapsed between the operation and the onset of the disease to indicate that the two conditions were unrelated), further emphasizes the concentration of the cases following operation as shown in Tables IV and V. One might reasonably include five of the cases listed in Table IV and two of the cases listed in Table V in this group.

TABLE VI

"SCATTER CASES" FOLLOWING TONSILLECTOMY AND ADENOIDECTOMY

Case 108932—Developed	spinal	poliomyelitis	5 weeks following operation
Case 194649—Developed	spinal	poliomyelitis	6 weeks following operation
Case 175114—Developed	bulbar	poliomyelitis	7 weeks following operation
Case 195734—Developed	spinal	poliomyelitis	8 weeks following operation
Case 196269—Developed	spinal	poliomyelitis	12 weeks following operation

It was thought that the type of paralysis occurring in the cases of bulbar poliomyelitis might bear some relationship to the presence or absence of the tonsils and adenoids. However, a study of Table VII does not confirm this impression. This may be due to the limited number of cases included in each group.

TABLE VII

DISTRIBUTION OF PARALYSIS IN BULBAR POLIOMYELITIS IN RELATION TO PRESENCE OR ABSENCE OF TONSILS AND ADENOIDS

BULBAR POLIOMYELITIS		
TONSILS AND ADENOIDS PRESENT	TONSILS AND ADENOIDS PREVIOUSLY EXCISED	FOLLOWING WITHIN 20 DAYS AFTER OPERATION
Pharyngeal 23 patients—57.50% Facial 6 patients—15.00% Respiratory 11 patients—22.50% Total No. patients—40	Pharyngeal 91 patients—77.00% Facial 13 patients—11.00% Respiratory 14 patients—11.80% Total No. patients—118	Pharyngeal 14 patients—77.8% Facial 3 patients—16.6% Respiratory 1 patient—5.5% Total No. patients—18

DISCUSSION

These clinical observations would give the impression that if the patient is harboring the virus at the time of the operation, traumatization of the tissues may enable it to gain entrance to the central nervous system either by way of the lymphatic system, the blood stream, or perhaps by direct neural extension. Furthermore, the high incidence of the bulbar form of the disease as compared with the spinal form suggested that it might be possible to reproduce this clinical condition in the monkey. However, suitable animal studies made in Dr. Lloyd Aycock's laboratory and under his direction produced uniformly negative results, as we were unable to produce the disease experimentally in monkeys by the direct inoculation of large amounts of a potent virus into either the tonsillar or peritonsillar tissues. The failure to reproduce the clinical condition in these animals may, however, be due to some anatomic difference between man and monkey and does not exclude tonsillectomy and adenoidectomy as possible factors contributory to the development of the infection in man.

The fact that one of the patients developed bulbar poliomyelitis following adenoidectomy (No. 108099, Table V) without tonsillectomy would indicate that it is not necessarily the latter operation that enables the virus to gain entrance to the central nervous system. This aspect of the problem, as well as the entire subject, requires further study before final conclusions can be safely made.

Abstracts of the patients included in this study are included.

We wish to acknowledge the helpful assistance of Dr. Lloyd Aycock of the Harvard Infantile Paralysis Commission, Harvard Medical School.

REFERENCES

1. Aycock, W. Lloyd: New England J. Med. **200**: 164, 1929.
2. Ayer, Wardner D.: Proceedings of Interstate Post-Graduate Medical Assembly of North America, 1928.

THE CONSTRUCTION OF AN EMERGENCY RESPIRATOR FOR USE IN TREATING RESPIRATORY FAILURE IN INFANTILE PARALYSIS

PHILIP DRINKER, M.D., AND EDGAR L. ROY, M.D., BOSTON, MASS.

ON FREQUENT occasions we have been asked to give directions for building respirators which would tide a patient over a day or a week, pending the arrival of a respirator of the type approved by the American Medical Association's Council of Physical Therapy.*

In Figs. 1, 2, and 3, constructional details of a wooden respirator which would answer such requests are given. The rubber collar is made by cutting a hole of suitable size from an inner tube of a moderate-size car.

The cover of the box is light and need not be hinged or fastened in any way (Figs. 1 and 3). The felt gasket is obtainable at any hardware store and is commonly used as weather stripping for leaky windows.

The vacuum pump shown at the right rear (Figs. 1 and 2) is the hand-size vacuum cleaner costing about $15.00 at any department store or electrical shop. The common household cleaners may pull a higher vacuum but are more expensive. The objectionable whining noise of the cleaner can be minimized by placing it in the next room and connecting it to the box by noncollapsible tubing (about 1 inch inside diameter). The length of tubing to be used should be determined by trial. If the tubing is too long, the cleaner cannot pull the required vacuum.

The observation window is made of double-thick (about ⅛ inch) window glass and should be about 6 inches square.

The frequency and depth of respiration are controlled by the hand-operated valve (Fig. 3), which is made from a piece of sole leather or of fiber. The valve hole in the box should be about 2 inches in diameter. If it is too small, the vacuum pump will maintain a slight negative pressure in the box, and then the patient cannot exhale easily. If the hole is too large, the valve will be difficult to work. This valve can be mechanized later by an experienced mechanic if the hand operation proves too arduous.

The pressure indicator may be a glass U-tube half full of colored water or a piece of straight glass tubing. If a U-tube is used, the arms should be about 12 inches to 15 inches long, while if a straight tube is preferred, it should be about that same length and dip vertically into a dish of water. One arm of the U-tube, or the upper end of the straight tube, should be connected by rubber tubing to the respirator box. A scale in

From the Harvard School of Public Health and Warren E. Collins, Inc., Boston, Mass.

*See J. A. M. A., May 9, 1931, p. 1580.

centimeters should be placed behind the manometer. The common type vacuum cleaner will lift water about 15 inches, although some cleaners are stronger. A vacuum of 8 inches (20 cm.) in the respirator box is probably the maximum that will ever be needed.

The dimensions of the box can be chosen to fit the patient, but the size of the head hole, viz. 9 inches, is important. The box in the illustration

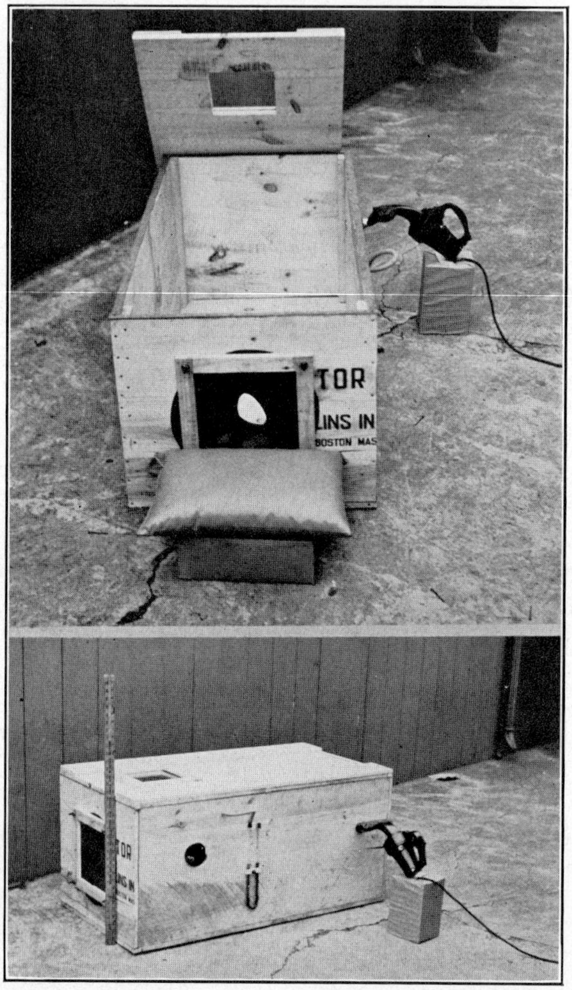

Figs. 1 and 2.—Wooden respirator, 43 in. × 22 in. × 21 in., with vacuum cleaner attached at rear right and hand-operated valve.

was made from ½ inch packing box material at hand and could be duplicated by an experienced carpenter in about two hours. If there is any choice of lumber we suggest matched spruce, tongued and grooved, of ⅝ inch to ⅞ inch thickness. For children's-size machines, the lighter wood is ample. If the wood is not straight and leaky cracks result, they are best stopped with adhesive tape. No painting is necessary.

A patient is placed in the machine by lowering him into the box, bending up his knees, if necessary. One person then stretches the rubber collar, and either one or two persons lift the patient and push his head through until the shoulders touch the head end of the box, as in the approved type respirator. The collar is then stretched to suit. In general, it is best to have the collar hole a bit too large; and the resulting leaks around the neck may be stuffed with cotton. Otherwise the sharp rubber edge from a freshly cut inner tube may irritate the patient's neck.

The lid is then placed on the box, the vacuum cleaner started, and the valve moved back and forth by hand so that the patient breathes about fifteen times a minute at about 15 cm. negative pressure on the manometer. If the patient is badly cyanosed, deeper and quicker breaths can be given by manipulating the valve.

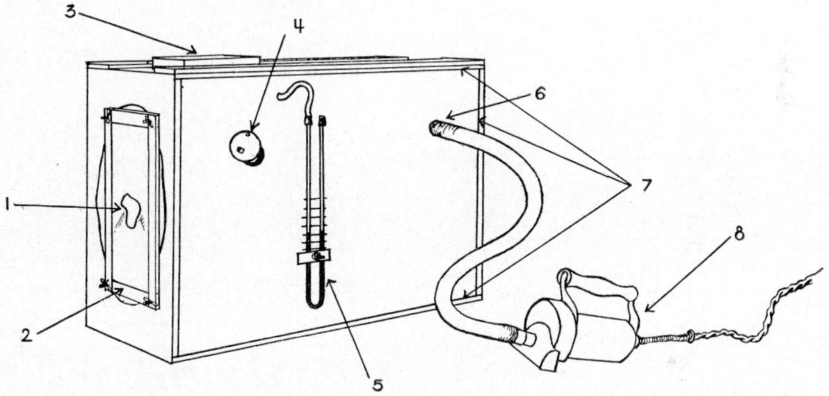

Fig. 3.—Measured perspective of wooden respirator. *1.* Rubber collar from inner tube 13 in. × 3 in. *2.* Collar frame fastened down with wing nuts on carriage bolts. *3.* Double-thickness glass window made tight with felt gasket. *4.* Valve port (2 in.) for hand-operable valve. *5.* U-tube manometer, 15 in. long, ¼ in. tubing. *6.* Hole, 1¼ in. *7.* Felt gaskets, tacked to frame. *8.* Vacuum cleaner.

A brief trial treatment on a healthy person, preferably a child, should be made by any group whose members have not used respirators. When the machine is running at about 15 cm. and 15 breaths a minute, speech will be interrupted when inhalation (negative pressure) is induced by the pump. Ask the subject to count out loud and the results will be evident immediately.

The objections to using such a makeshift apparatus are serious and perfectly definite. We have, therefore, misgivings in presenting this description. We would not offer the device for approval to the American Medical Association's Council of Physical Therapy. Nevertheless, when we receive emergency requests for help in building a machine for a few days' use, pending the arrival of a more satisfactory device, this is the type of equipment we recommend.

The objections to the emergency respirator are the following:

First, it is impossible to give any but small patients a semblance of the nursing care which is so vital in poliomyelitis. It is difficult to make the patient comfortable and to effect the postural changes so necessary in most patients with severe or even mild respiratory embarrassment. Even if the respirator works perfectly, it will not take the place of nursing care.

Second, such respirators made with the best cabinet-quality wood and by skilled cabinet workers have checked and cracked in an annoyingly short time. Such failure is probably caused by the rapid pressure changes and dampness within the respirator. It is, therefore, risky to use such a machine, put it in storage in the basement, and then expect it to be in working condition when the emergency arises. Theoretically, the wooden machines should last a long time. Practically, this has not proved to be the case.

MENTAL HYGIENE IN AN ORTHOPEDIC HOSPITAL

J. D. M. Griffin, M.D., D.P.M. (Eng.),
W. A. Hawke, M.D., M.R.C.P. (Lond.), and
W. Wray Barraclough, M.D., M.R.C.P. (Lond.)
Toronto, Canada

THE problems of the management of prolonged convalescence are different from those of acute illness. As the acute stage passes and the patient enters the phase of recovery, the psychologic factors of the situation become increasingly important. It is so easy for the patient who is spending months at a time in bed to become discouraged and depressed. Even more significant is the ease with which such a patient develops selfish attitudes and lazy habits of thinking. These psychologic factors, rather than any physical defects, frequently form the primary basis of a patient's unwillingness or inability to resume a full and active life.

In children these factors are doubly important. The child's mind is extremely sensitive to suggestion, and the sheltered environment and limitation of activities necessary in any long convalescence are almost bound to have harmful effects unless careful precautions are taken. Most of these harmful effects are directly conditioned by the attitudes and behavior of adults surrounding the patient.

In the recent epidemic of poliomyelitis in Ontario attention was drawn to this aspect of treatment in a very dramatic way. Several hundred patients, most of them children, sustained paralysis which made it necessary for them to undergo a prolonged convalescence. This article describes the efforts which were made to reduce the seriousness of psychologic factors in such an epidemic.

CONVALESCENCE IN CHILDREN

Parents who are confronted with sudden serious illness in their child are naturally apprehensive. When this illness has the reputation of leaving the victim badly crippled for life, their feeling of anxiety is greatly heightened. An epidemic of "polio," for example, with its scare headlines and daily mounting toll of fatalities and paralysis is a terrifying experience for the parents of young children. The child himself when stricken with illnesses of this type cannot help but be influenced by the fear of his parents. This emotional attitude determines his behavior all the way through convalescence.

When the child recovers from the acute phases of the illness and begins to feel well in every respect, the necessity of physical restraint is bound

From the Department of Psychological Medicine of the Hospital for Sick Children and the Department of Paediatrics in the University of Toronto, under the direction of Alan Brown, M.D., F.R.C.P.(C).

to be irksome. Impatience, together with feelings of uneasiness concerning the prognosis, combine to make a situation fraught with emotional tension. The child is not sure of anything. He does not understand clearly why he must remain quiet for so long. Vague adult explanations are often incomplete and alarming. The talk of lameness when he feels so well is likely to be confusing.

Meanwhile the parents' anxiety makes them oversolicitous for the child and overattentive to his every need; this increased attention, coupled with his own immobility, creates a demand for entertainment. Anything that will amuse the child, keep him quiet and comparatively contented, is utilized. Very rapidly the child becomes more demanding, increasingly fond of being the center of attention, and finally a veritable egotistic despot. The fact that every trifling complaint is regarded seriously encourages him to overplay the invalid role. If he does not get his own way at once, he is likely to become emotionally upset and display heart-broken tears or else tantrums of anger. Such a situation, in short, tends to "spoil" the child. It is very difficult for him to keep his wholesome personality.

Poliomyelitis is an outstanding example of a disease in which such emotional factors are exceedingly important. Furthermore, the writers believe that many of the children who have apparently had this disease, have really had polioencephalomyelitis, in which there is usually widespread involvement of the central nervous system. The possibility of organic damage to those centers in the brain which have to do with emotional control must therefore be considered. This is probably an additional factor accounting for the difficulty that many convalescent children have in controlling their tempers and their behavior. Some children of this type show very little else in the way of sequelae and, superficially, seem to have recovered completely. This makes it all the harder for such children to understand the necessity of even a short convalescence. Usually they have little insight into their emotional instability.

THE ONTARIO ORTHOPEDIC HOSPITAL

During the late summer and early autumn of 1937, an epidemic of poliomyelitis of primary importance swept through Ontario. In all 2,635 people were affected, and of these over 1,000 sustained paralysis sufficiently severe to warrant careful orthopedic treatment. In order to carry out this treatment, it was necessary in the majority of cases for the patients to be flat on their backs (usually on Bradford frames) for many months. At the beginning of the treatment it was not known exactly how long this physical restraint would have to be continued, but in some cases at least it was estimated that it would be six to eighteen months or even longer. In order to rest weakened or paralyzed muscles, the affected limbs were placed in special splints. Physiotherapy and good nursing care completed the physical aspects of the treatment.

The Provincial Department of Health in Ontario wished to make certain that every child paralyzed as a result of this epidemic would have a good start along the road to recovery. The department therefore undertook to supply, free of charge to all who wished, a short period of hospital treatment. The hospital arrangements varied according to the needs of the community. In Toronto, where the concentration of cases was greatest, the Department of Health took over a hospital building which had been used for several years as a nurses' residence;* and within a few days equipped it completely as an orthopedic hospital. The full details of this project are published elsewhere.† The chief purpose was to provide each child with at least three weeks' treatment in a carefully controlled environment. During this time the child was properly fitted with a Bradford frame and splints if necessary. Suitable physiotherapy was given. It was decided that the three weeks' stay in the hospital was sufficient to train the children to become accustomed to this treatment so that the regimen could be continued efficiently at home. In order to ensure this, the mothers of the children were brought into the hospital and carefully instructed as to the correct way of nursing and massaging the patients. Instruction was given by means of lectures, demonstrations, and practical work under supervision. It took place during the two days prior to each child's discharge.

The first children to be admitted to the hospital arrived on Sept. 27, 1937, and they were discharged in groups ranging in numbers from eight to twenty-four, twice weekly beginning three weeks later. The last group was discharged on Dec. 8, 1937. During the ten weeks in which the hospital was open, 283 children received treatment and training. The age and sex distributions of these children are shown in Table I. There were more boys than girls and nearly one-half (46 per cent) of the children were under six years of age. Many young adults were treated in the general hospitals of the city, and many patients were kept at home under the care of their family doctors. These figures, therefore, do not give a complete picture of the extent of the epidemic in Toronto. Of the children treated in the Orthopedic Hospital, 218 came from Toronto or the immediate environs. The other 65 came from widely scattered points in the province.

TABLE I

AGE (YR.)	BOYS	GIRLS	TOTAL
0- 3	20	20	40
3- 6	48	41	89
6- 9	40	23	63
9-12	23	18	41
12-15	15	19	34
15-18	15	1	16
	161	122	283

*The Grace Hospital, College and Huron Streets, Toronto.

†Report on Poliomyelitis in Ontario, 1937, published by authority of the Minister of Health, Toronto, Ontario, March, 1938.

Responsibility for the medical and surgical treatment of these children was given to the staff of the Hospital for Sick Children, Toronto. The supervision of their mental health was at once recognized as an important part of the general medical care. The recognized purpose of the Orthopedic Hospital was not only to minimize the extent of physical crippling, but also to prevent the development of any mental crippling. A detailed mental hygiene program was carefully prepared. The Deputy Minister of Health for Ontario collaborated in this project and through his generous support the plan as described below was put into action.

THE MENTAL HYGIENE STAFF

The mental hygiene staff consisted of a neurologist, psychiatrist, and psychiatric social worker from the Department of Psychological Medicine of the Hospital for Sick Children, together with four occupational therapists provided by the Provincial Department of Health. Friends or relatives were not allowed to visit the children because of the danger of concurrent infections. For this reason the early evenings, Saturdays, and Sundays might have been trying times. However, there was a sufficiently large full-time staff to enable two or three aides to be on duty during these times and at all other times when the children were not either busy with routine medical and nursing procedures or asleep.

The program in its final form would have been difficult had it not been for the voluntary assistance of many workers, including librarians, teachers, artists, and occupational therapy students. At one time the number of voluntary assistants, spending a definitely assigned time each week in the hospital, was over twenty.

THE WARDS

Two floors of the hospital were thrown open to patients. The wards were small, the largest having space for nine patients and the smallest, for only one or two. There were fourteen such wards on each floor. For several weeks an additional ward containing over thirty beds was also used. While everything was perfectly clean, it must be remembered that the building was old. The lighting in many of the wards was poor, and the walls were dull and unattractive. One of the first tasks was to brighten the atmosphere of the wards. Colorful posters were donated by the various travel agencies and foreign consulates in the city and were fastened high on the walls so that they could easily be seen. Later many of these were replaced by even more colorful pictures made by the children themselves.

The lack of adequate lighting presented a serious problem which was never completely solved. The danger of eyestrain in children who had to lie for long periods on their backs seemed to be a real one, especially when they tried to read in this position. In a few of the darker wards, however, suitable lamps were attached to the walls to provide indirect illumination of the correct intensity.

The number of small wards made the grouping of children relatively easy. Nevertheless the rapid turnover made the hospital population anything but static, and it was hard to keep any one ward limited to one particular type of child. In so far as it was possible, the children were arranged according to their age groups, as well as according to their sex and the extent of their disability.

PLANNED ACTIVITIES

The basic principle of the program of activities was very simple. It was decided that nothing would be included in the program which did not have positive, constructive, and, as far as possible, permanent value for the children. In other words, there was little place for that sort of entertainment which is merely amusing or exciting. Granted that the visit of the clowns from the indoor circus was a delight to both children and staff, such entertainment was not considered to be sufficiently constructive for a regular place on the long-term program.

Music.—Through the courtesy of radio manufacturers, twelve radios were lent or donated to the hospital. These were distributed among the older children's wards. In addition to the radios, two large phonographs and one portable phonograph were donated privately. An electrical company lent three record-players which could be attached to the radio loud speakers. With this equipment an excellent musical program was worked out.

It was realized at the outset that it would be a mistake to have the radios on all the time. This would be distracting and fatiguing. At certain times the children could select their own programs, but usually they were guided in their selection. Such programs as the Children's Symphony Hour with Walter Damrosch were featured. In addition to encouraging them to listen to good music, an effort was made to build up their musical background and help them to develop an interest in all aspects of music. Books were provided which told about the composers, the stories of the operas, etc. Interest was further fostered by the playing of many fine records which were purchased especially for the purpose.

Singing was an important part of the musical program. No matter how badly disabled a child may have been, he could always sing (or try to). Simple songs were taught to the younger children, while part songs were attempted by the older ones. Rhythm bands were organized among the younger children. The instruments were merely cheap rattles or homemade noisemakers, but the skill in their use acquired by some of the children was amazing.

Reading.—The problem of reading was a difficult one. All the children had to remain on their backs, most of them without a pillow.

Many of them had both arms in splints, and therefore could not hold a book or turn pages. As an emergency measure a stock model bed tray with an elevating top was adapted by making one or two minor changes. Reading material could be clamped securely to the top, and then held in position over the patient's head so that the text could be read easily.

The Toronto Public Library lent the hospital over one hundred books. The Junior League and other private agencies donated nearly two hundred more. By the time the hospital had been open two weeks, an excellent library was available, containing books suitable for children of all ages. It was often difficult to get the children to start reading. Most of them preferred the comics sent from home. These, with their small indistinct print and frequently fantastic plots, were but poor substitutes for good books. However, once the child developed an interest in a story or a book, it was relatively easy to keep him going. The volunteer librarians were a great help in this field. All the children loved having stories read to them. Often one child in a ward would undertake the responsibility of reading a story or even a full length book to the others. Sometimes the children in a ward would read a play, each child taking a different part. This seemed to bring unusual satisfaction. Some of the younger children actually made a start toward learning how to read, partly because of stimulation from the other children, partly because of the books provided, and partly by means of the various alphabet games which were available. The educational and cultural value of this part of the program was unlimited. Many of the children asked for their school books. No formal teaching of school work was attempted because the children were not in the hospital for sufficient length of time to warrant it. Nevertheless, by encouraging the reading of books which had some relationship to their school studies, the children maintained their interest in school. A teacher, assigned to the hospital as liaison officer by the local Board of Education, organized the extramural teaching of the children after they were discharged.

Motion Pictures.—A moving picture projector was borrowed from the Department of Psychology, University of Toronto, for the whole time that the hospital was open. After experimenting with one or two short films of the cartoon and comedy variety, it was obvious that this type of entertainment was too exciting and stimulating to be good therapy. Finally, however, some excellent nature films were borrowed from the provincial government. These proved to be valuable in many ways. They stimulated conversation about the nature and habits of animals and led many of the children to seek more information in reference books. Particularly valuable were the colored travel films, lent by several interested physicians. Great interest in geography and history was engendered by these pictures. Such remarks as, "they didn't tell us at school that they had such modern looking houses in Oslo!" were typical.

The films were shown to the older children three or four times a week, usually in the early evenings. It was discovered that if the pictures were projected high on the cream-colored walls near the ceilings, all the children could see perfectly without straining their eyes or moving their heads. Very little shifting of the beds was required in order that all could have a clear view.

Occupational Activities.—The occupational therapists showed great initiative in adapting their usual type of craft and occupational work to the special difficulties of these convalescent children. For example, suitable occupations had to be devised for the large number of 2- and 3-year-old patients. The program finally developed was surprisingly varied. Peg boards, blocks, large beads which could be threaded on a shoe string, and a wide assortment of toy animals and dolls were used for the very young patients. Balloons and toy airplanes strung up overhead were a special source of joy and interest. Cutting and pasting, leather work, weaving, sewing, knitting, making puppet heads and dresses, and making plasticine models were activities frequently seen among the older children.

Creative Activities.—The hospital had not been open long before some of the teachers from the Children's Art Center of the Art Gallery became interested in the work. They, with the assistance of graduates of the College of Art, were most generous with their time.* The timetable was arranged so that every child more than 4 years old had at least two periods a week of creative art. This included not only drawing and coloring pictures, but modeling, cutting figures from colored sheets of paper, and assembling all sorts of artistic projects such as miniature circuses, parades, etc. Even those children with both arms in splints could look on and offer advice and criticism. They were usually given some title to dignify their position, such as "Chairman of the Advisory Board" or "Chief Inspector and Critic of Art."

Free Time.—With all this program in action, one might wonder if the children did not have too much to do, too much stimulation, and far too much fuss made over them. This danger was foreseen at the start. The children's daily routine called for a two-hour rest period immediately after the midday meal. This rest period was carefully enforced. Blinds were drawn, windows opened, and both patients and nurses encouraged to be as quiet as possible. Most of the children slept during this time. In addition to this rest period each child had time during the day when he was left to his own devices. He was encouraged to do anything he wished, except call for help and attention. In this way a beginning was made towards the development in these children of some measure of independence.

*Acknowledgement is gratefully made to Mr. Arthur Lismer and Mr. J. deN. Kennedy for their interest and help in making the art program possible.

MENTAL HYGIENE WORK

The Children.—Every child more than 4 years old was seen by the psychiatrist or the psychiatric social worker, either during admission or as soon as possible afterwards. This interview was felt to be very important since in a five- or ten-minute chat it was possible to make the child feel that some one at the hospital was taking a special interest in him. The reason for the child's coming to the hospital, the nature of his disability, and the rationale underlying the prescribed treatment were explained in simple terms. If possible, he was told the approximate length of his stay. The fact that there could be no visitors was made quite clear, and the reason for this rule was explained. This first interview usually closed with a brief description of the sort of proceedings and activities which the child might expect at the hospital.

During subsequent interviews the child was made to understand that his convalescence must necessarily be prolonged. The same sort of treatment he was receiving in the hospital must be continued at home. There would be no skating or climbing fences that winter. Most of the older children wanted to know the chances of a complete cure, with return of power to the weakened muscles. These questions were always answered truthfully by saying that it was impossible to tell at the moment and that improvement took place slowly but steadily, sometimes for many months. The problem of the future gave the younger children no concern whatever. These talks with the children were always made as cheerful and optimistic as possible. It was pointed out that they would now have the opportunity to learn to do all kinds of interesting things at home, things they never had time to do before.

Occasionally children with emotional problems of one kind or another were found. There were several severe cases of homesickness. The commonest psychologic factor here was an abnormally strong attachment to the mother plus the fact that the child, in most cases, had never been away from home before, even for one night. There were several children who were emotionally unstable, showing either excessive crying or unusual lability of mood and excitability. Reassurance, cheerfulness, and gentle firmness usually helped the child to regain his self-control and sense of security.

The different types of paralysis in the children made individual work almost obligatory. The problem presented by a boy with paralysis of both legs was different from that of the girl who could move her legs but whose arms were completely useless. The latter type of child, however, could always participate in conversation, singing, and listening.

Work with the Nurses.—Naturally a program as intensive as this could not be attempted without gaining the full understanding and cooperation of the nurses. At the beginning of the project the nurses were assembled and the significance of the psychologic factors was fully explained to them. The proposed activities were outlined, and the necessity for maintaining an objective and optimistic attitude towards the children was urged. It was pointed out that the danger lay in allowing one's natural sympathies to get out-of-hand. The importance of helping these convalescent children to develop wholesome habits of behavior was emphasized.

Close contact with the work of the nurses was constantly maintained. Children with problems in behavior or adjustment were referred by them from time to time. Such children were usually interviewed privately. The problem was then discussed with the nurse, and a method of dealing with the situation was worked out. On several occasions, towards the end of the hospital project, the nurses handled situations of this kind themselves with admirable results. The interest shown by the nurses in the whole program was very gratifying.

Work with the Parents.—During the two-day training period for the parents time was set aside for an informal lecture and discussion on the important general principles underlying the subsequent training of the child at home. The dangers of too much sympathy and too much spoiling were pointed out. The importance of routine, of good habits of eating, sleeping, and elimination, and of consistent discipline was stressed. In order to make sure that the most important points were remembered, a multigraphed booklet was prepared for the parents. This contained instructions and suggestions calculated to be of help in looking after the children at home. In the discharge ward the parents were shown in detail how to help the child carry on many of the interesting things he had learned to do in the hospital. Displays of suitable books, games, occupational and creative material were set up, keeping in mind the fact that most of the homes to which the children would return were either in marginal financial circumstances or on relief.

As the work developed, more and more visiting nurses and social workers from various city and provincial organizations began to come to the lectures. Often there were more workers present than parents. The visiting teacher assigned to the hospital, being fully acquainted with the problems involved in the convalescent care of these children, was in a unique position to follow these children after they went home and to supervise their education. She made arrangements with those parents who had children of school age to visit their homes in order to carry on educational work.

THE FOLLOW-UP

The average stay of the children in the Orthopedic Hospital was a little over three weeks. On discharge most of them returned to their homes under the care of their parents. A few, who for one reason or another could not be cared for properly at home, were transferred to a special ward in the Toronto hospital for infectious diseases. The follow-up was in charge of the local, municipal, and county departments of health. In most centers special public health nurses were assigned to make frequent visits. Cooperating with the nurses were the visiting teachers, and physiotherapists. The local service clubs and the Ontario Society for Crippled Children provided reading racks and other materials where necessary. They also arranged to bring the children back to the Hospital for Sick Children at stated intervals for orthopedic and neurologic examinations.

RESULTS

The difficulty of appraising the results of this mental hygiene program is obvious enough. Mental health and wholesome attitudes are attributes which are not easy to measure quantitatively. By observing the change in the children during their three weeks' stay, however, and by observing them again on their return to the Hospital for Sick Children for re-examination, the writers were left with little doubt as to the efficacy of the measures employed. They were strikingly successful. This was reinforced by the spontaneous remarks and comments made by the many physicians who visited the Orthopedic Hospital and saw the program in action. It was further reinforced by the information obtained through informal chats with the parents when they returned with their children for re-examinations.

In the first place the hospital itself was an unusually cheerful place. There was never any effort to keep the wards very quiet except during the rest periods, and at certain times of the day shouting, laughing, and singing could be heard from almost all wards. The second noticeable feature was the spirit of unselfishness and the desire to help one another that was so frequently seen among the children. The third characteristic which was not so obvious to the casual observer but which was perhaps more important than the first two was the willingness to learn and the spirit of cooperation which these children developed. The visiting teachers reported later that never had they taught a more enthusiastic and interested group of children than those who had been in the Orthopedic Hospital. The following case summary is only one example of many that could be cited:

J. B., aged 13 years, an intelligent, attractive girl who lived in a small town thirty miles from Toronto, contracted a ''cold'' early in September. Within twenty-four hours her four limbs were completely paralyzed. There was also some involvement of her intercostal and back muscles. On the third day she was transferred to the Hospital for Sick Children because it was felt that she might need the respirator at any time. She survived the acute stage, however, without the ''iron lung.'' She was placed on a Bradford frame, with splints applied to immobilize her four limbs. About this time (sixteen days after the onset) she became very depressed and homesick. It was the first time she had ever been away from home. She also became increasingly irritable and difficult to nurse. She kept demanding to be allowed to go home. Her crying and her tempers upset the other children in the ward.

When the Orthopedic Hospital was opened, she was one of the first to be admitted. The psychiatrist chatted with her and allowed her to tell all her complaints in detail. She explained that she knew the doctors had lied to her. They had promised her that she would go home in two weeks and here it was nearly three. She knew they had lied to her about her paralysis, too. She was convinced that she would never be able to walk again.

Some time was taken to explain exactly what was going to happen at this new hospital and how the staff were really counting on her help to maintain cheerfulness in the ward. As soon as possible she was informed of the exact date of her discharge. Something of the girl's problem was explained to the nurses, and they took a special interest in her for a few days. By this time the other factors, such as the infectious cheerfulness and the full program of activities, had begun to take effect. She responded very well. She and a few other girls of about her own age developed little games they could play. Finally a small play was organized. She was particularly interested in stories which were read to her at first. Finally she achieved a technique so that she could read a book and turn the pages herself, using one of the reading stands.

After nearly five weeks she went home with her mother—a radiantly happy and cheerful girl. Contact was maintained by correspondence, and a steady improvement in her muscle power took place. Six months later (March, 1938) she returned to Toronto for re-examination. This showed marked improvement in all limbs except the left leg. However, her chances of being able to walk with the aid of some sort of brace were excellent.

Her mother stated that she maintained her cheerfulness and unselfishness at home. She has been working hard at her studies with the help of one of the teachers from the high school. One of the chief items of interest, however, was the fact that she had been responsible for the organization of a troup of Girl Guides among the friends she had made at the Orthopedic Hospital. This was accomplished entirely by correspondence.

The girl's attitude to herself and her illness is as fine as could be desired. She is optimistic and is not afraid. Her illness will not leave her with psychologic and emotional distortions.

The program in psychologic medicine introduced into the Ontario Orthopedic Hospital served a twofold purpose. Primarily organized to give the younger patients guidance in adjusting to a prolonged convalescence, the hospital was also used as a demonstration center. The results obtained, therefore, are not to be judged by the effect on the children alone. Physicians and nurses from all over the province were frequent visitors. The parents of the patients received instruction not only in physical management of the paralyzed patient, but also suggestions whereby psychologic problems could be anticipated and met. At the conclusion of the work in psychologic medicine carried out in this hospital, it was felt that the effort expended had produced a beneficial result.

DRUGS TRANSMITTED THROUGH BREAST MILK

II. Barbiturates

Ralph M. Tyson, M.D., Earl A. Shrader, Ed.D.,
and H. Harris Perlman, M.D.
Philadelphia, Pa.

In continuation of our study on drugs transmitted through breast milk[1] we proceeded with the barbiturates and submit here the results.

The literature contains very little in regard to barbiturates in connection with breast milk. Frensdorf[2] gave an epileptic woman 0.1 gm. of phenobarbital three times daily for a few days before and after labor. Her child, normal at birth, became gradually more and more sleepy but recuperated after the mother discontinued the drug. This would point to transmission although no chemical analysis of the milk is reported to confirm the passage of the drug in the milk.

Kwit and Hatcher,[3] on the other hand, gave barbital to each of two women in a dose of 325 mg. and to each of two others in a dose of 650 mg., and no evidence could be found of the presence of barbital in any specimen of milk.

EXPERIMENTAL

Patients in the maternity ward of Temple University Hospital having babies at the breast were used as subjects in this study. Four series were run using phenobarbital U.S.P. and phenobarbital sodium U.S.P. with each drug subdivided as to sedative and hypnotic effects.

During the first five days following delivery no medication in any form was given to either the mother or the nursling used in these tests. Following the administration of the drug, one-half ounce of milk was collected at each of the feedings during each day (6 A.M., 10 A.M., 2 P.M., 6 P.M. and 10 P.M.) and pooled for chemical analysis.

The chemical test used was that described by Beal and Czalkowski[4] in which the phenol group is converted into m-nitrobenzoic acid by heating with sulfuric acid and potassium nitrate. The reaction mixture is then made alkaline with ammonium hydroxide and reduced with ammonium sulfide. The m-diamino compound is formed with the production of a reddish-brown ring which diffuses through the liquid to an orange color. The ammonium sulfide is added without mixing, in order to produce the ring.

From the Departments of Pediatrics, Physiological Chemistry and Obstetrics, Temple University School of Medicine.

This study was made possible by a grant from Mead Johnson & Company, Evansville, Ind.

Samples of milk from mothers having no drug were negative, and samples (2 oz.) to which ½ grain of phenobarbital had been added gave positive reactions with this test. One-half ounce of milk was used in making the chemical test, thus detecting phenobarbital when present to the extent of ⅛ grain in the sample used. These served as controls for the application of the test on samples of milk tested in the series. The procedure of the drug administration will be described in connection with each series.

Series 1 consisted of 10 patients using phenobarbital. Beginning on the morning of the sixth day after delivery, one tablet containing ½ grain of phenobarbital (average dose) was administered to the mother by mouth at 7 A.M., 11 A.M., 3 P.M., and 7 P.M. Thus a total of 2 grains was given each day until the patient was discharged from the hospital.

Observations were made on mother and child as to the sedative effect of the drug, as well as effect on respiration, gastric disturbances, skin rashes, effect on temperature, and any unusual symptoms.

TABLE I

PHENOBARBITAL—SEDATIVE EFFECT

SUBJECT	USE OF SEDATIVES BEFORE ADMISSION	NO. DAYS RECEIVED DRUG	GRAINS PER DAY	CHEMICAL TESTS		SYMPTOMS	
				POSITIVE	NEGATIVE	MOTHER	CHILD
M. D.	None	4	2	3	1(2)	None	None
H. S.	None	5	2	4	1(3)	None	None
H. L.	None	4	2	3	1(3)	None	None
R. S.	None	4	2	1(2)	3	None	None
F. G.	None	1	2	0	1	None	None
A. W.	None	4	2	1(3)	3	None	None
E. G.	None	4	2	1(2)	2	None	None
J. K.	None	4	2	3	1(4)	None	None
G. B.	None	4	2	4	0	None	None
M. S.	None	4	2	3	1(2)	None	None

A total of thirty-seven day-samples having been collected, a positive reaction was obtained in 23 cases (62.16 per cent) and negative reaction in 14 (37.84 per cent). Of the 10 cases, 6 (60 per cent) showed more positive specimens than negative specimens (Table I). The small number in parenthesis refers to the day of drug administration when the exception was noted. No clinical evidence of transmission was noted in any case.

Series 2 consisted of 10 patients using phenobarbital; the hypnotic effect on mother and child was noted. The only change in procedure was to administer to the mother one tablet containing 1½ grains of phenobarbital at bedtime on the evening of the fifth day after delivery, and this was continued each night until the patient was discharged.

A total of forty day-samples having been collected, a positive reaction was obtained in 32 cases (80 per cent) and negative reaction in 8 (20 per cent). Of the 10 cases, 9 (90 per cent) showed more positive specimens than negative specimens, the other case being 50 per cent positive (Table II). The small number in parenthesis refers to the day of drug administration when the exception was noted. Only in the last case (E. B.) were any clinical symptoms manifest, as noted. The evident of rash on the child before drug administration cannot be deduced as being caused by the drug even though present the first day of the test.

TABLE II

PHENOBARBITAL—HYPNOTIC EFFECT

SUBJECT	USE OF SEDATIVES BEFORE ADMISSION	NO. NIGHTS RECEIVED DRUG	GRAINS PER NIGHT	CHEMICAL TESTS		SYMPTOMS	
				POSITIVE	NEGATIVE	MOTHER	CHILD
F. V.	None	4	1½	4	0	None	None
A. M.	None	4	1½	3	1 (1)	None	None
G. H.	None	4	1½	4	0	None	None
R. R.	None	3	1½	2	1 (1)	None	None
L. M.	None	4	1½	3	1 (1)	None	None
S. W.	None	4	1½	3	1 (2)	None	None
M. W.	None	4	1½	2	2 (1, 4)	None	None
M. D.	None	4	1½	4	0	None	None
C. S.	None	5	1½	3	2 (1, 5)	None	None
E. B.	None	4	1½	4	0	Temperature 103.2° F. 1st day. Herpes on lips 3rd day.	Rash 2 days preceding drug and only 1st day of drug.

Series 3 consisted of 10 cases and repeated Series 1 for the sedative effect; phenobarbital sodium was used in this series.

TABLE III

PHENOBARBITAL SODIUM—SEDATIVE EFFECT

SUBJECT	USE OF SEDATIVES BEFORE ADMISSION	NO. DAYS RECEIVED DRUG	GRAINS PER DAY	CHEMICAL TESTS		SYMPTOMS	
				POSITIVE	NEGATIVE	MOTHER	CHILD
F. S.	None	4	2	3	1 (4)	None	None
M. S.	None	5	2	5	0	None	None
M. B.	None	4	2	2	2 (1, 4)	None	None
A. O.	None	4	2	3	1 (4)	None	None
G. D.	None	3	2	2	1 (1)	None	None
M. M.	None	4	2	3	1 (2)	None	None
C. Z.	None	4	2	0	4	None	None
M. G.	None	4	2	2	2 (1, 3)	None	None
A. Y.	None	4	2	4	0	None	None
A. W.	None	4	2	3	1 (1)	None	None

A total of forty day-samples having been collected, a positive reaction was obtained in 27 cases (67.5 per cent) and negative reaction in 13 (32.5 per cent). Of the 10 cases, 7 (70 per cent) showed more positive specimen than negative specimens, 2 of the remainder showed 50 per cent positive, and only 1 was entirely negative (Table III).

The small number in parenthesis refers to the day of drug administration when the exception was noted. No clinical evidence of transmission was noted in any case.

Series 4 consisted of 11 cases and repeated Series 2 for the hypnotic effect; phenobarbital sodium was used in this series.

TABLE IV

PHENOBARBITAL SODIUM—HYPNOTIC EFFECT

SUBJECT	USE OF SEDATIVES BEFORE ADMISSION	NO. NIGHTS RECEIVED DRUG	GRAINS PER NIGHT	CHEMICAL TESTS		SYMPTOMS	
				POSITIVE	NEGATIVE	MOTHER	CHILD
M. M.	None	4	1½	3	1 (3)	None	None
E. T.	None	4	1½	4	0	None	None
P. C.	None	4	1½	3	1 (2)	None	None
R. B.	None	5	1½	3	2 (1, 5)	None	None
M. Cr.	None	5	1½	5	0	None	Hypnotic effect on 8th & 9th days. Sleepy and hard to awaken.
H. V.	None	5	1½	3	2 (4, 5)	None	None
C. H.	None	3	1½	2	1 (2)	None	Seemed toxic. Slept all the time, quite hard to awaken.
E. M.	None	4	1½	3	1 (4)	None	None
S. R.	None	4	1½	3	1 (2)	None	None
A. D.	None	5	1½	3	2 (2, 3)	None	None
M. Ch.	None	4	1½	3	1 (2)	None	None

A total of forty-seven day-samples having been collected, a positive reaction was obtained in 35 cases (74.47 per cent) and negative reaction in 12 (25.53 per cent). The 11 cases (100 per cent) showed more positive specimens than negative specimens (Table IV). The small number in parenthesis refers to the day of drug administration when the exception was noted. Two cases showed definite clinical evidence

TABLE V

DRUG	CHEMICAL TESTS ON SAMPLES OF MILK		CASES IN WHICH MAJORITY WERE		TOTAL CASES SHOWING TRANSMISSION PER CENT	CASES OF CLINICAL EVIDENCE
	POSITIVE PER CENT	NEGATIVE PER CENT	POSITIVE PER CENT	NEGATIVE PER CENT		
Phenobarbital (sedative)	62.16	37.84	60.0	40.0	90.0	0
Phenobarbital (hypnotic)	80.00	20.00	90.0	0.0	100.0	0
Phenobarbital Sodium (sedative)	67.50	32.50	70.0	10.0	90.0	0
Phenobarbital Sodium (hypnotic)	74.47	25.53	100.0	0.0	100.0	2

of the transmission of the drug with resulting symptoms of hypnotic effect, with deep slumber attended by some difficulty in awakening.

SUMMARY AND CONCLUSIONS

Barbiturates when administered to a lactating mother are transmitted by breast milk, as shown by chemical analysis.

Analyses of individual specimens of milk after administration of barbiturates in ½ grain doses at stated intervals, although amounting in the aggregate to 2 grains in a day, do not show as high a percentage of positive reactions as do similar specimens after the administration of 1½ grains at bedtime. Thus, concentrated doses seem to have more effect on transmission than do cumulative doses.

The individual cases show the same relationship as the individual specimens.

In only two of the forty-one cases was there any clinical evidence in the child, and thus there is the possibility that the child may be affected by the breast milk after medication of the mother with barbiturates. In this series the possibility is about 5 per cent and occurs in the hypnotic group.

REFERENCES

1. Tyson, R. M., Shrader, E. A., and Perlman, H. H.: J. Pediat. **11**: 824, 1937.
2. Frensdorf: München. med. Wchnschr. **73**: 322, 1926.
3. Kwit, N. T., and Hatcher, R. A.: Am. J. Dis. Child. **49**: 900, 1935.
4. Beal, J. D., and Czalkowski, C. R.: J. Am. Pharm. A. **23**: 18, 1934.

DRUGS TRANSMITTED THROUGH BREAST MILK

III. Bromides

Ralph M. Tyson, M.D., Earl A. Shrader, Ed.D.,
and H. Harris Perlman, M.D.
Philadelphia, Pa.

A THIRD part of our study on drugs transmitted through breast milk[1] consists of a series during the administration of sodium bromide to the lactating mother.

Holt[2] states that bromides, when long administered, may be eliminated in sufficient quantity to produce their constitutional effects on the child. Morse[3] mentions bromides as being transmitted through breast milk. Griffith[4] states that bromine passes into the milk to some extent and occasionally in such a way as to affect the infant seriously. Kwit and Hatcher,[5] after studying a number of drugs, found that none of them except sodium bromide was present in the milk in an amount sufficient to indicate that the continued use of such milk would injure a normal nursing child. After administering sodium bromide in single doses of 1 gm. and total doses of 15 gm., every specimen of milk, except the first in one case, and the first and second in another, yielded bromide.

Bucura[6] also definitely demonstrated bromides in breast milk. Van der Bogert[7] reported a case in a 6-month-old nursling in whom a painful papulopustular eruption occurred. The mother had been taking a bromide preparation for some time, and the breast milk contained more than traces of bromide.

Our tests were carried out to ascertain whether or not the clinical evidence of transmission of bromides would be confirmed by chemical analysis of the breast milk during the course of administration of the bromide to the lactating mother.

EXPERIMENTAL STUDIES

Patients in the maternity ward of Temple University Hospital having babies at the breast were used as subjects. During the first five days following delivery, no medication in any form was given to either mother or nursling used in these tests.

Beginning on the morning of the sixth day following delivery, one fluid dram of sodium bromide in peppermint water (average dose, 15 grains of sodium bromide in each fluid dram) was administered to the

From the Departments of Pediatrics, Physiological Chemistry and Obstetrics, Temple University School of Medicine.

This study was made possible by a grant from Mead Johnson & Company, Evansville, Ind.

mother. This was repeated every four hours (6 A.M., 10 A.M., 2 P.M., 6 P.M., 10 P.M., and 2 A.M.), and the medication continued each day until the mother was discharged from the hospital.

Observations were made on both mother and child as to the sedative action of the bromide, effect on respiration, gastric disturbances, skin rashes, effect on temperature, and any unusual symptoms.

At each feeding during the twenty-four hours, one-half ounce of breast milk was collected and pooled for analysis.

One ounce of breast milk was heated to coagulate the proteins and filtered. The filtrate was acidified with dilute sulfuric acid, a few drops of concentrated nitric acid were added, and carbon bisulfide was used as the solvent for any bromine liberated, a positive test resulting in a brown color. Three fluid drams of the bromide solution in peppermint water when added to 2 ounces of breast milk and 1

TABLE I

SODIUM BROMIDE—SEDATIVE EFFECT

SUBJECT	USE OF SEDATIVES BEFORE ADMISSION	NO. DAYS RECEIVED DRUG	GRAINS PER DAY	CHEMICAL TESTS		SYMPTOMS	
				POSITIVE	NEGATIVE	MOTHER	CHILD
A. G.	None	4	90	3	1 (4)	Not as nervous, slept well but not drowsy.	Less irritable
A. F.	None	4	90	4	0	Rested comfortably, slept well, not drowsy.	Less irritable
G. M.	None	4	90	4	0	Papulopustular rash on face, neck and other parts of body. Felt well, slept well, no drowsiness.	Rested quietly, did not cry frequently.
M. La.	None	4	90	4	0	Very drowsy, slept practically all the time.	Very drowsy, did not cry when disturbed. Slept continually but nursed well.
J. C.	None	4	90	4	0	No unusual symptoms. Rested and slept comfortably.	Less irritable.
M. P.	None	4	90	4	0	No unusual symptoms. Rested and slept comfortably.	Seemed sleepy. Not irritable. Rested quietly.
M. Le.	None	3	90	3	0	No unusual symptoms. Rested quietly.	Less irritable.
V. D.	None	4	90	4	0	Less irritable.	Less irritable.
J. Ch.	None	3	90	3	0	Less irritable.	Less irritable.
R. G.	None	5	90	4*	0	Papulopustular rash on face and neck.	Slight rash on face for 2 days.

*One sample lost due to breaking of bottle.

ounce of this prepared milk used for a control test gave positive evidence of bromide. The amount added to the control specimen represented 45 grains of bromide, or half the amount administered to the subject, and gave 22.5 grains in the amount taken to test.

Ten subjects were used in this series as shown in Table I.

A total of 38 specimens of milk were analyzed and 37 (97.37 per cent) gave positive results; only 1 (2.63 per cent) was negative, and that one specimen was the fourth taken on the first case. Clinical evidence of transmission was manifested in the child to a marked extent in four cases (Table I), although in every case there was a marked diminution in the irritability of the child as well as the mother.

CONCLUSION

We conclude, therefore, from both chemical and clinical evidence that sodium bromide is transmitted through breast milk in sufficient quantity to produce an effect upon the nursling.

REFERENCES

1. Tyson, R. M., Shrader, E. A., and Perlman, H. H.: J. Pediat. **11**: 824, 1937.
2. Holt, L. E.: Diseases of Infancy and Childhood, p. 143, New York, 1916, D. Appleton-Century Company, Inc.
3. Morse, J. L.: Clinical Pediatrics, Philadelphia, 1926, W. B. Saunders Company, p. 122.
4. Griffith, J. P. C.: The Diseases of Infants and Children, Vol. I, p. 106, Philadelphia, 1919, W. B. Saunders Company.
5. Kwit, N. T., and Hatcher, R. A.: Am. J. Dis. Child. **49**: 900, 1935.
6. Bucura, C. J.: Ztschr. f. exper. Path. u. Therap. **4**: 398, 1907.
7. Van der Bogert, F.: Am. J. Dis. Child. **21**: 167, 1921.

ERYTHEMA ANNULARE RHEUMATICUM

Clinical Significance in Rheumatic States of Childhood

Harold Abramson, M.D., and Arthur M. Tunick, M.D.
New York, N. Y.

THE attention of the clinician has always been attracted by the occurrence of cutaneous lesions, namely, purpura and erythema, in rheumatic states of childhood. For the most part, interest has centered in the varied manifestations of the exanthem erythema multiforme, particularly with respect to the annular, circinate, or marginate type. The latter form of eruption is generally referred to as erythema annulare rheumaticum and is of importance in connection with the diagnosis of rheumatic heart disease in children. As early as 1835, Rayer[1] described the lesion and suggested its relationship to rheumatic states. In 1881 Barlow and Warner[2] and again, shortly after, Barlow[3] observed that the eruption was frequently present in children with rheumatism and occasionally chorea. In 1889 Cheadle[4] discussed the exanthem in his monograph and stated that the marginate type of erythema which occurred in rheumatic fever was "not infrequently associated with endocarditis and pericarditis in the more serious cases." Thereafter brief references to the lesion were made in the literature. Cockayne[5] noted its association with rheumatism in childhood and described the various ring forms ranging from the more common annular morphology to that of the less frequent erythema iris and herpes iris. Poynton and Paine[6] then indicated that the cutaneous manifestations may occur before the appearance of the complete picture of rheumatic disease or as an isolated instance between recurrent attacks. In 1922 Lehndorff and Leiner[7] directed renewed attention to the significance of erythema annulare rheumaticum and stressed that the eruption is typical and affords conclusive evidence of the existence of organic heart disease of rheumatic origin.

In their description, Lehndorff and Leiner stated that the lesion occurs in children up to 14 years of age, but not among infants of the suckling period. The observers were of the opinion that erythema annulare rheumaticum occurs late in the course of rheumatic infection, not at the outset, and frequently is first noted in children already afebrile and exhibiting manifest signs of rheumatic endocarditis. It is also seen in association with chorea, but never in cases of malignant endocarditis or in endocarditis due to such conditions as gonorrhea, syphilis, or scarlet fever. The early lesions are described as being small, discrete, pink or blue rings, so pale as to be easily overlooked. They are macular,

From the Department of Pediatrics, Beth Israel Hospital, service of Dr. Herman Schwarz.

never papular, and usually appear on the trunk between the lower half of the chest and the upper half of the abdomen, as well as on the lateral thorax and the back. Less often the lesions are found on the extremities, favoring the inner surfaces of the thighs; the face and mucous membranes are never involved. Itching is absent and hemorrhage, edema, pigmentation, and scaling are not accompanying features. In the more severe form, the lesions grow in size and may become confluent. The duration of the eruption is very variable and may last but few hours or as long as several days.

The conclusions of Lehndorff and Leiner have been accepted by von Leichtentritt,[8] Abt,[9] Perry,[10] and others. The consensus of opinion is that the onset of the eruption is not simultaneous with the occurrence of joint symptoms, but that it becomes manifest after defervescence and when cardiac involvement is evident. It is also stated that the general characteristics of erythema annulare rheumaticum do not run parallel to the clinical severity of rheumatic infection. However, in agreement with the impressions of Poynton and Paine[6] and of Perry,[10] our observations have indicated that the above sequence of events does not always hold true. It is also our impression that at times the severity of the lesion and of the rheumatic infection may be of comparable intensity. We wish, therefore, to present two instances of erythema annulare rheumaticum illustrating these points. In Case 1 the eruption and arthritic symptoms occurred concomitantly, and signs of cardiac damage appeared subsequently. In addition, the severity of the rheumatism and the extent and duration of the eruption ran parallel courses. In the other, Case 2, the rash appeared before the signs of heart involvement, and joint manifestations were evidenced last. Fulminating pneumonia characterized the fatal termination of both cases in which the rheumatic infection represented initial attacks.

CASE REPORTS

CASE 1.—J. K., a 3-year-old white male, was admitted to the hospital with a history of difficulty in standing and fever of two days' duration. This was the boy's fifth admission, having previously been observed for acute laryngitis, hypochromic anemia, and upper respiratory infections. The past history and the family history were otherwise negative.

The present illness began suddenly two days prior to admission when the child complained of inability to stand. At the outset there were no joint pains, and the temperature was 101° F. But several hours later, both knees became swollen and tender, and motion became limited and painful. Two days later the temperature rose to 104° F., and a rash was noted in the right axilla. On admission, physical examination revealed an acutely ill boy in pain. He was dyspneic but not cyanotic. The temperature was 103° F., the pulse rate 128, and respiration rate 34. An irregular macular eruption was present in the right axilla, over both buttocks, and the thighs. The lesions were erythematous and annular with central areas of lighter hue. Herpes simplex was present at the angle of the mouth; the tonsils were enlarged and congested; and there was a marked postnasal discharge. General lymphadenopathy was noted. The lungs were clear. The heart was not enlarged and the point of maximal cardiac impulse was in the fifth left interspace medial to the midclavicular line. The heart rate was 156 per minute. The sounds were of fair quality and the second pulmonic sound was not unduly accentuated. No murmurs were heard. The blood pressure was 90/46. The liver edge was palpable below the costal margin, but not the spleen. Laboratory tests yielded the following data: the urine was negative; the blood revealed a hemoglobin of 70 per cent (Sahli) and a red cell count of 3,550,000 per cubic millimeter. The white cells were 15,450 per cubic millimeter of which 58 per cent were polymorphonuclear neutrophiles with two staff forms. The sedimentation rate of the blood was 46 mm. in forty-five minutes. The Wassermann reaction was negative, as were the Schick and tuberculin tests. A throat culture showed the presence of *Streptococcus viridans* and *Staphylococcus albus*. The blood culture was negative.

Clinical Course.—On the day following admission, the annular eruption on the buttocks and thighs and in the axilla became more apparent. The lesions varied in size from 2 mm. to several centimeters in diameter; some areas were confluent. As the lesions grew, the centers became paler, and considerable contrast developed with the peripheries. Both knees were swollen and exceedingly painful. On the sixth day of illness the skin eruption had spread over the trunk and lower extremities (Fig. 1). The heart rate remained rapid, but the character and quality of the sounds

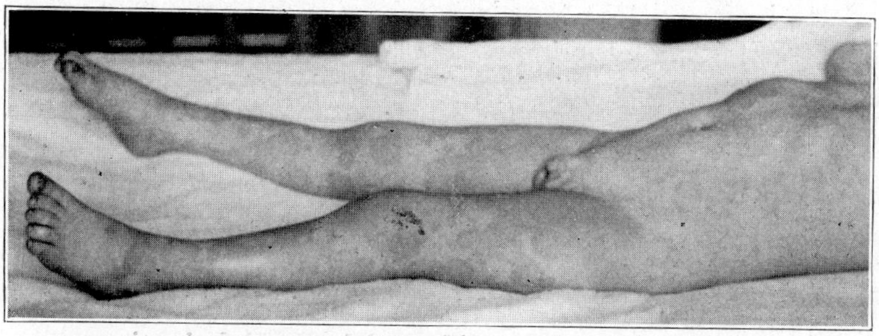

Fig. 1.—Case 1. Erythema annulare rheumaticum. Note the extent and distribution of the eruption and the discrete and confluent ring forms.

had not changed. On the seventh day a short soft systolic murmur was first noted in the fourth left interspace near the sternum. One day later the first mitral sound was replaced almost entirely by a blowing systolic murmur. The second mitral sound was loud and sharp and the second pulmonic sound accentuated. The sedimentation rate of the blood was then 70 mm. in forty-five minutes. On the tenth day of illness, the apical systolic murmur became high pitched and musical and the second sound dull and muffled. Roentgenographic examination of the heart showed an accentuation of the right and left borders and a contour indicating mitral valvular disease. An esophagogram showed a marked enlargement of the left auricle. The P-R interval of an electrocardiographic tracing was 0.20 sec. On the thirteenth day of illness the rash disappeared almost entirely. The subsequent clinical course was marked by rapidly progressive rheumatic heart disease. The heart increased in size considerably until the time of death of the boy. Clinically and roentgenologically evidence of pericardial effusion was present. On the day before death the child suddenly experienced marked respiratory distress and a pneumonic infiltration of the right upper lobe was found. During the course of the next twenty-four hours, the pulmonary consolidation spread to both sides and the child died in the seventh week of illness.

Post-Mortem Examination.—Necropsy by Dr. A Plaut showed the following.—*Heart:* About 200 c.c. of clear yellow fluid were present in the pericardial sac. The heart weighed 165 gm. and measured 8.5 cm. by 8.0 cm. by 6.0 cm. The tissues were soft and edematous throughout. The pericardial surface was hyperemic and exhibited many small and large hemorrhages, particularly over the right ventricle anteriorly where a thick bloody adhesion was seen. The outer surface of the aorta was similarly involved. All cavities of the heart contained large amounts of cruor. The pulmonary cusps were thickened. The endocardium of the right auricle was free of lesions. The left ventricle was enlarged and its endocardium diffusely thickened. Small, partly confluent hemorrhages occupied the base of the right aortic cusp. The aortic cusps also showed irregular thickenings but no definite verrucosities. The mitral valve and the endocardium of the left auricle likewise displayed many confluent irregular thickenings. The myocardium throughout was edematous. Microscopically, although no fully formed Aschoff bodies were seen, the heart showed partly diffuse and partly focal lesions characteristic of rheumatic inflammation. Little was found in the ascending aorta, but the pulmonary artery was the seat of severe rheumatic infiltration. A similar picture was evidenced in the pericardial tissues. Fatty changes were present throughout the myocardium.

Lungs: The pleural surfaces of both lungs showed many large, smooth, depressed cyanotic areas, alternating with smaller protruding pink portions. The right lung was adherent to the pleura at its upper lobe. The cut surfaces were homogeneously red. No focal lesions were found. The bronchi were intensely hyperemic. The lymph nodes were unusually large and soft and their cut surfaces smooth and glistening. Microscopically, the lungs showed hemorrhage, edema, and overgrowth of the capillary endothelium. The capillaries were distended with pale staining red cells. The alveoli contained large numbers of characteristic large mononuclear cells and some smaller cells with deeper staining nuclei.

Anatomic Diagnosis.—Severe rheumatic pancarditis; edema and hemorrhage in the lungs and hyperplasia of the lymphatic apparatus.

Summary.—This case illustrates a first attack of severe rheumatic infection in a three-year-old boy in which joint symptoms and erythema annulare rheumaticum characterized the onset of the disease. The exanthem was extensive, lasting about two weeks and reflecting the intensity of the rheumatic infection. Signs of cardiac involvement, as evidenced by the appearance of a murmur, were first noted on the seventh day of illness. The fatal termination of the case was characterized by severe and rapidly spreading pneumonic infiltration of the lungs. Post-mortem examination showed diffuse rheumatic pancarditis.

CASE 2.—M. B., 8-year-old white female, was admitted to the pediatric service complaining of fever and loss of appetite of two weeks' duration. The family history was irrelevant. The past history was of note in that one year prior to admission the girl had been hospitalized elsewhere for a purpuric eruption associated with bleeding from the gums and nose. A diagnosis of "thrombocytopenic purpura" was made. The clinical course was complicated by intercurrent attacks of varicella and of measles. Tonsillectomy and adenoidotomy were performed at three and one-half years of age. Upper respiratory infections were frequent.

The present illness began acutely two weeks prior to admission, being ushered in by malaise, nausea, vomiting, and fever ranging from 101 to 102° F. Eleven days after the onset of illness the child was brought to the outpatient department because of a rash on the legs and the back. Examination disclosed an annular erythematous eruption. The pharynx was congested and the spleen palpable. No evidence of cardiac involvement was noted. On the following day, the girl's temperature rose to

105° F., and headache appeared. On admission to the hospital, physical examination revealed a well-developed and well-nourished white female who did not appear to be very ill. There was no cyanosis or dyspnea. The skin of the left lower abdomen and of the buttocks showed erythematous lesions of annular morphology, about 1.5 cm. in diameter. The central areas were pale. There were no purpuric eruptions or subcutaneous nodules, nor was there any general or regional adenopathy. The lungs were clear. The heart showed the apical impulse in the fourth left interspace in the midclavicular line. The boundaries of the heart were normal to percussion and the sounds of good quality. Sinus tachycardia with a rate of 138 was present. At this time, two weeks after the onset of illness, a short, soft, localized systolic murmur was first heard at the mitral area. The second pulmonic sound was not accentuated. The pulses were equal, regular, and of good volume. The blood pressure was 88/46. The abdomen was soft, and no viscera were palpable. The deep and superficial reflexes were normal. There was no joint involvement. Laboratory tests showed the following: the urine was negative, but gave a four-plus acetone reaction; the blood showed 5,050,000 red cells per cubic millimeter and a hemoglobin of 88 per cent (Sahli). The white cells were 20,300 per cubic millimeter, and the differential count revealed 74 per cent polynuclear neutrophiles of which 6 per cent were staff forms. The sedimentation rate was 40 mm. in forty-five minutes. The Wassermann reaction was negative; the Shick test was positive; and the tuberculin reaction doubtful. A throat culture showed the presence of hemolytic streptococci and *Streptococcus viridans.* Blood culture showed no growth.

Clinical Course.—Two days after admission, the temperature rose to 104.6° F., and pain in the left knee joint appeared. On the seventeenth day of illness the left knee and ankle became swollen; motion was limited. The skin eruption was not now visible. Two days later, the murmur at the apex of the heart became more marked, and an acute involvement of the right knee joint with effusion appeared. The child was exceedingly ill, dyspneic, and cyanotic. An area of dullness was found over the right middle lobe. Bronchial breathing was present as well as numerous small moist râles. The heart was exceedingly rapid, and the systolic murmur was obscured. The pneumonic infiltration of the lungs spread rapidly to all lobes. The child's condition became rapidly worse, and death occurred on the twenty-first day of illness. Sputum cultures taken just prior to death showed the presence of pneumococcus Type XX, as well as hemolytic streptococci. Cultures were made of fluid aspirated post mortem from the pericardial and pleural cavities and from the right knee joint, but no growth of microorganisms was obtained.

Post-Mortem Examination.—Examination by Dr. A. Plaut revealed the following.—*Heart:* The heart weighed 565 gm. and measured 9.0 by 9.0 by 10.0 cm. The pericardium was smooth, and the sac contained a large amount of clear fluid. There were many subepicardial hemorrhages. The right auricle was enlarged. The left auricle appeared normal. A few small verrucae were seen on the aortic leaflet of the mitral valve; the chordae tendineae appeared thicker than normal and the webs well preserved. The other leaflet was peculiarly soft, and no definite verrucae were visible; the chordae were friable, and the corresponding papillary muscle unusually soft and yellow. The endocardium of the left auricle showed irregular, protruding, yellowish netlike markings. The myocardium was softer and thicker than normal and of yellowish hue. Microscopically, the endocardium of the left auricle was densely infiltrated with leucocytes and mononuclear elements in parallel rows. Many small necrotic areas were present. In addition, large cells with basophilic protoplasm were seen arranged in indistinct ovoid foci resembling Aschoff bodies. As is usually seen in rheumatic lesions, the connective tissue was homogeneous and structureless. Numbers of basophilic, medium sized, round and ovoid cells surrounded small blood vessels in the inner myocardial layers. Throughout the myocardium there were inflammatory areas containing mononuclear cells and leucocytes. The homogeneous change in the connective tissue was unusually conspicuous. The posterior mitral area showed very severe inflammation with necrosis at the base of the mitral valve, as well as characteristic Aschoff nodules in the superficial layers of the valvular tissue. Similar changes were present in the posterior papillary muscle, the aortic and mitral valves, and in the pulmonary valve. Other sections showed subendocardial hemorrhages. The myocardium also revealed severe fatty changes irregularly infiltrated. Sections from the thoracic and abdominal aorta showed mononuclear inflammatory foci, and the abdominal aorta contained hemorrhages under the adventitia.

Lungs: The pleural surfaces of the lungs were smooth. The cut surfaces were deeply cyanotic and oozed a large amount of frothy fluid. Microscopically considerable edema was present throughout, and many bronchopneumonic foci were present. Mononuclear elements were seen in the connective tissue around the smallest arteries.

Anatomic Diagnosis.—Rheumatic carditis; bronchopneumonia with severe stasis and edema of the lungs; parenchymatous and fatty change in the kidneys and liver.

Summary.—The foregoing case in an 8-year-old child is characterized by the occurrence of erythema annulare rheumaticum as an advance sign of very severe rheumatic infection. The eruption lasting one week, preceded by several days the initial signs of cardiac damage. Polyarticular symptoms appeared subsequently. The infection was fulminating in course and was complicated by severe terminal pneumonia. Necropsy studies revealed pathologic changes in the heart tissue characteristic of rheumatism.

COMMENT

One of the valuable clinical aids in the diagnosis of the various acute systemic diseases of childhood is the morphologic expression of associated cutaneous lesions. Among the great variety of these eruptions, probably the most commonly encountered in many unrelated disorders are the varied and bizarre configurations of the broad group, descriptively designated as erythema multiforme. From this nonspecific group of eruptions one form, namely, erythema annulare rheumaticum, has been set apart because of its characteristic features and because of its frequent association with rheumatism of childhood.

It is generally agreed by clinical observers that erythema annulare rheumaticum is a specific exanthem of significant value in the diagnosis of rheumatic states of childhood and that it is occasionally evidenced in the allied disorder, chorea. In its occurrence erythema annulare rheumaticum is also stated to appear typically either during the subsidence of rheumatic infection or between recurrent attacks of the disease. The opinion is likewise held that the general clinical characteristics of the eruption do not reflect the degree of severity of the rheumatic process and that its use as an index of prognosis is of questionable value.

However, it seems that the early observations of Poynton and Paine[6] have not been sufficiently stressed. These clinicians emphasized that the cutaneous manifestations may occur before the full picture of rheumatic infection develops. This observation is brought out by the cases cited above in which erythema annulare rheumaticum appeared as an advance sign of rheumatic disease concurrently with, or preceding, heart and joint involvement. In addition, the extent and duration of the cutaneous lesions in one case ran parallel in its clinical course to the severity of the rheumatism. In its duration, the eruption in the other case likewise appeared to indicate a fulminating clinical course. From the above observations, it seems then that at times the severity of erythema annulare rheumaticum may bear a close relationship to the final outcome of cases of rheumatic disease in childhood. Likewise, the clinical characteristics of the eruption may also indicate an unfavorable prognosis in the disease.

As a final note, it should be borne in mind that, although erythema annulare rheumaticum should strongly suggest existing or impending rheumatic infection, as an isolated sign its occurrence is not always pathognomonic of the disease. Annulare eruptions of erythematous nature may also occur in such conditions as Still's disease[11] and serum sickness.[10]

REFERENCES

1. Rayer, P.: Treatise on Diseases of the Skin, ed. 2, p. 101, translated by R. Willis, London, 1835, Tindall & Cox Baillière.
2. Barlow, T., and Warner, F.: Trans. Internat. Med. Congress, Section Pediatrics **4**: 116, 1881.
3. Barlow, T.: Brit. M. J. **2**: 509, 1883.
4. Cheadle, W. B.: The Various Manifestations of the Rheumatic State as Exemplified in Childhood and Early Life, Harveian Society Lectures, Lecture II: Erythema Exudativum: The Marginate and Urticarious Forms, p. 46, London, 1889, Smith, Elder & Co.
5. Cockayne, E. A.: Arch. Middlesex Hosp., Clinical Series No. XI **28**: 28, 1912.
6. Poynton, F. J., and Paine, A.: Researches on Rheumatism, p. 420, London, 1913, J. & A. Churchill.
7. Lehndorff, H., and Leiner, C.: Ztschr. f. Kinderh. **32**: 46, 1922; Lehndorff, H.: Wien. med. Wchnschr. **80**: 1449, 1930.
8. von Leichtentritt, B.: Ergebn. d. inn. Med. u. Kinderh. **37**: 1, 1930; Idem: Acute Articular Rheumatism: Special Forms of the Disease, in Pfaundler and Schlossman's Diseases of Children, English Translation by M. G. Peterman, Vol. 3, p. 359, Philadelphia, 1935, J. B. Lippincott Company.
9. Abt, A. F.: Am. J. M. Sc. **190**: 824, 1935.
10. Perry, C. B.: Arch. Dis. Childhood **12**: 233, 1937.
11. Smith, R. M., and Gallup, H. E.: Atrophic Arthritis, in Brenneman's Pediatrics, Vol. 4, p. 8, Hagerstown, Md., 1937, W. F. Prior Company, Inc.

1097 Madison Avenue

Critical Review

CONGENITAL SYPHILIS

Part II. Prevention and Treatment*

Dorothy V. Whipple, M.D., and Ethel C. Dunham, M.D.
Washington, D. C.

Prevention

CONGENITAL syphilis can be prevented by the adequate treatment of every syphilitic woman during each pregnancy. The first step in prevention is, therefore, the detection of every case of syphilis in women either before conception or soon after conception.

DIAGNOSIS OF SYPHILIS DURING PREGNANCY

Syphilitic infection is frequently masked by pregnancy so that it is often difficult to make a diagnosis of the infection in the ante-partum patient.[67] The diagnosis may be made (1) by the medical history of the patient, (2) by physical examination, and (3) by serologic examination of the blood.

History.—A history of infection with syphilis is often difficult to obtain. Ingraham[44] found that when a "woman was questioned alone, carefully and confidentially, with the thought of syphilis uppermost in mind," a "positive" history was obtained in 80 per cent of the cases at the first interview. He found, however, that without the constant awareness of syphilis and a sympathetic approach on the part of the physician the information was not obtained in half the cases. Dodds[28] obtained a history of syphilis in 64 per cent of a group of 73 cases showing a strongly positive Wassermann reaction. Boas, Gammeltoft, and Sieck[12] obtained a history of infection in 57 per cent of their cases, but Browne[15] was able to elicit a suggestive history in only 25 per cent of his cases. Previous obstetric history is of value, as shown by the fact that 40 to 80 per cent of multiparous syphilitic women give a history of pregnancies resulting in stillbirth, in births of infants who die in early infancy, or in births of syphilitic children.[6, 8, 40, 41, 80, 101] Belding and Hunter[9] were able to obtain histories suggestive of syphilis in 83 per cent of their patients. In 53 per cent of them the history given by the patient indicated syphilis, in 10 per cent the history of previous pregnancies led to a suspicion of syphilis, and in 20 per cent the husband's history was suggestive of syphilis.

Physical Examination.—The clinical signs and symptoms of syphilis are often absent during pregnancy. Welz and Van Nest[107] found during careful examination that among 147 pregnant women who were proved to be syphilitic 20 per cent had syphilitic skin lesions, 29 per cent absent or sluggish reflexes, 12 per cent Argyll-Robertson pupils, and 50 per cent

From the Division of Research in Child Development, Children's Bureau, United States Department of Labor and the Department of Pediatrics, School of Medicine, University of Pennsylvania.

*Part I (Incidence, Transmission, and Diagnosis) was published in this Journal, March, 1938.

a generalized adenopathy. Ingraham[44] found that 24 per cent of 239 syphilitic pregnant women showed syphilis on physical examination.

Serologic Examination of the Blood.—Since in many women the most searching physical examination fails to reveal any evidence of the existence of syphilitic infection, the best, and in many cases the only way to recognize its presence is by means of the routine use of the blood Wassermann test. Occasionally the Wassermann test is negative in a pregnant woman who is later found to be syphilitic. In such a case, in the absence of physical signs, it is manifestly impossible to make a diagnosis during pregnancy except on the basis of the history.[67] The routine use of the Wassermann test in *all* pregnant women, however, will detect the majority of cases of unsuspected syphilis.[110] For example, the reported incidence of syphilis was 5 per cent in 25 prenatal clinics in Philadelphia making routine serologic tests but only 1 per cent in 11 prenatal clinics employing the test merely "as indicated."[45]

In a study reported in 1936, the American Social Hygiene Association found that in 250 of 268 ante-partum clinics the Wassermann test was used routinely, in contrast to its use in only 15 of 37 clinics surveyed in 1925.[33] A study made in 1935 by the same group showed that only half of 82 practitioners made routine Wassermann tests of the blood of their private obstetric patients.[33]

Moore[67] states that pregnancy is *not* a frequent cause of false positive Wassermann reactions. The current consensus on this point is that although nonspecific positive reactions do not occur during the early months of pregnancy, they may appear very rarely in the later months of pregnancy.

FACTORS WHICH INFLUENCE THE FUTURE HEALTH OF THE CHILD OF A SYPHILITIC MOTHER

Factors which influence the health of a child of a syphilitic mother are those chiefly concerned with the therapy administered to the mother and with the stage and activity of the infectious process in the mother.

Therapeutic Factors.—Treatment given a syphilitic woman during pregnancy is directed primarily toward preventing or curing syphilis in the infant and only secondarily toward curing the mother. The therapeutic factors of importance from the point of view of the infant are (a) the amount and kind of therapy received by the mother during pregnancy, (b) the time during pregnancy when therapy was received, and (c) the amount of therapy received by the mother before conception.

A. Treatment During Pregnancy.—It is generally conceded that an arsenical should be used in treating the pregnant syphilitic woman. Bismuth or mercury is almost routinely used with the arsenical. The arsenicals which have been most commonly used with the best results are arsphenamine and neoarsphenamine. More important than the choice of arsenical is the amount of drug administered during pregnancy. There appears to be a direct correlation between the amount of drug given and the proportion of healthy children produced in a given number of pregnancies. McKelvey and Turner[60] used arsphenamine in the treatment of 382 pregnant syphilitic women. The ultimate clinical status of 271 children of these women was ascertained. When the mother had received prenatally less than 1 gram of the drug, 73 per cent of the children were nonsyphilitic; 1 to 2 grams, 80 per cent; 2 to 3 grams, 84 per cent; 3 to 4 grams, 88 per cent; and 4 to 6 grams, 100 per cent. Ingraham[44] also used arsphenamine and reported that among a group of syphilitic women receiving no prenatal treatment 20 per cent had nonsyphilitic children, those receiving less than 4 injections, 29 per cent; 4 to 8 injections, 52 per cent; 9 to 16 injections, 61 per cent; and more than 16 injections, 85 per cent.

Acetarsone or acetylarsan has been used in the treatment of syphilis in pregnant women, but reports of the results are not conclusive. Castallo and Rakoff,[19] for example, used acetylarsan in the treatment of 57 syphilitic pregnant women, 97 per cent of whose pregnancies resulted in live births. They compare these results with those of a similar series in which they used arsphenamine and obtained essentially the same results (95 per cent live births). Coppolino,[25] however, found the results with acetylarsan distinctly inferior to those with neoarsphenamine. Thirty-one syphilitic women treated during pregnancy with neoarsphenamine gave birth to 30 normal and only 1 syphilitic infant, while 39 syphilitic women treated with acetylarsan gave birth to 14 normal and 15 syphilitic infants.

Klaften[50, 51] has reported somewhat inconclusively on the use of malaria therapy during pregnancy in syphilitic women.

B. Time of Administering Treatment.—Treatment should be started before the fifth month of pregnancy if the largest number of fetuses are to be saved, since infection of the fetus probably takes place after the fourth month of gestation. The Cooperative Clinical Group[22] found that when treatment was started between the first and fifth months 22 per cent of the pregnancies of syphilitic women ended "disastrously" for the fetuses; when treatment was started between the fifth and tenth months 39 per cent ended "disastrously." McKelvey and Turner[60] found that the incidence of fetal and neonatal deaths was lowest when syphilitic women were given arsenicals during the last trimester of pregnancy, regardless of the amount of treatment previously received by them.

Treatment during the early months of pregnancy does not cure the mother of her infection, but the treatment protects the fetus from infection. If the concentration of the drug in the mother's tissues is not maintained throughout pregnancy, periodic invasion of the blood stream by spirochetes may occur resulting in infection of the fetus.

A questionnaire survey made by a committee of the Medical Women's National Association, aided by the American Social Hygiene Association, showed that, in 9 clinics serving 3,400 patients during 1923, 76 per cent of the pregnant women were first seen during the first six months of pregnancy.[75] In a similar but much larger series of cases studied by Exner[33] in 1935, it was found that conditions with respect to early attendance at ante-partum clinics had not changed materially. Of 142 clinics reporting, 62 stated that 50 per cent of their patients were seen before the middle of pregnancy. A survey[103] in the spring and summer of 1937 in Chicago indicated that in less than half the syphilitic pregnant women had the disease been detected before the fifth month of pregnancy, and among these women only 21 per cent had received adequate treatment.

C. Anteconceptional Treatment.—The question whether or not women who have once had syphilis should be treated in every subsequent pregnancy has been raised again recently by several workers. Reports made by McKelvey and Turner[60] and by the Cooperative Clinical Group[22] indicate that treatment received prior to pregnancy will be of definite advantage in a future pregnancy but that such treatment will not insure the birth of a healthy infant as often as does treatment during pregnancy. Birnbaum[10] reported the cases of 21 women with early syphilis who were given rigorous antisyphilitic treatment "to the point of complete cure." The author studied the 34 subsequent pregnancies of these women; none of them was treated during pregnancy, and all of the children were apparently healthy. Some of them have been examined as late as six years after birth. Ingraham and Kahler[45] contend that in the light of our present knowledge of the curability of syphilis the obstetrician takes an unwarranted risk in permitting such women to go through pregnancy without antisyphilitic treatment. The Cooperative Clinical Group (1938)[69] recommends that the syphilitic mother be given "early and adequate treatment throughout every pregnancy."

MATERNAL FACTORS INFLUENCING THE OUTCOME OF PREGNANCY IN SYPHILITIC WOMEN

The Cooperative Clinical Group studied the mother's serology before and during pregnancy in relation to the result of pregnancy. They found that 39 per cent of pregnancies ended disastrously for the infant among women whose Wassermann reactions were positive before and negative during pregnancy compared with 43 per cent when the Wassermann reactions remained positive during pregnancy. The results of the pregnancies were studied in relation to the stage of the maternal infection. It was found that the stage of the infection was apparently not a definite factor in the transmission of the infection to the child as long as the Wassermann reaction remained negative during pregnancy. When the Wassermann reaction was positive during pregnancy, however, those women with active syphilis transmitted the disease to their infants in 31 per cent of the cases, whereas those women with positive serology but a latent infection transmitted the disease to the offspring in only 19 per cent of the cases.[22]

Fordyce and Rosen[36] recommended in 1922 that all pregnant women be treated for syphilis on the mere suspicion of the presence of the disease. Barnett[4] treats a pregnant woman for syphilis when the only indication is the presence of the disease in the husband. Many workers (Barnett,[4] Macnicol,[61] Abraham,[2] and Spiegler[91]) recommend that women receive antisyphilitic treatment during every pregnancy if they have been known to have had the disease, regardless of the amount of therapy received and regardless of the Wassermann reaction.

Since reactions of the mothers to antisyphilitic therapy have been used as an argument against treating the syphilitic woman during pregnancy, the Cooperative Clinical Group[22] studied the toxic reactions to antisyphilitic treatment during pregnancy and concluded that arsenical treatment need never be withheld from a pregnant woman for fear of irritating the kidneys or causing arsenical reactions. Ingraham and Kahler,[45] on the other hand, found that the only death from arsphenamine occurring in the University of Pennsylvania Hospital in a series of 17,000 injections was in a pregnant woman. Kristjansen[54] reports a few serious reactions in pregnant women. However, there is almost universal agreement that the pregnancy is not a contraindication for vigorous antisyphilitic treatment.

Treatment of Congenital Syphilis in Early Infancy

It has been said that the best means of treating congenital syphilis is to prevent it. The methods of prevention are well known, but the fact that in this country 60,000 infants[76] each year are born with congenital syphilis shows that all syphilitic women do not receive adequate treatment during pregnancy. The problem of treating the infected newborn infant remains, therefore, an important part of the attack upon syphilis.

THE PROBLEM OF THE SELECTION OF INFANTS FOR THE ADMINISTRATION OF ANTISYPHILITIC TREATMENT

Infants of untreated or inadequately treated syphilitic mothers may or may not be infected. There is no problem in deciding whether to administer antisyphilitic treatment when infants show manifestations of syphilis at birth; but many syphilitic infants show no signs of the disease at birth,[3, 21, 46, 96] and it is difficult to decide whether or not to treat these infants. There are two main groups of authorities who hold different opinions on this matter. One group[3, 63, 65, 78, 85, 92, 98] advocates the treatment of all infants of syphilitic mothers, whether clinical signs of syphilis are present or absent in the infant. Another group[1, 11, 16, 25, 45, 67] advocates that no infant should be treated for syphilis until the diagnosis is established. The literature has been searched for evidences of the advantages of giving or withholding treatment of apparently healthy infants of syphilitic mothers, and the information has been briefly summarized as follows:

The reasons that have been advanced for treating all infants born of syphilitic mothers are:

1. It is often impossible to tell at birth which infants are infected with syphilis and which are not.
2. Treatment of the mother results in treatment of the fetus in utero, and the infant at birth, although infected, may show no evidence of the disease. The treatment of the infant should not be interrupted at birth.

   In cases in which the mother is treated throughout pregnancy, a course of treatment given to the infant postnatally may be necessary to supplement his prenatal treatment. (It is assumed that the infant's tissues are permeated by these drugs given to the mother.)
3. The incidence of late complications of syphilis in the infants of syphilitic women is decreased.
4. If a syphilitic infant, apparently healthy at birth, is not treated immediately after birth an unjustifiable risk is taken in that the disease may not be detected early and therefore treatment may be necessarily delayed.

The reasons that have been advanced for withholding treatment until a definite diagnosis of congenital syphilis in the infant has been established are:

1. If treatment for syphilis is begun it should be continued for a long period. (It is here assumed that the fetus does not receive antisyphilitic treatment administered to the mother.)

2. It is impossible to evaluate the results of therapy unless the diagnosis is established in each instance.
3. It is not justifiable to place the stigma of syphilis on a nonsyphilitic child.
4. It is a needless risk to submit a nonsyphilitic infant to the hazards of antisyphilitic therapy.
5. It is an unjustifiable expense to treat nonsyphilitic infants.

These differences of opinion are based upon differences in interpretation of the mechanism of prenatal treatment of the mother.

Almost all authorities agree that infection of the fetus does not take place before the fourth to fifth month of pregnancy.[38, 46, 52, 67, 77, 86] Therefore treatment of the mother started at this time or earlier probably prevents the infection in the fetus either by sterilizing the maternal blood stream or by preventing transfer of the organisms to the fetus by concentration of antispirocheticidal drugs in the placenta.[46, 67] There is agreement also that to prevent infection of the fetus it is necessary to continue treatment of the mother with arsenicals during the last months of pregnancy in order to insure a maintenance of the concentration of the drug in the maternal blood, in the placenta, or in both.[30, 82, 102]

Treatment of the mother begun even late in pregnancy materially reduces the incidence of infection of the offspring.[22, 60, 62, 83] It is in regard to the mechanism by which treatment of the mother begun late in pregnancy affects the welfare of the fetus that authorities have disagreed.

One group believes that the drugs used in the treatment of the mother late in pregnancy actually saturate the tissues of the fetus, which is already infected. The permeability of the placenta to the drug is said to be proved by the concentration of antisyphilitic drugs found in fetal tissues. Eastman and Dippel[31] found large amounts of arsenic in the meconium of infants born of mothers who received arsphenamine during pregnancy. Levy and Selter[58] detected bismuth in both placenta and fetuses of rabbits. Kraul and Bodnar[53] found bismuth in the human amniotic fluid after therapeutic doses had been given to the mother, and Caffey[17] detected bismuth in the bones of infants whose mothers received bismuth during pregnancy.

Another group considers that treatment of the mother late in pregnancy prevents infection of the fetus by concentration of the antisyphilitic drugs in the placenta or by a continuous sterilization of the maternal blood stream. The mechanism is exactly the same as that of treatment early in pregnancy. This group maintains that the placenta is relatively impermeable to antisyphilitic drugs administered to the mother. Voegtlin[106] and others found less arsenic in the embryo than in any maternal tissue. Vamos and Böhm[104] were unable to detect arsenic in the fetal organs of rabbits whose mothers had been given intravenous arsphenamine. Leonard and Love[57] could detect only very small amounts of bismuth in fetal tissue.

If the theory of the first group is accepted, that is, the infected fetus is treated in utero, there would seem to be a rational basis for treating all infants of syphilitic mothers; if the theory of the second group is accepted, that is, that treatment of the mother prevents infection of the fetus, these infants need not be treated until a diagnosis can be established.

Klaften[50] states that if the offspring of untreated syphilitic women are permitted to go without specific treatment for syphilis until they are clinically syphilitic, 56 per cent will die in the first three months of life, whereas if all are treated immediately after birth the mortality rate will be only 16 per cent.

Morgan[70] states that more than 90 per cent of the deaths from this disease occur in the first few months of life, and he concludes from his own research that 80 per cent of syphilitic infants can be serologically cured if treatment is instituted at birth. Sylvester[96] says: "My conviction is that the baby who is seen early and treated adequately and early, will become normal in every way and remain so for so long that it may be considered cured."

It has been found, moreover, that from 70 to 80 per cent of infants born of mothers who have received only one month or less of prenatal treatment, or of mothers whose syphilitic infection is recent and active, will develop congenital syphilis.[44]

THE PROBLEM OF TREATING SYPHILITIC INFANTS

The treatment of congenital syphilis in early infancy is complicated by the fact that the disease in its active form frequently produces a severe toxemia and that severe constitutional disturbances may result.[67] The aim of treatment is therefore twofold: to preserve the life of the infant and to cure the infection.

General pediatric care is of great importance in preserving the life of the congenitally syphilitic infant. Breast feeding is recommended by Stokes,[93] but he warns against permitting any one but the mother to nurse a syphilitic infant, whether the infant has obvious signs of syphilis or not, because of the possible danger of infecting a healthy woman. The mother should be under treatment during the period of lactation, and the infant will receive some benefits from antisyphilitic drugs transmitted through the milk. Most investigators think that such medication is of minor significance in treating the infant. Campbell and Frost,[18] however, recommend treatment of the infant by means of the mother's milk as the sole specific treatment in certain cases.

Syphilitic infants should be protected from respiratory and intestinal infection, since their ability to resist infection is decreased.

Mortality of congenitally syphilitic infants in the first few months of life, whether they are treated or not, is high. Sylvester[97] found that during the twenty-five years' period, 1901-1925, nearly all of a series of infants who showed definite clinical signs of syphilis within the first three weeks of life died. He noted no decrease in mortality for this age group during the decade, 1915-1924, when methods of general care and treatment of syphilis had greatly improved. Jones[47] found 100 per cent mortality among syphilitic infants who showed manifest lesions during the first month of life, a 17 per cent mortality among infants who did not develop signs of syphilis until the second to the sixth month, and an 8 per cent mortality among those who did not develop signs of syphilis until the second half of the first year. Smith,[89] in making a study of the records of 621 syphilitic infants, found that 91 per cent of the deaths directly attributable to syphilis occurred in infants under six months of age.

The severity of the lesions was found by Jones[47] to influence mortality. Severe syphilis was found in 34 per cent and mild lesions in 5 per cent of the children dying in the first year.

The amount of treatment was found by Smith[88] to influence mortality. Twenty-two per cent of the infants dying of syphilis had received no treatment, 12 per cent had received less than six injections, and 2 per cent had received more than six injections.

Many congenitally syphilitic infants die of causes not directly associated with syphilis. Respiratory diseases take a heavy toll during the first year. Fürst[37] found that of 702 congenitally syphilitic children more than half died, approximately one-third of the deaths being due to pneumonia.

TECHNIQUE OF THERAPY

1. *Drugs Used.*—The antisyphilitic drugs that have been used in the treatment of congenital syphilis and the usual routes of administration are as follows:

Arsenicals

Arsphenamine ---------- intravenous
Neoarsphenamine ------- intravenous (occasionally intramuscular or, rarely, intraperitoneal)
Sulfarsphenamine ------ intramuscular and subcutaneous
Mapharsen ------------- intravenous
Acetarsone ------------ oral

Heavy Metals

Bismuth --------------- intramuscular
Mercury --------------- inunction, oral, or intramuscular

Combination of Arsenical and Heavy Metal

Bismarsen ------------- intramuscular

2. *Routes of Administration.*—In pediatric practice the routes of administration of the antisyphilitic drugs and in some cases the ease of administration, rather than the efficacy of the drug, have often determined the type of therapy.

The technique of intravenous administration is difficult to use in young infants because of the small size of the veins and the lack of cooperation on the part of the patient. The cubital or jugular veins are commonly employed. Moore[67] warns especially against the use of the longitudinal sinus by way of the anterior fontanel because of the danger of infiltration of the brain substance.

Intramuscular injection is not a difficult technique for the physician, but it is sometimes painful for the patient, and some physicians feel that the obvious discomfort caused by such treatment interferes with the regularity with which mothers are willing to bring their infants to the clinic.

The oral route is free from all the difficulties and discomforts of any treatment "by needle." It is, however, a somewhat unreliable method of treatment, since the physician can never be sure how much of the prescribed drug is actually taken by the patient when the entire responsibility for its administration is left in the hands of the mother.

Intraperitoneal injection of neoarsphenamine has been advocated by Grulee, Sanford, and Waldo[39a] in cases in which rapidity of action is desired and the small veins make intravenous injection impossible. In a personal communication to the authors Sanford states that intraperitoneal therapy is now used only as "an emergency measure in florid cases to achieve rapid action."

3. *Intervals of Treatment.*—The treatments are usually given at weekly intervals. There are three different methods for giving courses of treatment. In the first, called continuous therapy, courses of arsenical and heavy metal follow each other without rest periods. In the second, intermittent therapy, courses of treatment are separated by intervals of varying lengths of time. In the third, intensive treatment, large doses of arsenical and heavy metal are given in a short period of time, followed by a comparatively long rest interval before the next phase of the treatment begins.

The Cooperative Clinical Group[95] has demonstrated that for adults continuous therapy is considerably superior to intermittent, irregular, or intensive treatment. Their findings are in accord with the theoretical explanation set forth by Moore and Keidel[68] in 1926 when they introduced into the Johns Hopkins Clinic the continuous treatment in which alternating courses of arsphenamine and heavy metal are given. No similar studies have been made for children. The results of the intensive method used in treating children have been reported by McBride,[59] by Schussler,[87] and by Kundratitz.[56] McBride's intensive treatment consisted of three injections of arsphenamine at forty-eight-hour intervals and in addition an injection of bismuth at the time of the first and third arsphenamine injections, followed by six weeks of treatment with mercury and chalk by mouth. The entire course was then repeated. Schussler's intensive course consisted of 8 doses of neoarsphenamine in three weeks, followed by 16 mercury inunctions in eight weeks and then a two-week rest period. Four such courses were given in the first year. Kundratitz has also reported the results of intensive treatment of infants.

These investigators might be considered to have used massive rather than intensive treatment in the sense used by Moore,[67] as no long rest periods without treatment were allowed between courses. The results obtained by them are shown below. It should be pointed out that the term "cured," as used by these authors, means freedom from clinical and serologic signs of syphilis for periods varying from a few months to two years.

AUTHOR	TOTAL CASES ADEQUATELY TREATED	PER CENT "CURED"
Schussler	13	100.0
McBride	19	100.0
Kundratitz	58	89.6

THE ARSENICALS

1. *The Arsphenamines.*—The general principle followed until recently in treating infants with congenital syphilis has been to use the same drugs used in treating adults and to make the dosage proportional to the weight of the infant. As knowledge of chemotherapy has advanced, however, it has been found that certain drugs are more suitable than others for treating infants.

Prior to 1922 almost all infants treated for congenital syphilis received either arsphenamine or neoarsphenamine. White and Veeder[108] were able to follow 22 infants who received an adequate amount of arsphenamine and mercury and found that only 59 per cent had been clinically and serologically cured. Morgan[70] found that 80 per cent of 75 syphilitic infants who were adequately treated with arsphenamine and bismuth and whose cases were followed for at least two years remained clinically and serologically free from syphilis. Smith[88] reported very similar results: 78 per cent cures among 49 children adequately treated with arsphenamine and bismuth.

Meyer[66] reported the results of the use of neoarsphenamine in the treatment of 127 syphilitic infants, 97 per cent of whom became serologically free from syphilis and continued free when examined from one to two years after the cessation of treatment. Fordyce and Rosen,[36] however, obtained only 55 per cent serologic and clinical cures after treating 55 syphilitic children with neoarsphenamine and mercury. Wile and Shaw[109] obtained disappearance of symptoms and serologic reversal in 90 per cent of children most of whom were treated with neoarsphenamine. Jones,[47] however, found no manifestations of syphilis in any of 13 infants who were adequately treated with neoarsphenamine and bismuth.

In 1922 Voegtlin, Johnson, and Dyer[105] discovered that sulfarsphenamine had a greater spirocheticidal property than either arsphenamine or neoarsphenamine and that experimental animals tolerated the drug well when it was administered intramuscularly. For the treatment of infants and children the advantages of a drug that could be administered intramuscularly soon became apparent.

Although the use of sulfarsphenamine for the treatment of syphilitic infants has received unqualified endorsement by the Clinical Cooperative group,[69] reports of the results of its use are few in number and not entirely satisfactory. Crawford and Fleming[26] used sulfarsphenamine combined with mercury in the treatment of 23 infants and 12 older children, but they reported that many of their patients remained Wassermann-fast. Boone and Weech[13] treated 21 infants and obtained good immediate results with no serious reactions, but they did not follow their cases long enough to obtain any data on the ultimate effect of the drug. Dunham[29] treated 5 infants and 23 older children with sulfarsphenamine combined with mercury. She concluded that the drug was not superior to neoarsphenamine for the treatment of syphilis but that its greater ease of administration gave it a place of value among the available antisyphilitic drugs. Atlee and Tyson[3] treated 106 infants with sulfarsphenamine combined with bismuth and observed no serious toxic manifestations; 98 of the infants became clinically and serologically free from syphilis and 8 remained serologically positive. It is important to point out, however, that some of the infants treated as syphilitic had as the only evidence of syphilis a positive Wassermann reaction of the cord blood.

Jeans and Cooke[46] and Moore[67] advocate the use of sulfarsphenamine in the treatment of congenital syphilis in early infancy because of its ease of administration and the low incidence of toxic manifestations.

2. *Acetarsone.*—This drug (a pentavalent arsenical) is known as acetarsone in the United States, as stovarsol in France, as spirocid in Germany, and as osarsol in Russia. It was first prepared by Ehrlich and Hata in 1908.

Acetarsone was used very little until about 1921, when a series of reports from France indicated that it was effective in the treatment of syphilis in children when given orally. Since that time there have been many reports, especially from Germany, on the value of acetarsone in the treatment of congenital syphilis. The drug has come into more or less common use in the United States in the past five years. The fact that acetarsone can be given by mouth, thus avoiding the difficulties of injections, accounts in part for its widespread use.

In spite of the fact that acetarsone has been in use since 1921 and that the literature contains about forty reports dealing with the treatment of more than 1,100 children, only four reports have been found in which sufficient follow-up has been made to evaluate the drug.

The dosage, method of administration, toxic effects, and immediate therapeutic value of acetarsone have received considerable attention. Acetarsone is a white crystalline powder conveniently dispensed in tablets containing 0.10 and 0.25 gram. It must be administered by mouth. The general opinion is that infants and children tolerate this drug best when it is given in small, gradually increasing doses. The size of the daily dose, the length of a course of treatment, and the total amount of drug given in a course have varied widely.

At the present time two plans of treatment are in comparatively frequent use in the United States. The more conservative plan is that devised by Bratusch-Marrain.[14] The dosage is based upon the weight of the child as follows:

First week	0.005 gram per kilogram daily
Second week	0.01 gram per kilogram daily
Third week	0.015 gram per kilogram daily
Next six weeks	0.02 gram per kilogram daily

The amount of acetarsone in grams consumed during one nine-week course by this system corresponds approximately to the weight of the infant in kilograms. For example, an infant weighing 6 kilograms would receive approximately 6 grams of acetarsone during one course of sixty-three days. This course of treatment is followed by a rest period of four to six weeks, and then the course of treatment is repeated until the Wassermann reaction, taken after every course, is negative three times in succession. An additional "safety course," given six months after the cessation of the regular course, is recommended even in the presence of a negative Wassermann reaction.

The plan of Maxwell and Glaser[63] is less conservative than that of Bratusch-Marrain. In this method of treatment the infant receives 14 grams of acetarsone in a forty-nine-day course, approximately twice as much acetarsone as that recommended by Bratusch-Marrain, and it is administered during a shorter period of time.

Both these methods of therapy call for continuous treatment during the course, followed by a six-week rest period between courses. Some German authors have advocated that treatment and rest follow each other at intervals of several days during the entire course of treatment. Baumbach[5] attempted to determine the relative value of these two plans of treatment. Equal doses of acetarsone were given to each of two groups of children, to one group in a six-week course, to the other in a twelve-week course (one week of treatment alternating with one week of rest). The conclusion reached was that the twelve-week intermittent course produced more reversals of the Wassermann reaction than did the six-week course. No further data have been found on this point. In this country almost all investigators administer acetarsone in continuous courses.

The question whether acetarsone is more efficacious when administered alone or combined with a heavy metal has also been commented upon in several reports. Baumbach[5] found that when mercury was given during the rest periods of the intermittent course (one week of acetarsone, one week of mercury) better results were obtained than when acetarsone was given alone. Rambar[80] gave mercury during the six-week rest periods, following the nine-week acetarsone phase of the Bratusch-Marrain plan of treatment. No better results could be detected than when acetarsone was given alone. Von den Steinen[92] and Joseph[48] both recommend bismuth injections alternating with acetarsone in an intermittent course (three days of acetarsone, three days of bismuth). Traisman[100] states that bismuth should be given during the six-week interval between continuous courses, especially to older children.

Reports of the effect of acetarsone on the lesions of syphilis in infants have been almost uniformly favorable. Pillsbury and Perlman[79] observed that spirochetes disappeared in seventy-two hours from lesions in which dark-field examinations were made at twenty-four-hour intervals.

In addition to the specific effect of the treatment, improvement in the general condition of syphilitic infants treated with acetarsone is frequently reported. Nedelmann,[74] Traisman,[99] and Huber[43] reported satisfactory gains in weight for syphilitic infants under treatment with acetarsone. Improvement in color, with a corresponding rise in hemoglobin content of the blood, has been noted.[34, 84, 92] Improved resistance to infection has been reported by Kiss,[49] Krombach,[55] and Menne.[64]

The effect of acetarsone upon the blood Wassermann reaction of infants has been reported to be satisfactory, but the reports are not convincing since many of the infants were not seen after completion of the treatment.

Comparisons of the immediate results of acetarsone therapy with the results of the older methods of treatment have been attempted. Davidson and Birt[27] reported, for example, that 14 of 23 children treated with acetarsone were "cured" in a two-year observation period as compared with only 6 of 27 patients treated with other drugs in a seven-year observation period. Bratusch-Marrain[14] reported that of 23 children under one year of age who were treated with acetarsone 14 were "cured" as compared with 6 of 27 children treated with neoarsphenamine. Pillsbury and Perlman[79] found that cutaneous lesions healed more quickly under acetarsone treatment than under bismuth treatment, but not so quickly as under arsphenamine treatment. Hom[42] states that the external symptoms of syphilis disappear during acetarsone treatment in the same time as under neoarsphenamine treatment, but that the visceral lesions respond more quickly to treatment with mercury, neoarsphenamine, and bismuth.

Toxic effects are produced in certain individuals by acetarsone as by other arsenical drugs. The majority of the reactions are mild, but since the introduction of the drug there have been 7 deaths reported among over 1,000 children which were directly attributable to its use. These deaths were reported to be due to "poisoning" of the central nervous system, "toxic dyspepsia," and "reactions of an exanthem nature." The mild reactions are controlled by discontinuing the drug for a brief time, during which the body eliminates accumulated arsenic after which acetarsone can usually be continued without any further untoward effects. The reported incidence of toxic reactions has varied. Traisman[100] feels that the size of the dose is directly related to the seriousness of the toxic reactions. He considers the dosage used by Maxwell and Glaser too high for many infants. He also states that rest periods between courses are essential to allow for the elimination of arsenic and to avoid reactions.

Most workers emphasize the fact that patients receiving acetarsone must be under constant medical supervision and should not be allowed to take long courses of the drug without a check-up by the physician, since many serious reactions can be avoided by detecting early signs of toxicity and temporarily discontinuing the drug.

From a review of these reports it is clear that at the present time it is impossible to draw any conclusion as to the optimum dosage and the system of administering acetarsone. Further controlled studies are needed to settle the present uncertainties.*

In a recent review, however, Yampolsky[112] states that he now considers acetarsone the drug of choice in treating congenital syphilis in young infants. Griffith and Mitchell[39] in the recent edition of their textbook report extensive use of acetarsone.

3. *Bismarsen (Bismuth Arsphenamine Sulfonate).*—An advantage of the use of this drug is that the therapeutic effects of arsenic and bismuth are combined in one drug. It was synthesized by Raiziss in 1925 and was first used for the treatment of adults in 1927 by Stokes and Chambers,[94] who reported very satisfactory results. Chambers and Koetter[20] and Reilly[81] used the drug for the treatment of congenital syphilis in children.

Bismarsen is given by the intramuscular route only. Stokes says that it should be used continuously for long periods and that the interval between injections should not be greater than three or four days. Chambers and Koetter gave bismarsen to children twice weekly in twenty injections, with rest intervals of two weeks between the first and second courses and of one month between the second and third courses. Therapeutic effects were good, but healing of lesions was not so rapid as under treatment with arsphenamine derivatives. Wassermann reversal was obtained in 91 of 100 children. Of the 91 children, 41 of whose cases were followed for twenty months, 5 showed "serologic relapse." Reilly gave bismarsen in weekly injections to 170 children; the serologic records of 61 patients were followed, and in 47 cases the reaction became negative. Ten of the 170 children suffered clinical relapses, and 8 suffered a serologic relapse after cessation of the treatment. It is possible that Chambers and Koetter obtained better results than Reilly because they administered the drug twice weekly and Reilly gave it only once a week.

Neither Chambers and Koetter nor Reilly encountered any serious toxic reactions in children in the course of over 9,200 injections. Mild reactions were found in about the same frequency as with the use of the other arsenical compounds. Yampolsky[112] says that in his experience bismarsen causes pain and therefore he has discontinued its use.

---

*Since this article went to press Dr. Pillsbury and Dr. Perlman, of the University of Pennsylvania, have furnished us with an unpublished manuscript giving the results of treatment with acetarsone of 187 syphilitic infants and children, using the Maxwell-Glaser plan of treatment. Toxic reactions occurred in 11 per cent of the children; in more than one-third of the toxic cases evidences of nephritis were found. In these cases the use of the drug was discontinued. Eighty-seven of the 187 children were observed for three years or more. In none of the cases did a clinical relapse occur; in only one case was there a serologic relapse.

4. *Mapharsen.*—This is the trade name for arsenoxide (meta-amino parahydroxy phenyl arsene oxide). Recent theoretical work lends support to the theory that arsenoxide is the agent in vivo which produces the spirocheticidal effect when the arsphenamines are injected. The suggestion has been made that, if this is true, the beneficial results of arsphenamine would be obtained by using arsenoxide for therapy and many of the complications of arsphenamine therapy would be avoided.

Reports on the use of this drug in infants and children are very few. Morgan[71] treated 39 syphilitic infants and children and kept them under observation for sixteen months. He compares the results of treatment in this series of cases with those of another series of children treated with other drugs during the past nineteen years. In giving 935 injections of mapharsen mild reactions were observed in 133 cases and a moderately severe reaction in 1 case. The dosage used was 0.5 mg. to 0.75 mg. per kilogram of body weight. He concludes that, although a complete evaluation of the drug is not yet possible, the results strongly suggest that mapharsen is a more powerful agent in effecting a serologic cure than any other arsenical compound previously used in his clinic.

Studies of the use of mapharsen are being made in several clinics at the present time.

THE HEAVY METALS

Two heavy metals (mercury and bismuth) are used for the treatment of syphilis in children. Mercury is one of the oldest known antisyphilitic remedies, but bismuth, which has come into use more recently, is rapidly replacing it.

1. *Mercury.*—In 1920 Findlay[35] said that treatment by mercury alone should be discarded. He reported that in a series of infants under three months of age who were treated with mercury alone the mortality was 71 per cent, while in two series of cases in which combined treatment with mercury and an arsenical was used the mortality was 37 and 26 per cent, respectively. There are, however, occasional reports in the recent literature of mercury being used as the sole drug in the treatment of congenital syphilis.

2. *Bismuth.*—Müller[73] reported the use of bismuth in the treatment of syphilis in children in 1922. Since that time there have been numerous reports of the use of bismuth alone or in addition to other therapeutic agents. Bismuth is said to stimulate the resistance of the host to invasion by the spirochete. It has, in addition, some direct antispirocheticidal properties which mercury does not have, although its action in this respect is not so great as that of the arsenicals. Bismuth is less toxic than mercury. Bismuth has been administered by several routes, but Stokes[93] says that the intramuscular route is the only practical one.

There are six preparations of bismuth in relatively common use at the present time and they vary according to the vehicle (water or oil) and the chemical constitution of the drug.

The water-soluble preparations require relatively frequent administration, two to three times per week; the oil-soluble preparations require less frequent administration, usually once a week.

The dosage of bismuth usually follows the Lomholt rule of 0.5 mg. bismuth metal per kilogram of body weight per day. It is usually considered good practice to allow rest periods of six to eight weeks between courses.

The clinical response to bismuth therapy has in general been reported to be satisfactory. Skin and mucous membrane lesions heal rapidly. Wright[111] found that the Wassermann reaction was reversed in some children when this could not be accomplished by other methods of treatment. Coppolino[24] reported good results with the use of bismuth in treating infants but found it less effective in older children. He does not consider it so useful a drug as acetarsone.

Some toxic reactions occur with intramuscular injections. They consist of anorexia, vomiting, and diarrhea with, occasionally, black deposits of bismuth sulphide in the mucous membranes. Occasionally cutaneous symptoms or generalized reactions take place, but they are rare. Beerman[7] studied the cases of fatal poisoning due to bismuth that were reported in the literature up to 1932 and concluded that intravenous administration (purposeful or accidental) was primarily responsible for sudden deaths.

PROGNOSIS

The tendency for syphilis to produce clinical signs or symptoms many years after the initial infection has led many syphilologists to give a very guarded prognosis of complete cure of syphilis even in children. Smith[88] has shown that the longer a group of children were under observation the larger was the number of relapses. In his series of children treated before the age of 2 years, relapses took place in 65 per cent of the cases five to twelve years after the child had been discharged from treatment. When these cases were followed for more than thirteen years after discharge it was found that relapses occurred in an additional 15 per cent of the cases. Smith[88] found that relapses were much more frequent in children whose blood Wassermann reactions remained persistently positive than in those whose Wassermann reactions became negative under treatment. The ultimate effect of treatment was found to depend upon the age at which treatment was begun and upon the amount and type of treatment given.

Smith reported that 9 per cent of children receiving "adequate" treatment suffered relapses, compared with 14 per cent of those receiving "inadequate" treatment. Jones[47] found that all infants were "cured" under "regular" treatment and only 50 per cent under "unsatisfactory" treatment.

Smith[88] found that, when treatment for syphilis was started before the third month of life, the relapse incidence was 6 per cent; between 4 to 6 months, 11 per cent; and between 7 to 12 months, 15 per cent. When treatment was delayed until some time during the second year, the relapse incidence was 19 per cent. White and Veeder[108] found that when treatment was started before the age of 2 months, 32 per cent of the children were "cured," compared with 25 per cent when treatment was started after the second month but before the second year.

The kind of antisyphilitic therapy used must necessarily influence the ultimate clinical outcome. Because of the large number of variables influencing the end results, however, it is not possible to obtain data regarding the most efficacious treatment. The amount and regularity of treatment, the age at which treatment is begun, the severity of the manifestations of syphilis, and the pediatric care of the infants are all perhaps as important as the selection of the drug or drugs used. There is a lack of controlled studies of the effect of different types of treatment.

In thirteen reports[32, 36, 46, 47, 56, 70, 72, 74, 87, 88, 90, 108, 109] of over 2,000 children diagnosed as syphilitic and treated by well-known methods before the age of 2 years, it was found that only one-fourth of the children were adequately treated and followed long enough to determine the results.

Fifty-five to 100 per cent of clinical and serologic cures are recorded in the various reports on this group, but no constant relation appears between the method of treatment and the percentage of cures.

It is impossible, considering all the variables in the statistics, to draw any conclusions concerning the relative therapeutic efficiency of the treatment systems used.

REFERENCES

1. Abner, L.: Should Seronegative Infants of Syphilitic Mothers Be Given Specific Treatment? Arch. f. Dermat. u. Syph. **167**: 315, 1933.
2. Abraham, J. J.: Some Comments on Syphilis in Women, Brit. M. J. **2**: 237, 1932.
3. Atlee, E. D., and Tyson, R. M.: Congenital Syphilis: Results of Early Treatment, Am. J. Dis. Child. **44**: 718, 1932.
4. Barnett, A. M.: Pregnancy and Syphilis, Urol. & Cutan. Rev. **32**: 796, 1928.
5. Baumbach: Experiments With Spirocid in Congenital Syphilis, Arch. Kinderh. **99**: 151, 1933.
6. Beck, Alfred C.: A Preliminary Report on the Treatment of Syphilis Complicating Pregnancy, Am. J. Obst. & Gynec. **2**: 416, 1921.
7. Beerman, H.: Fatalities Due to Bismuth in the Treatment of Syphilis, Arch. Dermat. & Syph. **26**: 797, 1932.
8. Belding, D. L.: The Effect of Treatment of the Syphilitic Pregnant Woman Upon the Incidence of Congenital Syphilis, Am. J. Obst. & Gynec. **12**: 839, 1926.
9. Belding, D. L., and Hunter, I. L.: The Wassermann Test. III. A Statistical Study of Clinical Syphilis and Fetal Deaths in Women with Positive Wassermann Reactions, Am. J. Obst. & Gynec. **8**: 22, 1924.
10. Birnbaum, G.: On the Curability of Syphilis and the Prevention of Congenital Syphilis Through Modern Treatment, Deutsche med. Wchnschr. **53**: 1893, 1927.
11. Boas, H.: The Prophylaxis of Congenital Syphilis. In Jadassohn's Handbuch der Haut-u. Geschlechtskr. **19**: 327, 1927.
12. Boas, H., Gammeltoft, S. A., and Sieck, K.: The Behavior of the Wassermann Reaction at Birth. Is the Venous Blood of a Parturient Suitable for Use? Arch. f. Gynäk. **128**: 537, 1926.
13. Boone, F. H., and Weech, A. A.: Treatment of Early Hereditary Syphilis With Intramuscular Injections of Sulpharsphenamin, Am. J. Dis. Child. **27**: 39, 1924.
14. Bratusch-Marrain, A.: Method and Value of Spirocid Treatment of Syphilis in Childhood, Archiv. f. Kinderh. **92**: 26, 1931.
15. Browne, F. J.: Neo-natal Death, Brit. M. J. **2**: 590, 1922.
16. Buschke, A., and Gumpert, M.: Congenital Syphilis, Klin. Wchnschr. **6**: 263, 1927.
17. Caffey, John: Changes in the Growing Skeleton After the Administration of Bismuth, Am. J. Dis. Child. **53**: 56, 1937.
18. Campbell, H. S., and Frost, K.: Indirect Treatment of a Presumably Syphilitic Child by Maternal Therapy During Lactation, California & West. Med. **32**: 231, 1930.
19. Castallo, M. A., and Rakoff, A. E.: An Analysis of 259 Cases of Syphilis Complicating Pregnancy, Pennsylvania M. J. **39**: 24, 1935.
20. Chambers, S. O., and Koetter, G. F.: Bismarsen in the Treatment for Congenital Syphilis, Arch. Dermat. & Syph. **25**: 1065, 1932.
21. Chargin, L., and Umansky, M.: Congenital Syphilis. Advantage of Early Treatment as Judged by the Wassermann Test, Am. J. Syph. **17**: 468, 1933.
22. Cole, H. N., and others: Syphilis in Pregnancy, Ven. Dis. Inform. **15**: 83, 1934.
23. Coppolino, J. F.: Bismuth Therapy Exclusively in Congenital Syphilis, Am. J. Dis. Child. **39**: 288, 1930. Discussion, 454.
24. Coppolino, J. F.: Acetarsone in the Treatment of Congenital Syphilis; a Comparison With Bismuth Therapy, Am. J. Dis. Child. **48**: 272, 1934.

25. Coppolino, J. F.: Prophylaxis of Congenital Syphilis, Am. J. Obst. & Gynec. **29**: 714, 1935.
26. Crawford, E., and Fleming, G. B.: A Note on the Use of Sulfarsenol in the Treatment of Congenital Syphilis, Lancet **2**: 700, 1921.
27. Davidson, A. M., and Birt, A. R.: The Treatment of Congenital Syphilis With Stovarsol, Canad. M. A. J. **34**: 33, 1936.
28. Dodds, G. H.: An Analysis of the Results of the Wassermann Reactions Obtained From 2,000 Consecutive Pregnant Women, J. Obst. & Gynæc. Brit. Emp. **34**: 779, 1927.
29. Dunham, E. C.: The Diagnosis of Congenital Syphilis in the Newborn, Am. J. Dis. Child. **43**: 317, 1932.
30. Eastman, N. J.: The Arsenic Content of the Human Placenta Following Arsphenamine Therapy, Am. J. Obst. & Gynec. **21**: 60, 1931.
31. Eastman, N. J., and Dippel, A. L.: The Passage of Arsenic Through the Human Placenta Following Arsphenamine Therapy, Bull. Johns Hopkins Hosp. **53**: 288, 1933.
32. Eckardt, F.: Spirocid in Congenital Syphilis, Jahrb. f. Kinderh. **141**: 278, 1934.
33. Exner, Max J.: Syphilis in Pregnancy, J. A. M. A. **106**: 488, 1936.
34. Fan, P. L.: Stovarsol Treatment of Congenital Syphilis in Chinese Children, Chinese M. J. **50**: 364, 1936.
35. Findlay, L.: The Treatment of Syphilis in Infancy and Childhood, Brit. M. J. **2**: 197, 1920.
36. Fordyce, J. A., and Rosen, I.: The Treatment of Antenatal and Congenital Syphilis, Arch. Dermat. & Syph. **5**: 1, 1922.
37. Fürst, K.: Treatment and Fate of Our Syphilitic Children, Jahrb. f. Kinderh. **119**: 335, 1928.
38. Gräfenberg: The Influence of Syphilis on Posterity, Arch. f. Gynäk. **87**: 190, 1909.
39. Griffith, J. P., and Mitchell, A. G.: Diseases of Infants and Children, ed. 2, Philadelphia, 1937, W. B. Saunders Company, pp. 1154.
39a. Grulee, C. G., Sanford, H. N., and Waldo, P. C.: Congenital Syphilis, Treatment by Intraperitoneal Injection of Neoarsphenamine: Report of Two Years' Work, Am. J. Dis. Child. **35**: 47, 1928.
40. Hall, Emmett R.: Treatment of the Syphilitic Expectant Mother, South. M. J. **18**: 757, 1925.
41. Halloran, C. R.: Syphilis and Pregnancy. Effect, Diagnosis, Treatment, and Complications with the Report of an Unusual Nitritoid Crisis, Am. J. Syph. **14**: 222, 1930.
42. Hom, J.: Results of Treatment of Congenital Syphilis With Spirocid as Compared with Those of Treatment With Neosalvarsan, Dissertation, Halle-Wittenberg, 1931.
43. Huber, H. G.: Two Years of Spirocid Therapy in Congenital Syphilis, Med. Welt **4**: 1331, 1930.
44. Ingraham, N. R., Jr.: The Diagnosis of Infantile Congenital Syphilis During the Period of Doubt, Am. J. Syph. **19**: 547, 1935.
45. Ingraham, N. R., Jr., and Kahler, J. E.: The Diagnosis and Treatment of Syphilis Complicating Pregnancy, Am. J. Obst. & Gynec. **27**: 134, 1934.
46. Jeans, P. C., and Cooke, J. V.: Prepubescent Syphilis, New York, 1930, D. Appleton-Century Company, Inc.
47. Jones, F. A., Jr.: A Study of the Results of Treatment of Congenital Syphilis in Infants Under Two Years of Age, Thesis, Yale, 1935 (Typewritten).
48. Joseph, B. M.: Stovarsol (Spirocid), Its Use in Congenital Syphilis. A Review of the Literature and a Report of 14 Cases, J. M. Soc. New Jersey **31**: 343, 1934.
49. Kiss, P.: The Present State of Oral Treatment of Congenital Syphilis, Jahrb. f. Kinderh. **126**: 211, 1930.
50. Klaften, E.: Fundamentals of Antisyphilitic Treatment of the Newborn Infant, Klin. Wchnschr. **7**: 458, 1928.
51. Klaften, E.: The Influence of Malaria Therapy of Syphilitic Women on the Product of Conception, Arch. f. Dermat. u. Syph. **157**: 280, 1929.
52. Klaften, E., and Priesel, R.: Bone Changes in Congenital Syphilis, Fortschr. a. d. Geb. d. Röntgenstrahlen **42**: 311, 1930.
53. Kraul, L., and Bodnar, L.: Influence of Antisyphilitic Treatment on Fetus, Arch. f. Gynäk. **128**: 238, 1926.

54. Kristjansen, A.: Antisyphilitic Treatment During Pregnancy and Results Obtained on the Basis of 118 Cases of Syphilitic Women Treated During Pregnancy, Hospitalstid. **70**: 97, 1927.
55. Krombach, K.: Treatment with Spirocid of Congenital Syphilis in Infants, Klin. Wchnschr. **7**: 1512, 1928.
56. Kundratitz, K.: Intensive Treatment of Congenital Syphilis, Arch. f. Kinderh. **91**: 21, 1930.
57. Leonard, C. S., and Love, R. B.: Studies in the Pharmacology of Bismuth Salts; the Permeability of the Placenta to Bismuth, J. Pharmacol. & Exper. Therap. **34**: 347, 1928.
58. Levy, S., and Selter, E.: Treatment of Congenital Syphilis With Spirobismol, Arch. f. Kinderh. **75**: 241, 1925.
59. McBride, R. H.: Congenital Syphilis. A Review of One Hundred and Ninety-Two Cases From a Rural Community With a Comparison of Two Methods of Treatment, Arch. Dermat. & Syph. **18**: 79, 1928.
60. McKelvey, J. L., and Turner, T. B.: Syphilis and Pregnancy: An Analysis of the Outcome of Pregnancy in Relation to Treatment in 943 Cases, J. A. M. A. **102**: 503, 1934.
61. Macnicol, M.: Methods at the Elsie Inglis Memorial Hospital, Lancet **2**: 206, 1931.
62. Marshall, C. H.: Prenatal Syphilis; Effects of Antepartum Treatment, J. A. M. A. **91**: 702, 1928.
63. Maxwell, C. H., Jr., and Glaser, J.: Treatment of Congenital Syphilis With Acetarsone Given by Mouth, Am. J. Dis. Child. **43**: 1461, 1932.
64. Menne, E.: Treatment of Syphilitic Infants with Spirocid. Thesis, Frankfurt-on-the-Main, 1931.
65. Mettenheim, H. V.: On the Peroral Treatment of Congenital Syphilis With Spirocid in Infancy, Med. Klin. **27**: 422, 1931.
66. Meyer, G.: Report on the Fate of Syphilitic Children Given Sufficient Treatment, Arch. f. Kinderh. **74**: 172, 1924.
67. Moore, J. E.: The Modern Treatment of Syphilis, Springfield, Ill., 1933, Charles C. Thomas.
68. Moore, J. E., and Keidel, A.: The Treatment of Early Syphilis. I. A Plan of Treatment for Routine Use, Bull. Johns Hopkins Hosp. **39**: 1, 1926.
69. Moore, J. E., and others: Management of Syphilis in General Practice. In press.
70. Morgan, E. A.: The Prognosis for a Serological Cure in Hereditary Syphilis, Canad. M. A. J. **23**: 811, 1930.
71. Morgan, E. A.: The Value of Mapharsen in the Treatment of Congenital Syphilis, Canad. M. A. J. **38**: 53, 1938.
72. Müller, E.: Spirocid Treatment of Congenital Syphilis and Its Results to Date, Arch. f. Kinderh. **91**: 108, 1930.
73. Müller, H.: Treatment of Syphilis With Bismuth, München. med. Wchnschr. **69**: 547, 1922.
74. Nedelmann, E.: Experiences With Spirocid Treatment of Congenital Syphilis, Jahrb. f. Kinderh. **134**: 89, 1931.
75. Parker, V. H.: A Study of Prenatal Clinics With Special Reference to the Diagnosis and Treatment of Syphilis in the Pregnant Woman, M. Woman's J. **34**: 330, 1927.
76. Parran, T.: Shadow on the Land, New York, 1937, Reynal & Hitchcock.
77. Pick, L.: Roentgen Examination as an Aid in the Diagnosis of Congenital Early Syphilis of the Bones, Deutsche Ztschr. f. d. ges. gerichtl. Med. **12**: 159, 1928.
78. Pillsbury, D. M.: The Prevention and Treatment of Prenatal Syphilis, Internat. Clin. **2**: 236, 1931.
79. Pillsbury, D. M., and Perlman, H. H.: The Treatment of Prenatal Syphilis With Acetarsone (Stovarsol). A Preliminary Report of Results in 73 Cases, Pennsylvania M. J. **38**: 327, 1935.
80. Rambar, A. C.: Syphilis and Prematurity With Special Reference to the Use of Stovarsal in Prophylactic and Curative Treatment of Congenital Syphilis, J. PEDIAT. **3**: 841, 1933.
81. Reilly, W. A.: Results of Treatment of Congenital Luetics With Bismuth Arsphenamine Sulfonate (Bismarsen) for Five Years, California & West. Med. **43**: 429, 1935.
82. Reinberger, J. R., and Toombs, P. W.: The End Results of Ten Years' Study of Treatment of Pregnancy Syphilis in Trimesters, South. M. J. **26**: 532, 1933.

83. Richter, W.: Result of Treatment of Syphilitic Pregnant Women With Regard to the Prognosis for the Child, München. med. Wchnschr. **76**: 735, 1929.
84. Rosenbaum, H. A.: A Survey of One Hundred Cases of Congenital Syphilis Treated With Stovarsol (Acetarsone), J. PEDIAT. **3**: 434, 1933.
85. Rutledge, W. V.: Congenital Syphilis, South M. J. **25**: 844, 1932.
86. Schneider, P.: Changes in the Organs in Congenital Early Syphilis, Centralbl. f. allg. Path. u. path. Anat. **43**: 11, 1928.
87. Schussler, H., Jr.: The Intensive Treatment of Congenital Syphilis (Final Report), California & West. Med. **23**: 446, 1925.
88. Smith, F. R., Jr.: Congenital Syphilis in Children: Results of Treatment in 521 Patients, Am. J. Syph. & Neurol. **19**: 532, 1935. Am. J. Syph., Gonor. & Ven. Dis. **20**: 45, 1936.
89. Smith, F. R., Jr.: Congenital Syphilis; The Results of Treatment in Children, J. A. M. A. **105**: 409, 1935.
90. Soldin, M., and Lesser, F.: Further Experiences With Spirocid in Syphilis of Infants, Deutsche med. Wchnschr. **54**: 958, 1928.
91. Spiegler, R.: Syphilis and Pregnancy, München. med. Wchnschr. **79**: 95, 1932.
92. von den Steinen, R.: Treatment of Infantile Lues with "Spirozid," München. med. Wchnschr. **74**: 1006, 1927.
93. Stokes, J. H.: Modern Clinical Syphilology, ed. 2, Philadelphia, 1936, W. B. Saunders Company.
94. Stokes, J. H., and Chambers, S. O.: Bismuth Arsphenamine Sulphonate: Clinical Observations on New Arsphenamine Synthetic in Treatment of Syphilis, J. A. M. A. **89**: 1500, 1927.
95. Stokes, J. H., and others: Cooperative Clinical Studies in the Treatment of Syphilis, Ven. Dis. Inform. **13**: 207, 1932.
96. Sylvester, P. H.: Observations on Congenital Syphilis, Boston M. & S. J. **193**: 393, 1925.
97. Sylvester, P. H.: Twenty-five Years of Congenital Syphilis in Boston. A Statistical and Comparative Study, J. A. M. A. **87**: 298, 1926.
98. Taylor, C. B.: Treatment of Syphilis in the Newborn, J. Oklahoma M. A. **23**: 301, 1930.
99. Traisman, A. S.: Treatment of Congenital Syphilis With Acetarsone (Stovarsol) by Mouth, Am. J. Dis. Child. **46**: 1027, 1933.
100. Traisman, A. S.: Further Observations on the Use of Acetarsone in the Treatment of Congenital Syphilis, J. PEDIAT. **7**: 495, 1935.
101. Turner, R. H.: The Value of the Obstetric History in Making a Diagnosis of Syphilis, M. Clin. North America **11**: 1211, 1928.
102. Underhill, F. P., and Amatruda, F. G.: The Transmission of Arsenic From Mother to Fetus, J. A. M. A. **81**: 2009, 1923.
103. Usilton, L. J., Hunter, H., and Vonderlehr, R. A.: Prevalence, Incidence and Trend of Syphilis in Chicago, J. A. M. A. **110**: 864, 1938.
104. Vamos, L., and Böhm, A.: Action of Arsenobenzol Preparations on the Fetus (Animal Experiments), Arch. f. Dermat. u. Syph. **176**: 245, 1937.
105. Voegtlin, C., Johnson, J. M., and Dyer, H.: Sulpharsphenamine. Its Manufacture and Its Chemical and Chemotherapeutic Properties, Pub. Health Rep. **37**: 2783, 1922.
106. Voegtlin, C., Smith, M. I., Dyer, H., and Thompson, J. W.: Penetration of Arsenic Into the Cerebrospinal Fluid, With Particular Reference to the Treatment of Protozoal Infections of the Central Nervous System, Pub. Health Rep. **38**: 1003, 1923.
107. Welz, W. E., and Van Nest, A. E.: Observations on the Treatment of Syphilis in Pregnancy in the Department of Health in Detroit, Am. J. Obst. & Gynec. **4**: 174, 1922.
108. White, P. J., and Veeder, B.: A Study of 443 Cases of Hereditary Syphilis With Especial Reference to Results of Treatment, Am. J. Syph. **6**: 353, 1922.
109. Wile, Udo J., and Shaw, J. W.: The Prenatal Treatment of Syphilis With Especial Reference to Early Syphilis in the Mother, J. A. M. A. **95**: 1791, 1930.
110. Williams, J. W.: The Influence of the Treatment of Syphilitic Pregnant Women Upon the Incidence of Congenital Syphilis, Bull. Johns Hopkins Hosp. **33**: 383, 1922.
111. Wright, Carroll S.: Bismuth in the Treatment of Congenital Syphilis, J. A. M. A. **89**: 424, 1927.
112. Yampolsky, J.: A Comparative Review of the Use of Antiluetic Drugs in the Treatment of Congenital Syphilis in Children, South. M. J. **31**: 406, 1938.

American Academy of Pediatrics

Proceedings

EIGHTH ANNUAL MEETING OF THE AMERICAN ACADEMY OF PEDIATRICS

HOTEL DEL MONTE, DEL MONTE, CALIF.

JUNE 9, 10, AND 11, 1938

Report of the Executive Board

I wish to submit the following report for the Executive Board of the American Academy of Pediatrics for the year ending May 1, 1938:

The meeting held in Evanston, Dec. 10 and 11, 1937, was the last one with the Executive Board consisting solely of the officers and the regional chairmen. At this meeting associate regional chairmen were appointed, Dr. Stanley Nichols for Region I, Dr. James Bruce for Region II, Dr. Edgar Martmer for Region III, and Dr. Hugh Berkley for Region IV. These associate chairmen in the future will meet with the board. The untimely death of Dr. Louis Schroeder, chairman of Region I, emphasizes the importance of the associate chairmen.

Thirty-three candidates were elected to Fellowship, twenty-four of whom were from Region I. Dr. Alfred J. Scott, Jr., was transferred to Emeritus Fellowship.

The change in the schedule of our annual meetings is significant. Beginning with 1939, the annual meeting will be held in the fall of the year, and the regional meetings in the spring of the year. In 1940 the International Congress of Pediatrics will meet in the United States for the first time. The meeting is to be held in Boston early in September. The close proximity of this meeting and our annual meeting was evident, and possible arrangements were discussed. The question of scheduling the regional meetings just before or after the American Medical Association meeting will have to be decided by the regional membership. Whether this change will increase or decrease the attendance of members of the Academy at the American Medical Association meeting is uncertain, but it is a question which deserves our very definite consideration.

The splendid reception which was accorded the published report of the Committee on Immunization Procedures within the Academy and without indicates the service the Academy can render in this and in similar fields.

The only other matter to which I wish to call attention is the increasing recognition which is being accorded the Academy by all organizations which deal with the child. Evidence of this is brought out by the many requests for cooperation which are received from these organizations.

HENRY F. HELMHOLZ, Vice-President.

Report of the Secretary

There are now 1,229 Fellows in the Academy.

The Secretary is sorry to have to record the death of six of the Academy Fellows during the past year:

Dr. Barnet E. Bonar, Salt Lake City, Utah
Dr. W. O. Colburn, Lincoln, Neb.
Dr. Sylvan D. Lazarus, Brooklyn, N. Y.
Dr. Gustave Lippman, St. Louis, Mo.
Dr. Louis C. Schroeder, New York, N. Y., Emeritus Fellow
Dr. LaFayette B. Mendel, New Haven, Conn.

Special mention should be made of the loss of Dr. Louis C. Schroeder whose devotion to the work of the Academy was in full measure responsible for the success in Region I. Dr. Schroeder was not only loved, but trusted, and his judgment was excellent. The Academy has lost more than it realizes in his death.

Besides the annual meeting, there have been four regional meetings: Region I at Boston, Mass., November 12 and 13; Region II at New Orleans, La., December 1 and 2; Region III at Chicago, Ill., October 14, 15, and 16; Region IV at Los Angeles, November 4, 5, and 6. The Secretary attended all of these meetings and can attest to the excellence of each.

The particular change in the administration of the Academy during the past year has been the elimination of the regional committees and their replacement with associate regional chairmen. This has expedited regional work materially and has also practically doubled the membership of the Executive Board. It is too early yet to say whether this will facilitate action or not, but it will certainly mean a better representation of the membership on that Board.

During the past year two new Committees have been added. The one on Contact Infections whose Chairman is Dr. Fairfax Hall, of New Rochelle, N. Y., has been organized to look into the situation regarding infection through school contacts, and contacts in the school and home especially with regard to teachers and domestics. The second is the Committee on Neonatal Morbidity and Mortality of which Dr. Harold C. Stuart of Boston, Mass., is chairman. This committee was started with Dr. Bonar as chairman, but his untimely death necessitated a revision of the committee which is to cooperate with a like committee from the American Pediatric Society and with the Children's Bureau in Washington.

The other committees have all been quite busy, especially the Committee on School Health and School Health Education, which has put out an excellent questionnaire, and also the Committee on Immunization Procedures, whose booklet you have already received and which has been very popular throughout the country. The Committee on Mental Hygiene has been revised and has decided to take some definite action to proceed with its work.

The Academy has received an offer from Mead Johnson & Company to provide money for a yearly prize. This is being considered by the Executive Board and doubtless will be accepted as soon as a few minor changes have been effected.

At the suggestion of the members of Region II, concurred in by the members of Region III, the Executive Board has recommended that hereafter the annual meeting be held in the fall and the regional meetings in the spring.

There is an ever increasing interest among the various state groups in the work that is being carried on in the states. This does not appear officially but is nevertheless a very important part of the work the Academy is doing and should be supported in every way by the members. It is surprising how much there is to do if we look for it. Oftentimes the states that have the smallest membership are the most active in getting things done. In many of the larger eastern states there has been a complacency which is certainly not justified.

In a recent letter, the American Medical Association offered to send typewritten lists of physicians who limit their practice, or give special attention to certain specialties. It is interesting that of the single groups, the first group is surgery with 13,696; the second group, internal medicine, 4,797; and the third group, pediatrics with 4,086. It is true that the group of specialists practicing both obstetrics and gynecology numbers 6,886; ophthalmology, otology, laryngology, and rhinology a total of 8,451. However, for the definite groups pediatrics ranks third and is just behind internal medicine.

Respectfully submitted,

CLIFFORD G. GRULEE, Secretary-Treasurer.

Report of Region I

In Memoriam

It is with sorrow and regret that Region I must report to the Academy the loss of its regional chairman, Dr. Louis C. Schroeder, of New York City, who had been chairman of Region I since the beginning of the Academy.

Dr. Schroeder gave a lifetime of devotion to the cause of child health in many fields. As chairman of Region I he was an inspirational leader and a friendly companion to every state officer and Fellow of the Academy.

It was characteristic of Dr. Schroeder that, when ordered by his physician, because of heart trouble, to give up all his general activities, he was quoted as saying to his secretary, ''Send in my resignations to all of my other positions, but maybe I can find a little time for the Academy work, as it means so much to me.''

Such a spirit cannot help but inspire all of the officers and Fellows of Region I to better service to the cause of child health. As a memorial to his untiring efforts and kindly leadership we will build a better structure because of the splendid foundation he has laid for us through the years.

Before presenting a bird's-eye view of the progress which has been made during the past year in each of the states and provinces of Region I, we would like to make a few observations as to the general pediatric situation in the region.

In all of our states and provinces there has been a steady growth of the influence of the Academy Fellowship in stimulating improvement in all forms of Child Health Service and bettering the medical status and pediatric knowledge of both the pediatrist and the general medical profession.

Section I of Article III of the Constitution of the American Academy of Pediatrics reads thus:

> ''The object of the Academy shall be to foster and *stimulate interest* in *pediatrics* and *correlate* all aspects of the work for the welfare of children which properly come within the scope of pediatrics.''

In other words, that the Academy shall—

(a) *stimulate* scientific pediatric knowledge

(b) *co-ordinate* Child Health Services in each state and province of the Academy.

We have listed below fifteen possible state academy activities, and we note by the reports of our state chairmen that in every state and province there has been, during the past year, a great deal of expansion in many of these fields. A much larger number of the Fellows of the Academy in each state are actively participating in the promotion of scientific pediatric knowledge and stimulating the various forms of better child health service. This is most encouraging evidence of sound growth and proves beyond doubt the continuing need of the leadership and guiding hand of the American Academy of Pediatrics in all of the facets of that evergrowing structure called ''child health service.''

Some of our states with larger membership have been able to develop most of these fifteen fields listed, while some states with fewer members have selected those activities which seemed to be most needed in their own districts. All have been active and are to be commended for their work and devotion to the general objectives of the Academy.

While it is not possible for a tail to wag a dog, it is perfectly possible and feasible for the American Academy of Pediatrics to be the "Thinking and Planning Child Health Lobe" of the brain and the "All-Seeing Child Health Eye" of the medical profession and governmental and welfare departments, as well as functioning similarly for nonofficial agencies dealing with some phases of child health.

Our national and state organizations of the American Academy of Pediatrics have proved their great value by providing leadership and active expert assistance in the coordination of the various child health services rendered by these several groups, and are the one medical body capable of doing this most important of all child health jobs.

How extensively this is being done in the various states and provinces in Region I, will be shown by the highlights of our state chairmen's reports covering the following list of Academy activities in some of our states.

It is clear that all of our state groups have realized the importance of *coordinating* and *stimulating* the *existing* official and nonofficial agencies dealing with Child Health and the *promotion* of pediatric knowledge among pediatrists, general practitioners and the public groups.

The most important single activity of any state Academy Fellowship is to act as the stimulating, coordinating keystone of child health development for both the state medical society and the state department of health. This is fully realized by our state chairmen. Most of the other important activities of the Academy can be built on this three-organization child health arch, when so erected.

With this clear understanding of our state chairmen of the objectives of the Academy and promotion of its ideals, Region I is looking forward to a year of increased usefulness to child health, by both improving the position of the pediatrist and rendering better child health service to the public.

State Activities

Outline of Academy Activities in Some of Our States and Provinces

A. Improving Pediatric Knowledge—

1. Helping our Fellows solve scientific pediatric problems
2. Helping our Fellows solve pediatric practice problems
3. Postgraduate education of
    a. Pediatricians
    b. General practitioners

B. Child Health Activities: Promotion and coordination of better child health service

4. Child Health activities in connection with state medical societies
    a. Maternal welfare section—
        Prenatal care
        Good obstetrics
        Maternal nursing
    b. Pediatric section—
        Care of the newborn infant
        Preschool age child
        School age child
        Adolescent

5. Child health activities in connection with state departments of health.
   a. Bureau of Child Hygiene and Maternal Health
6. Child health activities in connection with state welfare departments.
   a. Health of dependent, handicapped and neglected children, etc.
7. Child health activities in connection with state departments of education
   a. Health of school age child
   b. Mental hygiene
   c. Adolescent problems
8. Child health activities in connection with other state official and nonofficial groups dealing with some phases of child health work.
9. Contagious disease facilities in hospitals and pediatric facilities in hospitals.
10. Control of communicable diseases.
11. Promoting routine child health supervision by

a. Pediatricians b. Family physicians	during	infancy preschool age school age adolescence

12. Mental hygiene and adolescent problems.
13. Tuberculosis control in childhood.
14. Safety of children during childhood.
    a. Auto and home accidents, burns, poisons, etc.
15. Health of children in summer camps.

Report of Region II

A survey of the activities of Region II for 1937 and 1938 reveals that it has made some progress. Although the region reported only three applications for membership, it must be remembered that the number of those who are qualified is limited. At the present time we have 243 members, with the prospect of a few more; only 15 remain who have an American Board of Pediatrics certificate. The states of Arkansas, Alabama, Louisiana, Mississippi, Oklahoma, and Virginia will have no more prospects until some of the younger men are able to fulfill the requirements of the American Board of Pediatrics.

Every state chairman has been working with the established agencies throughout the states, the plan being to coordinate the various pediatric activities, to eliminate the weak ones, to assist the strong ones, and to attempt to interest those concerned with child health problems in certain definite projects, so that the work will not overlap. Each state in the South has a pediatric society, which is working in conjunction with the state medical society.

Refresher courses are being given in the majority of the southern states. Florida, Georgia, Kentucky, Mississippi, North Carolina, Oklahoma, South Carolina, Texas, Virginia, and West Virginia have well-established programs, either under control of the state medical society or the state health department.

As a complete résumé of the activities of this region is presented in THE JOURNAL OF PEDIATRICS, April, 1938, a more detailed description is unnecessary.

This region voted unanimously that the national meeting of the Academy be held at a separate place and at a separate time from that of the American Medical Association, also, that the regional meeting be held separately from that of the Southern Medical Association. It was the consensus that both the Academy and the respective sections would be benefited by this change. The members of the Academy of this region who were present pledged their allegiance to the pediatric sections of the American Medical Association and the Southern Medical Association; all felt that the Academy members should be the leaders in these sections. It was also the general opinion that the programs in these sections should be practical, arranged primarily for the general practitioner and others interested in pediatrics, rather than for the specialist in this field. Further, it was agreed that all those interested in pediatrics be invited to the meeting of Region II and that this program consist of clinics as well as round table and panel discussions.

During his six years in office the regional chairman has visited most of the states in the region. There seems to be harmony and a good spirit among the Academy members, although there is still a feeling that the "rank and file" do not have a sufficient part in Academy policies. Many of the members appear willing to allow a few to do all the work. This materially limits the possibilities of the group.

The chairman would recommend that there be a meeting of all the members of the Academy at least once each year in each state; that there be no program, but rather, a full, free discussion of all the pediatric problems in that state; that committees be appointed by the state chairman to see that every Academy member in that state has some active part in its work. When this is accomplished, there will be no difficulty in securing the fifteen eligibles in this region who are still not members of the Academy. Solicitation of members is believed to be a bad policy; the Academy should demonstrate by its accomplishments that it is of more value to any man than that man is to the Academy.

It is also recommended that the state chairmen request every man in the state to pass either favorably or unfavorably upon every applicant from that state. If this were done in writing, there could be no later criticism, as has occurred in many instances.

I believe the change from the regional board to an associate chairman was a happy solution of some of our difficulties. I am especially pleased with the selection of Dr. James Bruce, of Louisville, as associate chairman of this region. We have discussed in detail the policies of the region, and I feel that his counsel will be of great assistance to me as its chairman.

In closing, I believe it is being demonstrated throughout the entire United States that the Academy was organized for a good purpose. The principles of the organization are sound, and its possibilities will be unlimited when all members become actively interested.

I wish to thank the state chairmen for their cooperation during the past year.

Respectfully submitted,
E. C. Mitchell,
Regional Chairman.

Report of Region III

On Oct. 14, 1937, a meeting of the state chairmen of Region III was held at the Lake Shore Athletic Club, Chicago. Dr. A. Graeme Mitchell, Regional Chairman, presided. There were present the following: Dr. Franklin P. Gengenbach, Colorado; Dr. Maurice L. Blatt, Illinois; Dr. E. G. Padfield, Kansas; Dr. Edgar E. Martmer, Michigan; Dr. E. J. Huenekens, Minnesota; Dr. Park J. White, co-chairman from Missouri; Dr. Ralph E. Pray, North Dakota; Dr. Sterling H. Ashmun, Ohio; Dr. Goldie E. Zimmerman, South Dakota; and Dr. Abraham B. Schwartz, Wisconsin.

Dr. E. W. Hancock represented Dr. Clyde Moore, Nebraska, who was unable to attend. Dr. Frederick B. Miner, Flint, Mich., was present by invitation.

Several state chairmen presented reports of the activities in their states.

The following applicants were recommended by the regional committee to the Executive Board for election to membership:

Dr. James J. Donahue, E. St. Louis, Ill.
Dr. Clair L. Douglas, Detroit, Mich.
Dr. Ernest Ekermeyer, Xenia, Ohio
Dr. Faith F. Hardy, Grand Rapids, Mich.
Dr. Harold O. Lund, Middletown, Ohio
Dr. John W. Maroney, Detroit, Mich.
Dr. Mark F. Osterlin, Traverse City, Mich.
Dr. Thomas P. Saltiel, Chicago, Ill.
Dr. Clara D. Tigay, Chicago, Ill.
Dr. Dwight A. Weir, Mansfield, Ohio

There was discussion of the matter of applicants who did not confine their practice to pediatrics. It was moved by Dr. Martmer and seconded by Dr. Pray that it be recognized as a plan of Region III that no applicants should be recommended to the Executive Board who did not limit their practice to pediatrics unless such applicants were engaged in a type of work which, because of specific circumstances, demonstrated a direct contribution to pediatrics.

On motion by Dr. Martmer it was recommended that there be a suggestion from Region III to the Executive Board that the Academy of Pediatrics make some study, perhaps by the appointment of a committee, in regard to the thymus gland. It was suggested that this might take the form of a round table discussion or a panel discussion at one of the Academy meetings. It was felt that, if it were possible for some definite statement to be made, even if negative in nature, regarding symptoms produced by the thymus gland, it would be helpful.

Dr. Martmer invited Region III to Detroit in 1938 for the next annual meeting. This invitation was immediately accepted and it was decided that the time of the meeting would be settled by the Michigan group.

There was discussion of recommendations for associate regional chairman. The regional chairman stated that he would get the opinion of each state chairman by letter, and it was moved that he then take these recommendations into consideration and recommend directly to the Executive Board the names of two candidates, one of whom would then be chosen by the Executive Board as an associate regional chairman.

Dr. Krafft, of Chicago, was allowed the floor. He wished to call the attention of the regional committee and of the Academy of Pediatrics to the underprivileged (precriminal) child. He thought that contacts should be made with educational organizations and with lay societies and organizations; that the physicians as well as the laity should be educated in the problems involved; that all children should be examined annually; that efforts should be made to secure legislation concerning these subnormal persons. It was the opinion of those at the meeting that many of these contacts were already being made in different states and that no particular recommendation need be made by the regional committee to the Executive Board.

The regional chairman, after communication with the various state chairmen and upon the basis of this, recommended to the Executive Board the names of two candidates, one of whom was to be chosen by the Executive Board for associate regional chairman. Of these two candidates, the Executive Board chose Dr. Edgar E. Martmer for associate regional chairman.

Region III of the Academy will hold its regular meeting in Detroit on October 27, 28, and 29. The arrangements for this meeting are under the charge of Dr. Edgar E. Martmer of Detroit.

A. Graeme Mitchell
Regional Chairman

Edgar E. Martmer
Associate Regional Chairman.

Report of Region IV

The membership of Region IV has reached a fair degree of saturation. There are now 120 members including a very high proportion of those doing exclusively pediatrics.

This membership is well represented in all that is being done in pediatrics in the West, including the administration of child welfare activities supported by federal social security funds. In several of the states the directors of child and maternal welfare are members of the Academy.

The tragic and untimely death of Barnet Bonar is sincerely mourned by the entire Region. He brought great ability and kindly personality to the practice of pediatrics. His loss will be a great one to pediatrics of the West.

The annual regional meeting was held last fall in Los Angeles. About two-thirds of the regional membership was in attendance, a most interesting and well-arranged scientific program was presented and arrangements for the comfort and entertainment of visitors left nothing to be desired.

This year, in order to concentrate interest in the Del Monte meeting, there will be no additional meeting of Region IV. It is our sincere wish that the first western meeting of the Academy shall be so pleasantly remembered as to be soon repeated.

EDWARD B. SHAW,
Regional Chairman.

SPECIAL COMMITTEE REPORTS

Report of the Committee Appointed to Study the Age Limits of Pediatric Practice

The Committee Appointed to Study the Age Limits of Pediatric Practice submits the following report for the consideration of the Executive Board and membership of the American Academy of Pediatrics.

It is the consensus of your committee that it is impractical to establish a definite age limit for pediatric practice. The practice of pediatrics begins at birth and should extend through the adolescent period. In most instances, the termination of pediatric practice would be between the sixteenth and eighteenth years of life.

Respectfully submitted,

EDGAR E. MARTMER, Chairman
STERLING H. ASHMUN
PHILIP M. STIMSON
HAROLD C. STUART
MELDRUM K. WYLDER

Report of the American Board of Pediatrics

The members of the American Board of Pediatrics appointed by the American Academy of Pediatrics submit the following report of the work of the board for the year 1937-1938.

Five examinations have been held; at Atlantic City (June), Chicago (October), Los Angeles (November), Boston (November) and New Orleans (December). In all, 182 candidates were examined, of whom 69.34 per cent passed and have been certified; 21.87 per cent failed, and 8.79 per cent were conditioned. To date, May 1, 1938, 1,226 certificates have been issued by this board.

In addition to the six announced in last year's report, Dr. Hugh Berkley and Dr. Victor Stork, of Los Angeles, have been appointed official examiners for the board.

At the meeting of the Advisory Board for Medical Specialties held in Atlantic City in June, 1937, it was decided to obtain funds to make a general survey of graduate medical education in the United States. A foundation grant of $75,000 has been obtained, and the survey is under way. Dr. Blackfan is the pediatrician appointed to the committee in charge of the survey.

Boards have been organized and are at work in all the twelve special fields recognized in the agreement between the advisory board and the Council on Medical Education of the American Medical Association.

A proposed biographical directory of the licentiates of all twelve boards has been postponed, awaiting the completion of the on record certification of the Boards of Medicine and Surgery.

The American Board of Pediatrics is compiling an address booklet of their licentiates.

No changes have been made in the membership of the board.

Respectfully submitted,

Harold C. Stuart
Borden S. Veeder
Alfred A. Walker

Report of the Committee on Child Health Relations

During the past year the Committee on Child Health Relations of the American Academy of Pediatrics has pursued its policy of stimulating a close cooperation between members of the Academy in each state and those agencies administering the three phases of the Social Security Act with which we are chiefly concerned; namely, maternal and child health, child welfare, and the crippled children's program.

Representatives of this committee have been appointed in forty-five states. Your committee has requested the Children's Bureau to forward to each of its representatives pertinent data pertaining to activities of the social security program, and any other material concerned with maternal and child health which it seemed would be of interest and aid to members of the Academy in their work in these fields. From the expressions of appreciation coming from the various states, the committee feels that this has been a very definite service and wishes to express the thanks of the Academy to the Children's Bureau.

A résumé of the activities of the members of the Academy in matters of maternal and child health, particularly as related to the program made possible through the Social Security Act, is included in this report. So many requests have been received, asking about programs in other states, it was thought advisable to give these in some detail.

The reports, as a whole, indicate that the Academy is very definitely interested in the program and ready to cooperate in any way possible. In many instances, however, members have not taken the initiative but have waited until their services have been requested by the various state agencies. One gains the impression in reading these reports that in many states there seems little desire on the part of these agencies to enlist the aid and advice of the Academy. Your committee feels that the Academy should initiate a more active program in its efforts to guide the various federal and state agencies working in the maternal and child health fields.

There is practically no evidence of Academy activity in the child welfare and crippled children's programs.

The committee feels that there is great need for integration of the maternal and child health activities carried on by the various lay and professional organizations in the states. When such coordination has been attempted, very definite benefits have accrued. This is particularly true in the rural sections. The Academy might well be the motivating force in initiating such a program.

Respectfully submitted,

M. Hines Roberts, Chairman
Philip F. Barbour George M. Lyon
W. L. Crawford Stanley H. Nichols
Martha M. Eliot Oscar Reiss

Résumé of Activities

California.—Three physicians are members of the professional advisory committee on maternal and child health. Three meetings during the year were held.

May, 1937: General outline of activities, forms and literature of the Bureau of Child Hygiene. Revision of a first-aid kit for rural schools. Possibility of professional education discussed.

November, 1937: Progress and activities of staff in the field during past six months.

January, 1938: Discussion of May Day Child Health Day. Lay advisory committee convened in joint session to work out relationship between professional and lay groups in rural areas and to promote organization of county committees. Dr. Shaw, Dr. Sweet, and Dr. Reiss participated in perigrinating orthopedic clinics. Dr. Sweet will hold clinics in Idaho, April 27 to May 3. Dr. Shaw expresses need for medical agency to coordinate child health activities, lay and professional.

Colorado.—Dr. Friedman reports that he has not been called upon to render medical service by any of the state agencies.

Iowa.—Two members act as consultants to the department of health in planning and administering funds in rural areas. Three members serve on Committee on Maternal and Child Health of the Iowa State Medical Society. A plan of considerable interest is the establishment of stations for the care of premature infants at strategic centers. Advice in preparation of programs of lay organizations. Pediatric clinics for general practitioners.

Certain members are opposed to any attempt to bring all lay and professional groups together in an integrated state and county program.

Louisiana.—Refresher courses in pediatrics in Mississippi, Louisiana, and Florida.

Maine.—Dr. Foster is chairman of the Advisory Committee on Maternal and Child Health, serving with three other members of the Academy. Refresher courses in pediatrics, obstetrics, and orthopedics. Physicians apathetic to program.

Georgia.—Two physicians are on Advisory Committee on Maternal and Child Health. Activities in the main are directed toward stimulating action in child health and welfare councils through the state. These councils are composed of lay and professional groups concerned with maternal and child health. Dr. M. Hines Roberts is a member of Advisory Committee of Child Welfare program. One meeting was held. Dr. Roberts was recently appointed by president of the Medical Association of Georgia to serve as a member of the Technical Advisory Committee of the Crippled Children's Service. No meeting as yet.

Maryland.—Dr. Knox states that he has received assistance from members of the Academy from time to time in promoting maternal and child hygiene.

Michigan.—The Academy is represented on preventive and maternal health committee of the state medical society. Prepared standard immunization schedule for state use.

Postgraduate program in conjunction with Michigan State Medical Society, University of Michigan, and Wayne University. Refresher courses under sponsorship of state director. Radio programs.

Minnesota.—Refresher courses for physicians and public health nurses. Cooperation with the state department of health in coordinating maternal and child welfare projects motivated by various professional and lay groups.

Missouri.—Dr. Dwyer is on Advisory Committee of Child Health division of state department of health. His services have never been requested. The Academy has no representation on state medical association's committee on maternal and child health. No pediatrician on this committee. Cooperation with P.T.A. campaign for examination of every school child before admission to school. Every child examined by own physician for $2. Trying to dissociate medicine and schools. Avoid introducing persons to well-baby stations and dispensaries.

Montana.—Conference with state department of health on maternal and child health. Examination of all preschool and government nursery school children for past two years with cooperation of state department of maternal and child health. Considerable opposition within state medical society to program.

Nevada.—Advisory to maternal and child health program under state department of health.

North Carolina.—Dr. Root serves on Advisory Committee on Maternal and Child Health of state board of health. This committee meets quarterly. Certain representatives feel need for integration of maternal and child health activities of various professional and lay groups in the state and county.

New Hampshire.—Cooperation with lay groups in their programs. No official status of Academy members in the social security program is reported.

New Jersey.—Representation on public health committee and Advisory Committee on Child Health and Maternal Health of the medical society of New Jersey. Lectures on preschool age group arranged by members of Academy, financed by social security funds.

North Dakota.—Academy members on Committee on Maternal and Child Welfare of North Dakota State Medical Society. No close cooperation between this group and the state department of health.

Feel that an effort to coordinate program of various professional and lay organizations on maternal and child health is definitely needed.

Oregon.—Dr. Henricke is chairman of the Committee on Clinic and Institutional Medical Care of the state medical society; he works in close cooperation with Division of Maternal and Child Hygiene of the state department of health. Strongly favors closer coordination of child health and welfare activities of lay and professional groups. The apathy or opposition of the general practitioner makes the program difficult.

Pennsylvania.—Academy members in cooperation with the Pennsylvania Medical Society have initiated an extensive maternal and child health program. Under the auspices of the county medical societies 59 counties have organized child health work. All agencies concerned with child health in the county have been drawn into the program. The Academy group has attempted to cooperate with the department of health and the maternal and child health program of the Children's Bureau. It feels, however, that a simpler medium and program than that of the maternal and child health service of the Children's Bureau is needed.

South Dakota.—Academy members are not active in support of agencies administering the Social Security Act.

Tennessee.—No report received of official activities of Academy members in the social security program.

Texas.—Academy members cooperate in child health lectures.

Vermont.—Cooperation with state department. Lectures before county medical societies.

Virginia.—In cooperation with state medical society and pediatric society recommend legislation for adequate care of tuberculous children, better teaching facilities for the mentally subnormal, and more widespread immunization of the indigent. Offered services to state agencies, but they have not accepted such service.

Washington.—Members of Academy cooperate with Committee on Maternal and Child Health of the state medical association in conducting programs in various county medical societies. Two members of Academy made nutritional survey, receiving help from ''Aid to Dependent Children.'' State chairman of Academy is relieving physicians in charge of maternal and child health program of the state health department and organizing group to coordinate activities of various lay and professional organizations in matters of maternal and child health. Academy members assist in postgraduate lecture program.

West Virginia.—Four members of Academy serve on Committee on Child Health of the state medical association. This committee in close cooperation with state in developing refresher courses, preschool conferences and an educational program including posters, radio, etc. Approves effort to integrate activities of various lay and professional groups concerned with maternal and child health.

Wisconsin.—Dr. Peterman giving refresher courses in Montana.

Report of the Committee on Clinical Investigation and Scientific Research

The Committee on Clinical Investigation and Scientific Research has considered the generous offer of Mead Johnson & Company to donate funds yearly for prizes to be awarded to young research workers. Your committee concludes that the administration of this work is not one of its functions and believes that a special committee should be appointed by the Academy to perform these duties. The committee would like to draw the attention of the Academy to the fact that it would be to the advantage of the Council for Pediatric Research if the money thus donated passed through the hands of the council.

The committee further recommends that the proposed investigation as to the cause of rickets, etc., be turned over to the Council for Pediatric Research for administration of funds and direction of the research.

Respectfully submitted,

FRITZ B. TALBOT, Chairman
WILBURT C. DAVISON OSCAR SCHLOSS
HENRY F. HELMHOLZ FRANCES SCOTT SMYTH

Report of the Committee on Contact Infections

Pediatricians have always shown themselves willing and anxious to take an active part in a program designed to benefit the health of the community and that of their patients. Close association of a child with a person having an unrecognized communicable disease is a potential source of infection for that child. The adults with whom children are most constantly in contact are parents, other members of the family, school teachers, and domestic employees. Although parents are the most intimate associates of children, the employees in a home are the persons about whom the least is known from a health standpoint. When nursemaids and houseworkers are engaged to help with the care of children, it should be known, that they are free from transmissible infections.

The diseases not infrequently transmitted by adults to children in their environment are tuberculosis, syphilis, gonorrhea, typhoid by carriers, and respiratory and skin diseases. The most important and the most dangerous for children is tuberculosis. It is well known that a case of open pulmonary tuberculosis without proper control in a home will infect every child there. It is against this disease that the greatest amount of protection for children may be expected by a proper physical examination of the adults to whom they are exposed. Since a roentgenogram of the lungs will detect the presence of any existing pulmonary tuberculosis, even in an uninfectious stage, it is essential that this be a routine procedure in examining adults for the protection of children.

It is extremely important that parents have no infectious diseases, not only for their own sakes but for their children's. Moreover, in order to obtain the cooperation of a domestic worker in having a medical examination, it is always desirable that the employers should have had a similar examination themselves and hold a certificate from the family physician, so stating. It is often necessary to set this example and use it as an argument in order to persuade some domestics to be examined.

If any great number of adults are to provide themselves with periodic health examinations, or if servants are to be willing to do so at the request of their employers, a great deal of effort must be put forth. An intensive campaign of education is necessary. The employers of domestic workers must learn to be discriminating in regard to the health of servants they engage to assist in the care of their children. Publicity must be sufficient to reach the domestic class in order to overcome prejudice against being examined and obtaining health cards. It must be pointed out to workers that the advantages gained by periodic examinations are not of health value alone but economic as well. Public opinion must be created to make health references as commonly asked for, and furnished, as character references. Pediatricians know the need for this and are in a position to be the greatest influence towards its accomplishment.

Experience in Westchester County, N. Y., with a plan to make this possible has been very encouraging. It has been received favorably both by doctors and by parents who employ household help. Many of the more influential women's organizations, public health societies, Parent-Teachers' Associations, and men's service clubs have been active with the publicity and education campaign. The Metropolitan Life Insurance Company has offered to aid the campaign among its policy holders in Westchester County.

The principle of periodic health examination was acceptable to the Medical Society of the County of Westchester. The medical aspect of the program has been sponsored by the society and its public health committee has arranged a standardized examination form for domestics. The members of the society have been requested to make this examination at a low fee. Roentgenologists have agreed to take a single film exposure of the chest for $3, and the blood Wassermanns are done by the state laboratory free of charge.

Even in this locality there remains much to be done. The public should be made more fully aware of the advisability of periodic health examinations. There still is opposition toward the idea on the part of some servants, and more effort is needed to secure the cooperation of employment agencies. The pediatrists should be encouraged to continue this effort they have begun to safeguard their patients.

Much headway has been made with this campaign in Knoxville, Tennessee. In that city 12 cases of active tuberculosis and many syphilis and 5 typhoid carriers were found in routine examination of domestics in the past year, In Newark, N. J., health cards have been required for several years. In North Carolina and other parts of the south, this matter has been given serious attention.

The Committee makes the following recommendations to the American Academy of Pediatrics:

1. Acquaint the members of the Academy with the advisability of recommending a thorough periodic physical examination to all adults in close contact with children.

2. Attempt to influence parents to have periodic examinations themselves for the protection of their children and as an example to their employees.

3. Ask pediatricians also, to have physical examinations in order to set a proper example and to create the impression that they believe in what they advise.

4. Encourage the x-ray examination of the lungs of teachers and other school employees.

5. Take steps to initiate a campaign for the education of the public regarding the need for, and value of, such examinations. Develop public opinion to the point where it becomes customary for domestic workers to hold medical cards as a "health reference" as the result of having undergone the necessary physical examination.

6. Get the cooperation of employment agencies to encourage domestics, who work in families with children, to obtain "health cards."

7. Enlist the assistance of child health-minded organizations, in as many communities as possible throughout the country, to carry out this campaign.

8. Secure the cooperation of local and county medical societies throughout the country to adopt a standardized examination which will detect evidence of communicable disease. (An x-ray of the lungs is requisite.) The charge for these examinations must be sufficiently low as to be within the ability to pay, of all who need them.

9. It is further recommended that subcommittees be appointed in each regional district to carry on this work in their localities.

Respectfully submitted,

FAIRFAX HALL, Chairman
GAYLORD W. GRAVES
REGINALD A. HIGGONS
OLIVER W. HILL

Report of the Committee on Cooperation with Nonmedical Groups and Societies

At the beginning of the year 1938, Dr. Henry F. Helmholz found it necessary to relinquish the chairmanship of this committee owing to the pressure of other duties. The present chairman was named by the president, Dr. Philip Van Ingen, to fill Dr. Helmholz' unexpired term. It is regrettable that the original chairman found it impossible to continue in charge of the committee which was created at his suggestion and for which he envisoned an increasingly important role in the affairs of the Academy. It is the hope of the remaining members of the committee that they may, in some measure at least, be able to bring their activities to the plane of usefulness Dr. Helmholz had in mind.

During the year the Committee has continued its cooperative efforts with the American Camping Association. On December 11, Dr. Henry E. Utter attended a meeting of the New England Camp Directors' Association at Boston, and on December 18, the Conference of Consultants of the American Camping Association Research Committee at New York. Dr. George F. Munns attended a conference of the latter group at Ann Arbor in November in place of Dr. Albert D. Kaiser who was ill at the time. A third meeting which was scheduled to be held in Chicago in February was postponed to some future date. The purpose of the conferences was to develop a research program for the study of camp practices leading to the establishment of certain standards and codes. It was suggested that the Academy might be in a position to influence the diversion of some of the funds granted to states under Title V of the Social Security Act to assist in carrying out the study. However, since the postponed conference has not as yet been held, the committee has no conclusions or recommendations to offer at present.

Recently contact has been made with Dr. Lillian Smith, National Chairman of the Summer Round-Up of the National Congress of Parents and Teachers. The movement sponsored by this organization is of interest to all members of the Academy. As yet, the committee has no formal cooperative program to recommend, but a suggestion, which Dr. Smith felt would be of considerable value, might be made that each state chairman appoint a committee of Academy members to confer with state and local summer round-up officials. One of the urgent needs of this lay group is an effective means of interpreting its program to the medical organization. In the capacity of a go-between, with the lay officials on the one hand and the medical profession on the other, such a committee should be able greatly to facilitate and enhance the program of this important national organization. The committee would make the further suggestion that state chairmen who think the plan feasible for their states, notify the chairman of this committee in order that he may forward the names of the Academy members selected to Dr. Smith. She in turn will advise the state summer round-up officials of the personnel of the committee available for cooperation.

The only other activity undertaken by the Committee in the past year was the reviewing and submitting of criticism of a brochure entitled "A Health Program for Children in Foster Care," prepared by Dr. Florence A. Browne, pediatrician for the Child Welfare League of America. The brochure is a brief outline of the various parts which together make up a complete health program. It is intended as a guide to agencies harboring foster children in determining the adequacy or inadequacy of the health services available for their charges.

Respectfully submitted,

Lee Forrest Hill, Chairman
Dennis H. Kelly, Secretary
C. A. Aldrich — Albert D. Kaiser
James W. Bruce — Henry E. Utter
Margaret I. Handy — Norman C. Wetzel

Report of the Committee on Hospitals and Dispensaries

The Committee on Hospitals and Dispensaries has recently finished a report concerning the question of age limits in pediatric hospitals and in pediatric divisions of general hospitals.

This report represents a consensus of opinion with respect to this and related questions among twenty-eight men who head children's hospitals in this country and Canada. Data were received by the questionnaire method and the report will be published in detail later.

Respectfully submitted,

George F. Munns, Secretary
Clifford G. Grulee, Chairman
Murray H. Bass — Henry Dietrich
Laurence R. DeBuys — Lewis Webb Hill

Report of the Committee on Immunization Procedures

The secretary of the Academy has submitted a copy of the report of the Committee on Immunization Procedures to each member of the Academy. No member of this Committee feels that this report was perfect or that it represented the last word on the subject. Additions, corrections, modifications, and improvements will be necessary.

In this report, the last sentence under "Rabies" should be deleted and the following sentence substituted: "This, however, is not so important as the fact that recovery from this disease is rare."

The members of the Academy are requested to aid us and send any suggestions or criticisms they may have to any member of the Committee. Such data will be analyzed and evaluated in the light of available controlled evidence. If the data is voluminous, another preliminary report would be forthcoming either at the semiannual meeting of the Executive Board in December or at the annual meeting in 1939.

Respectfully submitted,

JOHN A. TOOMEY, Chairman
HORTON CASPARIS
E. J. HUENEKENS
CHARLES MCKHANN
BÉLA SCHICK
EDWARD B. SHAW

Report of the Committee on Infantile Paralysis

The Committee on Infantile Paralysis has not held a meeting since its last report, since there seemed to be no particularly good reason for it. The chairman of the committee, however has been in contact with Mr. Basil O'Connor, the president of the new National Foundation for Infantile Paralysis. Certain advice was given which at this stage related only to the fact that this new committee should have an advisory medical council. The recommendations or, rather, suggestions, were made concerning the personnel of this advisory committee.

Last year it was suggested that this Committee on Infantile Paralysis of the Academy cease to function. At the present moment it is suggested that it might be well to continue this committee since possibly it may have some function in the next year or two.

Signed,

A. GRAEME MITCHELL, Chairman

Report of the Committee on Medical Education

Postgraduate Education.—Reports were received from all but three of the states in regard to extramural postgraduate courses in pediatrics. Questionnaires were sent to all state chairmen and to all directors of maternal and child health.

An outstanding feature was that during 1937 there was a marked increase in the active interest of state chairmen and of individual Academy members in this activity. Discussions accompanying the returned questionnaires evidence a greater understanding on the part of state chairmen not only of the objectives of such programs, but also of the difficulties encountered in the mechanics of organization of such courses and their bearing on the degree of success subsequently achieved.

Programs of outstanding accomplishment during the year were conducted in Iowa, Minnesota, Michigan, Wisconsin, Mississippi, Virginia, Massachusetts, and Texas. Many other states initiated programs during the year, and still others, recognizing the weaknesses in their technic of organization, are now making improved plans directed toward a more effective interest and attendance in the programs to be attempted in the future.

It is apparent from the brief experience at hand that no one type of plan will be universally successful. It is equally apparent that no matter how good the instructor, the course cannot succeed as well as it should unless there is the proper organization preceding it. At the moment the chief problems confronting those attempting to develop such extramural postgraduate courses lie not in the selection of proper instructors, or in the content of material given, but in the selection of the proper type of course for the locality to be served, satisfying therein as well as possible those variables which may work for or against the success of the course and which are of almost equal importance in the matter of the development of an increasingly more effective organization and build-up. The most common adverse comments encountered in the replies received would seem to be fairly well covered by the implications embodied in the suggested outline for organization, which was prepared and submitted to all directors of maternal and child health and to all state chairmen of the Academy. Much is yet to be learned, however, in regard to methods of organization.

During the year there was increasingly more utilization of such interest-increasing techniques as (1) personal consultations, (2) check lists for demonstrations of clinical and therapeutic procedures, (3) informal out of hour discussion, (4) talks to lay groups in attempts to advance the understanding of child health protection locally, and (5) better preliminary organization and build-up with proper regard to specific local characteristics, such as number of physicians in district served, season of year, geographic and economic characteristics of the community, etc.

There seems to be an increased tendency at least in some states to integrate the program with that of the extension department of a medical school or of a state university. This is probably a logical and constructive procedure. It is certainly true that many state medical society committees on postgraduate education are not active enough to put over properly the organization and preliminary build-up generally so essential to a proper development of such courses. Some committees have not sensed the specific needs for, and objectives of, these courses, while others because they are of necessity only volunteer part-time workers, cannot devote to the program and its development the time and effort so necessary to make it successful. There is a logical reason why such state or regional committees can be expected to serve effectively in an advisory capacity, but it is not so logical to expect them to provide the personnel so essential for visiting local physicians, explaining to them the objectives and nature of the course, obtaining enrollment in course, etc. These essential details of the executive administration must have proper treatment. It has been repeatedly observed that it takes more than personal letters from the president of the state society, the president of the local county society and the chairman of the local committee to provide a preliminary build-up. Programs that depend primarily upon such a foundation for their build-up will generally not be very successful. There is real need for a definite executive agency being integrated with the program. The state health department does not seem to be the agency most ideally suited to the best execution of this part of the program.

Throughout the questionnaires a significant statement appears with amazing regularity. It is to the effect that the local chairman is the keyman in the success of such a program. It is intimated repeatedly that rarely can a course have a successful attendance unless the local keyman does provide the proper build-up preceding the course and provide proper assistance throughout the conduct of the course. He is the one who has had to be responsible for getting the attendance and he is the one to bring the instructor and physicians attending the course ever more intimately together. Unfortunately it is not always possible to have good keymen. It is therefore desirable to work out a procedure that is not dependent upon a local leader to put it across successfully, at least the local man must not have to do it all.

For those interested in developing such courses or for those acting as instructors, the committee has on file an interesting collection of letters, outlines, and brochures. From this data at all times the chairman will be glad to supply, on request, such aid as Academy members may desire.

Respectfully submitted,

George M. Lyon, Chairman
Horton Casparis
Hugh L. Dwyer

Report of the Committee on Mental Hygiene

The Committee on Mental Hygiene feels that the mental growth and development of the child and all of the factors which influence it favorably or unfavorably are as much the responsibility of the pediatrician as is the physical growth and development and all the factors which influence it favorably or unfavorably. The pediatrician is the sole consultant of parents concerning physical and mental health problems during the preschool period and should continue as the chief consultant during the remainder of childhood and adolescence.

Medical schools and training centers have, in general, failed to provide adequate training in mental growth and development and mental hygiene problems of children for medical students or pediatric interns and residents. Less than 50 per cent of the medical schools give any instruction in pediatric psychiatry. Very few hospitals give the pediatric intern and resident an opportunity to study the subject. The pediatrician loses, thereby, a valuable stimulus for active interest in mental hygiene and its problems. The committee feels that it should be its function and the function of the Academy as a whole to stimulate more adequate training and a more active interest. The committee further feels that the responsibility for these activities rests first with the chiefs of the pediatric departments of the medical schools and children's hospitals and, second, with pediatricians as a whole.

The committee therefore recommends:

I. Adequate training in medical schools as follows:
   1. Instruction during the first two years in medical school to include lectures on mental health.
   2. A formal course on mental growth and development, the mental aspects of various disease conditions, and common mental hygiene problems during the last two years of medicine. The chairman of the Educational Committee of the National Committee for Mental Hygiene suggests that such a course should be at least twelve hours in length.
   3. The use of a well-baby clinic as a means of teaching mental health to children.
   4. A mental health clinic in the pediatric department.
   5. Cooperation between the pediatric and psychiatric departments.

II. Adequate training of the pediatric intern and resident as follows:
   1. An opportunity to work in a mental hygiene clinic during a part of his internship or residency.
   2. An opportunity to attend seminars conducted by staff men qualified to give them the proper attitude towards mental health.
   3. An opportunity to study mental health and development in well-baby and older children's clinics.

III. In order to stimulate a more active interest in mental hygiene among pediatricians and to bring to their attention the valuable information found in medical literature, other than pediatric journals, it is suggested that a program be worked out for publication, extending over a period of several years, dealing with pertinent facts on mental health. These articles are to be published in THE JOURNAL OF PEDIATRICS. The Committee is now working on that program.

The committee welcomes suggestions from all members of the Academy and feels that the support and cooperation of all members is essential to the successful carrying out of the above program.

Respectfully submitted,

BERT I. BEVERLY, Chairman
C. A. ALDRICH
FREDERICK H. ALLEN
HORTON CASPARIS
BRONSON CROTHERS
GEORGE MOHR
ARTHUR H. PARMELEE
VICTOR E. STORK

Report of the Committee on Nursing Education in Pediatrics

While there has been no meeting of the entire committee, the chairman and secretary of this committee have been in conference. There has been consultation with Miss Corinne Bancroft, who is a member of the committee on the child in nursing education of the National League of Nursing Education. At this meeting there was discussed the question of the minimum requirements of instruction necessary in graduate training of nurses in pediatrics. No final decision was reached, and it was felt that the committee needed additional information. It was decided to request Miss Bancroft to secure a complete report of the opinion of the committee on nursing education of the National League of Nursing Education and subsequent meetings would then be held to discuss this material.

It was also thought that further study should be made of the requirements in undergraduate courses for nurses in pediatrics. Material will be gathered for this study and a report made later.

Signed,

A. Graeme Mitchell, Chairman

Report of the Committee on Revision of the Pharmacopoeia

This committee has presented a prospectus for a book on pediatric therapeutics and likewise has recommended that the Academy ask for formal application for membership in the United States Pharmacopoeia and National Formulary Convention, to be held in 1940.

Respectfully submitted,

Isaac A. Abt, Chairman
William N. Bradley
Bernard Fantus
H. H. Perlman
Louis W. Sauer

Report of the Committee on School Health and School Health Education

During the past year two new organizations concerned with school health programs have been formed by a reorganization of three groups. In June, by a merger of the American Physical Education Association and the Section on Health and Physical Education of the National Education Association, the American Association for Health and Physical Education was organized. This association is a department of the National Education Association. In October the American Association of School Physicians adopted a new constitution and by-laws and became the American School Health Association.

The American Association for Health and Physical Education has a very large membership of physical educators and a smaller active group of health educators, and it aims to develop active sections in other special fields such as medical and nursing services. It would seem that this association has an important function to perform particularly with reference to informing teachers, principals, and school administrators as to the progress of school health program development and in coordinating the various physical education activities with the health education and medical and nursing service activities in the schools.

The American School Health Association is a smaller organization including most of the state and city directors of school health and many school physicians. Its new constitution admits dentists, nurses, public health workers, nutritionists, mental hygienists, and health educators on the same basis as physicians, but requires adequate training in the basic medical sciences for membership. Conducting its annual meeting and activities as it does in close collaboration with the American Public

Health Association, it has a particular responsibility for the development and maintenance of professional standards for personnel and service through the coordination of the many special groups concerned with the various aspects of school health programs for which they were especially trained.

There is such a variety of other organizations who are concerned with some special aspect of the health of the school child that it is apparent that some organization is needed to coordinate the special services of various contributors to school health program development. Such organizations as the National Society for the Prevention of Blindness, the American Association for the Hard of Hearing, the National Organization for Public Health Nursing, the National Tuberculosis Association, the National Committee for Mental Hygiene, the American Heart Association, the American Dental Association, the American Society for the Promotion of Dentistry for Children, and other national groups continually give stimulus in developing standards and promoting interest in these special services. The American School Health Association through its relations with the American Public Health Association provides the facilities for coordination of these special contributions for the use of state, city, county and other public health officials.

The committee of the American Academy of Pediatrics feels that at the present time its function should be the interpretation of the viewpoint of the pediatric profession to these various groups and bring to pediatricians some of the trends and activities of school health associations and the contributing special organizations.

In our last report we pointed out the tendency of school and other professional leaders to expect that the school examination can meet the whole need for health examination. To correct this tendency there is need for our best pediatric leadership, and physicians who appreciate the importance of continued medical supervision of children must counteract such unsound trends. Your committee has had representatives attend meetings of the various national groups who influence school health program policies and have discussed this problem. The section, "Principles," in the last report of your committee was presented to the Committee on School Health of the Child Hygiene Section of the American Public Health Association and given such approval that it was incorporated in the report of the committee and published in the year book of the American Public Health Association with credit to your committee. We believe that many individual members of the Academy can influence school health program policy through the facilities of organized medicine in their community, through membership on boards of education and health, and through the organization of medical advisory councils for school programs. The following discussion is presented as a further indication of trends which our members can influence through community activity.

The emphasis upon periodic health examinations by the medical profession has, no doubt, had its influence in developing this excessive reliance upon the school medical service. A false sense of security from school examinations has resulted from a lack of sufficient medical guidance of the program. Too often physicians have been employed by school and health authorities merely to make examinations rather than to interpret the child's need and to act as medical advisors to the school authorities. The nonmedical professional leaders have accepted the health examination as important, but they have not recognized their own inability to judge the limitations of the service nor the possibilities of more adequate health supervision. They have not understood that the health examination "is not an isolated event purchasable wholesale in mechanized ways, it is important but only incidental to a well-rounded service of preventive medical care through life."

We may expect that school authorities will not develop an educational program that will protect the public against excessive reliance upon school examinations until we have given proper emphasis to the reasons for examinations by private physicians. The people who can afford health supervision by their own pediatrician certainly should have more education along this line through the schools. The New Jersey Fellows have prepared for distribution to parents a leaflet, ''A Study of the Minimum Desirable Standards for the Health Supervision and Care of Infants and Children,'' in which the frequency of health supervision visits for various age groups is considered. The average medical practitioner must recognize too the need for more thorough attention to health advice and educational procedure for those who do come to him for a health examination.

Another trend in schools that should be appreciated by the medical profession is the greater number of schools which give more time to the routine examination and who invite parents to attend the examination. As the rapid march-by inspections are replaced by more careful examinations in schools, the need becomes greater for education of the public regarding continued health supervision. The better the school service the more difficult it is for the school authorities and the public to interpret properly the limitations of the service and the advantage of personal or private preventive medicine. This tendency, no doubt, has led to some unwarranted fear on the part of a few practitioners that the schools would take over personal preventive health service and leave no opportunity for the development of this service by the private practitioner.

It must be recognized that it is natural for school authorities to want the public to appreciate the service provided through the school budget or through the cooperation of the education department, and so they themselves are likely to believe the service in their school is more adequate and complete than it is. It is not surprising that they should have a tendency to interpret the school medical service as offering more than is possible without any intent to exaggerate the value of the school service.

A proper evaluation of both school and private services is also made more difficult when no attempt is made to define the limitations of each particular school service to the educational authorities and to the public. Physicians have accepted the responsibility of examining large numbers of children in school without clearly differentiating the difference between such mass examinations and a private office service. We should recognize that private office health examinations have too often not met our best standards. So it is apparent that organized medicine must through advisory committees and through assistance on school problems gain sufficient influence that the limitations of the school service may be understood by the school authorities. The schools must in turn interpret the service properly to the public.

School authorities generally recognize the importance of education for proper attitudes and so may be led to understand the importance of educating both children and parents to want the kind of individualized service that is possible when the physician continues supervision over a period of time. No doubt the educator will thus appreciate the importance of the highest standards of continued service when he has had the service explained in connection with the care of his own children.

Of course, the problem will not be solved by limitations put upon the school service. More thorough study of each child by the school physician is essential for improving the advice given to teachers and parents in an educational program. In fact, an educational program by the school physician should provide no competition with a private office service. The physician who meets the parent in school can guide in the use of community medical resources, he can advise parents who might try unwisely to save on doctor's bills; he can increase the demand for preventive medicine; and he can point out the need for care of trivial ailments and the risk of ignoring the early signs of ill health. If the fundamental purpose of the service of the nurse and physician in the schools is to be education, we shall not restrict this educational program.

We should make clear that the physician can be more than an examiner in the schools. A school medical advisor can bring the contributions of the private practitioner to apply to the individual needs of his patient for guidance in the classroom. He can guide the teachers in training school children for improved attitudes about medical service. A medical advisor is needed to interpret the health education needs of pupils and parents to the teachers. The unreasonable fear of surgery, the superstitious belief in drugstore medication, the seeking for panaceas, the use of the physician as a last resort, and the failure to return to the physician when clinical study and diagnosis are needed are some of the common attitudes which every physician recognizes as neglected aspects of education. We should make clear to the school authorities and the public that more time could be used by the physician in the school without extending his service to those health examinations that could be more effective as a part of continued supervision by private physicians.

The summer round-up program of the National Congress of Parents and Teachers is an example of the critical situation needing organized pediatric guidance to determine future policies. Every physician is familiar with the round-up of children into a clinic by Parent-Teachers' Association members and the rapid file of children before a charitably minded physician who wished to help the mothers by looking for physical defects before school opens. One physician after another has become disgusted with the excessive demands for looking over large groups of children, but other physicians have taken their places. The Round-up was regarded as a demonstration, but after years of demonstration an advisory committee made up of experienced public health workers has advised the National Congress that the emphasis should be first upon immunization and then upon consultation with the private physician rather than an isolated wholesale procedure for finding deviations from a supposed normal child.

In many places this service has now been taken over by the school or as a part of the school medical service. It is not easy to turn the service back to the private physicians even if they are willing to give examinations in their private offices at reduced rates or free to the indigent.

The leadership in the National Congress of Parents and Teachers is urging local Parent-Teachers' Associations to seek and follow the advice of organized medicine. Parents need education as to the value of continued health supervision. Many local Parent-Teachers' Associations want guidance in modifying their summer round-up program. We should provide further leadership to use interest for sound public education.

Respectfully submitted,

Harold H. Mitchell, Chairman
Rockwell M. Kempton
Arthur E. Wade
M. Hines Roberts
Estella F. Warner
A. Clement Silverman
LeRoy A. Wilkes
Clifford D. Sweet

Report of the Council for Pediatric Research

The council opened its office a little over a year ago. Its first aims were to acquire information regarding research facilities and activities in clinics and laboratories throughout the country and to get in touch with possible donors of research funds, and acquaint them with the reason for the council's formation, its organization, and its proposed activities.

Information regarding laboratories and clinics has been gathered partly by personal visits of the secretary and partly by means of a questionnaire sent to quite a large list of institutions. By these means a fairly complete index has been built up of laboratories and clinics engaging in research bearing on pediatrics, their personnel and equipment, resources, special research interests, and investigations now in progress. This index will be amplified by other personal visits as opportunity arises. The secretary is aware that any such method of collecting data will miss some more or less independent investigators and would be glad to hear from any who have not been reached.

Contact with possible donors has been sought, both by letter and by personal visit to organizations known or supposed to be interested in subsidizing investigation. A complete list of such organizations is hardly possible, but various means have been used to reach at least the most likely prospects. Many contacts have been made; a number of commercial firms have sent representatives to the council's office to inquire into its purposes and methods, while others have expressed by letter sympathy with our ideas. Almost without exception the expressions of such organizations have been favorable.

These contacts with representatives of manufacturing firms have given the council a good deal of information regarding the problems with which it is attempting to deal. An obvious fact is that uncertainty regarding business conditions is very definitely limiting expenditures on research projects. This was to be expected. An apparent fear on the part of some less informed houses that the council may turn out to be "just another racket" is perhaps not surprising, but will probably be allayed in time. Two conditions of which we were aware will limit the possible scope of our activities. One of these is the fact that several of the larger houses have supervisors of research, quite capable of placing their research grants under most circumstances and having little need of the council's help. Another is the practice of making good-will grants on solicitation by clinics and laboratories. This is a nuisance to the manufacturers, but hard to check. The council may hope to have some effect on it in time and to divert some of this money to better purposes. There is also some evidence of what might be designated tacit opposition to the council on the part of investigators who seem to feel that they will have a better chance of obtaining large grants if they can deal directly with the grantors rather than through the mediation of the council. The council has no wish to interfere with established relationships between investigators and donors and sees no reason for this feeling.

Actually, we are just beginning to have definite projects brought to us which will probably result in research grants of some importance. Several of these are now in hand which we expect to handle successfully. Our experience has shown that, if we are to make a satisfactory showing during the two years of the grant from the Carnegie Corporation, we shall need assistance from Fellows of the Academy and others interested in what we are trying to do, in referring possible donors to us until we are better known. It is in this way that our best contacts have been made. It would seem that some commercial organizations need assurance of the disinterestedness and good faith of the council from their personal acquaintances in the profession.

In addition to its activities regarding the allocation of funds for research, the council is seeing some indications of other possible service within its scope. A number of the foundations have shown interest in our project from the start, and some of them have shown a desire to make use of the information we have been gathering which no one else seems to have. We have been approached also as to the possibility of our taking an active part in the direction of one quite ambitious long-term study, which if carried through, should be of considerable importance.

We have not yet had opportunity to make use of our information for the purpose, which seems very desirable, of coordinating research in certain fields, and helping to eliminate waste motion and duplication, which we have reason to know exists to a considerable extent.

Altogether, while we have not had such prompt success as we might have hoped, we feel that our idea is sound and that we shall have an increasing demand for our services. In the meantime, we may be said to be acquiring a technique in a rather difficult field.

Respectfully submitted,

THOMAS B. COOLEY, Executive Secretary

No reports have been made by the following committees:

Committee on Cooperation With Medical Groups and Societies

Committee on Legislation

(No matters have been referred to the above two committees during the past year.)

Committee on Neonatal Morbidity and Mortality

(Owing to the death of the chairman and reorganization of this committee, there is no report.)

SEVENTH ANNUAL MEETING OF THE AMERICAN ACADEMY OF PEDIATRICS

NEW YORK, N. Y., JUNE 3-5, 1937

Round Table Discussion on Anemia of the Newborn

Dr. Hugh Josephs, Baltimore, Md., Chairman
Dr. Thomas B. Cooley, Detroit, Mich.
Dr. Louis K. Diamond, Boston, Mass.

CHAIRMAN JOSEPHS.—Our present conception of anemia of the newborn is a merging of several lines of observation. First, there is the pathologic term ''erythroblastosis fetalis'' first applied to cases of hydrops and for long confined to pathologic literature, scarcely more than an obstetric curiosity. Second, there was ''icterus gravis'' long used for certain severe and usually fatal cases of jaundice and recognized as frequently occurring in successive pregnancies. Tissue erythroblastosis was described in cases of icterus gravis about 1916. Following this there developed a gradual realization that icterus gravis with erythroblastosis was closely related to hydrops of the newborn with erythroblastosis. Third, ''anemia of the newborn'' developed quite independently following Ecklen's description of a case in 1919, though ten years earlier Buchan and Comrie had described the condition. Both these reports describe easily recognizable cases of what is now called ''erythroblastosis fetalis,'' the condition that will form the principal topic of discussion today. Many of the cases reported as anemia of the newborn belong to this group, but the relationship to icterus gravis and erythroblastosis was unrecognized until 1931.

The first source of confusion then is in nomenclature: ''erythroblastosis,'' a term used to describe a pathologic picture also used to designate a disease entity;

"icterus gravis," a descriptive term used also as the name of a disease; "anemia of the newborn," another descriptive term, the vaguest of all, employed as if all the cases to which it could be applied belonged together.

These three terms are often used as if they meant the same thing; herein lies a second source of confusion, for they are not absolutely synonymous. As has been pointed out, icterus gravis, a purely descriptive term, is used as if it designated a disease. Erythroblastosis is, however, only one of the conditions associated with icterus gravis although probably the most common, especially in familial cases. Severe icterus may result from sepsis and severe liver damage of unknown cause, which may sometimes be familial. Anemia and some degree of erythroblastosis may occur in these cases, and it is sometimes difficult to decide where to classify a case.

Similarly there are many cases of anemia of the newborn which clearly do not belong to the erythroblastosis group, and there are others without erythroblastosis but with increased hemolysis; thus one may be in doubt as to how to consider them.

A third source of error arises from the fact that the distinction between normal and pathologic is not as sharply defined as we should like to have it. There is scarcely a thing that is considered characteristic of anemia of the newborn with icterus gravis and erythroblastosis that does not occur normally. The difference is rather quantitative than qualitative. Erythroblastosis is often present at birth normally and occasionally the numbers may increase to what is usually considered pathologic. The difficulty of distinguishing icterus gravis from physiologic icterus is, of course, well known; the speed with which the red cell count and the hemoglobin content fall after birth may vary within wide limits, and not a few cases of so-called anemia of the newborn may be considered an exaggeration of the normal with quite as much reason as something essentially pathologic.

Out of all this confusion there has been separated a group of cases in which the symptom pattern is repeated over and over again and which has received the name "erythroblastosis fetalis." We call this condition an entity and talk of it as a disease because the clinical course and the histologic picture are similar, but we have no reason to assume that the process giving rise to the clinical and pathologic picture is the same in all cases. It is of course well known that syphilis and sepsis may reproduce the picture of erythroblastosis fetalis in all details. What we call erythroblastosis fetalis is what remains after the cases with syphilis and sepsis have been excluded. The exclusion of cases for which some explanation has been found is no more than a convenience leading to the grouping of cases that still await explanation but unfortunately has led to the labeling of the unexplained cases as "primary." The tendency to consider a pathologic end result as a disease is an important source of confusion. This point will be considered more fully in the discussion of etiology.

In the discussion that follows, it will be convenient to treat "erythroblastosis fetalis" as a disease entity. It must be remembered, however, that we know little of the essential nature of the condition, i.e., of the processes which give rise to the pathologic changes or the etiological factors that influence these processes.

DR. DIAMOND.—The following discussion of the clinical aspects of anemia of the newborn is based upon personal experience with 80 cases of erythroblastosis fetalis, 35 cases of sepsis in the neonatal period of life, resulting in anemia, 4 cases of anemia without jaundice or erythroblastosis (that is, of the aplastic type) and a large but uncounted number of cases of anemia developing later in the newborn period.

To dispose first of the better known types of anemia in the newborn, that is, the last three mentioned above:

1. Anemia developing later in the newborn period, by which we mean after the third month of life, is fairly common and has been relatively well studied. The

chief causative factors are, first and foremost, infection; second, prematurity and multiple births; third, dietary deficiency in either the mother or her offspring; and fourth, congenital malformations of the gastrointestinal tract and other systems of the body. We may forego discussion of anemia due to these factors since they are relatively well understood.

2. Anemia without jaundice or erythroblastosis, and incidentally without splenomegaly or hepatomegaly, that is, an aplastic type of anemia, is the least common of the blood disturbances of this age group. Of the four cases seen by us, three were in infants who had an aplastic bone marrow, proved by biopsy, and who required regular transfusions for the preservation of a blood level consistent with life. They first showed evidence of deficiency in hematopoiesis in the third to fourth month after birth. None of them was anemic at, or immediately after, birth. These three infants have been kept alive now for a period varying between one and five years, by means of transfusions given every two months and have shown no tendency to improve. The fourth infant in this group had a malignant hemangioendothelioma invading the bone marrow and causing an aplastic anemia.

3. Anemia due to sepsis and infection is also fairly common in the newborn infant. This factor therefore should always be excluded before the diagnosis of erythroblastosis or of aplastic anemia is accepted. Congenital syphilis is very likely to resemble the symptom complex which has been designated erythroblastosis fetalis. We have seen eight infants who at birth showed jaundice which increased in severity later, marked splenomegaly and hepatomegaly, increasing anemia through the neonatal period, and tremendous numbers of immature erythrocytes and leucocytes. Roentgenograms, blood serology tests, and in a few instances post-mortem examination of the tissues, established the diagnosis of congenital syphilis as the cause of these abnormal findings. Since specific treatment, as well as transfusion, was indicated in such cases, it was highly important that this specific disease be considered when the symptoms grouped above appeared in the newborn infant. Of the less well-known infectious agents colon bacillus not infrequently causes severe anemia, enlargement of the liver and spleen, and anemia in the newborn. We have seen two instances of acute pyelonephritis with colon bacillus bacteremia and jaundice and anemia, ending fatally in the first week of life. On the other hand, nine such patients have recovered following the usual supportive measures, including transfusion. Streptococcus or staphylococcus omphalitis, peritonitis, and pneumonia have accounted for the remainder of the cases in this group, except two cases of malaria occurring in the second month of life in infants who had hemorrhagic disease of the newborn and had been transfused with blood from parents suffering from latent chronic malaria.

To turn finally to the symptom complex known as erythroblastosis fetalis: This gained increasing attention recently because it is a relatively new disease in point of view of general medical interest. Also, increasing numbers of cases are being recognized which have been previously overlooked or erroneously diagnosed. Finally, with improvement in diagnostic ability there has been a satisfactory decrease in the mortality, as earlier and more vigorous therapy has been adopted.

We have listed for discussion under this heading, universal edema of the fetus, familial icterus gravis, erythroblastosis fetalis as described by Schridde (that is, from the pathologists' viewpoint), and anemia of the newborn. The question arises immediately, Are these manifestations of a single disease process, and if so, why is there so much disagreement concerning this point? I firmly believe that if every physician who sees such cases could play the role of the family doctor and see the mother of the child during her period of gestation, know her history well, attend the delivery, and make observations in regard to the infant immediately after birth, as well as the placenta accompanying it, and then follow the blood changes as well as the changes in the tissues of the fatal cases, there would not be any question as to the identity of these symptom complexes. The difficulty has been that each specialist, that is, the obstetrician, the pathologist, and the pediatrician, has described that portion of the disease which has happened to come to his particular attention. The obstetrician has described the cases of universal edema of the fetus and familial icterus gravis with death in the first few days of life; the pathologist, the tissues of the stillborn infant with edema or of the infant with familial icterus gravis. The pediatrician, who usually does not see these two types of cases in the early stages and who rarely has the opportunity to examine the tissues in such cases, describes the later stages of the condition, when the anemia may be the most important symptom and the jaundice be either stationary or fading.

In our 80 cases we have been fortunate in having the cooperation of the obstetrical department under the supervision of Dr. Irving at the Boston Lying-in Hospital, of the pathology department under Dr. Wolbach, Dr. Farber, and Dr. Hertig, and of the pediatrics department under Dr. Blackfan and under Dr. Clifford at the Lying-in Hospital. Our observations, therefore, are a composite, not only of the opinions of all these individuals, but of the material available from before birth, through delivery, and into the neonatal life of the infant.

The typical picture of erythroblastosis fetalis in the moderately severe form may be as follows: In about one case out of three the mother may give a story of previous pregnancies ending in the birth of stillborn infants or infants dying with jaundice shortly after birth. In such cases an interesting corollary is the mother's story that fetal movements become lethargic and may even cease entirely in the last few days before delivery. At birth jaundice in the skin of the infant and occasionally a yellow orange hue to the vernix caseosa covering the infant may be noted. Also occasionally the placenta is enlarged one and one-half to two times the normal size. There may be a slight to moderate amount of edema demonstrable in the child's subcutaneous tissues. The liver and the spleen are both moderately enlarged. Occasionally petechiae appear spontaneously, and ecchymoses and free bleeding in the first few days may suggest hemorrhagic disease. The cord blood or blood from the capillary bed may show 50 to 100,000 or more nucleated erythrocytes. Anemia, though sometimes present at birth, more usually first appears in the first twenty-four hours after birth and becomes progressively more severe thereafter. In general, the slower this anemia in its appearance and development, the better the outlook, since such cases are relatively milder, with less jaundice, no edema, no petechiae, and fewer erythroblasts in the peripheral blood.

The milder types of this disturbance frequently escape notice during the first few days after birth and sometimes even during the first few weeks. Since icterus in such cases is either so mild and transitory that it passes for the ordinary icterus neonatorum and since blood examination for nucleated erythrocytes is not necessitated by the appearance of any other symptoms of the condition, the first sign of the disturbance may be the residual anemia which is present in all infants with the disturbance and which shows itself by a progressive pallor of the skin and mucous membranes. If a blood examination is not performed until the second or third week of life, there may be very few immature erythrocytes and merely an aplastic type of anemia.

A discussion as to pathogenesis and etiology is purposely avoided here. It is hoped, however, that the objective signs and symptoms which have been observed not only in these 80 cases but in the large number described in the literature will be explained by the later discussion. As a basis for this, certain other findings made in our personal contact with this disease will now be enlarged upon, and the obvious questions arising from this will be answered as far as possible.

As regards the inheritance of this condition, very little can be said until further studies like the recent one by Macklin have been made. I should like to call attention to the paper now in press by Hellman and Hertig on the subject of erythroblastosis as seen at the Boston Lying-In Hospital. Here an excellent discussion of the hereditary factor is given. In our own cases 35 per cent showed a positive family history. In general it may be said that a woman may have a child with erythroblastosis and yet have subsequent pregnancies result in normal children. However, after the birth of an infant with universal edema, the chances are better than 50 per cent for the recurrence of this abnormality. After the birth of two or more children with erythroblastosis and severe jaundice, the chances are better than 70 per cent for the recurrence. In such cases sterilization may be considered advisable.

The disappearance of erythroblasts from the peripheral blood is often very rapid. We have seen the number drop from 100,000 per cubic millimeter to 20,000 at the end of twenty-four hours and less than 1,000 at the end of forty-eight hours. With transfusion this disappearance may be even more rapid, so that following one transfusion no erythroblasts may be found.

The degree of icterus which develops in any given case is probably the result of several factors: the functional capacity of the liver to excrete bilirubin, the rapidity of destruction of abnormal cells, as well as the number of these cells. Therefore in an infant with a relatively mild degree of the condition in which the numbers of abnormal cells are not too great, their destruction not too rapid, and the functional capacity of the liver, which is notoriously poor at the time of birth, not too inefficient, no great degree of jaundice, that is, not much more than the normal child usually shows, need appear. However, on the basis of relatively few examinations in these milder cases it is our feeling that every case of erythroblastosis has an increase above normal in the bilirubin content of the blood. The hemorrhagic tendency has been found only in the severely affected patients, as those with universal edema and early and severe icterus gravis. In these cases it is associated not only with the prolongation of the bleeding and clotting times but also with lowered platelet count and pathologically with thrombi of nucleated red cells in the final capillaries. Anemia has been found in every case seen by us. It may vary from a level just below 3,000,000 per cubic millimeter to one less than 1,000,000. Although the anemia may not show itself in the first twenty-four hours, we should deny the possibility of a state of typical erythroblastosis existing with no anemia at any time. Some other cause for the erythroblastosis must be sought in such instances.

The cause of early death in the severe cases cannot be definitely stated at present. At post-mortem examination any one or a combination of the following may be blamed for it: free bleeding into the central nervous system and into the various cavities of the body; petechial hemorrhage in the brain due to thrombi of nucleated erythrocytes; extreme jaundice with toxemia, staining of the nuclei in the brain, and terminal convulsions; dilatation of the chambers of the heart and evidence of congestive heart failure; and anoxemia due to rapid development of severe anemia. Undoubtedly combinations of these are responsible for the early fatal cases rather than any one cause alone. As to the cause of death in the late cases, that is in patients dying after the first week of life, anoxemia due to profound anemia untreated by transfusion is the chief cause. Convulsions due to kernicterus may occur during the second and third weeks and may lead to death. Also intercurrent infection such as that produced by the colon bacillus in debilitated newborn infants or by any other pathogenic organism may occur at this time.

Spontaneous recovery probably occurs much more frequently than we realize, particularly in the group of infants who show no edema and very little jaundice in the first few days of life and who therefore are not suspected of having the disturbance. Recently by following the blood changes in offspring from families in which other cases have occurred, we have seen examples of the milder forms of erythroblastosis with a tendency to spontaneous recovery or at least an early recovery with only a single transfusion.

Kernicterus was the unfortunate result in 5 of our 60 living children. Each of these had had very severe jaundice shortly after birth and although the profound anemia which developed responded to treatment by transfusion, this unfortunate residual complication existed after the child's blood had returned to normal. Spasticity and imbecility were the final results in all of them. My knowledge of the reason for the nuclear damage or staining, or both, is too incomplete to permit of any conclusions in regard to kernicterus.

As regards treatment, it is our feeling that transfusion with matched whole blood, given directly into a vein, is most satisfactory at present. Theoretically and on the basis of a few cases reported in the literature, blood serum or blood plasma, again best given intravenously, may be of some assistance. But since, as we have stated, anemia exists in every case, the erythrocytes can do little harm and may be of great value when put into the circulation of the child with erythroblastosis. Transfusion should be repeated as frequently as necessary to control the anoxemia due to profound anemia and also for its beneficial effect in controlling the hemolytic tendency evidenced by increasing icterus and lethargy. In the milder cases a single transfusion may be sufficient to tide the patient over the period of hemolysis as well as the period of functional aplasia which follows this. However, in the more severe cases as many as 15 or more transfusions have been given before recovery has occurred. A word of warning here: It is not necessary to keep the blood level up to 4 or 5 millions per cubic millimeter by repeated transfusions. A level of 2,500,000 to 3,000,000 has usually been found satisfactory to carry on all the functions of the body as evidenced by good appetite and gain in weight. Too frequent transfusion may not only increase the hemolytic tendency unnecessarily, but also may prolong the period of functional aplasia of the bone marrow. We have noted this in a few of our earlier cases. It is our feeling that the disease tends to run a self-limited course with spontaneous recovery at the end of this and that transfusion is necessary to tide the patient over the period of abnormal blood production and destruction.

We have insufficient evidence at present to settle the question as to whether kernicterus is a less frequent complication in the cases so treated but certainly it is not more frequent due to our method of repeated transfusions.

Although there seems to be some evidence for the fact that following transfusion there may be an increase in hemolysis when previously it had seemed to be subsiding, transfusions cannot safely be omitted in the face of anoxemia due to severe anemia. One therefore has to steer a medium course as to the frequency of transfusion and amount of infused blood so that on the one hand hemolysis is not accelerated and on the other, dangerous anemia does not occur.

The theory has been offered that erythroblastosis fetalis, which shows so strikingly a macrocytosis in the first few days of life, is an infantile form of pernicious anemia and should therefore respond to treatment with liver extract. Such a theory, however, is not borne out by our observations and our trial with liver extract in large amounts both orally and parenterally. Splenectomy may offer a means of reducing the hemolytic tendency. However, the operation is fraught with so many dangers in the newborn infant as to render it unfeasible in the very case in which it is needed the most, that is the one- or two-day-old infant with severe icterus, anemia, and cardiac enlargement. Blood or blood serum intramuscularly may have some beneficial effect, but the need for blood is usually so urgent that waiting for its absorption from the tissue spaces is often hazardous. Iron in the form of small amounts of iron sulfate has seemed to benefit some of our patients late in the course of spontaneous recovery, when beginning cell regeneration appears. However, it is inadvisable to burden the infant's gastrointestinal tract with extra medication earlier in the course of the disease.

Finally, our conclusions as to the advisability of transfusion at properly spaced intervals in cases of erythroblastosis fetalis are based upon our accumulating statistical data. Excluding the infants with universal edema, all of whom have either been born dead or have died within the first few hours of life, our mortality rate during the first three years of our study was 33⅓ per cent, during the next three years 20 per cent, and during the last three years, 7 per cent.

DR. S. H. CLIFFORD (BROOKLINE, MASS.).—At the Boston Lying-in Hospital every baby born with yellow vernix is suspected of having erythroblastosis and is referred immediately to the Pediatric Service. In our experience only a small proportion of the babies with this so-called yellow vernix have actually been proved to have erythroblastosis. The most frequent cause of this staining has been found to be intrauterine asphyxia with the passing of meconium in utero which material stains the vernix and produces this color. I was of the opinion for a considerable period that by investigating the protective folds of the newborn, such as deep in the axilla, or in the folds of the groin, or in the region of the labia minora, or by retracting the prepuce on the boy babies, one could make the differential diagnosis between the yellow vernix of erythroblastosis and the staining due to some other factor. In other words, I felt that in erythroblastosis the yellow stain would penetrate to these areas, whereas, in meconium staining for instance, the vernix would still be white in the protected spots. I have since discovered that this assumption is not correct and I have recently seen a typical case of erythroblastosis with icterus gravus in which the vernix in the protected area was pure white while over the body it was golden yellow.

We are frequently confronted with the practical question as to whether a mother once having had an erythroblastic baby should necessarily avoid future pregnancy. When a given mother has had several babies with erythroblastosis, future pregnancies have been discouraged. When there have been other normal babies or when the baby with erythroblastosis occurs at the first pregnancy, the parents are advised that they have a greater chance of having an erythroblastic baby than a normal family, but, if they desire more children, they are encouraged to proceed. The reason for this is that, even though a second erythroblastic baby is born, the chances are all in favor of its not having a fatal hydrops type of the disease, and with immediate diagnosis and treatment, the prognosis should be favorable.

There remains a great deal to be done in the field of the congenital anemias. We are convinced that certain babies with congenital anemia are typical examples of erythroblastosis; yet there are other babies in whom this diagnosis is not tenable. We have seen several newborn babies with congenital anemia whose mothers have premature separation of the placenta or placenta previa, and we suspect that the separation of the placenta involved the fetal villi as well as the maternal and resulted in loss of fetal as well as maternal blood. This point has not as yet been proved.

CHAIRMAN JOSEPHS.—The incidence of the disease is of interest because of the discrepancy in numbers in the different cities, there being more cases reported in some sections than in others.

DR. DIAMOND.—I believe that the families become interested. The question of inheritance is not fixed.

CHAIRMAN JOSEPHS.—When the children recover, does the condition tend to recur?

DR. DIAMOND.—We have several patients who are now six to nine years old who are in good health. We have never known of a recurrence.

CHAIRMAN JOSEPHS.—What about the question of sterilization of the mother?

DR. DIAMOND.—We have two cases in which sterilization was recommended because in each succeeding child the condition was worse.

DR. H. M. GREENWALD (BROOKLYN, N. Y.).—I had an infant recently suffering from anemia of the newborn. Repeated transfusions and the administration of iron failed to bring about an increase either in the hemoglobin content or in the number of red blood cells. A hematocrit study showed the presence of a macrocytic anemia. Liver extract was given by injection and immediate improvement occurred. This was evident by an immediate and sharp rise in the hemoglobin content and in the number of red blood cells.

CHAIRMAN JOSEPHS.—How old was the infant when the treatment was started? What preparation did you use?

DR. GREENWALD.—Five to six weeks. A liver extract prepared by Lilly was used intravenously.

DR. DIAMOND.—We have used liver extract early in a few cases without success.

DR. C. H. SMITH (NEW YORK CITY).—We have had two cases in our hospital with no regeneration following transfusions and iron therapy. Liver extract was given orally and intravenously, and the children recovered.

DR. GREENWALD.—Hampson has used the injection of serum rather than whole blood in the treatment of icterus gravis neonatorum with excellent results. He believes that an antihemolytic substance which is probably absent in these cases is supplied when the parent's serum is injected and that this is responsible for the improvement. My own experience and the experience of others do not bear out the work of Hampson.

DR. COOLEY.—There may be a deficiency. When we use liver, we use the whole extract, and we feel that we get better results than with the P.A. extract.

DR. H. D. PASACHOFF (NEW YORK, N. Y.).—Dr. Diamond mentioned that erythroblastosis disappears early. In 1931 Dr. Leo Wilson and I reported a case of congenital anemia of the newborn, fatal on the fifth day, in which erythroblastosis was absent in the circulating blood. Post-mortem examination failed to show erythroblastosis. Two subsequent pregnancies in the same mother, both of which resulted in premature stillborn infants with universal edema, gave additional support to our diagnosis. There was no evidence of abnormal erythroblastic activity in these cases. We regard erythroblastemia as a secondary response to the anemia rather than as the underlying pathology in congenital anemia of the newborn.

DR. H. S. ALTMAN (NEW YORK, N. Y.).—Is there any advantage in giving transfusion to mothers of potential cases of erythroblastosis prior to the birth of the baby?

DR. PASACHOFF.—I would like to ask about your experience in prophylaxis in newborn infants by treating the mother. In one instance in which the mother was treated, her baby was normal; her three previous children had erythroblastosis. It may be a coincidence. I would like to ask Dr. Diamond how to explain an erythroblastemia at the time of recovery.

DR. DIAMOND.—Instances are on record in which whole liver extract has been given to these mothers, the birth of normal babies resulting. When the extract was stopped, subsequent pregnancies resulted in the birth of children with erythroblastosis; this is unconfirmed, however.

DR. COOLEY.—How great was the erythroblastosis at the time?

DR. PASACHOFF.—I had a case of a negro infant who showed a hemoglobin of 38 per cent on the eighth day of life, with one normoblast per 100 white cells counted. At twenty days the striking feature was the very marked evidence of regenerative activity present in the blood smear. There were 50 nucleated red cells per 100 white cells. We have had a number of such cases of congenital anemia of the newborn in which the erythroblasts in the circulating blood were few in number at the time of the most severe anemia, and with a considerable increase in their number at the time of recovery. The occurrence of this erythroblastemia late in the disease seems to corroborate the theory that erythroblastosis is a secondary feature rather than the basic disorder in this group of diseases.

DR. COOLEY.—I think the increase in erythroblasts may be due to a decrease in destruction.

DR. R. M. TYSON (PHILADELPHIA, PA.).—Are we to regard the extramedullary hematopoietic centers as cause or effect?

CHAIRMAN JOSEPHS.—This introduces a subject which is responsible for much argument, namely the mechanism of erythroblastosis. One group holds that the condition is essentially hemolytic and the erythroblastosis a response to the increased need. Opposed to this is the idea that the condition is essentially a disturbance in erythropoiesis and that hemolysis is a secondary phenomenon. Undoubtedly both hemolysis and erythropoietic disturbance are present more or less independently, and it is not unlikely that variations in their relative preponderance, as well as their varying duration, may go far toward explaining variations in the picture as well as apparent exceptions. I have no doubt that the erythroblastosis of the first few days is largely dependent on disturbance in erythropoiesis at least in the majority of cases. This disturbance, however, usually subsides relatively rapidly, and with it the majority of nucleated red cells in the blood. The hemolytic process is much slower to disappear, and it is not at all unlikely that the persistence of nucleated red cells may depend largely on the persistence of an increased need. At the time of beginning recovery there is often a moderate rise in the number of nucleated red cells accompanying a rise in reticulocytes—fairly clear evidence that now the erythroblasts are due to an increase in erythropoietic activity that heralds a return to normal. Why the rise in nucleated red cells at this time in Pasachoff's case should have been so much greater than usual I do not believe one can say. It seems likely enough that there may have been some residue of erythropoietic disturbance. This is, however, no more than a guess. The problem is too complex to admit of satisfactory discussion at the present time, but it is just such exceptions that Passachoff has brought forward that may lead to a better understanding.

DR. GREENWALD.—In answer to the question, "What is the earliest age at which a case of Cooley's anemia has been observed?" I may say this: It is quite likely that Cooley's anemia is not only a familial, but also a congenital disease; but the signs and symptoms of the disease cannot always be recognized until the child attains the age of five or six months. The following case may prove an exception. I have now on my service an infant who was born with a harelip and a cleft palate whose older brother and cousin died of Cooley's anemia. This infant was not icteric at any time. At two weeks of age a severe anemia and an enlargement of the liver and spleen were observed; the spleen and liver could be felt four fingerbreadths below the costal margin. The hemoglobin content at that time was 45 per cent and the red blood count was 2,000,000 with 21 per cent erythroblasts and 14 per cent reticulocytes. This anemia and the enlargement of the liver and spleen have persisted in spite of the usual treatment with liver, iron, and transfusions. The number of erythroblasts has decreased from time to time but they are never entirely absent. The reticulocyte count has been consistently high. Repeated roentgenologic examination of the long bones and the skull have failed to show the changes characteristic of Cooley's anemia. Of course, the question arises, Is this an anemia of the newborn of the erythroblastotic type, or is this an early case of Cooley's anemia? This is a difficult question to answer at this time in view of the negative roentgenologic findings, but the familial history leads me to suspect that this may be an early case of Cooley's anemia.

DR. DIAMOND.—We have a family now with three children with Mediterranean anemia; the youngest, who was followed from birth, first showed blood changes typical of this condition at two months of age.

DR. COOLEY.—What causes kernicterus fetalis?

DR. DIAMOND.—Either primary damage to the brain nucleus followed by staining or vice versa. In patients who die with kernicterus there is increased liver damage. No definite information is available at present to explain the exact cause of kernicterus.

DR. J. M. LEWIS (NEW YORK, N. Y.).—Is kernicterus ever found in conditions other than icterus gravis?

DR. DIAMOND.—Cases of congenital obstruction of the bile duct have been studied at necropsy, and no evidence of kernicterus was found. Kernicterus may be found in Wilson's disease. One case of sepsis resulted in kernicterus.

CHAIRMAN JOSEPHS.—We could find in literature no report of cases of kernicterus occurring in conditions other than icterus gravis.

DR. COOLEY.—We have noted a report of kernicterus in a case of acute yellow atrophy of the liver.

DR. TYSON.—Are there instances on record of erythroblastosis in premature babies born dead? May this symptom complex begin and end during pregnancy so that at term the infant may show only an anemia?

DR. DIAMOND.—Only one case has been seen in a premature infant. The last question cannot be answered definitely. The condition is most common in full-term infants.

DR. J. A. RITTER (PHILADELPHIA, PA.).—Does the condition occur more frequently in general hospital wards rather than in private practice? Is there a deficiency factor? Have gastric content studies been made in these cases?

DR. DIAMOND.—As many cases occur in private practice as in general wards. Estimations of gastric acidity have been made in the recent cases but not enough reports are as yet available to be conclusive.

DR. JOSEPH STOKES, JR. (PHILADELPHIA, PA.).—What studies in chemistry of mother's blood have been done?

DR. DIAMOND.—There was no evidence of anything abnormal in work done on two cases.

DR. CLIFFORD.—Dr. Irving and Dr. Minot followed two cases very closely and could find nothing abnormal.

DR. RITTER.—Is there any relation between the macrocytic anemia of pregnancy and the causation of erythroblastosis?

DR. DIAMOND.—There has been no relation in cases that we have studied.

CHAIRMAN JOSEPHS.—In a review of the literature I have been unable to find any relation between macrocytic anemia in the mother and erythroblastosis in the infant.

DR. RITTER.—When the erythrocyte count in newborn infants becomes low, is there any change in the blood type?

DR. DIAMOND.—No change has been noted.

DR. TYSON.—Is there any relationship in hemorrhagic disease of the newborn and erythroblastosis?

DR. SMITH.—Is the so-called anemia of the newborn related to erythroblastosis?

DR. COOLEY.—Not all anemias of the newborn are due to erythroblastosis. Anemias due to acute infections, sepsis, and syphilis have been mentioned. Hemorrhagic disease of the newborn is a definite entity, though of unknown etiology. There seems to be a group of deficiency anemias in the newborn period, and in these cases it is often found that the mother has been gravely anemic during the pregnancy. I think that the type of hemolysis may be a valuable diagnostic criterion. In the anemias due to infection and in the deficiency anemias, the blood smears give the picture of marked increase in fragmentation. In true erythroblastosis there is no increase in fragmenting forms, though there may be striking anisocytosis. Fragility is likely to be somewhat increased, and there is a strong suggestion of the type of hemolysis met with in hemolytic icterus. We think that the abrupt cessation of the hemolytic process and the rapid improvement of the blood picture observed in three cases after splenectomy are good evidence that the spleen plays a role here much like that in hemolytic icterus.

Pathogenesis.—I should like to suggest a theory of the pathogenetic process involved. In the first place, there are evidently two types of cases, grouped according to when hemolysis begins. In one, hemolysis has been marked before birth, the vernix and the amniotic fluid are pigmented, and the child is born jaundiced. The cases with hydrops belong with this early group. In the other type the babies are born to all appearances normal, but within the first few hours after birth sudden, extreme hemolysis occurs, with rapid development of pronounced icterus. I think that we have primarily a state of polycythemia, due to a constitutional exaggeration of the fetal type of hemopoiesis, possibly with production of abnormal, unusually susceptible erythrocytes. In the first type, the spleen has reacted to this condition by a hyperactivity similar to that spoken of as ''hypersplenism'' in hemolytic icterus; in the second type this hyperactivity does not develop until the added stimulus of the birth changes supervenes. In either case, the result is a hemolytic anemia. If the child survives, the extramedullary foci disappear, splenic activity gradually returns to normal, and after a more or less prolonged period of marrow hypoplasia the whole picture gradually clears up.

Though we think that we have demonstrated that prompt splenectomy has the same prompt curative effect here as in hemolytic icterus, we are inclined not to advise it except in obviously grave cases. The operation offers serious surgical difficulties in so young a patient, and statistics of results of less drastic treatment are very satisfactory.

DR. DIAMOND.—In cases in which hemolysis began after the first few days there was no evidence of enlargement of the spleen. However, after transfusion splenic enlargement was noted and hemolysis became a prominent factor. Excessive hemopoiesis comes first and is followed by hemolysis.

DR. COOLEY.—There may be excessive hemolysis of transfused blood if hemolysis occurs by fragmentation. The important point in arriving at a diagnosis of anemia in the newborn is the determination of what is going on in the hemopoietic system.

DR. RITTER.—In transfusing patients with erythroblastosis is citrated blood used?

DR. DIAMOND.—We use citrated blood only and do not have any increase in untoward reactions. Usually 10 c.c. of blood per pound of body weight is given. In children showing marked anemia 20 c.c. per pound may be used.

DR. T. B. GIVAN (BROOKLYN, N. Y.).—What veins are used?

DR. DIAMOND.—This depends on the skill of the operator. In Children's and Infants' hospital we never cut down on a vein. In most instances scalp veins are used. Difficulty seldom arises if the technique is mastered. We use a 24 gauge needle with a Kauffman-Luer side arm syringe and a pressure 20 c.c. syringe. We never give blood into the superior longitudinal sinus; the ankle veins or the femoral veins may be used. Blood is not given by the drip method ordinarily. The transfusion is stopped if any evidence of heart embarrassment occurs; the remainder of the blood may be given in divided amounts.

DR. COOLEY.—We never give more than 15 c.c. of blood per pound of body weight. Veins on the dorsal aspect of the hands may be used. There is no reason why the internal saphenous vein could not be cut down on. Blood should never be given by the intraperitoneal route. In debilitated or morbid infants the blood may remain unchanged or unabsorbed in the peritoneal cavity following transfusion by this route.

DR. H. G. PONCHER (EVANSTON, ILL.).—In severely jaundiced cases, does transfusion cause any ill effect, from products resulting from destruction of blood?

DR. DIAMOND.—You would have to have parallel cases to answer definitely.

CHAIRMAN JOSEPHS.—There is probably no doubt that transfusion does add to the jaundice, but do not withhold it on this account because transfusion does have a definite value.

DR. L. S. FRIEDMAN (CINCINNATI, OHIO.).—Would you give a prophylactic transfusion to a normal appearing infant at birth?

DR. DIAMOND.—We have always waited for changes to appear before giving a transfusion.

DR. COOLEY.—I doubt the wisdom of transfusion before the appearance of anemia. If transfusion is given before anemia manifests itself, greater hemolysis may result, or a troublesome polycythemia may be produced. I have seen one death which may have been the result of premature transfusion.

DR. FRIEDMAN.—Is irradiation of the spleen useful in cases of erythroblastosis?

DR. DIAMOND.—Effects of irradiation are too slow in this condition to be of any value.

DR. COOLEY.—Since changes in the spleen are usually temporary, there is no need for splenectomy or irradiation in most cases.

DR. WALTER LEVY (NEW YORK, N. Y.).—Have there been any necropsy studies of the mothers of children with erythroblastosis?

DR. DIAMOND.—None reported or known.

DR. GIVAN.—Is erythroblastosis ever associated with congenital defects?

DR. DIAMOND.—Erythroblastemia may occur with other congenital defects such as obliteration of the bile ducts and congenital cardiac anomalies.

CHAIRMAN JOSEPHS.—I may mention Passachoff's case in which in addition to congenital atresia of the bile ducts there was also a typical picture of erythroblastosis.

Before bringing the discussion to a close, I wish to say a few words regarding etiology. I have arranged in a table the principal factors, known and hypothetical, that should be considered in any discussion of anemia of the newborn. *Syphilis*, *sepsis* and *malaria* have already been thoroughly discussed. *Hemorrhage* as a cause of anemia is too obvious to need discussion, but I should like to emphasize one or two points. Purpuric manifestations and reductions of platelets are not at all uncommon in erythroblastosis. The case that Dr. Cooley cited earlier was particularly interesting because of the fact that thrombopenic purpura was present without any other of the manifestations of erythroblastosis fetalis, although from the family history we can be fairly sure that the condition was present. It has already been brought out that some of the cases of hemorrhagic disease of the newborn may have been cases of erythroblastosis with terminal hemorrhage.

Hemorrhage into the adrenals might be specially mentioned since it may go unrecognized, even when large enough to cause anemia. Recently I have seen a case with a cephalhematoma causing severe anemia. In these cases there may be jaundice and evidence of increased pigment excretion.

The rare possibility of leucemia and osteosclerosis need be no more than mentioned.

Congenital aplastic anemia has already been mentioned. A number of the reported cases of anemia of the newborn fall in this group, but, because of the relative slowness with which the anemia may develop, they may not be recognized until after the passage of several weeks. There is almost no literature on them. I can add two from my own experience to those which Dr. Diamond has mentioned. I should like to warn here against too indiscriminate diagnosis of aplastic anemia on the basis of absence of erythroblastosis and a low reticulocyte count. Cases with clear evidence of hemolysis may have no erythroblastosis, and normally there is a period in the second and third week of life in which the reticulocytes are at a very low point. The diagnosis of aplastic anemia should depend either on autopsy or on the continuance of the signs of aplasia beyond the third week. However, some degree of temporary hypoplasia may be a factor in cases without erythroblastosis, and even in some cases with erythroblastosis.

Congenital hemolytic jaundice has rarely been reported as a cause of anemia at birth; sickle-cell anemia never, to my knowledge. With regard to Mediterranean anemia I shall have to ask Dr. Cooley and Dr. Diamond what their experience has been.

So much for the etiological agents that are known to be capable of causing anemia at birth or shortly after birth. Since in the majority of cases with the clinical and hematologic picture of erythroblastosis these known etiological factors have been excluded, we are forced to turn to a consideration of more or less hypothetical possibilities. These are to be looked on not as cause of a disease, but as factors which may singly or in combination give rise to pathologic changes, the results of which are the syndromes that we call erythroblastosis or anemia of the newborn, or other names. There is evidence in favor of each of these possibilities as well as difficulties in the way of their acceptance, without making assumptions at present incapable of proof.

The first possibility is that of inherited defect affecting the baby. Of course, congenital hemolytic jaundice is just such a condition and is apparently capable of appearing at birth; it, or some other similar type of defect, may be present in some cases. In the majority, however, the complete recovery precludes this as a possibility. On the other hand, there are undoubted cases in which an inherited factor is clearly present, especially those in which the tendency to give birth to babies with erythroblastosis appears in several generations of the same family. What the nature of this inherited factor is and how and where it acts are entirely unknown. Moreover, only investigation of the future can determine how frequently it is to be considered a factor in these cases.

The second possibility is that of a failure in the development of the hemopoietic tissue, so that an earlier embryonic type of blood formation persists up to the time of delivery. This may be either constitutional or due to some factor associated with the pregnancy. It would be hard to understand a retardation that persisted for several months of intrauterine life followed by an acceleration sufficient to bring hemopoiesis to a normal level in three to four weeks of extrauterine life, unless the retardation has been caused by something closely associated with the pregnancy. Whether we are dealing with a failure to develop or a return to previous level due to something happening in the latter months of pregnancy, I do not believe can be decided at present. Because of the rarity of this condition in premature babies, as gathered from cases in the literature, I would personally incline to the latter view.

The third possibility, now almost universally abandoned, is that of some obscure infection. As a cause of erythroblastosis, anemia and jaundice in the newborn, of course, infection always remains a possibility; but, as a cause of the entity that we are discussing, infection is a very unlikely possibility. It would have to be something existing over a long period of time in the mother, without affecting her in any ascertainable way, and it would have to affect the baby at certain specific points. Actually syphilis is an infection capable of doing just this, and for this reason alone we cannot say that some other specific infection, at present unrecognized, is inconceivable.

The hypothesis that the condition is due to some intoxication associated with pregnancy, is at present the most widely held. It would explain some of the characteristics of the condition, such as its rapid disappearance after birth and its occurrence in successive pregnancies, as well as the pathologic picture. Also erythroblastosis has actually occurred in association with toxemia. Since in the majority of cases there is no evidence of toxemia in the mother to maintain this hypothesis we are forced to assume some hitherto undescribed intoxication which causes no damage except under conditions which exist on the fetal side of the placenta (e.g., anoxemia), or one arising from the placenta itself. This raises the question whether disease of the placenta itself may be a factor in these cases, a possibility that has not yet received sufficient attention in the literature.

Lastly we have the possibility that the condition is due to a deficiency. As in the case of intoxication we are compelled to make certain assumptions. In general, the baby develops at the expense of the mother, so that it is the mother and not the baby who gives evidence of deficiency. We may raise the question whether in these cases the placenta is impermeable, but, since these babies are not rachitic or scorbutic, the impermeability of the placenta must be selective. Or we may question whether the deficiency causes damage only under the condition existing in the fetus. It may thus be seen that to maintain the idea of deficiency leads to difficulties, but these difficulties are not very different from those encountered in maintaining the idea of an intoxication. On the other hand, the idea of a deficiency receives support from cases in which liver given to the mother during pregnancy has apparently prevented the occurrence of the condition in the baby.

This ends a rather sketchy discussion of etiology. Questions have been raised for which there is no answer today. Before we can begin to answer them we must know more than we do now concerning the placenta, not just the anatomic changes, but the physiology including such things as permeability and the part pathologic changes may play in the development of the fetus. We must also know more definitely the answers to questions raised today: the specific effect of transfusion, the relation of liver pathology to the picture, the effect of serum, the prophylactic effect of liver, and the influence of hereditary factors.

Benjamin Hoyer, M.D., Secretary.

The Journal of Pediatrics

Vol. 14 | August, 1938 | No. 2

Original Communications

SUBPHRENIC ABSCESS IN CHILDREN

With Special Reference to Roentgen Signs of Transphrenic Infection

William E. Anspach, M.D.
Chicago, Ill.

Although subphrenic abscess has held a prominent place in the literature for nearly a century, there have been relatively few articles devoted to a study of this disease as it affects children. Montgomery[1] and Ireland,[2] upon whose service most of the cases included in this report have been observed, have each made contributions to recent literature on this subject. LeWald[3] and Gleick[4] recently reported two instances of subphrenic abscess in children. Pancoast[5] included two children in a report of sixteen cases; Gatewood[6] in 1930 included only two children in a group of forty-one cases found in a study of patients of all ages at the Presbyterian Hospital over a ten-year period. The paucity of children in which this condition has been recognized is evident in all of the extensive literature upon subphrenic abscess. In the present report emphasis is placed upon transphrenic infection, as it has been almost constantly present in subphrenic abscess in children and as it usually produces a readily recognizable x-ray sign. Much can be gained from a study of serial roentgenograms made early and along the course of this disease, in which clinical symptoms and signs are likely to vary greatly. The acute symptoms coming on soon after an easily recognizable abdominal infection suggest subphrenic abscess, but cases seen for the first time at a later period are likely to be misdiagnosed as primary pulmonary disease. Too often abdominal findings, if not vague at the onset, are overshadowed later by pulmonary signs. As an increasing number of subphrenic abscesses in children are recognized, there remains little doubt about the prevalence of certain x-ray signs. In previous reports, mostly by surgeons, the atten-

From the X-Ray Department of the Children's Memorial Hospital.

Exhibited under "Roentgen Studies in Children" at the Fifth International Congress of Radiology, Chicago, Ill., 1937.

Read in part at the 1937 meeting of the American Academy of Pediatrics in Chicago.

tion has been directed principally to x-ray signs of "gas and fluid level" below the diaphragm. At this time I wish to pay special attention to roentgen ray signs above the diaphragm, which I have found to be present sooner or later in all subphrenic abscesses in children. Since x-ray is often the most useful single diagnostic procedure in this disease, a detailed report of ten consecutive cases, picturing the variation of roentgen appearances, should not be amiss. Illustrations of three additional cases are added to cover more completely conditions described in the text.

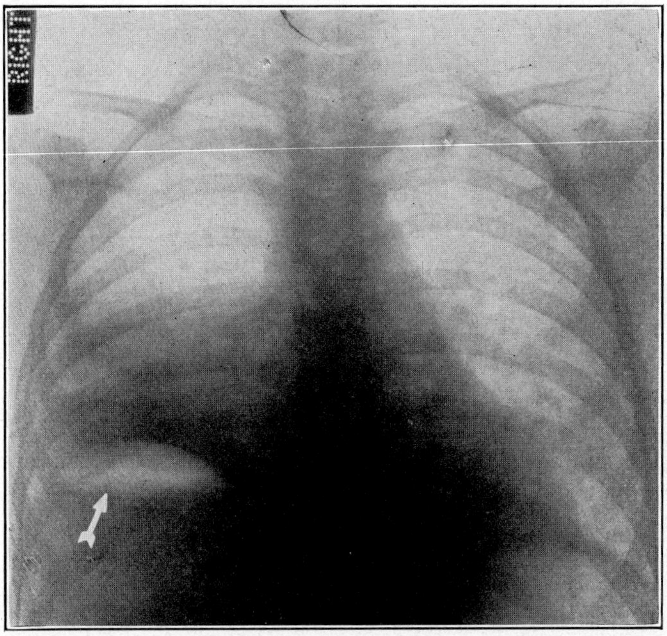

Fig. 1*A*.—Case 1. Chest roentgenogram showing gas and fluid level beneath right leaf of diaphragm. This was noted eight months after a diagnosis of appendicitis. At this time, patient was sent to hospital because of a diagnosis of pulmonary disease.

CASE 1.—Subphrenic abscess, right side, with gas and fluid level beneath.

K. B., a girl 9 years of age, was thought to have a ruptured appendix and was observed at the Cook County Hospital. Her symptoms seemed to improve and an operation was not performed. Later pulmonary symptoms developed, consisting of cough with profuse expectoration. The patient was examined in the dispensary of the Children's Memorial Hospital approximately eighteen months later. A roentgenogram showed gas and fluid level beneath the right leaf of the diaphragm and a moderately dense shadow at the base of the right lung with a fading horizontal upper border (Fig. 1*A*). At the time of admission the patient had clubbing of the fingers. The referring physician thought the patient had chronic pneumonia and endocarditis. She was also thought to have frequent colds and a rheumatic condition. The x-ray findings at this time were interpreted as evidence of a subphrenic abscess. A tube was inserted through the costophrenic angle into the abscess cavity without permitting the formation of a pneumothorax. There was almost immediate improvement in the pulmonary symptoms and the shadows at the base of the right lung partially disappeared (Fig. 1*B*). Drainage persisted through the tube for more than nine months. The patient has been observed for an additional three-year period and has regained her health, although for a considerable period it was thought clinically that a bronchiectasis might be present at the right base. Recent roentgenograms show complete clearing of the right lung. There is still slight elevation of the right leaf of the diaphragm.

CASE 2.—Subphrenic abscess, right side, in an infant.

C. H., aged 16 months, had diarrhea and fever for three days before entering the hospital. The stools contained slime, but no blood was noted. The thighs were kept flexed and the abdomen was somewhat resistant to pressure. No masses were palpated. The diarrhea disappeared promptly, but the temperature average of 103° F., and distention and moderate tenseness of the abdomen continued. There was an occasional cough and also reddening of the upper respiratory passages. The

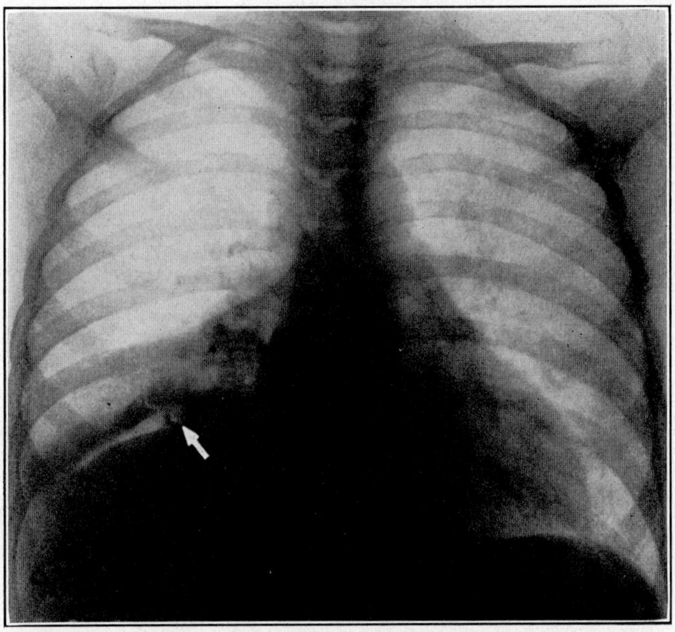

Fig. 1*B*.—Case 1. After drainage. Pulmonary signs considerably improved, but drainage continued for nine months.

appetite was poor and the child seemed to have frequent abdominal pain. A roentgenogram made on the seventh day of hospitalization showed air and fluid level beneath the right leaf of the diaphragm (Fig. 2*A*) with evidence of fluid in the costal pleura. A diagnosis of subphrenic abscess was made, and two days later, under a general anesthesia, a tube was inserted between the liver and the diaphragm. A large quantity of foul-smelling pus escaped. The exact source of the infection was not determined. The general condition of the patient improved immediately. The temperature dropped to 101° F.; the leucocyte count dropped from 28,000 to 12,800. A roentgenogram (Fig. 2*B*), made seven days after drainage, showed complete clearing of the abnormal densities in the chest (Fig. 2*C*). The tube was kept in place for thirty days, and then removed. An exacerbation of the symptoms occurred a few days later, and drainage had to be re-established for a few days. The convalescence from then on was uneventful. The child has been in good health for more than three years.

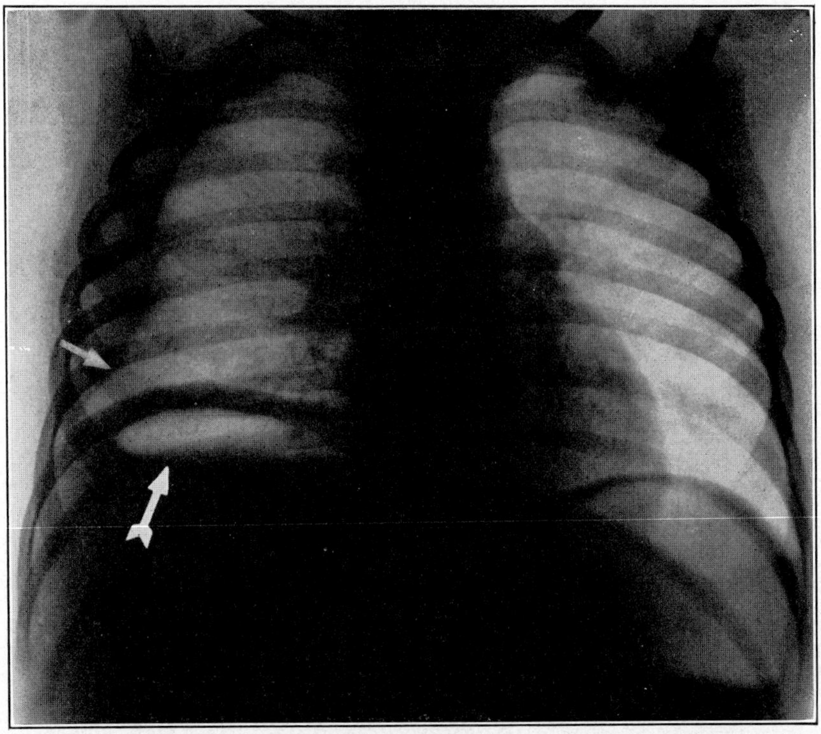

Fig. 2A.—Case 2. Gas and fluid level beneath right leaf of diaphragm. Note absence of retraction of the lung from the costophrenic angle. Early cementing together of the pleura at the diaphragm is a characteristic of subphrenic abscess.

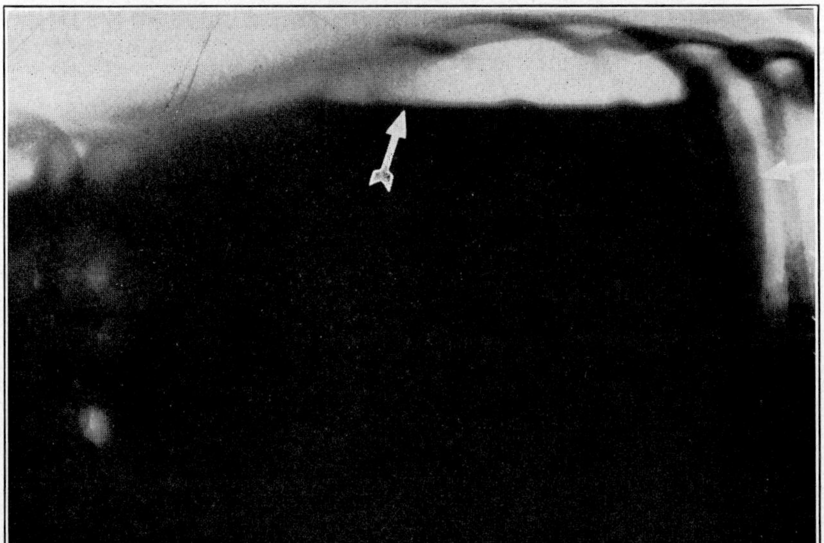

Fig. 2B.—Case 2. Showing extent of loculation with patient lying on left side.

CASE 3.—Absence of fluid level and gas beneath right leaf of diaphragm. Basal exudate.

J. P., girl aged 12 years, was admitted to the hospital on Dec. 28, 1932, because of abdominal pain of three days' duration. The throat was inflamed. There was marked muscular rigidity and tenderness over the right lower quadrant. A mass in the region of the appendix was thought to exist. Two days after admission the abdomen was opened over McBurney's point. A ruptured appendix was found but not removed. The peritoneal cavity seemed to be filled with pus. A drainage tube was left in place. The temperature, which on admission was 104° F., varied following drainage from 102 to 103.5° F. for twenty-three days. The leucocyte count on admission was 26,000. This dropped to 12,400 in twenty-four hours following drainage of the peritoneal cavity. A chest roentgenogram (Fig. 3*A*), taken eleven

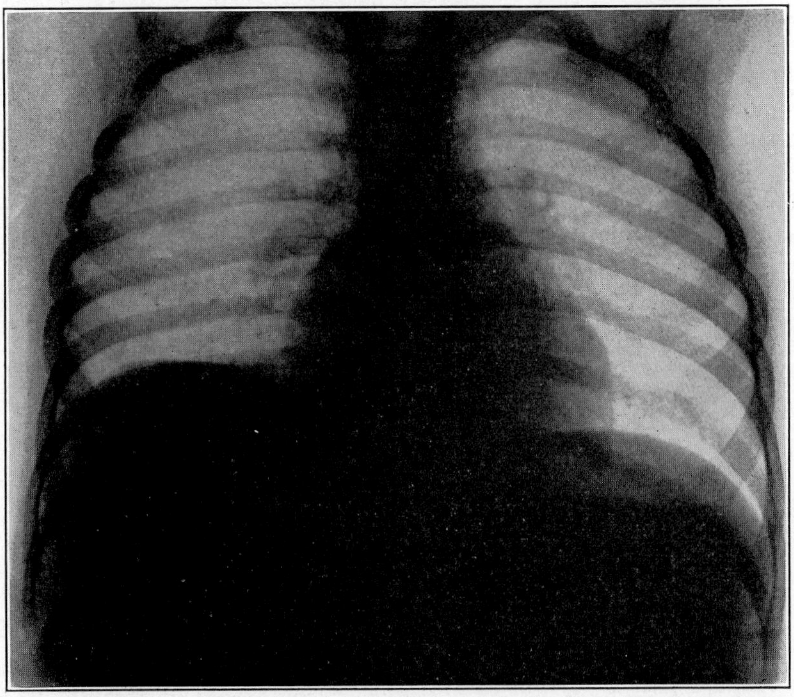

Fig. 2*C*.—Complete disappearance of pulmonary shadows one week after subphrenic drainage.

days after admission, was interpreted as showing an exudate at the base of the right pleural cavity, most likely secondary to subphrenic infection. Because of failure to improve, a two-stage operation for drainage was decided upon thirty-two days following the first operation. The first step consisted of marsupialization of the pleura in the costophrenic sinus in the posterior axillary line. Four days later a tube was inserted through the costophrenic sinus, draining a large quantity of foul-smelling pus. Air did not enter the pleural cavity. A cough, moist expectoration, and crackling râles in the base of the right lung since admission to the hospital disappeared within a few days. A roentgenogram of the chest (Fig. 3*B*), taken eleven days after the first, showed that the shadows of increased density at the base of the lung had disappeared. The temperature dropped following subphrenic drainage, but remained elevated approximately one degree for two weeks. Drainage continued and the right leaf of the diaphragm remained slightly elevated for several weeks. Complete recovery eventually occurred. Pulmonary symptoms completely disappeared with subphrenic drainage.

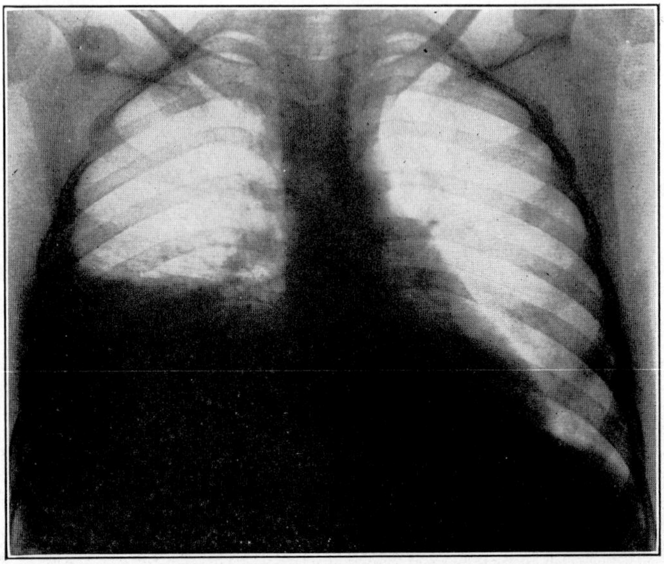

Fig. 3*A*.—Case 3. Shadow at right base with fading horizontal upper border due to transphrenic infection. No gas and fluid level beneath diaphragm.

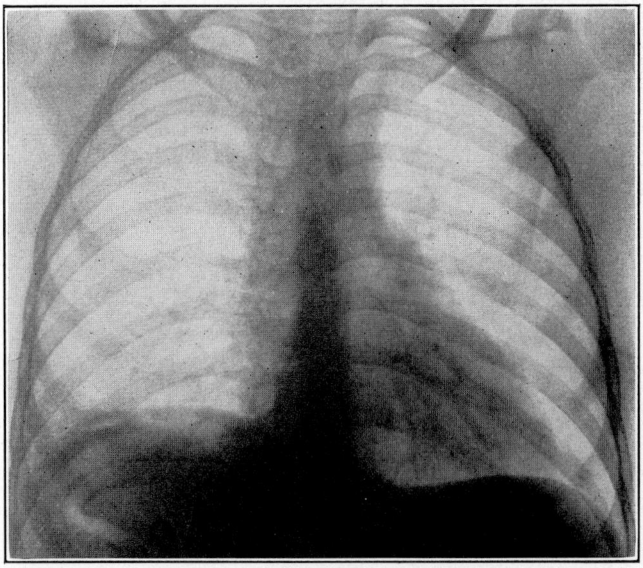

Fig. 3*B*.—Case 3. Eleven days after drainage of the abscess which followed preliminary marsupialization.

CASE 4.—Subphrenic abscess. Absence of "gas and fluid level."

J. P., female aged 5 years. The first symptom was severe cramplike pain in the lower right quadrant of the abdomen. This appeared and disappeared for almost a week, when the spasms of pain became very severe. The patient was then taken to the hospital where a diagnosis of appendicitis was made and the patient operated upon on the seventh day of illness. A sanguineous fluid was present upon opening the peritoneal cavity. The appendix was covered with a fibrinous exudate and was adherent to the lateral abdominal wall. After removal of the appendix, two large drainage tubes were left in place. The patient's temperature, which had been 102° F. before operation, receded for a few days, then fluctuated markedly from a little above normal to 105° F. There was tenderness and rigidity over the upper right quadrant. An x-ray of the chest (Fig. 4) taken two weeks after operation showed a diaphragmatic pleurisy and was interpreted as showing the early signs of a transphrenic infection. Transpleural drainage was established with a subphrenic abscess. The patient left the hospital thirty-three days after the operation, making an uneventful recovery.

CASE 5.—Subphrenic abscess with bronchial fistula and rest cavity, right side.

C. W., aged 10 years, a poorly developed and poorly nourished white boy, who was apparently not acutely ill, came to the hospital because of a cough of two years' duration. There was only slight expectoration and no hemoptysis or streaking of blood. The child had lost 15 pounds. There was vague tenderness in the abdomen at intervals. For the last five or six months the weight had remained stationary. The cough had been much worse for the preceding three weeks. There had been no colds, sore throat, or trouble with the ears, and no known abdominal trouble excepting for an occasional pain in the right side. Some impairment of resonance, suppression of breath sounds, occasional râles, wheezes, and decreased vocal fremitus were noted at the right base. No distention or rigidity was noted in the abdomen. The liver and the spleen were not palpable. On admission the presence of bronchiectasis or lung abscess was considered. The leucocyte count was 18,600.

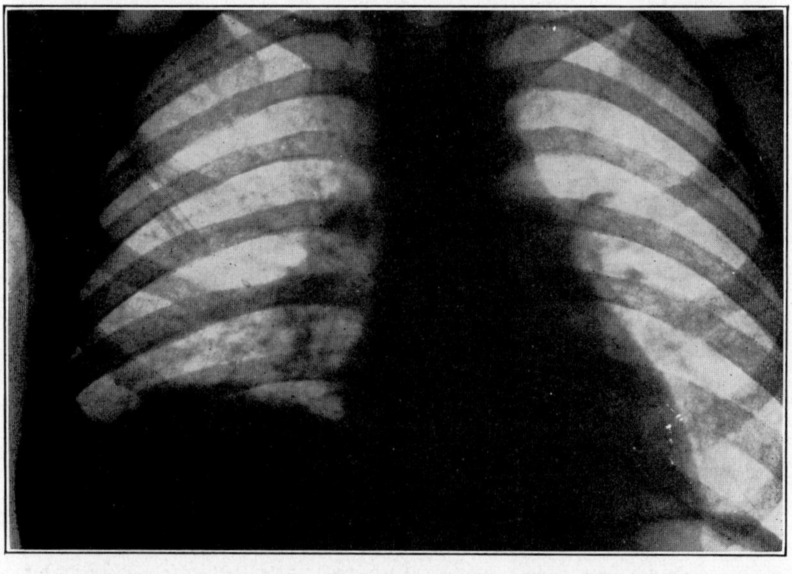

Fig. 4.—Case 4. Early signs of a diaphragmatic pleuritis following a ruptured appendix. Note ragged appearance of right leaf of diaphragm.

The following day Dr. Joseph Brennemann made the following pertinent note after examining the chest: "He has a succussion sound in the lower portion of the right chest—cannot tell if it is above or below the diaphragm." Later "succussion splashes" were frequently heard. The right leaf of the diaphragm showed no

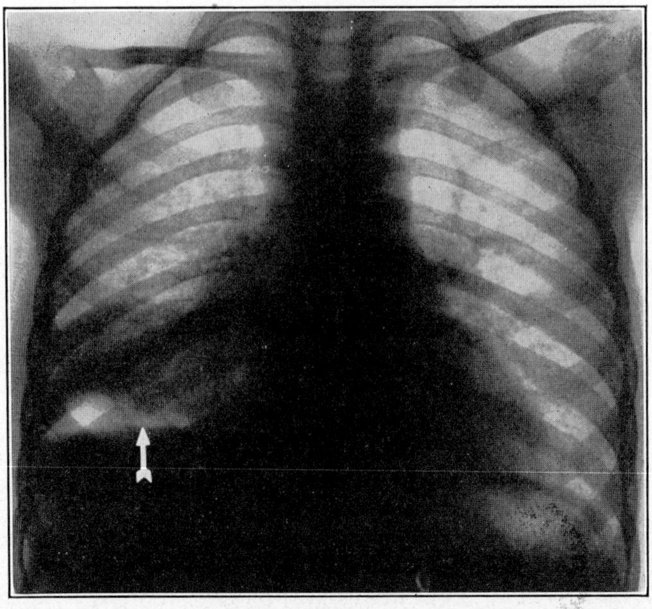

Fig. 5*A*.—Case 5. Large rest cavity at right base which developed following amoebic dysentery. The fluid could be drained through a bronchus by inverted posture. Clinically patient was thought to have bronchiectasis or lung abscess.

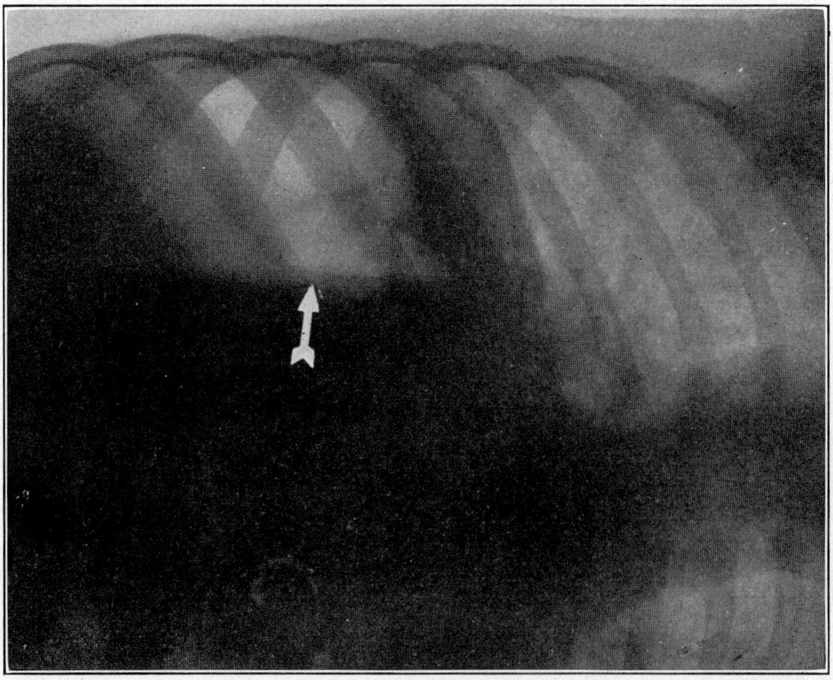

Fig. 5*B*.—Case 5. Left side down.

excursion. A chest roentgenogram (Fig. 5*A*) made the same day showed a hazy density apparently mistakenly thought to represent the elevated right leaf of the diaphragm, with gas and fluid level beneath. Additional films made with the patient

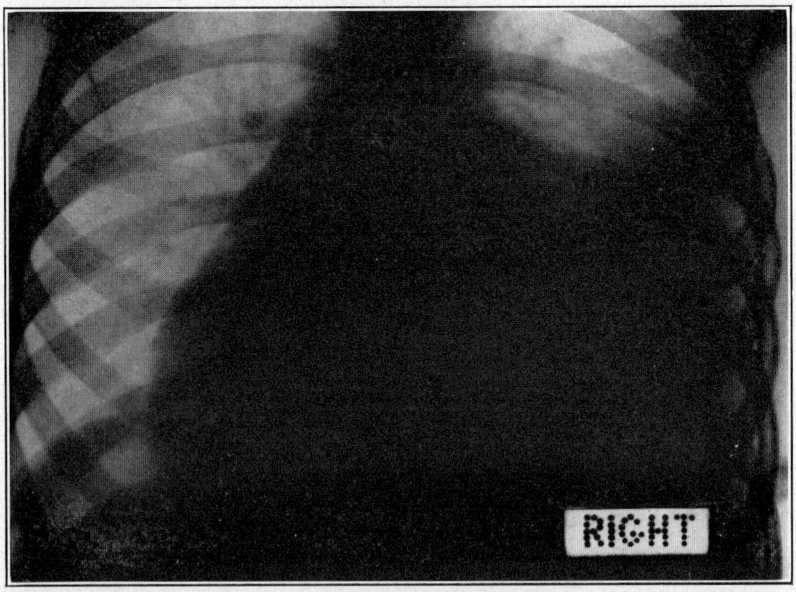

Fig. 6*A*.—Case 6. Clouding, right base, following appendectomy. There was a gradual accumulation of fluid for three weeks.

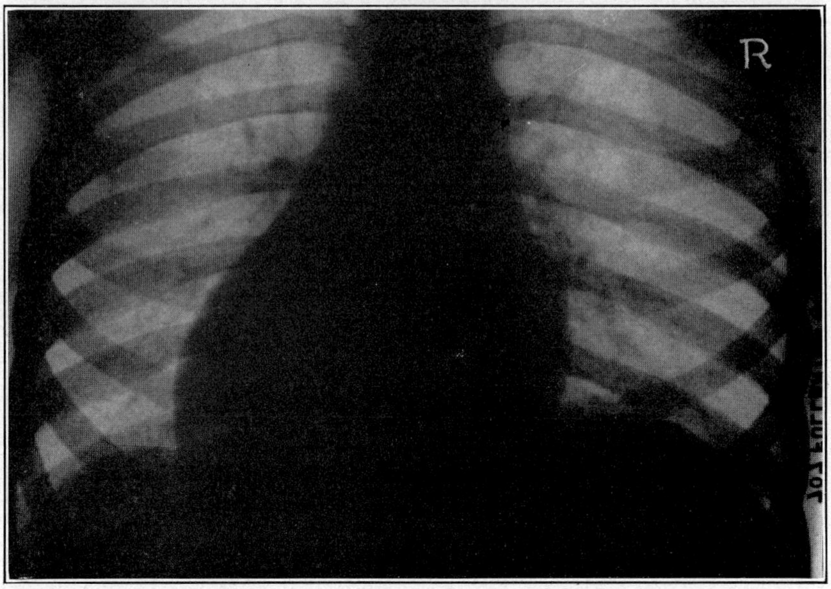

Fig. 6*B*.—Case 6. Drainage of subphrenic abscess was scheduled, but the fluid had suddenly disappeared.

lying on his side (Fig. 5*B*) proved the absence of gas below the diaphragm. There were hazy shadows along the bronchovascular markings at the right base and a suggestion of exudate in the pleural cavity. Because of frequent spells of productive coughing, films were made immediately before and immediately after assuming a face-down position with head lowered. Fifty c.c. of thick, foul-smelling pus came slowly and were expectorated while this position was resumed. After ten minutes of this procedure, the second film showed a substantial decrease in the fluid level, indicating a direct communication between the pus in the cavity and the bronchus. The temperature fluctuated only slightly, remaining about 1 degree elevated. Ten days later a tube was inserted through the chest wall draining a large quantity of pus. The patient withstood the operation under local anesthetic very well, but improvement was slow. The air and fluid level persisted after removal of the drainage tube. Finally a thoracoplasty was performed. Portions of three ribs were removed. A phrenicotomy was done on the right side at this time. Examination of the stool had shown the presence of amoebae, and it was thought that an amoebic abscess had penetrated the diaphragm. The patient left the hospital a year after admission to be watched in the outpatient department.

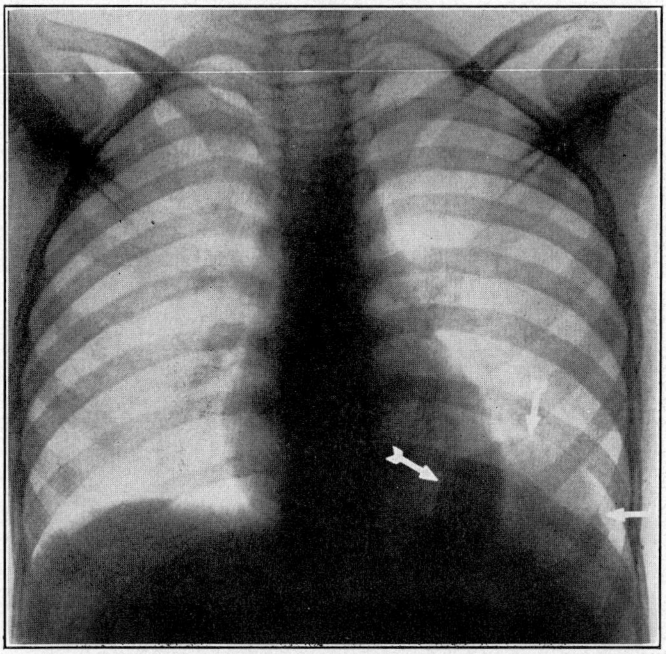

Fig. 7*A*.—Case 7. Density with convex outline left base following a local peritonitis.

A large rest cavity persisted on the right, which filled with fluid after the drainage wound healed. This rest cavity was present for more than a year after drainage. At present there are no amoebae in the stool. Three thoracoplasties have been necessary in an attempt to close the rest cavity. The patient has been free from pulmonary symptoms for the past year and the lung fields have shown no abnormal signs. The patient has gained 20 pounds in weight.

CASE 6.—Subphrenic abscess with spontaneous disappearance of pleural fluid. T. I., an 8-year-old white girl, was admitted to the hospital because of midabdominal pain and tenderness of three days' duration. The pain gradually spread to include the greater portion of the abdomen, especially the upper half. An appendectomy was performed. The appendix was not ruptured, but the abdomen contained serous fluid. The temperature rose from the admission temperature of 99 to 103° F. following the operation. An x-ray examination at this time showed

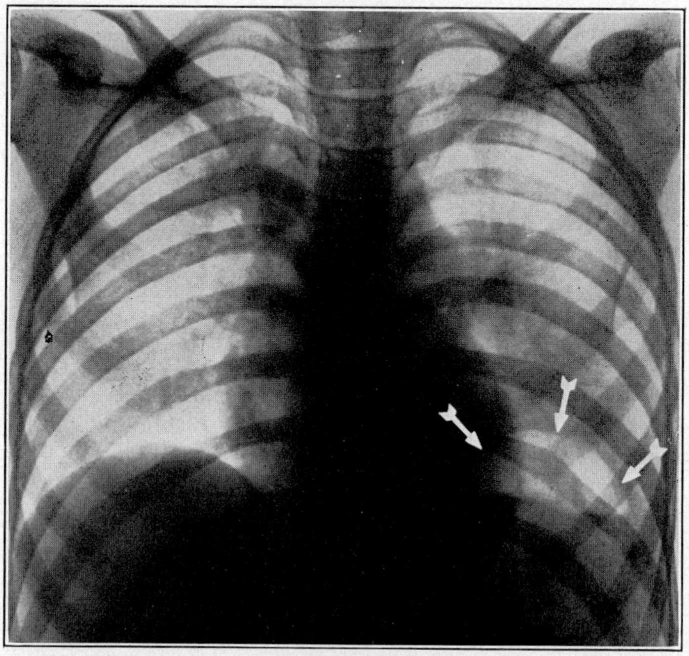

Fig. 7*B*.—Case 7. The pleural pocket has communicated with a bronchus and exchanged fluid for air. Here an adhesive diaphragmatic pleuritis has prevented separation of the pleura for more than a short distance.

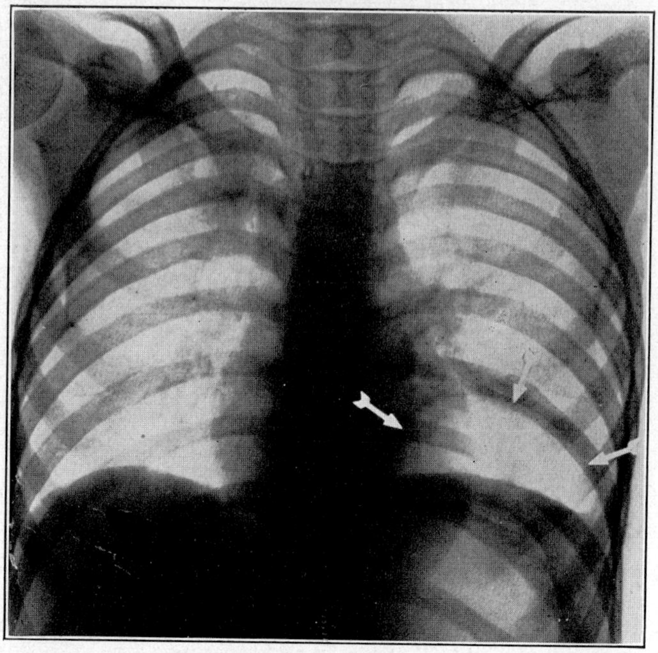

Fig. 7*C*.—Case 7. Following day, air containing cavity has ballooned out slightly but the surrounding visceral and diaphragmatic pleurae are still adherent to each other.

elevation and fixation of the right leaf of the diaphragm. There was no evidence of a diaphragmatic pleurisy. Two days later an x-ray film showed the appearance of a small quantity of fluid at the base of the right lung (Figs. 6*A* and 6*B*). Gradually there was an accumulation of fluid; then suddenly it disappeared. The patient left the hospital five weeks after admission and has been well for six months. The tuberculin test was negative.

CASE 7.—Subphrenic abscess, left side, bronchial fistula with spontaneous healing.

G. P., a white girl aged 12 years, was admitted to the hospital because of a large, tender mass, which was noted in the right flank following abdominal pain, nausea, and vomiting of three days' duration. A diagnosis of an appendiceal abscess was made. At operation a general peritonitis was thought to exist. Drainage of foul pus was profuse for ten days; then a fecal fistula developed. Three

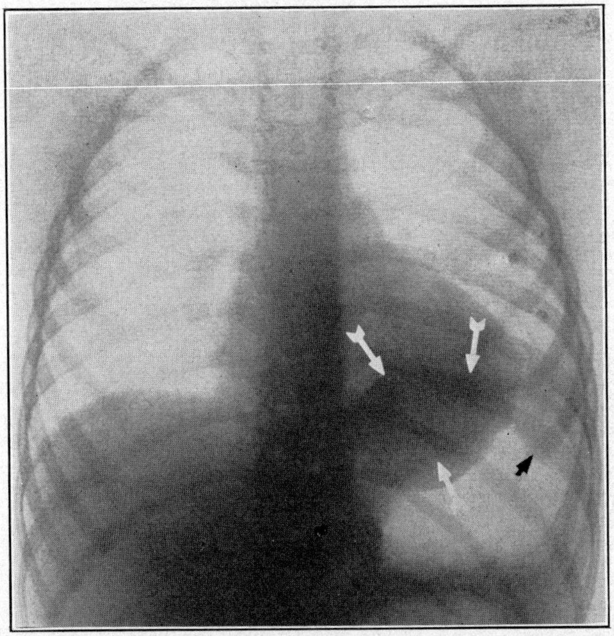

Fig. 8*A*.—Case 8. Haziness above left leaf of the diaphragm with widened "liver" (?) shadow directly beneath following a bacillary dysentery.

weeks after the operation, a roentgenogram of the chest, including the upper abdomen, was made. This showed a wide area of homogeneous density between the mesial portion of the air-filled fundus of the stomach and the elevated left leaf of the diaphragm. This was thought to be a subphrenic encapsulation of pus. This idea was confirmed by an anterior incision. A drainage tube was inserted and free drainage secured for several days. The general condition of the patient remained poor and two blood transfusions were given. After two months' hospitalization, another homogeneous density was noted in the region of the left leaf of the diaphragm. This shadow had a smooth convex upper border (Fig. 7*A*). It was thought to be encapsulated fluid between the stomach and the diaphragm or an exudate in the diaphragmatic portion of the pleural cavity. Dr. A. H. Montgomery, following this clue and believing the pus to be beneath the diaphragm, made a posterior approach but found only adhesions between the diaphragm and the fundus of the stomach. The density was not influenced by the operation. Four days later the leucocyte count showed a drop from 24,600 to 16,200. The child began to cough up foul-smelling pus, and a roentgenogram made at this time showed the replacement of the dense shadow at the left base by a similar shadow of decreased density (Fig. 7*B*), indicating that the fluid had drained through a

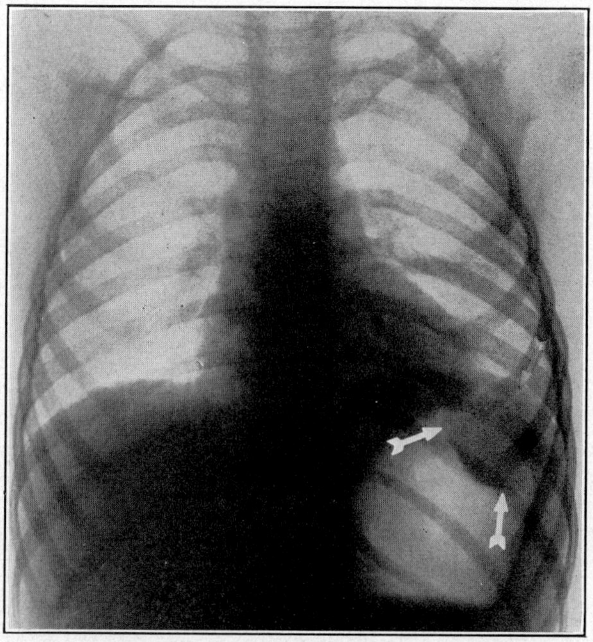

Fig. 8*B*.—Case 8. Oval mass encroaching upon stomach on earlier film thought to be the "head" of the spleen, but here it is more dense than previously and the "liver" shadow is smaller, suggesting connecting pockets of fluid below the diaphragm.

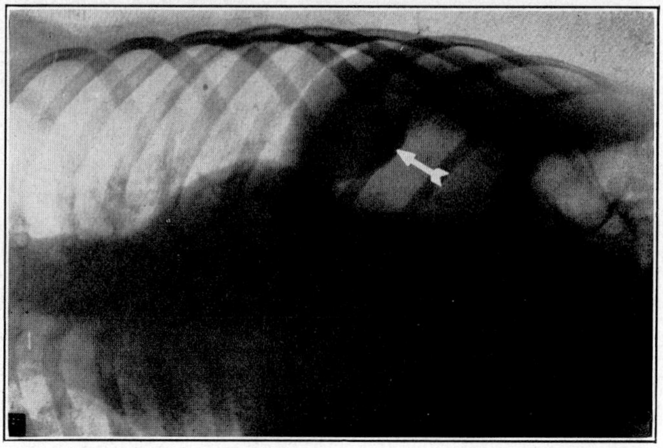

Fig. 8*C*.—Case 8. Patient lying on left side. Arrow indicates a loculation between the fundus and the diaphragm. This shadow was not present on films made after recovery.

bronchus and the encapsulated area had filled with air (Fig. 7*C*). Definite improvement with complete clearing of the pulmonary symptoms occurred in ten days. The temperature became normal and the child was well, excepting for a fecal fistula at McBurney's point which had persisted from the first operation. The child left the hospital six months after admission. The fecal fistula had closed and the patient gained considerable weight during her stay in the hospital. She has been well for more than a year.

CASE 8.—Subphrenic abscess, left side, recovery without drainage.

R. B., a 5-year-old white boy (patient of Dr. C. A. Aldrich). The first symptoms were noted ten days before entering the hospital. There were fever, vomiting, and convulsions, followed two days later by the finding of blood and mucus in the stools. Marked tenderness was present in the right upper quadrant for a few days and then the tenderness decreased in amount, and the fever, vomiting, and convulsions subsided. The return of fever ten days later with marked abdominal pain and also pain below the left shoulder caused the child to be brought to the hospital. At this time there was tenderness, dullness, and an indistinct mass slightly to the right of the midline in the upper abdomen. This seemed to be immediately beneath the liver. The leucocyte count was 26,300. Analysis of the stools before entering the hospital had resulted in a diagnosis of bacillary dysentery (Flexner type). A chest roentgenogram (Fig. 8*A*), made on admission to the hospital, showed elevation of the left leaf of the diaphragm and an oval density apparently between the left leaf of the diaphragm and the stomach (see also Figs. 8*B* and 8*C*). On the second day of hospitalization the patient began to cough up mousey-smelling, yellow sputum, which continued for twenty-four hours and then subsided. The child remained in the hospital for eight days, during which time the temperature dropped from 103° F. to normal. The constant pain in the abdomen and occasional pain under the left shoulder gradually disappeared, as did the mass in the abdomen. A friction rub had been present for a few days at the base of the left lung but disappeared at the time the subdiaphragmatic mass disappeared. The stools became negative for dysentery. More recent roentgenograms have shown complete disappearance of the oval density between the left leaf of the diaphragm and the stomach. The patient has been well for two years.

CASE 9.—Subphrenic abscess, left side, following perforation of gastric ulcer in a young child.

M. C., a white girl 2 years of age, came to the hospital because of severe pain in the abdomen, which seemed to come on definitely at 2:00 P.M. On admission the child seemed very ill, and a few moments after the examination was begun the patient had a clonic convulsion lasting ten minutes. Later other convulsions seemed to follow intense pain in the abdomen, at which time the child would scream out. The stools, three or four a day, were green and jellylike. They contained no visible blood. The abdomen seemed pliable and soft at first, but on the eighth day of hospitalization it was moderately rigid all over, but rigidity seemed slightly more marked on the left. Four days later a well-circumscribed mass could be palpated in the midline of the epigastrium. The skin surface over the mass appeared hyperemic, and there was some crepitation. An incision was made over the mass, and 200 c.c. of brownish-yellow pus was secured from the abdominal cavity. Following this, bile and material from the intestinal lumen were noted in the drainage material. A tube was left in position. A roentgenogram failed to show evidence of gas free in the abdominal cavity but showed a dense triangular shadow through the left heart shadow, suggesting the presence of a collapsed left lobe and exudate in the pleural cavity. The patient began vomiting, lost ground, and died two weeks after admission. The temperature had varied between 101 and 104° F., subsiding slightly after the operation.

At necropsy a healing penetrating ulcer of the posterior wall of the stomach was found. There was a thin layer of exudate with adhesions between the left leaf of the diaphragm and the stomach, also between the diaphragm and the base of the left lung, besides a local peritonitis. The exudate had surrounded the left lower lobe of the lung, causing it to become indurated on the surface. The shrinking in size was due to atelectasis. The latter accounted for the triangular density seen on the roentgenogram (Fig. 9), which displaced the heart toward the affected side.

CASE 10.—Subphrenic abscess, left side, following trauma.

W. B., male aged 12 years (patient of Dr. William Beck and Dr. Carl Beck) was struck by the fender of an automobile in the left upper quadrant of the abdomen. The patient was brought to the hospital and was able to walk unassisted into the hospital. There was marked tenderness over the left upper quadrant where the superficial tissues were bruised. Six hours later the chest was fluoroscoped and film exposed because of a possible injury to the left leaf of the diaphragm. There was decreased excursion of the diaphragm, but the lung fields were clear. Repeated similar examinations failed to show any change until the fourth day when a fuzzy shadow appeared above the diaphragm. This was interpreted as evidence of a transphrenic infection producing a diaphragmatic pleuritis (Fig. 10*A*). The amount of exudate in the pleural cavity gradually increased until at the end of three weeks' hospitalization, the left lung field was almost completely obliterated on the regular chest roentgenogram (Fig. 10*B*). An overexposed film showed air

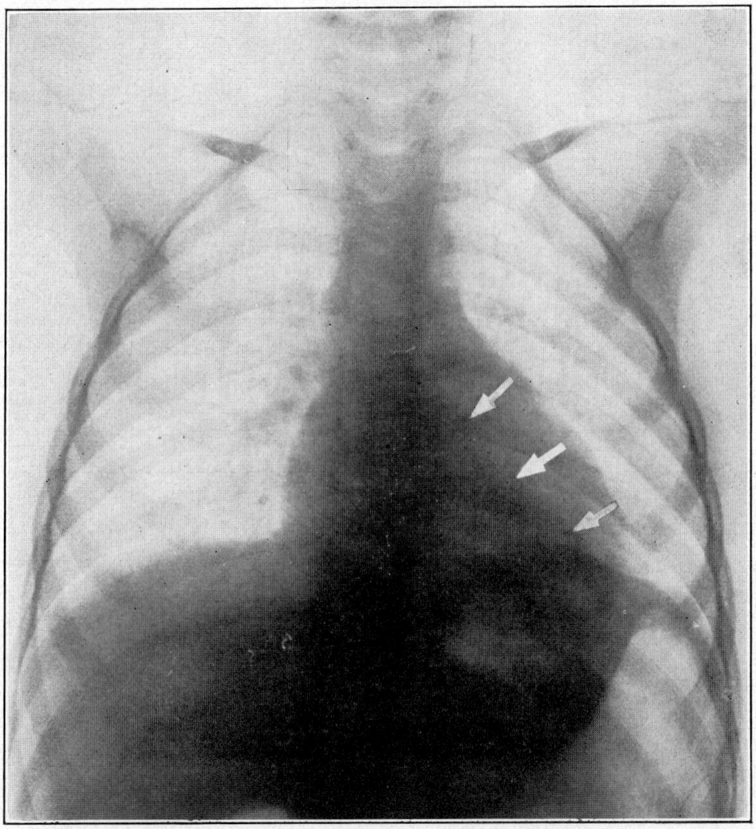

Fig. 9.—Case 9. Atelectasis of left lower lobe seen as a triangular shadow back of heart shadow caused by transphrenic infection following a perforated gastric ulcer. Necropsy.

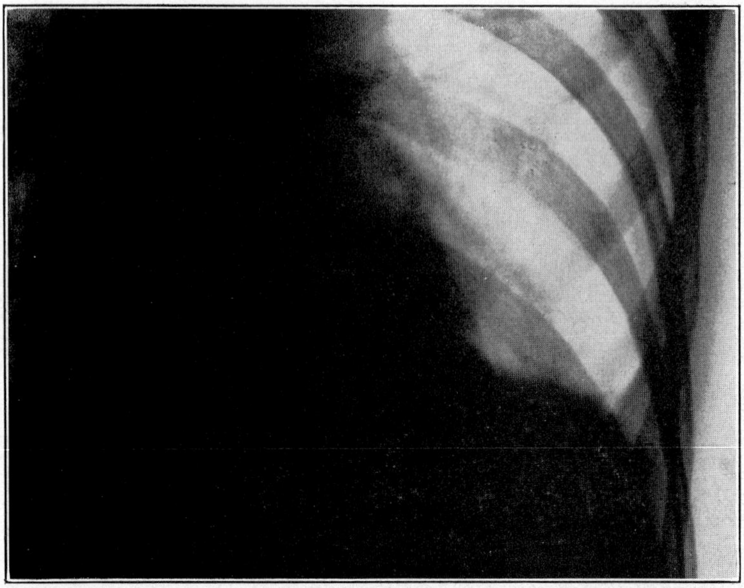

Fig. 10*A*.—Case 10. (Patient of Dr. William Beck and Dr. Carl Beck) Diaphragmatic pleurisy following injury to left upper quadrant of abdomen. Note fuzzy outline to diaphragm. This film was made on the fourth day following injury.

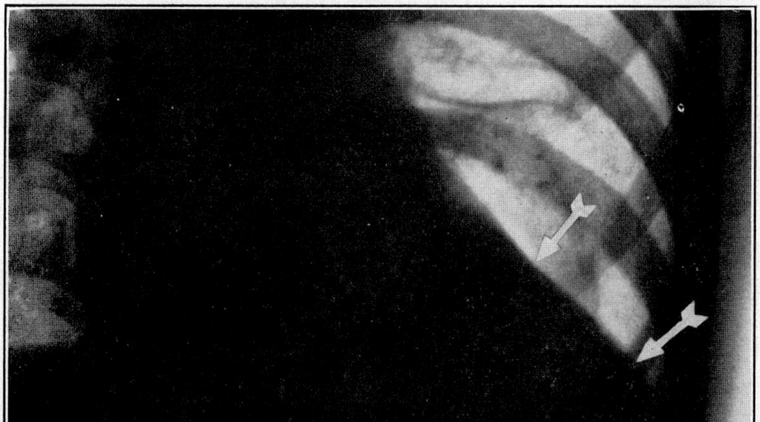

Fig. 10*B*.—Case 10. Infection has penetrated the lower lobe, occluding the bronchi and bringing about collapse. The dense shadow of the lower lobe cannot be distinguished from the heart shadow. Later the fluid increased and blotted out the lung field.

in the left lower lobe with the base of the lung and the diaphragm making normal contact with each other. There was separation of the visceral and costal pleurae above the costophrenic angle. Posterior subdiaphragmatic drainage was established, removing considerable pus and old blood. The fluid in the left pleural cavity completely disappeared within a few days (Fig. 10*C*). The source of the infection in the lesser peritoneal cavity was never ascertained. The patient has been well for one year.

ROENTGEN SIGNS

The first sign made evident by the x-ray examination in subphrenic abscess is fixation or limitation of motion of one leaf of the diaphragm. The leaf on the affected side is usually elevated. The elevation and fixation are especially noticeable at the end of deep inspiration because

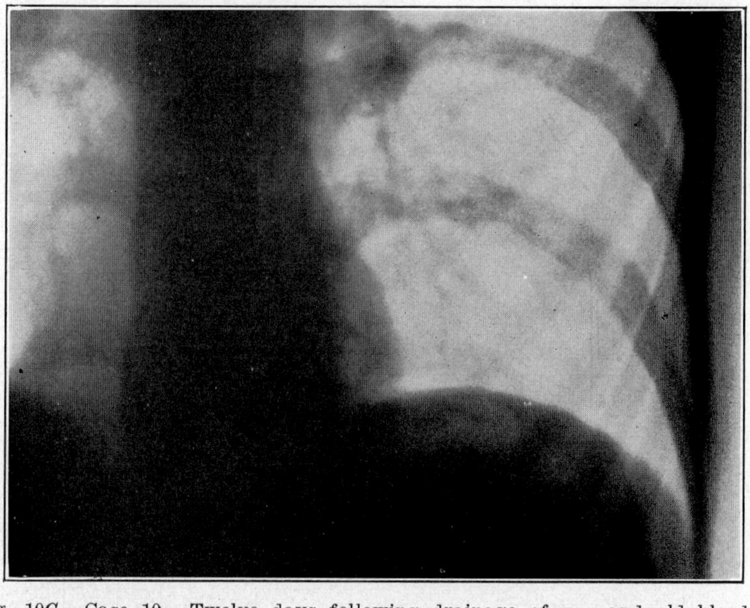

Fig. 10*C*.—Case 10. Twelve days following drainage of pus and old blood from lesser peritoneal cavity. Note complete clearing. There is now no evidence of obliteration of the costophrenic sinus or evidence of fluid.

of a depressed leaf on the opposite side. Although these signs most often represent the presence of infection, direct and indirect trauma also have been known to immobilize the diaphragm. The next sign, the first pulmonary sign, is a fuzziness of the upper surface of the diaphragm on the affected side (Cases 4 and 10). This appears as the infection passes upward through the diaphragm producing an adhesive pleuritis. This must not be confused with concentration of linear markings due to the elevated leaf of the diaphragm. Later, there is a slow gradual accumulation of exudate, which early partially and later completely obliterates the base of the lung field and frequently presents a fairly well-defined horizontal upper margin as time goes on (Cases 1, 3, 6 and in Fig. 11). Occasionally an irregular semitransparent shadow is seen which outlines a portion of a fissure (Case 2). This occurs as the exudate tends to separate the surfaces of the pleurae. The exudate, as a rule, is sealed off from a portion if not all of the diaphragmatic pleural space of the lower lobe for several days, often for weeks, during which time the exudate in neighboring portions of the pleural cavity is not large in amount. Only occasionally does the fluid become sufficient in amount to separate the visceral and costal pleurae over a wide area. Rarely do the visceral and diaphragmatic pleurae separate without showing signs of neighboring pleural adhesions (Case 7). The normal

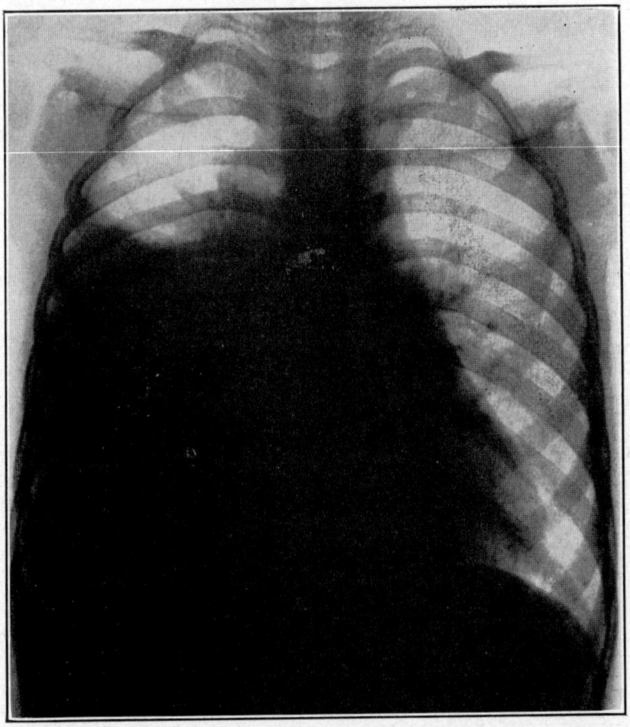

Fig. 11.—Additional case. Subphrenic abscess showing marked tendency to maintain a horizontal upper margin to the basal shadow, even when fluid is large in amount. This disappeared after subphrenic drainage.

relationship maintained at the base is the result of the adhesive quality of the exudate early, and local induration and fibrous adhesions later.

The changes so far described seem to represent the general trend in this disease in children. They have been present in all of our cases of transphrenic infection observed early. In extremely far-advanced or long-standing progressive cases, the pleural exudate may finally become large in amount and the lung field obliterated to a high degree (Fig. 11), but even here there is a noticeable tendency for the basal shadow to maintain a horizontal upper margin in the absence of pneumothorax, and an almost normal relationship at the base. The slow accumulation of exudate and tendency to seal off the base of the pleural cavity is an outstanding characteristic of transphrenic infection. When the fluid is large in amount, the differentiation from empyema, following primary pulmonary disease, is difficult or impossible from a single x-ray examination. However, the type of infection common in these cases seems to bring about considerable shrinking of the lung, and consequently there is less contralateral displacement of the mediastinal structures than in the usual empyema. The early, almost universal, adherence of the lung to the diaphragm also aids in preventing displacement. Often an overexposed film will show evidence of air in the lower lobe otherwise obscured by the fluid and reveal the base of the lung contacting the diaphragm as normally, or it may reveal the dense triangular shadow[7] caused by the collapsed lower lobe (Cases 9 and 10). These findings are less often found following the type of primary infection of the lung ordinarily confused in the diagnosis of subphrenic abscess. In empyema following pneumonia, there is nearly always retraction of the lung base from a portion of the diaphragm.

Pneumonitis is occasionally present above the diaphragmatic pleuritis or basal exudate (Case 7). This is seen as a secondary faint shadow which seems to follow the general course of the bronchi, gradually extending toward the hilus. These signs are often seen just preceding the development of a bronchial fistula, and one cannot easily differentiate pneumonitis from a small tonguelike shadow of fluid in the fissure.

When a fistula develops, spontaneous clearing may take place (Fig. 7*B*), but often it persists over a long period and a rest cavity remains (Fig. 5). The latter is seen as a partially filled air and fluid cavity or as a local pneumothorax (Case 7). Pus is formed constantly, and even though a bronchial fistula may drain the cavity, healing does not readily occur because of a constant supply of infection filtering up through the diaphragm. In addition, there is soon a complicating infection and accumulation of secretion from the bronchial tree. Early healing of the bronchial fistula, frequently met with in this disease, seems to depend mostly upon early clearing of the source of the infection beneath the diaphragm, possibly slightly to the ability of the neighboring lung to expand and other local factors which keep the cavity from becoming large and remaining so over a long period. The greater tendency for a rest cavity to form in this disease than in primary pulmonary disease seems to be due to the marked trend to firm pleural adhesions and constant peripheral invasion of the infection into the lung. The latter produces thick secretions in the smaller bronchi, occluding them and leading to atelectasis. Atelectasis, in decreasing the volume of the involved portion of the lung, prevents the re-expansion necessary to fill in the local pneumothorax. Actually atelectasis tends to increase the size of the cavity. The tendency toward basal infiltration and shrinking of the lung was evident throughout this study. Extensive atelectasis, markedly shrinking the lower lobe, occurred in two of these cases (Cases 9 and 10).

After fairly firm diaphragmatic adhesions have been formed, infrequently there is development of a loculation between portions of the visceral and diaphragmatic pleura. This may be seen as a shadow of increased density just above the diaphragm (Fig. 7*A*), often with a convex upper border which may be erroneously taken for the diaphragm. Later the exudate may break through into other portions of the pleural space or rupture and drain through a bronchus. The cavity, thus formed, may refill with air (Fig. 7*B*) and become a local positive pressure pneumothorax (Fig. 7*C*).

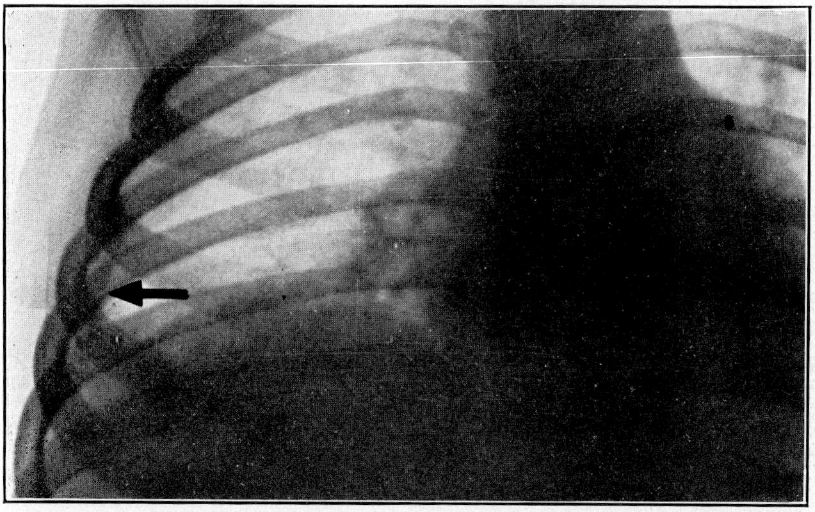

Fig. 12.—R. S. Evidence of slight separation of the visceral and costal pleura (arrow). The appearance remained unchanged over a period of six weeks. In the interim a laparotomy failed to disclose evidence of infection below the liver. Later 8 ounces of pus was drained transpleurally from the sulcus between the right leaf of the diaphragm and the liver. Rapid recovery.

The preceding description has dealt mainly with pulmonary signs or signs noted above the diaphragm on regular chest roentgenograms. They are the signs presented by all cases to a varying degree in which infection passes upward through the diaphragm, i.e., the signs of pulmonary complications. While these have been universal, in approximately one-half of the patients, there are also x-ray signs below the diaphragm, primary signs, which may make the diagnosis unassisted or aid greatly in making the diagnosis of an intraperitoneal abscess. These shadows are caused by the contents of the abscess or by displacement of the neighboring structures by the abscess or adhesions. If gas is present in the abscess, it is usually recognizable because of its contrast in density and unchanged appearance at successive x-ray examinations. The ''typical'' x-ray finding of subphrenic abscess, which has been often described, is "gas and fluid level" beneath the diaphragm (Cases 1 and 2). The presence of these changes just beneath the right leaf of the diaphragm, generally thought not to exist except in an abscess, unfortunately are present in only approximately one-fourth of the children known to have this disease. Frequently the gas in the stomach and intestine delineates to quite a dependable degree a fluid-containing abscess. This is noted on the left when a collection of pus separates the fundus of the stomach from the diaphragm (Case 7). It is also observed frequently on the right because of the displacement mesially or downward of the colon or small intestine. By means of a careful study of abdominal roentgenograms made with the patient in different

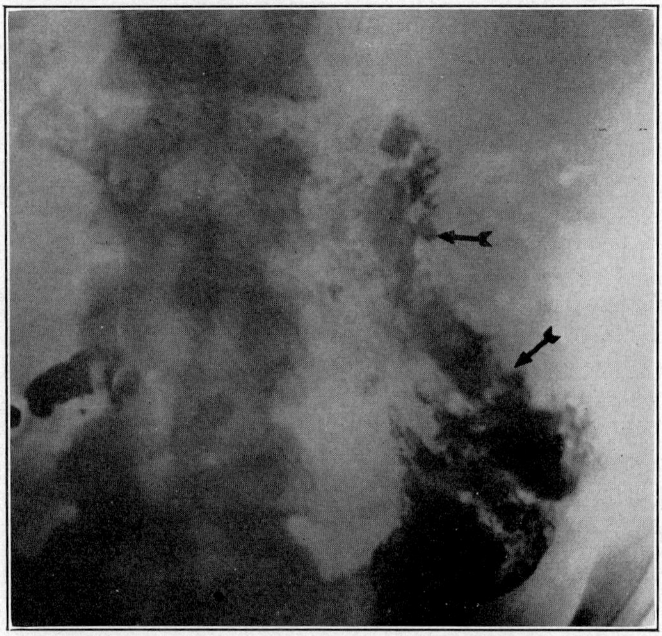

Fig. 13.—Case illustrating mesial displacement of the colon by intraperitoneal abscess. A preliminary chest roentgenogram showed a small collection of fluid at the base of the lung on the affected right side and suggested the presence of subphrenic abscess. The patient was treated conservatively without surgery and made an uneventful recovery. (Patient of Dr. George Fitzgerald of St. Joseph's Hospital.)

positions, with or without the aid of barium, the location of loculations and intercommunicating pockets of pus can often be determined. This aids greatly in making the diagnosis in late cases, in which the pulmonary signs are likely to predominate if not entirely overshadow abdominal signs. In one instance we were aided in a puzzling case by an intravenous pyelogram, which revealed the displacement of the right ureter by an appendiceal abscess. In another the barium entered a fixed segment of colon within the abscess with great difficulty (Fig. 13).

Only one patient in six has left-sided subphrenic abscess, according to reports of a large number of cases in the literature. However, in our experience approximately one-third have been left-sided. These have shown a marked tendency to heal without drainage. Because of spontaneous healing it would seem that a higher percentage of left-sided cases exist than the literature would indicate, especially if penetrating ulcers of the stomach in adults are carefully studied.[8] A more or less unusual and circumscribed dense shadow in the sulcus between the fundus of the stomach and the left leaf of the diaphragm, associated with the evidence of a diaphragmatic plastic pleuritis, should strongly suggest a left-sided subphrenic abscess. Multiple pockets may communicate with each other and the size of one density may decrease as the fluid escapes into the other by change in position or by change in pressure (Fig. 8). If the shadow is at all inconstant and there is doubt about the diaphragmatic pleurisy, a barium enema or barium meal may be necessary to rule out the presence of loops of bowel, but often one gets a clue from a single film of the abdomen. Gas, associated with fluid level, has not been seen, as a rule, on the left as it has been on the right. If present, it is not so readily differentiated from intestinal patterns.

COMMENT

Ireland,[2] recently in writing about subphrenic abscess said, "There are few diseases which cause more uncertainty in the diagnosis," and the late Dr. Beye,[9] in an early excellent description of this disease, made the observation that "subphrenic abscess is seldom stumbled onto as a diagnostic accident." The diagnosis of subphrenic abscess has been most confusing in the past, and, while now it is generally recognized in early postoperative cases, the vague clinical signs still cause mistaken diagnoses in small hidden perforations of viscera and in extremely late postoperative cases, especially in children, if the patient is being seen for the first time. The fuller use of the x-ray, it seems, is largely responsible for the improvement in diagnosis. One can prophesy that regular chest roentgenograms taken at periods of a few days in a suspicious case will not only decrease still further the diagnostic errors, but will prove of great assistance in the choice of treatment and the time of administering such treatment.

Certain clinical observations should be emphasized in considering this disease. One of these is the frequently long period between an initial abdominal ailment and the later pulmonary signs. The two conditions are prone to be considered in no way related to each other. A history of an earlier attack of appendicitis, with or without operation, is often an important lead in the consideration of subphrenic abscess. Also the fetid or mousey odor of the sputum of a child, with fairly sudden onset of a productive cough, should cause subphrenic abscess to be considered.[9] Often the case is not seen until secondary pulmonary symptoms are well established, and bronchiectasis or lung abscess is mistakenly thought to exist. Also the associated finding of x-ray signs suggesting pleuritis or fluid immediately above the diaphragm, in the absence of earlier acute pulmonary symptoms and in the presence of definite local or vague abdominal signs, should arouse suspicion of an existing loculation beneath the diaphragm.

Because of the possibility of eventration of the diaphragm, one author[10] has recently suggested that the x-ray diagnosis of subphrenic abscess should possibly be limited to cases showing a gas dome and fluid level beneath the diaphragm. Eventration is such a rare condition that ordinarily it should not complicate the diagnosis of transphrenic infection. There is no evidence of diaphragmatic pleurisy or of exudate above the unusually elevated leaf of the diaphragm, and usually clinical signs do not suggest the presence of an infection.

Janz[8] has recently been quoted as saying that "the existence of a basal pleurisy on the same side renders the roentgenologic differentiation impossible." On the contrary, a primary basal pleuritis should always arouse suspicion of a transphrenic infection, especially if associated with previous or present abdominal symptoms. While pleurisy may rapidly follow a pyogenic pneumonic process, lung tissue adjacent to the diaphragm is not the common site of an invisible focus of consolidation producing a diaphragmatic pleuritis. The absence of a latent basal pulmonary shadow in the presence of elevation of a relatively fixed diaphragm indicates the absence of infection directly beneath the diaphragm and favors the presence of a loculation at some distance from the diaphragm.

Early in the disease the x-ray evidence of subphrenic and perinephritic abscess is often similar, as fixation of the diaphragm may be the only visible sign. Later the signs of transphrenic infection favor subphrenic abscess. I have seen only one case of transphrenic infection in a perinephritic abscess and believe it to be unusually rare. Likewise, an intraperitoneal infection is infrequently a complication of perinephritic abscess. In my experience the intestines have not been matted together, and the barium-filled intestines could be displaced to either side of the retrocolic mass at fluoroscopy in perinephritic abscess. The upward direction of flow in the lymphatics seems to account for pulmonary complications.

The differentiation between an early tuberculous effusion and an early transphrenic infection is most difficult and may be impossible to determine from x-ray evidence alone. However, abdominal signs, tendency to fixation of the diaphragm, and negative tuberculin tests support a transphrenic infection. The early changes in the pleura following tuberculosis rarely fix the diaphragm, and often other characteristic signs of phthisis are present. The temperature is usually higher and more irregular and symptoms more pronounced in subphrenic infection.

Hemorrhage into the pleural cavity from trauma to the thoracic wall can usually be readily differentiated from transphrenic infection, as there are almost immediately signs of fluid free in the pleural cavity and no unusual tendency for the base of the lung to maintain its normal relationship with the diaphragm. The peripheral portion of the base of the lung is displaced from the costophrenic sinus.

During this study, three cases of rapid involvement of the pleural cavity were encountered following acute abdominal symptoms. All were rapidly fatal within a few days. All came to necropsy where the hemolytic streptococcus was found scattered throughout all tissues, these findings favoring a diagnosis of septicemia rather than subphrenic abscess, although the exudate appeared older below the diaphragm than above, and histologic sections of the diaphragm suggested the passage upward of the infection.

A word of caution must be given against making a diagnosis from x-ray evidence alone. While strongly suggestive signs may be present at the first x-ray examination, careful watching at subsequent examinations and close correlation with the history and physical findings should be made before subphrenic drainage is undertaken.

The x-ray signs of subphrenic abscess in young children are not materially different from those seen in adults. Adults are prone to have a perforated viscus, which produces quite characteristic symptoms of a peritonitis. Loculations, in both children and adults, on the right side most often follow a rupture of the appendix. Those on the left side in adults, as a rule, follow a perforation of a gastric ulcer. Although one case (Case 9) has been included in this report, gastric and duodenal ulcers are generally rare in children. Left-sided subphrenic abscess seems to occur more often in children than in adults following a ruptured appendix. A serious liver abscess seems to be less frequently present in children, while minute perforations of the intestines, following diarrhea, intussusceptions, and diverticulitis (Meckel's), are more frequent. The site of the perforation is more likely to vary greatly in children, and the infection contacts the diaphragm more often. The difficulty experienced in obtaining subjective signs in infants and young children and frequently the absence of rigidity in the presence of a peritonitis make the clinical diagnosis more difficult. Judging from reports in the literature and my own experience, I find spontaneous healing occurs more often in children than in adults. It is possible that some of the cases thought to be empyema following primary pulmonary disease, in which only the pleural cavity was drained, really cleared because of spontaneous healing of the infection in the abdomen.

The lack of increasing x-ray signs is not a reliable criterion upon which to base an opinion of arrested progress of this disease, but the disappearance of x-ray signs has gone strikingly hand in hand with clinical improvement and recovery. The absence of clearly defined x-ray signs does not rule out a subphrenic abscess, but the abscess that does not eventually show x-ray signs in children is the exception and not the rule.

Watchful waiting for several days, sometimes for weeks, until a clearly defined loculation is demonstrable by the x-ray, seems to be the proper treatment in a large number of cases. If, for any reason, moderate delay, which has seemed to aid all of our cases, should seem hazardous in the absence of roentgenologic signs at the base of the lung, a subpleural, rather than transpleural, approach should be anticipated. The persistent fixation of the diaphragm, with no evidence of infection passing upward, has indicated most often a lesion removed from the diaphragm, such as perinephritic abscess, subhepatic abscess, rarely liver abscess or trauma temporarily decreasing the excursion of the diaphragm, still more rarely the presence of a neoplasm or hematoma. All cases of subphrenic abscess in the present group had an average of eight x-ray examinations before surgical drainage, although the diagnosis was often quite definite at the time of the first examination.

In this group the type of surgical attack was decided upon only after a thorough roentgenographic study. An attempt was made to go directly to the abscess, after signs of basal pleurisy had been present for several days or weeks. A one- or two-stage transpleural approach was the usual procedure. A tube was inserted directly through the costophrenic sinus and diaphragm following a primary needle puncture. When there was evidence of separation of the costal and visceral pleurae, or no local shadow on the roentgenograms suggesting the presence of well-formed adhesions, a two-stage operation was chosen. Marsupialization preceded the second stage by a period of a few days. Both types of operations were successful in draining the abscess in all but one case. In this instance rapid complete absorption of the pleural exudate had occurred just preceding the operation. Only one patient (Case 9) failed to recover. One case of bronchial fistula (Case 7) cleared spontaneously. Another patient (Case 5) has had three thoracoplasties in an attempt to close a long-standing rest cavity.

If the pleural cavity only is drained, the period of convalescence is often unusually long. I have observed this in adults, as well as in children. The drainage of the pleural cavity above apparently has little effect, if any, upon the course of the abscess beneath the diaphragm. Fistula formation and chronic rest cavities seem to be more common complications in the neglected cases of several months' duration than in empyema following primary pulmonary disease.

SUMMARY

Ten cases of subphrenic abscess in children are reported in detail, illustrations of three additional cases are included. The x-ray examination is an important adjunct to the history and clinical findings and seldom fails to offer important evidence in this disease, often making the diagnosis almost singlehanded. Fixation of the diaphragm is the earliest roentgenographic sign, the evidence of diaphragmatic pleurisy

TABLE I

CASE	AGE	SEX	SIDE	SOURCE OF INFECTION*	"GAS AND FLUID LEVEL" IN ABSCESS	X-RAY SIGNS OF BASAL PLEURITIS OR FLUID	SURGICAL DRAINAGE OF SUBPHRENIC ABSCESS	TYPE OF DRAINAGE	CONVALESCENT PERIOD
1	9 yr.	F	R	Unknown, appendicitis? 18 mo. earlier	Yes	Yes	18 mo. after first abdominal symptom	Transpleural diaphragmatic	Well after 9 months
2	16 mo.	M	R	Unknown, diarrhea for 3 days	Yes	Yes	12 days after first abdominal symptom	Transpleural diaphragmatic	Well after 40 days
3	12 yr.	F	R	Ruptured appendix	No	Yes	32 days after first operation	Transpleural diaphragmatic	Well after 66 days
4	5 yr.	F	R	Appendicitis 7 days	No	Yes	14 days after first operation	Transpleural diaphragmatic	Well after 33 days
5	10 yr.	M	R	Unknown, pain in abdomen for 1 yr. (amebic dysentery)	No	Yes	2 years after first abdominal operation	Transpleural	Well after 1 year. Fistula right base still open (2½ years)
6	8 yr.	F	R	Peritonitis	No	Yes	None	Spontaneous absorption	Well after 5 weeks
7	12 yr.	F	L	Ruptured appendix	No	Yes	None	Spontaneous absorption and through bronchus	Well after 6 months. Fistula over McBurney's Point 9 months
8	5 yr.	M	L	Unknown, bacillary dysentery	No	Yes	None	Spontaneous absorption	Well after 21 days
9	2 yr.	F	L	Perforated gastric ulcer	No	Yes	12 days after first operation	Midline abdominal	Died 24 hours after second operation
10	12 yr.	M	L	Peritonitis following trauma	No	Yes (4th day)	Third week	Left subdiaphragmatic	Well after 5 weeks
Totals		4 M 6 F	6 R 4 L		2 Yes 8 No				1 died 8 perfectly well 1 has surface fistula but otherwise in excellent health

*The exact source of infection remains unknown in 6 cases; evidence of peritonitis was present at operation in 7 cases; 3 cases that cleared spontaneously were thought clinically to have had a definite peritonitis.

next, then the signs of a small accumulation of fluid which tends to remain small in amount, and later, even in neglected cases with extensive empyema, the evidence of an almost normal contact of the visceral and diaphragmatic pleurae (in overexposed films). The x-ray signs, which are almost pathognomonic of this disease, are the shadows of "gas and fluid level" beneath the right leaf of the diaphragm. However, these latter signs were present in only one-fourth of this group of children. The x-ray signs of pneumonitis and collapse of the lower lobe are occasionally associated findings as the infection invades or surrounds the lung tissue. A local basal pneumothorax is prone to follow a bronchial fistula, with or without spontaneous healing. A rest cavity is more common than in primary pulmonary disease. The majority of cases follow appendicitis. Small perforations in other viscera are thought to account for most left-sided cases. These have a greater tendency to heal spontaneously than right-sided cases. Waiting for definite x-ray signs of a loculation before establishing drainage seems to be judicious treatment.

CONCLUSIONS

1. The so-called characteristic signs of "gas and fluid level" are infrequently seen in subphrenic abscess in children.

2. There is frequently a long period between the first abdominal symptom and the first pulmonary sign, often with apparent return of health in the interim.

3. Diarrhea and appendicitis often precede subphrenic abscess in children. Gastric and duodenal ulcers are rarely an etiological factor.

4. The sudden onset of pulmonary symptoms and the coughing up of "mousey-smelling" sputum should arouse suspicions of a subphrenic abscess.

5. Early cementing of the base of the lung to the diaphragm, sealing off a portion of the pleural space, is a characteristic of subphrenic abscess.

6. Infection after contacting the under surface of the diaphragm will usually show x-ray evidence of pleuritis or a small quantity of fluid just above the diaphragm within four or five days.

7. Left-sided involvement may follow appendicitis but more frequently follows perforation of other viscera.

8. The lack of increasing pulmonary x-ray signs is not a dependable criterion upon which to base prognosis, but the disappearance of pulmonary signs occurs rapidly following the disappearance of the source of infection in the abdomen.

9. Spontaneous recovery without drainage occurred in one-third of the cases here reported.

10. Few diseases require more careful correlation of clinical and roentgen signs for correct diagnosis and for the choice of proper treatment.

11. The presence of a diaphragmatic pleurisy which arises in the course of a vague or definite abdominal complaint should arouse suspicion that a transphrenic infection is present. It is the most constant and, therefore, the most useful roentgenologic sign in the diagnosis of subphrenic abscess in children.

REFERENCES

1. Montgomery, A. H.: Brennemann's Practice of Pediatrics, Chap. 6, Vol. 3, Hagerstown, Md., 1937, W. F. Prior Company, Inc.
2. Ireland, J.: Surg., Gynec. & Obst. **159**: 789, 1934.
3. LeWald, L. T.: Arch. Surg. **10**: 544, 1925.
4. Gleick, M.: Arch. Pediat. **43**: 732, 1926.
5. Pancoast, H. K.: Am. J. Roentgenol. **16**: 303, 1926.
6. Gatewood: Am. J. M. Sc. **180**: 398, 1930.
7. Anspach, W. E.: Am. J. Dis. Child. **47**: 1011, 1934.
8. Janz, G.: Arch. f. klin Chir. **178**: 482, 1933.
9. Beye, R. H.: J. Thoracic Surg. **1**: 655, 1932.
10. Hailes, W. A.: Australian & New Zealand J. Surg. **4**: 3, 1934.

Additional References

11. Bogart, L. M.: Am. J. Surg. **26**: 467, 1934.
12. Cabot: New England J. Med. 227, 1934.
13. Cahen, J., and Cogniaux, F.: J. de chir. et ann. Soc. belge de chir. **33-31**: 365, 1934.
14. De Lario, A. J.: Am. J. Roentgenol. **31**: 177, 1934.
15. Doherty, W. D., and Rowlands, R. P.: Brit. M. J. **1**: 168, 1931.
16. Faranda, G.: Rinasc. med. **9**: 441, 1932.
17. Harrington, S. W.: S. Clin. North America **14**: 625, 1934.
18. Heckmann, K., and Altenburger, E.: München. med. Wchnschr. **82**: 1800, 1935.
19. Harper, F. R., and Thomas, C. A.: J. A. M. A. **105**: 1267, 1935.
20. Hodges, F. M.: J. A. M. A. **80**: 1053, 1923.
21. Lemoine, G.: J. de chir. et ann. Soc. belge de chir. **31-29**: 181-189, 1932.
22. Marille, J., and Lacroix, P.: J. de chir. et ann. Soc. belge de chir. **33-31**: 425-430, 1934.
23. Palma, R.: Riforma med. **51**: 909, 1935.
24. Russell, T. H.: Ann. Surg. **90**: 238, 1929.
25. Sauret, C.: Ann. de Hosp. de Santa Creu i Sant Pau **8**: 171, 1934.
26. Schwartz, J.: Arch. Surg. **20**: 317, 1930.
27. Sperling, R.: Ztschr. f. Kinderh. **39**: 122, 1925.
28. Stein, J. L., and Wolfson, W. L.: Am. J. Dis. Child. **48**: 580, 1934.
29. Von Szacsray, I.: Beitr. z. klin. Chir. **160**: 591, 1934.
30. Vaslenko, L. D.: Soret, Klin. **19**: 213, 1933.
31. Van der Muilen. Nederl. tijdschr. v. geneesk. **78**: 278, 1934.
32. Weasler and Jackes: Clinical Roentgenology of Diseases of the Chest, pp. 489-499, Troy, N. Y., 1923, Southworth Co.

PNEUMATOSIS OF THE INTESTINE IN INFANCY

Thomas W. Botsford, M.D., and Cecil Krakower, M.D.
Boston, Massachusetts

PNEUMATOSIS of the intestine is considered to be a rare pathologic condition. It was first clearly described in a human by Bang[1] in 1876. With the advent of abdominal surgery in the latter part of the nineteenth century, instances of this disease noted at operation and post mortem have steadily been reported up to the present. Turnure[2] in 1913 collected 50 cases; Mills[3] in 1925, 100 cases; and Memmi[4] in 1934 brought the total to 154. Twenty-one additional cases, not included in the above, have been found. These comprise reports by Silverstone,[5] Lamont,[6] Sawada,[7] Moore,[8] Tung and Ngai,[9] Pybus,[10] Kemal,[11] Nimet,[12] Bsteh,[13] and Englund and Wahlgren.[14] Of these 171 cases, there have been only 5 authentic cases in childhood and infancy. Schnyder[15] in 1917 observed gas cysts in the intestinal lymphatics, mesentery, and mesenteric glands in a 5-year-old child who died of diphtheria. Moore[8] in 1929 reported four cases in infants of 2 weeks to 14 months of age. Of the six instances that we are reporting, five were observed during the period of approximately one year.

CASE REPORTS

Case 1.—(A-26-15.) This 4-week-old, white, premature male infant was brought to the hospital because of failure to gain in weight. Subsequently he developed attacks of cyanosis and physical signs of pneumonia. He died two weeks after entry.

Necropsy was performed six hours post mortem. The anatomic diagnoses were acute suppurative bronchopneumonia, acute bronchial lymphadenitis, and pneumatosis of the colon.

Gross Examination.—The upper portion of the ileum was markedly injected, but there were no areas of ulceration. In the descending colon there were many small air blebs, varying from 1 to 3 mm. in diameter. The mucosa was mildly injected in this portion of the large bowel.

Microscopic Examination.—*Jejunum:* There was intense vascular congestion throughout the mucosa. The glandular lumina were frequently dilated but free of inspissated mucoid contents. Goblet cells were moderately in excess. There was striking diminution in the number of mitoses. The tunica propria was cellular with excessive numbers of polymorphonuclear leucocytes, particularly at the tips of villi. The submucosal blood vessels were greatly dilated and congested. There were no lymphoid aggregates. The serosa was edematous. There were dilated submucosal lymphatics.

Ileum: The sections were similar to the jejunum with the exception that there was somewhat less polymorphonuclear cell infiltration in the tunica propria of the mucosa. There were dilated lymphatics in the submucosa.

Colon: The mucosa was moderately thinned and compressed. There was fairly marked vascular congestion throughout the tunica propria. The glands assumed

From the Department of Pathology, the Children's Hospital.

varied appearances. In instances their lumina were dilated, containing inspissated mucus or necrotic cellular elements. The lining cells were in places flattened and atrophic. Elsewhere, the epithelial cells were tall but laterally flattened with variable amounts of mucus, but practically never of the full goblet type with flattened basal nucleus. Mitoses in glandular epitheliums were relatively infrequent. There were occasional mucosal gas cysts. The muscularis mucosae was thinned, more markedly so where forming the wall of a distended submucosal gas cyst. There were occasional small submucosal lymphoid nodules. The whole of the submucosa otherwise was replaced by numerous gas cysts. These possessed no specific endothelial lining. There were no giant cells. There were dilated perivascular lymphatics in the muscular and serosal coats.

CASE 2.—(A-36-19.) This 9-month-old white male infant was readmitted because of persistent edema and an upper respiratory infection. Three months previously a diagnosis of nephrosis had been made at his first admission. There had been no improvement in his condition in the interim. For the first week during this second admission, he did fairly well. Vomiting and diarrhea then supervened. He died a week later.

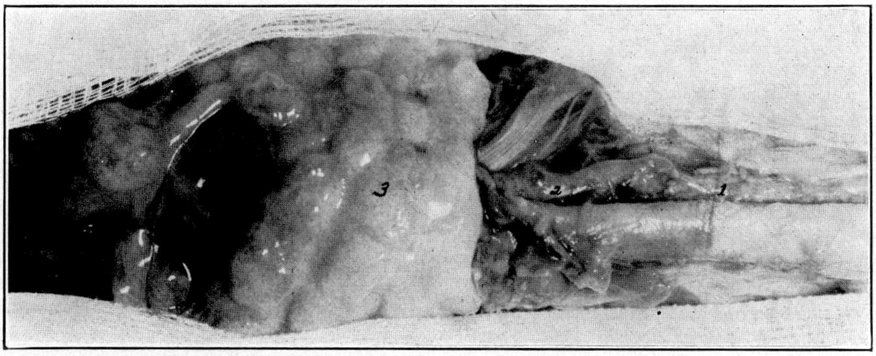

Fig. 1.—Case 2. *1,* Thoracic duct; *2,* cisterna chyli; *3,* mesenteric lymph nodes. Note marked emphysema of lymph nodes and distention of cisterna chyli and thoracic duct with gas.

Necropsy was performed one hour post mortem. The anatomic diagnoses were subacute glomerulonephritis; bronchopneumonia with interstitial emphysema; nonobstructive biliary cirrhosis (mild); acute otitis media, bilateral; acute mesenteric lymphadenitis; pneumatosis of ileum, ascending and pelvic colons, mesenteric lymph nodes, cisterna chyli, and thoracic duct.

Gross Examination.—The pharyngeal mucosa was reddened and thickened. The esophagus and stomach were not remarkable. The jejunum was distended with gas, and there were occasional areas of emphysematosis over the mucosal aspect. The entire inner surface of the ileum was a mass of frothy-appearing gas cysts, distributed irregularly toward the ileocecal valve. None of these cysts contained fluid. There were no frank areas of ulceration. The mucosal surface of the intestine, particularly in the emphysematous regions, had a dry granular and bright pinkish appearance. The mucosal aspect of the cecum, descending, and pelvic colon was likewise emphysematous. The colon was distended with gas. The mesenteric lymph nodes were enlarged and replaced in many instances by numerous gas cysts. The cisterna chyli and the proximal half of the thoracic duct were distended with gas. There was, however, no evidence of air embolism.

Microscopic Examination.—Esophagus and stomach were normal.

Duodenum: The tunica propria was cellular but not exceptionally vascular. The glandular lumina were dilated, with occasionally low and atrophic epithelium. There were diminished numbers of mucous-secreting cells. There were moderately frequent mitoses. Brunner's glands were normal.

Jejunum and Ileum: The mucosa was variably thinned. There was glandular atrophy both in areas overlying cysts as well as in uninvolved zones. The glandular lumina were dilated and frequently contained inspissated mucus, desquamated epithelial cells, occasional polymorphonuclear leucocytes, and wandering cells. The epithelial cells were to a varied degree atrophic, and occasionally necrotic. Goblet cells and the varied phases of pre- or postsecretory mucous cells were rare. There were fairly frequent mitoses. The stroma was quite markedly hyperemic and cellular. There were increased numbers of polymorphonuclear leucocytes and phagocytic monocytes, particularly close to the surface of villar folds and interglandular areas. In the involved areas, there were occasional mucosal gas cysts. The muscularis mucosae was greatly thinned. There were numerous cysts that distended the submucosa. These infrequently appeared to have an endothelial-like lining; usually they were bordered by collagen alone. There were no giant cells. The adjoining stroma was often edematous and cellular, with rare polymorphonuclear leucocytes and more frequent monocytes, lymphocytes, and plasma cells. There were flattened bands of lymphoid tissue bordering the cysts in juxtaposition to the muscularis mucosae. Nerve cells and fibers were stretched and distorted within the involved portions of submucosa. There were dilated submucosal lymphatics, containing lymphocytes and polymorphonuclear leucocytes in instances. There was evidence of dissection of gas through the muscular coat into the serosa along the perivascular lymphatics, where endothelial lining membranes were clearly definable. The serosa was generally thin, but there were instances where it was thickened, edematous, infiltrated by round cells, and contained occasional gas cysts.

Mesenteric Glands: The peripheral lymphatics were dilated. The gas cysts were diffusely disseminated throughout the lymph nodes. There was apparent lymphoid depletion with accentuation of the reticular stroma and perivascular fibrosis. The sinusoids revealed endothelial hyperplasia and contain lymphocytes and polymorphonuclear leucocytes.

CASE 3.—(A-36-34.) This 7-month-old white male infant was admitted to the hospital for cough and fever of one week's duration. He was cyanotic and presented signs of patchy pneumonia. Two weeks before death he developed persistent vomiting and diarrhea. The patient died five weeks after entry.

Necropsy was performed four hours post mortem. The anatomic diagnoses were bilateral bronchopneumonia; acute bilateral otitis media; cerebral edema; fatty infiltration of the liver; pneumatosis of ileum and mesenteric lymph nodes; and acute mesenteric lymphadenitis.

Gross Examination.—About 145 cm. from the ileocecal valve there was a raised irregular, frothylike area of emphysematosis, measuring 1.5 by 0.5 cm. Proximal to this area, and continuous with it, there was a column of air terminating in an apical point, where there was seen to be a small pin-point aperture. The appearance of the whole lesion suggested forceful injection of air through a very narrow mucosal aperture which dissected its way in a straight but ever broadening path until it finally broke up into a number of large submucosal cysts. In other areas throughout the length of the small intestine there was diffuse reddening but no ulceration. The colon presented a moderately reddened but nonulcerated mucosa.

Microscopic Examination.—Esophagus: There were small recent ulcers with underlying acute inflammation.

Stomach: There was cystic dilatation of some of the glands.

Jejunum and Ileum: In sections of uninvolved portions of the jejunum and ileum there were evident mucosal changes. These were characterized by thinning in some instances, hyperemia in all instances, broadening and flattening of the villi and interglandular areas, and increased cellularity and fairly marked polymorphonuclear leucocytic infiltration, particularly toward the surface. The glandular lumina were dilated and contained inspissated secretion and cellular debris in some areas. Occasionally there was quite marked atrophy of the glandular epithelium with few goblet cells. In some sections there were fairly abundant, incompletely filled, mucous-containing cells. There was decreased mitotic activity. There was very little lymphoid tissue in the submucosa. There were occasional dilated submucosal lymphatics.

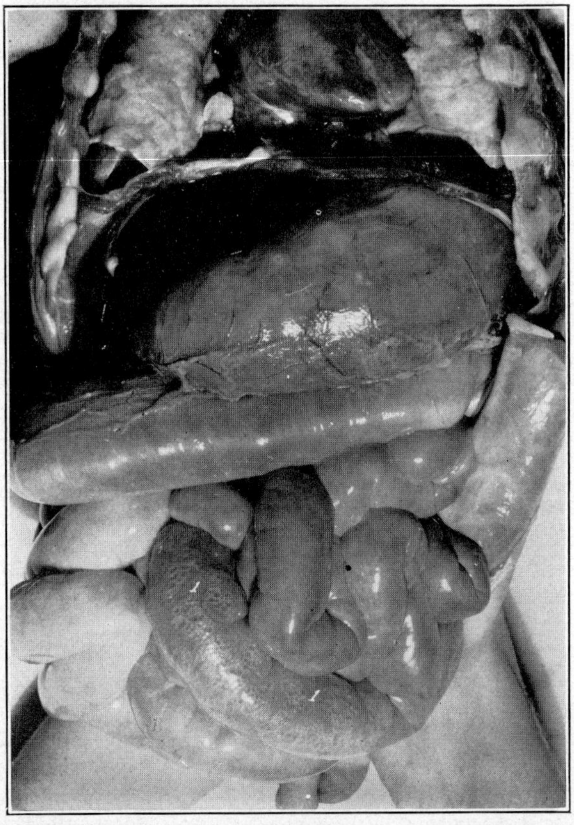

Fig. 2.—Case 4. Pneumatosis of loop of jejunum, *1*.

In the involved portions of the intestine the gas cysts were practically confined to the submucosa. In areas they appeared to be lined by endothelial cells. There were no giant cells, but in a few areas some polymorphonuclear leucocytes and monocytes were in apposition to the inner cyst wall. In the adjoining stroma there were occasional areas with apparent increase in fibroblasts and rarely some polymorphonuclear reaction.

Mesenteric Lymph Nodes: There were several small gas cysts. The peripheral and medullary sinusoids were widened and contained many polymorphonuclear leucocytes and proliferated endothelial cells. There was relative depletion of lymphoid tissue.

CASE 4.—(A-36-56.) At 2½ months of age this male child was admitted to the hospital for jaundice of two weeks' duration. There were no unusual symptoms accompanying the onset of jaundice. Physical examination revealed a jaundiced infant with liver palpable 3 cm. below the costal margin. On the twelfth hospital day he developed diarrhea and vomiting. The diarrhea persisted until the time of death on the twenty-sixth hospital day.

Necropsy was performed four and one-half hours post mortem. The anatomic diagnoses were nonobstructive biliary cirrhosis; pulmonary congestion; pneumatosis of jejunum and mesenteric lymph nodes; acute mesenteric lymphadenitis; rickets, mild; and scurvy, mild.

Gross Examination.—Pharynx and esophagus were not remarkable. The stomach was distended with gas. There was pneumatosis of the jejunum, extending 40 cm. from the pylorus for a distance caudad of 30 cm. The cysts were small, averaging 0.3 to 0.5 cm. and were grouped in clusters. There were no areas of ulceration. The mucosa of the small and large intestine elsewhere was pinkish gray.

Microscopic Examination.—*Esophagus and stomach* were normal.

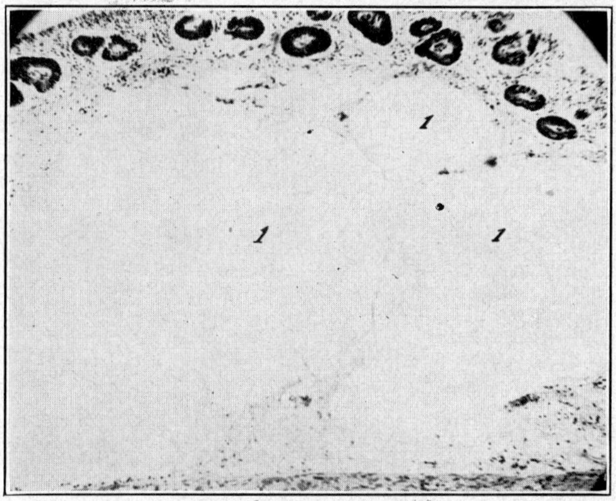

Fig. 3.—Case 4. Microscopic section of jejunum with emphysema. *1.* Note compression and thinning of mucosa with glandular dilatation and epithelial desquamation.

Duodenum: There was moderate mucosal vascular congestion. The glandular lumina were dilated. The epithelium was moderately reduced in height, distinctly atrophic, and almost flattened in instances. There were diminished numbers of complete goblet cells and increased numbers of polymorphonuclear leucocytes in areas.

Jejunum (nonemphysematous portion): There was quite marked mucosal vascular congestion, particularly in the inner third. There was considerable polymorphonuclear leucocytic infiltration, especially close to the surface and within the villi. The reticular stroma was loose and edematous. Whereas there was probably some increase in the spacing between glandular bases, the villi and intervillar areas appeared thick and cellular. The glands were irregularly tortuous. The lumina were frequently mildly dilated, and a few contained epithelial debris and infrequent polymorphonuclear leucocytes. The epithelium in the more dilated glands was low and of irregular shape. There were rare goblet cells, but many with small amounts of mucus of nongoblet form (stages of secretion). Within epithelial cells there were many oval, slightly basophilic structures surrounded by a halo which resembles an inclusion body; but they were probably products of secretion. There were frequent mitoses and necrotic epithelial cells. There were a few dilated submucosal lymphatics, but little lymphoid tissue.

Jejunum (emphysematous portion): The mucosal changes resemble those of the nonemphysematous areas and were, in all, less marked. The gas cysts were restricted to the submucosa. There was no clear-cut endothelial lining. There was mild lymphocytic and monocytic reaction with occasional polymorphonuclear leucocytes about, and adjoining the inner membrane of the cyst wall. There were dilated lymphatics in the noninvolved portions of the submucosa and in the serosa.

Mesenteric Lymph Nodes: The peripheral lymphatics were wide and cystic. One small lymph node was honeycombed with gas cysts. Two others contained one and six cysts, respectively. The sinusoids were wide and active with many phagocytic endothelial cells, abundant polymorphonuclear leucocytes, and scattered red blood cells. There were many eosinophiles throughout the depleted lymphoid tissue. There was apparent proliferation and, certainly, increase in size and activity of the reticular cells. There was also fibroblastic proliferation within the lymph nodes, capsule, and mesenteric tissues.

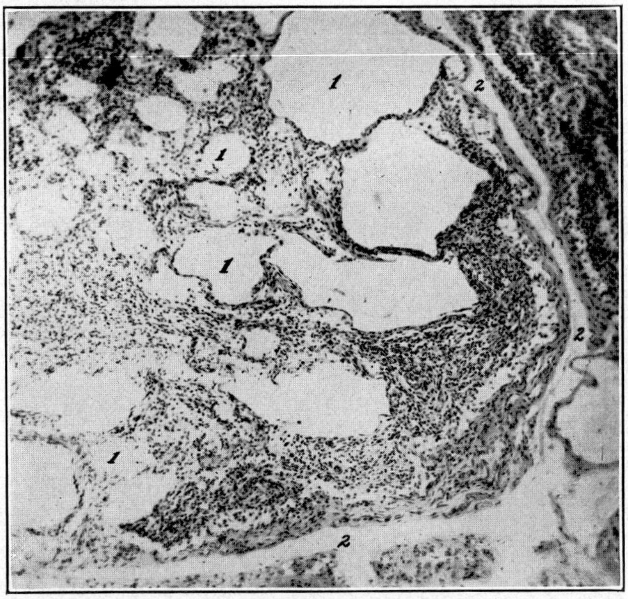

Fig. 4.—Case 4. Microscopic section of mesenteric lymph node with emphysema, *1*. Note dilated peripheral sinusoids, *2*.

CASE 5.—(A-36-84). This 3½-month-old male infant was admitted to the hospital because of vomiting and watery diarrhea of eighteen hours' duration. He was one of twins. (The other twin was admitted about the same time with similar complaints. He died a week later, but at autopsy no intestinal emphysema was encountered.) Physical examination revealed a malnourished, irritable infant with bilateral otitis media. Vomiting and diarrhea continued unabated up to the time of death, sixteen days after entry.

Necropsy was performed three hours post mortem. The anatomic diagnoses were bronchopneumonia, mild; nonobstructive biliary cirrhosis, mild; emphysematosis of ileum; acute otitis media, bilateral; and acute mesenteric lymphadenitis.

Gross Examination.—The pharynx was mildly injected. There was vascular congestion and edema of the lower half of the esophagus, but without ulceration. The stomach was distended with gas and its mucosa moderately congested. There was intense vascular congestion of the mucosa of the small intestine, without ulceration. Approximately 30 cm. from the ileocecal valve there was an area of emphysema, 3 cm. in length, over the antimesenteric aspect of the ileum. The emphysema was largely limited to the submucosal coat with no appreciable involvement of the mucosa. Throughout the large intestine vascular congestion similar to that of the small intestine was noted. The mesenteric lymph nodes were not emphysematous.

Microscopic Examination.—Esophagus and stomach were normal.

Duodenum: The mucosa was very cellular with many infiltrating polymorphonuclear leucocytes, especially close to, and within, the villi. The glandular lumina were widened, and in many the epithelium was of lower columnar type than usual. There was desquamated epithelium and debris within the lumina of some glands. There were numerous mitoses and fair numbers of goblet cells.

Small Intestine: Here again, there was polymorphonuclear leucocytic infiltration within the mucosa, more or less intense in varied sections, with accompanying marked hyperemia. There were either catarrhal epithelial changes with many pregoblet cell forms, fewer mitoses, and epithelial desquamation; or there was a marked scarcity in mucus-secreting cells with epithelial necroses, many mitoses, cystic dilatation of the glandular lumina, and varied atrophy of the epithelium. There was very little submucosal lymphoid tissue. There was moderate edema of the submucosa.

In the *terminal ileum* and *colon* there were marked catarrhal changes. The glandular lumina were widened, frequently cystic, and filled with mucus and epithelial debris. The lining epithelial cells were of low columnar form and, at times, almost flattened, with poorly defined striate borders. There were abundant mucus-filled cells, and many of these had complete goblet characters. There were fairly frequent mitoses.

Ileum (emphysematous): There were mucosal changes similar in character to those of the nonemphysematous portions of bowel, plus pronounced thinning and atrophy over the larger submucosal gas cysts. As in the other cases, the latter varied in size and were separated by edematous connective tissue with very little evidence of inflammatory reaction. There were no giant cells and practically no specific lining cells. There were, however, distinctly dilated lymphatics within the submucosa. In addition, there were several gas cysts.

Mesenteric Lymph Nodes: The sinusoids were greatly widened. There was marked endothelial proliferation with very active phagocytosis. There were also fair numbers of polymorphonuclear leucocytes and lymphocytes. There were no microscopic gas cysts.

CASE 6.—(A-37-5.) This 2-week-old male infant was admitted to the hospital because of blisters over hands, feet, and body, of twelve days' duration. Physical examination revealed a poorly developed and poorly nourished, hypertonic infant with large excoriated lesions of feet, hands, face, left groin, and back. The skin lesions failed to respond to a variety of local applications. Intermittent vomiting and diarrhea appeared and persisted. He died on the thirty-seventh hospital day. Stool examinations were consistently positive for occult blood.

Necropsy was performed one hour post mortem. The anatomic diagnoses were epidermolysis bullosa; bronchopneumonia, bilateral; acute otitis media; acute mastoiditis, bilateral; acute enteritis, marked; pneumatosis of colon; acute mesenteric lymphadenitis; and aberrant pancreas in wall of stomach.

Gross Examination.—The small intestine was moderately distended with gas. There were several small areas of mucosal congestion but no ulcers. The colon likewise was moderately distended with gas. The mucosal surfaces of the cecum and ascending colon were not very remarkable, although there was considerable adherent sticky mucus. The wall of the transverse colon was considerably thickened, and its submucosa and serosa were honeycombed by numerous gas-filled cysts. Here too, the mucosa was covered by tenacious mucus, which when removed left an irregular surface both smooth and granular in character.

Microscopic Examination.—Esophagus: There was evidence of recent epithelial regeneration with subepithelial vascular dilatation and the formation of small contracted newly formed blood vessels.

Stomach: There was an island of aberrant pancreas in the submucosa.

Small Intestine: The mucosa was cellular and heavily infiltrated by polymorphonuclear leucocytes, particularly close to the surface. There was rounding and broadening of the interglandular surface portions with poorly defined villi. There was little vascular congestion, but some of the vessels near the surface were thrombosed. The glands shared in the inflammatory reaction and were often compressed. The lining cells were low and almost flattened. Here and there the lumina were dilated and filled with cellular debris. Portions of the glandular epithelium were entirely ulcerated, and there were inflammatory cells in the lumen. The elongated, flatter cells had the appearance of being of recent regenerative character, yet mitoses were rare. There were fair numbers of goblet cells. There were rare small lymphoid follicles in the submucosa. In the latter, there were rare vascular thrombi, edema, and lymphangiectasis. In the serosa there were dilated endothelial-lined lymphatics and areas of fibrosis, vascularization, edema, and round, cell infiltration.

Colon (nonemphysematous): A thick layer of mucus covered the mucosa. The glands were practically made up of large goblet cells with wide cryptic openings where, in particular, there was considerable epithelial desquamation. The interglandular stroma was free of active inflammatory reaction. The submucosa and serosa were of the same character as in the ileum, poor in lymphoid tissue in the former, fibrosed and cellular in the latter, and with dilated irregular lymphatic channels in both.

Colon (emphysematous): The mucosa resembled that of the nonemphysematous portions of the large bowel but was thinned over larger cysts. The submucosa was riddled by numerous gas cysts. Occasionally they extended through the muscular coat. Frequently they formed honeycombed areas in the serosa. The cysts in the submucosa possessed no specific lining except for rare, questionable, endothelial cells. In the serosa the smaller ones were more clearly of dilated lymphatic character. There was no cellular exudate within or adjoining the cysts. There were no giant cells. The submucosal stroma was, however, frequently mildly edematous. The muscularis mucosae was intact and thickened in all instances.

Mesenteric Lymph Nodes: There were greatly dilated and tortuous pericapsular lymphatics filled with a granular precipitate. The peripheral and medullary sinusoids of the lymph nodes were very wide and contained numbers of polymorphonuclear leucocytes and proliferated endothelial cells.

DISCUSSION

The varied factors associated with the production of intestinal emphysema are yet poorly understood. Of the prevailing etiological theories, the mechanical one has gained general acceptance. This theory implies that the gas from the intestinal lumen penetrates the intestinal wall through gross or microscopic mucosal defects. It is believed that the gas may form local cysts or may permeate the intestinal wall and form cystic aggregates at some point distant from the site of entrance.

Increased intragastric or intraintestinal pressure is probably of importance in initiating, and peristaltic activity in determining, the site of intestinal emphysema.

In partial substantiation of this viewpoint is the fact that there have been gastric or duodenal ulcers, often with stenosis, in more than 50 per cent of the cases in adults. In many of the others there have been ulcers, strictures, or obstruction occasioned by intrinsic or extrinsic factors, in other portions of the intestine. However, experimentally, Tung and Ngai[9] failed to produce local intestinal emphysema in dogs following injection of air into the intestinal wall, although they observed its passage into the mesenteric lymphatics. Likewise, when they produced artificial gastric ulcers and then distended the stomach, air bubbles were found in the serosal lymphatics of the stomach and omentum but failed to form local or distinct intestinal gaseous cysts. Similarly, we failed to reproduce the condition in healthy rabbits and cats by injection of air into the submucosa. The gas would invariably escape into perivascular, serosal, and mesenteric lymphatics, forming cysts in the mesentery and retroperitoneal tissues but not locally in the intestinal wall. It would seem that under normal conditions the bowel wall can rid itself of the entering gas through patent lymphatics.

It is of interest that in the somewhat similar disease in swine there is a constant catarrhal enteritis. In infancy, enteric symptoms such as diarrhea and vomiting are very common but most often are unaccompanied by anatomic change in the intestine. Intestinal pneumatosis is very rare as far as we know. This does not preclude the possibility, however, that enteritis may be an important factor in the pathogenesis of the condition. Very little attention has been paid to the uninvolved portions of the intestine, and it is felt that in these areas there may be functional as well as anatomic changes. In all of Moore's cases there was an intense enteritis and a macroscopic ulcer in one. In five of our patients persistent vomiting and diarrhea, or diarrhea alone, were present. In the intestines of all of these there were glandular changes and inflammatory reactions in the small intestine, but there was no gross ulceration. These findings were constantly present in distant areas, as well as in the emphysematous regions. With these changes present, especially hyperemia and hyposecretion of mucus, minute fissures in a relatively dry and friable mucous membrane could allow the continued entrance of gas. Certainly disturbances in peristalsis and intraintestinal gaseous pressures could coexist with the enteritis. In addition, increased or disturbed lymphatic drainage, as evidenced by the fairly frequent finding of dilated lymphatics in the intestinal wall and dilated active sinusoids in the mesenteric lymph nodes, would facilitate the diffusion or accumulation of gas. That the latter permeates lymphatic channels is well known. Not only were the mesenteric lymph nodes the seat of gas cysts in three of the six cases, but in one the cisterna chyli and thoracic duct were also involved.

The presence of giant cells and fibroblastic proliferation about the gas cysts commonly reported in adults is evidence of chronicity, as indicated by the experimental injections of gas into subcutaneous tissues by Wright,[16] where such reactions about gas-filled spaces were noted only after several days. Giant cells were entirely absent in the present cases. There was little evidence of fibrosis, although there were occasional areas of mild inflammation. This would indicate that, in the early establishment of the emphysema, the reaction may be minimal and that here the disease process is quite recent.

It is also of interest that in three cases there were evidences of injury to the liver. In Case 4, a nonobstructive biliary cirrhosis was the chief anatomic finding.

It is conceivable that, with ulcers or inflammation of the intestinal tract, small amounts of gas may enter the intestinal wall and rapidly be disposed of by diffusion and absorption. It is true that the condition is overlooked clinically, but there may be temporary symptoms suggesting appendicitis, peritonitis, or intestinal obstruction. It is known that following laparotomy the gas cysts have disappeared spontaneously. Of recent years Bonnamour, Badolle, and Beaupere[17] and Graberger[18] have stressed the possibility of the recognition of the disease by x-ray examination.

CONCLUSIONS

Six cases are added to the four examples of intestinal pneumatosis in infancy and childhood reported in the literature. Five of these were observed over the period of approximately one year.

It is believed that in the absence of ulcers or obstruction as commonly occur in the adult, enteritis and accompanying functional changes are probably important factors in the initiation and evolution of the disease.

REFERENCES

1. Bang: Nord. Med. Ark. **8**: 18, 1876; quoted by Nitch: Brit. J. Surg. **11**: 714, 1924.
2. Turnure, P. R.: Ann. Surg. **57**: 811, 1913.
3. Mills, H. W.: Surg. Gynec. & Obst. **40**: 387, 1925.
4. Memmi, R.: Policlinico (sez. chir.) **41**: 408, 1934.
5. Silverstone, J.: Lancet **1**: 129, 1928.
6. Lamont, D.: Tr. Roy. Med.-Chir. Soc. Glasgow **23**: 113, 1928-29.
7. Sawada, B.: J. Orient. Med. **9**: 66, 1928.
8. Moore, R. A.: Am. J. Dis. Child. **38**: 818, 1929.
9. Tung, P. C., and Ngai, S. K.: Chinese M. J. **47**: 1-14, 1933.
10. Pybus, F. C.: Brit. J. Surg. **21**: 539, 1934.
11. Kemal, M.: Deutsche med. Wchnschr. **59**: 1707, 1933.
12. Nimet, B.: Zentralbl. f. Chir. **61**: 1986, 1934.
13. Bsteh, O.: Arch. f. klin. Chir. **181**: 707, 1935.
14. Englund, F., and Wahlgren, F.: Acta chir. Scandinav. **76**: 601, 1935.
15. Schnyder, K.: Cor.-Bl. f. schweiz. Aerzte. **47**: 289, 1917; quoted by Mills.
16. Wright, A. W.: Am. J. Path. **6**: 87, 1930.
17. Bonnamour, Badolle, and Beaupere: J. de. radiol. et d'electrol. **10**: 164, 1926.
18. Graberger, G.: Acta radiol. **16**: 439, 1935.

THE SIGNIFICANCE OF THE CONDITIONS OF EXPOSURE IN THE STUDY OF MEASLES PROPHYLAXIS

An Added Criterion in the Evaluation of Measles Prophylactic Agents

Samuel Karelitz, M.D., Assisted by Ruth F. Karelitz
New York, N. Y.

Considerable difference of opinion is noted in the literature when one seeks to evaluate the various substances used in the prophylaxis of measles. Some observers note excellent results using convalescent serum, immune adult serum, or placental globulins, while the results reported by others are less favorable. I believe that in addition to the question of correct dosage of the prophylactic agents, much of the difficulty lies in the failure of most investigators to consider the conditions under which exposure of the susceptibles was assumed to have occurred.

Thus the presence of a child with measles, whether it is in the schoolroom, in a trolley car or bus, in a nursery, at play outdoors, in a dining room of a school, at a party, or in a hospital ward, is regarded by most investigators as adequate evidence that all of the susceptible children present at the same time are exposed to measles and that such an exposure is equivalent to one of a sick sibling at home, and is so regarded for the evaluation of a measles prophylactic serum.

In studies reported with Schick,[1] we called attention to the fallacy of this assumption. While testing the efficacy of various doses of serum obtained from measles-immune adults, it became apparent that the results were strikingly dependent on the conditions of exposure of the susceptible child. The conclusions drawn from these studies were: (1) that hospital and institution wards are usually inadequate for the evaluation of a measles prophylactic substance because of the uncertainty and difference of exposure of the susceptible child; (2) that the percentage of exposed susceptible children who completely escaped measles varied with the intensity and the duration of the exposure. The greater number of so-called complete protections occur in those home in which facilities make possible isolation of the sick child at an early stage of the disease; (3) that in homes where the early isolation of the patient is impossible, better results can be expected in the exposed contacts by increasing the dose of serum injected; (4) that the dosage of infection with measles acquired within a period of a few days determines in large measure whether the disease will develop in susceptible children.

From the Department of Pediatrics, Mount Sinai Hospital, New York.

These conclusions are significant, first, because they must be considered for proper evaluation of the prophylactic value of sera and, second, because they imply a conception of the nature of the measles infection different from that still held by many.

In view of the importance of the above statements, I believed it necessary to fortify my earlier observations by further experience. I have therefore analyzed 314 additional cases treated prophylactically with various placental products and with globulin of immune adult serum and have extended the study to a number of individuals in whom the contact was even more casual than those of the earlier group. I have compared results with measles prophylactic substances in homes and hospitals, in homes of good and bad hygiene, and these results in turn with their use in children who were presumably exposed in classrooms, in streetcars and busses, at parties, and while at play indoors or outdoors. Actually these studies amount to a comparison of the results obtained with different periods of exposure beginning with the very equivocal exposures in hospital to those which, besides being doubtful, are less than seven hours (school, busses, parties, and at play) and to those lasting from four to eight days.

COMPARISON OF RESULTS OBTAINED IN HOMES AND IN HOSPITALS

The results are presented in four tables: analysis of Table I shows that with conditions of study alike except for location of contact there is a vast difference in the percentage of protections obtained in home and hospital contacts. Thus with 6 c.c. of adult serum administered alike to children from 2 to 10 years of age, 83 per cent of the contacts in hospital escaped measles, and 17 per cent developed modified measles, whereas in home exposures only 29 per cent escaped measles, 22 per cent developed modified measles, and in 49 per cent no noticeable amelioration of symptoms resulted.

In the second series of cases I used placental extract, or placental fluid, in doses equivalent to 10 c.c. and occasionally 15-20 c.c. of immune adult serum. In this series both the expected results and those obtained were recorded, the expected results being those which might have followed the use of equivalent dosages of immune adult or convalescent serum under comparable conditions.

It was observed in the earlier studies that a large percentage of the presumably exposed hospitalized children remained well. In the later work I attempted, therefore, to obtain only modification of measles in the hospital contacts by giving small doses of serum. Nevertheless, almost all children failed to develop measles. The difference in results in hospitals and home exposures in this series is therefore more striking than in our first studies.

TABLE I

COMPARISON OF RESULTS IN MEASLES PROPHYLAXIS CARRIED OUT IN HOMES AND HOSPITALS

AUTHOR	AGE, YR.	DAYS EXPOSED	SERUM	TYPE OF EXPOSURE	CASES	NO MEASLES OR PROTECTED	MODIFIED	FAILURE
Karelitz and Schick Series 1930-31	2-10	5 or less	6 c.c. A.S.	Hospital	69	83%	17%	0
				Home	65	29%	22%	49%
			8 c.c. A.S.	Home	75	46%	43%	11%
			12-25 c.c. A.S.	Home	54	57%	20%	23%
Morales and Mandry	½-10	6 or less	10 c.c. A.S.	Home	138	41%	?	?
			15-30 c.c. A.S.	Home	321	58%	22%	20%
			4-6 c.c. C.S.	Home	120	84%	11%	5%
Karelitz, present series 1933-37	1-12	3-6	Pl. Ext. equivalent 10 c.c. A.S.	Hospital	27	85%	11%	4% Obt.
						0	100%	0 Exp.
				Home	146	31%	55%	14% Obt.
	1-12	3-6	Same as above			30%	61%	9% Exp.
Park and Freeman		5 or less	5-10 c.c. C.S.	Hospital	652	91%	7%	2%
				Home	226	52%	42%	6%
McKhann and Coady			Pl. Ext.	Hospital	95	97%	3%	0
Robinson and McKhann			Pl. Ext.	Hospital				
				Home	1628	69.9%	25.6%	4.5%
Eley, 1935			Pl. Ext.	Intimate exposure	299	57.4%	36.1%	6.5%
				Home	174	60.9%	32.2%	6.9%

Obt.—obtained
Exp.—expected

A.S.—adult serum
C.S.—convalescent serum

Pl. Ext.—placental extract

NURSERY EXPERIMENTS

As further evidence of this important difference in exposure in institutions, I have analyzed two nursery epidemics, using adult serum in one and placental extract in the second (Table II). In the first epidemic, seventeen children between 1 and 2 years of age, housed in one large

TABLE II

COMPARISON OF RESULTS IN MEASLES PROPHYLAXIS CARRIED OUT IN NURSERIES AND UNDER OTHER CONDITIONS, SCHOOLS, PARTIES, ETC.

AUTHOR	AGE YR.	DAYS EX-POSED	SERUM	EXPOSURE	CASES	NO MEASLES OR PROTECTED	MODIFIED	FAILURE	
Karelitz, present series	½-2	4	Pl. Ext. equivalent 10 c.c. A.S.	Nursery	11	73%	27%	0	Obt.
				Controls	11	73%	0	27%	
	1-2	4	6 c.c. A.S.	Nursery	17	82%	18%	0	Obt.
						0	100%	0	Exp.
				Controls	4	100%	0	0	
	3-12	Less than 7 hr.	Pl. Ext. & C.S. 5-12 c.c.	Outdoor play Schoolroom Bus, etc.	13	77%	23%	0	Obt.
						0	100%	0	Exp.
	3-12	Less than 7 hr.	Pl. Ext. & C.S. 5-12 c.c.	Indoor play Parties, etc.	34	82%	15%	3%	Obt.
						0	100%	0	Exp.
McGavran 1936		2-6	Pl. Ext.	Intimate contact	57	33%	64%	3%	
				Casual contact	20	60%	30%	10%	
Levitas 1935			Pl. Ext.	Intimate contact	13	0	100%	0	
				Moderate contract	2	100%	0	0	

Pl. Ext.—placental extract C.S.—convalescent serum Exp.—expected
A.S.—adult serum Obt.—obtained

ward and exposed to a child ill with measles for four days, were each injected with 6 c.c. of immune adult serum, a dosage only sufficient for modification of measles, and insufficient to suppress measles entirely. Fourteen (82 per cent) remained free of measles, and only three developed modified measles. Four babies who were not treated remained well. Seven of the fourteen treated children who remained well after the first exposure developed modified measles two weeks after exposure to the three cases of modified measles.

In the second measles epidemic at the same nursery, eleven children between 9 months and 2 years of age were injected with placental extract on the fourth day of exposure. Six infants under 6 months and eleven between 1 and 2 years of age were left untreated. Three of the treated children developed modified measles, and three controls of the 1- to 2-year group developed mild measles. Of the six younger than 6 months, one child each of 2, three, and four months developed mild measles. The measles was so slight that it might easily have been regarded as modified, had treatment been given. The observations made in this nursery, just as those in hospitals, show how difficult it would be to attempt to determine the efficacy of the serum or placental extract under such conditions except for the relative severity of the measles which developed among the treated and untreated children.

In Tables I and II, I have included the published data of McKhann and his co-workers[2-4] and Eley,[5] as well as those of McGavran[6] and Levitas,[7] because these investigators have followed our recommendation to divide their cases according to the type of exposure. In the first report on placental extract, McKhann and Chu treated forty hospitalized children prophylactically with placental extract, without a single failure. In a later report McKhann and Coady state that in ninety-five hospitalized children placental extract prevented measles in 97 per cent and modified the measles of the remaining 3 per cent. In more recent publications Robinson and McKhann and Eley referred to the difference in degree and intensity of exposure and in their late reports separated the cases accordingly. Thus they have confirmed our findings, in that their results varied considerably with the type of exposure. Instead of 97 per cent protections and 3 per cent modifications as reported earlier by McKhann and Coady, Eley and McKhann more recently reported for intimate contacts, 57.4 per cent protections, 32.2 per cent modifications, and 6.9 per cent failures.

CAN RESULTS IN HOMES BE IMPROVED BY INCREASING THE SERUM DOSAGE?

The results following the use of 8 c.c. of adult serum in one group of children and doses of 12 to 25 c.c. (varying with the age of the contact) in another (Table I), and the data of results following the use of serum globulins in doses equivalent to 15 to 30 c.c. of adult serum (Table III), indicate that under similar conditions an increasing per cent of protections can be obtained in home contacts by increasing the dosage of adult serum. Morales and Mandry's results[8] with increasing doses of adult serum in home contacts are so similar to our own, that they lend confirmatory evidence to our findings. Park and Freeman's data[9] show that the difference in results in hospitals and homes exists even when using convalescent serum.

STUDIES OF CASUAL CONTACTS AT PLAY, IN BUSSES, SCHOOLS, AT PARTIES, ETC.

In Table II are recorded results obtained with children who presumably were infected with measles while at school, while riding in a bus, or playing outdoors with children who were in the prodromal stage of measles. In the latter group, as in the next, comprised of children who were supposedly exposed to measles because they attended an indoor party or played indoors where a playmate had prodromal symptoms of measles, I injected only modifying doses of placental extract or of convalescent serum. Even though smaller doses of serum were injected, the results were far better than expected. The percentage of children who did not get sick was almost the same as in the group of hospital ward exposures. In the first group 77 per cent escaped measles and 23 per cent developed modified measles, and in the second group 78 per cent escaped and 18 per cent developed modified measles. Only one child developed ordinary measles. In hospital exposures my results were 85 per cent protection, 11 per cent modification, and only 4 per cent failure. From the above reports it may be concluded that in the exposures of susceptible contacts under such conditions a relatively small percentage of the children are infected, just as in hospitals and nurseries. The results obtained under such conditions are, therefore, generally not comparable to those obtained after exposure for longer periods, such as those in homes.

McGavran's data reproduced in Table II further corroborate the difference in results obtained when the contacts were intimate as compared to those which were casual. Those of Levitas show how difficult it is to protect children at home with small doses of placental extract.

COMPARISON OF RESULTS IN HOMES OF GOOD AND BAD HYGIENE

To this point the studies made in private homes have been classified merely as home exposures, but, as has been previously pointed out, there is a great difference in the conditions of exposure in homes. I have therefore separated the homes according to the accomplishment in isolation of the child sick with measles from his well siblings. Considering the factor of isolation alone, I have referred to a home of good hygiene, one where, at the first recognition of illness, the sick child is completely isolated from his well siblings, as compared with the home of poor hygiene where, either because of lack of facilities or because of lack of cooperation and understanding, the sick child and well contacts are permitted to mingle until the rash appears or throughout the illness.

In the home designated as having good hygiene, exposure lasts for one or two days, occasionally three, whereas in the home of poor hygiene the exposure is usually more intimate and lasts at least until the rash appears on the fourth day or for the entire period during which the sick child is infectious. Table III consistently shows the greater difficulty in protecting a child of a home of poor hygiene from measles, regardless of whether adult serum, placental extracts, or globulin extracts of adult blood were used. Whereas the complete protection exceeded our expectations in homes of good hygiene, they fell short of our expectations in homes of poor hygiene. The latter results varied with the dosage and potency of the preparation used. The better the preparation, the more nearly did the results obtained approximate the expected results in homes of good hygiene. On the other hand, the smaller the injected dose of serum, the more striking was the difference in the results between homes of good and bad hygiene. That is especially evident when the results using 6 c.c. of adult serum, as recorded in Table III, are compared with those in which placental extract was injected in doses equal to 10 to 20 c.c. of immune adult blood serum, and blood serum globulin preparations given in amounts equivalent to 15 to 30 c.c. of adult blood serum.

TABLE III

HOMES OF GOOD AND BAD HYGIENE

AUTHOR	AGE YR.	DAYS EXPOSED	SERUM	TYPE OF EXPOSURE	CASES	PROTECTED	MODIFIED	FAILURE
Karelitz and Schick Series 1930-31	2-6	2-5	6 c.c. A.S.*	Home, good hygiene	32	58.0%	23.0%	19.0%
				Home, bad hygiene	26	0	27.0%	73.0%
				Hospital	48	83.0%	17.0%	0
Karelitz Present Series 1933-37	1-12	2-6	Pl. Ext. equivalent 10 c.c. A.S.	Home, bad hygiene	12	17.0% 0	17.0% 75.0%	66.0% Obt. 25.0% Exp.
				Home, good hygiene	87	50.5% 11.5%	41.5% 87.0%	8.0% Obt. 11.5% Exp.
				Hospital	27	85.0%	12.0% 100.0%	3.0% Obt. Exp.
	1-10	2-6	Serum Glob. equivalent to 15-30 c.c. A.S.	Home, good hygiene	10	90.0% 50.0%	10.0% 50.0%	0 Obt. 0 Exp.
				Home, bad hygiene	70	51.4% 70.0%	44.0% 30.0%	4.6% Obt. 0 Exp.
	1-12	2-6	Commercial Glob. Ext.	Casual	9	100.0%	0	0
				Home	33	33.0%	22.0%	45.0%

*See footnote at bottom of Table I.

COMPOSITE DATA OF SECOND SERIES OF CASES

Table IV presents composite data of our entire present series of 314 cases. On examination of Table IV certain figures stand out prominently. These confirm the conclusions drawn from earlier studies when comparison was made of the results obtained in homes of different hygiene. These data indicate that the percentage of modifications accomplished was almost the same for both groups but that the difference occurred in the percentage of protections and failures. In the homes of good hygiene 54.6 per cent escaped measles, and only 42.6 per cent remained well in homes of poor hygiene. In the homes of poor hygiene, 22.6 per cent developed ordinary measles against only 7.3 per cent in the homes of good hygiene. The results in hospitals, as noted in our earlier studies (Table I), were much better than expected.

It is significant, however, that in the second series of hospitalized children (Table IV) only modifying doses of serum were given, yet 85 per cent did not develop the disease.

TABLE IV

COMPOSITE ANALYSIS OF PRESENT SERIES OF 314 CASES

EXPOSURE	CASES	NO MEASLES OR PROTECTED	MODIFIED	FAILURE
Homes of good hygiene	97	54.6%	38.1%	7.3%
Homes of bad hygiene	115	42.6%	34.8%	22.6%
Hospital	27	85.0%	12.0%	3.0%
Nurseries	28	78.6%	21.4%	0
Play outdoors	13	77.0%	23.0%	0
Play indoors	34	82.0%	15.0%	3.0%
Combined hospital, nurseries, play indoor and play outdoor groups	102	82.3%	15.7%	2.0%

The results in the play group in the hospital and in the nursery were so much alike that it seemed justifiable to pool those small groups of 27, 28, 13, and 34 cases into one of 102. If that is done, the composite results show 82.3 per cent protections, 15.7 per cent modifications, and 2 per cent failures. These results are very similar to those of any one component of this group. It seems fair to deduce from these data that the presumed exposures at play, in school, at parties, etc., are as doubtful and as variable in intensity as they are in hospital and nursery wards, and therefore are equally unsuited for the evaluation of a measles prophylactic substance.

DISCUSSION

A total of 583 children susceptible and exposed to measles were treated prophylactically with various preparations. The criteria used for determining dosage were the age, size, and health of the child, the period of exposure, and the potency of the preparation. These were analyzed to determine the importance of the type or the circumstances of the exposure, as an added criterion in the evaluation of measles prophylactic substances.

The analysis of the results, as well as the confirmatory published data presented in the charts, shows that exposure to measles may be a variable quantity, and, depending on its size, a given amount of measles prophylactic substance may or may not be adequate. Thus it establishes the necessity for considering the type of exposure to measles in attempting to evaluate the efficacy of any preparation used for prophylaxis. Failure to consider this factor probably explains much of the discrepancy in results reported by various workers using similar substances.

These observations, I believe, indicate also that one of the fundamental principles of bacterial infection applies also to the virus disease of measles, that is, that the dosage of bacteria (in this study of measles virus) with which a susceptible contact becomes infected and the number of times he becomes reinfected within a period of time influence the incidence rate of the disease. These observations also suggest very strongly that the nature of spread of measles is primarily by direct contact and to some degree via the air at a relatively short distance from the source of infection.

Top,[10] in an analysis of the 1935 measles epidemic in Detroit, found very little difference in the incidence rate of measles when the exposure was eight-child days or sixteen- or twenty-four-child days, that is, exposure to one child throughout the eight days of infectivity or exposure to two or three sick children simultaneously for the same eight-day period. Top's conclusion was that intensity of exposure does not appreciably influence the secondary attack rate among susceptibles at risk. This would seem to disagree with my findings. Nevertheless, when the periods of exposure in Top's cases are compared to those in my group, it presents an obvious explanation for this difference. I have compared the results in prophylactically treated children whose exposure varied from doubtful to exposure for a few minutes to six hours, and to exposure of one to three days, and to those exposed intimately for a maximum of eight-child days. I found that the ability to prevent measles with a given amount of serum diminished as the period of exposure became more certain or more intimate and longer. These findings, I believe, permit the inference that the incidence rate of measles rises with increasing intensity and duration of exposure from those lasting minutes or hours to those lasting four to eight days. Top's finding that intensity of exposure does not appreciably influence the secondary attack rate of measles would seem to be correct only when the minimum exposure is a severe one, eight-child days. In fact, under such conditions Top found that the secondary attack rate was 83 per cent, whereas it is known that in hospitals it is usually about 25 per cent.

The aforesaid may be elaborated upon by the following: The exposures in hospitals, nurseries, playgrounds and schools may vary from doubtful to intensive, but because of the low secondary attack rate they may be included in the category of indeterminate or mild infection. Exposures in homes of good hygiene may vary from a few hours to two or three days and might be considered moderate infection; in homes of bad hygiene exposure is close and repeated for four to eight days and may be classified as intensive or severe. An increasing difficulty in preventing measles as well as an increasing secondary attack rate was noted as exposure increased from the indeterminate or mild to the moderate, to the severe type.

It is generally accepted that the incidence rate of measles is usually less than 100 per cent, even with seemingly sufficient exposure. Top has shown that if susceptible contacts, after eight days of exposure to measles, are re-exposed for an equal period, 37.5 per cent of them develop measles. If, therefore, some children who have not had measles require repeated infection with measles or continuous infection for a longer period of time before they succumb, it seems quite reasonable to believe, or at least to suggest, that infection acquired through casual contact or short period might be overcome by a larger number of susceptible children. On further analysis the results presented in this report can be interpreted in only two ways, either the larger percentage of children who were exposed in hospitals, nurseries, and play groups did not become infected at all, or, if they did, the relatively small dose of infection was neutralized so that no manifestations of the disease appeared. Since only small doses of serum were used in these groups, doses which were ineffective when the exposure to measles was intensive, it must be concluded that if the contacts became infected at all, they were able to withstand the measles virus both because of the small dose of the infection and because of the serum, rather than because of the serum alone.

Further evidence that intimacy of contact and dosage of infection are significant in the incidence of measles may be assumed from the experiences noted by various workers, among them Halliday[11] and Debré and Joannon.[12] Those authors found that the incidence rate of measles is greater among the working classes in Glasgow and Paris, or in the sections of those cities where the dwellings are so constructed that there is closer and more frequent communication both among members of one family and among members of neighbors' families. They also found that measles occurs at an earlier age period (in infancy and in the preschool period) in a larger percentage of children living in more congested sections of Glasgow and Paris, whereas it is more prevalent in children of school age among the better housed inhabitants of those cities. As further confirmation, these authors cite a greater mortality rate from measles among the poor, which they correctly ascribe to the fact that measles among the poor occurs more commonly during infancy and early periods of life when measles is known to be associated with severe complications and therefore with the highest mortality. These studies also indicate that distance between contacts and susceptibles is important or that air transmission of the virus must be limited.

Added support for the viewpoint that dosage of infection with the measles virus is important may be drawn from knowledge about other infections. Powell and Clowes[13] in their studies of the common cold found that smearing cold virus on the nasal mucosa of human adults only once did not produce colds, whereas, after the applications were repeated several times, colds developed.

My experience with scarlet fever, mumps, and pertussis has caused me to believe that in these conditions, as in measles, the prophylactic value of sera and the secondary attack rate are influenced by the type of exposure. That is, the incidence of secondary cases of these diseases is greater when the contact is more intimate and is lower when contact is casual. Second attacks of whooping cough are not rare in adult life, but they usually develop after intensive exposure, as for example, to one's own child.

Measles is considered to be an air-borne disease. When measles breaks out in a ward it is assumed, therefore, that it infects all contacts within the hospital ward and perhaps those beyond the room of the measles patient. The virus is believed to travel through open windows and through open doors. It has been reported that it traveled through a chimney flue[14] to infect susceptibles on an upper floor. There is sufficient evidence for the belief that measles is an air-borne disease, but, since the measles virus is so very vulnerable, being destroyed very rapidly outside the human body, it seems likely that measles will be transmitted through the air only as far as it is propelled by a cough or a sneeze, in a moist state, whether that be 12 to 30 feet in quiet atmosphere or further in a room with greater air motion. Transmission of the virus through the air to remote distances seems very unlikely. This view seems to be borne out in the papers of Halliday, and Debré and Joannon, and I believe is also suggested in the following observations.

Experience has shown that in a large hospital ward when measles breaks out, usually only about 25 per cent of the susceptible patients develop measles within the next fourteen-day period. The remaining susceptible patients are then more likely to be infected because of the increase in the infectious cases. In the next fourteen-day period another group of cases develops measles. In the third fourteen-day period the remaining susceptibles develop the disease. Thus, an epidemic of measles in a ward to which no new susceptible patients are admitted usually runs a course of about two months, an observation made by Schick[15] and others long ago. The fact that only about 25 per cent of the patients of a hospital ward develop measles after the first contact is discovered, even though no prophylactic sera are used, is very suggestive supportive evidence that all children in the ward are not necessarily infected. This belief is further supported by the fact that, when measles breaks out in wards, the children nearest to the measles patient usually are the first and the most likely ones to develop the disease. It is also strengthened by the fact that in very small wards or in those where the children are permitted out of bed, or where there is no cubicle system or other form of isolation, a higher incidence rate of measles (more nearly like that in private homes) might and usually does occur.

Finally a report has been called to my attention by Dr. Jean Broadhurst of New York Teacher's College which bears out my findings even though it concerns a very small group of cases: On April 1, 1917, a child, D. R., arrived in a small town in New York from Ohio. There was no measles in this town in New York state. On April 15 she developed a typical measles rash. It was recalled that while on the train on April 1 D. R. played with a child who was coughing and sneezing a great deal and in the prodromal stage of measles. The health officer of the town traced all of her contacts between April 1 and April 15. M.T. and R.P., children who played with D. R. on the street, did not develop measles, nor did A. G. and D. C. who took their meals in the same boarding house dining room, nor did F. A., who passed her in the street; but S. F. J. and A. B. J., who played with D. R. in her home repeatedly, developed measles on April 30, 1917. The health officer, L. W. Hubbard, concluded that the history of these cases was interesting because of the apparent necessity for rather close contact to convey the disease.

CONCLUSIONS

1. The measles virus, like many other infectious agents, usually infects by direct contact, the spread of the disease through the air being limited by several factors, of which the distance between contacts is important, and the ease with which the virus is destroyed.

2. The dosage of virus or the frequency of infection acquired within a given time or the intimacy or duration of exposure to the disease determines in large measure both the incidence rate of measles and the efficacy of a given dosage of any measles prophylactic measure.

3. Hospital and institution wards are usually inadequate for the evaluation of a measles prophylactic substance because of the uncertainty and difference of the intensity and duration of the exposure of the susceptible children.

4. Exposures presumably consummated in nurseries, at school, in busses, in playgrounds, at parties, and at play indoors are no more certain than in hospitals and vary in intensity and duration, as in hospitals, and are, therefore, just as unreliable as hospital wards are for the study of measles prophylaxis.

5. The percentage of completely protected cases in homes varies with the hygiene, the greater number of protections being recorded in homes of better hygiene or in those in which facilities make possible isolation of the sick child at an early stage of the disease.

6. The percentage of complete protections in homes of poor hygiene increased progressively with corresponding increase in the serum dosage or potency.

7. The criteria for determination of dosage of a given preparation in measles prophylaxis should be modified to include the type or condition of the exposure.

REFERENCES

1. Karelitz, S., and Schick, B.: J. A. M. A. **104**: 991, 1935.
2. McKhann, C. F., and Chu, Fu Tang: Am. J. Dis. Child. **45**: 475, 1933.
3. McKhann, C. F., and Coady, H.: South. M. J. **27**: 20, 1934.
4. Robinson, E. S., and McKhann, C. F.: Am. J. Pub. Health **25**: 1353, 1935.
5. Eley, R. C.: New England J. Med. **213**: 195, 1935.
6. McGavran, E. G.: J. A. M. A. **106**: 1781, 1936.
7. Levitas, I. M.: J. A. M. A. **105**: 493, 1935.
8. Morales, E. G., and Mandry, O. C.: Bol. Asoc. méd. de Puerto Rico **22**: 217, 1930.
9. Park, W. H., and Freeman, R. Jr.: J. A. M. A. **87**: 556, 1926.
10. Top, F. H.: Presented before the Third Session of the Epidemiology Section of the Am. Pub. Health Assoc., New York City, Oct. 8, 1937.
11. Halliday, James L.: Great Britain Privy Council Medical Research Council, Special Report Series, 1927-1929.
12. Debré, R., and Joannon, P.: La Rougeole, Epidemiologie, Immunologie, Prophylaxie. Paris, 1926, Masson & Cie.
13. Powell and Clowes: Proc. Soc. Exper. Biol. & Med., 1926. Personal communication with Dr. Powell.
14. Moro: Von Pfaundler und Schlossmann Handbuch der Kinderheilkunde, Vol. II, 1923.
15. Schick, B.: Von Pfaundler und Schlossmann Handbuch der Kinderheilkunde, Vol. II, 1923.

1127 PARK AVENUE

ATELECTASIS OF THE LUNGS IN THE NEWBORN BABY, RESULTING FROM LESIONS OF THE NERVOUS CENTERS

ROBERT DEBRÉ, JULIEN MARIE, MAURICE LAMY, AND DE FONT-RÉAULX
PARIS, FRANCE

FOR a long time atelectasis of the lung was considered a rather frequent anatomic condition, a post-mortem finding detected in the vicinity of hematose, congestive, or emphysematous areas. A few years ago this lesion became included in clinical work.

If a fairly extensive area is involved (as the pulmonary lobe or even the entire lung), it is fairly easy to detect the clinical and radiologic symptoms, the most important of which show a modification of the statics of the thorax, the result of the retraction of the lungs, indrawing with increased slanting of the ribs, cardiomediastinal retraction, and raising of the diaphragm.

In adults and older children atelectasis is caused in most instances by an obstruction or compression of the bronchial tubes. At first sight the mechanical theory of atelectasis seems clear and logical and appears to have been completely confirmed by experimental studies. Clinical pathology shows demonstrated cases of atelectasis to be due to the presence of foreign bodies in the bronchi. Further, by reason of the good results obtained by bronchial aspiration in acute postoperative atelectasis, the lead of Chevalier Jackson is followed in detecting its causes in a bronchial obstruction.

Experimental work which has been chiefly the product of American surgeons appears to be equally convincing. By experiments with a bronchial foreign body, by cauterization of the bronchial mucosa, or by ligature of the bronchial tubes, it is possible to produce atelectasis in the corresponding area of the lung.

However, it is impossible from these facts to form the conclusion of a unique etiology or a general pathologic theory. It is certain that in a number of histories, bronchial obstruction is doubtful and even nonexistent. It is doubtful in many cases of acute postoperative atelectasis, in which nothing is obtained by aspiration, but in which a spontaneous recovery occurs in the course of the following days; and also it is doubtful in posthemoptoic atelectasis.

Above all, bronchial obstruction cannot be incriminated in cases in which atelectasis occurs after a subdiaphragmatic operation performed under local anesthesia, a thoracic traumatism (Bradford), a diaphragmatic paralysis (W. Pasteur), or a lesion of the cervical medulla (Churchill).

It is in early infancy that atelectasis seems to be especially frequent and of particular interest. The history of the following case which relates the clinical and anatomical findings and results helps throw a light on the origin of atelectasis in infancy, and at the same time contributes to the study of this lesion.

M. L., born Jan. 3, 1936, premature (8½ months), weighed 2,350 gm. Confinement was normal, without extraction. The respiration was immediately normal. For a period of eight days the baby was breast fed and remained in perfect condition. On January 10 the child began coughing and coughed slightly during the following days. He had frequent hiccoughing after feedings and even during the night. However, he developed normally, weighing 2,530 gm. at twenty days.

On January 24 the mother took him to a baby clinic where a mustard poultice and half a teaspoon of syrup containing a minute dose of morphia were prescribed. In the evening the mother noticed a slight cyanosis and irregular respiration.

On January 25 at 4 A.M., she found the child looking purple, cold, and apparently not breathing. It was only after one-half hour of brisk rubbing that the respiration returned gradually. During the morning these attacks of apnea with cyanosis occurred. In the afternoon the child was admitted to the hospital, the same condition continuing after admission.

On January 26 the respiration was irregular with quick breathing followed by short pauses; weight 2,470 gm.; no fever. Examination was negative except for a few telangiectases on the upper eyelid. Palpation of the cranium showed a periscissural softening and a positive Chvostek sign. The child was given ten drops of irradiated ergosterol and, by stomach tube, 5 gm. of calcium chloride. This latter medication was discontinued on February 4, when blood calcium was found to be 163 mmgr.

The condition remained stationary during the following days, the increase in weight being very slow. An x-ray film of the chest on January 27 showed a normal thoracic picture. A lumbar puncture on February 3 yielded a perfectly clear fluid containing 6 to 8 leucocytes per cubic centimeter and 0.40 of albumin.

On February 2, after gavage, dyspnea with cyanosis recurred without convulsive movements.

On February 6, arrhythmic respiration was more noticeable at first inspection. The child had periods of tachypnea during which the rate, difficult to count, ran to more than 150 per minute. Each inspiration was brusque and spasmodic and accompanied by noticeable infrasternal and only slight suprasternal recession. These fits of tachypnea lasted for variable lengths of time, usually about 10 seconds. They both began and ended suddenly; they were separated by intervals of 4 to 5 seconds and sometimes for as long as 30 seconds. At certain moments the respiratory rhythm was practically normal; the transition from one rhythm to another occurred without any apparent reason.

The cough persisted with no particular characteristics. Clinical examination of the lungs proved negative, but radioscopy and radiography from the front and in profile showed the existence of an opaque focus of the right superior lobe and medium parahilar region; also the shadows of the heart and mediastinum were displaced to the right.

During the following days, the condition of the child remained unchanged, the respiratory disturbances continuing. Each day when breathing was particularly difficult, the child was placed for half an hour under an artificial respirator of carbogene; then the rhythm became normal quickly and the child breathed normally and easily. The feeding was not easy; the child sucked with difficulty, and coughing caused frequent vomiting. Weight remained stationary.

Ophthalmic examination showed normal eye grounds. On the right side there was a noticeable congenital peripapillary pigmentation.

On February 11 both radioscopy and radiography showed that the opacity of the right lung had extended to the upper two-thirds of the hemithorax. The heart and the mediastinum were very much drawn to the right; the trachea was quite deviated towards the same side. The diaphragm was mobile but in place. There was no definite modification of the ribs or intercostal spaces.

Pulmonary examination showed slight dullness of the right apex, back and front. On this level, there were numerous faint bullous râles. With the exception of the fits of apnea and cyanosis the facies of the child remained excellent; there was none of the painful and ''pushed'' breathing of bronchial pneumonia. There was no throbbing of the alae nasi, and no fever.

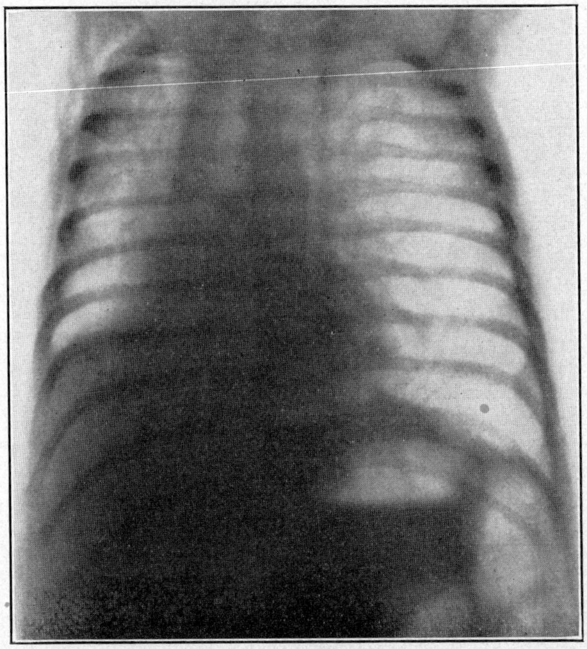

Fig. 1.—February 11. Heart and mediastinum drawn to the right. The right diaphragmatic cupola is raised

An attempt at bronchoscopy was decided upon in the hope of discovering some foreign body or, in case of resorption of any obstacle of organic nature, to discover any phenomenon of subsequent inflammatory edema. The operation was performed February 14 by Dr. Marcel Ombredanne. Bronchoscopy revealed a slight congested aspect of the right bronchus. Aspiration produced neither secretion nor foreign body.

On February 15 and 16 arrhythmic respiration was still as noticeable. Periods of apnea were disquieting by their frequency and duration, and the child had to be almost continuously under the influence of carbogene. He took with difficulty bottles of breast milk which had to be given under the respirator for fear of a fit of apnea. It should be noted that oxygen had practically no action on the arrhythmic respiration, and after several tries it was necessary to return to carbogene, which always had a regulating effect on the respiratory rhythm.

Physical and radiologic examination revealed no change in the lung condition. The film showed a typical aspect of atelectasis of the right lung. The child lost a little weight.

On February 17 it was decided to perform an artificial pneumothorax on the right side in the hope of counteracting the cardiomediastinal displacement. The initial intrapleural pressure oscillated between -2 and -18 (average -10) in the respiratory movements of normal amplitude, but largely surpassed these limits when the respiration was amplified. An injection of about 50 c.c. of oxygen rapidly raised the pressure to +2 to +10 (average +6). Under the screen a small gas ball was detected on the extreme apex.

Immediately after the operation symptoms of mild shock were noted, and the patient had to be replaced under the carbogene respirator. The rest of the day and night were good; respiratory rhythm seemed a little more regular; feeding was easier; and carbogene was only given at intervals.

On February 18, another pleural puncture was made. During a phase of polypnea the manometer oscillated very faintly around –8. In deep respiration initial pressure was +14 to -24 (average -5). About 75 c.c. of air were injected rapidly without our being able to measure the terminal pressure.

On February 22 a third intrapleural injection of about 75 c.c. of air was given, the average terminal pressure being +10 (0 to +20). The child was very cyanotic, respiration was slow, and he had to be returned rapidly to the respirator. Films showed complete pneumothorax of the big cavity. The superior lobe was the most flattened. Heart and mediastinum were almost in normal position.

These intrapleural injections coincided with a comparative regularity of the respiratory rhythm. The mother, especially, found that the baby drank more easily. In fact he gained 250 gm. in weight between February 20 and 25. At the same time, 50 gm. of glucose solution were given daily by clysis.

After February 25 the spells of apnea became more frequent; often after taking a little milk with a spoon (he refused to take a bottle), the baby became cyanotic. Respiration stopped at times for one-half to one minute. Each spell ended with long and deep respiratory movements. There were no convulsions. At other periods, polypnea was more apparent, and there was a little throbbing of the alae nasi.

On February 29 the film showed complete opacity of the right pulmonary field. The shape of the main bronchi and also some faint bronchial arborizations alone could be detected by transparence. The trachea, the heart, and the mediastinum were again markedly deviated to the right. Auscultation, which was negative after pneumothorax, now, after resorption of air, revealed big humid râles and an inspiratory souffle. Temperature rose slightly to around 37.5 and 38° C. The weight chart was irregular with no increase.

On March 2 after the child had lost 70 gm. of weight since the previous day, it was decided to try a new insufflation of air in the hope of facilitating the ingestion of food, this method having proved successful before. After an injection of 100 c.c. of air, terminal pressure was around +5. The child, who seemed not to suffer from shock, was put back under the carbogene respirator. Five minutes later he was livid, inert, and had ceased breathing. In spite of prolonged artificial respiration and lumbar intraspinal injection of lobeline and intracardiac injection of adrenalin, death followed rapidly.

At post-mortem examination on March 4 no anomaly of the thorax was found. After removal of the costoscapular breastplate and exposing the contents of the thorax, the left lung was seen to occupy the greater part of the thoracic frame. The right lung, quite small, was flattened and retracted. Its color, pale and whitish, contrasted to that of the opposite lung. There were a few hemorrhagic suffusions under the pleura. The heart was horizontal in normal position. The mediastinum occupied a middle position, and the right hemidiaphragm did not seem raised abnormally.

The whole content of the thoracic frame was removed in one piece. The right lung was completely thick and stiff on pressure, excepting an anterior tongue of the superior and middle lobes. Cutting showed great density with no air. A portion of tissue removed sank immediately in water. The left lung was normal except for the posteroinferior portion of the inferior lobe, which was of an abnormal consistency and sank also. The bronchial ramifications starting from the trachea were opened methodically. Two centimeters from the right hilus, against the bronchia of the inferior lobe, a small nodule the size of a pea, which appeared to be a ganglion, was discovered, but there was no intrabronchial foreign body and no extrinsic compression. Histologic examination of the atelectatic lesions showed clearly the charac-

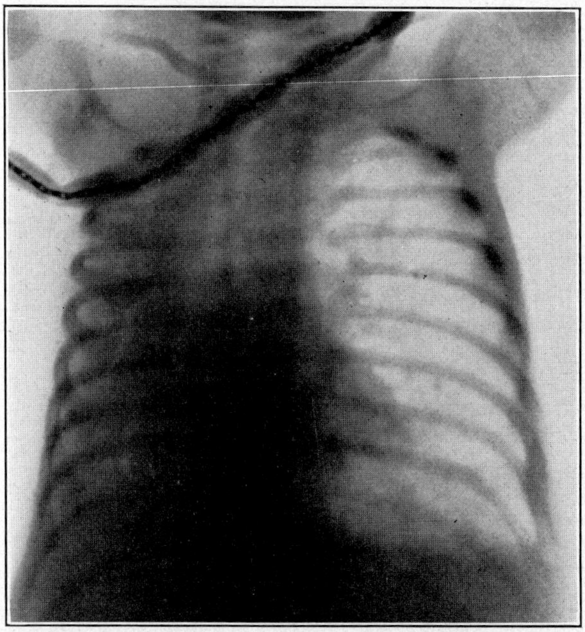

Fig. 2.—February 29. Atelectasis of the right lung. Cardiomediastinal deviation to the right.

teristic lesions of the lung (E. Normand): flattening of the alveolar cavities which had become unrecognizable, thickening of the walls with vascular distention, and tumescence of the large endothelial cells which were difficult to detect from other mononuclear elements which filled these cavities.

The mediastinum was normal, and thymus was not enlarged.

On opening the cranium, the cortical substance of the brain appeared normal. There was no trace of blood in the subarachnoidal spaces. But as the brain was lifted progressively from front to back and as the nerves of the base were cut, a large hematoma was discovered in the bulboprotuberential region. It adhered to, and could be removed with, the brain and was certainly of long standing, as it was already partially organized. It was proved to be a meningeal peribulbar median hemorrhage, encircling the anterior and lateral surfaces of the bulb, overlapping on to the protuberance after having filled the bulboprotuberential groove, and ending on a level with the occipital duct.

Summary.—A newborn premature infant showed a respiratory syndrome beginning on the seventh day after birth with a cough and on the twenty-first day with a fit of apnea.

Disturbances of the respiratory rhythm increased till they reached a very serious dyspnea characterized by fits of tachypnea during which the rhythm surpassed 150 per minute. Each inspiration was brusque and spasmodic and was accompanied by a strong subcostal recession and only a slight substernal recession. These spells lasted for varying lengths of time, usually about 10 seconds. They began and ended suddenly. They were separated by intervals sometimes as long as one-half minute.

X-ray findings showed atelectasis of the right lung. Attempts were made at bronchoscopy to clear the right bronchi and therapeutic pneumothorax to replace the heart and mediastinum in proper position.

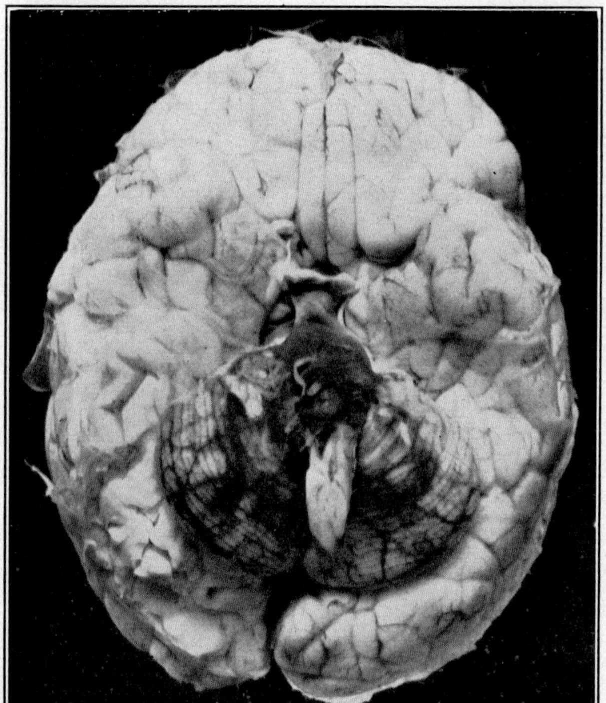

Fig. 3.—Bulboprotuberantial hemorrhage. The limits of the clot of blood are well defined. The clot is attached to the brain below the pia mater. It fills the anterior surface of the protuberance, the upper portion of the bulb and spreads over the inferior surface of the cerebellum.

Finally, at the age of 59 days the child died without showing (which is to be carefully noted) the slightest obvious disturbance of the nerve functions or any symptoms of meningeal origin (the spinal fluid having kept its normal, clear aspect, containing no red cells). Post-mortem examination showed, on one hand, an atelectatic collapse of the whole of the right lung (except for the inferior tongue of the superior and middle lobes) in contrast to the normal appearance of the left lung (except for an atelectatic zone on the posteroinferior region of the inferior lobe) and, on the other hand, an absence of bronchial obstruction or compression, so that the cause of atelectasis would have remained unknown if the meningeal hemorrhage, which the plate showed to be considerable, were not present to give the necessary explanation. The meningeal clot was of long standing; its limits were defined under the pia mater and adherent to the nerve centers at the level of the protuberance and the bulb, with a diffused area extending over the inferior surface of the cerebellum.

Through this interesting history we are in possession of the following data: A meningeal hemorrhage of the bulboprotuberential region with no clinical findings but those of a progressive atelectasis of the lung, coughing, and grave disturbances of the respiratory mechanism, was the cause of the death of a newborn infant at the age of 59 days.

These anatomical clinical findings throw light on certain cases we had observed formerly, but in which the mechanism appeared to us particularly obscure. We will report briefly on them, as their histories are incomplete. In the first of the three cases the baby died, and autopsy of the cranium was refused by the family. The two other patients recovered without subdural puncture through the fontanel. We have no proof of the central origin of these two cases of atelectasis, which were accompanied by serious respiratory disturbances, with sudden and unexplainable onset. We simply report these facts to draw attention to them. Subdural puncture should be performed through the fontanel in order to find the etiology of such cases. The three histories have been published at length in French.

The first case is that of an infant, born at term after normal labor who, until seen in the hospital, was perfectly healthy. On the twentieth day cough and dyspnea appeared suddenly without any seeming cause; in the following days these disturbances became more intense and were accompanied by suffocating spells with cyanosis. The frequency and the imperious and noisy form of coughing and the intensity of dyspnea were in vivid contrast with the good general condition and the total apyrexia. Roentgenograms showed the formation and the progressive extension of atelectasis of the right lung, which finding was confirmed by autopsy (complete atelectasis of the right lung, reducing it to the size of a fetal lung).

The second was a definite case of atelectasis, clinically primitive, apyretic, entirely inexplicable in its etiology, showing only intense coughing accentuated by feeding, in a child 5 weeks old, whose recovery was complete.

The last case is particularly interesting because it reproduces the disturbances of the respiratory rhythm noted in our principal case report. In a baby 13 days old, in perfect health until that day, apneic spells suddenly appeared, with serious disturbances of the respiratory rhythm, loss of consciousness, and lack of muscular resistance; all these symptoms disappeared by degrees after three weeks. This alarming condition was accompanied by the appearance of râles on auscultation of the lung and some opaque zones on the film. These findings allow the diagnosis of atelectasis in spite of faintness of the characteristic symptoms, such as displacement of the mediastinum, raising of the diaphragm, and sinking of the intercostal spaces.

Formerly we should have classified two of these histories as "atelectasis of unknown origin in the newborn" (and should probably have incriminated, without proof, some foreign body from the alimentary tract), and the third case as "apneic spells in the newborn." Are we not right in connecting all these observations and in laying stress on the interesting association of spells of apnea, serious disturbances of the respiratory rhythm, spasmodic paroxysms of coughing, and even hiccoughing (M. Lelong) with that of an atelectatic picture? All these details combine to show, as we have already demonstrated in the history published above, that these troubles have their origin in the nerve centers. Up to the present we had very little knowledge of the subject of clinically primitive pulmonary atelectasis in the very young child. However, similar cases have been observed and, if not studied, at least mentioned by various authors (Iorg, quoted by Rilliet and Barthez and more recently by Kundrath and by Blanco and Paperini). In spite of the uncertainty of the indications given, they admit the possibility of the connection between cerebral hemorrhage of the newborn and atelectasis.

On the other hand, spells of apnea in the newborn, clearly described by Rilliet and Barthez, have since been observed by numerous authors, as Marfan, D'Astros, Gardère, Still, Rohmer, and Ribadeau-Dumas and his pupils. Ribadeau-Dumas lays stress on the frequency of meningeal hemorrhage. One of his histories (meningeal hemorrhage of the inferior vermis and the fourth ventricle) is typical, and he concludes, quoting Waitz, that cerebromeningeal hemorrhages should first be taken into consideration in cases of apneic spells in the newborn.

In any case these observations oblige us to consider pulmonary atelectasis of the newborn or of the very young child, not as a purely local phenomenon, but as a sequel to a cerebral lesion or, more exactly, to a meningeal hemorrhage. But is it the result of a motion at a distance, a reflex, or does the central lesion, moved by a different mechanism, modify the respiratory rhythm and consequently the pulmonary ventilation?

The point is that the lungs are not merely inactive masses with their motility always and exclusively actioned by the surrounding walls; on the contrary, they are endowed with a certain autoregulation and independent activity. Pulmonary atelectasis may therefore be considered as an *active phenomenon,* the result of contraction of the lung proper under diverse reflex influences.

A direct explanation of this theory is not easy: certainly the richness of the lung in elastic fibers, shown by anatomy, proves the possibility of an activity proper to the lung, to be compared relatively with that of the bladder or the spleen. But in our ignorance of the normal and pathologic physiology of pulmonary innervation, there is too much margin for the hypothesis.

Research workers have seldom inquired into the nervous mechanism of atelectasis, previously cited by Mendelssohn. W. Pasteur attempted to provoke atelectasis by sectioning the phrenic nerve to prove the theory which made paresis of the diaphragm the principal factor of atelectasis. He obtained a chance result, as did Schroeder and Green and, more recently, Briscoe.

This line of research was almost abandoned until the study of Fontaine and Hermann on pulmonary innervation. These authors, experimenting on dogs, succeeded in sectioning the extrinsic nerves of the lung by extirpating the star ganglion with Vieussens' annulus and sectioning the vagosympathetic nerve for a length of a few centimeters. They ascertained that no microscopic or macroscopic alterations were present in the denervated lung after the operation. But chance allowed them to observe an instantaneous and fatal atelectasis on the operated side two days later. Benedetti and Lasdhy obtained negative results with the same operation.

On the other hand, Pari, experimenting on a frog, obtained a permanent atelectasis by sectioning the pneumogastric nerve, and in amphibians and cold blooded animals Carlson and Luckardt describe the appearance of a permanent retraction of the lung following a sectioning of the pneumogastric nerve or excitation of the sympathetic nerve.

In spite of these experimental, uncertain, partial, and, for the most part negative, results, the school of Bologna with Viola and Benedetti believed that they could define the physiology of pulmonary innervation; their conviction is that a disturbance of the pulmonary tonus plays an important part in the pathogenesis of atelectasis. Their theory is that the pleurointerlobulary smooth muscular system innervated by the sympathetic is antagonistic to the bronchial muscular system innervated by the parasympathetic system.

Excitation of the vagus creates a condition of pulmonary expansion, a definite diastole, while excitation of the sympathetic causes contraction capable of reaching a stage of atelectasis. They base this theory on a series of clinical observations of unequal values, of which the principal ones are thoracic dilatation and homolateral emphysema in a case of paralysis of the cervical sympathetic; pulmonary distention with bronchial spasms in conditions presenting a vagal predominance, such as asthma or an anaphylactic shock; and increase of atelectatic functional disturbances after an injection of atropine.

Once the active retraction of the lung is admitted and considered as being caused by a reflex, the source of the reflex is found to vary, being sometimes intrapulmonary, such as atelectasis following endobronchial irritation or a thoracic wound. Or it may be in the vicinity, as in cases of postoperative atelectasis, of which the frequency after operation in the subdiaphragmatic region is a consequence of the quantity of nervous fibers spreading under the cupola and grouped in the region of the solar plexus. Or, finally, the nervous mechanism is still more evident when atelectasis is consecutive to a medullar or bulbar lesion in the case that we have reported above.

Moreover, this nervous reflex mechanism can be understood in various ways. We have given weight to the active pulmonary retraction which seems the most obvious, but we cannot underestimate the rôle of hypoventilation. This can also be the consequence of a local factor as "prolonged decubitus, immobilization due to pain, diaphragmatic paralysis," or it may depend on a central, cerebral, and especially bulbar mechanism. We must not forget that the infant who suffered from a peribulbar hemorrhage showed a respiratory arrhythmia with impressive spells of apnea.

Sante was wise in laying stress on the part played by respiratory insufficiency, by functional inhibition, in causing pulmonary atelectasis. And lastly Binet, and Jaulmes, experimenting with the aid of a special technique on an isolated, rhythmically ventilated and artificially perfused lung, were able to obtain at will, if not atelectasis, at least a partial or massive collapse by varying the intensity of pulmonary ventilation.

In any case it is our opinion that in the newborn or early infancy certain cases of atelectasis, of apnea, and of serious disturbances of the respiratory rhythm have been caused by a meningeal hemorrhage. It is well to remember that these hemorrhages, the etiology of which is obscure, are not very rare; their clinical explanation is difficult, and particularly in hemorrhages of the eyeground, may not be forthcoming. It is also important to remember that the spinal fluid drawn by lumbar puncture may be normal, whereas the puncture of the dura mater sometimes produces an hemorrhagic or a xanthochromic fluid (Debré and G. Semelaigne). This simple method is without danger and should therefore be applied in all cases where either isolated disturbances of the respiratory rhythm are observed or when symptoms show definite or suspected atelectasis.

In conclusion, the diagnosis of pulmonary atelectasis resulting from a nervous lesion indicates the employment of a particular therapy for stimulating the respiratory centers, i.e., inhalation of carbogene, the efficiency of which has been proved on several occasions.

SUMMARY AND CONCLUSIONS

1. Pulmonary atelectasis in a very young infant may be caused by cerebral hemorrhage.

2. This atelectasis may be accompanied by serious disturbances of the respiratory rhythm, fits of apnea, phases of polypnea, Cheyne-Stokes respiration, and paroxysmal coughing, due to the same lesion.

3. Meningeal hemorrhage in such cases may be latent, the spinal fluid remaining normal. Under such conditions, recourse should be made to puncture of the dura mater which may produce a tinted liquid.

4. The mechanism of these pulmonary atelectases in early infancy is obscure. There is a possibility that it may be the outcome of a distant activity, a reflex. The nervous lesion may also be activated by a different mechanism, by modifying the respiratory rhythm, and consequently by decreasing pulmonary ventilation.

5. Hyperpnea caused by inhalations of carbogene constitutes the most effective treatment in these cases of nervous reflex atelectasis without bronchial obliteration.

REFERENCES

Adams, W. E., and Livingstone: Arch. Surg. **23**: 500, 1931.
d'Astros: Marseille-méd. Dec. 15, 1901; Jan. 12, 1902.
Benedetti, Piero: Paris méd. 425, 1929.
Binet, Léon, and Jaulmes, Ch.: Bull. et mém. Soc. méd. d. hôp. de Paris **52**: 1556, 1936.
Blanco, Vélasco, and Paperini, Humberto: Arch. am. de med. 1926.
Bradford, John Rose: Bull. et mém. Soc. méd. d. hôp. de Paris, 719, 1917.
Briscoe: Quart. J. Med. **23**: 293, 1920.
Carlson and Luckardt: Quoted by Benedetti.
Churchill: Quoted by Benedetti.
Coryllos and Birnbaum: Arch. Surg. **16**: 501, 1928.
Debré, Robert, Marie, Julien, Lamy, Maurice, and de Font-Réaulx, P.: Bull. et mém. Soc. méd. d. hôp. de Paris, 1606, 1936.
Fontaine and Hermann: Lyon chir. **25**: 29, 1928.
Jackson, Chevalier, and Lee: Tr. Am. S. A. **13**: 723, 1925.
Kundrath: In Traité de Médecine des Enfants, of von Pfaundler and Schlossmann.
Marfan: Clinique des Maladies de la Première Enfance, 557, 1926.
Mendelssohn: Der Mechanismus der Resp. und Zirkul, Berlin, 1845.
Nissen: Deutsche Ztschr. f. Chir. **179**: 160, 1923.
Pari: Quoted by Benedetti.
Pasteur, W.: Am. J. M. Sc. **100**: 292, 1890; and Lancet **1**: 1428, 1914.
Ribadeau-Dumas: Encyclop. médico-chir. Pédiatrie, Vol. II, p. 606.
Ribadeau-Dumas and Guédé: Semaine d. hôp. de Paris, p. 9, 1932.
Ribadeau-Dumas, and Melle. Spire-Weil: Bull. Soc. de pédiat. de Paris, Jan. 15, 45, 1935.
Rohmer: Traité de Méd. des Enfants, Vol. I, p. 374.
Sante: Am. J. Roentgenol. **20**: 213, 1928.
Schroeder and Green: Am. J. M. Sc. **123**: 196, 1902.
Viola: Bull. d. sc. med. **4**: 20, 1928; and **5**: 354, 1928.
Waitz: Thèsis: Paris, 1931.

SERUM TREATMENT OF PNEUMONIA IN CHILDHOOD

Rosa Lee Nemir, M.D.
New York, N. Y.

THE use of antipneumococcus serum in the treatment of pneumonia during childhood was begun at Bellevue Hospital on the Children's Medical Service in January, 1932. The first eighty-two patients treated were reported in 1933.[1] Following the use of Types I, XIV, VII, and V sera, the duration of the disease was shortened by several days, with dramatic precipitation of crisis in most instances. No appreciable effect on the low mortality rate of lobar pneumonia was demonstrated by the administration of antipneumococcus serum in this first group. It was pointed out that type XIV is the most frequent pneumococcus in pneumonia occurring in infants less than 2 years of age and in the runabout age group, and is usually associated with severe pneumonia.

The present report comprises an additional study of sixty-nine infants and children treated with antipneumococcus serum and one hundred twenty-eight untreated patients during the period from Sept. 15, 1933, to June 1, 1936. Cases due to Type XIV were not treated after April 1, 1936, as the serum was exhausted at that time. The types for which serum was used were I, II, IV, V, VI, VII, IX, XIV, XVIII, and XIX. The present study corroborates the findings of the previous report regarding the effect of serum upon the severity and course of disease, and throws additional light on its influence on mortality rate and on the development of empyema.

There are certain differences between pneumonia in adults and in children. It has been pointed out that the pneumococcus types associated with pneumonia differ. In adults Types I and II pneumococcus infections account for approximately one-half the cases of lobar pneumonia. In children, slightly less than one-half the lobar pneumonia cases were associated with Types I, XIV, and VI.[2] Pneumococcus II pneumonia is rare in patients less than 12 years old. The pediatrist dealing with pneumococcus pneumonia has a more complicated and diversified bacteriologic and, hence, clinical picture to study.

From the Department of Pediatrics, New York University, and the Children's Medical Service, Bellevue Hospital, and the Bureau of Laboratories, Department of Health, New York City.

This investigation was made possible by a grant from the Commonwealth Fund to the New York University, Department of Pediatrics, for research in pneumonia during 1931 to 1933. Assistance was also given during the first year by the Altman Foundation and during the year 1934-35 by the Metropolitan Life Insurance Company.

This study was made under the direction and advice of Dr. William H. Park, director emeritus of the Bureau of Laboratories, Department of Health, New York City, and Dr. Charles Hendee Smith, director of the Children's Medical Service, Bellevue Hospital and Professor of Pediatrics, New York University. The author wishes also to thank Dr. Julia Vinograd for her conscientious work in the bacteriologic typing throughout this study.

In addition to the differences in bacteriology, the severity is decreased and the mortality is lower in lobar pneumonia in children than in adults. With the same type of pneumococcus infection the severity of pneumonia in infants less than 2 years old occupies an intermediate position between the relatively milder disease found in older children and the severe disease with the higher death rate among adults. Cardiac failure, even in fatal cases, is rare in infants and children. It becomes apparent that the results of antipneumococcus serum therapy in adults cannot be directly compared with those for children and that a separate study may also contribute information concerning Types XIV and VI particularly.

METHOD

Choice of Material.—In this report only infants receiving antipneumococcus serum before the sixth day of disease and children treated before the fifth day are included in the serum group. Pneumonia in infants was several days longer than in older children with the same type of pneumococcus infection. During the last year of this study members of the house staff, encouraged by results of serum therapy in previous cases, administered serum late in the disease. These patients have not been included in the serum study group but will be referred to later in the paper. No patient admitted after the fourth or fifth day of disease has been included in the untreated control group. Approximately alternate patients in whom pneumonia was diagnosed early and on whom prompt bacteriologic typing was obtained received treatment. Some patients, mildly ill, were not diagnosed with certainty until a roentgenogram was obtained, and this was often too late for serum therapy. Crisis occurred in a number of patients before the pneumococcus typing was obtained; these patients were added to the untreated control group. It is apparent that the untreated control group necessarily was larger than the serum-treated group and contained many more mild cases. In the last year of the study many mildly ill patients were deliberately not treated with serum even though they were seen early in the disease. These facts should be kept in mind in evaluating the results as they indicate that the untreated patients were not as severely ill as those receiving treatment.

Most of the patients receiving serum had lobar pneumonia; the bacteriologic study of the majority of patients with bronchopneumonia did not reveal pneumococci for which therapeutic sera were available. The diagnosis of lobar pneumonia was made as previously outlined[1] on the basis of the well-known clinical picture and x-ray evidence of consolidation. Smith[3] has given the criteria for the diagnosis of the various types of pneumonia as used on the Children's Medical Service of Bellevue Hospital, which were followed in this study.

Method of Typing.—As soon as a diagnosis of pneumonia was suspected, a laryngeal culture was obtained by means of a long cotton swab[4] and was put into a tube of plasma broth. In obtaining the swab it is important to have the child cough several times before taking the swab or, in an infant, to irritate the throat several times and remove the tongue depressor to enable the baby to cough up mucus. Another cough is thus provoked, and the foamy mucus is caught on the Neufeld (quellung) reaction as adapted originally by Sabin[5a] for tongue depressor.

The material so obtained was studied bacteriologically by three methods. 1. A blood agar streaked plate was made, using the original swab. 2. A mouse was injected with the inoculated plasma broth after incubation. Pneumococcus typing was determined both from the peritoneal exudate and from the blood of the mouse's heart by the Sabin slide agglutination technique.[5] 3. A rapid direct typing was made for the Neufeld (quellung) reaction as adapted originally by Sabin[5a] for immediate typing of pneumococci from sputum. Centrifuged inoculated plasma broth was used for this study as described by Vinograd, Nemir, and Park.[4]

A typing was usually obtained within eight to twenty-four hours. If two few pneumococci were found for typing within twelve hours, another swab was taken. Repeat cultures were taken from all patients who failed to show pneumococci and from all patients having pneumococci III, VI, and XIX or any of the higher numbered types which are rarely seen in patients with pneumonia (XIII, XXI, XXIII, XXX, and XXXII). Types III, VI, and XIX were found in patients with pneumonia, as was verified in some cases by cultures of these types from pleural exudate, blood culture, spinal fluid, or post-mortem lung suction culture. Nevertheless, these organisms occurred so commonly in healthy infants and children that repeated studies were necessary to evaluate their significance in the laryngeal culture; they might have been accidental pharyngeal inhabitants and not the causative factor of pneumonia. Andrews,[6] in her bacteriologic study of patients with pneumonia and their contacts with the Children's Medical Service, Bellevue Hospital, illustrates this observation.

SERUM ADMINISTRATION

Concentrated refined horse sera were furnished by the Bureau of Laboratories of the Department of Health, New York City, by courtesy of the late Miss Georgia Cooper. Concentrated serum varying in potency from 400 to 2,000 units per cubic centimeter was used. Each patient before treatment received an intracutaneous injection of 0.1 c.c. of a 1:10 dilution of the serum to be administered and also received one drop of this dilution in the eye. A patient with either a positive skin test or ophthalmic test within twenty minutes was not treated.

Only four patients of about seventy tested had a positive skin test, and none showed a positive eye test. Acetylsalicylic acid was given to patients with a temperature over 104° F. one-half hour before treatment to prevent excessive hyperpyrexia in the event of a thermal serum reaction. We do not recommend acetylsalicylic acid routinely for high fever in pneumonia. Patients were more uncomfortable during fluctuations of temperature. A blood culture was taken from most patients immediately before the first treatment.

No patient with eczema or known allergic history was treated, nor were the few with a positive skin test.

The initial dose of serum (test dose for sensitivity) was never greater than 2 cc. for patients less than 2 years old and frequently only 1 c.c. The serum was diluted to 10 c.c. with normal saline solution in order to facilitate slow administration. The initial dose for patients more than 2 years old was from 2 to 4 c.c. diluted to 10 c.c. Adrenalin was always at hand during the injection, to be used if indicated.

The first dose of serum was given intravenously and *slowly,* requiring one minute for the first cubic centimeter of the above diluted serum, and the entire administration consumed *at least five minutes,* as carefully timed by an assistant. Serum must be given slowly and should always be *timed with a watch,* since reactions are likely to follow rapid serum administration. Lord and Heffron[7] described precipitation of the serum after dilution, but we have never observed it. In infants the intravenous injection was best given into a scalp vein by a fine needle. Intravenous therapy by means of the jugular vein requires more handling and restraint of the baby.

Subsequent treatments were given at four- to six-hour intervals, intravenously if the temperature was still high and the patient was still very sick, otherwise, intramuscularly (undiluted). An intramuscular or intravenous injection was always given after the temperature, pulse, and respiration had been normal from six to eight hours. If this is not done, recurrence of symptoms is likely to occur. The amount of the subsequent dosage was dependent upon the response to the first injection. If definite marked improvement occurred, as was often the case, the same dosage was used, otherwise the initial dose was doubled. No more than 10 c.c. of serum was ever given at one time.

A crisis was observed following only three or four injections of serum (12 to 20 c.c., approximately 25,000 to 35,000 units) in two-thirds of the patients. Many of these patients showed marked improvement after a single treatment.

Regularity of treatment is very important. It seems much more desirable to give the same dosage in three or four injections at four-to six- or even eight-hour intervals than to divide the amount into two large doses at twelve-hour periods. In this series no patient was treated longer than forty-eight hours.

The total amount of serum needed depended on several factors. As in adults, when the blood culture is positive, more serum is required. The severity and duration of the disease at the time of treatment, the extent of pleurisy and alveolar exudate, i.e., number and extent of lobes involved, all influence the amount of specific antibody needed. Patients treated very early in the disease seemed to require less treatment. For these reasons it is difficult to formulate a rule for the amount of serum required. It cannot be administered with the accuracy of digitalis. Clinical judgment for each individual patient is always important.

Failure to show distinct improvement after three or four injections in twenty hours (for Types I and XIV, certainly, and perhaps also in Types V and VII) should always suggest one of the following factors: (1) error in bacteriologic type or mixed bacteriologic infection (other pneumococci or streptococci); (2) error in clinical diagnosis; (3) presence of some complication, e.g., empyema, otitis media, pyelitis, a bacteriemia, etc. One infant who was treated with Type XIV serum before the x-ray picture was received and failed to show improvement was found to have influenzal meningitis. In patients failing to respond to treatment, a careful examination with the aid of fluoroscopy and x-ray pictures (using lateral, eccentric and anteroposterior views) and a search for other causes of disease or complications were made. The laryngeal swab was repeated, blood agar streaked plates being used, to verify the bacteriologic diagnosis of the disease.

Cases 1 and 2 illustrated the importance of this procedure. A comparison of the results with the temperature charts of patients 3 to 12 is interesting.

CASE 1.—J. C., a 21-month-old infant, was admitted because of high fever, chill, and rapid respiration of three days' duration. Signs of consolidation were found over the right upper lobe, confirmed by a dense x-ray shadow. The patient was acutely ill on admission when a laryngeal swab was taken, and in eighteen hours pneumococcus Type VI was cultured from the mouse's heart's blood and peritoneum. Treatment with Type VI serum was begun at once, but, as customary in Type VI pneumonia, another laryngeal culture was immediately taken.

No change in the clinical picture was observed after five doses of serum (25,000 units), two intravenously and three intramuscularly. At this time the second swab revealed both pneumococcus Types I and VI in the mouse's heart's blood and peritoneum. The apparent failure of serum in this patient was really a failure to make the correct etiological diagnosis. Pneumococcus I, if not the sole etiological agent, was at least the most important factor, and Type VI was either the normal inhabitant of the throat or only partially responsible for the pneumonia.

Type I pneumococcus when cultured from the swab of a patient with pneumonia was always etiologically related to the disease, as was often evidenced by cultures from other body fluids. Conversely, Type VI was probably an accidental inhabitant of the throat and not responsible for the lung infection in certain cases.

CASE 2.—L. O., an infant 11½ months old, was admitted on the second day of illness from pneumonia. For seven days the baby had "cold and a little fever"; the day before admission the fever became very high. The infant was severely ill, and signs of right upper lobe consolidation were confirmed by x-ray pictures. The first laryngeal swab revealed pneumococcus Type IX from the mouse's heart's blood. Three injections of serum, two intravenously and one intramuscularly, of 13 c.c. (6,500 units) were given with no apparent clinical improvement. From the second

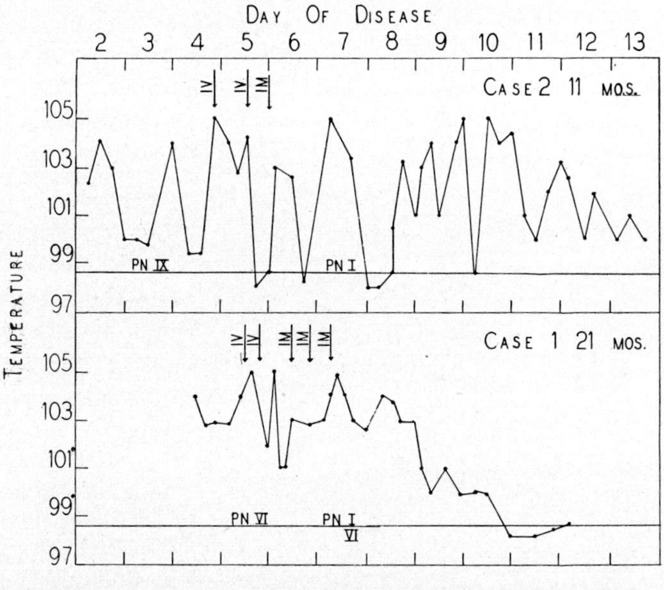

Chart 1.—Temperature curves of 2 patients failing to show the usual response to serum therapy; see text for description of cases. Both patients had unsatisfactory response to therapy because of error in etiological diagnosis. Serum injections are represented by arrows; IV means intravenously; IM, intramuscularly.

swab only pneumococcus Type I was cultured, and Type IX was not found either in the mouse or on the blood agar plate. Type IX seems to have been the throat inhabitant, and Type I, the cause of the pneumonia.

The importance of attempting to evaluate the presence of the higher numbered types and the pneumococci commonly found in the normal respiratory passages is apparent in Cases 1 and 2. Repeated cultures are advised in all such instances, as well as in those in which response to serum administration is unsatisfactory.

Serum Reactions.—Immediate anaphylactic reaction was not seen during the three years covered by this report in the eighty-one patients receiving serum. One patient developed generalized urticaria after the first injection of 2 c.c. of antipneumococcus serum intravenously. The preliminary ophthalmic test was negative, but by error an intracutaneous test was not done.

Serum sickness was seen in two of seventy-nine patients, ten of whom were treated too late to be included in the study of serum efficacy. One case of serum sickness occurred in an infant 23 months of age who had received four injections, totaling 11 c.c. of serum. The second patient, a 6-year-old child, showed an accelerated reaction consisting of edema of the eyes and urticaria four days after treatment with six injections. This patient had received antipneumococcus serum two years previously.

Febrile reactions following serum in the past three years were rare. A few patients had a rise in temperature of 2 to 3° F. with chills, dyspnea, and occasional cyanosis, occurring from one-half to one hour after the serum administration. Rapid serum injections may produce even earlier reactions. One of these occurred as early as twenty minutes after the first dose of serum. The treatment for this type of reaction is the same as for any hyperpyrexia. Adrenalin is not helpful.

RESULTS

There were 128 untreated control patients with lobar and bronchopneumonia and sixty-nine who received specific antipneumococcus serum. Therapeutic sera for Types I, IV, V, VI, VII, IX, XIV, XVIII, and XIX were used. Each serum should be evaluated separately since the clinical picture associated with each type of pneumococcus differs in severity, complications, and response to specific serum. Types I, XIV, and VI were the predominant organisms associated with lobar pneumonia, accounting for almost half of the cases of lobar pneumonia in this series. As previously shown,[2] Type I pneumococcus was the predominant organism in the older children with pneumonia and Type XIV in the pneumonia of infants less than 2 years of age.

The distribution of the sixty serum-treated patients with lobar pneumonia by age group and pneumococcus types is shown in Table I. The untreated control group of one hundred seventeen patients with lobar pneumonia included more mildly ill patients as noted previously. Crisis occurred in a moderate number of these patients before a bacteriologic typing was obtained, so that a choice of treatment could not be made.

A therapeutic agent may show its efficacy by (1) reducing the mortality rate, (2) reducing the incidence of complications, and (3) its effect upon the clinical course of the disease.

Because of the relative benignancy of lobar pneumonia in children, the case fatality rate can only be used as a criterion of the value of serum when hundreds of cases are treated. In the young infant with lobar pneumonia the mortality rate is higher. The failure of serum to show a reduction of the mortality rate in our series may be due to the small number of patients.

TABLE I

DISTRIBUTION OF PATIENTS WITH LOBAR PNEUMONIA BY AGE GROUP AND PNEUMOCOCCUS TYPE

(Sept. 1, 1933, to June 1, 1936)

	SERUM-TREATED PATIENTS							UNTREATED CONTROL PATIENTS							
	UNDER 2 YR.			2-12 YR.				UNDER 2 YR.			2-12 YR.				
TYPE	PATIENTS	EMPYEMA (CASES)	DEATHS	PATIENTS	EMPYEMA (CASES)	DEATHS	TOTAL	PATIENTS	EMPYEMA (CASES)	DEATHS	PATIENTS	EMPYEMA (CASES)	DEATHS	TOTAL	GRAND TOTAL
I	3	0	0	20	1	0	23	8	0	0	41	7	0	49	72
II	0			2*	0	0	2	0			8*	2	0	8	10
IV	0			1*	0	0	1	0			2*	0	0	2	3
V	0			3*	1	0	3	0			4*	0	0	4	7
VI	3	0	0	0			3	10	0	1†	0			10	13
VII	1	0	0	6	0	0	7	0			12	0	0	12	19
IX	2‡	1§	1§				2	1‡	0	0	0			1	3
XIV	13	0	1	5	0	0	18	21	2	2	10	1	1	31	49
XVIII	0			1	0	0	1	0			0			0	1
	22	1	2	38	2	0	60	40	2	3	77	10	1	117	177

*No patients included for 1933 to 1934 or 1935 to 1936, because there were no treated cases.

†This baby at autopsy had a combination of lipoid pneumonia and broncholobular pneumonia. Pneumococcus VI cultures from the post-mortem lung puncture were made immediately after death.

‡No patients included for 1934 to 1935 or 1935 to 1936.

§This patient had a positive blood culture at the time of initial treatment.

In considering the cases of pneumonia which probably do not fall into the group of lobar pneumonia, it may be well to mention the tentative classification of pneumonia we are using at present: (1) lobar, or pneumococcus pneumonia (alveolar or croupous pneumonia, etc.); (2) lobular pneumonia, a patchy alveolar exudate with no bronchopneumonia (often due to aspiration in young infants); (3) broncholobular pneumonia, a combination of these two, with peribronchial infiltration and patchy lobular exudate. The amount of these two elements is extremely variable, and the disease may begin in either form. We believe at present that a virus may cause the peribronchial exudate, while the alveolar inflammatory reaction is probably due to pneumococcus or other bacteria.

In cases of bronchopneumonia, many of which were probably of the broncholobular variety, a significant reduction in the fatality rate apparently occurred in the serum-treated group (Table II), when bronchopneumonia was associated with pneumococci for which sera were available. Although the number of patients in this group was small, the results were consistent for both periods studied. When patients with bronchopneumonia associated with pneumococcus XIV or I were treated with specific sera, they were benefited clinically and apparently sufficiently to enable more of them to recover than those in a similar untreated group. Even though these types of pneumococci may not have been the sole etiological agent of bronchopneumonia, they were certainly sufficiently responsible for some of the toxicity to warrant treatment with serum. The response to serum of patients with bronchopneumonia differed from that of patients with lobar pneumonia. There was no prompt crisis, but a loss of toxicity, a drop in temperature, often to normal, and a loss of respiratory difficulty was noticed after twenty-four hours' treatment. These patients were treated arbitrarily for only forty-eight hours (about seven or eight injections of serum).

Table II

Mortality Rate of Serum-Treated and Control Patients With Bronchopneumonia (Broncholobular) Types I, XIV, and XIX

AGE	SERUM-TREATED CASES			UNTREATED CASES	
	TYPE	PATIENTS	DEATHS	PATIENTS	DEATHS
Under 2 yr.	I	2	0	0	0
	XIV	4	0	5	1
	XIX	2	1	5	3
2-12 yr.	XIX	1	0	1	0
Total of all types					
Present report		9	1	11	4
Previous report		12	6	24	17
Grand total (1932-1936)		21	7 (33.3%)	35	21(60%)

The mortality rate for untreated patients with Type XIV lobar pneumonia was higher than for those with Type I, probably to a large extent because of the frequent occurrence of Type XIV infection in patients less than 2 years of age, a period when the disease is more fatal, even with the same type of pneumococcus. The serum-treated group was much smaller than the control untreated group, and the patients were more seriously ill. There were three deaths among the forty-three treated patients, the same mortality rate as in the untreated control group. Two infants less than 1 year old died during serum treatment in the first year of the study; one immediately following the first intravenous injection and the other immediately following the second intravenous administration of serum. We believe the deaths were due to rapid serum administration and, therefore, were preventable. Both patients were acutely ill. They had negative skin and eye tests for horse-serum sensitivity.

Of the forty-five patients with pneumococcus Type I lobar pneumonia treated with serum during the five-year period, none died. There was one death among the seventy-nine untreated control patients.

No deaths were observed in the small serum-treated group with Types II, IV, V, VI, or VII and only one in the untreated series; the death occurred in an infant whose laryngeal swab revealed pneumococcus Type VI. At autopsy lipoid pneumonia was discovered, thus minimizing the etiological significance, if any, of pneumococcus VI in this patient.

The frequency of empyema differed with the type of infecting pneumococcus. Type I infections, regardless of treatment, showed a high incidence of empyema as reported in a five-year study.[2] Of the 142 patients with Type I pneumonia, regardless of treatment or time of admission to the hospital, 30 (21 per cent) developed empyema. In the present report 12.6 per cent of the 79 untreated control patients during the past five years had empyema. When antipneumococcus serum was administered early in the disease, only 1 (2.2 per cent) of the forty-five serum treated patients developed empyema (Table III).

TABLE III

INCIDENCE OF COMPLICATIONS AND MORTALITY IN LOBAR PNEUMONIA PATIENTS LESS THAN 12 YEARS OLD

PNEUMOCOCCUS TYPES I, XIV, AND V

(Jan. 1, 1932, to June 1, 1936)

TYPE		SERUM-TREATED PATIENTS*			UNTREATED CONTROL PATIENTS		
		PATIENTS	EMPYEMA (CASES)	DEATHS	PATIENTS	EMPYEMA (CASES)	DEATHS
I	Present series	23	1	0	49	7	0
	Previous report	22	0	0	30	3	1
	Total	45	1 (2.2%)	0	79	10 (12.6%)	1 (1.3%)
XIV	Present series	18	0	1	31	3	3
	Previous report	25	0	2†	34	1	2
	Total	43	0	3 (7%)	65	4 (6.1%)	5 (7.7%)
V	Present series	3	1	0	4	0	0
	Previous report	3	0	0	6	2	0
	Total	6	1	0	10	2	0
Grand total		94	2 (2.1%)	3 (3.2%)	154	16 (10.4%)	6 (3.9%)

*Only those treated on or before the fifth day of disease in children, or the sixth in infants.

†Both deaths probably due to serum accident in the first year of study. Both babies had negative skin and eye test for sensitivity; one died immediately after the first injection and the other immediately after the second.

Note there was no reduction in the mortality rate in the two groups, but there was an apparent effect on the incidence of empyema.

The figures cited above for the percentage of deaths and empyema in the untreated control patients do not represent the true mortality or empyema incidence because this group excludes (1) all patients admitted late in the disease, who are usually extremely ill; (2) children dying at the time of admission; and (3) those having empyema when admitted.

Patients with Type XIV pneumonia, regardless of type of therapy, had a much lower empyema rate than those with Type I pneumonia. In the previous study[2] only fourteen (8 per cent) of 174 patients with

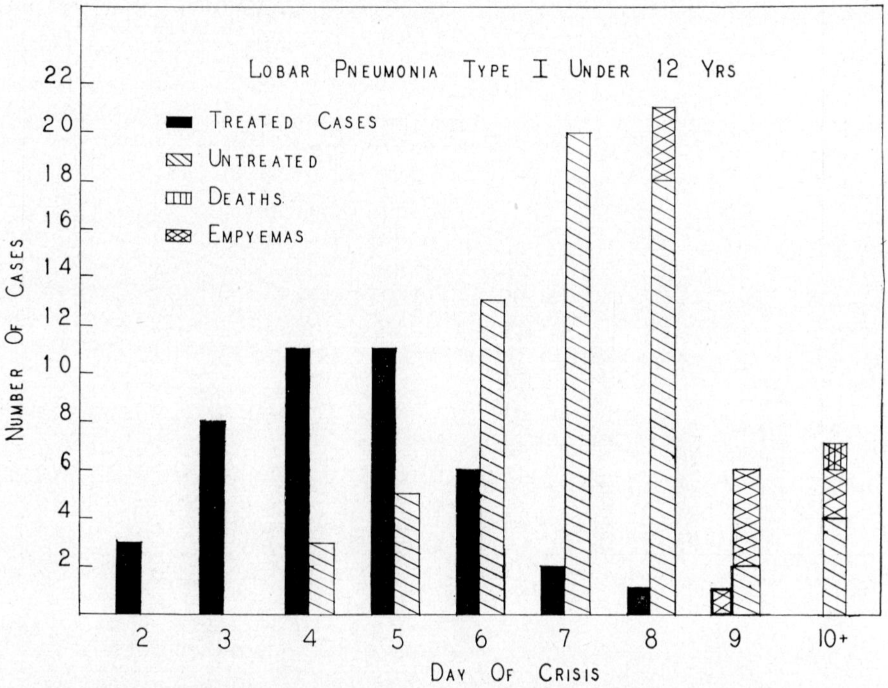

Chart 2.—Duration of Type I pneumococcus pneumonia in 43 patients treated with Type I serum compared with 75 untreated patients. Seventy-six per cent of the patients receiving serum had a crisis on or before the fifth day of disease, and only 11 per cent of the untreated group had such an early crisis.

pneumococcus XIV pneumonia developed suppurative pleurisy. In the present study none of the 43 patients treated early with type XIV serum developed empyema as compared with 4 (6.1 per cent) in the 65 untreated control patients. That late administration of serum did not seem to affect the incidence of empyema was readily seen in the fate of twelve patients treated after the fifth day of disease, six with Type XIV, and six with Type I. Four of each of these two groups developed empyema, and two of these infected with Type XIV subsequently died. However, one baby, desperately ill with Type XIV bacteriemia and pneumonia, survived. One previously reported patient with Type V pneumonia was treated late and also developed empyema.

Empyema was rare in Type VI pneumonia patients even though this was a frequent type of pneumococcus in the pneumonia of infancy and early childhood. Similarly uncommon was Type VII empyema. None of the patients in either group of treated or untreated patients developed empyema with Types VI or VII.

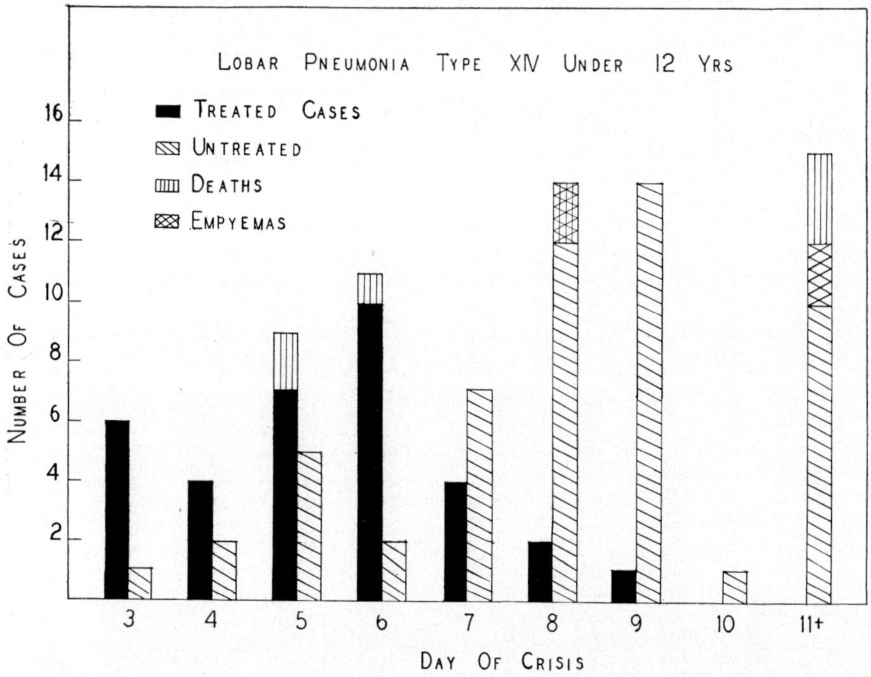

Chart 3.—Duration of Type XIV pneumococcus pneumonia for 37 patients treated with serum compared with 61 untreated control patients. The early crisis in this group is also apparent; 16.4 per cent of the untreated patients had a crisis on or before the sixth day of disease as compared with 73 per cent of those receiving serum.

The effect of specific antipneumococcus serum upon the course of the disease was so dramatic and was so regularly observed following the administration of certain types of sera (I, XIV, VII, and V) as to preclude chance association. The few cases of Type II pneumonia which were treated showed similar results. Of the untreated control patients with Type I lobar pneumonia, 11 per cent had a crisis on or before the fifth day as compared with 76 per cent of the treated group. The figures illustrating the shortening of disease were equally as impressive for Type XIV pneumonia; only 16.4 per cent of the untreated control patients had a crisis on or before the sixth day of disease as compared with 73 per cent of those receiving antipneumococcus serum

(Charts 2 and 3). In the majority of patients within twelve to twenty-four hours the temperature, pulse, and respiratory rate dropped to normal, and signs of toxicity practically disappeared. A low-grade temperature occasionally persisted if another infection was present (e.g., otitis media, as commonly occurred in infants suffering with pneumonia), but the patient no longer presented the typical picture of pneumonia, with rapid pulse and respiration and general signs of toxicity. (Charts of Cases 3 through 11 illustrate the usual response to serum.)

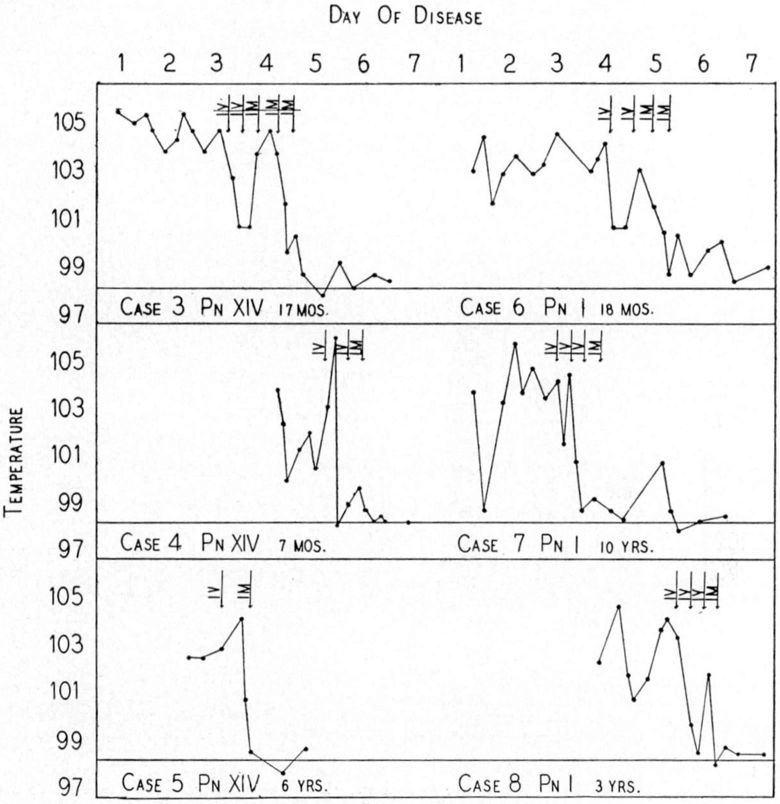

Chart 4.—Selected temperature charts of patients with lobar pneumonia treated for Type I and XIV pneumonia at different ages, showing the usual prompt response to therapy and the number and frequency of treatment. The total dosage for cases given was as follows: Case 3, 12 c.c. or 9,600 units; Case 4, 11 c.c. or 33,000 units; Case 5, 7 c.c. or 10,500 units; Case 6, 13 c.c. or 52,000 units; Case 7, 20 c.c. or 30,000 units; Case 8, 22 c.c. or 33,000 units. The variability in number of doses and amount of serum is shown, illustrating the importance of clinical judgment.

Precipitation of crisis as described above was so irregularly observed after the use of serum in Type VI pneumonia that this serum cannot be recommended at present (Cases 12 and 13). Several explanations were possible: (1) This pneumococcus commonly present in normal individuals may not have been the etiological factor in the disease;

(2) the sera may not have been sufficiently potent; and (3) pneumococcus Type VI pneumonia on the whole is so mild that shortening of the disease is difficult to demonstrate. We have used antipneumococcus Type VI serum for treating three patients with meningitis and bacteriemia and for two others with bacteriemia alone, all of whom died. Undoubtedly Type VI was the etiological organism in these patients.*

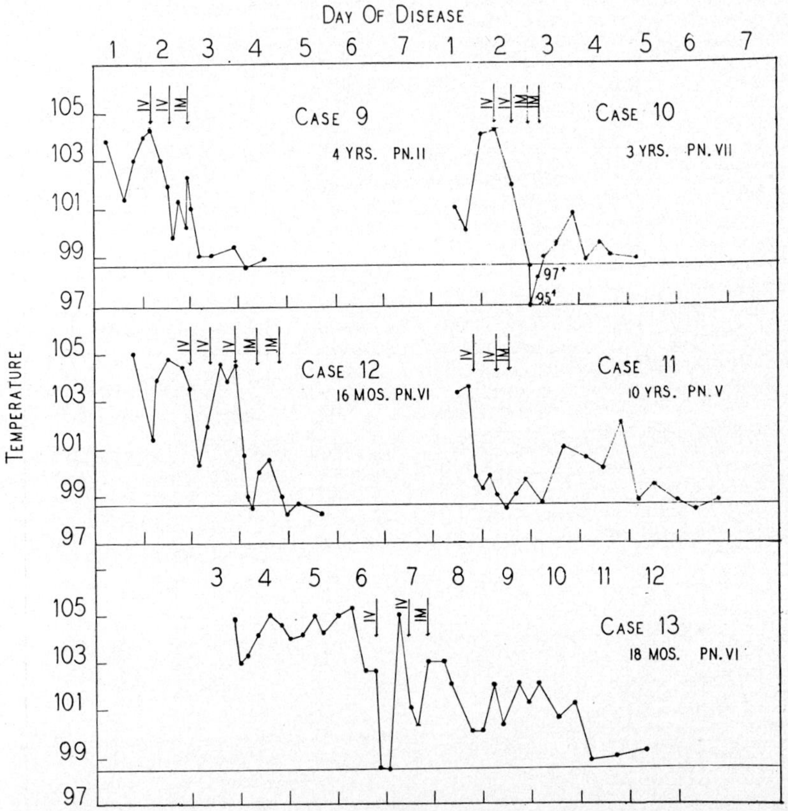

Chart 5.—Selected temperature curves of patients with lobar pneumonia for Types VII, V, II, and VI. Serum injections are represented by arrows, IV means intravenously; IM means intramuscularly. The amount of serum given in each case was as follows: Case 9, 13 c.c. or 19,500 units; Case 10, 14 c.c. or 21,000 units; Case 11, 10 c.c. or 15,000 units; Case 12, 12 c.c. or 18,000 units; Case 13, 11 c.c. or 17,600 units. Response to Types VII, V, and II was comparable to that seen with Types I and XIV; on the other hand, Type VI did not regularly show the prompt improvement seen with these types. Note drop of temperature to 95.4° F. in Case 10, accompanied by cyanosis and symptoms of shock for twelve hours. This reaction was also seen in several other cases, all not treated with serum.

COMMENT

Both statistical evidence and clinical observations of individual cases in a large series of patients convince us that Types I and XIV sera

*During 1938 one 3-month-old patient severely ill with Type VI bacteriemia was treated with homologous serum and recovered.

are valuable and effective aids in the treatment of pneumonia in children. In a smaller series Types VII, V, and II (the latter on a very few patients) are shown to be similarly valuable.

Bullowa,[8] working also in New York City, reported his experience with Type XIV sera both in children and adults and showed definite results in the reduction of mortality, particularly in cases with bacteriemia, and in shortening the course of the disease. Kereszturi and Hauptmann[9] similarly showed the value of Types I and XIV sera in the treatment of pneumonia in children in another section of New York City.

Even though dramatic response to serum therapy may be obtained, other considerations are important prior to the decision to use antipneumococcus serum in children. Since the mortality rate of lobar pneumonia is low in children more than 2 or 3 years old, a specific therapeutic agent is not imperative. Although pneumococcus serum administration involves a minimal sensitization to horse serum,* it is a consideration to be kept in mind in deciding to use this type of treatment. Sensitization has not been demonstrable in several cases as shown by skin and eye tests at a later time. Two patients were treated a second time, one three to four weeks later, and the other one year later without any reaction in the first and an accelerated serum sickness in the second.

Treatment of patients with serum late in the disease is probably useless in patients less than 12 years old since it appears to affect mortality only slightly and complications not at all. However, in the presence of a bacteriemia, even though discovered late, sera shown to be effective (in our experience I and XIV, certainly, and VII, V, II, probably) are advised. Bacteriemia, a rare complication in children, when present indicates very severe and overwhelming infection. Most workers with antipneumococcus serum have constantly emphasized the importance of early treatment. Cecil,[10] combining his cases of Type I pneumonia with those of Bullowa, Heffron, and Rogers, has recently emphasized and demonstrated in a very interesting way the value and importance of very early serum treatment. Cole[11] has similarly shown the greater effectiveness of serum the earlier treatment is instituted; the mortality rate for those treated after the fifth day was 19.5 per cent and declined rapidly, with earlier treatment, to 4.8 per cent for those receiving serum during the first three days of illness. Rosenbluth and Block[12] likewise found a decline in mortality rate from 26 per cent in those treated from the third to the seventh

*During the period of study here reported only horse serum was used. At present a limited amount of rabbit's serum, Type XIV, is being supplied through the courtesy of Lederle Laboratories.

day as compared with 5.4 per cent for those whose treatment was started during the first three days after the onset of pneumonia.

Infants severely ill with Type XIV pneumococcus pneumonia should receive homologous serum early in the disease, since in this age group (less than 2 years old) the mortality rate is high.

The use of a combined nonspecific serum (e.g., Types I and XIV, or I and II) in the treatment of a severely ill infant or child before obtaining a pneumococcus typing on the swab is not recommended. The frequency of the two most effective types, I and XIV, does not justify the procedure, particularly in view of the fact that a typing can be obtained in from eight to twelve hours.[4] Types I and XIV occurred in 30.5 per cent of our 1,033 patients during a five-year period. In patients with lobar pneumonia Type I caused 23.9 per cent of the cases of pneumonia in patients 2 years of age or older. In those less than 2 years old Type XIV was cultured from 36 per cent of the patients with pneumonia. Our experience has repeatedly shown that serum is effective only for the specific type associated with the disease.

Although the efficacy of serum has been demonstrated previously, we advise its use only for those severely ill patients whose cases are diagnosed early, and for young infants, in whom the mortality rate is high. Indiscriminate utilization of serum for moderately or mildly ill patients is inadvisable because of the sensitization to horse serum and the consequent interference with subsequent therapy with the use of horse serum. It is urged, however, that every patient with pneumonia receive a pneumococcus typing as early as the diagnosis is made; the organism often serves as a guide to the course and duration of disease, incidence of complications, particularly empyema, and chances of fatality. Also the isolation of a hemolytic streptococcus or a pneumococcus Type III may well suggest the therapeutic use of sulphanilamide.

CONCLUSIONS

During a five-year study from Jan. 1, 1932, to June 1, 1936, of the value of antipneumococcus serum in the treatment of pneumonia in infants and children, one hundred fifty-one patients were treated and compared with 253 untreated control patients.

Type I was the predominant infecting organism in lobar pneumonia in patients more than 2 years old, and Type XIV the most frequent pneumococcus in patients less than 2 years of age.

The mortality rate for lobar pneumonia was low in both groups, and in this small series the administration of serum showed no reduction.

The incidence of empyema in patients with Types I, XIV, and V lobar pneumonia receiving serum early in the disease was reduced.

Late administration of serum in severely ill patients was obviously valueless in preventing or reducing the development of this complication.

A dramatic precipitation of the crisis was observed in the majority of patients treated with specific antibody within twelve to eighteen hours after the first treatment.

REFERENCES

1. Nemir, R. L.: J. Pediat. 3: 827, 1933.
2. Nemir, R. L., Andrews, E. T., and Vinograd, J.: Am. J. Dis. Child. **51**: 1277, 1936.
3. Smith, C. H.: Proc. Interstate Post-Grad. M. A., North America, October, 1935.
4. Vinograd, J., Nemir, R. L., and Park, W. H.: Am. J. Dis. Child. **51**: 782, 1936.
5. Sabin, A. B.: J. Infect. Dis. **46**: 469, 1930.
   a. Idem: J. A. M. A. **100**: 1584, 1933.
6. Andrews, E. T.: Am. J. Dis. Child. **54**: 1285, 1937.
7. Lord, F. T., and Heffron, R.: Lobar Pneumonia and Serum Therapy, New York, 1936, The Commonwealth Fund.
8. Bullowa, J. G. M.: J. Clin. Investigation **14**: 373, 1935.
9. Kereszturi, C., and Hauptmann, D.: J. Pediat. **4**: 331, 1934.
10. Cecil, R. L.: J. A. M. A. **108**: 689, 1937.
11. Cole, R.: Ann. Int. Med. **10**: 1, 1936.
12. Rosenbluth, M. B.. and Block, M.: Arch. Int. Med. **58**: 102, 1936.

MYOTONIA CONGENITA

Report of a Case Treated by Quinine

William A. Hawke, M.D., M.R.C.P. (London)
Toronto, Ont.

Myotonia congenita was first described in 1876 by Thomsen. About twenty cases had occurred in four generations of this physician's family, and to many this condition is better known as Thomsen's disease. The etiology is unknown; it was considered at first to be familial, but many cases have since been recorded with a negative family history. The essential conditions are slow contractions, and relaxations of the voluntary musculature. The disease has been investigated recently by the electromyograph, and Lindsley and Curnan[3] believe the primary factors are hyperexcitable sensory nerve endings in the affected muscles, producing the myotonic reaction through reflex activities. Kennedy and Wolf,[2] on the other hand, believe that the site of the disease lies in the myoneural junction. Contrasting myotonia with myasthenia, they consider that some abnormality in the metabolism of acetylcholine is probably the primary condition.

The affected muscles usually show gross hypertrophy, and microscopically there is no evidence of fibrous or fatty infiltration. The diameter of the individual fibers varies from 60 to 145 microns, in contrast to a normal variation of from 20 to 65 microns. There is an associated increase in the sarcolemmal nuclei and some loss of transverse striations.

The condition of myotonia usually appears in childhood, though in certain cases it may not be noticed until maturity. The characteristic features lie in the slow, clumsy, movements, the slow initiation of muscle contraction, and extremely slow relaxation. These factors are increased by fatigue, cold, and hunger and are decreased by warmth and exercise. The myotonic patient may approach normal activity if the movements are repeated, as this "warming up" seems to abolish the myotonia. The degree of myotonia varies from inconvenience to immobilization. It may be generalized or localized and, if the latter, is most commonly seen in the legs. In severe myotonia the patient cannot run, is barely able to walk, and loses his balance easily; the grasp is slow and takes several seconds to relax, and mastication and

From the Department of Paediatrics, University of Toronto, and the Hospital for Sick Children.

Read at the combined meeting of the sections of Paediatrics, and Neurology and Psychiatry, Academy of Medicine, Toronto, Nov. 18, 1937.

speech may be difficult. Upon examination the myotonic muscles may show hypertrophy. There is no alteration in sensation or in mentality. The reflexes often present a peculiar phenomenon. The muscle belly when tapped shows a deep groove of contraction which remains for several seconds. Upon faradic or galvanic stimulation a tense contraction of the muscle occurs, which persists several seconds longer than the stimulus.

Myotonia as a form of muscular reaction is not confined to myotonia congenita. A similar condition may be seen in myotonia atrophica, in which the myotonia is accompanied by atrophy of the facial, sternomastoid, or quadriceps muscles, and is associated with endocrine disturbances. It has also been reported by Krabbe,[1] following an acute illness, presumably peripheral neuritis, and by Moore[4] following severe trauma. The myotonic reaction may be confused with the rigidity of striatal disease, and in children the condition is often mistaken for the early stages of pseudohypertrophic muscular dystrophy.

Until recent years the treatment was extremely varied and had very little success. In 1936 Wolf presented a preliminary study of four cases treated by quinine therapy[7] and followed this with a further report in 1937.[2] Smith[6] in 1937 reported the successful treatment of three siblings with quinine. The mode of action is unknown, though Kennedy and Wolf[2] believe that quinine inhibits the formation of acetylcholine at the myoneural junction. When given intravenously as the dihydrochloride, it abolishes the myotonic reaction within ten minutes. Oral doses of 10 grains three times daily alleviate symptoms in most cases.

Case Report.—G. M., a 7-year-old boy, was brought to the outpatient neurological clinic in May, 1937.

As a child he had been clumsy, and at 2 years of age his parents noticed that his movements were stiff compared with those of his brother. This awkwardness had never left him but had gradually increased until he had been forced to give up many games. At first it seemed only the left leg was affected, but recently both arms and both legs showed the condition.

The boy complained of stiffness which was worse after resting but would go away upon limbering up. When beginning a game he was awkward and would stumble and fall since he could not maintain his balance and could be easily pushed over. When he ran races, his legs would drag; he would be behind at first but occasionally would catch up if the race was long enough. There was a definite difficulty in climbing stairs, which was more marked after resting. His fingers were stiff, and he became unable to catch a baseball. He never complained of weakness but maintained that his disability was due to stiffness of his limbs.

His birth was a normal, noninstrumental delivery at full term (weight, 6¾ lb.). He walked at 14 months of age, talked at 18 months, and at the age of 7 years was in the junior second class. In 1936 he had a tonsillectomy following mild attacks of measles and pertussis. His only sibling, a brother eight years old, has shown no myotonic phenomena, and there is no family history suggestive of this condition.

He was a well-developed, well-nourished boy with no defects except those of the nervous system. The cranial nerves were normal, motor power was good, but there was a definite slowness in movement, particularly after resting. This seemed most marked in both legs and in the left arm but disappeared rapidly upon exercise, when the movements became more normal. Definite hypertrophy was seen in the gastrocnemii and glutei. Sensation was normal. The deep reflexes were present, active and equal, and the plantar responses flexor. When the gastrocnemii, deltoids, glutei, or abdominal muscles were tapped, the resulting contraction lasted for several seconds. The muscular contraction to faradic current lasted 3 to 5 seconds longer than the stimulus.

Blood calcium was 9.3 mg. per 100 c.c. of blood. Urinalysis and complete hematologic examinations were normal. A biopsy of the left gastrocnemius showed no evidence of fatty or fibrous infiltration. The majority of the fibers were normal in size, but many were larger, reaching 75 microns in diameter. These larger fibers were round with tense sheaths and showed an increase in the sarcolemmal nuclei. Scattered about were a few small foci of lymphocytic infiltration.

In view of the history, physical examination, electrical reactions, and biopsy, there was no doubt about the presence of myotonia. Even in the absence of a positive family history it would be classed as myotonia congenita or Thomsen's disease.

The patient was given quinine sulfate, 5 grains t.i.d. with a definite improvement in symptoms. A severe headache and enuresis developed during the first week, and the quinine was stopped with a return of symptoms. Quinine was again commenced, and 10 grains t.i.d. gave almost complete relief. If the dosage was reduced to 15 grains daily, some stiffness returned; at least 30 grains a day was necessary to produce a satisfactory result. The last dose had to be after supper in order to prevent stiffness upon arising. On several occasions when the quinine has run low, the myotonia has returned immediately. The patient, followed for nine months, has shown consistent relief obtained from quinine therapy.

CONCLUSIONS

A case of myotonia congenita in a 7-year-old boy has been reported and the favorable result of quinine therapy described.

REFERENCES

1. Krabbe, K. H.: Brain **57**: 184, 1934.
2. Kennedy, F., and Wolf, A.: Arch. Neurol. & Psychiat. **37**: 68, 1937.
3. Lindsley, D. B., and Curnan, E. C.: Arch. Neurol. & Psychiat. **35**: 253, 1936.
4. Moore: Report, Philadelphia Neurological Society, May, 1935.
5. Oppenheim: Text Book of Nervous Diseases, Edinburgh, 1911, Schultze.
6. Smith, W. A.: J. A. M. A. **198**: 43, 1937.
7. Wolf, A.: Arch. Neurol. & Psychiat. **36**: 382, 1936.

RIPE BANANA AS A COMPLEMENTARY FEEDING IN INFANTS

A Study of 444 Cases

John Dorsey Craig, M.D.
New York, N. Y.

About seven years ago the introduction of ripe banana as the first solid food for infants 6 weeks of age and older was made a routine practice in this hospital and has continued as such with only short periodic omissions to the present date. The following analytical study of 444 cases taken at random from the hospital records is an attempt to evaluate the results of this complementary feeding.

METHOD OF PROCEDURE

The physicians ordering the administration of ripe banana always specified the quantities in inches, that is, one or two inches a day, etc.* It is obvious that an inch of banana at the end of the "finger" will have less bulk than an inch taken from the middle of the fruit. Nevertheless, generally speaking, an inch of banana will yield approximately eighteen to twenty calories in food value (18 to 20 gm. or 0.6 to 0.7 oz.). The infants were all started with one inch of the fruit which was increased inch by inch according to their desire for it. Only ripe, mashed fruit was given, and it was fed separately from the milk formulas. The mode of administration was by spoon or by the use of a tongue depressor used in a similar manner, or the banana was pushed off into the mouth with a second depressor. The infants were not given any other solid foods, as it is practically impossible to ascertain the value of any single solid when more than one is being fed.

In all cases in both groups orange juice was given as the antiscorbutic agent. Antirachitic agents of various kinds, especially cod-liver oil, were used in all the cases. Viosterol was not given.[1-4]

Table I includes the normal and underweight institutional patients with and without complicating illnesses. No patients with symptoms referable to the gastrointestinal tract are included as these are discussed under a separate heading.

Table II lists the complicating illnesses occurring during the period of observation of the Cases in Table I, Groups 2, 4, and 6.

The average period of observation of this group of cases was from one to two and one-half months, the lowest being four weeks, while

From the New York Foundling Hospital.

*At present banana is given in teaspoon amounts (4.7 gm. or 0.17 oz.) to facilitate accuracy in dosage.

TABLE I

INSTITUTIONAL PATIENTS (GROUPS)	NUMBER OF PATIENTS	RANGE IN AGE WHEN BANANA FEEDING WAS STARTED	AVERAGE AGE WHEN BANANA FEEDING WAS STARTED	RANGE IN NO. WK. OBSERVED	AVERAGE NO. WK. OBSERVED	RANGE IN AMOUNT OF BANANA EATEN DAILY	AVERAGE AMOUNT OF BANANA TAKEN DAILY	AVERAGE WEIGHT WHEN BANANA FEEDING WAS STARTED	AVERAGE WEIGHT GAIN WEEKLY (OZ.)	AVERAGE NUMBER OF STOOLS DAILY	AVERAGE CALORIES PER POUND OF BODY WEIGHT IN FORMULAS	TYPE MILK FORMULA FED	CASES
1. Normal weight with no complications	62	5 wk. to 2.7 mo.	1.52 mo.	5-10	5.5	1 in. to 1 whole banana	2-3 in.	8′ 13″	3.6	1-2 yellow firm	48	1. Powdered whole lactic acid milk	54
												2. Milk and karo	6
												3. Evaporated milk and karo	1
												4. Breast	1
2. Normal weight with complicating illnesses	48	5 wk. to 6.5 mo.	2.1 mo.	4-15	7.7	1 in. to 1 whole banana	3 in.	10′ 7″	2.8	1-2 yellow firm	50	1. Powdered whole lactic acid milk	23
												2. Milk and karo	24
												3. Breast	1
3. Less than 15 per cent underweight—no complications	75	1-5 mo.	2.0 mo.	4-11	6.5	1 in. to 1 whole banana. 1 case 3 mo. old (9.8) took 2 bananas daily for 4 wk.	2-4 in.	8′ 10″	3.1	1-2 yellow firm	64	1. Powdered whole lactic acid milk	56
												2. Milk and karo	9
												3. Milk and dextrimaltose	8
												4. Evaporated milk and karo	1
												5. Lactogen	1
4. Less than 15 per cent underweight with complicating illnesses	84	4 wk. to 6 mo.	2.3 mo.	4-15	7.4	1 in. to 1 whole banana	2-3 in.	8′ 8″	2.9	1-2 yellow firm	60	1. Powdered whole lactic acid milk	48
												2. Milk and karo	19
												3. Milk and dextrimaltose	15
												4. Buttermilk	2
5. More than 15 per cent underweight—no complications	41	2-7 mo.	3.1 mo.	4-13	7.3	1 in. to 1 whole banana	2-3 in.	8′ 7″	4.2	1-2 yellow firm	62	1. Powdered whole lactic acid milk	33
												2. Milk and karo	7
												3. Evaporated milk and karo	1
6. More than 15 per cent underweight with complicating illnesses	83	1½ to 8 mo.	4.0 mo.	5-27	9.76	1 in. to 1 whole banana	2-3 in.	8′ 8″	3.8	1-2 yellow firm	63	1. Powdered whole lactic acid milk	48
												2. Milk and karo	23
												3. Milk and dextrimaltose	7
												4. Evaporated milk with karo	4
												5. Lactogen	1

one case was observed twenty-seven weeks (Table I, Group 6). The stools in all the groups numbered one to two daily and were firm and singularly regular. Generally speaking, the dosage was two to three inches of banana daily, and in each group some infants took as high as a whole banana daily. One 3-month-old infant (Table I, Group 3) weighing 9 lb. 8 oz., took two whole bananas daily for four weeks. This added feeding did not cut the appetite for the regular formula.

TABLE II

	GROUPS		
	2	4	6
Upper respiratory infection	26	25	21
Upper respiratory infection with bilateral otitis media	7	19	12
Generalized furunculosis	3	8	7
Bronchitis	3	5	8
Bronchopneumonia	2	1	
Upper respiratory infection with purulent otitis media	2	12	12
Lobar pneumonia	1		
Furunculosis, head	1	6	1
Tetany	1		
Congenital syphilis	1		
Pertussis	1	3	5
Varicella with bilateral purulent otitis media		1	
Impetigo		1	1
Thrush with bilateral purulent otitis media		1	
Furunculosis with bilateral purulent otitis media		1	5
Bronchitis (tuberculous?) Mantoux positive and mother with positive tuberculin test		1	
Prematurity			5
Thrush and furunculosis			2
Follicular tonsillitis			1
Peritonsillar abscess			1
Pylorospasm			1
Gonorrheal vaginitis			1

The infants with no complications gained on an average more than those with complicating illnesses, and those underweight for age, gained more than those of normal weight. The more underweight the infant was, the higher the average gain; and those more than 15 per cent underweight for age (Table I, Group 5) with no complicating illnesses showed the highest average gain in weight. The average weight gain of the entire group of patients was low.

In Table III all patients observed had had diarrhea or other gastrointestinal upsets immediately preceding the institution of banana as a complementary feeding, and none had complicating illnesses.

It is significant that none of these thirty-five patients had a recurrence of the gastrointestinal symptoms on starting the solid fruit feeding. The weight gain of the normal weight patients was markedly lower than that in the two underweight groups.

TABLE III

NORMAL AND UNDERWEIGHT PATIENTS WHO HAD GASTROINTESTINAL DISORDERS PRECEDING THE FEEDING OF BANANA AS A COMPLEMENTARY FEEDING

INSTITUTIONAL PATIENTS	NUMBER OF PATIENTS	RANGE IN AGE WHEN BANANA FEEDING WAS STARTED	AVERAGE AGE WHEN BANANA FEEDING WAS STARTED	RANGE IN NO. WK. OBSERVED	AVERAGE NO. WK. OBSERVED	RANGE IN AMOUNT OF BANANA EATEN DAILY	AVERAGE AMOUNT BANANA TAKEN DAILY	AVERAGE WEIGHT WHEN BANANA FEEDING WAS STARTED	AVERAGE WEIGHT GAIN WEEKLY (OZ.)	AVERAGE NUMBER OF STOOLS DAILY	AVERAGE CALORIES PER POUND OF BODY WEIGHT IN FORMULAS	TYPE MILK FORMULA FED	CASES
1. Normal weight for age	7	6 wk. to 6 mo.	2.1 mo.	4-5	4.5	1-4 in.	2-3 in.	11′ 11″	1.1	2-3 yellow firm to pasty	52	1. Powdered whole lactic acid milk 2. Milk and karo	6 1
2. Less than 15 per cent underweight for age	19	4-8 wk.	2.1 mo.	--	6.7	2 in. to 1 whole banana	2-4 in.	7′ 14″	3.6	1-2 yellow firm	61	1. Powdered whole lactic acid milk 2. Milk and dextrimaltose 3. Milk and karo	11 5 3
3. More than 15 per cent underweight for age	9	2.5 to 5 mo.	3 mo.	5-17	11	2 in. to 1 whole banana	4 in.	7′ 4″	3.9	2-3 yellow firm	63	1. Powdered whole lactic acid milk	9

GASTROINTESTINAL UPSETS AND DIARRHEA OCCURRING DURING THE COURSE OF COMPLEMENTARY BANANA FEEDING

In the 444 cases reviewed, there were sixteen cases of gastrointestinal upsets and diarrheas representing an occurrence of 3.5 per cent. In spite of the fact that these were institutionalized patients, many of whom were markedly underweight and had complicating illnesses, this figure compares favorably with the incidence I have observed in two series of normal, outpatient babies without complications showing an incidence of 3 per cent[5] and 7 per cent,[6] respectively.

Of these sixteen infants, ten had gastrointestinal upsets, of which six were associated with parenteral infection, and six were cases of diarrhea, four of the parenteral type. The six patients with gastrointestinal upsets due to parenteral infection had upper respiratory infections except one, who had an associated right acute otitis media. These patients had four or five loose, yellow, semisolid stools daily during the infection; all were fed powdered whole lactic acid milk, and banana was continued throughout. In seven to ten days the stools returned to normal. The average age of these infants was 2 months; the average weight 8½ lb.; and the average amount of banana taken per day, two to three inches. The average age in weeks when banana feeding was started was 5.6, and the average weight gain was 2 oz. a week.

The other four patients with gastrointestinal upsets had no complicating illness. Three were fed powdered whole lactic acid milk, and one, milk and dextrimaltose. These patients, after having normal stools, reverted to three to 5 yellow, semisolid stools daily for eight to ten days and returned to normal with the reduction of the carbohydrate in the formula. Banana was fed throughout the period, the average amount taken being two to three inches daily. The average age of the infants was 3 months; the average weight, 9 lb.; and the average period of observation, eight and one-half weeks.

Four of the six cases of diarrhea were parenteral in type, two being associated with upper respiratory infections, one with bronchopneumonia, and one with purulent bilateral otitis media. In all cases the stools were watery, yellow to green in color, and five to eight a day in number. Banana feeding was discontinued at the onset of the diarrhea and started in all but one of the cases after cessation of the symptoms, with no recurrences.

The other two patients with diarrhea had no associated illness but spontaneously had five or six yellow to green watery stools daily. Banana was stopped during treatment and in six and eight days, respectively, after diarrhea was controlled was started again with no recurrences. The average age of these six patients was 3.1 months and the average weight was 8 lb. 10 oz. The average number of weeks of banana feeding before the diarrhea started was five, and the average amount ingested daily, two inches.

In reviewing these cases it is apparent that the banana feeding had nothing to do with the onset of diarrhea, and there were no recurrences after its reinstatement in the dietary regime. In the simple gastrointestinal upsets banana feeding was continued throughout with no ill effects.

DISCUSSION AND REVIEW OF THE LITERATURE

As early as 1910 Pritchard advocated the addition of mashed banana to the milk mixtures of artificially fed infants. He began giving small quantities when the infant was no more than a week or 2 old. Johnston[8] and von Meysenbug[9] in 1927 and Scriver and Ross[10] in 1929 obtained good results in feeding banana as a complementary food, the two latter starting it when the patient was 3 months old and the former at 6 weeks. Thursfield[11] was enthusiastic about its use as a complementary food for marantic infants. These are the only other similar series of cases in the literature since in the others banana was given in addition to other solids.

Digestibility of Banana.—Taking into consideration the extreme malnutrition of many of these patients, the fact that they were institutionalized, and the fact that the feeding was started at such a young average age, the low incidence of gastrointestinal upsets is sufficient clinical evidence of the easy digestibility of banana. Probably the most commonly known clinical proof of its digestibility is its ability to control coeliac disease dietetically. This phenomenon was first shown by Haas[12] in 1924 and since then substantiated by many others.[13, 16] MacLean and Sullivan,[17] Badenoch and Morris,[18] Haas,[19] and Nelson[20] have offered various explanations of this observation; however, there is no agreement in the theories. Higgins[21] showed the diabetic child has a better tolerance for banana than for any other form of carbohydrate. His findings were substantiated by Herlitz[22] and von Noorden.[23]

Amount Fed.—The average amount of banana taken by these infants was two to three inches daily. As stated before, it was not forced, the desire of the infant for the fruit being the guide as to the amount given. The smallest amount taken was one inch daily and the largest, two whole bananas. This was taken (Table I, Column 3) by a 3-month-old infant weighing 9 lb. 8 oz.

In the entire group the youngest infant fed the fruit was 33 days old, weighing 7 lb., while two other babies weighing 6 lb. 8 oz. and 6 lb. 12 oz., respectively, took it without upset following and with apparently perfect assimilation.

Weight Gain.—In order to give a fair comparison, only those babies who had no complicating illnesses are included in Table IV.

TABLE IV

AVERAGE WEIGHT GAINS OF ALL INFANTS HAVING NO COMPLICATING ILLNESS	NUMBER OF INFANTS	GAIN PER WEEK (OZ.)
Infants of normal weight	62	3.6
Infants less than 15 per cent underweight	75	3.1
Infants more than 15 per cent underweight	41	4.2

The largest average gains were in the infants underweight for their age; however, they did not approach the gains reported by Thursfield[11] probably because his group was small in number. The general averages are similar to those reported by Scriver and Ross[10] in a smaller series of cases.

The impression I received in summarizing the charts was that the average weight gain was not in keeping with the added calories in the form of banana in addition to the milk formula. The question arises: Is the carbohydrate of banana utilized in the body in the same manner as other carbohydrates used in modifying the milk formula? Thursfield,[11] in a manner, recognized this discrepancy in stating that the good effects of added banana feeding cannot be due to the mere addition of carbohydrate because in one of his infants who did well, the total carbohydrate intake was actually diminished in substituting the banana sugar for another. He further suggested that the benefit was due not to any known peculiarity of the banana, but possibly to some unidentified element. A coworker investigated the point without discovering any new element.

Stools.—In these cases the majority of the stools numbered one or two daily, were yellow in color and firm to pasty in consistency; however, in the group observed following gastrointestinal disturbances, there were two or three stools a day of the same consistency.

These findings generally corroborate the observations of Scriver and Ross.[10] They found the fruit neither constipating nor laxative in action.

No notes were recorded concerning the size of the stools in this series, although other workers[9, 21, 24-26] have noted an increase in the bulk on the introduction of banana into the child's diet. It is obvious in reviewing the literature that the increase in size of the stools is in the children fed the largest amounts of banana.

GASTROINTESTINAL UPSETS AND DIARRHEA

Banana was not used therapeutically in any case of diarrhea. The cases in Table III are interesting because other workers have found the banana useful as the first solid used in a transition diet after apple therapy for diarrhea cases and as a means of making the apple therapy diet more palatable. Utilized in the transition diet as the first solid, good results have been obtained by Giblin,[27] Tompkins,[28] and Boyd.[29] Such a result would be expected since the literature is becoming richer in articles showing banana alone is effective as a therapeutic agent in the diarrheas of childhood. Joslin,[30] Brubaker,[31] Fanconi,[32] and Baumann[33, 34] reported good results in feeding both ripe banana and banana powder as a therapeutic agent in acute diarrheal disorders in infants.

Scheuer[35] from this same institution, reporting on summer diarrheas in the months of July and August, 1931 to 1934, showed only one case of diarrhea in this period in the infants fed powdered whole lactic acid milk. He ascribed the cut in rate to this type of feeding, as the decrease in diarrhea coincided with its inclusion. Since the routine feeding of banana was started about the same time, it would be interesting to observe a control group on lactic acid mixtures alone to determine the influence of the ripe fruit in preventing diarrhea.

SUMMARY

Four hundred forty-four bottle-fed infants were fed ripe mashed banana as a complementary feeding beginning at the age of 6 weeks. The majority of these infants were either underweight or had complicating illnesses. Tangible, reportable evidence of the advantage of this complementary feeding demonstrates that (a) because of the banana's digestibility, it acts as an ideal first solid to offer infants to make them accustomed to solid food; and also (b) when given with cod-liver oil increases the ease of administering the oil to small infants. Although it is merely clinical observation and opinion, as no criterion except personal judgment is available, some at this institution share the belief that the turgor in the banana fed infants is better. Citing the small average amount of banana taken, others deny the possibility of affecting turgor; however, all agree on the ease of assimilation.

Considering the large number of undernourished and sick infants reported, the incidence of gastrointestinal upsets is low (3.56 per cent), and this may be due to the fact that a little less carbohydrate can be used in the formula when the infant is getting a complementary banana feeding.

Until a group of control infants who are not given complementary feeding is studied at the same time as those fed banana, these controversial opinions cannot be settled.

A group of infants fed mashed ripe banana immediately after the cessation of diarrhea assimilated the fruit with ease and showed no recurrences.

CONCLUSIONS

1. Ripe mashed banana is easily digested by infants 6 weeks of age or older, regardless of complicating illnesses or degree of malnutrition.

2. Ripe mashed banana is easily assimilated as the first solid food given after the treatment of diarrheal disorders in infants.

3. The effect of complementary banana feeding on the weight curve of infants was that of control rather than increase.

I wish to thank Dr. John Giblin for allowing me to report these cases, many of which were from his service.

REFERENCES

1. Hess, A. F., and Lewis, J. M.: J. A. M. A. **97**: 369, 1931.
2. Barnes, D. J., Brady, M. J., and James, E. M.: Am. J. Dis. Child. **39**: 45, 45, 1930.
3. DeSanctis, A. G., and Craig, J. D.: J. A. M. A. **94**: 1285, 1930.
4. Lewis, J. M.: J. PEDIAT. **10**: 155, 1937.
5. DeSanctis, Adolph G., Craig, J. D., and Stringfield, Oliver: J. PEDIAT. **1**: 704, 1932.
6. DeSanctis, Adolph G., Craig, John D., and Fales, Helen: J. PEDIAT. **3**: 891, 1933.
7. Pritchard, Eric: Brit. M. J. No. 2598: 1145, 1910.
8. Johnston, Joseph A.: J. Am. Dietet. A. Vol. 3, September, 1927.
9. Von Meysenbug, L.: New Orleans M. & S. J. **30**: 180, 1927.
10. Scriver, J. B., and Ross, S. G.: Canad. M. A. J. **20**: 162, 1929.
11. Thursfield, H.: Arch. Dis. Childhood **2**: 49, 1927.
12. Haas, Sidney V.: Am. J. Dis. Child. **28**: 421, 1924.
13. Griffith, J. P. Crozer, and Mitchell, A. Graeme: The Diseases of Infants and Children, page 610, Philadelphia, 1935, W. B. Saunders Company.
14. Holt, L. Emmett, Jr., and McIntosh, Rustin: Holt's Diseases of Infancy and Childhood, page 215, New York, 1933, D. Appleton-Century Company, Inc.
15. Kerley, Charles G., and Craig, H. R.: Am. J. Dis. Child. **28**: 520, 1924.
16. Nelson, Martha van Kirk: Am. J. Dis. Child. **39**: 76, 1930.
17. MacLean, Aubrey B., and Sullivan, Ruth C.: Am. J. Dis. Child. **38**: 16, 1929.
18. Badenoch, Eleanor, and Morris, Noah: Quart. J. Med. **5**: 240, 1936.
19. Haas, Sidney: Arch. Pediat. **48**: 248, 1931.
20. Nelson, Martha Van Kirk: Am. J. Dis. Child. **39**: 76, 1930.
21. Higgins, Harold L.: Am. J. Dis. Child. **46**: 446, 1933.
22. Herlitz, C. W.: Acta paediat. **18**: 1, 1935.
23. Von Noorden, Carl: Alte und neuzeitliche Ernährungsfragen, page 96, Vienna, 1931, Julius Springer.
24. Brown, Alan, and Courtney, Angelia M.: Canad. M. A. J. **21**: 37, 1929.
25. Fanconi, G.: Deutsche med. Wchnschr. **56**: 1949, 1930.
26. Russell, Hollis K.: Life and Health (The National Health Journal), 8, 1935.
27. Giblin, John, and Lischner, M. D.: Arch. Pediat. **52**: 355, 1935.
28. Tompkins, Charles A.: J. Indiana M. A. **38**: 278, 1935.
29. Boyd, Julian D.: J. PEDIAT. **8**: 234, 1936.
30. Joslin, C. Loring: Southern M. J. **29**: 1007, 1936.
31. Brubaker, Earl W.: J. Michigan M. Soc. **36**: 40, 1937.
32. Fanconi, G.: Monatschr. f. Kinderh. **49**: 232, 1931.
33. Baumann, T.: Hippokrates **8**: 857, 1937.
34. Baumann, T.: Die Wirkung der Rohobstdiat auf den kindlichen Organismus, Berlin, 1936, S. Karger.
35. Scheuer, Lewis A.: J. PEDIAT. **7**: 468, 1935.

THE TREATMENT OF TUBERCULOSIS OF THE SPINE BY SPINAL FUSION

Results in 309 Children Less Than 10 Years of Age

Walker E. Swift, M.D.
New York, N. Y.

The familiar first aphorism of Hippocrates seems to me to be appropriate as an introduction to this paper. It has been translated as follows: "Life is short, and the Art long; occasion is fleeting; experience is fallacious, and decision difficult. The physician must not only be prepared to do what is right himself, but also to make the patient, the attendants, and externals cooperate."

The subject of the treatment of tuberculosis of the spine by fusion operation is a long and complicated one, and I am not going to enter into a lengthy statistical exposition. It is more to my purpose to relate as plainly as I can the theoretic conception of treatment by the fusion operation, how it has been carried out, some of the difficulties, and some of the results which have been obtained. These matters have been the subject of observation and study by the staff of the New York Orthopaedic Dispensary and Hospital for the past twenty-six years, during which time fusion of the spine has been performed on more than 800 patients who had vertebral tuberculosis. As a representative of these men, I think I am expressing their unanimous opinion when I say that the fusion operation is their treatment of choice for children and adults who have tuberculosis of the spine.

I should like to state a few things about which I think all will agree, but which are most important to keep in mind when talking about what can be and what has been accomplished in treating this disease.

1. Tuberculosis of the spine is not a primary nor a solitary lesion. Its presence means that the patient is suffering from a serious, chronic, general disease which will require all his and all his physician's resources to keep in check.

2. Tuberculosis of the spine is a most serious complication of the general disease.

3. There is a real difference in the constitutional powers of individuals to overcome and control tuberculous infection and toxemia.

4. The actual pathology of tuberculosis of the spine varies greatly as to location, degree, and extent.

5. The aims of treatment of a patient with tuberculosis of the spine are: to assist him in obtaining a subsidence of the activity of the lesion,

---

From The New York Orthopaedic Dispensary and Hospital.

Read at the regular monthly meeting of the Orthopedic Section of the New York Academy of Medicine, Oct. 15, 1937.

to protect him from possible deformity, to assure him that the particular lesion will not return to plague him, and to enable him to return to a relatively normal life. I might add that the more quickly and economically these aims can be accomplished, the better. I know it is said that time is the least important element, but I can never forget that, to an individual who has the constant threat of tuberculosis hanging over him, a matter of several years spent in an institution may seem and actually be more important than to the rest of us who fully expect to live out our threescore years and ten.

The operation of fusion for the treatment of tuberculosis of the spine was devised by Dr. Russell A. Hibbs with the full understanding of these factors. It is not, and never has been thought, a specific remedy for tuberculosis in the sense that diphtheria antitoxin is a specific remedy for diphtheria. It is thought of simply as a means of assisting the patient to use his own recuperative powers to the best advantage. It is considered the best possible means of applying the most effective remedy which anybody knows for tuberculosis in any part of the body, namely, rest. Just how or why rest makes it possible for the local tissues to carry out their protective functions nobody can say until more is known of the physical and chemical changes in the environment of tuberculosis and the intricate chemistry of the products of the tubercle bacilli themselves. But rest and the removal of trauma are accepted as essential for the healing of a tuberculous focus. There are three main factors which make it practically impossible to give complete rest to one or more diseased vertebrae if only simple recumbency, a brace, a plaster jacket, or a hyperextension frame is used. First, because with every act of respiration, the vertebral joints move to a certain extent, and this motion is transmitted to the vertebral bodies. Second, because contraction of the abdominal and spinal muscles transmits stress and motion to the area of vertebral disease. Third, because if there is any loss of bone substance due to the disease, all of these motions and stresses will become exaggerated. If, on the other hand, the posterior intervertebral joints and laminae are fused, the motions due to respiratory and muscular contractions will be eliminated over the area fused. This being understood, it is apparent that the primary theoretic reason for performing this operation is to give the diseased part the greatest possible amount of rest.

Another theoretic reason for employing fusion in this disease is to supply a strong bony support over the involved vertebrae, the intention being to lessen, if not entirely to prevent, the forward collapse of the bodies which have been more or less destroyed. One has only to turn to a study of scoliosis, in which it has been amply proved that a solid fusion will support the spine against severe muscle pulls and weight thrusts, to realize that the same thing can be applied to forward bending of the spine.

The Hibbs type of fusion is the operation which has been used on all the patients treated at the New York Orthopaedic Hospital since 1911. It seems to us to give the best form of intervertebral stabilization, and I shall not take the time to explain the reasons for this belief nor to describe the technique. There are a few things to say about it, however. The operation is not easy to do well and requires a great deal of attention to details. If it is done well there is relatively little difficulty and relatively little shock. The most important thing about spinal fusion, whatever the method, is that it must succeed in order to be of the slightest value. That the operation does not always succeed in producing a continuous fusion should be obvious to anyone who is familiar with surgical procedures and knows that none are perfect. Failure of fusion does occur, and in the series of operations done at the New York Orthopaedic Hospital for tuberculosis of the spine a pseudarthrosis was found in about 10 per cent of all operations. This fact is one to be emphasized, not to condemn the operation, but so that anyone who doubts the value of fusion because of poor results which he may have seen should be urged to restudy the results to determine whether or not there was actually complete fusion present. The benefits of spinal fusion for tuberculosis should not be judged except in patients in whom a successful fusion has been obtained. It has been our experience that a pseudarthrosis is probably present when the clinical signs and symptoms continue for a longer period than expected, when the deformity is found to be increasing more than is expected, and when the roentgenograms show evidence that the activity of the disease is not subsiding as is expected. Should these circumstances arise, a secondary operation should be done and a pseudarthrosis repaired if it is found, because it is obvious that a fusion which is incomplete at any point cannot perform the functions for which it was intended.

Another essential part of the operation is that the area fused be long enough, and this means including two vertebrae above and two below those recognized as being diseased. It is our belief that many disappointments may have occurred because of failure to immobilize a sufficient number of vertebrae. Not infrequently we have had to perform a secondary operation, adding one or two vertebrae above or below the fusion when it became evident that the original area was too short, either because of a mistake in identifying the vertebrae at the time of operation or failing to recognize the true extent of the disease.

In any surgical procedure there is the danger of operative mortality and operative infection. Both of these risks can be minimized by the exercise of sound judgment in deciding when and on whom to operate and the practice of scrupulous technique in the handling of tissues as well as instruments. The operative mortality at the New York Orthopaedic Hospital has been 1.3 per cent in the primary and secondary operations performed on tuberculous spines, and the percentage of infections has been something under 1 per cent. These are real hazards, the importance of which must be weighed against the ultimate value of the procedure.

The experience of operating upon a patient and then seeing him steadily lose ground owing to continuing active tuberculous disease is most distressing. The number of such occurrences may be decreased by sound medical judgment in attempting to estimate the true extent of the disease in each particular patient and his particular powers of resistance against tuberculosis, before advising surgery. It is a most difficult problem, but it is important to say that the presence of one or more other tuberculous foci in an individual is not in itself a reason for deciding against a fusion operation. Frequently it has been noted that with the subsidence of activity of a vertebral lesion after a successful fusion, there has occurred improvement in other distant areas of disease. On the other hand, patients have been encountered who obtain a successful fusion and show evidence of subsiding activity of the spinal lesion, yet they succumb to tuberculosis. This does not seem to indict the spinal fusion operation but rather our ignorance of how to help a person whose constitutional capacity to resist tuberculosis is either inadequate or exhausted.

Difficulties arising from tuberculous abscesses and sinuses as a result of spinal disease can be troublesome, whether they were present before operation or appeared later. It is our expectation, based on many clinical examples, that a successful fusion will hasten the disappearance of an abscess or the healing of a sinus rather than cause them to appear as complications, as has been reported by some surgeons. The answer to this problem seems to us to be linked with the question of whether or not the fusion was really complete and was performed soon enough.

The fear which is often mentioned of the possible dissemination of a generalized tuberculous infection as a result of surgery on a spine is one which we believe may be discounted almost completely. Although a number of our patients have died of tuberculous meningitis fairly soon after a spinal fusion operation, it has not been possible to establish definitely a cause and effect relationship. On the other hand, the actual number of cases of meningitis has declined markedly in the period of years during which fusion has been used, when compared with the preceding period of conservative treatment. We feel that this problem is linked with the patient's general resistance, the duration of the disease, and its extent at the time of operation rather than with the direct effects of the surgery.

RESULTS

As is only too apparent, the complexity of presenting an understandable analysis of the results of operations on 800 patients is enormous, so I

Fig. 1.

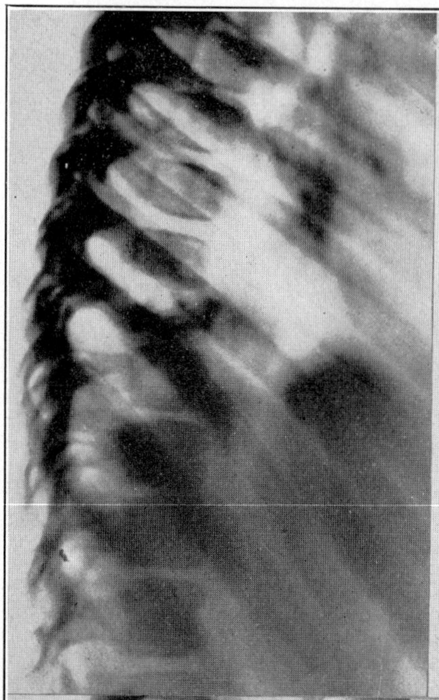

Fig. 2.

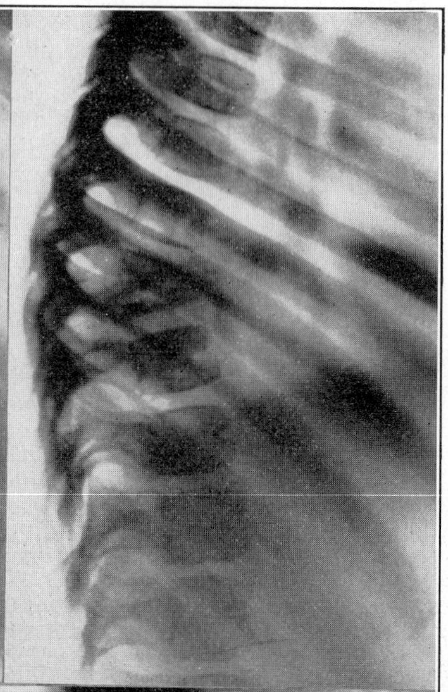

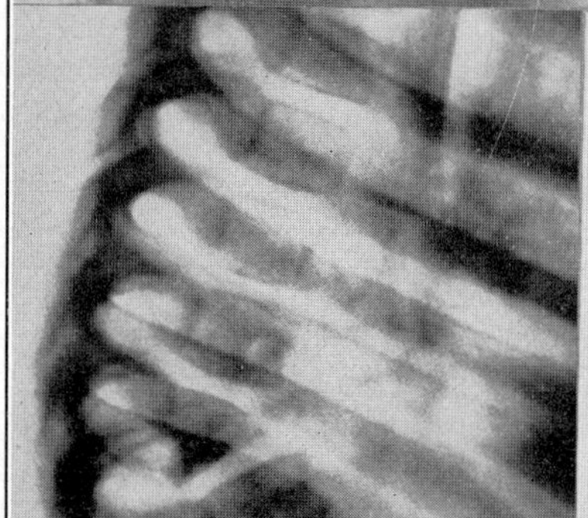

Fig. 3.

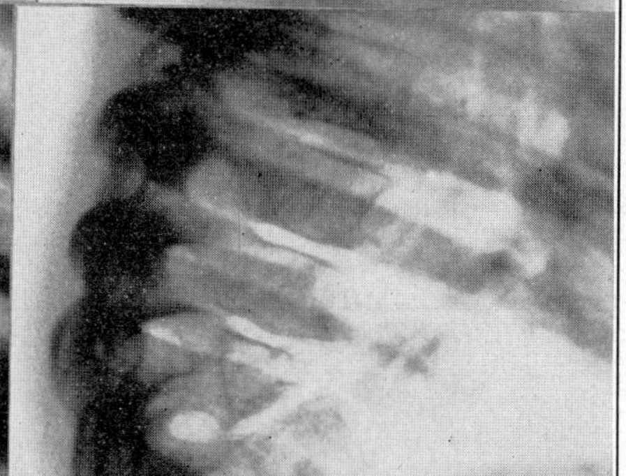

Fig. 4.

Fig. 1.—CASE 1, *A*. Lateral view of lesion one month before operation. Girl, 4 years old when admitted in November, 1929, had a short history of symptoms and presented few physical signs, but x-ray films showed an active tuberculous lesion involving the eighth and ninth dorsal vertebral bodies. Fusion was done from the sixth to the eleventh dorsal vertebrae in December, 1929. She had a good convalescence, wore a spinal brace for three months after operation, and was allowed to be up four months after operation, with no signs nor symptoms. As will be noted, there was a rapid collapse of the diseased vertebrae while the child was in bed wearing a brace.

(*Continued on facing page*)

shall limit myself to a group of children ten years of age or younger who were operated upon at the New York Orthopaedic Hospital during the years 1911 to 1932. There are 309 children in this group for whom we have long and adequate follow-up observations. They are not a selected group, except as one may call the patients who come to this hospital a selected group, because with very few exceptions all the children who were seen with tuberculosis of the spine were considered to be suitable for this form of treatment. The exceptions were patients who were in such condition that no one's surgical judgment could be stretched to the point of thinking them operable. Many of them had had no previous treatment; many of them had had varying forms of so-called conservative treatment. All of them were considered to have active disease, although there was great variation in the degree of activity of the lesions. The operation was not necessarily denied because of the presence of abscess, sinus, or pulmonary lesion, but the children who had such complications or were otherwise in poor health were kept in our Country Branch Hospital for a period of observation until they had gained sufficiently to be able safely to undergo the operation. It has been amazing to observe how well children of all ages withstand a spinal fusion operation and how relatively little postoperative shock is suffered. Two or three weeks after operation the children were sent back to the Country Branch Hospital, where they continued their convalescence in the best environment which we have been able to supply.

The observations made on these children during their convalescence and long follow-up periods have been extremely interesting and form the basis for our continued enthusiasm for spinal fusion.

As a result of examinations made when secondary operations have been performed, it is known that a successful spinal fusion will be firm enough to arrest respiratory motion in the diseased area by the third or fourth week after operation. Therefore, the benefits of complete rest will begin at this very early date in the course of treatment.

Roentgenographic evidence of subsidence of activity of the disease in the bone and soft tissues may be seen as early as the second month. It depends entirely upon the degree of activity and the extent of the original lesion, the more virulent infections taking longer periods of time, but it has been our experience that fusion definitely turns the tide in favor of repair at a very early date.

Compare the preoperative film *A* and film *B* made four months after operation. Today such a child would be given a longer period of recumbency. However, she has continued in excellent health, is now 12 years old, has grown well, and shows no apparent handicap.

Fig. 2.—Case 1, *B*. Lateral view of lesion four months after operation. There has been a collapse of the involved vertebral bodies, but the activity of the lesion appears to be subsiding.

Fig. 3.—Case 1, *C*. Lateral view of lesion ten months after operation. No further increase in deformity, and the diseased vertebral bodies appear to be fusing with the activity of the lesion subsided.

Fig. 4.—Case 1, *D*. Lateral view of lesion six years after operation. It shows no increase in deformity, the bodies fused, the lesion apparently cured, and growth of the vertebral bodies.

A kyphos may remain at its preoperative position, but usually there will be some increase of the angulation. This again will depend on the character of the individual lesion and on the fact that active disease does continue for a short time. During this period there may be absorption of bone and consequent slight increase of deformity. The fusion mass will take several months to reach a state of maturity such that it will resist the tendency to deformity, and it cannot be depended upon to hold apart a gap in the vertebral bodies. However, as the activity of the disease tends to diminish quickly, it has been our experience that after fusion there is definitely less loss of bone substance and hence less kyphos increase than would be the case without opera-

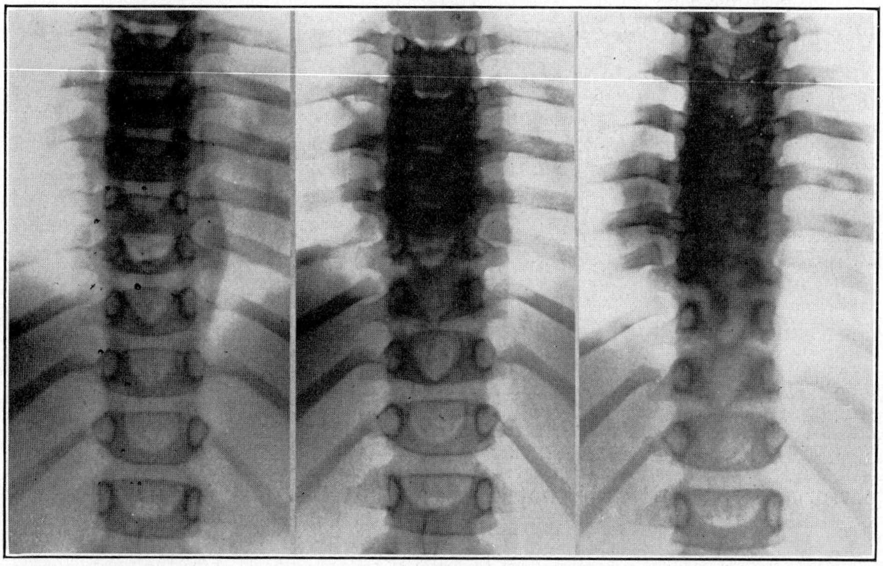

Fig. 5. Fig. 6. Fig. 7.

Fig. 5.—Case 1, *E.* Anteroposterior view of lesion one month before operation. It shows an abscess around the diseased vertebrae.

Fig. 6.—Case 1, *F.* Anteroposterior view of lesion four months after operation. It shows almost complete disappearance of the abscess, indicating subsidence of activity of the lesion.

Fig. 7.—Case 1, *G.* Anteroposterior view of lesion ten months after operation. It shows complete disappearance of the abscess and firm fusion.

tion. Once repair is established and the vertebral bodies are in contact or close to contact, the fusion will prevent further increase of deformity.

Soft tissue abscesses around the lesion will sometimes tend to increase in size for a time, but often they will be found to be decreasing at a time coincident with the roentgenographic evidence of subsiding activity in the vertebrae. It has been our experience that fusion has a very definite tendency to hasten the disappearance of abscesses and thereby adds a factor of tremendous importance to the well-being of the patient.

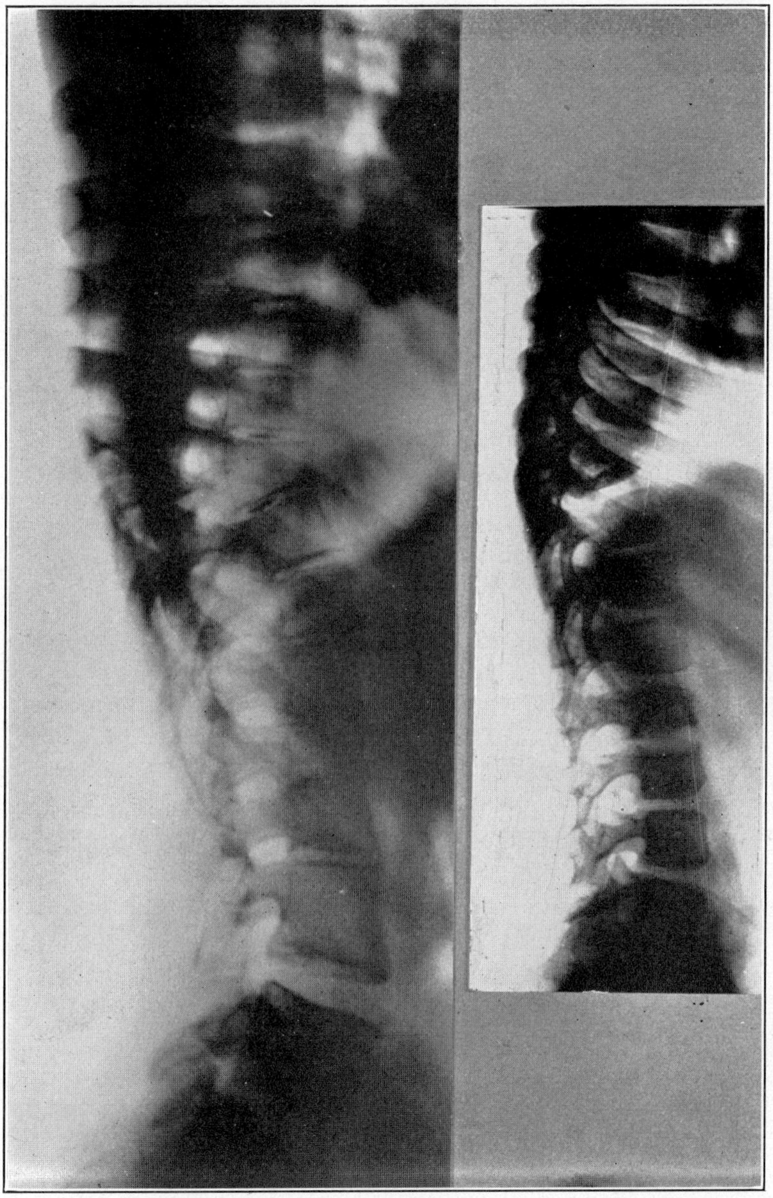

Fig. 8.—Case 2. Boy, 3 years and 3 months old when admitted in April, 1925, had symptoms and signs for six months with no treatment. Fair condition. Small insert on right shows at that time a double tuberculous lesion, ninth to tenth dorsal and second to third lumbar. Fusion was done in two stages in April and June, 1925, from sixth dorsal to fourth lumbar. A brace was worn for three months after operations, and the child was ambulatory six months after operations. The film on the left was made twelve and one-half years after operations. Comparison with the original film shows both lesions apparently cured, excellent growth of the vertebrae, and little deformity. The child has developed normally, is very active, and has no apparent handicap. He is 64 inches tall, the spine having grown approximately 9 inches. The two reproductions are on the same scale.

Within four to six months after fusion the child should show unmistakable evidences of repair and subsidence of activity of the disease, with the fusion of sufficient strength so that he may become ambulatory. In another few months of observation, the changes initiated by the fusion progress steadily toward healing, and, on the average, the patient will be able to go home safely after a total of ten to twelve months in the hospital.

I have just described the course of a child who obtains a primary solid fusion and who was in reasonably good condition and had a satisfactory resistance to tuberculosis. In the group of 309 children, this course was followed by approximately 45 per cent of the 74 per cent who obtained good results and is intended to show the result of spinal fusion at its best. It shows a child returned to a relatively normal life after only ten months of hospital treatment. It is a course which may seem inconceivable to anyone who has not actually seen it happen, and yet I repeat it was the course followed by approximately 45 per cent of this group of children.

Obviously many children do not follow this extraordinary course and will be delayed in their healing because of pseudarthrosis requiring a second operation, or because of having had very extensive disease, or because they took longer to build up resistance to the general toxemia of tuberculosis. Of this group many will eventually be classed with the good results, and I may say that their average stay in the hospital is two years and two months.

Other children will not do well at all and will continue a downhill course in spite of what we may do. Some will develop paraplegia and a certain number will die, usually of some form of tuberculous disease. These delayed and poor results are not minimized in any way, but I am not going to make an analysis of them now for fear that the actual proved benefits of a successful fusion will be overlooked.

Table I gives the final results which have been obtained by the fusion operation in 309 children less than 10 years old.

CONCLUSION

Three hundred and nine children less than 10 years of age who had active tuberculosis of the spine have been treated by spinal fusion, and 74 per cent of them have had good results. By a good result we mean that to all intents and purposes the child is well, leading an active normal life for his age, and is without danger of return of the disease at the original area. There are no symptoms or physical signs referable to the spine other than the deformity and limitation of motion which may be present. Furthermore, roentgenograms show a completely subsided lesion with a progressive tendency to show healthier texture in the soft tissue and bone, whether or not there is complete bony union of the vertebral bodies. We believe that the activity in these lesions will not recur. A time will come when the site of the former lesion can be called healthy if examined roentgenographically. It is at this point that one seems justified in saying that this particular tuberculous lesion is cured in the sense that it will not recur. The patient is not necessarily freed of other tuberculous foci, but the local spinal lesion may properly be said to be cured. It is not denied that a recurrence may conceivably happen in a rare instance, but we do not expect it, and not one has been met with in our experience after this roentgenographic appearance of health has been obtained. The longest follow-up periods for this observation are twenty years. It is our belief that this status is the expected result after fusion but is almost unknown after so-called conservative treatment.

TABLE I

RESULTS OF SPINAL FUSION OPERATION ON 309 CHILDREN LESS THAN 10 YEARS OLD (1911 TO 1932)

Average stay in bed, all patients	8 months
Average stay in hospital, all patients	2 years
Average stay in bed if normal fusion, no complications	4 to 6 months
Average stay in hospital if normal fusion, no complications	10 months
Average stay in hospital with pseudarthrosis	2 years, 2 months
Average stay in hospital with delayed union	2 years, 4 months
Good result: 74 per cent	Dead: 15 per cent
Poor result: 11 per cent	Operative mortality: 0.64 per cent
Pseudarthrosis: 15 per cent	

Approximately 45 per cent of the children with good results have followed an optimum course after fusion and completed their hospitalization and need for support in ten months. It is our belief that this course may be expected in a child with tuberculosis of the spine if treated by a successful fusion operation early in the course of the disease but that it cannot possibly be anticipated with so-called conservative treatment. As the time comes when tuberculosis of the spine is recognized and attacked earlier, more and more children will be found in this present fortunate group of 45 per cent.

For many years the medical profession has accepted and followed the teaching that tuberculosis of the spine will go through a certain cycle in its evolution toward healing and that nothing can be done to change or hasten this cycle after one has put the patient at rest, exposed him to sunshine, and given him good food. It should now be evident that something else can be done. Whether the patient with tuberculosis of the spine is a child or an adult, the spinal fusion operation does change the cycle, not only hastening the expected repair, but also resulting in a more complete and permanent healing.

American Academy of Pediatrics

Proceedings

EIGHTH ANNUAL MEETING OF THE AMERICAN ACADEMY OF PEDIATRICS

HOTEL DEL MONTE, DEL MONTE, CALIF.

JUNE 9, 10, AND 11, 1938

General Meeting

The general meeting of the American Academy of Pediatrics was held at Hotel Del Monte, Del Monte, Calif., on Saturday morning, June 11, 1938, at 9:45 A.M. President Philip Van Ingen presided.

While the membership stood in silence, the secretary read the list of those members who had been lost through death, during the past year:

Dr. Barnet E. Bonar, Salt Lake City, Utah.
Dr. W. O. Colburn, Lincoln, Neb.
Dr. Sylvan D. Lazarus, Brooklyn, N. Y.
Dr. Gustave Lippman, St. Louis, Mo.
Dr. Louis C. Schroeder, New York, N. Y.

Emeritus Fellow

Dr. LaFayette B. Mendel, New Haven, Conn.

Report of the Treasurer

STATEMENT OF RECEIPTS AND DISBURSEMENTS

June 1, 1937, to June 30, 1938 (13 Months)

Balance, June 1, 1937				$ 6,267.05
Transferred from Savings Account (For Bonds—see below)			$ 2,000.00	
Receipts:				
Dues		$23,402.10		
Exhibits		3,410.00		
Interest on Bonds		355.00		
Council for Pediatric Research		500.00		
Report of Committee on Immunization Procedures		33.80	$27,700.90	$29,700.90
				$35,967.95
Disbursements:				
Office				
Salaries				
Secretary	$5,400.00			
Stenographer	1,950.00			
Office	455.00	$ 7,805.00		

Rent		650.00	
Subscriptions		6,015.00	
Annual Meeting, 1937		2,833.15	
1938		3,620.39	
Balance on Bonds		2,985.51*	
Executive Board Meeting		947.83	
Travelling Expense		574.23	
Printing		757.52	
Postage		639.04	
Office Supplies		135.97	
Treasurer's Bond		62.50	
Certificates		44.80	
Telephone and Telegrams		50.19	
Exchange on checks		56.83	
Tax on checks		2.01	
Refunds (Initiation Fees)		270.00	
Miscellaneous		11.63	$27,461.60

Amounts Brought Forward

Receipts		$35,967.95
Disbursements	$27,461.60	

Regional Expense:

Region I	$ 489.56	
II	220.55	
III	352.17	
IV	187.12	$ 1,249.40

State Expense:

Region I		
New Jersey		$ 92.32
Region II		
Alabama	$ 24.00	
Florida	31.00	
Georgia	27.07	
Mississippi	18.00	
North Carolina	10.00	
Oklahoma	4.25	
Tennessee	40.00	$ 154.32
Region III		
Illinois	153.63	
Michigan	88.62	
Ohio	27.00	
Wisconsin	28.00	$ 297.25

*Purchased: $5,000 City of Chicago Municipal T. B. Sanitarium TAW 2.375 per cent 1937 Levy $5,030.46
Matured: $2,000 City of Evansville 4.75 per cent 2,044.95

Balance $2,985.51

Region IV			
Washington	13.33	$ 557.22	
Committees:			
Mental Hygiene	$ 218.21		
Immunization Procedures	134.15		
Nonmedical Groups	56.87		
Age Limit of Pediatrics	41.20		
Child Health Relations	30.00		
School Health	22.22		
Contact Infections	8.43	$ 511.08	$29,779.30

Balance, June 30, 1938 $ 6,188.65

Audited and found correct.

Clifford G. Grulee
Treasurer.

Report of the Executive Board

The Report of the Executive Board was given by Dr. Henry F. Helmholz. Each item was discussed as read.

The following applications for membership were approved:

Region I

Dr. William Leslie Bradford, Rochester, N. Y.
Dr. Louis Fischer, New York, N. Y.
Dr. John P. Hubbard, Boston, Mass.
Dr. Hugh Francis Leahy, Albany, N. Y.
Dr. Edith M. Lincoln, New York, N. Y.
Dr. Claire Cutten Manwell, Northampton, Mass.
Dr. John Jacob Slavens, Toronto, Ont., Canada.
Dr. Pearl Summerfeldt, Toronto, Ont., Canada.

Region II

Dr. William H. Bradford, Dallas, Texas.

Region III

Dr. Julian D. Boyd, Iowa City, Iowa.
Dr. Jeannette Hork, Chicago, Ill.
Dr. Kenneth B. McDonough, Madison, Wis.
Dr. James D. McKinney, Champaign, Ill.
Dr. Wilfred S. Nolting, Detroit, Mich.

Region IV

Dr. Carl G. Ashley, Portland, Ore.
Dr. Harry F. Dietrich, Beverly Hills, Calif.
Dr. Harry H. Horwitz, Oakland, Calif.
Dr. Donald C. Shelby, Los Angeles, Calif.
Dr. Brick Pomeroy Storts, Tucson, Ariz.

Dr. Maurice L. Blatt (Chicago, Ill.) presented the advantages of Chicago as a meeting place.

The recommendation of the Executive Board that the next meeting be held in Cincinnati in the fall of 1939 was approved.

The appointment of Dr. Harold C. Stuart of Boston, Massachusetts, as a member of the American Board of Pediatrics was unanimously approved.

Discussion of the Report of the Committee on Contact Infections

The report of the Committee on Contact Infections was read by Dr. Fairfax Hall of New Rochelle, N. Y.

Since pediatricians have always shown themselves willing and anxious to take an active part in every program designed to benefit the health of the community and the health of their patients, we hope this program will have your support.

It is an obvious fact that for a child to be in close contact with a person having an unrecognized communicable disease is a potential source of infection for that child. The adult persons with whom children are most closely associated are parents, other members of the family, school teachers, and domestic employees. Although parents are in the most intimate contact with their children, the employees in a home are the persons about whom the least is known from a health standpoint. It is essential, therefore, when houseworkers are engaged to help with the care of children, that they be free from transmissible infections.

The diseases not infrequently transmitted to children by adults in their environment are tuberculosis, syphilis, gonorrhea, typhoid by carriers, respiratory and skin diseases. The disease of greatest danger to children from this source is tuberculosis. A case of open pulmonary tuberculosis in a home, without proper control, will eventually infect every child there.

It is against this disease that the greatest amount of protection can be afforded children by a proper physical examination of the adults to whom they are exposed. Since an x-ray examination of the lungs will detect the presence of any significant existing pulmonary tuberculosis, even in an uninfectious stage, it is essential that this should be a routine procedure in the examination of adults for the protection of children.

It is extremely important that parents have no infectious diseases, not only for their own sakes, but for that of their children. Moreover, in order to obtain the cooperation of a domestic worker in having a medical examination, it is always desirable that the employers should have had similar examinations themselves and hold certificates from the family physician, so stating. It is often necessary for this example to be set and used as an argument, in order to persuade some domestics to be examined. Their resistance to having health examinations is often very hard to overcome.

If any great number of adults are to provide themselves with periodic health examinations or if servants are to be willing to do so at the request of their employers, a great deal of effort must be put forth. An intensive campaign of education is necessary. The employers of domestic workers must learn to be discriminating in regard to the health of servants they engage to assist in the care of their children. Publicity must be sufficient to reach the domestic class in order to overcome prejudice, on their part, against being examined and obtaining health cards. Domestic workers must be shown that the advantages gained by periodic examinations will be not of health value alone, but economic as well, and that they will enable them to secure better positions with higher wages.

Public opinion must be created to make health references as commonly asked for, and furnished, as are character references. Pediatricians know the need for this, and the Academy of Pediatrics is in a position to be a great influence towards its accomplishment.

Much headway has been made with such a campaign in Knoxville, Tenn. (Dr. Oliver Hill of this Committee). In that city during the past year, twelve patients with active tuberculosis, many syphilitics, and five typhoid carriers were found by routine examination of domestics.

In Newark, N. J., domestic servant health cards have been required by local statute for several years. In the state of North Carolina and other parts of the South this matter has been given serious attention.

In Westchester County, New York, experience with a program designed to make sure of the good health of adults in contact with children has been very encouraging. It has been favorably received by doctors and by the parents who employ servants to assist in the care of their children, but not so favorably received by some of the servants.

When this idea was approached on the voluntary basis, many of the influential women's organizations, parent-teachers' associations, men's service clubs, and the public health societies joined actively in the publicity and educational campaign. The Metropolitan Life Insurance Company has offered to aid the campaign among its policy holders in the county.

The Westchester County Medical Society has sponsored the medical aspects of the program by arranging a standardized examination form to be used for adults in contact with children. The members of the Society have been asked to make this examination at a low fee. The blood Wassermann tests are done by the state laboratory, free of charge. Most important of all, the radiologists have agreed to take a single film exposure of the chest for $3.00. (The total cost of financing is $1.00 a month.)

We feel that a plan similar to this, modified to meet local conditions, can be put into operation in any part of the country. In order to bring this about the backing of those interested in child health, particularly the backing of pediatricians, is required.

The Committee makes the following recommendations to the Academy of Pediatrics:

1. That the attention of the members of the Academy be called to the advisability of recommending thorough periodic physical examinations for all adults in close contact with children.
2. That parents be influenced to have such examinations as an example to their employees.
3. That pediatricians, themselves, should have physical examinations, in order to set a proper example and to show that they believe in what they advise.
4. That the x-ray examination of the lungs of teachers and other school employees be encouraged (as in Minneapolis, where eight active cases of tuberculosis were found in the schools).
5. That steps be taken to initiate a campaign for the education of the public regarding the need for and value of periodic health examinations of adults in contact with children; that public opinion thereby be developed to the point where it becomes customary for domestic workers to hold medical cards as health references because they have undergone the necessary physical examination.
6. That the cooperation of employment agencies be secured to encourage domestics who work in families with children to obtain "health cards."
7. That the assistance of organizations interested in child health be enlisted in as many communities as possible throughout the country to aid in this campaign.
8. That nationwide cooperation of local and county medical societies be secured to adopt a standardized form of examination which will detect evidence of communicable disease in adults contacting children. (An x-ray examination of the lungs is requisite.) The charge for these examinations must not be in excess of the ability of all to pay.
9. It is further recommended that subcommittees be appointed in each regional district and each state to carry on this work in their localities.

DR. HENRY F. HELMHOLZ (ROCHESTER, MINN.).—I do not believe we should pass this by without some discussion. I know the importance of this from the tubercular infection in the family of one of my conferees in Rochester, where unquestionably the infection occurred through one of their employees. It occurs all the time and yet we just haven't done anything about it.

This committee has presented something that we can definitely take with us and put into practice, and I know of nothing that has come up in the Academy that calls for such definite action on the part of each and every one of us as this problem. Here is a question that concerns all patients directly.

We do not need anything from the report of the Academy. We can start in, each one of us, in our community. I think the headline in the San Francisco newspapers this morning about the dangers of contact infection is a step in the right direction. When we go home we can see that it is published in our own local newspapers. I do not think that there will be any trouble in our getting all the organizations interested, such as the women's clubs, for we have one or two examples in every city that can show the importance of this kind of work. I have not seen anything recently that is such a direct challenge for each and every one.

DR. CLIFFORD D. SWEET (OAKLAND, CALIF.).—I am on a special committee which, with the Chamber of Commerce, is working along this line. I would like to include, however, a health card for the grandparents.

Frequently we find an elderly person infecting other members of the family. I have found a practical way of overcoming this in my own practice. Tuberculosis tests are made for the children, and when a child 6, 8, or 10 years old shows positive tuberculosis, I tell the patients that this is not necessarily a danger signal, but it does mean one thing, that we must investigate that child's environment and find out whether or not he is in contact with anyone wtih active tuberculosis. That is a distinct lever in getting everyone in the family examined.

These tests keep one informed as to whether or not the child is infected and examination of the family, or every one with whom the child is in contact, leads sometimes to the source of infection.

DR. ANDREW J. THORNTON (SAN DIEGO, CALIF.).—All the school children in San Diego have an examination every year, including a Wassermann test for $1.50.

PRESIDENT VAN INGEN.—The Committee is emphasizing that this really be one of the activities of the Academy, and that means it is another job for our state chairmen. After all, it is a state program and it is up to the regional chairmen to encourage our state chairmen to organize in their own state a campaign of this sort. It will be interesting to see, if we decide to do it, what we accomplish before our next meeting.

DR. ELMER W. BARRON (BOSTON, MASS.).—Would it not be more acceptable for the Academy to go on record as approving these procedures in making it more effective for us so that when we try to organize these efforts, we can say this is approved by the National Association? Rather than merely accepting the report, would it not be better that we go on record as approving such a procedure?

PRESIDENT VAN INGEN.—It would seem that is cumbersome. We accepted the recommendations and those recommendations are a part of that report; that is what we are accepting as one of our obligations.

DR. EDWIN G. SCHWARTZ (FORT WORTH, TEXAS).—I felt that this was one of the most pertinent things I could see in these reports. Naturally, the country has been publicized during the last few months on the syphilis campaign, and I think this would follow up at a pertinent time. I do not think any part of the country has not been publicized and been informed on the syphilis campaign and I believe it is most important for this to follow it up.

There is a question in my mind as to the means of following it out, and I believe the state chairmen can appoint committees throughout the states. I feel also that it is a campaign where no one could accuse the pediatrician of having any ulterior motives, and, frankly, this campaign is such that it could and would be carried out by other clubs. It is also an effort where the general practitioners would not feel that we were crossing them, but rather that we were boosting their type of work.

DR. HAROLD H. MITCHELL (ASTORIA, N. Y.).—Nothing has been said about the possibilities of getting the public health, the educational, and the tuberculosis associations to back this. I think the action and leadership on the part of the Academy is going to be a great stimulus, and undoubtedly these other organizations are going to stand behind us.

PRESIDENT VAN INGEN.—Evidently there is not going to be any trouble in arousing interest on the part of the tuberculosis associations throughout the country.

DR. FAIRFAX HALL (NEW ROCHELLE, N. Y.).—I would like to speak on the question of classing this as ''food-handling associations.'' The public health authorities do not favor routine food-handling organizations. What one gets from food-handling is typhoid, and typhoid carriers are very hard to detect. If this is put in the public health associations' hands, examinations are not certain. They do not include x-ray examinations. I have no doubt but that means a great many of cases of tuberculosis, at least, the latent cases. If this thing can be done through organized medicine and county medical societies and kept in the hands of the local practitioner, I believe it is going to be more practical.

DR. WILLIAM WESTON (COLUMBIA, S. C.).—I will amend my own motion that it be the sense of this meeting that the state chairmen be instructed to make this an integral part of their public health program and to promote it in their several states.

When the amendment to the motion was accepted by the member seconding it, the following discussion was held:

DR. HORTON CASPARIS (NASHVILLE, TENN.).—I am going to present this matter to the National Tuberculosis Association in Los Angeles, the week after next. The subject is going to be brought up there in a symposium, and I am going to present the Academy viewpoint.

DR. MAURICE L. BLATT (CHICAGO, ILL.).—I would like to say a word in support of this measure and against the matter of putting this through as a law or increasing the responsibility of our public health authorities.

As has been stated before, it is most important that the pediatrician, in order that his influence be evident, extend to the general practitioner every effort possible. This thought, expressed by Dr. Hall, is a great opportunity to do so. There is not any one of us who has been practicing pediatrics for any length of time who has not had experiences with tuberculosis similar to those cited here this morning. Those families who have had trouble influence other families of the better type to have their help examined, and there is no question but that many of them will pay the examination fees. Many of the families I have will gladly pay the price.

The responsibility will not fall on the individual employee, and many of the employees not previously examined will be examined.

I would like to ask a question: Has anything been done on hospital cross-infections which in any way corresponds to this report?

PRESIDENT VAN INGEN.—That should be a function of our Hospital and Dispensaries Committee.

DR. FLORENCE A. BROWNE (NEW YORK, N. Y.).—I wish to bring out the work to be done for dependent children. I have been going across the country and visiting a good many institutions for children and also home organizations, and in different cities across the country the men practicing pediatrics are not sure of the health program for these children. Routine tuberculosis testing is very scant, and it seems to me that it is time that this program be extended to dependent children in institutions and homes as well as to the employees, the nuns in institutions, etc.

I think it would be well for the Academy to go on record as favoring this program for dependent children also.

DR. HARRY BAKWIN (NEW YORK, N. Y.).—I have checked this idea with others and find that in most cases the employees are willing to accept an examination. The difficulty has been in the changing of nurses for the children. Usually they change several times before they find one they like, and that is where one loses out. I think this organized effort of Dr. Hall ought to be extremely valuable.

The motion, having been made and seconded, was unanimously carried, that the report be accepted and that the state chairmen be instructed to make this matter an integral part of their public health program and promote it in their several states.

Discussion of the Report of the Committee on Mental Hygiene

The Report of the Committee on Mental Hygiene was unanimously approved. It was recommended that this Committee be continued and instructed to proceed with this work.

DR. HELMHOLZ.—The Chairman, Dr. Beverly, is not here but perhaps Dr. Casparis might say a few words.

DR. HORTON CASPARIS.—We have had a meeting of this committee and have gone into the situation very carefully. There are three aspects of training that are stimulating interest in pediatricians; one of them, of course, concerns adequate training in medical schools, and we have recommended this training or teaching in mental growth development by starting in at the beginning in the medical school and continuing it throughout the curriculum.

Another aspect is to give better training to those who are being trained to be pediatricians and the stimulation of interest in those already graduated, by adding more papers on this subject approved by the medical board. We feel, if the committee is continued, that we are going further, and formulate actual teaching programs in connection with the Mental Hygiene Association for inclusion in the curriculum of the schools, urging that more time be given to this subject.

PRESIDENT VAN INGEN.—It seems that this report recommends that this be made a part of the undergraduate or medical school work, and it seems to me that if the Academy approves of that being done it should express it by a definite motion, that the report of this committee be put into effect as far as the Academy is concerned.

Discussion of the Report of the Committee on School Health and School Education

DR. HELMHOLZ.—The Report of the Committee on School Health and School Health Education was unanimously approved.

PRESIDENT VAN INGEN.—Dr. Harold Mitchell is here and I will ask him if he will say a few words to us about the work of his committee which, as I have already expressed to you, is in my opinion an extremely valuable one.

DR. HAROLD H. MITCHELL.—Dr. Van Ingen has emphasized the question of school health programs in reference to the many people concerned; physical educators, nurses, teachers, and school boards, and at our round table discussions in the last few days there was a general impression that the pediatricians could do something about it. In fact, it is safe to predict that if the pediatricians do not take more interest in school affairs in the next twenty years than they have in the last twenty years, there's going to be a definite change in policy in regard to the school health programs.

The educators are very much concerned about having medical service that includes diagnosis and treatment in the schools. They are not concerned about having doctors on salary at all. Fortunately, the idea still prevails in schools that the school health program should be fundamentally educational; and that is an idea which offers the best developments along sound lines.

A good example is what has been done in Seattle where 90 per cent of the members of the pediatric group are members of the American Academy of Pediatricians. Recently they have been influential in having a pediatrician put on for the first time as advisor in their school health program. That can be done if the pediatricians, or the organized medical profession through communities, take up the matter of the kind of program that is going on, with regard to the examinations and inspections, rather than medical guidance and health recreation. If you recognize that educators tend to distrust a practitioner unless he approaches them, first, from the standpoint of structure or improving quality of the program (we all know there is room for improvement in the procedure in the schools), so that the educators realize that there is no ulterior motive in attempting to improve the quality, you are certain such matters as competition and lack of interest will be eliminated in following the advice of the practitioner. That will take care of itself.

The survey we made last year showed truly how much dissatisfaction and how many complaints there were about competition coming through school health programs. In general, that is not a large problem at all, but there is a strong tendency among educators to demand a strong kind of service; I think the suggestions about improvement of quality will lend the kind of influence necessary to make it possible to overcome the kind of thing we want to avoid.

The motion was made, seconded, and unanimously carried that this report be accepted and approved.

Discussion of the Report of the Committee on Age Limits of Pediatric Practice

The report of the special committee appointed to study the age limits of pediatric practice was discussed at length. It was moved and seconded that the report of the Committee be accepted with the provision that the last paragraph of the report be changed so as to read,

> "The practice of pediatrics begins at birth and extends well into adolescence and in most cases it would terminate between the sixteenth and eighteenth year of life,"

instead of the paragraph as given in the report. The motion was unanimously carried.

Dr. Martmer, the Chairman of that committee, was called upon to speak.

DR. EDGAR E. MARTMER (DETROIT, MICH.).—This report is the outcome of a meeting of the state chairmen last year in response to a request made at that time that there be a definite stand on the part of the Academy as to what would constitute an age limit of pediatric practice.

It was necessary to check and define the word "pediatric" and "pediatric practice." I think most of us have very definite ideas as to what that constitutes, but when you try to find what wording is to be put down in print, it is not very easy to do.

The White House Conference had many ideas along those lines, and dictionaries are of no benefit whatsoever. We began with a questionnaire sent throughout the country. On a program of this type it would be impossible to contact every member of the Academy so we used a method of canvassing the various parts of the country. Responses to the questionnaire were splendid. Out of 117 questionnaires which were sent out, we had a response of more than 90 per cent, and I think the committee, as a whole, wishes to express its appreciation for the effort of those men who took the time to fill out the questionnaires and return them.

They were made short and to the point, and we had a great deal of satisfaction in going over them, realizing that the men who responded had given considerable thought before answering. Obviously, having established a definition as we did, the question answered itself in that it is practically impossible to set a definite age at which pediatric practice shall terminate. So many features are involved that it is impossible to say when the pediatric practice should terminate, whether at the sixteenth year or the seventeenth year of life, or any other particular point.

For that reason we have submitted the report which is published and which you have read. For your benefit, I will read the last portion of that report which has been changed and now reads:

> "The practice of pediatrics begins at birth and extends well into adolescence, and in most cases it would terminate between the sixteenth and eighteenth year of life."

PRESIDENT VAN INGEN.—It means that we accept the definition as the Academy of Pediatrics.

The motion was made, seconded, and unanimously carried that the report be accepted.

DR. HERBERT L. MOON (SEATTLE, WASH.).—In view of the fact that the Social Security Act has definitely made the statement that children shall be considered as such up to the age of 21 years (that has been the federal law for some time under Section 5, Article I), I think we have been conservative in this matter. I think that it is a proposition that we should get behind.

DR. HELMHOLZ.—If I may, I'd like to make a change and speak of the resolution of the Brooklyn Academy because it concerns this topic.

The resolution presented by the Brooklyn Academy of Pediatrics, regarding the requirements for applicants in the American Board of Obstetrics and Gynecology, was read to the Board and a lengthy discussion was had thereon. Several suggestions were offered, whereupon it was moved and seconded that the Brooklyn Academy of Pediatrics be informed that the Executive Board, to whom their resolution was referred, is in sympathy with the principles of their resolution and will take such action as seems most probable of producing results along the lines suggested, and that a committee shall be appointed to further continue our fight to have this injustice corrected.

The motion was unanimously carried.

DR. HELMHOLZ.—I might say that this concerns the care of the infant during the first year by the obstetrician. If I may, I'd like to say one word in that regard as to what has been done by the American Board of Pediatrics:

Ever since its inception, the Board has recognized that if a pediatrician is not allowed to practice obstetrics because he has passed the American Board of

Pediatrics, the obstetrician should not be allowed to practice pediatrics because he has passed the Board of Obstetrics and Gynecology.

There are many obstetricians in favor of the pediatrician's point of view, but there are a number on the Board still controlling the vote, so it has been impossible up to this time to have this changed. I think a great many obstetricians are favorable to our point of view.

The question arose of changing the time of our meeting to the fall. That is the time when the other Academies meet. It was decided at the Executive Board meeting last December to change our time of meeting, so that it will be held in the fall instead of in the spring, and we would like to have the approval of the membership on this change.

It was moved and seconded that this change be made.

PRESIDENT VAN INGEN.—I would like to call your attention to the fact that this change of date was originally suggested at a meeting of Region II, in New Orleans, and it was also approved by Region IV, with the proviso that we do everything we can at the same time to stimulate the pediatric section of the American Medical Association.

DR. EDITH BOYD (MINNEAPOLIS, MINN.).—A meeting in the fall is hard for those of us who teach. That is the most difficult time of the year for a teacher to get away for classes are just starting.

PRESIDENT VAN INGEN.—No matter what time we meet, it is difficult for someone to get away.

DR. BOYD.—If it is far enough into the fall so that classes have already started it is easier.

DR. HELMHOLZ.—That matter has been considered. The meeting has been set for some time between October 15 and November 15.

The motion was unanimously carried.

DR. HELMHOLZ.—It is the feeling of the Executive Board that the meetings of the Academy have not had the amount of publicity which they should have received, and often the actions taken have not received any publicity at all.

Considerable discussion was had regarding the employment of someone to handle the publicity for the Academy, and a letter was read from Mr. Richard Smith, Publicity Expert, proposing to handle the publicity for the organization for a period of twelve months at $200 a month, including all expenses.

The secretary stated that this was the only person who had been contacted, and after further discussion it was decided that this need not be taken up further until the first of the year. The secretary was instructed to continue further with the investigation of this subject and endeavor to have something more definite to report at the fall meeting of the Executive Committee.

PRESIDENT VAN INGEN.—In this paper it says $200 a month including all expenses. There is nothing additional, but that is not the point.

The Executive Board would like to have the approval of the Academy of the proposition of spending some of the Academy funds for publicity in connection with our meetings and in furthering our work. This service, if in force now, would be brought in on this question of household servants on the contact infection program. We would have the services of a publicity man which would save us trouble and would give us better results. The general principle of whether or not the Academy should spend funds for publicity is before you.

It was moved and seconded that authority be given the Executive Board to take such action as it deems proper.

DR. GILBERT J. LEVY (MEMPHIS, TENN.).—I think it would be well for the Academy to be wisely guided in spending this money so as not to spend any excessive amount for this purpose. I think the amount suggested is almost prohibitive. I think an agency could be secured for as little as $50 per month. I think we should provide that if one should be secured, the amount to be expended should not exceed $50 or $75 a month.

DR. FRANCIS SCOTT SMYTH (SAN FRANCISCO, CALIF.).—It is not a matter of expenses but I should like to say this:

I have developed a strong feeling that as a profession, we have reached the stage where we are being pushed—demands are being made of us in that when research work is being carried on, with a possible implication to the laity, and we are asked to handle a program that is almost prohibitive, I do think we can afford, at any cost, to supervise the publicity so that we will not have a backfire.

PRESIDENT VAN INGEN.—All we are asking is that the Academy approve of further investigation in this matter and then we will act if the Executive Board feels it is necessary.

I can assure you of one thing, that the Board, in my two years' experience on it, is extremely tight-fisted and it does not grant an unlimited expenditure of funds to the secretary and, I might say, the secretary is one of the most tight-fisted men I have met when it comes to spending money on the Academy.

I agree with Dr. Smyth but all we are talking about is what the Academy has definitely decided to do. I think there has been something spent in getting publicity for this meeting and I know that everything that has gone out concerning this meeting has been seen in advance and has been approved by somebody from the office of the Academy. We would like to have further discussion.

DR. EDGAR E. MARTMER.—The question as to the advisability of having a publicity expert has been pretty well answered by an examination of the San Francisco papers since the beginning of this meeting.

The American Psychiatric Association is having a meeting in San Francisco which has been thoroughly and fully plastered all over the newspapers. Our meeting has had a considerable amount of publicity but in proportion to that devoted to the American Psychiatric Association, I don't think we have had anywhere near the same amount of publicity.

The American Psychiatric Association has had a man working on this for the past year. Therefore, he has been able to formulate a program, and when the proper time arose he has been able to transmit to the newspapers medical information in a manner in which it can be utilized by the newspapers.

For a newspaper reporter to sit in on this meeting and then go out and write a story is almost impossible, but a publicity man can take the material we have under discussion and prepare it for the newspapers and see that it receives the distribution which it requires. To carry out such a program requires that he not be present at any meeting but that he have the matter in mind during the entire year. Things come up at meetings which have considerable news value, and which would be beneficial if properly presented, but if a publicity man attends one meeting a year, nothing is accomplished. This one program on contact infections, if carried out, is enough material to fill a large scrapbook.

If you have preliminary announcements and then follow them up not only in that immediate vicinity, but throughout the country, I think it would be a wise thing to do. I do not know of any man in the profession of medicine who would be able to produce such material for release. The only man who can do that is a publicity man who knows his business. I do not think you will get anywhere on this proposition if you try to limit the Board to a definite amount they may or may not spend, providing you approve it in principle. They will not spend your money foolishly, as they have proved time and time again. I think we should approve this and leave it to the Board as to the amount they should spend.

DR. CLIFFORD G. GRULEE.—This suggestion comes from me because I have been faced with it every time we have had a meeting, for it has been very galling to me to see the x-ray men, the dermatologists, and so forth, featured on the front page, whereas the pediatricians have been very glad to get something under the Castoria advertisement.

I have not looked thoroughly into the subject. It was put in as a tentative subject by me for discussion by the Executive Committee. I have had only this one proposition put up to me. I have no idea whether there are people who will do it for less, but personally I don't want to have it done at all unless it is done right. You can do a lot more harm than good by having poor advertising, and if it costs too much for us, let's don't do it at all; but if it has to be done, let's do it right.

DR. CLIFFORD D. SWEET.—I should like at this time to express my entire willingness to leave this matter in the hands of the Executive Committee, feeling certain that it will be done well, better than any of us can do it.

DR. THOMAS B. COOLEY (DETROIT, MICH.).—Dr. Smyth said almost what I was going to say. I have had considerable experience with the Executive Board of this Society. They are a surprisingly wise group of men. I should feel perfectly safe in leaving it to them. I have as much horror as Dr. Smyth has regarding bad type of publicity, but I feel that this matter can safely be left to the Executive Board.

The motion was unanimously carried.

DR. HELMHOLZ.—Discussion was had concerning the pediatric award offered by Mead Johnson & Company, and it was the recommendation of the Board that this award be accepted with the understanding that the award does not necessarily have to be given for work published in the year of the award.

I would like to say with regard to the Mead Johnson award, that this is to be given annually, consisting of two prizes: the first prize to be $500 and the second prize $300. These awards are to be given annually for the best work in pediatrics by men who have been out of medical school not longer than fifteen years. The object of this award by Mead Johnson & Company is to stimulate research of a clinical as well as a laboratory nature, and I think this is an expression of the appreciation of pediatric research by Mead Johnson & Company.

PRESIDENT VAN INGEN.—I think also it is an expression of confidence in the judgment of the Academy in deciding which research investigation is valuable, and I think Mead Johnson & Company, who are giving this as a memorial for the founder of the fund to be known as the "E. Mead Johnson Memorial" are giving it as an expression of confidence. We have practically accepted this award, but we would like to have your approval before going further in this matter. It has been published in the JOURNAL so you have a chance to express your approval.

It was moved and seconded that the action of the Board be approved. The motion was unanimously carried.

In view of the offer of the American Speech Correction Association to stage a demonstration of the work they are doing, during the annual meeting of the Academy, the secretary was instructed to reply to this and inform them that the Board is in keen sympathy with their work but that the next meeting of the Academy will not occur until a year from next fall; he should add, however, that this feature may be worked in with the program at that time.

The necessity of cooperation with all organizations doing work for the child and the interest shown last year by the members of the Academy aroused the feeling that it was desirable to have such demonstration. No action was deemed necessary on this matter at present.

The request of Mead Johnson & Company regarding an investigation of x-ray diagnosis of rickets was brought to the attention of the Board, and after careful consideration of the correspondence relating thereto, it was found that that company is willing to undertake to defray the cost of publishing and distributing the report of the Academy on this subject but that they will not pay for the costs of the investigation. It was moved and seconded that Mead Johnson & Company be informed that the Academy is not in a position to make this study. The motion was unanimously carried.

DR. HELMHOLZ.—Discussion was had regarding the request of the California Society for the promotion of medical research, having to do with the vivisection laws in California, and it was moved and seconded that the secretary send a copy of the resolution which has been adopted at former meetings on this subject and that a letter accompany said resolution. The motion was unanimously carried.

DR. HELMHOLZ.—It was moved and seconded that when the meetings of the American Board of Pediatrics are held in conjunction with those of the American Academy of Pediatrics, we invite applicants to attend our meetings.

The motion was unanimously carried.

DR. HELMHOLZ.—The matter of the International Congress of Pediatrics to be held in Boston in 1940 was discussed at some length, particularly with regard to the Academy's part in financing such meeting and the manner in which the meeting might be financed. The estimate of $20,000 needed by the Congress for such purposes was discussed, as well as the purposes for which such a sum would be required. No program having been definitely decided upon, it was found difficult to allocate specific sums to the carrying out of such matters as entertainment, translations, and publishing costs, etc.

It was moved and seconded that following the invitation of the Academy of last year, which has been accepted, the Executive Board recommend that a special assessment, not to exceed $5.00 per year, per member, be levied for two years. This assessment would be to cover the dues to the Congress, each member to receive a copy of the transactions and a ticket entitling him to attendance. The motion was unanimously carried.

With regard to the International Congress, first of all, I will try to give you a budget of costs. I have obtained from the Swedish Congress as well as from the Congress in Rome, some of their figures. The Swedish Congress cost about $13,000, with an attendance of only about 600. Considerable part of the cost was defrayed by the government, which is not included in these estimates.

The Italian Congress cost 300,000 lira, which amounts to about $17,000, but the question is, will $17,000 purchase in the way of entertainment, etc., what 300,000 lira purchased? I don't believe it will, so we have placed the figure at $20,000, as a possible minimum. It is difficult to determine.

I was talking with Dr. O'Leary. They intend to hold the International Dermatological Congress in New York at the same time. They are figuring on $35,000. They have levied $5.00 per year for three years on their membership of about 1,000, and their figure does not include admission to the Congress, which I understand is to be $15.00.

In this report, for the money levied, we are giving the membership admission to the Congress, and each Fellow will receive a copy of the transactions whether he attends or not.

I have tried to make out a budget but find it is extremely difficult.

I have taken it up to $17,000, with a note of $2,500 for arrangements with the Bell Telephone Company regarding translation into other languages. That will require translators of considerable ability and a complete set of earphones for a large group. The International Urological Association will meet in New York in 1939 and they are hoping to put on their program in a similar way. This is a smaller group, and I question whether the equipment they have will be sufficient for our needs, but it will give us an opportunity to see.

The difficulty of an International Congress is that a portion of the audience understands only one language; then it must be translated into three or four other languages which slows up the meeting to such an extent that one very easily loses interest. So we are trying to introduce this method of translation to an International Congress, which I feel will add a great deal, not only to the pleasure of the Congress, but to the possibilities of a real international discussion.

I might say that the Urological group are assessing themselves $50.00 per member.

PRESIDENT VAN INGEN.—I would like to call your attention to one thing in that resultion; it says, ''not to exceed $5.00 per year, per member.'' I think, unless I am very much mistaken, that the Board felt that if that money was paid and we had any money from other sources that that money would be rebated in the way of dues.

DR. HELMHOLZ.—When we considered an assessment of $5.00 with regard to defraying part of the expenses, that was in the form of a guarantee.

PRESIDENT VAN INGEN.—This Academy approved of inviting the International Congress to come here. Perhaps they did not recognize the fact that it would cost money to do this, but we are in it now, and it seems to the Board that the only thing that we can do so long as we are in it is to do it well and spread the expenses out among the Fellows of the Academy. The amount admits every member to the Congress, and in any event they will receive a copy of the transactions which will be well worth having.

DR. HUGH K. BERKLEY (LOS ANGELES, CALIF.).—Is it the intention of the Academy to meet in conjunction with the International Congress at the same time?

PRESIDENT VAN INGEN.—That is the intention of the Academy, to hold its meeting in Boston in connection with the International Congress.

DR. OSCAR REISS (LOS ANGELES, CALIF.).—I think as in all matters that have preceded this last part of the report, a vote of confidence in the wisdom and integrity of the Committee is in order. I think they have given this matter every effort and thought, and an effort will be made on their part to secure funds wherever possible, and a vote on the part of the Fellowship is shown in the invitation for the Congress to be held in America. I think all of us should be anxious and willing to contribute.

DR. T. S. WILDER (PHILADELPHIA, PA.).—I make a motion that we approve the action of the Executive Board in this matter and I personally feel that if we are able to entertain the International Congress for $10.00 apiece, Dr. Grulee is not only Scotch but Pennsylvania Dutch as well.

The motion was seconded and unanimously carried.

PRESIDENT VAN INGEN.—I want to call on some of the special committee chairmen; I wonder if Dr. Weston will speak to us about the Committee on Cooperation with Medical Groups.

DR. WILLIAM WESTON (COLUMBIA, S. C.).—I wish to say that we feel it is of the utmost importance, if the standard of the Section on Pediatrics is to continue to be high, that you give it your support.

We feel that if you have any grievances against the American Medical Association, its management and control, or affairs, and particularly the crisis which it confronts, it is your part to make your grievances known. We feel that those men have sufficient influence, in a way at least, to carry out your demands.

DR. CLIFFORD G. GRULEE (EVANSTON, ILL.).—One of the cardinal principles put down as one of the fundamental things this Society was to do was to further the Section of Pediatrics of the American Medical Association. This Society has never deviated from that course, but I think we ought to have a vote of thanks, seconding Dr. Weston's remarks, and to say that we are wholeheartedly back of the Section of Pediatrics of the American Medical Association.

The motion was seconded and unanimously carried.

PRESIDENT VAN INGEN.—The work of the Council for Pediatric Research has been followed with interest.

It was the hope that something might be done in this line. Nearly two years ago the Council was appointed and funds obtained from outside resources for investigation and research. We were fortunate enough to get Dr. Cooley to make this investigation and act as executive head of the Council. We would like to have Dr. Cooley give us a few remarks about the hopes and ambitions of that Council.

DR. THOMAS B. COOLEY (DETROIT, MICH.).—I do not know whether or not I shall discuss all that the Council hoped to accomplish. I have suspected before that a surprisingly large portion of the money going to support pediatric research and investigation comes from the commercial firms who manufacture and sell things for use in pediatrics. This money is not all very wisely spent. I think all of us appreciate that. It has been done largely by direct requests from the investigators and laboratory workers as individuals, and not in what I would call a dignified way; things of that sort are always open to a certain suspicion.

There has been an attempt to find out what kind of work the various laboratories and clinics in the country are qualified to do well, what their personnel and equipment is, and what things they are particularly interested in, so that if a manufacturer has a product that he wants examined, and many of them are anxious to get these things thoroughly studied before they make any attempt to put them on the market, they will know where to go.

Sometimes they do it the other way; they market it first and then have it examined after it is on the market. In the year during which we have been at work, it has been impossible to get an adequate directory of the clinics and laboratories which are in a position to do real work, so that we can refer these people to them and then act as an intermediary on the subject.

We have had in mind the idea that we might be able to coordinate the research going on in certain lines.

Five years ago, I estimated if such a thing as this Council were well established what it might have done with a study on rickets. I think we might perhaps save the people money who are backing those causes.

There is one thing we want to do, but we have not gone very far as yet, and that is to find out from the various investigators for what particular lines or promising items they want money, and we will be able to tell them where to get that money. So far, we have been feeling our way. We are just beginning now to have projects brought to us, which may result in research grants of no little importance.

An interesting thing has come up and that is the rather elaborate study on adolescence. This particular study will call for quite a large amount of money, and we have been asked as a council for research to take a more or less advisory part in that study, and probably to take for them the money that they receive and supervise its expenditures. This, we think, is in our province and is a very fine thing for us to foster. These are things we hope to be able to do.

It is very hard for us to get the publicity we would like, and it isn't very easy to locate all of the people who may be putting money into this sort of thing. We would like to have the members of the Academy when they know of anything of that kind to refer them to the Council. So far everything coming to us has come, not as a result of the publicity we have had in pediatric journals, but as the result of the interest of some individual who sent the particular man to us as the proper place to come.

PRESIDENT VAN INGEN.—I had hoped we would be able to call on all committees to report besides those who already have reported, and there are four more in this Academy who do a great deal more than many of the Fellows realize; they are the four regional chairmen. I had hoped to ask each of them to say a word but I will ask if any of them have anything they would like to say especially?

I want one more statement. We have with us Dr. Bierman, as the personal representative of Dr. Elliott of the Children's Bureau, and she wants to say a word as to the new legislation now before Congress.

DR. JESSIE M. BIERMAN (HELENA, MONT.).—The legislation which is before Congress now calls for an amendment for Title 5, Part I of the Social Security Act, governing maternal and child health, for an increase in appropriation. The purpose is to afford one means of combating and attempting to lower the excessive maternal and neonatal mortality, which you all know has not decreased, especially since we have been keeping mortality statistics. Very little progress has been made in the neonatal period, and as you know, in maternal mortality. The continuing high mortality is becoming increasingly a matter of concern, particularly in view of our declining birth rate.

It does not involve any changes in the present law except that money will be made available for the actual payment of qualified, local practicing physicians for giving obstetric and pediatric care. The plan is to provide for an obstetric and pediatric consultation service to the physicians who are giving the care. Most of this program, of course, is designed to be carried out in the rural areas. There are more than a quarter of a million women in this country who have no medical care of any kind during childbirth. The purpose is to provide medical care for this group and also to give aid to the practicing physician in rural areas, to give him help and also to provide hospitalization where there are certain types of emergencies, and where now it is impossible because of financial reasons to obtain such care. There is no thought of putting a full-time man out in the field to do this work. The plan is to utilize the practitioners in their own local communities. Every state will have the opportunity because now it has to develop its own program according to its own needs.

PRESIDENT VAN INGEN.—I am going to call upon Dr. Nichols, an active member on our Committee of Child Health Relations, to say a word.

DR. STANLEY H. NICHOLS (ASBURY PARK, N. J.).—Dr. Bierman is here representing Dr. Elliott, Dr. Hines Roberts is absent and has asked me to present a word, as he has worked closely with the Children's Bureau along this line. He presents in his report, as you have noticed, the fact that in many instances, members have not taken the initiative but have waited until their services have been requested by the various state agencies. Only a part of these agencies enlist the aid and service of the Academy. The Committee feels that the Academy should initiate a more active program in its efforts to guide the various federal and state agencies working in the maternal and child health fields.

The last recommendation that Dr. Roberts' committee made was that there was a great need for integration of the maternal and child health activities carried on by the various lay and professional organizations in the states. The Academy might well be the motivating force in initiating such a program.

The Committee made every effort, with Dr. Bierman representing Dr. Elliott, to discuss the needs of our state chairmen. It is very clear that our Fellowship from each state should be in three groups: state medical society, the state board of health, and the state health agency dealing with the various phases of child health.

At this meeting we discussed how this might be done, and Dr. Bierman said that in the state welfare group the reason they got so far was that the President, at Mr. Adair's request, requested each state department of health along these lines; and each state department of health appointed representatives of Dr. Adair's obstetrics and gynecology organization. That is the machinery of the whole matter, and she states that it has been effective in forty-eight states in getting this done. So, along this line, while it goes back to the Executive Board, I would like to present the three concrete suggestions our Committee passed on yesterday:

1. We recommend that the President of the American Academy of Pediatrics write the president of each state medical society asking that child health leaders be used and child health committees be appointed, enclosing a list of the state Fellowship in each state.

2. We recommend that the President send similar letters to each state Board of Health, enclosing such list.

3. We suggest that each state chairman make a list of the child health societies in his state and ask one of his Fellows to be present or serve on each of these groups in order that the Fellowship of this Academy might lead the child health progress by our participation. It is true that this will take time.

In New Jersey it took us four years to make the State Medical Society child-health-minded. It can be done. It can be done by concentration of the Fellowship in each state, whether they have two Fellows or 200.

DR. CLIFFORD G. GRULEE.—Every state health department several years ago was apprised of the fact that there was such a thing as an Academy. The names of the state chairmen were sent to the organizations in each state, but we did not get any reply. I doubt very much if such an effort on the part of the President will help because you have to pull from within and not from without.

DR. HARVEY F. GARRISON (JACKSON, MISS.).—I have been delighted to hear the report of Dr. Nichols. I think that everything said by that Committee certainly is appropriate at this time.

It seems to me that the Academy could take some active steps or probably offer an extended hand to Dr. Bierman and her department in the way of cooperation with any plan they may have which looks to the best interest of child health in every state. I think the suggestions made by the Committee are probably sufficient, but it seems to me that a motion now to the effect that the Academy go on record as favoring hearty cooperation with the Children's Bureau and all its activities towards child health, and extending our willingness to help from each state, is in order.

The motion was thereupon seconded.

PRESIDENT VAN INGEN.—This Academy has gone on record several times as endorsing the activity in the Children's Bureau. This is for the benefit of every pediatrist in the country, and I think it will be well for this Academy to go on record as not being in opposition to the bill before Congress by reiterating our hearty wish to cooperate with the Children's Bureau.

The motion was unanimously carried.

PRESIDENT VAN INGEN.—There is one thing more for you to act upon as an Academy—the action of the Nominating Committee. They have nominated as president, Dr. Henry F. Helmholz; for vice-president, Dr. Joseph B. Bilderback, of Portland, Ore.; for chairman, Region IV, Dr. Edward B. Shaw, San Francisco; and for chairman, Region I, Dr. Stanley H. Nichols, Asbury Park, N. J., for one year to fill out the unexpired term of Dr. Schroeder. That report is submitted to you by a comittee of four members of the Academy, no one of whom is on the Executive Board, as required by the Constitution.

The motion was made, seconded, and unanimously carried that the recommendation of the Nominating Committee be approved, as read.

PRESIDENT VAN INGEN.—Article II, Section 4, an amendment adding Porto Rico to Region II and Alaska to Region IV.

It was moved, seconded, and unanimously carried that this action be taken.

PRESIDENT VAN INGEN.—Article VII to be amended so that the words "until the 1932 annual meeting" are deleted.

It was moved, seconded, and unanimously carried that such amendment be made.

PRESIDENT VAN INGEN.—I retire happy, realizing that the Academy is in the hands of Dr. Helmholz and happy in the interest you have shown this morning in attending this general session.

DR. HELMHOLZ.—I am highly appreciative of the honor that you have done me in electing me as president, but I am also conscious of the great responsibility that you have placed in my hands to carry on the work of the Academy for this next year. The high standards that have been set by our past presidents are such that I am fearful whether I can carry on in the same way. But I am encouraged by this meeting and I want to congratulate Dr. Van Ingen on the success of the meeting that we have had this morning. I have a feeling that we have gotten together. I have a feeling that we feel we are working for a common purpose in a way that I have never seen in one of these annual meetings before, and I have attended most of them. I am hopeful from the spirit that I have seen exhibited this morning that we are all in accord with the ideals of the Academy, and that as members of the Academy, as officers of our Fellowship, but more particularly as individual members of the Academy, we will put our shoulders to the wheel and carry on.

DR. WARREN W. QUILLIAN (CORAL GABLES, FLA.).—I am sure that I express the sentiment of all the visiting members of the Academy in expressing to Dr. Shaw, as Regional Chairman, and to the Fellowship of Region IV, our thanks for their serving as hosts at this meeting.

We appreciate the generous hospitality and the opportunity to visit the state of California. I express this sentiment as a member from Florida.

The motion was duly seconded and unanimously carried.

DR. WESTON.—I feel that we would be remiss if we did not thank the retiring President for the splendid and progressive administration which he has given the Academy and above all for establishing upon a permanent basis a feeling of sound and delightful fellowship among our members.

The motion was seconded and unanimously carried by a rising vote.

EIGHTH ANNUAL MEETING OF THE AMERICAN ACADEMY OF PEDIATRICS

DEL MONTE, CALIF., JUNE 9, 10, AND 11, 1938

Round Table Conference on Vaccine Prophylaxis of Whooping Cough

Chairman: Dr. Harold K. Faber, San Francisco, Calif.
Assistants: Dr. L. J. Schermerhorn, Grand Rapids, Mich.
Dr. John J. Miller, Jr., San Francisco, Calif.
Dr. Charlotte H. Singer-Brooks, San Francisco, Calif.

CHAIRMAN FABER.—The discussion today will deal mainly with the active prophlyaxis of whooping cough by vaccine, especially by vaccine of the so-called Phase I type. The subject was debated a year ago at the last annual meeting of the Academy, when a diversity of views on the value of vaccine was evident. Disagreement is still general, and it would be well to acknowledge at once that well-conducted studies are available in support of both sides of the controversy. At the present time it is fair to say that one who unreservedly adopts either side apparently cannot justify himself without disregarding important evidence against it. By ''unreservedly,'' however, I refer only to the absolute concepts of no protection at all, on the one hand, and of an almost perfect protection on the other. A brief review of the more important studies and a consideration of the criteria on which the various conclusions are based will, I believe, show that the truth of the matter lies somewhere between the two extremes of opinion. For the purposes of the practicing pediatrician the important question to solve is, not so much whether vaccine affords absolute protection under all conditions, but whether it affords enough protection to be of service to his patients.

In judging the value of immunization for pertussis we are at present almost entirely dependent on statistical criteria. Such biologic tests as are available are either too cumbersome for general use, or are unreliable or of unproved value. Analysis and comparison of most of the published series involve the attack rate and the communicability rate: the former being the proportion of a given population that acquires the disease; the second, the proportion of individuals who acquire the disease after known exposure to it. Both methods are liable to serious errors, which make comparison of the rates in different series dangerous and misleading unless several variables are clearly stated and taken into account. This will be more fully discussed by later speakers, but I believe it is fair to say that the communicability rate is on the whole a more reliable index of immunity than the attack rate, unless the latter is calculated by refined methods of analysis. Such methods have only exceptionally been used in the published studies. Even when alternation is employed, every other child being vaccinated, it is difficult to be sure that identical conditions of exposure have existed in both groups, or to know how large the groups should be to avoid errors of random sampling in respect to exposure. The attack rates in published series vary from 5 per cent to 98 per cent in unvaccinated susceptible persons. In respect to the communicability rate, we have at least the fact of exposure to the disease on which to depend. Granting that intensity of exposure, continuance of exposure, period of the disease in the source of the exposure, age of the exposed, and certain other conditions introduce variables of importance, nevertheless, it seems fair to assume that most exposures serve to introduce *Hemophilus pertussis* into the exposed individual's respiratory system and that the appearance or nonappearance of the disease depends on the absence or presence of specific immunity to it.

We have a number of data on the proportion of children who develop whooping cough after contact with the disease. Biedert, in 1885, reported a rate of 91 per cent in susceptible children in a village population in Germany. In Madsen's report, 98 per cent of unvaccinated individuals in the isolated, rural population of the Faroe Islands developed the disease, the rate being so high that we must assume universal exposure and susceptibility. Kendrick reported a rate of 75 per cent in unvaccinated children in Grand Rapids, all being less than 3 years of age. Wheeler reported from a rural community in New York State rates of about 93 per cent in patients less than 4 years old; 88 per cent, between 5 and 14 years old; and 38 per cent, between 15 and 19 years of age. From Cleveland, Green reported rates of 71 per cent in patients less than 4 years old and only 12 per cent, between 10 and 14 years old, indicating the spontaneous acquisition of immunity during childhood in urban populations. It will be noted that in young children generally and in older children and even adults in rural or isolated communities whooping cough is contracted after exposure in 70 per cent or more of the cases. It is therefore particularly interesting to note the communicability rate in children who have been vaccinated. Sauer, in Evanston, reports a rate of 4.7 per cent; Kendrick and Eldering, of 13.5 per cent; Daughtry-Denmark, of 10.9 per cent. In the report of Doull, Shibley and McClelland, who on the basis of the attack rate concluded that vaccine is of no value, fourteen of the vaccinated control patients escaped the disease after exposure, while none of the unvaccinated controls escaped. All these studies dealt with young children. The contrast is therefore quite striking and uniform between the vaccinated and the unvaccinated; particularly so in the study of Kendrick and Eldering, who selected children by alternation for vaccination and found the incidence of pertussis after exposure about six times greater in the untreated group than in the treated.

The studies just mentioned have dealt with children at normal life. Two studies remain to be mentioned in which the children were in institutions: one in a sanitarium for tuberculosis, the other in an orphanage; in both places epidemics of whooping cough occurred and subjected the children to prolonged, intimate, and presumably rather intense exposure. The first report is that of Siegel and Goldberger, in which sixty-four children less than 6 years old were exposed during the epidemic. Of these, thirty-six had not had pertussis; sixteen had a definite history of the disease, and twelve had a doubtful history. Of the thirty-six without any history of pertussis, seventeen were given vaccine; of these, five, or 27 per cent, developed typical whooping cough, and four more, mild or doubtful attacks. The remaining nineteen were not given vaccine, and of these, ten, or 53 per cent, developed typical whooping cough, and one had a mild or doubtful attack. Of the sixteen who had a definite history of the disease and were not vaccinated, 5, or 31 per cent, developed typical whooping cough, as compared with five patients, or 50 per cent, in the twelve who had a doubtful history and were not vaccinated. While this report has been generally considered as casting doubt on the value of vaccine, it would appear that the vaccinated susceptible children showed a significant difference from the unvaccinated susceptibles in the severity of the disease; and also that the vaccinated children showed a response to exposure very similar to that of those who had already had the disease.

The other study, by Kramer, of an outbreak in an orphanage with twenty-nine children exposed, shows very similar results, but in greater individual detail, the day-by-day course of the disease in each child being separately plotted. Twelve of the children had no history of the disease and were not vaccinated; all developed typical pertussis, none had less than five weeks of coughing, and all could be classed as having moderately severe cases. Nine children had no history of pertussis and had been given vaccine two years before. Of these, six had mild cases averaging three weeks in duration; one coughed only one week, one only a single day, and one escaped the disease entirely. There were eight children who had a previous history of whooping cough and were not vaccinated; all caught the disease, and six of them coughed for an average period of three weeks, and two only one week. Here, as in the report of Siegel and Goldberger, the relative mildness of the attacks in the vaccinated group is brought out, and the similarity of the vaccinated group to the group with a positive history of previous attacks is striking.

I have gone into the last two reports in detail because institutional epidemics, with their conditions of prolonged and intimate exposure, give a more severe and crucial test of the value of immunization than do noninstitutional exposures where, even when pertussis is prevalent in the home, the children usually spend a good deal of time out of doors and are not so continuously exposed. There are, I believe, certain features of these institutional reports which offer clues to the solution of the problem under discussion today. First, it is obvious that the immunity supplied by prophylactic injection of *Hemophilus pertussis* vaccine is not, and cannot be expected to be, absolute. Second, contrary to earlier belief, the immunity derived from a previous attack of the disease itself is also far from absolute. Third, in both cases it tends to break down when exposure is intimate and prolonged. Fourth, under less drastic conditions of exposure both the artificially and the naturally induced immunity appear to afford protection in a large proportion of cases, and in general the protection from both sources appears to be approximately equal. Fifth, there is evidence of partial protection when the immunized individual does acquire the disease, as shown by briefer and milder symptoms.

It is clear, I think, from the evidence that I have reviewed that many problems need further study. We need more field studies. We need a practicable clinical test for immunity. Dosage may need revision, perhaps upward. The optimum intervals between injections may be greater than one week. We do not as yet know how long immunity lasts or the rate at which it declines. There may be strains of *Hemophilus pertussis,* such as the one which Bradford has recently noted, in about 5 per cent of cases, which should be included in the vaccine in order to increase the number of protected individuals.

A Report on the Progress of The Grand Rapids Pertussis Immunization Study

L. J. Schermerhorn, M.D.

Since the discovery of *Bacillus pertussis* in 1906 there have been too few clinical studies directed toward the control of pertussis, a disease which leads the contagious group as a cause of death in patients less than 5 years of age. While this apparent failure or reluctance to apply the results of Bordet's[1] and subsequent bacteriologic studies in pertussis control cannot be entirely justified, it must be admitted that broad application of control measures cannot be expected until the reporting of satisfactory results in controlled studies over a period of years. Satisfactory studies of this type on pertussis control have accumulated slowly. Reports of studies indicating that inoculations with potent antigen confer protection on a high percentage of young children, have only in late years contained controlled data approaching the criteria of scientific truth necessary before wide application can be expected. That certain features of pertussis lend themselves poorly to controlled experimental methods does not entirely account for this lag in the reporting of pertussis control studies. Probably the most important single factor has been our inability to clearly define and meet the requirements for antigenic uniformity in the vaccines used. As recently as 1931 the reporting of conflicting and irregular results due to this factor caused commercially prepared pertussis vaccines to be dropped from the list of new and nonofficial remedies.[2] Nevertheless, such careful reports as those of Madsen[3] and later Sauer's studies[4] presented sufficiently encouraging results to justify further investigation. The Grand Rapids pertussis immunization study was started in 1932 to aid in hastening general application of any promising control measures, already too long delayed, by presenting evidence gathered from a sufficiently large, carefully planned, and adequately controlled study, which, it was hoped, would withstand critical analysis.

Dr. Pearl Kendrick, associate director of the Michigan Department of Health Laboratories, working in the Western Michigan Division Laboratory in Grand Rapids, planned and actively directed this study. While I worked with Dr. Kendrick in the clinical aspects of the study during its inauguration and early years, a prolonged illness required my withdrawal from active participation. Only because of Dr. Kendrick's inability to attend this meeting have I consented to make a report of the progress made, as requested by Dr. Faber.

The program of this study included, in addition to the clinical problems, an exhaustive bacteriologic study of morphologic, cultural, biochemical and serologic aspects of *Bacillus pertussis,* which clarified older studies and extended our knowledge of this organism. These studies led to the formulation of methods for the preparation of pertussis vaccine, convalescent serum, and hyperimmune serum for later clinical trial. Details of these bacteriologic studies by Dr. Kendrick and Miss Eldering will be found in the literature.[5, 6] Our clinical interest in these studies for the moment centers about, first, the demonstration of the practicability of cough plates in diagnosis and release from quarantine of pertussis patients by health departments, and second, the description of methods for the preparation of uniformly potent therapeutic agents for clinical use.

Cough Plate Studies

In clinical studies, inaccurate diagnoses must be reduced to the minimum. The value of the bacteriologic diagnosis of pertussis was studied and found to be of sufficient aid to play an important part in our efforts to insure correct diagnoses. *Bacillus pertussis* could be isolated from enough pertussis patients to make the results diagnostically significant. The data on several thousand cough plates, including about 1,500 patients with pertussis, indicate that as the technique approaches perfection positive findings early in the disease approach 100 per cent. In fact, many patients with mild pertussis demonstrated clearly that diagnosis often depends upon bacteriologic methods. The organism was found in patients with the mildest symptoms. Dr. Kendrick found that about 75 per cent of the cultures taken during the first week of pertussis were positive; 70 per cent, the second week; 60 per cent, the third week; 30 per cent, the fourth week; and 15 per cent, the fifth week. The Health Department of Grand Rapids cooperated with Dr. Kendrick in this study, obtaining cough plates on all reported, suspicious, and contact individuals. The actual exposure of the plates was carried out by nurses from the Bureau of Public Nursing who were each responsible for definite districts of the city. At the request of a private physician, school physician, or health department officials, cough plates were secured for diagnosis, with the laboratory reporting the results to both the physician requesting it and the health department. The local health department has found the cough plate to be very valuable in the handling of pertussis contagion, especially in decisions involving patients with light symptoms. It has also made it possible to place release from quarantine on a more rational basis. In Grand Rapids, pertussis quarantine is lifted after two consecutive negative cough plates have been obtained, the first one taken not earlier than twenty-one days after onset of symptoms. There would appear to be no excuse for the wide differences in length of quarantine now prevailing in different parts of the country today if the results of this cough plate study are reliable, and I believe that they are because I have seen how carefully the work has been done. A report on the length of quarantine for pertussis in twenty-eight of the largest cities in the United States shows five cities require two weeks, six cities require three weeks, nine cities require four weeks, two cities require five weeks, and six cities require six weeks.[7] It would seem that the end of the fifth week, with only 1 per cent of the children showing positive cough plates, should be a safe period of quarantine. The nurses report no difficulty in obtaining the cough plates, and health officials have experienced no hardships in the administration of a cough plate service.

Preparation of Vaccine and Sera

The following brief descriptions indicate the salient points in the preparation of biologic products used in the clinical studies.

TABLE I

PRINCIPAL CONSIDERATIONS IN THE PREPARATION OF PERTUSSIS VACCINE AS DESCRIBED BY KENDRICK AND ELDERING AND USED IN THIS STUDY

Choice of Cultures.—Five to seven cultures are selected for each lot of vaccine. *All* cultures *must* exhibit immediately before use: Phase I (Leslie and Gardner) characteristics with typical colony appearance on Bordet-Gengou medium, including hemolysis of red cells; typical morphology and staining reactions; agglutination with Phase I antiserum in high (essential) titers (1:10,000 to 1:25,000); capacity to produce a high agglutinating titer in a rabbit for smooth strain cultures; and the typical skin reaction of hemorrhagic necrosis in the rabbit.

Culture Medium.—Bordet and Gengou's potato blood agar modified with 1 per cent proteose-peptone and the addition of sheep blood to a final concentration of 15 per cent.

Technical Factors.—Cultures harvested after seventy-two hours incubation. One washing with normal saline.
Chemical killing agent, either merthiolate 1:10,000 or phenol 0.5 per cent.
Standardized with ten billion organisms per cubic centimeter.

Bacillus Pertussis Vaccine.—All *Bacillus pertussis* cultures used in the preparation of vaccine must be Phase 1 cultures, the term used by Leslie and Gardner[8] to describe the antigenic state characteristic of cultures just isolated from patients with pertussis. These Phase 1 characteristics must be demonstrated just prior to use in vaccine preparation. The cultures used must be capable of producing a certain degree of induration and necrosis when injected into the skin of a rabbit. At least five to seven cultures were used in each lot of vaccine prepared. The organisms were grown on Bordet-Gengou media to which proteose-peptone was added to make a more luxuriant growth. Sheep blood was also added in sufficient quantity to make a final concentration of 15 per cent. The organisms were grown for seventy-two hours at 37° C. They were washed once in saline solution and filtered through cotton and gauze. After filtration the saline suspension was centrifuged, and the organisms were resuspended in saline solution containing 1:10,000 merthiolate or 0.5 per cent phenol. The chemical killing which takes place was assured by storage for one week in the cold room. After tests for sterility and purity, standardization of the suspension to ten billion organisms per cubic centimeter was carried out. The final product must show agglutination with Phase 1 antiserum in titers of at least 1:10,000 or higher and demonstrate capacity to produce a high agglutinating titer in a rabbit, at least 1:10,000 for smooth strain cultures. Safety tests on 300 gram guinea pigs inoculated with 0.5, 1.0, and 1.5 c.c., respectively, must show all pigs alive and having regained their weight by the end of two weeks.

Bacillus Pertussis Convalescent Serum.—The blood donors were required to have had pertussis within the past year. The blood was processed according to established convalescent serum preparation methods.

Bacillus Pertussis Hyperimmune Serum.—Adults giving a definite history of pertussis during childhood were inoculated with *Bacillus pertussis* vaccine. A total dosage of 7 to 20 c.c. of vaccine distributed over a period of weeks was used. Ten days after the last injection of vaccine, blood was collected and processed similar to the methods used in convalescent serum preparation, including a Mandler filtration. The serum thus obtained was required to show agglutinins for *Bacillus pertussis* and a very strong opsonic reaction.

Definition of Terms

Before outlining the plan and results of clinical studies, it is necessary to define certain terms. While the difficulties of accurately describing exposure and severity in pertussis either qualitatively or quantitatively were well recognized, the need for such information in this study is apparent. Consequently, exposures have been classified somewhat arbitrarily into definite, indefinite, and unknown. A definite exposure is described as an intimate indoor contact with a child having pertussis of less than three weeks' duration. It may occur in a family or in a household outside the family. Indefinite exposures include many types of reported contacts which cannot be classified as definite. Unknown exposure is the type occurring in children who contract pertussis but for whom there is no knowledge of any exposure to the disease. To indicate the severity of the disease the terms severe, typical, light, and very light are used. A patient has severe pertussis if paroxysms are unusually frequent and violent, persisting more than six weeks and associated with weight loss and often complications such as bronchopneumonia. Uncomplicated pertussis of five to six weeks' duration, having a characteristic whoop, is referred to as typical. A patient with only an occasional whoop or vomiting of less than four weeks' duration and no obvious interference with nutrition has light pertussis. Very light pertussis shows no whooping and vomiting but a cough which lasts for more than one week in conjunction with a history of definite exposure or positive cough plate finding.

Clinical Studies

1. A study was made of the comparative value of convalescent serum and vaccine given before the onset of symptoms to directly exposed children in the prevention of pertussis.

TABLE II

COMPARATIVE VALUE IN THE PREVENTION OF PERTUSSIS OF CONVALESCENT SERUM AND VACCINE GIVEN BEFORE THE ONSET OF SYMPTOMS TO DIRECTLY EXPOSED CHILDREN*

TYPE OF PREVENTIVE THERAPY	NUMBER OF PATIENTS PER GROUP	NUMBER OF PATIENTS DEVELOPING PERTUSSIS	PERCENTAGE OF PATIENTS DEVELOPING PERTUSSIS
Convalescent serum	30	8	27%
Vaccine	27	9	34%
No therapy	29	24	82%

*A direct exposure is defined as an intimate indoor family exposure.

The health department and city physician referred all patients with pertussis in families on relief to us for study. As soon as reports were received an investigation was made, and each family with two or more children, one of whom had pertussis, was placed in one of three groups: the convalescent serum group, the vaccine group or the control group, by Dr. Kendrick in the order in which they were reported. In as much as I did the field work and Dr. Kendrick placed patients in the various groups, there was no chance of selecting desirable patients for any one group.

A positive diagnosis of pertussis, either by typical symptoms or cough plate in one member of a family, along with at least one or more other children who had not yet contracted the disease, was required before placement of a family in any group. At least two calls were made on these families each week for six weeks, with careful watching to see if the exposed children developed any symptoms of pertussis and, if so, how severe they were. No effort was made in any of the groups to keep the contact cases away from the other children. Living quarters for the most part were crowded, and isolation was impossible. To the directly exposed children of families in the first group 20 c.c. of pertussis convalescent serum was given intramuscularly, followed by a second injection ten days later of 10 c.c. To the directly exposed children of families in the second group 1 or 1.5 c.c. of pertussis vaccine was given every other day until the total dosage reached 8 c.c. To the directly exposed children of the families in the third group no therapy of any kind was given, although they were watched carefully with visits twice each week. Table II shows the results of this study.

In the convalescent serum group there were thirty children injected, less than five years old, who had had direct exposure to pertussis but who had not developed symptoms of the disease. In this group of thirty children, twenty-two, 73 per cent, did not develop pertussis. Eight children, or 27 per cent, developed pertussis. Twelve children of this group who had already developed symptoms of pertussis were given convalescent serum, and as far as I was able to determine it was of no value. There were twenty-seven children in the vaccine group who were given repeated doses of pertussis vaccine. In this group, eighteen children or 67 per cent did not develop pertussis. There were nine children, 33 per cent, that did develop pertussis. In the control group there were twenty-nine children, with five children, or 18 per cent, that did not develop pertussis.

2. A study was made to determine the preventive value of pertussis hyperimmune serum in a selected group of twenty-two directly exposed babies less than 1 year of age.

All twenty-two babies were directly exposed, and eight babies were less than 1 month old. Of this group seventeen received an injection of 10 c.c. of hyperimmune serum as soon after exposure as possible, and this dosage was repeated in ten days. Of the seventeen patients injected, eleven were given the hyperimmune serum before symptoms developed. Nine of these eleven patients given hyperimmune serum early did not develop pertussis; one developed only a light attack, and one baby developed light to typical pertussis. The pertussis patients to which these eleven babies were exposed numbered twenty-two, with eight classified as severe, seven typical, six light, and one as very light. The six babies given hyperimmune serum after the onset of symptoms showed no apparent benefit from the serum. In the control group of five babies given no therapy there were two newborn babies, two 8 weeks old and one baby 6 months old. All five babies were directly exposed to pertussis in their families. Three of these five babies given no therapy developed severe pertussis, two of the three being critically ill; the fourth developed typical pertussis, while the fifth escaped infection. The mother of the baby that escaped infection made a most decided effort to keep him well isolated. It is doubtful if this baby had an adequate exposure, even though living in the same home with a pertussis patient. While the number of patients in this study is too small to offer any basis for conclusions, it is encouraging to note that in the group of eleven exposed babies who received hyperimmune serum before the onset of symptoms, only two developed pertussis. We believe there may be a place for such a serum in the prevention of pertussis in exposed babies and those older children in whom its occurrence would be greatly feared. We feel that further work should be attempted with hyperimmune serum by those who have facilities for studying this method of pertussis prevention.

3. A study is being made of the comparative incidence of pertussis following exposure in children previously given pertussis vaccine and children given no preventive therapy. It has been in progress since 1932. The late Dr. W. H. Frost of Johns Hopkins University and others have consulted freely with Dr. Kendrick in this study. The program required the cooperation of school physicians, city health department physicians, and many private physicians. Nursing personnel was supplied by the Bureau of Public Nursing which placed twenty-five nurses at Dr. Kendrick's disposal. In 1933, at the end of the first year of work, the study was made a government project under the F. E. R. A. Since that time there have been as many as sixteen of the study's personnel, including nurses and other workers, provided by the P. W. A.

Children from 8 months to 5 years of age were included in the study. None of the children had pertussis and none had ever received any pertussis preventive therapy. They were assigned either to the group destined to receive pertussis vaccine or to the control group receiving no preventive therapy. A special effort was made to leave children of both groups in each family when possible. The two groups were comparable in regard to age and time of selection. Pertussis immunization clinics were held in the schools. Children in the vaccine group were given the four injections of pertussis vaccine at weekly intervals by the school physician. A schedule to insure uniformity of dosage and sites of injection was employed: the first injection of 1 c.c. was given subcutaneously in the region of the left biceps; the second of 1.5 c.c. was given in the region of the right triceps; the third of 1.5 c.c. was given in the region of the left triceps; and the fourth of 1.5 c.c. injected into both the right and the left deltoid regions. Aside from an occasional fever and restlessness during the twenty-four hours after inoculation, there was little reaction. Nurses made regular home calls on the children in both the vaccine and the control group at about two-month intervals. These nurses were especially trained to obtain complete histories of each child's health, being especially on the alert for histories of exposures and those symptoms suggestive of pertussis. In addition to these frequent interval histories of each child obtained by the nurses, information often was obtained from the files of the health department and the laboratory's cough plate files. It was almost impossible for a child in either group to have pertussis and not have such information recorded on our records.

Two interval progress reports have previously been published.[9, 10] The last report summarized the study's data to Aug. 20, 1935. At that time there were 1,592 patients under observation, with 712 in the vaccine group and 880 in the control group. In the vaccine group there were sixty patients with exposures of various types and four patients with pertussis, two of whom had no known exposure. In the control group there were eighty-four exposures and sixty-three patients with pertussis, eleven of whom had no known exposure. Six per cent of the patients exposed in the vaccine group developed pertussis and 75 per cent of those exposed in the control group developed pertussis.

Two months later, on Oct. 22, 1935, a summary indicated that there were 1,763 patients under observation, with 814 in the vaccine group and 949 in the control group. In the vaccine group there were seventy exposures and six patients with pertussis. In the control group there were ninety-four exposures and seventy patients with pertussis. Eight per cent of the patients exposed in the vaccine group developed pertussis and 74 per cent of those exposed in the control group developed pertussis.

TABLE III

THE INCIDENCE OF PERTUSSIS FOLLOWING DIRECT, INDIRECT, AND UNKNOWN EXPOSURES IN CHILDREN PREVIOUSLY GIVEN VACCINE AND CHILDREN GIVEN NO PREVENTIVE THERAPY*

Summary of data to Oct. 22, 1935, approximately a three-year interval, with 1,763 patients under observation.

NUMBER OF PATIENTS PER GROUP	NUMBER OF EACH TYPE OF EXPOSURE		NUMBER OF PATIENTS DEVELOPING PERTUSSIS AFTER EACH TYPE	PERCENTAGE OF EXPOSED PATIENTS DEVELOPING PERTUSSIS
Given vaccine therapy: 814	Direct	29	3	
	Indirect	39	1	
	Unknown	2	2	8.7%
	Total	70	6	
Given no preventive therapy: 949	Direct	41	35	
	Indirect	42	24	
	Unknown	11	11	74.5%
	Total	94	70	

*Direct exposure is defined as an intimate indoor home exposure.

Indirect exposure is defined as a reported exposure occurring outside the home. The development of pertussis in a child without a known contact is classified as unknown exposure.

TABLE IV

THE INCIDENCE OF PERTUSSIS FOLLOWING DIRECT, INDIRECT AND UNKNOWN EXPOSURES IN CHILDREN PREVIOUSLY GIVEN VACCINE AND CHILDREN GIVEN NO PREVENTIVE THERAPY

Summary of data to March 1, 1936, approximately a three and one-half-year interval, with 2,018 patients under observation.

NUMBER OF PATIENTS PER GROUP	NUMBER OF EACH TYPE OF EXPOSURE		NUMBER OF PATIENTS DEVELOPING PERTUSSIS AFTER EACH TYPE OF EXPOSURE	PERCENTAGE OF EXPOSED PATIENTS DEVELOPING PERTUSSIS
Given vaccine therapy: 1,002	Direct	58	9	
	Indirect	51	3	
	Unknown	3	3	13.4%
	Total	112	15	
Given no preventive therapy: 1,016	Direct	67	54	
	Indirect	51	27	
	Unknown	23	23	73.8%
	Total	141	104	

On March 1, 1936, a summary indicated that there were 2,018 patients under observation, with 1,002 in the vaccine group and 1,016 in the control group. In the vaccine group there were 112 exposures and fifteen patients with pertussis. In the control group there were 141 exposures and 104 patients with pertussis. Thirteen per cent of the patients exposed in the vaccine group developed pertussis, and 73 per cent of those exposed in the control group developed pertussis. At the time of this summary there had been only three pertussis patients in the vaccine group with unknown exposures, while twenty-three pertussis patients in the control group had unknown exposures.

TABLE V

THE INCIDENCE OF PERTUSSIS FOLLOWING DIRECT, INDIRECT AND UNKNOWN EXPOSURES IN CHILDREN PREVIOUSLY GIVEN VACCINE AND CHILDREN GIVEN NO PREVENTIVE THERAPY

Summary of data to Oct. 1, 1936, approximately a four-year interval, with 3,102 patients under observation.

NUMBER OF PATIENTS PER GROUP	NUMBER OF EACH TYPE OF EXPOSURE		NUMBER OF PATIENTS DEVELOPING PERTUSSIS AFTER EACH TYPE	PERCENTAGE OF EXPOSED PATIENTS DEVELOPING PERTUSSIS
Given vaccine therapy: 1,573	Direct	75	12	
	Indirect	71	3	
	Unknown	5	5	13%
	Total	151	20	
Given no preventive therapy: 1,529	Direct	92	77	
	Indirect	57	30	
	Unknown	33	33	76%
	Total	182	140	

On Oct. 1, 1936, a summary listed 3,102 children under observation, with 1,573 in the vaccine group and 1,529 in the control group. In the vaccine group there were 151 exposures and twenty patients with pertussis. In the control group there were 182 exposures with 140 patients with pertussis. Thirteen per cent of the patients exposed in the vaccine group developed pertussis and 76 per cent of those exposed in the control group developed pertussis.

TABLE VI

COMPARATIVE INCIDENCE OF PERTUSSIS FOLLOWING EXPOSURES IN CHILDREN PREVIOUSLY GIVEN VACCINE AND CHILDREN GIVEN NO PREVENTIVE THERAPY

Summary of data to Sept. 1, 1937, approximately a five-year interval, with about 4,000 patients under observation.

NUMBER OF PATIENTS PER GROUP	NUMBER OF PATIENTS EXPOSED, ALL TYPES	NUMBER OF PATIENTS DEVELOPING PERTUSSIS	PERCENTAGE OF EXPOSED PATIENTS DEVELOPING PERTUSSIS
Given vaccine therapy: 2,000 (approximate)	295	40	13.5%
Given no preventive therapy: 2,000 (approximate)	358	270	75.0%

On Sept. 1, 1937, the summary data are incomplete because our records have been turned over to the Committee on Administrative Practice of the American Public Health Association who are making a critical analysis of this study. However, about 1,971 children were found in the vaccine group, and only forty children developed pertussis compared with 270 children developing pertussis in the control group.

These analyses made at intervals during this study would seem to indicate that about 13.5 per cent of the children who have been actively immunized to pertussis with vaccine will develop pertussis after an exposure to the disease. Approximately 75 per cent of the children who have not been actively immunized will develop pertussis after exposure.

An attempt has been made to determine the difference in severity of the disease in the vaccine-treated group and the control group. In the analysis of October, 1935, there had been six patients with pertussis in the vaccine group, with four of

TABLE VII

COMPARATIVE SEVERITY OF PERTUSSIS IN CHILDREN PREVIOUSLY GIVEN VACCINE AND IN CHILDREN GIVEN NO PREVENTIVE THERAPY

DATA COMPILED	TYPE OF THERAPY	PATIENTS WITH SEVERE PERTUSSIS	PATIENTS WITH TYPICAL PERTUSSIS	PATIENTS WITH LIGHT PERTUSSIS	PATIENTS WITH VERY LIGHT PERTUSSIS	TOTAL PERTUSSIS PER GROUP
Oct. 22, 1935	Given vaccine	0	0	4	2	6
	Given no therapy	12	45	8	5	70
Mar. 1, 1936	Given vaccine	0	4	4	7	15
	Given no therapy	20	63	13	8	104
Oct. 1, 1936	Given vaccine	0	5	6	9	20
	Given no therapy	27	84	18	11	140

them showing light pertussis and two of them very light pertussis. In the control group there had been seventy pertussis patients, with twelve of them severe, forty-five typical, eight light, and five very light pertussis. In the vaccine group 100 per cent had been light or very light pertussis, while in the control group only 18 per cent had been light or very light.

In the March, 1936, analysis, with fifteen pertussis patients in the vaccine group, eleven were light or very light and four were typical pertussis. In the control group of 104 pertussis patients there had been twenty severe pertussis, sixty-three typical, thirteen light, and eight very light pertussis. Seventy-four per cent of the vaccine-treated patients were light or very light pertussis while only 20 per cent were light or very light pertussis in the control group.

Another analysis was made in October, 1936. There was no severe pertussis in the vaccine group, only five typical, six light, and nine very light pertussis. In the control group there were twenty-seven severe pertussis patients, eighty-four typical, eighteen light, and eleven very light pertussis. Seventy-five per cent of the patients wtih pertussis in the vaccine group were either light or very light, while only 21 per cent could be classed as light or very light in the control group.

TABLE VIII

INCIDENCE OF PERTUSSIS IN CHILDREN WHO WERE EXPOSED DURING THE FIRST 4-MONTH INTERVAL, 4TH TO 12TH MONTH-, AND 12TH TO 24TH MONTH-INTERVALS OF TIME FOLLOWING VACCINE ADMINISTRATION

INTERVALS OF TIME FOLLOWING VACCINE ADMINISTRATION	PATIENTS EXPOSED DURING EACH TIME INTERVAL	PATIENTS DEVELOPING PERTUSSIS DURING EACH TIME INTERVAL
0 to 4th month	58	10
4th to 12th month	77	9
12 to 24th month	16	1

In the analysis of September, 1937, about 75 per cent of the forty pertussis patients in the vaccine-treated group were light or very light pertussis, while 20 per cent of the 270 pertussis patients in the control group could be so considered.

While it is difficult to determine the severity of pertussis, with our classification the field workers have little uncertainty in placing patients in the right group. Approximately 50 per cent of the vaccine-treated cases were placed in the very light group. That means half of the pertussis in the vaccine-treated group had been called pertussis and yet the patients had never whooped or vomited. Another 25 per cent of the patients with pertussis in the vaccine-treated group have had an occasional whoop, a short duration of illness, and no other constitutional symptoms. In contrast to these, workers have placed only 8 per cent of the control group in the very light group and another 12 per cent in the light group. It would appear that vaccine must protect, at least partially, even those children who do not completely escape the disease.

An attempt has also been made to determine when children develop their immunity after *Bacillus pertussis* inoculations. Considerable work has been done in testing for agglutinins and opsonins during the course of vaccine injections. A relatively high level is reached in most cases after the third injection or very soon after the fourth injection. These circulating antibodies may not mean protection; however, they show a response to injections which is similar to that induced by the disease. The analysis made in October, 1936, in which there were 151 exposures followed by twenty patients with pertussis showed that two patients exposed less than one month after injections were given did not develop pertussis. During the first two months after injections four patients out of thirty-two exposed developed pertussis. During the third and fourth months there were six pertussis patients out of twenty-four exposures. During the fifth and sixth months there were no pertussis patients following twelve exposures. During the period from six months to one year there were nine pertussis patients following sixty-five exposures. During the next year there was one patient with pertussis following sixteen exposures. While nothing definite can be concluded from this study, it would suggest that immunity may develop very shortly after the injections are completed.

COMMENTS

The vaccine used in this study differs somewhat from vaccines described in similar studies. Dr. Sauer refers to the cultures used in his vaccine as ''young'' cultures. He replaces the cultures when they are sixty days old with fresh cultures obtained from a patient with pertussis. The cultures for his vaccine are grown on a medium containing 10 per cent blood. He explains the failure of some of his vaccine in 1934 and 1935 on the fact that two commercial laboratories that made the vaccine did not change cultures every three or four weeks but used the same cultures for many months. He reports that this practice has now been corrected. If a medium containing only 10 per cent blood is used to make subcultures, the organisms will not stay in Phase I. Dr. Kendrick and others have shown that the minimum amount of blood that can be used for subcultures, and permit retention of Phase I characteristics, is a final concentration of 15 per cent. Had these cultures been tested for Phase I characteristics and had the organisms been injected into the skin of a rabbit to test their capacity to produce characteristic necrosis reactions, then I do not believe there would have been failures reported with Sauer's vaccine in 1934 and 1935. Cultures have been kept in Phase I during this study for two years without any changes as far as could be detected. As far as I know all Phase I *Bacillus pertussis* organisms are identical. Although five to seven cultures were used in all lots of the vaccine in this study there is no reason to believe that multiple cultures make a better vaccine than a single culture. Dr. Sauer uses human blood in preparing culture media. Sheep's blood has been entirely satisfactory in this work. Dr. Sauer does not wash his vaccine. He feels that a certain portion of the vaccine is lost in the washing. Dr. Kendrick feels that it is better to lose a little of the antigen quantitatively than it is to have blood and media in the final product. This point of difference is probably not important as far as the efficiency of the vaccine is concerned. There are two or three points of difference between the vaccine used in this study and the vaccine used by Dr. Doull in Cleveland.[11] Dr. Doull used about twice as much blood in preparing his media as was used in this study. He washed his organisms at the end of forty-eight hours in distilled water. In this study it has seemed that the organisms are at their height by the end of seventy-two hours and not forty-eight hours. However, this probably would make no difference in the value of the vaccine. The fact that the cultures were washed in distilled water and not in normal saline solution might make a tremendous difference. It is a known fact that certain antigens or fractions of antigens are soluble in distilled water and not soluble in saline solution. This might or might not be the reason that the Cleveland vaccine failed to produce active immunization. One per cent formalin or 0.5 per cent phenol or 1:10,000 merthiolate have been used as preservatives. Experiments would seem to show that merthiolate is less destructive to the antigen than formalin or phenol. Merthiolate has been the preservative of choice in the Grand Rapids study. One group of workers gave 8 c.c. in three injections. We gave 7 c.c. in four injections. I don't think that this difference in technique makes any difference in the end results, but perhaps it might.

Up to June 1, 1937, Dr. Kendrick had isolated ten cultures which resembled *Bacillus pertussis,* but did not conform to all its characteristics. Over 1,500 cough plates on upper respiratory infections other than pertussis did not give a similar culture. These cultures were isolated from patients severely ill with what appeared to be typical pertussis. While the original cough plates were typical of *Bacillus pertussis* for the first two or three days, the colonies then became large and unlike *Bacillus pertussis* colonies. They grew readily on plain agar and broth. They cannot be told from *Bacillus pertussis* by their morphology or staining reactions. They agglutinated in low dilution with *Bacillus pertussis* agglutinating serum. They agglutinated to a high titer with *Bacillus bronchisepticus* agglutinating serum but they were nonmotile. Dr. Kendrick has called these organisms *B. parapertussis.* I mention that study because these organisms would probably be of no value even though fresh, in producing *Bacillus pertussis* vaccine.

SUMMARY

This study has shown:

1. The use of cough plates by health departments is practical in the diagnosis of pertussis and also in release from pertussis quarantine.
2. Convalescent serum given in sufficient dosage will passively immunize about 70 per cent of the infants and young children exposed to pertussis but not yet showing symptoms.
3. Convalescent serum is of no preventive value after symptoms have developed.
4. Pertussis vaccine may be of value for the immunization of young children exposed to pertussis if given before symptoms develop.
5. Hyperimmune serum may be of value for passive immunization of infants that have been exposed to pertussis if given before symptoms develop.
6. Pertussis vaccine, produced according to the standards described in this paper, will actively immunize about 85 per cent of young children who have not been exposed to pertussis.
7. Fifteen per cent of vaccine-immunized children that later develop the disease will have a milder attack than children who have not received the vaccine.

References

1. Bordet, J., and Gengou, O.: Ann. de l'Inst. **20:** 731, 1906.
2. Council on Pharmacy and Chemistry; Report: J. A. M. A. **96:** 613, 1931.
3. Madsen, P.: J. A. M. A. **101:** 187, 1933.
4. Sauer, L. W.: J. A. M. A. **101:** 1449, 1933.
5. Kendrick, P., and Eldering, G.: Am. J. Pub. Health **24:** 309, 1934.
6. Kendrick, P., and Eldering, G.: Am. J. Pub. Health **25:** 147, 1935.
7. Emerson, Haven: Supplement, Am. J. Pub. Health **27:** 6, 1937.
8. Leslie, P. H., and Gardner, A. D.: J. Hyg. **31:** 423, 1931.
9. Kendrick, P., and Eldering, G.: Am. J. Pub. Health **26:** 1, 1936.
10. Eldering, G., and Kendrick, P.: Am. J. Pub. Health **26:** 5, 1936.
11. Doull, James A., Shibley, Gerald S., and McClelland, Joseph E.: Am. J. Pub. Health **26:** 1097, 1936.

A Controlled Study in Pertussis Immunization

John J. Miller, Jr., M.D.
San Francisco, Calif.

At the Stanford University School of Medicine Children's Clinic a small controlled study in pertussis immunization has been going on since October, 1935. I wish to report our findings to date. A more detailed report will be published later. Since the above-mentioned date we have injected every month a few babies in our well baby clinic and followed a similar number of babies as controls. The great majority of injected, or tested, babies and control babies were 6 to 10 months of age when injected or placed in the control group. A few ranged up to 30 months of age.

The vaccine used was Phase I *Hemophilus pertussis* vaccine, kindly supplied by the Cutter Laboratories, Berkeley. This product is made from strains isolated at the cough plate stations in San Francisco. Freshly isolated strains fulfilling the characteristics of the first Phase of *Hemophilus pertussis* are grown on human blood agar, harvested without washing, and killed with merthiolate and phenol. A total dose of eighty billion cells were used throughout. This was divided at first into six injections and later into only three injections of twenty, thirty, and thirty billions of bacteria. Injections were given intramuscularly at weekly intervals. No child was considered to have entered the test group until the day the last injection was given.

We have seen four systemic reactions to the vaccine with fever lasting twenty-four hours. No local reactions beyond an occasional mild inflammation have been observed.

We have recently reinjected a number of children who were vaccinated more than two years ago. A dose of forty billions has been used. It so happens that none of these children have been exposed since the reinjections. Table I summarizes our findings to date.

TABLE I

	TOTAL NUMBER	BOYS	GIRLS	EXPOSURES			CASES	ESCAPES	COMMUNICABILITY RATE %	CRUDE ATTACK RATE %
				KNOWN	UNKNOWN	TOTAL				
Test	206	112	94	26	1	27	8	19	29.6 ± 8.8	3.9 ± 1.3
Control	181	92	89	19	13	32	29	3	90.6 ± 5.2	16.0 ± 2.7

There have been twenty-seven exposures in the test group, twenty-six known and one unknown. An unknown exposure is one which must have occurred when a child contracts pertussis without known exposure. These twenty-seven exposures were followed by eight cases of pertussis and nineteen escaped infection.

There have been thirty-two exposures in the control group, nineteen known and thirteen unknown. Twenty-nine cases have occurred, and three exposed control infants escaped. The far greater number of unknown exposures in this control group suggests that many more than one unknown exposure actually also occurred in the test group. Such additional exposures, if known, would have tended to lower the communicability rate. The communicability rate, which is simply the ratio of disease to exposure, was 29.6 per cent (8/27) in the test group and 90.6 per cent (29/32) in the control group. The probable errors for these rates have been computed. It is seen that the probable errors are less than one-third of the rates in each case, which indicates that the rates are statistically significant.

The difference between the communicability rates in the two groups is also significant. Nine more escapes occurred in the test group than might have by chance (delta equals 9), and Yule's Q comes out 0.91, which indicates a correlation between vaccination and escape.

The crude attack rates in the two groups also show significant differences.

TABLE II

ANALYSIS OF ESCAPES

	DURATION OF EXPOSURE			INTERVAL AFTER VACCINATION FOR 19 ESCAPES (MONTHS)
	FOR 1 WEEK OR MORE	LESS THAN 1 WEEK, MORE THAN 1 DAY	1 DAY OR LESS	
Test	9	1	9	5 9 13 20 5 12 16 20 6 12 16 20 6 12 18 21 8 18 22
Control	0	0	3	

Table II tabulates those who escaped infection after known exposure. Nine injected children were exposed to pertussis for one week or more and yet escaped the disease. Evidently these nine individuals had a high degree of immunity. It is of interest to note that one-half of those who escaped were children who had had vaccine more than one year previously.

TABLE III

TIME IN WHICH CASES OCCURRED AFTER VACCINATION

	SEVERE	MODERATE	MILD
Test Group		14 mo. 18 mo. 20 mo.	20 days 1 mo. 4 mo. 9 mo. 11 mo.
	0	3 cases	5 cases
Control Group	2	18 cases	9 cases

Table III summarizes the relative severity of the cases which have occurred. The number of cases is probably too small to warrant comment.

It happened that the five patients with mild cases had had their vaccine within a year. Two of the mild cases tested (1 month and 9 months) are somewhat questionable, as positive cough plates were never obtained. One of these children coughed only seven days.

Our conclusions are:

1. This vaccine is a potent antigen. It seems to confer complete protection on some children and partial protection on many of the others. If we had used a larger dose the degree of protection might have been increased.

2. Until a simple test for immunity has been developed, proper dosage can only be determined by clinical trial. Undoubtedly there is marked individual variation in the dose required. Undoubtedly there exist some individuals who will fail to be protected by even massive doses.

Our observation of the two moderately severe cases of pertussis in children vaccinated more than one year previously suggests to us the advisability of reinjection at yearly intervals, for which we employ a dose one-half of the original. To date, however, we have only reinjected children after an interval of two years or more.

A Controlled Study of Pertussis Prophylaxis

Comparison of Phase I Hemophilus Pertussis Vaccine With Undenatured Bacterial Antigen

Charlotte H. Singer-Brooks, M.D.
San Francisco, Calif.

In March, 1935, an investigation of pertussis prophylaxis was undertaken by a member of the Pediatric Staff of the University of California Outpatient Department.*

Purpose.—The purpose of this investigation was critically to evaluate pertussis prophylaxis by careful control of a small series and by conducting an intimate follow-up, the nature of which would not be permitted by a large group. We wished to determine: (1) Whether the injection of pertussis antigen would protect against the disease in children who were exposed; (2) whether the course of pertussis was altered favorably in children who were not completely protected; and (3) if protection were conferred, the duration of this protection, if possible.

Plan and Method of Study.—1. Children included in this study were those referred from the well baby and general pediatrics clinics of the University of California Outpatient Department, who did not have a history of a previous attack of whooping cough or known direct exposure to whooping cough.

2. Immunizing injections were to be given to children who were more than 5 months of age.

3. Sibling controls were to be used rather than alternate cases in order to provide the best clinical test of protection conferred by the immunizing injections.

4. An educational program was organized to enlist the cooperation of parents for follow-up visits over a period of years. No charge was made either for the prophylactic injections or the subsequent follow-up visits.

5. Definite appointments for follow-up visits were given at regular intervals of three to four months. Upper respiratory infections developing between the appointments were checked by clinic visits to rule out atypical whooping cough. Known exposures occurring between visits were requested to be reported immediately. A careful history of the character (distance between contact and child, in or out of doors, and duration) of each exposure was taken. In addition, the contact patient was visited for the purpose of taking cough plates and thus determining whether the contact was in the communicable phase of the disease.

As our study progressed, we found that we were unable to attain the ideal of sibling controls for all of the treated children. A number of the children referred to us were either an only child or the only sibling of the family who did not have a previous attack of pertussis. We expected to follow our groups for a period of five years. The possibility that chance exposure might not occur before additional members were added to the family group seemed to justify our giving the only child member of the family prophylactic injections, and using the subsequent members as sibling controls. We have also used as controls children whose parents objected to prophylactic measures.

Criteria for Exposure.—1. In the group where siblings were available, exposure comprises contact with the child suffering with pertussis (proved bacteriologically).

2. For children where siblings were not available, exposure comprises:

a. Known close contact (at play, parties, meals, etc., during which time frequent coughing occurred) with a child who has whooping cough, and who has been proved by cough plates to be in the communicable phase of the disease.

From the Department of Pediatrics of the University of California Medical School and The Hooper Foundation for Medical Research.

This study was made possible by a grant from the Christine Breon Fund.

*Acknowledgment is hereby made to John J. Miller, Jr., who organized the early part of the investigation.

b. If the exposure is reported to have taken place outside of San Francisco, over week ends or other visits, cough plate follow-up on the contact is not possible. When this occurs our criteria for direct exposure are based upon the history of typical whooping cough developing in the susceptible contact patient who was exposed at the same time, in the same manner, and for the same duration of time as the child reported in our group.

c. The development of clinical pertussis (proved bacteriologically) without a history of known exposure to pertussis.

By application of these criteria, we were able to determine whether direct exposure occurred and to eliminate the instances of indirect and improbable exposure. Inasmuch as pertussis cases are seldom isolated, daily contact with children in the communicable phase of the disease occurs with considerable frequency. While, perhaps, this is not equal to exposure by sibling, nevertheless, it serves as a good control for the injected children who do not have sibling controls and who were exposed in this manner. These criteria for exposure to pertussis are severe tests, and it is possible that more exposures occurred than are reported.

During a period of three years observations were made upon ninety-five children injected with undenatured bacterial antigen,* 272 children injected with Phase I, H. pertussis vaccine,† and 256 noninjected children who served as controls for the treated groups.

Undenatured bacterial antigen was used as a prophylactic agent between March, 1935, and December 31, 1935. During this nine-month period ninety-five children were given injections of this antigen. Each of ninety-five children received a total dose of 10 c.c. The total dose was divided and given at three visits, at weekly intervals. Part was given subcutaneously and part intracutaneously. Seventy seven of these children were controlled with siblings, and eighteen did not have sibling controls.

Phase I, H. pertussis vaccine was used as a prophylactic agent from September, 1935, to the present time. During this period 272 children were injected with this antigen. Except for ten who did not return after the first injection (dose ten billion), all of the 272 children received a total dose of eighty billion Phase I, H. pertussis organisms. One hundred and sixty-two of these children were controlled with siblings, and 110 did not have sibling controls.

The control group has been under observation since March, 1935. This group comprises 256 nonimmunized children who serve as controls for both injected groups. Two hundred and seven of these children are siblings,‡ and forty-nine are not siblings.

When siblings are used as controls, rather than alternate patients, it is not possible to have the same number in each age group represented. In our series 65 per cent

*Supplied by Eli Lilly and Company. Undenatured bacterial antigen is the protein filtrate obtained after mechanical disruption in a ball mill of a suspension of the living Phase I, H. pertussis cells. Merthiolate 1:100,000 is added to the filtrate as a preservative.

†Supplied by the Cutter Laboratories. Phase I, H. pertussis vaccine is prepared from four to six recently isolated local strains supplied by the author and others. Each culture is tested, not only for hemolysis, but also for toxicity and specific agglutinability. Only those cultures which conform to the Phase I grouping of Leslie and Gardner are used. The cultures are grown on Bordet-Gengou human blood media. The vaccine is an unwashed suspension of Phase I organisms, killed with 1:20,000 dilution of merthiolate and diluted with 0.5 per cent phenol saline solution. Two concentrations of vaccine were used in this study, standardized to contain (1) ten billion organisms per cubic centimeter and (2) twenty billion organisms per cubic centimeter.

‡In a number of instances these siblings serve as controls for both vaccine and undenatured bacterial antigen. Between September and December, 1935 (a four-month period during which both antigens were used), in families of three or more children, one child was injected with antigen, one with pertussis vaccine, and the third or remaining children served as controls for both injected children.

of the children injected with undenatured bacterial antigen, 87 per cent of the children injected with pertussis vaccine, and only 44 per cent of the control children were less than 3 years of age. Thus it would seem that the possibility of exposure was greatest in the control series, since a large number of these children were in the preschool and school age group. But the fact that older children may be less susceptible should also be considered, and this factor may have favored our control group. A high percentage of the injected children were in the more susceptible age groups, and consequently the possibility of developing pertussis after exposure was greater in these children than in the control group.

For comparison of the findings in the three groups the results of each are summarized in Table I.

TABLE I

SUMMARY OF RESULTS OVER A THREE-YEAR PERIOD OF OBSERVATION OF PERTUSSIS PROPHYLAXIS

Three groups of children were observed: (1) Children injected with undenatured bacterial antigen, (2) Children injected with Phase I, H. pertussis vaccine, and (3) Noninjected control children.

GROUP	TOTAL NUMBER	EXPOSURES	CASES	RATE OF* COMMUNICABILITY	ESCAPES	RATE OF* PROTECTION	RATE OF* ATTACK	ESTIMATE OF CLINICAL COURSE (CASES)	
1. Undenatured bacterial antigen	95	34	28†	82.3%	6	17.6%	29.4%	Severe	6
								Moderately severe	11
								Moderate	8
								Mild	3
2. Phase I H. pertussis vaccine	272	42	7‡	16.6%	35	83.4%	2.5%	Severe	0
								Moderately severe	1
								Moderate	4
								Mild	2
3. Control	256	71	62†	87.2%	9	12.6%	24.2%	Severe	10
								Moderately severe	22
								Moderate	24
								Mild	6

*Rate of: Communicability refers to the percentage of exposed children who developed pertussis.

Protection refers to the percentage of exposed children who escaped.

Attack refers to the percentage of the total number (both exposed and nonexposed) who developed pertussis.

†One child had two attacks.

‡Two of these children received only one injection (dose, ten billion organisms).

The following observations of the seven cases of pertussis, which developed in the injected children of the Phase I vaccine group, are of interest:

1. Four months after a total dose of eighty billion organisms one of the patients developed a nonparoxysmal cough of three days' duration, and it may be assumed that he had an abortive attack of pertussis, even though clinical and bacterial diagnosis were lacking. A week after this ''mild cold'' cleared up, the 5-week-old sister, who had no other possible source of exposure to pertussis, developed a cough, and positive cough plates were obtained. The infant had a severe attack of pertussis, and, although the older brother was in daily contact with his sister throughout the entire course of the disease, he developed no further symptoms.

2. One of the seven patients was subjected to two intimate exposures. The first exposure occurred four months after vaccine injection (dose, eighty billion). At this time the patient was intimately exposed (daily for a ten-day period) to a foster child who was in the coryzal and early paroxysmal stage of whooping cough. No symptoms developed. Two years later (two years and 4 months after vaccine injection) this patient was again intimately exposed in another foster home, and after this exposure he developed a moderate attack of pertussis (proved bacteriologically).

3. One of the seven patients subjected to familial exposure, six months after injection of pertussis vaccine (dose, eighty billion), developed a moderate attack of pertussis.

4. Another of the patients, an only child, was exposed outside of the family twenty-seven months after injection of pertussis vaccine (dose, eighty billion), and this child developed a moderately severe attack.

5. The fifth patient, after being subjected to repeated nonfamilial exposure, developed a mild attack of pertussis about two and one-half months after injection. Paroxysmal coughing lasted two weeks; there was no whoop or vomiting.

6. Two of the patients received a total dose of only ten billion organisms. Approximately eighteen months after each injection of vaccine, each of these children developed typical whooping cough. The attacks were moderate.

In comparing the findings in each of the groups (Table I), it will be noted that there is a difference of only 4.9 per cent between the communicability rate of the group injected with undenatured bacterial antigen and the control group. On the other hand, a comparison of the group injected with pertussis vaccine and the

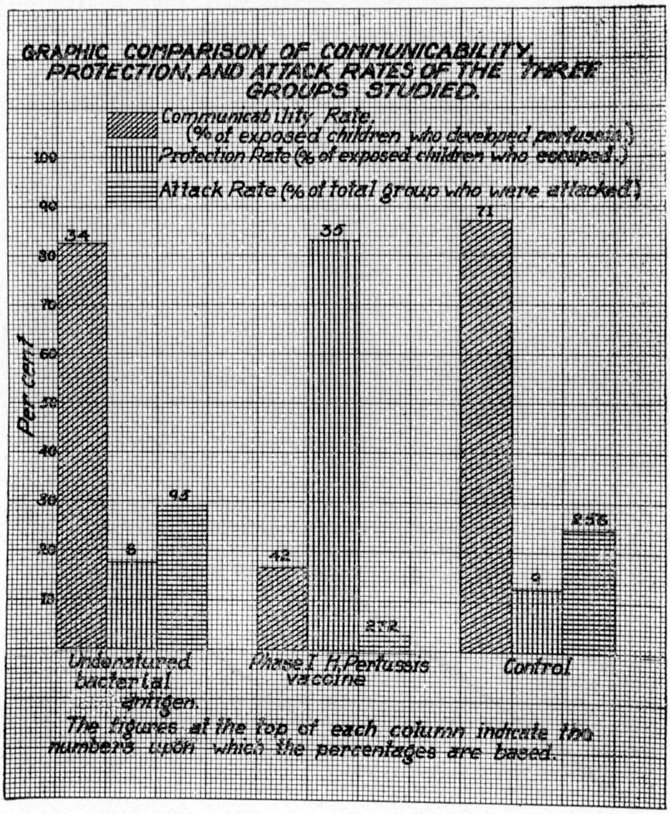

control group shows a difference of 70.6 per cent in the communicability rate. Noteworthy difference is also observed in connection with the attack rate. In the case of the undenatured bacterial antigen group and the control group, there is a difference of 5.2 per cent. But between the pertussis vaccine group and the control group there is again the more striking difference of 21.7 per cent. These differences are shown graphically in Fig. 1.

In the short period of time that our groups have been under observation, we have encountered two children who had second attacks occurring approximately one year apart. During the observation of the ninety-seven cases of pertussis which occurred in the children of the three groups studied, we have encountered, in addition, six cases in adults (parents) who had histories of having had whooping cough during childhood. These six attacks were mild (paroxysmal coughs for short duration without whoops) and undoubtedly would have escaped notice if cough plates had not been taken.

Conclusion.—In a controlled study of pertussis prophylaxis the demonstrable immunity conferred by injection of undenatured bacterial antigen was found to be negligible. In our Phase I, H. pertussis vaccine series 83.4 per cent of the children who were directly exposed to living H. pertussis organisms did not develop the disease. It would seem that immunity to pertussis is not absolute, but relative, and that it may be influenced, not only by lapse of time, but also by intensity and frequency of exposure to infective dosage.

DISCUSSION

DR. J. W. ROSENFELD (PORTLAND, ORE.).—I understand that recurrent paroxysmal pertussis coughs do not produce positive cough plates. I would like to learn the experience of this group on that question. How easy is it to obtain a positive cough plate in pertussis cases? How long should quarantine be continued?

CHAIRMAN FABER.—There are reports in the literature of positive cough plates in second attacks of pertussis.

DR. MILLER.—I have seen positive plates in six cases.

DR. SCHERMERHORN.—Three cases.

DR. E. E. MARTMER (DETROIT).—I have seen twenty-five positive cases in adults with a history of previous attacks during childhood.

DR. V. E. STORK (LOS ANGELES).—How long after onset is whooping cough communicable?

DR. SCHERMERHORN.—Seventy-five per cent of the cases will give positive cough plates the first week, seventy per cent the second week, 60 per cent the third week, 30 per cent the fourth week, 15 per cent the fifth week, and about 1 per cent the sixth week. The period of isolation varies considerably in different cities. I feel that pertussis cases should not be released from quarantine for six weeks.

DR. LEE COHN (SAN FRANCISCO).—What is meant by quarantine? Who foots the expense of this study? Is it practical? How useful is the cough plate?

DR. SCHERMERHORN.—In Grand Rapids the premises of whooping cough cases are placarded. The study has cost between $50,000 and $100,000 with the help of P. W. A. workers. A similar study should be made in another community. This study was financed by the Public Health Department, the P. W. A., the city, and by private individuals.

DR. ROSENFELD.—Is the paroxysmal cough of a later upper respiratory infec-fection infectious with pertussis organisms?

DR. MILLER.—We have found one or two convalescent carriers.

DR. SCHERMERHORN.—The use of the cough plate is advantageous for releasing from quarantine. I have seen positive cases lasting eight to ten weeks without a cough.

DR. MILLER.—Later whooping subsequent to pertussis cases is of frequent occurrence but is probably usually not due to pertussis but occasionally one may be.

DR. D. C. SHELBY (LOS ANGELES).—What is the technique for making a test cough plate? How do you make the child cough?

DR. SINGER-BROOKS.—A cough can sometimes be excited by placing a cotton applicator in the ear, or by making pressure with the finger in the suprasternal notch, or by getting the child to breathe deeply. One does not need much of a cough. Hold the plate about six inches from the mouth.

DR. MILLER.—It is a good idea to wash out the mouth first with cold water. To excite a cough a lighted cigarette held in front of the child's face is helpful.

DR. SHELBY.—Is there less danger of contracting pertussis out of doors than indoors?

CHAIRMAN FABER.—It is generally agree that indoor exposures are more severe. In institutions the exposures are likely to be prolonged and severe, as they are also in a house with family contacts.

DR. C. B. HILLS (BERKELEY, CALIF.).—What about the time for immunization and the question of repeating?

DR. W. L. CRAWFORD (ROCKFORD, ILL.).—What dosages?

DR. SHELBY.—What is the age limit for the use of the prophylactic vaccine?

DR. L. M. EARLE (LOS ANGELES).—To what age do you plan to continue the practice of yearly injections?

DR. SCHERMERHORN.—Immunize at 6 months of age. Dosages vary. We use five single injections, 1 c.c. plus, to 8 c.c. We repeat a small revaccination in two or three years. There is no reaction. The vaccination is usually given to children less than 5 years old, but it could be given later.

DR. MILLER.—We reinject every year but do not know just what amount should be used. We have not decided how long these yearly reinjections will be continued, but probably through elementary school. There is no vaccine which protects for many years.

DR. SINGER-BROOKS.—We have given no reinjections but believe that the protection does not last much longer than eighteen months.

DR. E. R. MURPHY (SALT LAKE CITY).—Is there any serious objection to injecting the newborn infant? I have, with infants whose mothers had pertussis.

DR. J. M. FRAWLEY (FRESNO, CALIF.).—There is danger of fatality in the newborn infant. Madsen has reported two cases.

CHAIRMAN FABER.—There were other explanations for those cases. They were cases of one physician, more than a year apart. However, Madsen now advises against it. He waits two or three months.

DR. CRAWFORD.—Dr. Sauer has immunized at two to three weeks. He believed the effects were temporary and repeated the injections at one year. I used 8 c.c. of Sauer's vaccine previous to 1935, and had no failures. I then had three failures at one time. Since then I have been using 10 c.c. and seem to be getting better protection. I give 1.5 c.c. in each arm, 1.75 c.c. in each arm, and 1.75 c.c. in each arm. Because of Sauer's experience, I am reluctant to give the injections at six months. However, the proper time seems uncertain.

DR. MARTMER.—Why inject the vaccine intramuscularly instead of subcutaneously?

DR. MILLER.—Local reactions are less likely to occur.

DR. JOHN MEAD (BAKERSFIELD, CALIF.).—Do you ever get local reactions severe enough to discontinue further injections?

DR. SCHERMERHORN.—We give 3 c.c. or thirty billion bacteria and never have had severe reactions. I think one is more likely to get severe reactions with the Sauer vaccine.

DR. MEAD.—Is there any advantage in using concentrated vaccine?

DR. SINGER-BROOKS.—We are using concentrated vaccine and get no severe reactions, but we often give divided doses of aspirin, giving one grain for each year of the child's age.

DR. MEAD.—Is the concentrated vaccine as potent?

DR. SCHERMERHORN.—Yes, entirely.

CHAIRMAN FABER.—Because the concentrated vaccine requires half the number of injections, there is less psychic trauma, and in my experience it causes no greater reactions.

DR. MORTON (SANTA ANA, CALIF.).—My results with Eastern vaccine were not as good as were those with the Cutter vaccine. Is the distance an element? I have been having better results with concentrated vaccine the past year.

DR. MILLER.—We haven't evaluated the results with vaccine of ten billion and twenty billion content. There should not be any difference between local and imported vaccine effects.

DR. SCHERMERHORN.—Sauer is now getting his cultures from Chicago. There should be no difference in what locality cultures are made. I do not see what difference dilution should make in the effects.

CHAIRMAN FABER.—Dr. Morton's experience probably was with the 1934-35 Sauer vaccine. The trouble of that time has been corrected.

DR. G. RICHARDA WILLIAMSON (NEW ORLEANS).—When is immunity established?

CHAIRMAN FABER.—Sauer says that the immunity is at maximum after four months. Dr. Schermerhorn's study indicates an earlier immunity.

DR. H. E. LONG (BERKELEY, CALIF.).—If there is a break in the weekly injections of the prophylactic vaccine so that the series is incomplete, how does one proceed?

CHAIRMAN FABER.—I am not convinced that one week is the optimum interval. It may be two weeks. I should go ahead with the series if the break is not more than two weeks.

DR. SCHERMERHORN.—It makes little difference how the injections are spaced so long as the total quantity is given. The effect depends upon the number of organisms injected.

CHAIRMAN FABER.—It might even be better to wait a month and then give another injection.

DR. MEAD.—Should older children have more?

DR. SCHERMERHORN.—They probably require more. It will often take from 7 to 25 c.c. to work the agglutination titer up to 25,000.

DR. MILLER.—It seems reasonable to give older children twenty billion bacteria or more to be safe. When we get a really good test for protection, that should be used.

CHAIRMAN FABER.—I think Dr. Sauer advocates larger doses for older children, 12 c.c. (120 billion bacteria).

DR. SHELBY.—Do you keep the vaccine in the icebox or at room temperature for a time before giving it?

DR. SCHERMERHORN.—The importance of refrigeration is more to prevent growth than to preserve the antigen. The antigen is very stable; it can be boiled.

CHAIRMAN FABER.—I would emphasize the great danger of keeping any vaccine at room temperature for any length of time.

DR. SCHERMERHORN.—It is interesting to note that sometimes immunity can be built up rapidly after injection. In some cases apparently the vaccine can be given effectively after exposure.

DR. R. P. SEITZ (SAN FRANCISCO).—If immunity is developed rapidly, how early in the first year can the vaccine be given?

DR. SINGER-BROOKS.—The very young infant has an immature mechanism for developing immunity. Dr. Sauer gave the vaccine very early but observed a higher incidence of infection.

DR. SEITZ.—In that respect then it is comparable to smallpox vaccination.

DR. STORK.—What is the optimum age to attempt immunization?

DR. SINGER-BROOKS.—After five months.

CHAIRMAN FABER.—Dr. Schermerhorn, what do you consider the optimum age?

DR. SCHERMERHORN.—My personal feeling is that the injections should be given between the sixth and eighth months, about the sixth month.

DR. E. H. CHRISTOPHERSON (SAN DIEGO, CALIF.).—In the report of the Committee on Immunization Procedures of the Academy it is stated that immunization may be started any time after the child is 3 months old. What is the basis for this statement?

DR. G. J. LEVY (MEMPHIS, TENN.).—I asked Dr. Sauer if the fourth month was a satisfactory age for immunization, and he said it was.

DR. SCHERMERHORN.—I would say that if the injections are given as early as that, they should be repeated early in the second year.

DR. CHRISTOPHERSON.—Will you please state the technique to be used when a child has been already exposed?

DR. SCHERMERHORN.—Give 1 c.c. the first day and 1.5 c.c. every other day, up to a total of 8 c.c.

DR. CHRISTOPHERSON.—Has not the tone of opinion regarding the effectiveness of prophylactic vaccination changed in the last two years?

CHAIRMAN FABER.—Decidedly, in favor of the vaccine. Recent favorable reports and others soon to appear are in sharp contrast to some which appeared previously. One will run into some failures, but it now appears that we will protect 80 per cent to 90 per cent and that failures will have mild attacks as a rule. As a matter of fact these results are nearly as good as are those with diphtheria.

DR. SCHERMERHORN.—We feel that the results will depend largely on how careful the laboratories are in keeping the organisms in Phase I.

CHAIRMAN FABER.—There is a sharp contrast between the Cleveland reports and the reports heard today. Today's reports seem convincing. The Cleveland report did not indicate the communicability.

DR. SCHERMERHORN.—An explanation for the failure at Cleveland was that the vaccine was washed in distilled water instead of saline solutions. We feel that some soluble antigen may be lost in the distilled water.

DR. MILLER.—Recently we washed one lot in distilled water, one in saline, and one was unwashed. Mouse protection tests are being carried out, but they are not yet completed. Both distilled water and saline washings contain precipitable proteins which contain the antigen. This fails to explain the great discrepancy between the Cleveland and the Grand Rapids results. We do not wash our antigens at all. The Cleveland results are unexplained.

DR. S. H. ASHMUN (DAYTON, OHIO).—How is one to make certain of obtaining a dependable supply of vaccine? The Cleveland requirements for exposure were very severe. I do not believe that their report is seriously discouraging. Are intracutaneous injections of value?

DR. SCHERMERHORN.—Reports in the literature do not show much advantage.

DR. MILLER.—In Blatt's recent report intracutaneous injections were given. The doses must be smaller.

DR. ASHMUN.—I mean injecting the first drop into the skin.

DR. MILLER.—That is an unnecessary refinement.

CHAIRMAN FABER.—In summing up I feel that we can express a definitely favorable opinion, with the limitations which have been stated, as to the efficacy of this prophylactic procedure.

Secretaries.

ORVILLE BARBOUR, M.D., *Peoria, Ill.*

VICTOR STORK, M.D., *Los Angeles, Calif.*

Academy News

Region III of the American Academy of Pediatrics will hold its eighth annual meeting Oct. 27, 28, and 29, 1938, at the Hotel Statler, Detroit Mich.

The scientific program will be given at morning and afternoon sessions on Thursday, October 27, Friday, October 28, and Saturday morning only, October 29. The program has been arranged so that discussions will be held at the end of each session. At this time it is hoped the members will enter into a free discussion of the various papers.

The session on Thursday morning will be devoted to the newborn period. The session on Saturday morning will be presented by members of the staff of the University of Michigan, from Ann Arbor. Drs. W. C. C. Cole, David J. Levy, Joseph A. Johnston, Thomas B. Cooley, and D. Murray Cowie will be chairmen of the sessions.

There will be a reception followed by dinner on Thursday evening. The members of the Detroit Pediatric Society will be hosts. Wives of members and guests are especially invited.

There will be a meeting of state chairmen at luncheon on Friday in the Judge Woodward Room, Hotel Statler.

Transportation has been arranged for members to attend the Illinois-Michigan football game at Ann Arbor on Saturday, October 29. Tickets for the game must be arranged for not later than 12:00 noon on Thursday, October 27.

News and Notes

The following men have been certified by the **American Board of Pediatrics** since the last report.

Edward Campion, M.D., San Francisco, Calif.
Paul F. Dwan, M.D., Minneapolis, Minn.
Louis Fischer, M.D., New York, N. Y.
George Sherman Frauenberger, M.D., Denver, Colo.
Samuel George Henricke, M.D., Portland, Ore.
Albert Lyon Hill, M.D., Los Angeles, Calif.
Clarence Ballard Hills, M.D., Berkeley, Calif.
Harry R. Lusignan, M.D., Monterey, Calif.
John Johnston Miller, Jr., M.D., San Francisco, Calif.
Harry A. Towsley, M.D., Ann Arbor, Mich.

Dr. Samuel Jennings Roberts, Miami, Fla., has been elected to Fellowship in the Academy.

Book Review

Tuberculosis Among Children and Young Adults. By J. ARTHUR MYERS, M.D., Chief of Medical Staff and Director of Tuberculosis Activities, Lymanhurst Health Center, and Professor of Preventive Medicine, University of Minnesota. Ed. 2. Springfield, 1938, Charles C. Thomas, Publisher, price $4.50.

Those who have followed the writings and teachings of Dr. Myers will recognize in this volume of some 390 pages a final summing up and condensation of the newer concepts of tuberculosis which have been put forth by the Lymanhurst group during the last fifteen years. So rapid has been the increase in tuberculosis knowledge during that period that this edition is a marked revision over the first edition published eight years ago. Longitudinal study of thousands of children, of students of medicine, of nurses, and of college students has given the author first-hand information which has made him one of the world's outstanding authorities on tuberculosis.

The book is divided into three parts: the first deals with tuberculosis in infancy, the second with tuberculosis in childhood, and the third with tuberculosis in young adults, with several additional chapters in which latency, family nature of tuberculosis, and tuberculosis among aged people are discussed. Each chapter is summarized and is followed by a generous list of references which obviously facilitates greatly the task of anyone desiring further information upon a particular point. The work is well illustrated with charts, x-ray plates, and pictorial diagrams.

Controversial questions, such as the relation of allergy to immunity, the relations of first infections to the later development of reinfections, regional tuberculosis, and the like, are all thoroughly discussed. The reviewer was particularly interested in Dr. Myers' viewpoint regarding the reason why the reinfection type of chronic pulmonary tuberculosis does not make its appearance until puberty.

The volume is easy to read, logical, and should be of great value to anyone interested in tuberculosis work.

Erratum

Dr. Minnola Stallings wishes to correct a statement in the round table discussion on whooping cough, which appeared in the April, 1938, issue of the Journal. On page 542 the paragraph beginning with line 17 should read as follows:

"The only manufacturers producing the Sauer pertussis vaccine strictly according to the specifications of Dr. L. Sauer and supervised and marketed under a permit granted by Northwestern University Medical School are Parke, Davis and Company and Eli Lilly and Company."

The Journal of Pediatrics

Vol. 13 | September, 1938 | No. 3

Original Communications

THE RECOGNITION OF COARCTATION OF THE AORTA (ADULT TYPE) DURING CHILDHOOD

George Eisenberg, M.D.
Chicago, Ill.

THE diagnosis of coarctation of the aorta at any age during life used to be considered quite a feat until King,[1] Blackford[2] and Abbott[3] gave impetus to its clinical recognition. The diagnosis of the condition in childhood, however, is still a rare occurrence. For instance, Blackford,[2] in 1928, wrote that about seventy-eight cases were recognized clinically up to that time, of which four were in children. The youngest of these four was 5 years of age. Between 1928 and the present time there are in the literature[4-25] about forty more authentic cases recognized in adults from the ages of 17 to 66 years. Two of these cases were reported by Walker,[26] dealing with occurrence of coarctation of the aorta in a father aged 49 years, and son, 18 years old. On the other hand, during this same period the number of coarctations recognized in children was only eleven. These children ranged from the ages of 5 to 14 years. It is clear, therefore, that the findings of coarctation of the aorta in children are yet not widely understood.

The usual picture of coarctation presented in the literature concerns adults, and stress is laid on observation for pulsating vessels of the chest wall and x-ray evidence of erosions of the ribs. These striking findings are likely to be absent in the child; they develop only over a period of many years. To depend upon such evidence will mean the oversight of instances of coarctation which might have been discovered early in childhood.

GENERAL REVIEW OF THE LITERATURE

As early as 1907, Carpenter[27] gave a good account of how coarctation of the aorta might be diagnosed. The condition was first described anatomically by Morgagni in 1760. It is a constriction of a varying degree of the aorta at or just distal to the insertion of the ductus

From the cardiac service of Children's Memorial Hospital, and the pediatric cardiac clinic of St. Luke's Hospital, Chicago.

arteriosus. The ductus arteriosus may be patent or obliterated without influencing the condition. The heart's structure in the so-called adult type of coarctation is normal except for the presence of a bicuspid aortic valve in 25 per cent of the cases, according to Abbott.[3] The adult type is compatible with long life as contrasted to infantile coarctation. Infantile coarctation is the occurrence of extensive and marked narrowing of the aortic arch, with congenital anomalies of the heart making the condition incompatible with life. In 1898 Reynaud considered the constriction to be due to developmental defects of the left fourth and fifth aortic arches. Because of the constriction, collateral circulation occurs which must apparently be already well established when the child is born. Collateral circulation takes place between the left subclavian and innominate arteries and the internal mammary, intercostal and dorsal scapular arteries. The internal mammary connects with the deep epigastric artery and with the aorta. Lewis[28] stressed the interesting facts that despite the resulting hypertension, cardiac hypertrophy is unusual and there is no increased arteriosclerosis demonstrable in the arteries of the upper extremities. He also pointed out how commonly one could feel or see, in adults, the enlarged collateral vessels of the chest wall.

Woltman[29] is credited by Blackford[2] as having first used the absence of femoral pulsations as an aid in diagnosis.

Meckel, according to Fray,[4] is said to have first described the groove-like erosions of the ribs from the enlarging intercostal arteries. This finding can be demonstrated in practically every adult by x-ray evidence. Lombardi reported[30] and I, likewise, report erosion of the ribs in a 5-year-old child, which is the earliest so far in the literature. Fray[4] and others, too, described the x-ray picture of the heart, pointing out the absence of the aortic knob in a postanterior view and the presence of a defect in the aortic arch in the left oblique view. Abbott,[3] in her classic article on coarctation of the aorta, presents a most detailed account of symptoms and physical findings as well as statistics on 200 autopsied patients. Some of the things she pointed out were these: 74 per cent died before they were 40 years old; 60 of the 200 died of congestive heart failure, 38 of rupture of the aorta, 26 of cerebral accidents due to leakage or rupture of an aneurysm of the circle of Willis; and 14 of subacute bacterial endocarditis. The remainder died of miscellaneous causes, two of heart rupture. Lewis[28] warned that individuals with coarctation might come to a physician first because of symptoms of early cardiac failure.

A REVIEW OF CASES REPORTED IN CHILDREN SINCE 1928

I believe I have here every report of coarctation of the aorta recognized in children during life since Blackford's[2] study; and since that time no one has reported more than a single instance of coarctation.

Poynton and Sheldon[31] wrote of an 8-year-old child with the condition, who succumbed from an ulcerative aortitis. The diagnosis was verified by autopsy. Thomson and Lamb[32] reported the occurrence of the condition in a 5-year-old child who died suddenly. Autopsy was not permitted of the head, which probably would have revealed the cause of death, since none was found in the organs of the chest and abdomen. Hampson[33] recognized the condition in a boy 12 years old. Wolffe[34] reported an instance discovered in a 7-year-old child, whose case he followed for ten years. At 17 years the youth was well and without symptoms. As a child this boy also had rheumatic fever. Montcrieff[35] reported a boy 6 years of age in whom coarctation was recognized. At the time the report was in print, the child was suspected also of having subacute bacterial endocarditis. Lichtenberg[36] gave details of a 12-year-old girl from our clinic who survived after a very severe cerebral accident followed by hemiplegia. Even now at the age of 19 years she is well and has been working as a nursemaid. She has recovered completely from the hemiplegia.

Vega Diaz et al.[37] reported the occurrence of the condition in a 13-year-old child who apparently was well and without symptoms. Purks[18] reported coarctation in a 14-year-old negro boy who was apparently well and without symptoms. Ferris[19] reported a cerebral death from coarctation diagnosed in a child aged 11 years. The period of observation was just a few weeks. Lian et al.[20] reported a 13-year-old child with apparently no trouble from the condition. Lombardi[30] recognized one case of coarctation in a 5-year-old child.

CASE REPORTS OF COARCTATION OF THE AORTA RECOGNIZED IN CHILDREN, AGED 2½, 3, AND 9 YEARS

CASE 1.—M. H., a girl born April 21, 1935, came to us September, 1937, at the age of 2 years and 5 months because of a severe upper respiratory infection and was admitted to the hospital. She had been seen occasionally in our clinics from the age of 5 months for such conditions as impetigo and mild colds, yet nothing abnormal about the heart was recorded.

Examination revealed a well-nourished girl with no disproportionment in development of lower and upper parts of the body. Her heart was normal in size. A rather loud, somewhat harsh murmur was best heard over the base of the heart at the second left interspace. The murmur was easily heard in the left axillary region and over the left back area. The feet felt distinctly colder than the hands. The femoral pulsations were not palpable. Blood pressure reading in the right arm was 124/86; in the left arm, 128/100. No pressure readings were obtainable in the legs.

An x-ray film failed to reveal erosions of the ribs. The electrocardiogram revealed a marked left axis deviation with a diphasic QRS in Lead II.

CASE 2.—G. H., a boy born June 13, 1934, came to us June, 1937, at the age of 3 years. He was diagnosed as having a congenital heart abnormality from the age of 8 months. There was no history of cyanosis, and the boy had no physical complaints, He was normally active.

Examination revealed a well-nourished and well-developed boy. His heart was not enlarged. A murmur was best heard at the apex, rather loud, but not widely transmitted. It was easily heard over the back, especially near the left scapular region. Pulsations in the groin and blood pressure readings in the legs were not obtainable. The blood pressure reading in the right arm was 140/70; in the left arm, 145/105.

An x-ray picture taken in June, 1937, showed a heart of about normal size, somewhat flask-shaped. There was no erosion of the ribs. The electrocardiogram showed a diphasic QRS complex in Leads I and III. There was no evident heart preponderance.

CASE 3.—R. M., born July 18, 1928, came to us first in March, 1933, at the age of 4½ years for a general examination. At this time, he apparently had no symptoms. About April, 1937, at the age of 9, he began to complain of marked pain in his legs after walking short distances and occasionally of pain beneath the ribs on his left side. Although he was seen every three months in the cardiac clinic, coarctation of the aorta was overlooked for about five years.

Examination revealed a robust looking boy of high color. The heart was not enlarged. There was an apical heart murmur described as soft but suggestive of rheumatic origin. Extrasystoles were present from time to time. Femoral pulsations were absent. The blood pressure reading in the right arm was 140/80; in the left arm, 154/100. No readings were obtainable in the legs.

An x-ray film taken when the patient was 5 years old showed early erosions of the lower margins of several ribs, but no one recognized the nature of the findings in the plate until he was properly diagnosed. At the age of 9 years these erosions were far more evident. The heart was normal in size in both plates.

The electrocardiogram showed left heart preponderance and ventricular extrasystoles.

COMMENT

I do not believe it can be overemphasized that the diagnosis of coarctation of the aorta was made correctly in the aforementioned children because the possibility was kept in mind. Before these cases were found, only one had been discovered in our clinics in the past ten years. The far more common reports of the condition in adults would indicate that it was being overlooked in childhood.

One should become aware of the fact that in children, with few exceptions, no symptoms are created by the adult type of coarctation. But when symptoms are present, they may be distinctive, as in Case 3. Intermittent claudication should suggest the possibility of coarctation.

The general physical examination will practically never disclose anything unusual. Each of these three children looks normal externally. In retrospect it is easy to attach significance to the heightened color of R. M.'s (Case 3) face and the definite colder feel of M. H.'s (Case 1) legs as compared to her arms. The pulsating, tortuous vessels seen on the chest walls of adults with coarctation take years to develop.

Heart enlargement will not be present because of coarctation. There must be some other cause to account for any dilatation or hypertrophy which is present. And I do not believe that the heart murmur one hears in a child with coarctation may be described as typical. Perhaps the most characteristic thing is that the murmur is heard in the back over the left scapular region, although this was not true in Case 3. By different examiners, the murmur in Case 1 was labeled functional and congenital. By every examiner the murmur in Case 3 was labeled as possibly rheumatic in origin. In all three cases the notes about the murmurs indicated that the examiners were a little puzzled as to the exact nature of the heart sounds.

The simplest and most direct method of making the diagnosis in a suspected instance of coarctation is to feel for femoral pulsations. I palpated for the femoral arteries in every new case referred to the heart clinic. Normally, the pulsations of the femoral artery in a child are very easily found. In the presence of a constriction of the aorta these pulsations are absent or, at least, are very difficult to obtain. To my surprise, I discovered Cases 1 and 2 within a few months of each other by noting the absence of femoral pulsations. In a like manner, Dr. Mandel L. Spivek diagnosed the condition of R. M. (Case 3).

Blood pressure readings when elevated will also give one a clue. Furthermore, in coarctation of the aorta the blood pressure readings of the arms are always higher than those of the legs. Normally, the reverse exists. Most frequently, no readings at all are obtainable in the legs as is true in the three cases I have reported.

X-ray pictures probably will not show erosions of the ribs from the intercostal arteries if the diagnosis is made as early in life as 3 years of age. In these three children, only the oldest had demonstrable erosion of the ribs. Fortunately, an x-ray film of the heart was taken of Case 3 when the patient was 5 years old, and in that picture the telltale erosions were definite, although very slight.

The electrocardiogram is no aid in diagnosis.

I have come to consider palpation for femoral pulsations just as much a part of a routine cardiac examination as palpation of the apex beat or percussion of the heart borders. The employment of this simple procedure in heart examinations will, I am sure, increase the number of instances of coarctation of the aorta recognized in childhood.

REFERENCES

1. King, J. T.: Arch. Int. Med. **38**: 69, 1926.
2. Blackford, L. M.: Arch. Int. Med. **41**: 702, 1928.
3. Abbott, M. E.: Am. Heart J. **3**: 392 and 574, 1928.
4. Fray, W. W.: Am. J. Roentgenol. **24**: 349, 1930.
5. Blumgart, H. L., Lawrence, J. S., and Ernstene, A. C.: Arch. Int. Med. **47**: 806, 1931.
6. Hodann, C.: Ztschr. f. Kreislaufforsch. **23**: 97, 1931.
7. Ernstene, A. C., and Robins, S. A.: Am. J. Roentgenol. **25**: 243, 1931.
8. Ulrich, Henry L.: Am. Heart J. **7**: 641, 1932.
9. East, T.: Proc. Roy. Soc. Med. **25**: 796, 1932.
10. Dock, W.: J. A. M. A. **99**: 2024, 1932.
11. Evans, Wm.: Quart. J. Med. (N. S.) **2**: 1, 1933.
12. Shapiro, M. J.: J. A. M. A. **100**: 640, 1933.

13. Eppinger, E. C., and Midelfart, P. A. H.: Am. J. M. Sc. **185**: 528, 1933.
14. Puyo Villafane, A., and Braun Menendez, E.: Rev. Asoc. méd. argent. **48**: 1294, 1934.
15. Hesdorffer, M. B.: Journal-Lancet **54**: 658, 1934.
16. Pierce, W. F.: J. A. M. A. **103**: 830, 1934.
17. Henri: Soc. de méd. mil. franç., Bull. mens. **29**: 273, 1935.
18. Purks, W. K., and Robert, W. P.: South. M. J. **28**: 158, 1935.
19. Ferris, H. A.: Canad. M. A. J. **32**: 276, 1935.
20. Lian, C., Abaza, A., and Frumusan, P.: Bull. et mém. Soc. méd. d. hôp. de Paris **52**: 782, 1936.
21. Cookson, H.: Lancet **2**: 623, 1936.
22. Blegen, E.: Norsk. mag. f. laegevidensk. **97**: 927, 1936.
23. Wolke, K.: Acta radiol. **18**: 319, 1937.
24. Goodson, W. H., Jr.: New England J. Med. **216**: 339, 1937.
25. Gitlow, S.: New York State J. Med. **37**: 155, 1934.
26. Walker, W. G.: New England J. Med. **211**: 1192, 1934.
27. Carpenter, G.: Proc. Roy. Soc. Med. **2**: 275, 1908-1909.
28. Lewis, Thomas: Heart **16**: 205, 1933.
29. Woltman, H. W., and Shelden, W. D.: Arch. Neurol. & Psychiat. **17**: 303, 1927.
30. Lombardi, Q.: Semana méd. **2**: 1004, 1936.
31. Poynton, F. J., and Sheldon, W. P. H.: Arch. Dis. Childhood **3**: 191, 1928.
32. Thomson, A. P., and Lamb, F. W. M.: Arch. Dis. Childhood **4**: 377, 1929.
33. Hampson, A. C.: Proc. Roy. Soc. Med. **25**: 420, 1932.
34. Wolffe, J. B.: Arch. Pediat. **49**: 100, 1932.
35. Montcrieff, A.: Proc. Roy. Soc. Med. **25**: 720, 1932.
36. Lichtenberg, H. H., and Gallagher, H. F.: Am. J. Dis. Child. **45**: 1253, 1933.
37. Vega Diaz, F., Albert, C., Irigoyen, A., and Suils, E.: Arch. cardiol. y hemat. **16**: 450, 1935.

THE RELATION BETWEEN PLASMA ASCORBIC ACID CONCENTRATION AND DIET IN THE NEWBORN INFANT

Rowland L. Mindlin, M.D.
Boston, Mass.

VITAMIN C is not usually added to the diet of the artificially-fed infant until the second or third month of life. According to Holt and McIntosh,[1] "infants who are fed on sterilized or pasteurized milk should always be given orange juice or some other antiscorbutic food from the second month onward." A League of Nations commission[2] has recently recommended that vitamin C should be "given as from the age of three months," with no differentiation between breast and artificial feeding. The purpose of this paper is to present evidence of the close relation, in newborn infants, between the dietary supply and plasma concentration of ascorbic acid.

That woman's milk contains a significant amount of ascorbic acid is evident not only from clinical observations, but also from experimental investigation by Selleg and King[3] and others; scurvy is rare in the breast-fed infant. Similar observations indicate that the pasteurized, boiled, or evaporated cow's milk usually used for the preparation of infant feeding mixtures has a low ascorbic acid content.[4, 5, 6] There has been in the past no direct measurable chemical evidence that the vitamin requirement differs in breast-fed and artificially fed infants. Consequently, it seemed probable that the ascorbic acid reserve of the infant would begin to be depleted from the inception of a dietary regime which is lacking in vitamin C substance, and that this depletion might be reflected by a diminution of its concentration in the blood plasma.

The plan of study herein reported was as follows: Fifty normal, full-term infants were selected for study at the end of the first two weeks of life. Group I was composed of twenty-one infants who were satisfactorily nursed at the breast. Group II contained nineteen infants who were entirely artificially-fed for the last four or more days because of an abrupt cessation of breast feeding. The artificial feeding was a twice-pasteurized cow's milk-karo-water mixture.* Group III consisted of ten infants similar to those in Group II, but who received daily supplements of ascorbic acid for the duration of artificial feeding.† Three infants were given 20 mg. of ascorbic acid daily, three, 30 mg. daily, and four, 75 mg. daily. Ten or 25 mg. of ascorbic acid were added to the feeding

From the Departments of Pediatrics and Obstetrics of the Harvard Medical School, the Infants' and Children's Hospitals, and the Boston Lying-In Hospital.

*The composition was: milk (2 per cent or 4 per cent) 12 oz., water 5 oz., karo 1 oz.

†The ascorbic acid was supplied by Merck & Co., Inc., Rahway, N. J.

mixture two or three times daily, about fifteen minutes before it was given to the infant. During this time complete solution occurs, but the oxidative loss of ascorbic acid is less than 5 per cent.

METHOD

The plasma ascorbic acid concentration was determined by the micromethod of Mindlin and Butler.[7*] This procedure measures colorimetrically, by means of a photoelectric microcolorimeter, the amount of reduction of 2, 6-dichlorophenol indophenol caused by the ascorbic acid in 0.1 c.c. of plasma. Blood samples were collected at varying intervals with respect to the previous feeding. This procedure is justified because it has been found[9] that the small amount of ascorbic acid ingested by a two-week-old infant in a single feeding of breast milk (5 mg. or less) does not result in a rise in the plasma concentration. However, in no instance was a sample taken from an infant who received 10 or 25 mg. of ascorbic acid in a feeding mixture within sixteen hours of the last dose.

RESULTS

The experimental results are presented in Tables I, II and III. The average plasma ascorbic acid concentration in Group I (normal, breast-

TABLE I

PLASMA ASCORBIC ACID CONCENTRATION IN BREAST-FED INFANTS

GROUP I

CASE NO.	AGE (DAYS)	PLASMA ASCORBIC ACID (MG. %)	REMARKS
1	14	1.6	
2	13	1.3	
3	14	1.2	Cesarean section
4	13	1.2	Cesarean section
5	14	1.1	
6	13	1.1	
7	13	1.1	
8	13	1.1	
9	13	1.1	
10	13	1.1	
11	13	1.0	
12	14	0.9	
13	13	0.9	
14	13	0.9	
15	14	0.8	
16	13	0.8	Complementary feedings, 5th to 7th days
17	13	0.7	
18	13	0.7	Complementary feedings, 6th to 8th days
19	13	0.7	
20	13	0.6	
21	13	0.6	
		Average: 1.0	

*Recent work[8] has shown that the use of potassium cyanide in this determination is unnecessary and may under certain conditions introduce error. Under the conditions prescribed by the method, the error in plasma values due to the additions of potassium cyanide may vary from 0.0 to 0.1 mg. per cent and is therefore insignificant.

TABLE II

PLASMA ASCORBIC ACID CONCENTRATION IN ARTIFICIALLY-FED INFANTS

GROUP II

CASE NO.	AGE (DAYS)	ARTIFICIAL FEEDING (DAYS)	PLASMA ASCORBIC ACID (MG. %)	REMARKS
1	12	5	0.7	
2	12	5	0.6	
3	13	6	0.5	
4	13	5	0.5	
5	13	4	0.4	Complementary feedings for 4 days before breast feedings discontinued.
6	13	7	0.4	
7	13	7	0.4	
8	15	8	0.4	
9	14	9	0.4	
10	15	5	0.3	
11	13	8	0.3	
12	20	7	0.3	
13	13	5	0.2	Complementary feedings for 6 days.
14	13	6	0.2	Complementary feedings for 2 days.
15	13	8	0.2	
16	8	8	0.2	
17	14	9	0.2	
18	13	13	0.2	
19	19	19	0.1	
			Average: 0.3	

TABLE III

PLASMA ASCORBIC ACID CONCENTRATION IN ARTIFICIALLY-FED INFANTS RECEIVING DAILY ASCORBIC ACID SUPPLEMENT

GROUP III

CASE NO.	AGE (DAYS)	ARTIFICIAL FEEDING (DAYS)	ASCORBIC ACID SUPPLEMENT (MG. PER DAY)	PLASMA ASCORBIC ACID (MG. %)
1	14	8	20	0.4
2	13	7	20	0.5
3	13	6	20	0.6
4	13	8	30	0.6
5	13	7	30	0.7
6	13	7	30	0.8
7	13	7	75	0.7
8	13	8	75	0.6
9	13	8	75	0.8
10	13	9	75	0.7

fed infants at the age of about 2 weeks) was 1.0 mg. per cent, with a range from 0.6 to 1.6 mg. per cent. Similar determinations on infants who had received pasteurized artificial feedings for varying periods of time (Group II) revealed considerably lower values; i.e., in fourteen infants who had received no breast milk for five to nine days, the average plasma ascorbic acid concentration was 0.4 mg. per cent. Those who were artificially fed for longer periods had still lower concentrations. One infant, 19 days of age, artificially fed from birth, had 0.1 mg. per cent of ascorbic acid in the plasma. The infants who were artificially fed and received daily supplements of ascorbic acid (Group III) had somewhat higher plasma ascorbic acid concentrations than those in the unsupplemented group (II) who had received artificial feedings for the same period of time.

DISCUSSION

The significance of low plasma ascorbic acid concentrations is not clear. From the work of Ingalls[10] it is evident that in infantile scurvy the amount of ascorbic acid in the plasma is so small that it approaches the limit of accuracy of the determination. However, there is a wide range in normal individuals. With increasing experience with the *method,* it has been found that for normal individuals the ascorbic acid content of the plasma gives a reliable index of the dietary intake of the vitamin. On this basis a standard has been established for normal children and adults: with optimal vitamin C intake the plasma ascorbic acid concentration is 0.6 mg. per cent or higher; with suboptimal and deficient intakes the concentration falls below this level to an extent dependent upon the degree and duration of the deficiency; with clinical scurvy it approaches zero.

Although the correlation between the depletion of the bodily store of ascorbic acid, as measured by its concentration in the plasma, and pathologic physiology and histologic change has not been established, nevertheless, it is probable that the optimum state for the individual is one of abundance rather than one of paucity. The numerous tests for "saturation,"[11] based upon the measurement of the urinary excretion of ascorbic acid, and the absence of a syndrome of hypervitaminosis C indicate that the substance is readily excreted and is nontoxic.

The data presented show that breast-fed infants, at least for the first two weeks of life, have an ascorbic acid intake sufficient to maintain a plasma concentration which is considered optimal for older children and adults. The artificially-fed infants of the same age group do not maintain this concentration when the dietary supply of ascorbic acid is deficient. These infants do not have scurvy. Infantile scurvy is a clinicopathologic entity with characteristic signs and symptoms, all of which were absent from this group. But these infants are receiving scorbutogenic diets and are in, or are approaching, a state of asymptomatic ascorbic acid deficiency which is the forerunner of clinical scurvy. The addition of sufficient ascorbic acid to the diet of the artificially-fed infant abolishes this state and restores the optimal concentration of ascorbic acid in the plasma.

The plasma concentrations in the artificially-fed infants who received ascorbic acid are near to the lower limit of the optimal range. These low values may be related to the sixteen-hour interval between the last administration of ascorbic acid and the taking of the blood sample. The breast-fed infants received a small amount of ascorbic acid with every feeding, that is, at intervals of four hours. Hence they were never subject to a sixteen-hour depletion period, which in the very young infant may cause a slight fall in the plasma level.

For optimal nutrition it seems indicated that newborn infants who are fed pasteurized artificial feedings should receive a daily supplement of ascorbic acid from the beginning rather than after two or three months.

SUMMARY

1. The plasma ascorbic acid concentration of normal two-week-old infants on breast feeding averages 1.0 mg. per cent.

2. The plasma ascorbic acid concentration of normal two-week-old infants on artificial feeding for about one week averages 0.4 mg. per cent. Lower values result from longer periods of artificial feeding.

3. The addition of sufficient ascorbic acid to the diet prevents the fall in plasma concentration invariably found with pasteurized feeding.

I wish to thank Dr. A. M. Butler and Dr. A. T. Shohl for their valuable criticisms and suggestions during the course of this work.

REFERENCES

1. Holt, L. E., and McIntosh, R.: Holt's Diseases of Infancy and Childhood, ed. 10, p. 166, New York, 1933, D. Appleton-Century Company, Inc.
2. Quart. Bull. Health Organ., League of Nations **6**: 291, 1937.
3. Selleg, I., and King, C. G.: J. Nutrition **11**: 559, 1936.
4. Hess, A. F., and Fish, M.: Am. J. Dis. Child. **8**: 385, 1914.
5. Chick, H., Hume, E. M., and Shelton, R. F.: Lancet **1**: 1, 1918.
6. Waugh, W. A., and King, C. G.: J. Dairy Science **17**: 489, 1933.
7. Mindlin, R. L., and Butler, A. M.: J. Biol. Chem. **122**: 673, 1938.
8. Cushman, M., and Butler, A. M.: Personal communication.
9. Mindlin, R. L.: Unpublished studies.
10. Ingalls, T. H.: J. PEDIAT. **10**: 577, 1937.
11. Harris, L. J., Ray, S. N., and Ward, A.: Biochem. J. **27**: 2011, 1933.

VITAMIN C CONTENT OF THE BLOOD IN NEWBORN INFANTS

Arthur W. Fleming, M.D., and Heyworth N. Sanford, M.D.
Chicago, Ill.

LABORATORY methods for the estimation of the vitamin C content of the blood now make it possible to study the amount of this vitamin under various conditions. Studies that have been made on the vitamin C content of the blood of the newborn infant show dissimilar values. The majority of these have been made on cord blood. Abt, Farmer, and Epstein[1] showed almost identical values of cord blood vitamin C and blood obtained from the mother. Nielsen[2] has found more in the fetal blood than in the maternal blood. These represent the two extremes, and other determinations will be discussed later. It seemed to us that the blood values for the newborn infant should be determined throughout the newborn period, and, if possible, these values should be correlated with those of the mother.

PROCEDURE

Almost all methods of determination of vitamin C depend upon its reducing power, even in an acid medium. Some methods also estimate the entire vitamin rather than the reduced vitamin. Values obtained for either of these quantities will be different and will account for different results obtained.

After various trials of different methods of blood vitamin C determinations, it was decided to use the method of Abt and Farmer. We do not wish to enter into any discussion of the various methods of determination for this vitamin. It was sufficient for us that this method gives constant values for all individuals who should have a constant vitamin C blood value, that is to say, individuals who have had adequate vitamin C intakes. Individuals who have had inadequate vitamin C intakes consistently show lower values, and in the one case of proved infantile scurvy that we had an opportunity to study the blood vitamin C value was lowest of all.

Both the micro- and macromethods were used. In the mothers and other adult cases both methods were used on each patient. In the infants both interval determinations were made by the micromethod, with the macromethod used as a check on one interval or the other. It was found that the average difference between the two methods was approximately 0.1 mg. per cent. Blood was drawn from the newborn infants on the second and eighth days of life, and on the same days from their mothers. These estimations were made immediately after withdrawal of the blood.

From the Department of Pediatrics, Rush Medical College, and the Presbyterian Hospital, Chicago.

TABLE I

BLOOD VITAMIN C VALUES

	VITAMIN C IN MG.								VITAMIN C AVERAGE OF TOTAL
	0.4	0.5	0.6	0.7	0.8	0.9	1.0	1.1	
123 infants	3%	14%	12.5%	18%	27%	13%	8%	4%	0.753 mg.
105 mothers	0	7%	12%	15%	27%	14%	9%	10%	0.884 mg.
51 adults	6%	10%	6%	19%	12%	8%	10%	29%	0.990 mg.

RESULTS

Table I shows the results obtained on the vitamin C blood values of fifty-one dispensary patients, from 6 to 60 years of age, presumably on an adequate diet. The members of this group, however, who were under 0.6 mg. per cent showed an interesting dietary history. The three mem-

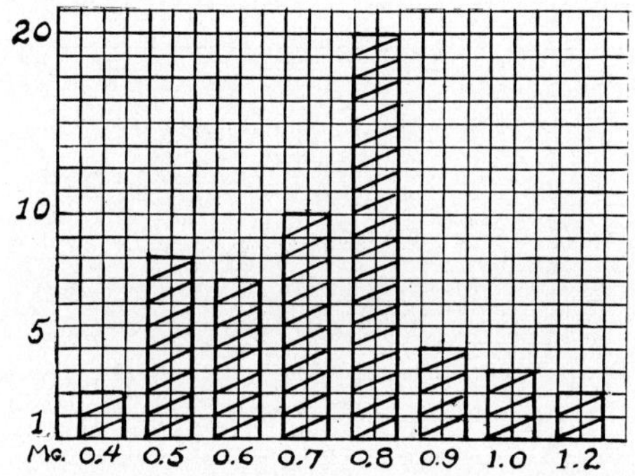

Fig. 1.—Vitamin C values of the blood in newborn infants.

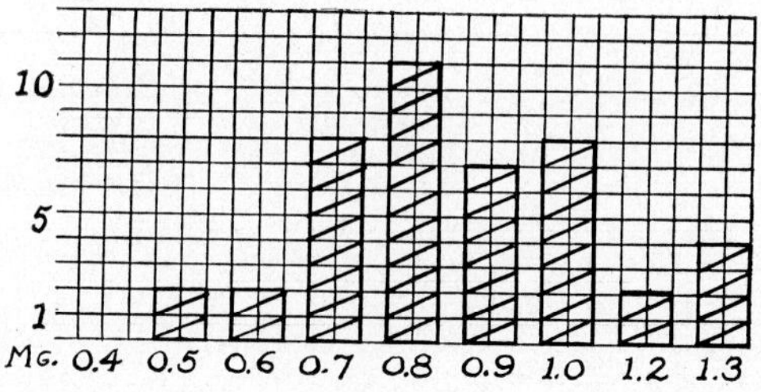

Fig. 2.—Vitamin C values of the blood in post-partum mothers.

bers whose blood values were under 0.5 mg. per cent were negro males from 44 to 50 years of age. Dietary history revealed they never ate oranges and rarely had fruit of any kind. The six members of the group between 0.5 mg. and 0.6 mg. per cent were white males, between 38 and 58 years of age. Their dietary history was that they ate fruits and oranges only occasionally. As a matter of interest, all of these individuals came to the clinic because of irritability, nervousness, and poor appetite of years' duration. They were all markedly thin, and the negroes were undernourished. However, these patients did not come to the dispensary for dietary management. They had no definite symptoms of scurvy, and we felt that in all fairness to the study they should be included in the average of the general control group. The average blood vitamin C value for this group was 0.99 mg.

Table I also shows vitamin C blood values of 123 infants and 105 mothers. These mothers are of moderate economic circumstances and pay a set fee for their entire hospital service. Their vitamin C intake is discussed in Table VIII. It may be considered on the whole as adequate. The average blood vitamin C values of these mothers was 0.884 mg. and of the infants, 0.753 mg. Figs. 1 and 2 show that the infant tends toward the same value as his mother.

Table II shows the direct comparison of the blood vitamin C values for

TABLE II

BLOOD VITAMIN C VALUES OF MOTHERS AND INFANTS

Mothers' vitamin C 72 mothers	0.5 mg. to 0.6 mg.	0.7 mg.	0.8 mg.	0.9 mg.	1.0 mg.	1.1 mg.
Percentage of infants in group 72 infants	21%	14%	28%	15%	11%	11%
Average vitamin C of infants	0.59	0.68	0.77	0.85	0.89	1.06

TABLE III

INFLUENCE OF BLOOD VITAMIN C ON BREAST MILK PRODUCTION

Mother—vitamin C value	0.5 mg.	0.6 mg.	0.7 mg.	0.8 mg.	0.9 mg.	1.0 mg.	1.1 mg.
Percentage of mothers	5.5%	15%	14%	28%	15%	11%	11%
Breast milk—ounces	30	48.8	40.1	45.8	37.8	36.3	45

TABLE IV

INFLUENCE OF BLOOD VITAMIN C OF MOTHER ON BIRTH WEIGHT OF INFANT

	BIRTH WEIGHT OF BABY IN LB.				
	5 to 6	6 to 7	7 to 8	8 to 9	9 to 10
Percentage of infants	1.5%	8%	49%	33%	7%
Average vitamin C of infant	0.95	0.81	0.74	0.85	0.80

72 individual mothers and their infants. This shows that each individual baby has practically the same vitamin C blood value as its mother. Table III compares the amount of breast milk produced by each mother and her blood vitamin C value. There is no correlation between the amount of blood vitamin C and the amount of breast milk produced. Table IV compares birth weight and the blood vitamin C of the infants. There is no correlation for the normal infant, but Table V, giving the values for seven premature infants, shows that for the majority of these infants the blood vitamin C value is lower than the expected average for normal infants.

TABLE V

BLOOD VITAMIN C VALUES IN PREMATURE INFANTS

AGE	WEIGHT	BIRTH WEIGHT	VITAMIN C (MG.)
1 day	4 lb. 10 oz.	4 lb. 10 oz.	0.40
5 days	5 lb.	5 lb. 2 oz.	0.53
5 days	4 lb. 12 oz.	5 lb. 2 oz.	0.88
8 days	4 lb. 9 oz.	4 lb. 13 oz.	0.63
13 days	3 lb. 15 oz.	3 lb. 15 oz.	0.55
26 days	5 lb. 8 oz.	5 lb. 6 oz.	0.75
27 days	6 lb. 2 oz.	4 lb. 15 oz.	0.58

Table VI compares the amount of breast milk received and the blood vitamin C values for the infants on the second day, with their range during the week. These infants received nothing but mother's milk and water. This shows that there is a slight gain with increasing breast milk, and a slight loss if the breast milk is insufficient.

TABLE VI

EFFECT OF BREAST MILK RECEIVED ON BLOOD VITAMIN C VALUES OF 72 INFANTS (ESTIMATIONS MADE ON THE SECOND AND EIGHTH DAYS)

Mother's milk in ounces (6 days)	0 to 30	30 to 40	40 to 50	50 to 60	60 to 70
Number of infants	13	17	19	16	6
Number of infants gaining vitamin C	2	7	12	10	5
Amount vitamin C gain in mg.	0.035	0.075	0.099	0.157	0.175
Number of infants losing vitamin C	11	10	7	6	1
Amount of vitamin C loss in mg.	0.177	0.129	0.067	0.066	0.017

Table VII shows the vitamin C blood values in infants who were diagnosed as suffering from cerebral hemorrhage and in their mothers.

TABLE VII

BLOOD VITAMIN C VALUES IN MOTHERS AND IN INFANTS WITH CEREBRAL HEMORRHAGE

NO.	MOTHERS VIT. C	INFANTS VIT. C	RESULT
1	0.63 (diabetic)	0.46	Recovered
2	0.66	0.62	Died—Autopsy showed cerebral hemorrhage
3	0.77	0.50	Recovered
4	0.70	0.57	Recovered
5	0.80	0.60	Recovered
6	0.70	0.47	Recovered
7	0.82	0.55	Recovered
8	0.76	0.60	Recovered

Table VIII shows the effect of citrus fruit or adequate vitamin C intake during pregnancy on the blood vitamin C value of the mother after delivery. In the group designated as "excellent," the intake was equivalent to one orange a day; "good," three oranges a week; "fair," one orange a week, and "poor," barely any citrus fruits at all. This table needs no further explanation, and the results are quite striking.

TABLE VIII

EFFECT OF DIET ON THE BLOOD VITAMIN C OF POST-PARTUM MOTHERS

	EXCELLENT	GOOD	FAIR	POOR
	1.62	0.75	0.65	0.46
	1.85	1.75	0.76	0.50
	2.40	0.68	0.56	0.63
	2.10	1.21	0.74	0.58
	2.50	0.75	0.72	0.65
Citrus fruit intake	1.16	0.80	0.81	0.61
	1.50	0.76	0.75	0.55
	1.87	1.25	0.78	0.45
	1.93	0.76	0.67	0.49
		0.88	0.83	
		0.99		
		1.05		
Average vitamin C value	1.88	0.969	0.727	0.546

DISCUSSION

In the control adult group, the limits of blood vitamin C were between 0.4 mg. and 1.8 mg. These individuals were presumed to have adequate vitamin C intakes, but the dietary history of the members of this group below 0.6 mg. per cent has been discussed. Since 76 per cent of this group have blood vitamin C values between 0.5 mg. and 1.2 mg., we may assume that these figures are the average blood vitamin C values for the normal individual. In individuals with inadequate vitamin C intakes the blood value always fell below 0.65 mg., and in the one infant with proved infantile scurvy the blood vitamin C value was 0.4 mg. The limits of blood vitamin C values for the maternal group were between 0.5 mg. and 1.4 mg. Since 72 per cent of these values are between 0.8 mg. and 1.2 mg., these figures may be assumed to be the average for post-partum mothers. In the newborn infant the blood vitamin C values were between 0.4 mg. and 1.2 mg. Since 78 per cent of these values are beween 0.5 mg. and 0.9 mg., this may be assumed to be the average for this group. The general average for the mothers is slightly below that of the adults, and the average for the infants is similar to the mothers. The figures show graphically that the general tendency of the blood vitamin C value of the infant is similar to that of the mother.

While the above results will show a general tendency in comparison with blood vitamin C values, they are not of as much value as the comparison of the values for each individual mother and child. This is shown in Table II, where it will be observed that in almost every case the newborn infant, with few individual variations, has a blood vitamin C value similar to that of his mother. Besides the authors mentioned before, Wahren and Rundquist[3] obtained higher blood vitamin C values for the newborn infant than for the mother. The average blood vitamin C value in seventeen mothers was 0.158 mg. and in the infant, 0.347 mg. A different method of determination of blood vitamin C was used (photometric methylene blue). Nielsen, using a similar method, found the blood vitamin C in forty-one mothers to be lower than in nonpregnant women, and in fetal blood a value eight times higher. By the same method, Braestrup[4] found the cord blood values to be 0.9 mg. in seventy-five infants, while the mothers blood vitamin C values averaged 0.36 mg.

There are two possible explanations for these differences between their results and ours: First, the estimations on the mothers' bloods were made during labor, and there is considerable evidence that labor, among other factors, temporarily reduces the amount of blood vitamin C. Second, the difference in method. Fujita and Ebihara,[5] who have made a comparison of the different methods for determining blood vitamin C content, state that with methylene blue titration a smaller quantity of blood may be used but that it always gives lower values than other methods, such as titration with 2:6-dichlorphenol indophenol. This might well explain the results obtained by Abt in the five mothers and their infants, whom he studied. These values were obtained on cord blood. The values he obtained for individual mothers and infants are quite similar to ours.

We are unable to find that the amount of blood vitamin C in the mother had any effect on the amount of milk that she produced. There is no particular reason that it should do so. An adequate vitamin C intake by the mother might affect the quality of her milk but not the quantity.

In the normal baby there was no correlation between the size of the baby and his blood vitamin C value, that is, a larger baby does not have a higher blood vitamin C value than a smaller one. In the findings of the few small babies studied, we were interested to discover comparatively high blood vitamin C values. For this reason the blood vitamin C values were determined on seven premature infants on different days of life. Instead of being higher, they were considerably lower than the average. Giraud[6] found that the younger the fetus, the higher the vitamin C content of its tissues. Rohmer[7] found the content of the cerebrospinal fluid to be about twice as high in six premature infants as six full-term infants. Certainly in the human fetus, as judged by the blood vitamin C in the premature infant, there is no tendency to store up vitamin C in fetal life.

There is a slight but definite increase in blood vitamin C value of the newborn infant throughout the first week of life, with sufficient mother's milk. Obviously this milk should be from a mother who has an adequate vitamin C intake. If a newborn infant has an adequate blood vitamin C value and obtains adequate milk from a mother on an adequate vitamin C intake, the infant should be amply protected from vitamin C deficiency. This has been found also by Widenbauer and Kuhner.[8]

We present our findings of the low blood vitamin C values in cerebral hemorrhage of the newborn infant but do not wish to draw any conclusions on such a small number of cases. We do feel, however, that the fact that eight newborn babies with a diagnosis of cerebral hemorrhage, whose mothers' blood vitamin C values are, like their infants, below the average, is worthy of note. It may be argued that the diagnosis of cerebral hemorrhage is questionable. We can only prove one case, which came to autopsy, but by the usual methods of making such a diagnosis we believe these infants suffered from such a condition. One mother had a very inadequate intake of vitamin C. She suffered from diabetes. After low blood vitamin C values had been found consistently in several cases, we made it a practice to give all infants with a diagnosis of cerebral hemorrhage cevitamic acid after the blood vitamin C was taken. The fact that these infants recovered proves nothing, as the other infants before this recovered without this treatment. We do feel that the factor of a vitamin C adequate intake in the mother may have some bearing on the condition of the child at birth. Could not a low blood vitamin C be a factor in the fragility of the cerebral capillaries if any extra strain was put on the system?

Finally, we arrive at the question of what all these findings mean. Certainly all of these infants were clinically normal. We never see clinical signs of scurvy before six months of life, and even then an infant on an inadequate vitamin C intake may not develop scurvy. However, there have always been factors in infantile scurvy that were never completely understood. May it not have been that those infants who began with a higher blood vitamin C value were better protected at a later time? How can we give a newborn infant an adequate vitamin C blood value? It clearly depends on the blood vitamin C of the mother, and this can be controlled by her vitamin C intake. As shown in Table VIII, the blood vitamin C of the mother can be tripled by an adequate citrus fruit intake, and this blood vitamin C value may be imparted to her child.

CONCLUSIONS

In 123 infants the average of two determinations made on the second and eighth days of life was 0.753 mg. In 105 mothers of these infants the average was 0.884 mg., and in fifty-one miscellaneous adults the average was 0.99 mg. In a comparison of seventy-two mothers and their infants, it was found that the amount of vitamin C in the infant's blood is directly determined by the mother's blood vitamin C value, and the infant's blood will be, on the average, similar to the mother's. The amount of vitamin C in the mother's blood has no influence on her production of breast milk, on the gain or loss of the infant, or any influence on the infant's birth weight. The birth weight of the infant does not influence the amount of its blood vitamin C, but, providing the mother has an average amount of blood vitamin C, a gain in weight by the infant taking her breast milk is followed by a small gain in the infant's vitamin C blood content.

Mothers having a liberal vitamin C intake during pregnancy will show a high vitamin C blood content after delivery, and this decreases in proportion as the mother's diet is deficient in vitamin C.

These findings indicate that the amount of vitamin C existing in the mother's blood depends on her diet during pregnancy, and this amount determines the quantity of vitamin C in the blood of her infant. The normal infant tends to the same vitamin C content of the blood as its mother. Seven infants suffering with a cerebral hemorrhage had blood vitamin C values of below 0.62 mg. In certain mothers with a low or threshold value of blood vitamin C, the infant may show a blood vitamin C value that is lower than is consistent with accepted normal values.

REFERENCES

1. Abt, A. F., Farmer, C. J., and Epstein, I. M.: J. Pediat. **8**: 1, 1936.
2. Nielsen, H. E.: Bibliot. f. laeger. **130**: 20, 1938.
3. Wahren, H., and Rundquist, O.: Klin. Wchnschr. **16**: 1498, 1937.
4. Braestrup, P. W.: Acta paediat. **19**: 328, 1937.
5. Fujita, A., and Ebihara, T.: Biochem. Ztschr. **290**: 172, 1937.
6. Giraud, A., et al.: Compt. rend. Soc. de biol. **123**: 1038, 1936.
7. Rohmer, P., Bezssonoff, N., and Stoerr, E.: Compt. rend. Soc. de biol. **121**: 987, 1935.
8. Widenbauer, F., and Kühner, A.: Ztschr. f. Vitaminforsch. **6**: 75, 1937; Widenbauer, F.: Monatschr. f. Kinderh. **68**: 360, 1937.

952 North Michigan Avenue

THE INCIDENCE OF HEMOLYTIC STREPTOCOCCI IN THE TONSILS OF CHILDREN AS RELATED TO THE VITAMIN C CONTENT OF TONSILS AND BLOOD

Albert D. Kaiser, M.D., and Betty Slavin
Rochester, N. Y.

SINCE methods have been devised for the accurate determination of vitamin C (ascorbic acid) in the urine and in the blood, numerous reports have been published dealing with the vitamin C content of urine and blood in a number of diseases.

In 1934 Rinehart and Mettier[1] cited experimental, epidemiologic and clinical data in favor of a theory that vitamin C deficiency may be a necessary accompaniment of rheumatic fever. In 1936 Abbasy, Hill, and Harris[2] reported on vitamin C studies in 107 children with active rheumatic fever. Their interpretation of the results is that with the infection which underlies rheumatic fever there is a greatly increased metabolic use of vitamin C and a correspondingly lowered degree of "saturation" of the body tissues. Other studies, notably those of Sendroy and Schultz,[3] do not agree with these observations. It does appear, however, that vitamin C deficiency may play some part in the course of certain infections as well as being the causative factor in scurvy.

In view of the fact that hemolytic streptococci have been associated with the causative factors in rheumatic infections, and that vitamin C metabolism may be influenced by infections, it seemed worth while to study the relationship of the incidence of hemolytic streptococci of the tonsils with the amount of vitamin C found in the blood and in the tonsils of these subjects. If subclinical scurvy can be recognized by a lowered content of vitamin C in the blood, as has been suggested by Abt,[4] it was proposed that there might be some measurable increase of infection in the individuals who show deficient amounts of vitamin C in the blood. The present study was undertaken to determine if any relationship in children exists between the level of vitamin C stored in the blood and the presence of hemolytic streptococcus infection in the tonsils.

A group of 123 children was utilized for this purpose. They ranged in ages from 6 to 16 years. They had been selected by school physicians for various reasons to have their tonsils and adenoids removed. All were admitted to the hospital the afternoon before operations were to be performed. Soon after admission to the hospital 5 c.c. of blood were withdrawn from the vein of each patient. This was examined the following morning for a quantitative determination of vitamin C. This

From the Department of Pediatrics, University of Rochester School of Medicine and Dentistry.

Aided by a grant from the Fluid Research Fund of the University of Rochester.

procedure was adopted after it was ascertained that practically no vitamin C was lost by keeping the blood cooled for fifteen hours. The tonsils were sent to the laboratory immediately after the operation and were prepared for study within three hours after removal. A quantitative determination of the vitamin C of the tonsils was made in a similar way to that of the blood. To determine the presence or absence of streptococci in the tonsils, the surface of the tonsil was seared and then cut with a sterile knife. Loops were taken from this cut surface and streaked on blood agar plates. Subcultures were made to determine the type of streptococci present in the tonsils. Intraperitoneal injections into mice were later made to determine the virulence of these streptococci. The following method utilized by Stephens and Hawley[5] was employed in determining the content of vitamin C of the blood and of the tonsils: To 2 c.c. samples of whole blood were added 2.5 c.c. of 20 per cent acid (18 per cent trichloracetic plus 2 per cent metaphosphoric acid) and 5.5 c.c. of distilled water. The deproteinized filtrate was used for the estimation of ascorbic acid. The ascorbic acid content of the filtrates obtained was determined by rapid titration against a standardized solution of 2:6-dichlorphenolindophenol. The titrations were completed within thirty seconds and were always made in duplicate. Results were expressed as milligrams of reduced ascorbic acid per 100 c.c. of whole blood. In the case of the tonsils, they were rinsed in distilled water, cut into small pieces, and a gram of tissue weighed out. This amount was ground with very fine sand in a mortar, and 5 c.c. of a 20 per cent solution containing 18 per cent trichloracetic acid plus 2 per cent metaphosphoric acid were added. This mixture was shaken for five minutes, then 15 c.c. of distilled water added and the whole mixture shaken again for ten minutes. It was then filtered through No. 1 filter paper, and the clear filtrate titrated against a known quantity of 2:6-dichlorphenolindophenol to determine the amount of vitamin C contained in 100 gm. of tonsillar tissue.

As noted in Table I, the vitamin C content of the blood varies from 0.50 mg. per cent to 1.08 mg. per cent. Similarly the vitamin C content of the tonsils varies from 18.6 mg. to 53.7 mg. per cent. None of the children on whom these determinations were made were acutely ill. More than half of them came from families who were on relief, while the remainder came from homes that were classed in the lower economic strata. It was possible to observe 96 of these 123 children for a period of six months or more after their tonsillectomy to determine something about the amount of vitamin C they obtained in their diet. During this period following the tonsil operation it was also possible to record the incidence of throat and respiratory infections in the children.

A careful study of the figures noted in Table I shows marked variations in the vitamin C values of the blood and of the tonsils. In Charts 1 and 2 this range from low to high is more easily recognized. The presence of hemolytic streptococci in the tonsil was demonstrated in

TABLE I

NO.	PATIENT	AGE	SEX	MONTH	VIT. C OF BLOOD IN MG.	VIT. C OF TONSIL IN MG.	PRESENCE OF HEM. STREP. IN TONSIL	MOUSE VIRULENCE TEST	DIET VIT. C	DICK TEST	HISTORY OF RESPIRATORY INFECTION SINCE TONSILLECTOMY
1	M. R.	9	F	July	0.70	18.6	Positive	Non-vir.	Inadq.	Neg.	Negative
2	J. B.	8	M	July	0.60	19.5	Negative	—	Inadq.	Neg.	Negative
3	R. D.	9	F	July	0.69	30.6	Negative	—	Inadq.	Pos.	Few colds
4	M. C.	11	F	July	0.57	26.6	Positive	Virulent	Adq.	Pos.	One cold
5	E. V.	9	M	July	0.70	30.6	Positive	Non-vir.	Adq.	Neg.	Negative
6	K. G.	7	F	July	0.70	33.6	Positive	Non-vir.	Inadq.	Neg.	Negative
7	H. B.	10	M	July	0.70	40.8	Negative	—	Adq.	Neg.	Negative
8	D. W.	13	M	July	0.91	36.6	Negative	—	Adq.	Neg.	Negative
9	G. B.	13	F	Sept.	0.80	32.6	Negative	—	Inadq.	Pos.	Two colds
10	B. S.	12	F	Sept.	0.60	26.6	Positive	Non-vir.	Adq.	Neg.	Negative
11	R. H.	9	F	Sept.	0.80	30.6	Negative	—	Adq.	Pos.	Negative
12	G. B.	10	F	Oct.	0.75	23.7	Positive	Virulent	Inadq.	Pos.	Negative
13	T. G.	9	M	Oct.	0.63	26.6	Positive	Non-vir.	Adq.	Pos.	Negative
14	T. P.	13	M	Oct.	0.75	26.6	Positive	Non-vir.	Adq.	Pos.	Negative
15	C. A.	13	M	Oct.	0.83	20.0	Negative	—	Inadq.	Neg.	Negative
16	A. S.	11	M	Oct.	0.92	27.0	Negative	—	Adq.	Pos.	Negative
17	F. B.	8	F	Oct.	0.72	39.0	Negative	—	Inadq.	Neg.	Few colds
18	E. S.	11	F	Oct.	0.69	46.5	Negative	—	Adq.	Neg.	Negative
19	A. C.	12	F	Oct.	0.68	29.4	Negative	—	Inadq.	—	Two colds
20	J. C.	12	F	Oct.	0.65	40.0	Negative	—	Inadq.	Pos.	Negative
21	C. A.	10	M	Oct.	0.71	32.6	Negative	—	Inadq.	Neg.	Negative
22	G. S.	8	F	Oct.	0.64	27.1	Negative	—	Adq.	Pos.	Negative
23	N. S.	11	M	Oct.	0.82	36.6	Positive	Non-vir.	Adq.	—	Negative
24	K. M.	9	F	Oct.	0.73	35.1	Negative	—	Adq.	Pos.	Negative
25	D. P.	13	F	Oct.	0.82	26.5	Positive	Virulent	Adq.	Pos.	One cold
26	L. S.	13	M	Oct.	0.67	39.9	Negative	—	Adq.	Pos.	Many colds
27	R. D.	11	M	Oct.	0.78	30.6	Positive	Non-vir.	Adq.	Pos.	One cold
28	M. P.	8	F	Oct.	0.66	45.0	Positive	Non-vir.	Adq.	Neg.	Many colds
29	M. G.	10	F	Oct.	0.64	43.6	Positive	Virulent	Adq.	Neg.	Sore throats
30	B. M.	11	F	Oct.	0.69	35.1	Positive	Virulent	Inadq.	Neg.	Sore throats, colds
31	L. D.	13	F	Oct.	0.67	44.1	Positive	Non-vir.	Inadq.	Neg.	Many colds

TABLE I—CONT'D

32	C. A.	10	M	Oct.	0.80	36.6	Negative	—	Inadq.	Neg.	Negative
33	J. L.	12	M	Oct.	0.93	26.5	Negative	—	Adq.	Neg.	Few colds
34	L. M.	8	M	Oct.	0.76	28.0	Positive	Non-vir.	Inadq.	Pos.	Negative
35	J. H.	9	M	Oct.	0.83	30.6	Positive	Non-vir.	Inadq.	Neg.	Discharging ears
36	L. D.	9	F	Nov.	0.80	35.1	Positive	Non-vir.	Adq.	Neg.	Many colds
37	J. T.	13	M	Nov.	0.82	23.7	Positive	Non-vir.	Inadq.	Pos.	Negative
38	M. L.	13	F	Nov.	0.89	32.7	Negative	—	Adq.	Neg.	Negative
39	C. H.	10	M	Nov.	0.80	23.7	Negative	—	Adq.	Neg.	Many colds
40	G. S.	11	F	Nov.	0.71	39.9	Positive	Non-vir.	Adq.	Neg.	Negative
41	J. G.	13	M	Nov.	0.69	33.6	Positive	Non-vir.	Adq.	Neg.	Negative
42	R. M.	15	M	Nov.	0.62	35.1	Positive	Non-vir.	Adq.	Neg.	Negative
43	S. L.	8	M	Nov.	0.85	49.4	Negative	—	Adq.	Pos.	Few colds
44	F. S.	9	M	Nov.	0.88	46.5	Negative	—	Adq.	Pos.	Negative
45	S. L.	11	M	Nov.	0.93	44.1	Negative	—	Adq.	Neg.	Negative
46	C. B.	9	F	Nov.	0.89	35.1	Negative	—	Inadq.	Neg.	Negative
47	H. S.	11	M	Nov.	1.08	26.5	Negative	—	Adq.	Neg.	Negative
48	C. B.	10	M	Nov.	0.93	36.6	Negative	—	Adq.	Pos.	Health improved
49	J. C.	10	F	Nov.	0.77	32.6	Negative	—	Adq.	Neg.	Hoarseness
50	R. M.	9	M	Nov.	1.05	39.9	Positive	Virulent		Pos.	Negative
51	S. P.	10	F	Dec.	1.02	34.4	Negative	—	Inadq.	Neg.	One cold
52	T. V.	9	F	Dec.	0.91	29.4	Negative	—	Adq.	Neg.	Negative
53	A. M.	11	F	Dec.	0.96	39.8	Negative	—	Adq.	Neg.	Many colds
54	A. P.	14	M	Dec.	1.02	32.4	Negative	—	Adq.	Neg.	Slight colds
55	J. C.	14	M	Dec.	0.69	31.8	Negative	—	Inadq.	Neg.	Slight colds
56	P. A.	13	M	Dec.	0.58	35.1	Positive	—	Inadq.	Neg.	Negative
57	W. W.	11	M	Dec.	0.57	18.8	Positive	—	Inadq.	Pos.	Negative
58	H. C.	10	F	Jan.	0.72	25.0	Positive	Non-vir.	Inadq.	Neg.	Colds
59	A. C.	9	F	Jan.	0.60	18.7	Positive	Non-vir.	Inadq.	Neg.	Negative
60	J. N.	8	F	Jan.	0.71	22.5	Negative	—	Adq.	Neg.	Negative
61	A. W.	13	M	Jan.	0.50	26.2	Positive	Non-vir.	Inadq.	Neg.	Negative
62	W. K.	12	M	Jan	0.69	38.2	Negative	—	Inadq.	Neg.	Slight colds
63	G. R.	13	M	Jan.	0.49	31.5	Positive	Non-vir.	Inadq.	Neg.	Negative
64	M. D.	13	F	Jan.	0.76	35.2	Negative	—	Adq.	Pos.	Negative
65	R. D.	10	F	Jan.	0.62	26.9	Negative	—	Adq.	Pos.	Negative
66	J. V.	13	M	Jan.	0.84	35.2	Negative	—	Adq.	Pos.	Negative

TABLE I—CONT'D

NO.	PATIENT	AGE	SEX	MONTH	VIT. C OF BLOOD IN MG.	VIT. C OF TONSIL IN MG.	PRESENCE OF HEM. STREP. IN TONSIL	MOUSE VIRULENCE TEST	DIET VIT. C	DICK TEST	HISTORY OF RESPIRATORY INFECTION SINCE TONSILLECTOMY
67	E. B.	12	M	Jan.	0.68	32.7	Negative	—	Adq.	Pos.	Negative
68	A. L.	14	F	Jan.	0.72	41.6	Negative	—	Inadq.	Pos.	Sore throats, colds
69	V. D.	13	F	Jan.	0.58	32.7	Negative	—	Adq.	Neg.	Negative
70	G. A.	7	F	Feb.	0.76	23.3	Negative	—	Adq.	—	Sore throats, colds
71	V. T.	11	M	Feb.	0.71	26.8	Negative	—	Inadq.	—	Negative
72	L. B.	12	M	Feb.	0.98	31.6	Positive	Non-vir.	Adq.	Neg.	Negative
73	M. R.	10	F	Feb.	1.01	32.5	Negative	—	Adq.	Neg.	Sore throat
74	J. V.	11	M	Feb.	0.75	41.3	Negative	—	Adq.	Pos.	Negative
75	W. R.	11	M	Feb.	0.90	25.5	Negative	—	Adq.	Pos.	Negative
76	B. K.	9	F	Feb.	0.65	29.8	Negative	—	Adq.	Pos.	Negative
77	C. D.	13	M	Feb.	0.94	29.8	Negative	—	Adq.	Pos.	Colds
78	H. G.	9	M	Feb.	0.79	38.3	Positive	Non-vir.	Adq.	Neg.	Negative
79	H. D.	10	F	Feb.	0.85	38.3	Negative	—	Adq.	Neg.	Negative
80	A. P.	12	F	Feb.	0.94	35.8	Negative	—	Adq.	Pos.	Negative
81	I. S.	11	F	Feb.	0.97	48.8	Negative	—	Adq.	Neg.	Negative
82	L. P.	12	F	Feb.	0.93	35.8	Negative	—	Inadq.	Neg.	Negative
83	H. D.	16	M	Feb.	0.87	29.8	Negative	—	Inadq.	Pos.	Negative
84	J. P.	13	M	Feb.	1.05	53.7	Negative	—	Inadq.	Neg.	Negative
85	W. D.	12	M	Feb.	0.94	48.8	Negative	—	Inadq.	Pos.	Bronchitis
86	R. I.	10	M	Feb.	1.05	41.3	Positive	Non-vir.	Inadq.	Neg.	Negative
87	J. M.	13	F	Feb.	1.01	38.3	Negative	—	Adq.	Neg.	Occasional cold
88	F. H.	12	M	Mar.	0.87	41.3	Negative	—	Inadq.	—	Negative
89	E. N.	16	M	Mar.	0.87	41.3	Positive	Non-vir.	Inadq.	—	Negative
90	T. L.	11	F	Mar.	0.97	29.8	Negative	—	Inadq.	—	Negative
91	D. U.	10	M	Mar.	0.84	38.3	Negative	—	Adq.	Neg.	Negative
92	D. M.	9	F	Mar.	0.82	35.8	Positive	Non-vir.	Adq.	—	Colds
93	V. S.	11	F	Mar.	0.89	35.1	Negative	—	Adq.	Neg.	Negative
94	E. M.	12	F	Mar.	0.96	31.3	Negative	—	Inadq.	Neg.	Colds
95	J. M.	11	M	Mar.	0.86	27.3	Negative	—	Adq.	Neg.	Sore throats, colds
96	E. S.	11	M	Mar.	0.96	30.6	Negative	—	Inadq.	Pos.	Negative

about 50 per cent of the children. An inadequate vitamin C intake in the diet was noted in about 40 per cent of the children. With these variations in the findings of apparently healthy children it became im-

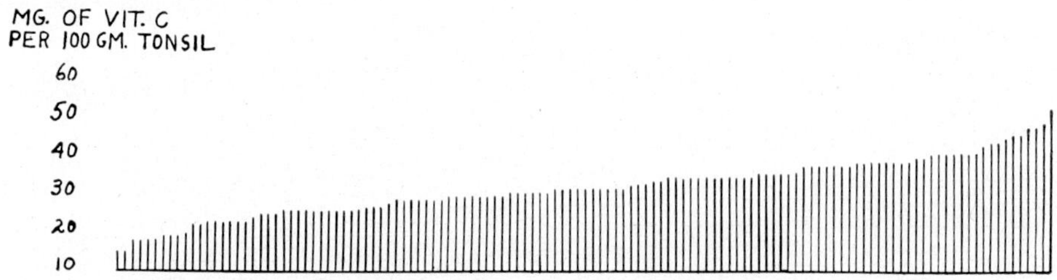

Chart 1.—Vitamin C values in milligrams per 100 gm. of tonsillar tissue from 125 pairs of tonsils.

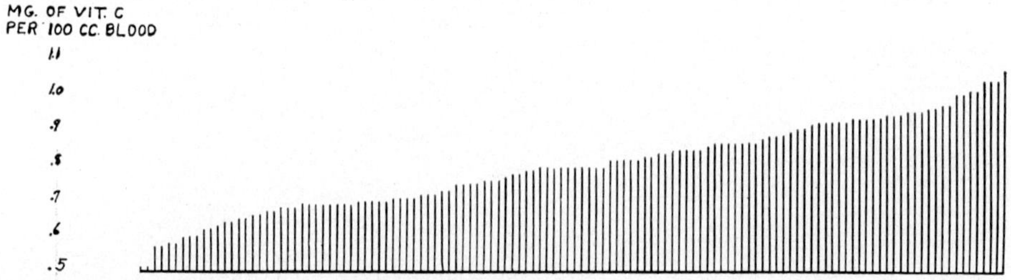

Chart 2.—Vitamin C values in milligrams per 100 c.c. of whole blood from 125 children.

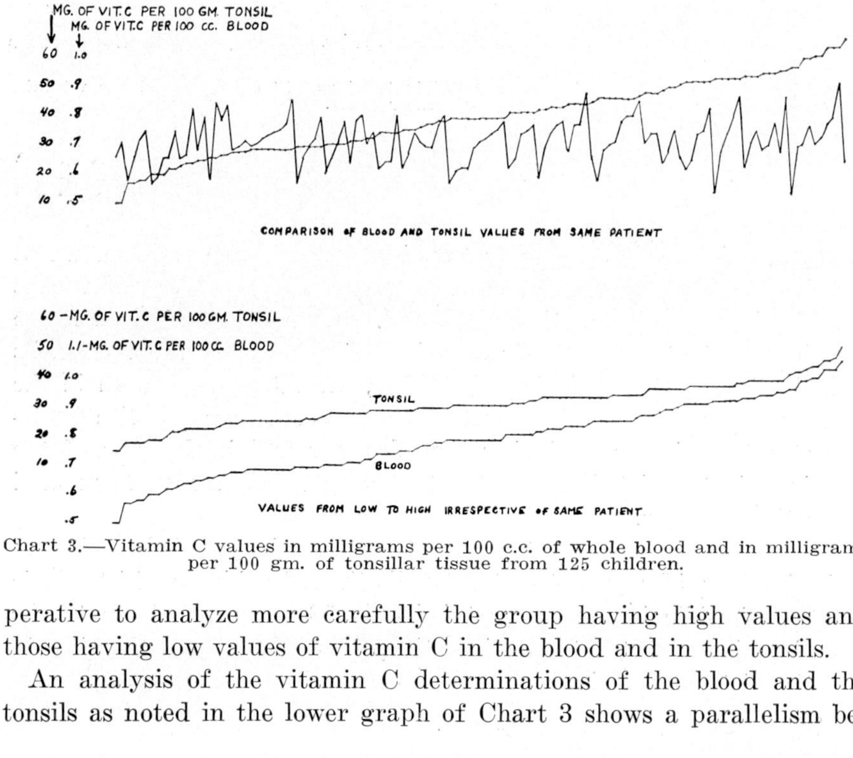

Chart 3.—Vitamin C values in milligrams per 100 c.c. of whole blood and in milligrams per 100 gm. of tonsillar tissue from 125 children.

perative to analyze more carefully the group having high values and those having low values of vitamin C in the blood and in the tonsils.

An analysis of the vitamin C determinations of the blood and the tonsils as noted in the lower graph of Chart 3 shows a parallelism between the variations in the vitamin C values. Approximately one-third of the children showed low values of vitamin C in the blood and in the tonsils. The middle third represents the average values and the upper third the high values. When, however, the vitamin C values of the blood and the tonsils from the same patient are plotted as is noted in the upper graph of Chart 3, it is obvious that the high and the low values do not always occur in the same patient. In other words, children whose vitamin C blood levels were low frequently showed average or above average amounts of vitamin C in the tonsils. Similarly, patients with high vitamin C values in the tonsils frequently showed low vitamin C values in the blood. There is therefore no constant relationship between the amount of vitamin C of the blood and of the tonsils.

Inasmuch as complete follow-up data were obtained on only ninety-six of the 123 children, this number was divided into three groups, the

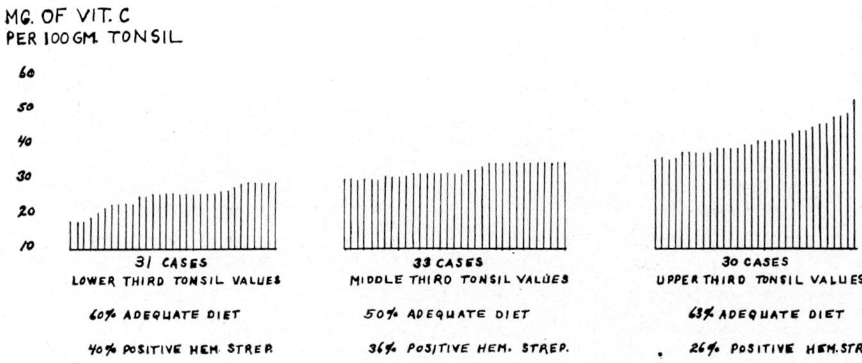

Chart 4.—Incidence of hemolytic streptococci in tonsils of 94 children and the vitamin C intake in their diets.

lower third having the lowest values of vitamin C in the blood and in the tonsils, a middle third which represented the average values, and an upper third with the highest values of vitamin C.

An analysis of Chart 4 shows that in the thirty-one children whose vitamin C content of the tonsils was low, 40 per cent of the tonsils showed evidence of hemolytic streptococci. In the thirty children whose vitamin C content of the tonsils was high, only 26 per cent of the tonsils showed evidence of hemolytic streptococci, while the 33 children in the middle group showed an incidence of 36 per cent infected with hemolytic streptococci. In analyzing the adequacy and inadequacy of the vitamin C in the diet, it was noted that no great difference was found in the three groups.

A similar analysis of Chart 5 shows that in the lower third of vitamin C blood values, 55 per cent of the tonsils showed evidence of hemolytic streptococci while in the upper third only 10 per cent of the tonsils showed evidence of streptococci infection. The adequacy of the vitamin C in the diet was noted with equal frequency in all three groups.

It appears from these observations that apparently healthy children, some of whom are receiving an adequate ration of vitamin C in their diet while others are not, have a considerable range of storage of vitamin C both in the blood and in the tonsillar tissue. There is a significant difference in the percentage of hemolytic streptococci found in the tonsils in these children. Based on the vitamin C content of the blood it is evident that hemolytic streptococci were found five times as often where the blood values were 0.7 mg. per cent or less, than when the blood values were 0.85 mg. per cent or more.

In order to more accurately determine if there is any significant difference in the incidence of hemolytic streptococci in the tonsils when there is a variation in the vitamin C of the blood and the tonsils further

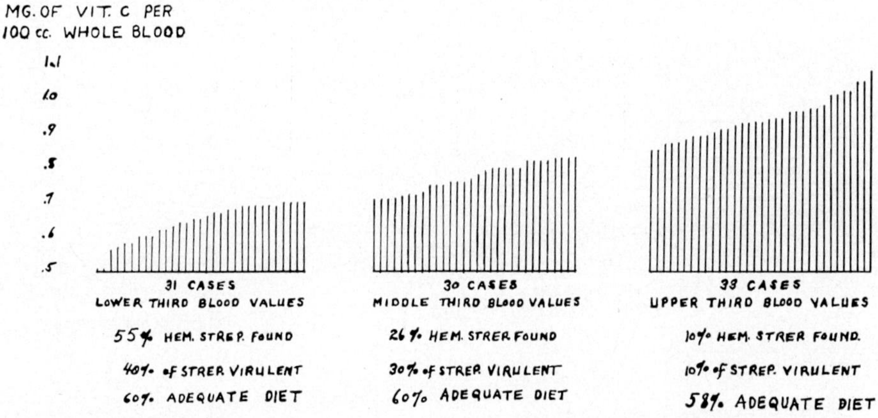

Chart 5.—Incidence of hemolytic streptococci and their virulence found in the tonsils of 94 children, based upon the vitamin C content of the blood of these children.

analyses were made. The entire group of 123 children was utilized. The mean values and the reliability of this mean were ascertained utilizing σ, the standard deviation; $\frac{100\ \sigma}{m}$, the coefficient of variability, and ϵ, the probable error of the mean.

TABLE II

COMPARISON OF THE GROUPS WITH AND WITHOUT HEMOLYTIC STREPTOCOCCI IN THE TONSILS

VITAMIN C. OF TONSILS	NUMBER	MEAN	σ	ϵ	$\frac{100\ \sigma}{m}$
No streptococci	77	34.32	7.78	0.604	22.7
Streptococci	46	30.44	7.49	0.754	24.6

Difference of means: 3.88 ± 0.965 – significant.

VITAMIN C. OF BLOOD	NUMBER	MEAN	σ	ϵ	$\frac{100\ \sigma}{m}$
No streptococci	77	0.8201	0.1328	0.0103	16.2
Streptococci	46	0.7544	0.1445	0.01452	19.1

Difference of means: 0.0657 ± 0.0178 – significant.

It appears from these calculations that the vitamin C content of the blood and of the tonsil is significantly lower in children whose tonsils contain hemolytic streptococci than in those whose tonsils do not contain hemolytic streptococci.

It is also possible to divide the observations into four groups: Those with vitamin C of blood and of tonsils both below the mean; those with vitamin C of blood and of tonsils both above the mean; those with vitamin C of blood above and vitamin C of tonsils below the mean; and those with vitamin C of blood below and vitamin C of tonsils above the mean. When this is done for the groups with and for those without streptococci in the tonsils, the diagram of Fig. 1 results.

PER CENT INFECTED

Blood ↑		
high	37.7	21.1
low	53.2	41.7
→ tonsils	low	high

Also, the correlation coefficient, r, between the vitamin C of the tonsils and the vitamin C of the blood was determined: In cases without streptococci in the tonsil, $r = 0.197 \pm 0.0739$; in cases with streptococci in the tonsil, $r = -0.0217 \pm 0.0995$. Only the former is significant.

In the case of determining the adequacy of vitamin C in the diet, it was found difficult to know when a child was receiving an inadequate amount. Inasmuch as the chief source for these children is from the citrus fruits, tomato juice and pineapple juice, the determinations were made on the parents' response as to the daily or periodic ingestion of one or more of these sources. No accurate information was obtained as to the diet of these children other than that of the fruit or vegetable juices mentioned. Based on this incomplete dietary information, no relationship could be found between low vitamin C values and an adequate vitamin C intake.

The significance of finding hemolytic streptococci in the tonsils is not clear. In the majority of the children in whom the organisms were found, no recognizable symptoms were present. An effort was made to determine the degree of virulence of these streptococci. Intraperitoneal injections of mice were made. Using control mice it was felt that some estimate of the virulence of the streptococci could be determined. An analysis of the virulence tests shows that 40 per cent of the streptococci found in the tonsils of children that had the lowest values of vitamin C were virulent; 30 per cent were virulent where the vitamin C values were average and only 10 per cent were virulent where the vitamin C values were above average. These findings suggest that not only are streptococci less likely to be found in tonsils where the blood values are high but if they are present, they are seldom virulent.

A clinical history of the children was tabulated to determine if the children harboring streptococci in the tonsils were more liable to upper respiratory infections than those whose tonsils did not show the presence of hemolytic streptococci. A few of the 96 children had been operated on for nine months, but most of them for less than six months. Such a period is obviously too short to observe the clinical course of these children. A number of the children have had attacks of sore throat, adenitis, and ear infections. Most of them showed streptococci in the tonsils. It is obviously unfair to pass any opinion on so few cases observed over such a short period of time.

Dick tests were performed on all of these children to determine if a positive Dick test was present more frequently in children with hemolytic streptococci in the tonsils and with low vitamin C values in the blood. No significant relationship could be found between a positive Dick test and the presence or absence of hemolytic streptococci in the tonsils, nor was any relationship noted in the cases of low vitamin C content of the blood in these children.

DISCUSSION

The various clinical reports on the influence of vitamin C on infections, notably rheumatic fever and tuberculosis, suggest that there might be some inhibitory influence of ascorbic acid on certain organisms. Before studying this relationship in the human body a series of experiments was undertaken to show the effect of vitamin C on certain organisms in vitro. The inhibitory effect of various dilutions of ascorbic acid was studied in the case of hemolytic streptococci, pneumococci, staphylococci, typhoid bacilli, coli bacilli, pertussis bacilli, and influenzae bacilli. It was found that the groups of virulent hemolytic streptococci were completely inhibited in twenty-one consecutive experiments, while in all instances the controls grew freely. Similar results were obtained using pneumococci and pertussis bacilli and influenzae bacilli. In the case of the coli bacillus, typhoid bacillus and staphylococcus, no inhibition was obtained. To obtain these results it was necessary to maintain a pH of from 3.4 to 4 with a solution of ascorbic acid of 1-100. A less acid solution did not completely inhibit these organisms. Other acids such as hydrochloric acid and acetic acid in the same dilution were also employed. They rarely inhibited the growth of hemolytic streptococci in vitro. These experiments suggest that ascorbic acid in adequate amounts with a pH of 4 exercised a definite inhibitory effect on certain organisms, especially hemolytic streptococci. A series of experiments was also conducted in vivo to determine if various amounts of ascorbic acid protected laboratory mice from hemolytic streptococci infections. The experiments in mice that received intraperitoneal injections of a virulent strain of hemolytic streptococci were less conclusive, but a considerable number escaped death where vitamin C was injected simultaneously with the lethal dose of hemolytic streptococci.

These observations prepared us for a study of the hemolytic streptococci found in the substance of the tonsils of children. It was not surprising, therefore, to find a higher incidence of streptococci in the tonsils of such children who showed low values of vitamin C or ascorbic acid in the blood.

If we can assume, as has been suggested by some authors, notably Abt, Farmer and Epstein,[4] that the vitamin C content of the blood is an index to the amount of vitamin C stored in the tissues, there should be some relationship to the ability of hemolytic streptococci to live in tissues where varying amounts of vitamin C are found. The tonsils were known to be well supplied with vitamin C, as has been shown by Clayton and Keith.[6] The amount of vitamin C found in the tonsils compares favorably with the amounts found in the adrenals and in the liver. Frequently, as is shown in our studies, the vitamin C content of the blood and of the tonsils bears a parallel relationship, though there are some variations which cannot be explained. The incidence of hemolytic streptococci in the freshly operated tonsils is definitely higher in the individual in whom the content of the vitamin C is low in the blood and in the tonsils, and it is low in such children where the vitamin C of the blood and the tonsils registers higher values. Inasmuch as the study of the streptococci was made from operated tonsils, no further study could be made of the lymphoid tissue even after the child had been saturated with vitamin C. Such studies would be helpful if an increase in the blood values of vitamin C would bring about a diminution in the number of hemolytic streptococci in the tonsils. The evidence at hand suggests that an adequate amount of vitamin C in the blood influences the incidence of hemolytic streptococci found in the tonsils. However, it is also possible that infection of the tonsil causes a lowering of the vitamin C content. Insufficient evidence is at hand to venture the opinion that when the amount of vitamin C falls below a certain level in the blood the individual is more liable to become infected with hemolytic streptococci. Other factors undoubtedly play a part in this mechanism.

The amount of vitamin C found in human blood is probably determined by the amount of this vitamin obtainable from certain foods. The daily ingestion of a reasonable amount of orange juice does not assure a high level of vitamin C in the blood in all instances according to the data obtained in this group of children. On the other hand, where generous amounts of vitamin C are taken daily in the form of orange juice, tomato juice, or pineapple juice, the vitamin C blood levels are uniformly high or in the average zone. It would seem therefore that the metabolism of vitamin C varies in children. This is known to be the case in the presence of infection and may be so in the absence of infection. The definite evidence of finding fewer hemolytic streptococci in the tonsils of children with average or better than average vitamin C content suggests an inhibitory relationship in the human body. Certainly from the clinical point of view it is desirable to supply the children with more than the minimum amount of vitamin C in their diets.

REFERENCES

1. Rinehart, J. F., and Mettier, S. R.: Am. J. Path. **10**: 61, 1934.
2. Abbasy, M. A., Hill, N. G., and Harris, L. J.: Special article, Lancet **2**: 1413, 1936.
3. Sendroy, Julius, Jr., and Schultz, Mark P.: J. Clin. Investigation **15**: 369, 1936.
4. Abt, Arthur F., Farmer, Chester J., and Epstein, I. M.: J. PEDIAT. **8**: 1, 1936.
5. Stephens, D. J., and Hawley, E. E.: J. Biol. Chem. **115**: 653, 1936.
6. Clayton, Mary M., and Keith, John D.: Science **84**: 377, 1936.

16 NORTH GOODMAN STREET

VITAMIN C IN TUBERCULOSIS

The Effect of Supplementary Synthetic Vitamin C on the Urinary Output of This Vitamin by Tuberculous Children

T. S. Bumbalo, M.D., and W. W. Jetter, M.D.
Buffalo, N. Y.

IN A recent publication[1] the authors observed the constant occurrence of hypovitaminosis C in active tuberculosis in children, determined by the subnormal excretion of the vitamin in the urine. In the study of thirty-seven cases in the Buffalo City Hospital an average excretion of 5.7 mg. per twenty-four hours was noted (reducing power as determined by the dichlorophenol indophenol method) on a daily ration of 55 to 65 mg. of vitamin C, whereas twenty-five normal, healthy children on approximately the same diet averaged 29.2 mg. per twenty-four hours. The present study was conducted to determine the approximate number of milligrams of synthetic vitamin C required to establish and maintain normal excretory levels of the vitamin in these tuberculous children.

METHOD

A group of ten tuberculous children taken from the larger group previously reported was selected. The diet for these children, considered to be high in vitamin C, contained approximately 55 to 65 mg. daily. Following a period to determine the basic vitamin C elimination level, 50 mg. of synthetic vitamin C in tablet form were added to the daily diet until normal excretory levels were established and maintained. A single case was then observed daily after discontinuance of the added vitamin, the diet returning to the basic intake of 55 to 65 mg. daily. Also, the urinary vitamin C output of the other nine patients was determined two weeks after discontinuance.

As a control the basic vitamin C elimination level of six normal, healthy children in middle-class American homes was established. As far as could be ascertained these children had an average vitamin C intake comparable to that of the tuberculous group, namely 55 to 65 mg. daily. Subsequently the diet of this group was also augmented by the same 50 mg. synthetic vitamin C tablet until the maximal increase in urinary output was obtained. The supplementary vitamin was then discontinued, and the results noted. The chemical technique used for the determination of vitamin C in urine was a modification of the dichlorophenol indophenol method of Harris and Ray, as previously described.[1]

From the Departments of Pediatrics and Pathology of the Buffalo City Hospital and the University of Buffalo Medical School.

CLINICAL MATERIAL

All ten of the tuberculous children had pulmonary involvement, cavitation being present in seven patients and a positive sputum in six.

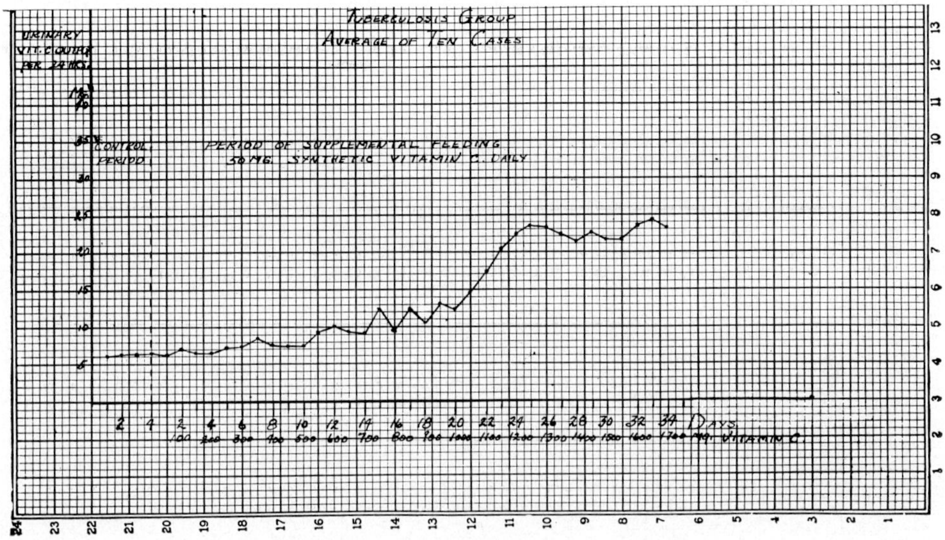

Fig. 1A.

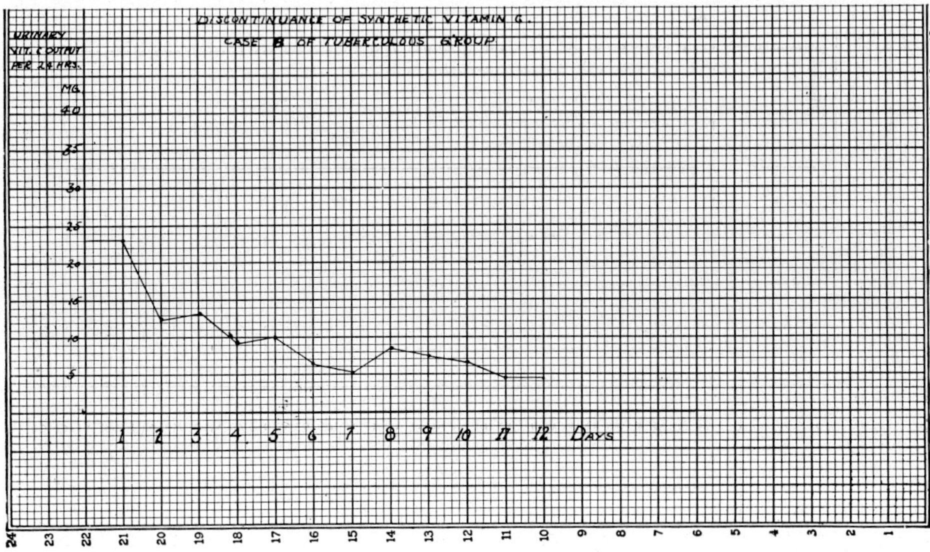

Fig. 1B.

Two showed associated involvement of the spine. The nutrition was considered poor in two cases and fair in eight. Eight were bed patients, and the other two were partially ambulatory.

TABLE I

TUBERCULOUS GROUP

DAYS	MG. FED	MILLIGRAMS EXCRETED PER 24 HOURS										AVERAGE
		CASE 1	CASE 2	CASE 3	CASE 4	CASE 5	CASE 6	CASE 7	CASE 8	CASE 9	CASE 10	
Control Period												
1		0.5	1.9	6.8	6.7	8.0	5.5	5.5	7.1	6.1	8.1	6.12
2		5.5	2.1	9.7	2.4	10.1	6.5	6.5	7.2	7.2	5.1	6.23
3		7.2	9.7	6.5	2.7	6.9	4.5	6.2	7.4	3.4	8.3	6.28
4		6.4	6.8	9.5	6.6	6.5	6.8	5.3	6.1	5.5	7.2	6.67
Period of Supplementary Feeding of 50 Mg. Daily of Synthetic Vitamin C												
1	50	8.1	5.2	7.5	5.2	5.6	6.4	6.8	6.0	6.5	6.1	6.34
2	100	5.8	7.4	8.2	6.5	6.5	7.2	7.2	7.5	7.9	8.5	7.07
3	150	6.4	6.8	9.5	5.2	8.4	5.9	5.9	8.2	8.3	3.8	6.84
4	200	7.2	5.2	6.5	8.4	3.9	8.7	7.5	5.5	6.4	9.5	6.88
5	250	6.1	3.1	5.6	9.5	8.5	9.2	8.2	8.3	8.3	6.8	7.36
6	300	6.5	4.8	9.5	8.6	4.2	6.4	9.1	9.1	9.4	7.2	7.48
7	350	3.0	8.5	10.1	6.9	6.5	10.1	6.8	7.2	9.5	9.3	8.79
8	400	6.8	9.2	8.2	7.8	10.4	9.3	7.5	6.8	8.4	4.9	7.93
9	450	7.5	6.5	5.4	6.5	10.1	8.4	8.2	6.5	3.9	6.8	7.98
10	500	5.5	8.8	6.9	5.2	9.5	6.1	6.8	7.5	9.5	7.1	7.29
11	550	8.3	7.2	6.3	9.0	15.8*	6.8	7.9	9.1	5.5	8.1	9.40
12	600	6.4	10.1	10.5	8.9	24.7	7.3	9.5	9.8	6.2	9.0	10.24
13	650	5.4	8.5	13.2	7.0	20.5	8.0	8.8	8.2	5.9	10.1	9.56
14	700	6.5	9.1	12.1	6.6	18.7	8.2	6.8	7.4	8.7	8.2	9.23
15	750	7.5	14.4	15.0	6.5	32.2	8.4	8.8	10.4	8.7	11.1	12.30
16	800	6.3	10.5	10.0	8.7	25.2	9.6	6.9	6.9	6.3	8.3	9.82
17	850	12.5*	24.0*	12.0	14.3	20.5	8.2	7.4	8.2	8.1	9.1	12.43
18	900	15.0	18.5	9.4	7.5	21.2	6.5	7.5	6.4	7.7	7.2	10.69
19	950	21.4	20.5	12.0	9.5	25.5	8.5	10.1	5.9	10.5	6.8	13.13
20	1000	22.4	19.5	16.0*	10.1	19.5	6.2	9.4	8.5	8.5	6.2	12.63
21	1050	25.5	17.5	18.0	10.8	25.2	9.5	11.5	10.1	12.5	9.2	14.98
22	1100	24.3	16.0	21.2	12.5	26.5	10.1	16.9*	19.5*	13.0	12.9	17.29
23	1150	21.4	20.1	20.0	15.5*	28.7	12.5	25.5	29.5	15.0*	18.1*	20.63
24	1200	28.7	16.8	72.5	20.1	30.1	15.5*	29.4	18.2	18.0	24.5	22.38
25	1250	27.2	18.0	20.5	18.2	27.2	17.5	35.5	28.5	21.5	19.9	23.40
26	1300	23.3	24.0	24.7	22.5	24.3	16.5	27.2	25.3	27.0	17.8	23.25
27	1350	19.5	18.7	17.0	19.5	21.2	20.4	25.2	30.1	18.5	18.5	22.86
28	1400	22.4	17.5	15.0	22.5	19.4	21.3	28.5	26.1	19.0	20.5	21.22
29	1450	25.4	21.2	21.0	19.6	30.5	18.7	30.1	20.5	16.5	23.8	22.73
30	1500	22.0	21.5	22.4	18.6	23.0	16.4	28.5	22.5	26.8	17.5	21.92
31	1550	25.2	27.6	28.3	21.5	19.5	19.3	25.2	19.8	13.2	19.8	21.94
32	1600	28.4	25.5	24.2	22.0	27.8	23.5	26.1	16.8	19.5	24.2	23.80
33	1650	21.5	27.5	25.0	27.0	20.4	20.4	22.2	24.8	23.5	19.8	24.41
34	1700	27.2	22.8	21.0	25.0	22.4	24.3	20.0	21.3	28.7	20.0	23.27

*Indicates day of significant rise.

RESULTS

In the tuberculous children the basic excretion on the diet of 55 to 65 mg. was 6.4 mg. per twenty-four hours as determined over a period of four days (Table I and Fig. 1*A*). In only one instance a result was found more than 10 mg. (10.1 mg. in Case 5 on the second day). Upon addition of the synthetic vitamin to the diet, an average total of 750 mg. over a period of fifteen days produced a rise in urinary output to levels slightly over 10 mg. per twenty-four hours and a total of 1,050 mg. in twenty-one days to 15 mg. per twenty-four hours. On the twenty-fourth day, after 1,200 mg. had been given, the average excretion had risen to 23 mg. per twenty-four hours. Continued feeding for another ten-day period showed a maintenance of this latter level, but there was no further rise. A typical case (Case 8) was studied after discontinuance of the supplementary vitamin. As shown in Fig. 1*B*, basic levels of 6 to 7 mg. per twenty-four hours occurred on the sixth day and were maintained for the remainder of the study, that is, eight more days. In only one instance (Case 5) was there considerable variation from the average.

TABLE II

NORMAL CONTROL GROUP

DAYS	MILLIGRAMS EXCRETED PER 24 HOURS						AVERAGE
	CASE 1	CASE 2	CASE 3	CASE 4	CASE 5	CASE 6	
Control Period							
1	54.0	36.0	18.5	37.0	30.5	31.5	34.6
2	58.0	24.0	20.5	33.0	31.0	34.0	34.6
3	41.5	31.0	41.0	37.0	24.5	21.5	33.4
4	40.5	36.0	27.0	39.0	28.0	40.0	35.1
5	28.0	35.0	27.5	32.0	28.5	30.0	30.2
Period of Supplemental Feeding of 50 Mg. of Synthetic Vitamin C							
1	49.5	39.0	44.0	44.0	42.0	35.0	42.3
2	79.0	60.0	70.0	68.0	64.0	82.0	70.5
3	84.0	68.0	68.0	79.0	81.0	78.0	76.4
4	92.0	77.0	72.0	84.0	71.0	69.0	77.5
5	83.0	74.0	65.0	80.0	82.0	75.0	77.5
6	74.0	80.0	69.0	72.0	73.0	69.0	73.0
Period of Discontinuance of Synthetic Vitamin C							
1	64.0	58.0	50.0	59.0	68.0	54.0	58.8
2	56.0	43.5	39.0	35.0	38.0	24.0	35.9
3	30.0	42.0	32.5	32.0	38.0	30.0	34.2
4	35.0	38.0	36.0	37.0	49.0	28.0	37.2
5	38.0	30.0	29.0	30.0	25.0	35.0	31.2
6	38.0	24.0	30.0	35.0	31.0	32.0	31.7

In this case 600 mg. over a period of twelve days were sufficient to produce an output of 24 mg. per twenty-four hours, while the highest excretion was 32 mg. per twenty-four hours. This was clinically the least severe of all of the cases. In the other nine patients, all with severe involvement, little variation in response to supplementary feeding was noted.

In the healthy control patients, on approximately the same basic diet, a five-day preliminary examination to establish a base line (Fig. 2 and

Table II) showed an average excretory level of 30 to 35 mg. per twenty-four hours. Upon supplementary feeding of 50 mg. of the same synthetic vitamin daily, a sharp increase promptly resulted, averaging 70 mg. per twenty-four hours on the second day after a total of 100 mg. had been taken. The maximum of 77.5 mg. per twenty-four hours was noted on the fourth day, after which time continued feeding for two more days revealed a maintenance but no further increase in the excretion of vitamin C. Upon discontinuance of the supplementary vitamin, the urinary output fell rapidly, the previous basic level of 30 to 35 mg. per twenty-four hours being reached on the third day.

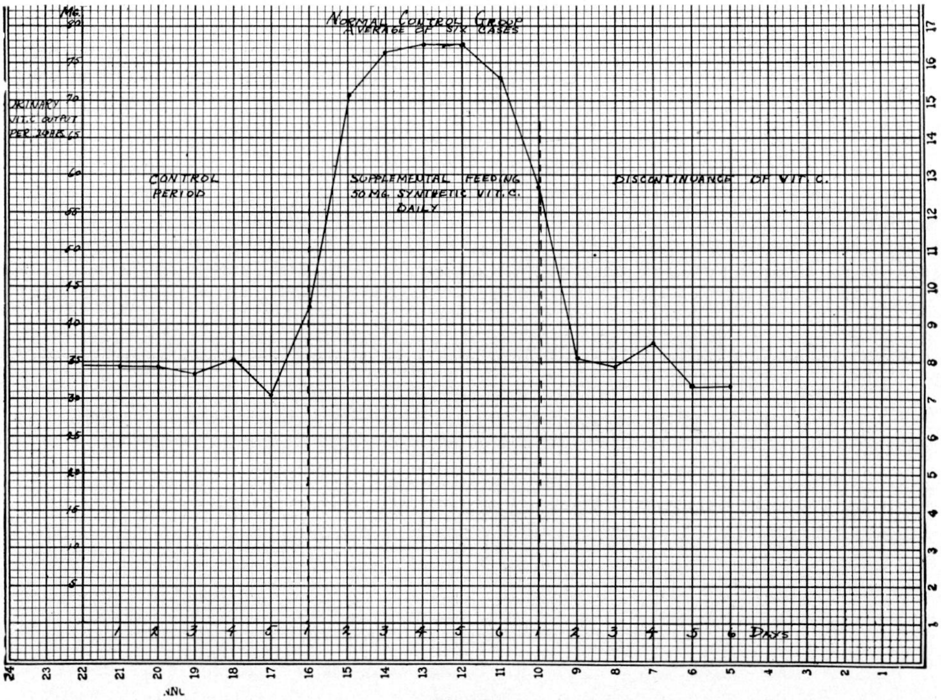

Fig. 2.

DISCUSSION

A comparison between the tuberculous and the control groups revealed certain significant differences. In the first place, the average basic level of the urinary excretion of vitamin C in the two groups varied considerably. The tuberculous group consistently excreted less than 10 mg. per twenty-four hours, the average of 6.4 mg. per twenty-four hours being below the accepted minimal normal levels of from 10 to 15 mg. per twenty-four hours.[2] On the other hand, the control groups of healthy children, with an average of 30 to 35 mg. per twenty-four hours, was definitely above this minimal normal level. As far as could be ascertained, the vitamin C intake of this latter group was approximately similar to that of the tuberculous group, showing that such a diet in a healthy child is adequate, but in one with a chronic infection, such as existed in the tuberculous group, it was insufficient.

Additional corroboration of the fact that the basic diet was adequate in the healthy children and inadequate in the tuberculous ones was offered by the results obtained from supplementary feeding of the vitamin. Additional feeding to the normal group resulted in a prompt rise of the vitamin excretion, with a maximal recovery of 84 per cent of the added vitamin. This would point to a ''spilling over'' of the excess vitamin into the urine, vitamin C being generally considered a threshold substance,[3] and would indicate saturation of the tissues. On the other hand, supplementary feeding did not cause a comparable rise in the tuberculous children. An average of 750 mg. in fifteen days was necessary to produce an excretion of 10 mg. per twenty-four hours and 1,050 mg. in twenty-one days for a level of 15 mg. per twenty-four hours. Thus, hypovitaminosis may be said to have existed in this group. Furthermore, assuming that vitamin C saturation of the body tissues was reached when the urinary excretion varied between 10 and 15 mg. per twenty-four hours, saturation could then be said to have been present in the tuberculous group somewhere between the fifteenth and twenty-first days. The average amount of vitamin C necessary to produce saturation could also be placed somewhere between 750 and 1,050 mg. Direct proof of saturation at this latter time might have been obtained by recovery, in high percentage similar to that found in the normal group, of an additional dose of vitamin C, for example, 100 mg. Unfortunately, this procedure was not performed. However, indirect proof was afforded by the comparatively sharp increase from 15 mg. per twenty-four hours to 23 mg. per twenty-four hours, which occurred from the twenty-first to the twenty-fourth day following continuation of the supplementary feeding. The less spectacular increase in the urinary excretion in the tuberculous group at this time, when compared to the normal group, could be explained by the hypothesis that nearly all of the supplementary vitamin was required for the maintenance of saturation. Further proof would seem afforded by the fact that continued feeding for another ten-day period (twenty-fourth to thirty-fourth day) showed no increase in the excretory level, indicating that the combined total of vitamin, namely 105 to 115 mg., was only slightly above the amount required for the maintenance of saturation in the tuberculous children.

Only one patient (Case 8) was studied following withdrawal of the supplementary vitamin. This patient showed a decline in excretion to the previous basic level, that is, 6 mg. per twenty-four hours in seven days. A check of the other nine patients, two weeks after discontinuance of supplementary vitamin, showed a similar return to the same basic level. This would seem additional proof of unsaturation.

As already mentioned, only one patient (Case 5) showed much variation from the average, requiring only 600 mg. per twenty-four hours to reach a urinary output of 24 mg. per twenty-four hours, while the highest excretion was 32 mg. per twenty-four hours. This patient showed clinically the least involvement of any of the tuberculous children. The other nine patients clinically exhibited a greater degree of involvement, but no significant variation in severity in any given case could be noted. On such a disproportionate division it is perhaps unwise to draw conclusions, but it would appear that increased demand for vitamin C was in direct relation to the severity of the tuberculous process. No attempt, in this study, has been made to evaluate the therapeutic effect of the production of vitamin C saturation in the tuberculous group because of the comparatively short period for observation. However, reports are to be noted in the literature[4] in which clinical improvement in the tuberculous process has been noted following augmented vitamin C intake. This would seem logical, as the tendency to hypovitaminosis in active tuberculosis appears pronounced.

SUMMARY AND CONCLUSIONS

A study comparing the vitamin C urinary excretion of a group of tuberculous and normal children, both on approximately the same basic vitamin C diet, that is, 55 to 65 mg. daily, was made, after which 50 mg. of synthetic vitamin C was added to the daily diet. An immediate rise was noted in the normal group, whereas the tuberculous group, in whom the average basic excretion was 6.4 mg. per twenty-four hours, required an average of 750 mg. in fifteen days to produce a rise in excretion to 10 mg. per twenty-four hours. The maximal output (23 mg. per twenty-four hours) was obtained on the twenty-fourth day after 1,200 mg. had been ingested. Subsequent feeding produced no further increase. Upon discontinuance of the added vitamin, the excretion of the tuberculous group promptly fell to the previous subnormal levels. This study points to hypovitaminosis C in active tuberculosis and suggests increased vitamin C intake as a therapeutic measure.

REFERENCES

1. Jetter, W. W., and Bumbalo, T. S.: Am. J. M. Sc. **195**: 362, 1938.
2. Abbasy, M. A., Hill, N. Gray, and Harris, Leslie J.: Lancet **2**: 1413, 1936; Harris, Leslie J., and Ray, S. N.: Lancet **1**: 71, 1936.
3. Faulkner, J. M., and Taylor, F. H. L.: J. Clin. Investigation **17**: 69, 1938.
4. Petter, Charles K.: Journal-Lancet **57**: 221, 1937; Radford, Molly, DeSavitsch, Eugene, and Sweany, Henry: Am. Rev. Tuberc. **35**: 784, 1937.

THE EVALUATION OF SEROLOGIC TESTS FOR CONGENITAL SYPHILIS

With Special Reference to the Neonatal Period

John A. V. Davies, M.D.
Boston, Mass.

THE recognition of congenital syphilis in the neonatal period often presents formidable difficulties. Definite clinical signs of syphilitic infection at birth are relatively rare. The longer the interval since the mother's infection (Kassowitz' law) and the more specific treatment she has received, the greater are her chances of giving birth to an apparently healthy infant. Treatment that is inadequate[1] may fail to protect the offspring and yet be sufficient to postpone and mask signs of infection in the newborn infant.

Some clinics rely, during the early months of infancy, on x-ray pictures of the long bones, but these often fail to reveal unequivocal signs of infection. McKelvey and Turner[2] found 69.3 per cent of the syphilitic infants in their series negative roentgenologically. If it were feasible to obtain films at frequent intervals, the number of cases of congenital syphilis discovered by this method undoubtedly would be higher. Pathognomonic changes shown in the films of the long bones of infants[3, 4] afford a sound basis for a positive diagnosis and are especially valuable in confirming a diagnosis based on clinical or serologic evidence. However, recent studies by Christie[5] point out pitfalls in the interpretation of films of the long bones.

Some of the traditional views regarding the reliability of serologic tests for syphilis in the newborn infant are in need of revision because, in many instances, these views are based on the results of tests which were relatively inefficient. True positive reactions were missed, and false positive reactions were relatively frequent. The recent evaluation of serodiagnostic tests for syphilis conducted under the auspices of the U. S. Public Health Service,[6] has brought into striking relief the wide differences in the efficiency of the participating laboratories.

A single qualitative blood test in the newborn infant, whether positive or negative, is by itself no criterion of the presence or absence of syphilitic infection. Recent workers[7, 8, 9] have suggested that a reaction in the blood of the newborn infant, which is quantitatively of higher titer than that of the mother, indicates actual syphilitic infection of the infant. Additional experience is desirable in order to confirm this impression. Even in the presence of a transmitted infection, many fac-

From the Departments of Pediatrics and Obstetrics, Harvard Medical School; the Wassermann Laboratory, Harvard Medical School; the Infants' and Children's Hospitals; and the Boston Lying-in Hospital, Boston, Mass.

tors, such as the immunologic immaturity[10, 11] of the infant, late intra-uterine infection, or treatment of the mother, may delay the production of sufficient syphilitic reagins in the blood of the newborn infant to be demonstrable by even the more sensitive tests. On the other hand, enough specific reagins may be transmitted from the serologically positive mother to give an uninfected infant a positive blood test (Fildes' law). The phenomenon of the passive transmission of antibodies and reagins in utero[12] is not unusual. To call this reaction a "false positive" is doing the test an injustice in most instances. A specific serologic test reports the presence or absence of syphilitic reagins and not the presence or absence of *Treponema pallidum.*

The importance of not making a diagnosis of congenital syphilis at birth on the basis of a single positive blood test is being recognized by an increasing number of physicians. Although the incidence of congenital syphilis is probably greater among the seropositive newborn infants than among the seronegative infants,[13] one would not be justified in making a diagnosis nor in starting treatment on the basis of this probability alone. Cregor and Dalton[14] found that if all the infants of syphilitic mothers in their series were treated, 91 per cent would be treated needlessly; and if all the newborn infants with a positive Wassermann reaction were treated, 69 per cent would be subjected to this procedure needlessly.

Using the Wassermann (complement fixation) reaction, Dunham,[7] Faber and Black,[8] and Christie[9] have titrated the specific serologic reactions in newborn infants over a period of weeks and months. According to them, a falling titer of syphilitic reagins presumably indicates a passively transferred reaction, whereas a reaction that is stronger than that of the mother at the time of delivery or one that increases progressively in titer indicates congenital syphilis. Christie extended the period of observation beyond that of Faber and Black and thereby was able to demonstrate that the mere decline or disappearance of a "pseudopositive" reaction does not prove that the infant has escaped the disease. A true positive reaction may be late in developing even though congenital infection is present. This time factor has been taken into account in evaluating the results of the neonatal serologic reactions in this study.

The purpose of this study was to follow the course of the serologic reactions of a series of infants born in 1935 and 1936 of syphilitic mothers. These infants were born in the Boston Lying-in Hospital, with the exception of a pair of twins who were admitted to the hospital soon after birth because of their small size. Although not all the infants of these mothers were brought to the attention of the investigators, eventually fifty-six were available for the survey. The first forty infants had been delivered at least twelve months, the next twelve infants from six to twelve months, and the last four from four to six months before the study closed. The final statistics were obtained May 1, 1937, four months after the last infant in the series was born.

The infants were given a careful physical examination at birth and on discharge from the maternity hospital, through the cooperation of the staff of the Boston Lying-in Hospital and the staff of the Infants' and Children's Hospitals. An attempt was made to secure a regular Hinton test for syphilis and x-ray films of the long bones within the first week after birth. Occasionally a cord blood specimen was sent to the Wassermann Laboratory for a Hinton and a Wassermann test. Placentas were examined by a competent pathologist, but no scrapings were made of the umbilical veins for *Treponema pallidum*.

Previous studies on the titration of the strength of the early positive reaction of infants born of syphilitic mothers[7, 8, 9] employed serial dilutions of serum obtained by venepuncture of the infant. In this study the strength of the serologic reactions of the infants was determined by the capillary Davies-Hinton test,[15] which is a micromodification of the Hinton flocculation test. This microtest requires merely 0.05 c.c. of serum, and the blood specimens were obtained by puncture of the infants' great toes. In an evaluation series conducted under the auspices of the U. S. Public Health Service in 1935,[6] this test attained a sensitivity of 91.9 per cent and a specificity* of 100 per cent. In the same series, the Hinton control test was rated 88.8 per cent sensitive, the Kahn control test 75.5 per cent, the Kline diagnostic control 88.8 per cent (and 99 per cent specific), and the Kolmer (complement fixation) Wassermann control 59 per cent sensitive. Because of the small amount of blood necessary for the test and the relative ease with which each specimen was obtained, it appeared feasible to take several samples of blood during the neonatal period. In most cases a similar test was made of the mother's capillary blood within a few days after delivery.

Although it is possible to titrate the strength of the capillary Hinton reaction by dilutions of the serum with Hinton-negative nonsyphilitic serum, the simpler routine capillary method was adopted. In this test the strength of the reaction is estimated in a mixture of equal parts of inactivated serum and Hinton antigen or indicator.† Thus no special dilutions were necessary. Experience enables one to estimate fairly

TABLE I

REACTION AT THE MENISCUS	RATING
Firm, cohesive disc or cone	4 plus
Disc easily broken into large and small aggregates	3 plus
Medium-sized, discrete aggregates	2 plus
Small, definite aggregates	1 plus
Negative	-

*Absence of false positive reactions.

†In actual practice a tube containing a mixture of one part serum to five parts Hinton antigen was also set up.

consistently the strength of the reaction at the meniscus in the tube after centrifugation. Designations which were used are given in Table I.

Ten newborn infants, aged 1 to 10 days, whose mothers had negative Hinton tests and were considered free from syphilis, served as controls. Their capillary Davies-Hinton tests were negative.

Congenital syphilis was detected in only one infant of the fifty-six in the series during the neonatal period. The baby was placed under treatment immediately and is now in excellent condition. The others were directed, upon discharge from the maternity hospital, to one of the Boston clinics or to their private physicians for suitable follow-up examinations.[16]

The plan adopted at the Infants' and Children's Hospitals was to examine each infant at the approximate ages of 6 weeks, 3 months, and 1 year. In special cases the intervals between visits were shortened. At each examination a blood specimen was taken for either a regular Hinton or a capillary Davies-Hinton test. X-ray films were ordered when serious doubt arose as to the condition of the child. Tables II, III, and IV summarize the results of the study. In spite of special efforts to secure the return of all the infants for periodic examinations, only twenty-two (including two that died of pneumonia) out of the forty who were born a year or more before the final statistics were obtained were considered to have satisfactory follow-up records. As the result of the first examination after discharge from the maternity hospital, a second infant (No. 55) was found to have syphilis.

Further studies with careful observation over a period of at least one year are necessary in order to determine the minimum length of time during which infants born of syphilitic mothers should receive periodic examinations in order to rule out the possibility of congenital infection. In this way only can the prognostic significance of early serologic tests be determined accurately. Most infants with congenital syphilis will probably develop positive blood tests by one of the more sensitive methods within four months after birth.[5] Infants and children with evident signs of syphilis are almost all serologically positive, according to Jeans and Cooke.[17] In order to rule out infection that is slow in developing it would seem that, in our present state of knowledge, infants of syphilitic mothers should be kept under observation for at least one year. At the end of this time they should be clinically and serologically free from all evidence of the disease.

It may be noted that the titer of the second specimen was sometimes higher than that of the first, particularly if the first specimen was taken shortly after birth. The cause of this preliminary rise is not clear. Some of these infants were moderately dehydrated at the time of the first test and had high hematocrit readings and icteric serum. In the single case of congenital syphilis detected during the first two weeks

TABLE II

INFANTS BORN CONSECUTIVELY AT LEAST ONE YEAR BEFORE CONCLUSION OF THE STUDY

NEONATAL BLOOD TESTS POSITIVE

	NEONATAL PERIOD															FOLLOW-UP PERIOD							MOTHER		
	CAPILLARY HINTON TESTS																								
SERIAL NUMBER	RESULT	DAY	RESULT	DAY	RESULT	DAY	RESULT	DAY	CORD HINTON	HINTON TEST	DAY	WASSERMANN	DAY	X-RAY OF L.B.	DAY	LAST POSITIVE	BLOOD TEST	FIRST NEGATIVE	BLOOD TEST	LAST NEGATIVE	BLOOD TEST	X-RAY NEGATIVE	SYPHILIS	CAPILLARY HINTON	REMARKS
122	-	3	-	7	+	11	+++	17						-	3	3m	*CH	7m	H	14m	CH	3m	A		Normal infant
7	++++	9	++++	11	+++	14								-	2								A	++++	No follow-up
13	++	9	++++	12						Pos.	12			+	11	3m	HW	8m	H	18m	H		A	++++	Congenital syphilis
12	++	1	+	4	-	5	-	12		-	5			-	1	4d	CH	5d	CH	1m	CH	1m	C	+++	Incomplete follow-up†
35	++	2	++	4	+	10	-	13		-	5			-	2	3m	H						A	++++	Congenital syphilis
21	++++	2												-	4	40d	*CH	8m	CH	18m	CH		A	++++	Normal infant (Col.)†
39	++	1	+++	2	+++	5	+	9		-	11	-	11			9d	CH	4m	CH	13m	CH		C	++++	Normal infant
J	+	3	+	4	-	7				-	3			-	3	4d	CH	7d	CH	8m	CH		A	+++	Incomplete follow-up
59	++	1	-	3	-	18			-					-	1	2d	CH	3d	CH	12m	CH		A	++++	Normal infant (Col.)
46	++	3	-	5					-	-	2	-	2	-	2	3d	CH	5d	CH	9m	H		A		Incomplete follow-up
71	+++	1	++++	2	+++	6	++	10		-	2	-	2	-	2	10d	CH	3m	H	3m	H	3m	C	++++	Died, pneumonia†
54	++	1	-	3					-	-	2			-	2	1d	CH	3d	CH	13m	CH		C?	++++	Normal infant
55	++	2	-	9						-	2	-	2	-	2	2d	CH	9d	CH	12m	CH	2m	C	+++	Normal infant
68	++	2	++++	6	-	9				-	10	-	2	-	5	6d	CH	9d	CH	14m	CH		C	++++	Normal infant
76	+	1	-	4	+	11						-	5	-	1	11d	CH						A	++++	No follow-up
I	++	1	++	5	+	8				-	1	-	1	-	2	8d	CH	50d	CH	6m	CH		A	++++	Incomplete follow-up
58	++	1	+++	7	-	12			-	-	2	-	2	-	2	7d	CH	12d	CH	5m	HW		A	++++	Incomplete follow-up
75	++	2	-	10	-	12								-	1	2d	CH	10d	CH	12d	CH		A	++++	No follow-up

H—Hinton test
W—Wassermann test
HW—Hinton and Wassermann tests
*2 plus reaction.
†Born one month before term.

CH—Capillary Hinton test
K—Kahn test
Day—Days after birth

L.B.—Long bones
m—Months after birth
d—Days after birth

A—Acquired syphilis
C—Congenital syphilis
- —Negative
Col.—Colored

of life (Table II, No. 13), the titer of the capillary reaction rose sharply to a maximum by the twelfth day, and the regular Hinton test and x-ray films of the long bones were also positive. The delayed rise in the titer of the first blood in the series (Table II, No. 122) cannot be attributed entirely to failure to inactivate the serum in the first two specimens nor to inexperience in making the readings.

Since the capillary Davies-Hinton readings were made under the low power of the microscope, it was possible to detect minimal reactions not visible to the naked eye in the regular Hinton test. Therefore, it is not surprising to find the Hinton tests negative in most of the infants, even in those whose capillary tests were positive.

Six infants in the series were colored, including a pair of dizygotic twins (Table III, No. 23a and 23b) whose blood tests were at all times negative. The other four colored infants gave early positive reactions (Table II, No. 21, 59 and Table IV, 101, and 106).

The two cases of congenital syphilis (Table II, No. 13 and 35) which were detected are instructive. They may be briefly summarized as follows:

Case 13.—A full-term infant, weighing 8 pounds and 4 ounces, appeared vigorous and free from stigmas of disease. The placenta was normal. The mother, aged 31, was a white, married, secundigravida who had had no treatment prior to this pregnancy. During the last two months of this pregnancy she received ten intravenous injections of an arsenical preparation. Her capillary ''Davies-Hinton'' test was 4 plus. The sibling was syphilitic. A capillary test of the infant obtained on the ninth day was 2 plus. Three days later it was 4 plus, and the regular Hinton test and x-ray films of the long bones were strongly positive. Hinton tests repeated when the infant was 17 days old, one month old, and at three months were all positive. This infant did well under specific treatment.

Case 35.—The infant was born by cesarean section four weeks after the calculated time at which it was due. Its weight was 4 pounds and 8 ounces, length, 19 in. There were no stigmas of syphilis. The placenta was normal. The mother, aged 25, was a white, married, secundigravida whose first pregnancy six years previously had terminated in a miscarriage at three months. She had had no treatment, with the exception of two intravenous injections of an arsenical preparation during the last two weeks of this pregnancy. Her capillary test was 4 plus. The infant gained slowly while in the maternity hospital. X-ray films of the long bones taken on the second day were equivocal. The Hinton test on the fifth day was negative. The capillary blood test on the second day was 2 plus, on the tenth day 1 plus, and on the thirteenth day, negative. When the infant was 14 weeks old the mother took it to the clinic where she was being treated. No record was kept at this clinic of the general condition of the child at this time, but the Hinton and Wassermann reactions were positive then and again a week later. No x-ray pictures were taken. A diagnosis of congenital syphilis was made, and the infant was placed under treatment at once. This case illustrates the fact that the mere ''washing out'' of the early transmitted reaction from the mother does not preclude syphilis in the infant.

A rough correlation between the strength of the serologic reactions of the mothers and the incidence of positive reactions in the infants during

TABLE III

INFANTS BORN CONSECUTIVELY AT LEAST ONE YEAR BEFORE CONCLUSION OF THE STUDY
NEONATAL BLOOD TESTS NEGATIVE

SERIAL NUMBER	NEONATAL PERIOD								FOLLOW-UP PERIOD							MOTHER		REMARKS
	CAPILLARY HINTON TESTS NEGATIVE DAYS AFTER BIRTH	CORD HINTON	HINTON	DAY	WASSERMANN	DAY	X-RAY L.B.	DAY	AGE	TEST NEGATIVE	AGE	TEST NEGATIVE	AGE	TEST NEGATIVE	X-RAY NEGATIVE	SYPHILIS	CAPILLARY HINTON	
H	6 8 11		-	16			-									A	++++	Died after 1 mo., pneumonia
15	1 5 9	-					-	3	2m	H	9m	CH	13m	CH		A	++	Normal infant
14	1 4 12		-	0			-	1	17m	CH						A	-	Normal infant
23a	1 4 12						-	1	3m	CH	12m	CH				A		Normal girl } Twins†
23b	1 4 12						-	1	3m	CH	12m	CH				A		Normal boy } (Col.)
30	3 6						-		9m	CH					9m	A	++++	Developed scurvy
29	8						-	4	8m	CH	19m	CH				?C		Normal infant
44	12	-					-	11	8m	CH						A	-	Care of private physician
28	3 7		-	3			-	4	2m	CH	2m	H	12m	CH		A	+++	Normal infant
19	1 4		-	2			-	4	5m	HW	8m	HW	14m	HW		A	+++	Normal infant
51	4 6						-	1								A	++++	No follow-up
34	2 4	-					-	3								A	+	No follow-up
50	3 6 11								1m	CH	6m	CH	17m	CH		A	+++	Normal infant
B	2 4 19 24						-	2								C	++++	No follow-up*
F	5 7						-	4	2m	CH	9m	CH	15m	CH	2m	C	++++	Normal infant
38	1 5						-									?C	++	Care of private physician
A	3 5		-	5	-	5			2m	CH						A	+++	Follow-up incomplete
E	1 4		-	2	-	2	-	1	3m	CH	9m	HWK				A	-	Apparently normal
45	2 6 16		-	1	-	1	-	1	44d	CH	5m	CH	16m	CH	44d	A	++++	Normal infant
69	4 11		-	2	-	2	-	1	1m	CH	5m	CH	13m	CH		A	+	Normal infant
60	1 7	-	-	1	-	1	-	1	7m	CH						A	++	Nutritional anemia
64	1 3	-	-	1			-	1	2m	CH	3m	CH	16m	CH		A	+++	Normal infant

*Born two months before term. Capillary Hinton test negative, 12/28/37.
†Born one month before term.
See Table II for legend.

TABLE IV

INFANTS BORN CONSECUTIVELY FOUR TO TWELVE MONTHS BEFORE CONCLUSION OF THE STUDY

	NEONATAL PERIOD															FOLLOW-UP PERIOD					MOTHER		
	CAPILLARY HINTON TESTS																						
SERIAL NUMBER	RESULT	DAY	RESULT	DAY	RESULT	DAY	RESULT	DAY	CORD HINTON	HINTON	DAY	WASSERMANN	DAY	X-RAY L.B.	DAY	AGE	TEST NEGATIVE	AGE	TEST NEGATIVE	X-RAY NEGATIVE	SYPHILIS	CAPILLARY HINTON	REMARKS
86	+++	2	+++	6						–	2	–	2	–	2						A	++++	Care of private physician
67	–	3	–	5						–	3	–	3	–	3	6m	H				A	+++	Apparently normal
70	–	1										–	2	–	0	6m	HWK				A		Apparently normal
85	–	1	–	6						–	1	–	1	–	1	7m	H			7m	A	+++	Apparently normal
97a	–	8	–	10										–		3m	H				?C		Twins, apparently normal
97b	–	8	–	10						–		–		–		3m	H				?C		
91	–	4	–	6						–	3	–	3	–	3						A	++++	Physical exam. neg. 11m
89	–	3	–	5						–	2	–	2	–	2	2m	HW				A	++++	Physical exam. neg. 4m
98	+++	2	–	5												4m	H			4m	A	++++	Apparently normal
100	++	6	++	9						Pos.	6	–	6	–	2	4m	H				A	++++	Apparently normal
102	+	8	+	11	++	22															A	++++	No follow-up in 6m
106	++	2	++	5						–	2	–	2	–	2						C	++++	No follow-up (Col.)
104	–	4	–	6						–	2	–	2	–	2	3m	H				A	++	Apparently normal
117	+++	3	+++	5	+	7	+	11 20		Pos.	1	Pos.	1	?	1	1m	CH	2m	CH		A	++++	HW positive on 7th day
109	–	2	–	5										–	2						A	+++	No follow-up in 4m
101	++	3	+	5	++	13	–	18		–	3			–	1						A	++++	No follow-up in 4 m (Col.)

*Born at home one month before term.
See Table II for legend.

the neonatal period was attempted (Table V). In both instances of congenital syphilis detected, the reaction in the serum of the mother was strongly positive (4 plus).

TABLE V

COMPARISON OF THE STRENGTH OF THE REACTION IN THE MOTHER'S BLOOD WITH THE NEONATAL REACTION IN THE INFANT (CAPILLARY "DAVIES-HINTON" TEST)

		MOTHER		
		4 PLUS	3 PLUS TO 1 PLUS	NEGATIVE
Infant	Positive	21	2	0
	Negative	8	15	3
	Total	29	17	3

From the foregoing study of the serologic reactions of a series of infants whose mothers have had syphilis, certain observations appear to be justified:

1. The stronger the positive reaction in the mother the greater the likelihood of a positive reaction in the newborn infant (Table V).

2. Although in most instances the transmitted positive reaction in the blood of the infants diminished or disappeared entirely within two weeks after birth, in one case (Table II, No. 122) it was detectable by the sensitive method employed for at least three months after birth and in another case (Table II, No. 21) for at least forty days. Both infants were kept under observation for more than one year and at the end of this time were discharged as nonsyphilitic.

3. In one case (Table II, No. 35) the transmitted positive reaction disappeared before the development by the syphilitic infant of specific reagins demonstrable in the blood.

4. Eleven infants whose neonatal blood tests were positive were followed clinically and serologically for six months or more. Two of these were recognized as having congenital syphilis. Nine were symptom-free at the end of one year.

5. Of the nineteen infants followed for at least six months, whose neonatal blood tests were consistently negative, none developed evidence of congenital syphilis. Twelve of these nineteen were followed for one year or more.

6. Employing a sensitive serologic test for syphilis, almost one-half (25 out of 56) of the infants in this series had positive neonatal blood tests, and yet congenital syphilis was detected in only two.

7. Seven infants born of mothers with congenital syphilis gave early positive serologic reactions. One died at 3 months of age, apparently nonsyphilitic; one was negative at 1 month of age and was not seen again; and one was not examined after leaving the maternity hospital. Four of the seven infants were kept under observation for over one year and at the last examination were clinically and serologically negative.

CONCLUSIONS

1. The results support Fildes' law that the neonatal positive reaction may simply reflect the existence of a positive reaction in the mother and is not of itself* a criterion of syphilitic infection of the infant nor an indication for treatment.

2. Infants born of syphilitic mothers whose neonatal blood tests are positive are more likely to develop evidence of congenital syphilis than those infants whose early blood tests are negative, and, therefore, the seropositive infants should be kept under particularly close observation.

3. The diminution in strength or the disappearance of the early positive reaction does not necessarily mean freedom from infection.

4. The age at which one should cease to discount the early positive reaction and at which a strongly and consistently positive reaction points to congenital syphilis is probably between 3 and 4 months after full-term birth.

5. The development of two or more strongly positive blood tests at any time after a negative test points strongly to actual infection and is an indication for energetic search for confirmatory evidence.

6. Unless a diagnosis of congenital syphilis has already been established, every infant born of a syphilitic mother should have periodic examinations, including efficient blood tests, for at least six months and preferably for one year.

SUMMARY

A series of fifty-six infants born of syphilitic mothers were studied by means of physical examinations and repeated "Davies-Hinton" micro-flocculation tests on serum obtained by skin puncture, together with x-ray films of the long bones and supplementary tests on blood obtained by venepuncture. An estimate of the strength of the reaction in the infant and in the mother was made. Twenty infants, including two in whom congenital syphilis was detected, were kept under observation for at least one year. Syphilis was recognized in one of these infants by serologic tests and x-ray films of the long bones before the development of outward evidence of the disease; in the other infant no physical signs were recorded. The length of time the transmitted positive reaction persists in the newborn infant and the apparent significance of a rising and a falling titer were noted. The study demonstrates the importance of a rigid follow-up system and lends support to the public health measures already being inaugurated.

Mrs. M. H. Walter and Mrs. R. S. Field were of great assistance in securing the return of the infants for follow-up examinations. Mrs. Walter helped prepare the material.

*A possible exception is a titer in excess of that of the mother, which may indicate syphilis in the infant.

REFERENCES

1. Cole, H. N., et al.: J. A. M. A. **106**: 464, 1936.
2. McKelvey, J. L., and Turner, T. B.: J. A. M. A. **102**: 503, 1934.
3. McLean, S.: Am. J. Dis. Child. **41**: 130, 363, 607, 887, 1128, 1411, 1931.
4. Vogt, E. C.: Am. J. Roentgenol. **26**: 96, 1931.
5. Christie, A.: Personal communication.
6. Parran, T., et al.: Ven. Dis. Inform. **18**: 4, 1937; Am. J. Pub. Health **27**: 15, 1937.
7. Dunham, E. C.: Am. J. Dis. Child. **43**: 317, 1932.
8. Faber, H. K., and Black, W. C.: Am. J. Dis. Child. **51**: 1257, 1936.
9. Christie, A. U.: Am. J. Dis. Child. **55**: 979, 1938.
10. Baumgartner, L.: Yale J. Biol. and Med. **6**: 403, 1934.
11. Davies, J. A. V.: J. Immunol. **33**: 1, 1937.
12. Cooke, J. V.: Am. Rev. Tuberc. **6**: 127, 1922.
13. McCord, J. R.: J. A. M. A. **105**: 89, 1935.
14. Cregor, F. W., and Dalton, J. E.: Arch. Dermat. & Syph. **35**: 580, 1937.
15. Davies, J. A. V.: J. Lab. & Clin. Med. **22**: 959, 1937; Ven. Dis. Inform. **18**: 187, 1937.
16. Caffey, J.: Congenital Syphilis. Nelson's Loose-Leaf Medicine. Vol. II, p. 330 D, 1937.
17. Jeans, P. C., and Cooke, J. V.: Am. J. Syph. **6**: 569, 1922.

101 Bay State Road

DIPHTHERITIC POLYNEURITIS

A Report of Nine Cases

Jay M. Arena, M.D., and Lester P. Rasmussen, M.D.
Durham, N. C.

During 1937 twenty-five children with diphtheria were admitted to Duke Hospital, nine of whom had polyneuritis due to their infection. A total of ninety-two cases of diphtheria had been admitted from 1930 to 1937, yet only five of these patients had postdiphtheritic paralysis.

It is generally stated that some form of neuritis develops in from 10 to 20 per cent of all cases of diphtheria. Paralysis may occur in treated cases of diphtheria as well as in those in which the nature of the throat infection has not been recognized. In treated cases, the earlier the antitoxin is given the less likelihood there is of paralysis developing. In Rolleston's large series,[1] only 3.6 per cent of the patients receiving antitoxin on the first day subsequently developed paralysis, whereas when antitoxin was not given until the third day, 21.4 per cent developed paralysis, and when specific therapy was delayed until the sixth day, 27.1 per cent developed some form of neuritis.

It seems to be well established that paralysis following diphtheria is due to the production of a neurotropic toxin which is absorbed by the blood stream and carried throughout the body. Walshe,[2] analyzing the mechanism of diphtheritic paralysis as a result of a study of wounds infected by the diphtheria bacillus, divided the neuritis into three groups: (1) the local, or regional, (2) the specific, and (3) the general. The local paralysis is well demonstrated by the involvement of the palate due to the direct action of the toxin. The paralysis of the ciliary muscle is called specific because it is peculiar to diphtheria and may occur even in the absence of general paralysis. Finally, generalized paralysis or polyneuritis is due to the presence of toxin in the blood stream. The investigations of Abel[3] on the pathways by which tetanus toxin reaches the nervous system would seem to apply with equal force to the diphtheritic toxin.

The sequence of the paralysis is quite uniform, the local, specific, and generalized type of paralysis following in the order named. The paralysis of the palate is usually the first and may be the only involvement. This is generally seen at the end of the second week of the illness, but

From the Department of Pediatrics, Duke University School of Medicine, and Duke Hospital.

may appear sooner. The later it appears, the less likely is the paralysis to be widespread. At about the same time, paralysis of the muscles of the pharynx and larynx may be noted. The ocular palsies appear about the third week, involving mainly the muscles of accommodation and less frequently the extraocular muscles. General paralysis rarely develops before the fifth week. Palsies of the lip or of the facial muscles and of the vesical and rectal sphincters may also occur at this period. These may be involved alone or in combination. Respiratory paralysis is seen late in the course of the disease and only in severe cases. It is due mainly to involvement of the phrenic nerves, although paralysis of the accessory muscles of respiration may also be a complicating factor. The deep reflexes, especially the knee jerks, are frequently abolished, even when the process is mild, but the superficial reflexes are retained, unless the neuritis is widespread.

Our patients were all seen late, and local as well as generalized paralysis had developed. Six of the nine children had such mild attacks of diphtheria that they were not recognized as such and therefore not treated. The three treated children received only 10,000 units of diphtheria antitoxin late in the course of the disease, one as late as the sixteenth day.

Of the nine children, three were referred to the hospital with a diagnosis of acute anterior poliomyelitis, two as having brain abscesses, and one with Bell's palsy; the remaining three were correctly diagnosed. Two of the nine children died with myocardial failure. Seven recovered in periods ranging from one to four months.

One child with a preceding history of membranous pharyngitis had only a facial paralysis and absent knee jerks; the child was referred to the clinic with a diagnosis of Bell's palsy. On investigating the ten cases of Bell's palsy on file in the record room it was interesting to note that all of them occurred during the months of November, December, and January—the diphtheria months. Perhaps on closer observation some of these palsies may have had a diphtheritic origin.

Seven of the nine patients still had positive culture for the Klebs-Löffler bacillus when admitted; unfortunately, virulence tests were not done. The Schick tests were uniformly negative. The spinal fluid findings on four patients were entirely normal. Six patients were studied electrocardiographically, but only one had any evidence of myocardial damage. This finding does not correspond with the results obtained by Burkhardt et al.[4] Sixty-five per cent of their large series of patients presenting electrocardiographic changes had peripheral nerve palsies of various degrees. The one child who had electrocardiographic changes died on the sixth hospital day. The only other fatality occurred in a boy with a generalized paralysis and physical signs of myocardial damage, who was moribund when admitted to the hospital and died soon afterwards.

As soon as the diagnosis was clarified, six of the patients received 10,000 to 20,000 units of diphtheria antitoxin without apparent benefit. The daily intravenous injection of 5 or 10 per cent glucose did not appear to influence the course of the disease. The weakened extremities were treated with heat, massage, and passive motion. Immobilization was necessary in only three cases. In the main, treatment consisted of complete bed rest, sedation, and gavage feedings if the pharyngeal paralysis was sufficient to interfere with swallowing. The Drinker respirator was lifesaving to the child with the complete respiratory paralysis, and because of the unusual features of this case it is reported in detail.

CASE REPORT

History.—B. M., a five-year-old white girl entered Duke Hospital on Feb. 26, 1937, because of weakness of the extremities of five weeks' duration. During the latter part of November, 1936, she developed sore throat, and a diagnosis of tonsillar diphtheria was made. She was given 10,000 units of diphtheria antitoxin and made what was apparently a complete recovery. On Jan. 15, 1937, she complained of being tired, lost her appetite, and became constipated. Two weeks later the parents noticed a definite weakness of the lower extremities which progressed to involve the upper extremities also. The past history was interesting in that the patient had been immunized one year previously against diphtheria.

Physical Examination revealed a well-developed, poorly-nourished 5-year-old girl who was lying quietly in bed. She was able to move only her left hand. Respirations were normal. Her voice was soft, but she spoke clearly and distinctly. The cervical and inguinal nodes were moderately enlarged. The pupils were equal and reacted well to light and accommodation. The tonsils were enlarged and hyperemic, and there was a mucopurulent discharge in the posterior pharynx. The heart and lungs were clinically negative. The upper extremities were extremely flaccid. She could extend her arms but could not flex them. There was limitation of both abduction and adduction, and she was able only slightly to flex and extend her fingers. Extension and flexion of the lower extremities were markedly limited. The periosteal radial reflexes were equal and active. No other reflexes could be obtained. The cranial nerves were intact except for the sixth (limitation of lateral deviation).

Laboratory Tests.—The blood count showed the following: Hb. 15 gm. (97 per cent, Sahli); red blood cells 4,940,000; white blood cells 6,100, with normal differential. Throat culture was negative for the Klebs-Löffler bacillus. Urinalysis and stool examination were both negative. Spinal fluid revealed normal cytology and dynamics. Glucose tolerance test was normal. Wassermann, Schick, and Tuberculin (0.1 mg. with old tuberculin) tests were negative.

Course.—The patient received 20,000 units of diphtheria antitoxin soon after admission, and 100 c.c. of 10 per cent glucose were given intravenously daily for the first nine days. There was no improvement following the above therapy. Two weeks after entering the hospital it was noted that the patient had developed a thoracic type of breathing. Fluoroscopic examination of the chest showed the lungs to be clear, but the diaphragms, which were smooth in outline, failed to move.

During the next eight days the involvement became more pronounced until on March 20, 1937, the respiratory distress became alarming and the patient was removed to the Johns Hopkins Hospital where she could be placed in a respirator. She remained in the respirator for two months, by which time the diaphragmatic paralysis

TABLE I

SUMMARY OF NINE CASES OF DIPHTHERITIC PARALYSIS

AGE	SEX	RACE	PRECEDING RESPIRATORY INFECTION	ANTITOXIN		THROAT CULTURE	SCHICK TEST	SPINAL FLUID	EKG	PARALYSIS AND COMMENT
				HOME	HOSPITAL					
6	M	W	Yes	0	10,000	Pos.	0	Neg.	Normal	Generalized muscular weakness, more marked on left. Apparent recovery by the end of three months.
1	F	W	No	0	10,000	Pos.	0	Neg.	--	Flaccid paralysis of the left leg. Improved over a period of two months.
7	M	W	Yes	Yes; 16th day; am't unknown	10,000	Pos.	0	--	Myocardial damage	5th, 7th, 9th, 11th, and 12th cranial nerve. Marked generalized weakness of muscles. Died on 6th hospital day.
10	M	W	Yes	0	0	Pos.	0	--	--	Bell's palsy with absent knee jerks. Recovery in three months.
4	M	W	Yes	0	10,000	Pos.	0	Neg.	Normal	Facial, laryngeal paralysis and generalized weakness, more marked on left, absent deep reflexes. Was considered to have brain abscess. Marked improvement in one month.
2	M	W	Yes	0	0	Pos.	--	--	--	Laryngeal, palatal, and generalized flaccid paralysis. Died soon after admission to the hospital.
3	M	W	Yes	0	0	Neg.	--	--	Normal	Palatal, facial, and generalized flaccid paralysis. Discharged day after admission against advice.
5	F	W	Yes	Yes; am't unknown	20,000	Neg.	0	Neg.	Normal	Facial, palatal, and diaphragmatic, with ascending paralysis of Landry type. Four months in respirator. Recovered.
4	M	W	Yes	Yes; 4 days after ill.	20,000	Pos.	0	--	Normal	Palatal, generalized flaccid paralysis which showed marked improvement in one month.

had cleared entirely. At the same time there was marked improvement of the paralysis of the extremities, and only a weakness of the dorsiflexors of the feet remained. When last heard from the patient had made a complete recovery.

CONCLUSION

1. Nine cases of diphtheritic paralysis occurring during the year 1937 are recorded.

2. The etiology, types, course, and treatment of diphtheritic paralysis are discussed.

REFERENCES

1. Rolleston, J. D.: Arch. Pediat. **30**: 335, 1913.
2. Walshe, F. R. M.: Quart. J. Med. **12**: 14, 1918.
3. Abel, J. J., Hampil, B., and Jonas, A. F.: Bull. Johns Hopkins Hosp. **57**: 343, 1935.
4. Burkhardt, E. A., Eggleston, C., and Smith, L. W.: Am. J. M. Sc. **195**: 301, 1938.

THE TREATMENT OF MENINGOCOCCUS MENINGITIS

Intraspinal Use of Antimeningococcus Serum at Bellevue Hospital, 1928 to 1936

Nils W. Bolduan, M.D.
Forest Hills, N. Y.

THE final test of any therapeutic procedure or substance is the benefit obtained by the patient, either in the saving of his life or in the rapidity of his convalescence from a serious disease. It is well known that meningococcus meningitis is just such a serious disease with a high case fatality rate and is attended by serious sequelae for those who survive. In the evaluation of its treatment several criteria are available, chief among which is the case fatality rate. Any form of treatment which can bring about a marked reduction in the rate in a large series of cases must be acknowledged as extremely desirable.

The purpose of this paper, dealing with the experience in the intraspinal use of antimeningococcus serum at Bellevue Hospital, is to demonstrate the value of such use as reflected in the course of the case fatality rate from 1928 through 1936. The results obtained will be seen to confirm the idea that the proper use of a potent antimeningococcus serum intraspinally is an adequate and valuable method of treatment. No attempt will be made to elucidate the nature of meningococcus meningitis; whether it is primarily a systemic disease with local manifestations in the nervous system or a local disease of the nervous system with systemic manifestations will not be discussed. However, since the pathologic changes occurring in acute meningococcus meningitis involve mainly the nervous system, and since the sequelae are most frequently manifestations of these changes (deafness, blindness, cerebral damage), treatment should be aimed at preventing their occurrence. This report is concerned with the treatment by intraspinal administration of a potent antimeningococcus serum.

Scope.—This study deals with the records of 191 patients from infancy to 12 years of age, admitted with meningococcus meningitis to the Children's Medical Service of Bellevue Hospital from 1928 through 1936. The data obtained from an analysis of the bedside records are presented in Tables I to V. Practically all the patients were seen or attended by one of the observers who contributed the summaries.

From the Department of Pediatrics, New York University and Children's Medical Service, Bellevue Hospital, N. Y.

This paper is based on summaries compiled by resident physicians on the Children's Medical Service: Dr. Julian Price, for the years 1912 to 1928, Dr. Norman Coward, 1928 to 1932, Dr. Dorothy Geib 1932 to 1935, and the writer, 1935 to 1936. Credit and thanks are due them for the excellency of their abstracts.

METHOD OF TREATMENT

During the years 1928 to 1932 the majority of the patients received serum intraspinally once every twenty-four hours, while from 1932 to 1936 serum was given intraspinally every twelve hours for the first few days. On admission to the hospital a patient suspected of having meningitis underwent lumbar puncture. If the spinal fluid was at all cloudy, as much of it as possible (usually 20 to 30 c.c.) was withdrawn, and 20 c.c. of antimeningococcus serum (prepared by the New York City or New York State Health Department) was allowed to run in by gravity. A specimen of the spinal fluid was examined for: cell count, sugar, protein, and organisms, by smear and culture.

The administration of serum intraspinally was continued at daily or twelve hour intervals until definite improvement was noted. The criteria for discontinuing serum therapy were as follows: (1) decrease of spinal fluid pleocytosis to about 500 cells or less; (2) normal or rapidly falling blood leucocytosis; (3) rising spinal fluid sugar; and (4) persistent negative spinal fluid culture.

From the practical standpoint it is well to emphasize the value of the first two laboratory factors in arriving at a decision. Both can be rapidly determined at the bedside, and it has been our experience that their answer is usually confirmed by the subsequent report of a negative culture and by the recovery of the patient. In our series of patients, if the above criteria had not been attained after four or five days of treatment, a change in the type of serum (from City to State or vice versa) was made, often with a happy outcome.

RESULTS

In the whole series of 191 patients on whom we are reporting there were forty-eight deaths, a *crude* case fatality rate of 25 per cent. This includes one patient who died of a secondary streptococcus meningitis and eighteen patients who received either no treatment at all (diagnosis post mortem) or who died within twelve hours of the initiation of therapy. In the group of 191 patients there were also some who were admitted with residual signs of a previously treated meningitis and who required no active specific therapy.

In all then, there were 169 patients treated, of whom twenty-nine died, a case fatality rate for the whole nine year period of 17 per cent. Before going on to a more detailed consideration of this rate, a brief summary of the more salient clinical features will be given.

Age Distribution.—A study of the age distribution (Table I) of the 191 patients shows that there were forty-one (22 per cent) less than 2 years old, seventy-three (38 per cent) more than 2 and under 7 years old, and seventy-seven (40 per cent) more than 7 and less than 12 years of age. In the years 1928 to 1929 there were relatively more infants, 25 per cent under 2 years of age, while in 1935 to 1936 about 16 per cent of the patients were in this age group. This change in age distribution from 1928 to 1936 has a definite bearing on a change in case fatality to be discussed later. That the disease tends to attack a somewhat older age group in more recent years has also been noted in New York City as a whole.

TABLE I

MENINGOCOCCUS MENINGITIS AT BELLEVUE HOSPITAL

		1928	1929	1930	1931	1932	1933	1934	1935	1936	Total
Number of cases		77	32	14	11	4	5	1	29	18	191
Number of cases treated		67	27	11	10	3	4	1	28	18	169
Males		29	17	7	7	1	1	1	21	9	93
Females		22	15	7	4	3	4	0	8	9	72
Less than 2 years old	cases	18	8	4	1	0	2	0	4	4	41
	deaths	15	2	2	1	0	1	0	1	0	22
2 years old and less than 7	cases	25	11	8	6	3	2	0	11	7	73
	deaths	6	3	1	1	2	0	0	1	2	16
7 years old and less than 12	cases	34	13	2	4	1	1	1	14	7	77
	deaths	7	2	0	0	0	0	1	0	0	10
Deaths, all cases		28	7	3	2	2	1	1	2	2	48
Deaths, in treated cases		18	4	1	1	1	0	1	1	2	29

Sex Distribution.—In the whole series there were 165 records on which sex was indicated, and from Table I we see that ninety-three (57 per cent) were males, and seventy-two (43 per cent) were females. This is in line with other studies showing a preponderance of males among the victims of the disease.

DURATION OF DISEASE ON ADMISSION AND INITIAL SYMPTOMS

From Table II we see that 133 (70 per cent) of the patients were admitted before the fourth day of illness. In the earlier years (1928 and 1929) this percentage is somewhat lower and in the later years (1935 and 1936) somewhat higher.

TABLE II

DURATION OF DISEASE ON ADMISSION

		1928	1929	1930	1931	1932	1933	1934	1935	1936	Total
Under 1 day	cases	30	11	4	4	1	2	0	14	6	72
	deaths	6	1	1	1	0	1	0	1	0	11
1 to 3 days	cases	21	8	5	5	2	1	1	9	9	61
	deaths	13	4	1	1	1	0	1	0	0	21
Over 3 days	cases	26	13	5	2	1	2	0	6	3	58
	deaths	9	2	1	0	1	0	0	1	2	16

The usual clinical features were noted: A rather abrupt onset with headache, vomiting, drowsiness, and nuchal stiffness were the outstanding signs and symptoms. A rash, usually petechial, occasionally purpuric, infrequently macular or morbilliform, was noted in ninety-seven or about 50 per cent of the patients. Among these ninety-seven patients there were twenty-five deaths. Among ninety-four patients without a rash there were twenty-three deaths. This confirmed our clinical impression that the presence of a rash is no indication of the severity of the disease. As a matter of fact, there was no definite sign, symptom, or group of signs or symptoms which helped in determining the prognosis when the patient was first seen. Some patients who looked very sick on admission recovered uneventfully, while others who seemed only moderately ill died.

TABLE III

		1928	1929	1930	1931	1932	1933	1934	1935	1936	Total
Rash on admission	cases	37	12	5	5	3	4	0	20	11	97
	deaths	12	4	1	1	2	1	0	2	2	25
Positive spinal fluid, culture or smear		60	24	8	5	3	5	1	24	16	146
Complications	eye	8	7	1	0	0	0	0	1	2	19
	ears	13	4	4	2	0	1	0	4	4	32
	joints	3	4	1	0	1	0	0	4	3	16

Complications.—From 35 to 40 per cent of the patients developed one or more complications. The more frequent complications encountered were arthritis, otitis media and mastoiditis, nerve deafness, ophthalmitis, and blindness (Table III).

Positive cultures.—The meningococcus was found in the spinal fluid by smear or culture in 146 (74 per cent) of the 191 cases studied. The remaining 26 per cent, with negative or doubtful smear or culture, showed either unequivocal clinical features or a rapid response to specific treatment, so that the diagnosis was not at all doubtful.

TABLE IV

TREATMENT

		1928	1929	1930	1931	1932	1933	1934	1935	1936	Total
Intraspinal administration	every 24 hr.	63	27	10	10	3	2	0	0	1	116
	every 12 hr.	4	0	1	0	0	2	1	28	17	53
One treatment or none		10	5	3	1	1	1	0	1	0	22
Intravenous serum	cases	10	3	2	1	0	2	1	21	8	48
	deaths	3	1	0	0	0	2	1	1	2	10
Average amount serum per patient (c.c.)		157	150	180	125	–	–	–	165	165	125-180
Serum sickness, cases		26	16	8	6	2	3	0	15	12	88

TREATMENT

Average Amount of Serum Used.—In 1928 and 1929 about 155 c.c. of serum were used per patient, and in 1935 and 1936 this average was 165 c.c.—a difference that is not remarkable. It shows that not much more serum needs to be used for each patient when treated twice daily than when treated only once.

Serum disease.—Serum disease as evidenced by an urticarial eruption, sometimes with fever and joint symptoms, was noted in about 48 per cent of the cases. No immediate anaphylactic severe or fatal serum reaction was noted. The serum disease usually occurred from four to seven days after initiation of treatment. A point to be noted here is the occasional difficulty of differentiating serum arthralgia from a complicating arthritis due to the meningococcus. The latter usually can be definitely established by aspiration.

Intravenous serum.—Of forty-eight patients between 1928 and 1936 who received serum by the intravenous as well as by the intraspinal route (usually 20 to 30 c.c. intravenously) ten (21 per cent) died. Among those who did not receive intravenous serum we find 143 patients with thirty-eight deaths, a case fatality of 26 per cent.

Case fatality.—During 1928 and 1929 and again during 1935 and 1936 the disease was prevalent in New York City in epidemic proportions. As a result these years give us an adequate number of cases for comparison of case fatality. From Table I we can abstract the following:

TABLE V

	1928-1929	1935-1936
Number of cases treated	94	46
Number of deaths	22	3
Case fatality	23%	7%

We believe that the case fatality for 1935 and 1936 of forty-six patients with but three deaths is ample confirmation of our faith in the orthodox method of therapy. At Post-Graduate Hospital Dr. Charles J. Leslie has noted correspondingly good results (personal communication).

TABLE VI

		1928*	1929-1932	1933-1937
Post-Graduate Hospital	cases	44	49	23
	deaths	14	12	3
Case fatality		32%	24%	13%
Bellevue Hospital	cases	67	51	51
	deaths	18	7	4
Case fatality		27%	14%	8%

*De Sanctis: Am. J. Dis. Child. 38: 730, 1929.

There was only one essential difference in the method of treatment at Bellevue Hospital from that at the Post-Graduate Hospital, namely, in the frequency of dosage. At Bellevue, in 1933 to 1936, the serum was given every twelve hours, while at the Post-Graduate Hospital the twenty-four-hour interval was employed. The sera used were the same in both hospitals, the hospitals drew patients from the same type of population, and the characteristics of the disease were the same in the two places.

Before taking the remarkable reduction in case fatality at Bellevue from 23 per cent to 7 per cent (Table V) at its face value, we should remember the influence of a greater proportion of infants in 1928 and 1929. Since the fatality rate in that age group was 68 per cent in those years, an unduly high figure, it is only fair to compare the older age groups without regarding the fatality in infants.

TABLE VII

CASE FATALITY IN AGE GROUP OF PATIENTS MORE THAN 2 YEARS OLD

	1928-1929	1935-1936
Cases	83	39
Deaths	18	3
Case Fatality	22%	8%

The difference between the two periods becomes slightly less when regarded from this standpoint.

A second factor to be noted in comparing 1928 and 1929 with 1935 and 1936 is the slightly longer duration of illness before diagnosis and treatment in 1928 and 1929. In those years 74 per cent of the patients received treatment before the fourth day of illness, while in 1935 and 1936 82 per cent of the patients were treated before the fourth day.

Both of these considerations modify the reduction in case fatality from 1928 and 1929 to 1935 and 1936 in the sense that it is somewhat smaller than would at first appear.

TABLE VIII

HOSPITAL STAY

	1928	1929	1930	1931	1932	1933	1934	1935	1936	Total
Less than 1 week, including deaths	21	8	2	1	1	1	0	3	1	38
1 week and less than 2	9	3	2	3	1	1	1	12	6	38
2 weeks and less than 4	28	13	7	6	2	2	0	9	9	76
Over 4 weeks	19	8	3	1	0	1	0	5	2	39

HOSPITAL STAY

During 1928 and 1929, of eighty patients who survived one week, sixty-eight (85 per cent) stayed longer than two weeks in the hospital. In 1935 and 1936, of forty-three patients who survived one week, only twenty-five or less than 60 per cent stayed longer than two weeks. In other words, in 1928 and 1929 less than two out of ten survivors left before the second week was over, while in 1935 and 1936 more than four out of ten left the hospital before their fourteenth hospital day.

DISCUSSION

In seeking a cause for the marked reduction in the case fatality rate and in the period of hospitalization from 1928 through 1936 in our series of patients, we felt at first that the twelve-hour interval of serum administration used in the latter years (1935 and 1936) was largely responsible. However, two other possibilities had to be considered, namely, a change in the virulence of the organism and an increase in the potency of the serum used.

For New York City as a whole the following figures were obtained from the New York City Health Department.

TABLE IX

MENINGOCOCCUS MENINGITIS, NEW YORK CITY

	1928	1929	1935	1936
Cases	1102	1000	529	538
Deaths	540	486	244	226
Case fatality	49%	49%	46%	42%

It seems fair to conclude that the organisms responsible for the 1935 and 1936 outbreak were quite as virulent as those in 1928 and 1929.

Since the reduction at Bellevue Hospital in the case fatality rate was paralleled, albeit at a somewhat higher level, by one at another hospital using the same type of sera, it is fair to conclude that a part of the reduction in case fatality must be ascribed to an increase in the potency of the sera used. Nevertheless, we still feel that the twelve-hour interval in dosage contributed in part to the reduction. This conclusion is based on a fatality rate at Bellevue Hospital about one-third lower than that at the Post-Graduate Hospital during a similar period.

SUMMARY

Our belief is that the intraspinal administration of a potent antimeningococcus serum every twelve hours for the first few days gives better results than when given at longer intervals. The case fatality rate is lower, the hospital stay is shortened, and the total amount of serum used is not much, if any, greater. Further reduction in case fatality is to be sought in earlier diagnosis and in the use of as potent a serum as can be manufactured. The reasons outlined in the beginning of this paper for intraspinal administration of antimeningococcus serum, rather than the intravenous use of antitoxin alone, we believe to be supported by our results.

GAUCHER'S DISEASE IN EARLY INFANCY

Review of Literature and Report of Case With Neurological Symptoms

Arturo J. Aballi, M.D., and Katsuji Kato, M.D.
Chicago, Ill.

In 1924 Reuben[39] called attention to the relative frequency of Gaucher's disease occurring in childhood, and in addition pointed out the relationship existing between age of onset and duration of the disease. Three years later Oberling and Woringer[33] reported on the outstanding difference between the manifestations of the disease in infancy, on the one hand, and in adults and older children, on the other. They observed four cases in infants occurring in the same family and all of which, in addition to the usual splenohepatomegaly, showed a remarkable neurological syndrome. Each of these four patients had a retraction of the head with rigidity of the neck, opisthotonus, spastic extremities, laryngeal spasms, dysphagia, trismus, strabismus, and a tendency to maintain the arms in certain positions for long periods of time. Three of these patients gave evidence of progressive loss of sensation and complete lack of interest in the environment. At autopsy of these cases pronounced changes were observed in the cerebral cortex, but the remaining portions of the brain were spared.

Prior to the appearance of the above mentioned case reports, Rusca,[41] Kraus,[23] Kohn,[22] Pick[34] and Nauwerck,[32] and Reber[36] had published cases in which this neurological syndrome existed to a greater or lesser extent, but upon which these observers placed no particular stress. Meyer,[29] collecting fourteen of such cases from the literature and adding one of his own, gave an elaborate description of the neurological picture which he considered to be a pseudobulbar syndrome. In this country, Hoffman and Makler[18] were the first to report a case of Gaucher's disease with neurological symptoms, but in some respects their case is exceptional. Winter[47] presented a fairly typical case of the disease, but he erroneously reported it as Niemann-Pick's disease. Rowland[40] gave a complete review of the subject and introduced the term "acute Gaucher's disease," by which term he excluded practically all except the neurological cases.

The present authors have collected from the literature a total of seventeen cases of Gaucher's disease occurring in infancy, and the predominating neurological symptoms of these cases are summarized in Table I. In addition to these, there are in the literature ten reported cases in which the onset of the disease had taken place during the first year of life but in which neurological manifestations were totally absent. With one exception these latter infants were past six months of age

TABLE I

CASES OF GAUCHER'S DISEASE WITH NEUROLOGICAL MANIFESTATIONS

AUTHOR (YEAR)	SEX	AGE OF ONSET	FIRST SEEN	AGE AT DEATH	FAMILY HISTORY	NEUROLOGICAL MANIFESTATIONS	SPLEEN	LIVER	HEMOGRAM AND BLOOD CHEMISTRY	OTHER FINDINGS
Rusca (1921)	M	6 mo.	11 mo.	12 mo.	–	Rigid neck; strabismus, hypotonia.	237 gm.	390 gm.	R.B.C. 3.10; Hb. 40% W.B.C. 10,000	Slight discoloration of skin; involvement of tracheobronchial, cervical, and inguinal nodes; femur and rib marrow affected.
Kraus 1921	F	6 mo.	7 mo.	12 mo.	–	Hypertonicity; convergent strabismus; mental retardation.	70 gm. To level of umbilicus	240 gm.		Premature; slight discoloration of the skin; mesenteric and peribronchial nodes affected.
Kohn (1921)	F	Since birth	9 mo.	9 mo.	–	Some neurological involvement.	310 gm.	–		
Pick-Nauwerck (1922)	M	–	8 mo.	8 mo.	–	Not mentioned.	80 gm.	Not enlarged		
Reber 1–(1924)	M	6 mo.	6 mo.	8 mo.	+	Neck rigidity; dysphagia; laryngeal spasm; hypertonicity; increased deep reflexes.	Markedly enlarged	Markedly enlarged		Diagnosis at autopsy; fever present.
Reber 2–(1924)	F	5 mo.	6 mo.	7 mo.	+	Neck rigidity; hypertonicity; increased deep reflexes; spasmodic cough unassociated with lung lesions.	Down to iliac crest	2 fingers below costal margin	R.B.C. 4.00; Hb. 62% W.B.C. 11,800	Pigmentation in spots over dorsum of fingers; febrile attacks.
Oberling-Woringer 1–(1927)	M	5 mo.	5 mo.	8 mo.	+	Opisthotonus; convergent strabismus; choking spells with convulsions; very marked apathy and sensory loss.				Abdomen prominent and indurated.

TABLE I—CONT'D

AUTHOR (YEAR)	SEX	AGE OF ONSET	FIRST SEEN	AGE AT DEATH	FAMILY HISTORY	NEUROLOGICAL MANIFESTATIONS	SPLEEN	LIVER	HEMOGRAM AND BLOOD CHEMISTRY	OTHER FINDINGS
Oberling-Woringer 2–(1927)	F	6 wk.	5 mo.	11 mo.	+	Strabismus; catatonia; apathy; dysphagia; laryngeal spasm; opisthotonus; marked hypertonicity; increased deep reflexes; trismus; mental and physical retardation.	To pelvis	To right iliac crest	R.B.C. 5.19	Slight cervical lymphadenopathy; sudden death; symptoms progressed in spite of antisyphilitic treatment
Oberling-Woringer 3–(1927)	F	6 wk.	5 mo.	11.5 mo.	+	Opisthotonus; laryngeal spasm; very marked hypertonicity; apathy; poverty of movements; trismus; convergent strabismus; increased deep reflexes; clonic convulsions; dysphagia; sensory loss.	1 finger above pubis	2½ fingers below costal margin	R.B.C. 4.40; Hb. 54%; W.B.C. 6,300; platelets 66,500.	Apparent death from asphyxia on several occasions; pallor.
Oberling-Woringer 4–(1927)	M	4 wk.	1 mo.	1 mo.	+	Apathy and poverty of movement.	Slightly enlarged	Enlarged	R.B.C. 4.35; Hb. 75%; W.B.C. 5,700	Marked pallor
Dienst-Hamperl (1927)	F	2 mo.	3 mo.	5 mo.	+	Opisthotonus; strabismus; hypertonicity; laryngeal spasms.	2 fingers below costal margin	3 fingers below costal margin	Hb. 50 %; increased urobilin in urine; cholesterol, 240.	Yellow discoloration of skin; diaphragmatic breathing; reported as Niemann-Pick's disease by Dienst; autopsy by Hamperl demonstrated Gaucher cells; sister of Stransky's patient.
Hoffman-Makler (1929)	M	–	17 mo.	17.5 mo.	–	Neck rigidity; hypertonic extremities; increased reflexes.	To umbilicus	Below umbilicus	R.B.C. 4.00; Hb. 70%; W.B.C. 26,000; cholesterol, 80; total fat 349.	Generalized lymphadenopathy; diagnosis by biopsy of lymph node.

TABLE I—CONT'D

Stransky (1930)	M	4 mo.	5 mo.	6 mo.	+	Opisthotonus; hypertonicity; stridulous breathing; stupor.	To iliac crest	3 fingers below costal margin	Phosphatides 9.5; R.B.C. 2.40; Hb. 58%; cholesterol, 135.	Continuous fever; brownish yellow tint of face.
Moncrief (1930)	M	10 wk.	10 wk.	4 mo.	–	Opisthotonus; hyperactive deep reflexes.	2 fingers below costal margin	Not enlarged		Examination of liver showed Gaucher cells despite absence of enlargement.
Meyer (1932)	F	6 mo.	7 mo.	9.5 mo.	–	Dysphagia; opisthotonus; convergent strabismus; laryngeal spasms; catatonia; poverty and slowness of movement; hemiplegia.	2 fingers below costal margin	2 fingers below costal margin	R.B.C. 3.00; Hb. 62%; W.B.C. 9,400; platelets, 80,000.	Febrile attacks; clinical diagnosis confirmed by splenic puncture.
Winter (1932)	F	3 mo.	4 mo.	8 mo.	+	Unable to look to one side (left); unable to take feedings; opisthotonus; hypertonicity.	3 cm. below costal margin	2 cm. below costal margin	R.B.C. 4.00; Hb. 80%; W.B.C. 7,600; platelets 80,000	Splenic puncture showed Gaucher cells, but case reported as Niemann-Pick's disease.
Meyer (1934)	F	4 mo.	4 mo.	7.5 mo.	+	Opisthotonus; rigidity of neck; poverty and slowness of movement; strabismus; catatonia; laryngeal spasms.	2 cm. above iliac crest	3 cm. below costal margin		Fifth member of family studied by Woringer and Oberling.
Authors (observed in 1937)	F	1 wk.	2.5 mo.	4.5 mo.	–	Opisthotonus; neck rigidity; hypertonicity; strabismus; dysphagia; laryngeal spasms; catatonia of extremities.	To iliac crest	3 cm. below costal margin	R.B.C. 4.85; Hb. 65%; W.B.C. 11,600; cholesterol, 129.	Cervical lymphadenopathy; discoloration of skin; febrile attacks; clinical diagnosis confirmed by finding Gaucher cells in sternal marrow material.

when the first symptoms appeared, in contrast to the group displaying neurological symptoms and wherein the onset occurred in the first half year of life. In both groups, however, the course was rapid with fatal termination. The salient features of the cases occurring under six months are summarized in Table II. The nature of the case here reported establishes it as belonging to the group of Gaucher's disease indicated in Table I.

REPORT OF CASE

C. R., a white female infant, was born at term of a low forceps delivery at the Chicago Lying-In Hospital on Dec. 13, 1936. She appeared normal at birth, weighed 3,015 gm. and measured 50 cm. in length. Both parents were American born, non-Semitic, and in good health except for a history of renal glycosuria on the part of the mother. There had been no other children and no miscarriages nor stillbirths. There was no family history of deaths from splenomegaly with neurological signs in the first year of life.

The baby did well in the hospital and was discharged on Dec. 22, 1936, weighing 3,250 gm. Shortly after she was taken home, the parents noticed that she tended to keep her neck retracted and had a slight squint. She continued to gain weight, however, and at the age of 2 months, up to which time she had been breast fed, weighed 5,000 gm. Towards the early part of the third month, after she had been weaned because of insufficient breast milk, the infant began to take feedings poorly; the amount taken at each feeding decreased to about 2.5 oz. whereas previously she had taken 5 to 6 oz. At times she choked and had attacks of difficult breathing unassociated with intake of food.

On Mar. 2, 1937, the baby was brought to the Infant Welfare Clinic of the Bobs Roberts Hospital because of a cold, difficulty in feeding, and constipation. The parents also inquired as to the strabismus and the tendency to keep the head retracted. Examination showed pallor, a slight strabismus, and a palpable spleen (one to two fingers below the costal margin). No definite neurological manifestations were observed. The weight was 4,300 gm. The blood examination revealed the hemoglobin to be 40 per cent (Sahli), leucocytes 5,300 with a differential picture of 19 per cent neutrophils, 72 per cent lymphocytes, 7 per cent monocytes, and 2 per cent eosinophils. The urine was negative. The child was given iron for the anemia, steam inhalation and nasal drops, and the formula was changed. The patient returned on April 10, 1937, unimproved, with a definite retraction of the neck and opisthotonus. She looked pale and showed a pronounced convergent strabismus. The spleen was very large and the liver also palpable (two fingers below the costal margin). Hospital admission was advised.

Physical Examination.—On admission (April 13, 1937) the patient was found to be an undernourished white female infant weighing 3,900 gm. and with a tendency to keep the head retracted and the back arched in opisthotonus (Fig. 1*B*). It is noteworthy that the neck could be bent forward without difficulty. The arms were elevated to the level of the shoulder with flexion at the elbow and adduction, so that the hands fell into position over the lower part of the face (Fig. 1*A*). The legs were in a position of flexion. The infant tended to maintain these positions for long periods of time. She did not appear acutely ill, and the temperature was entirely normal. The skin had a pasty pallor; there were no eruptions or desquamations. The head measured 38 cm. in circumference. The anterior fontanel was open (2 by 3 cm.), and there was no separation of the cranial sutures. The ears were negative. Examination of the eyes showed a convergent strabismus with a rapid fine nystagmus. The pupils reacted well to light and the fundi were normal. The child appeared to perceive light but did not follow objects with her eyes. There was no facial asymmetry, but the expression was peculiar. The nose, mouth, and throat revealed no significant findings. The cervical lymph nodes were moderately enlarged. The chest was symmetrical, the lungs clear, and the heart normal. The abdomen was not distended, even though the liver was enlarged two fingerbreadths below the costal margin and the spleen reached down to a centimeter above the left iliac crest. The splenic notch could be felt plainly; the organ was firm to touch and extremely movable. There was a reducible protrusion of the umbilicus. The genitals were normal. The deep reflexes were brisk but not definitely increased. There was no clonus, but the lower extremities were slightly spastic. The plantar reflexes were both in extension. The Oppenheim sign was positive. Abdominal reflexes could not be elicited.

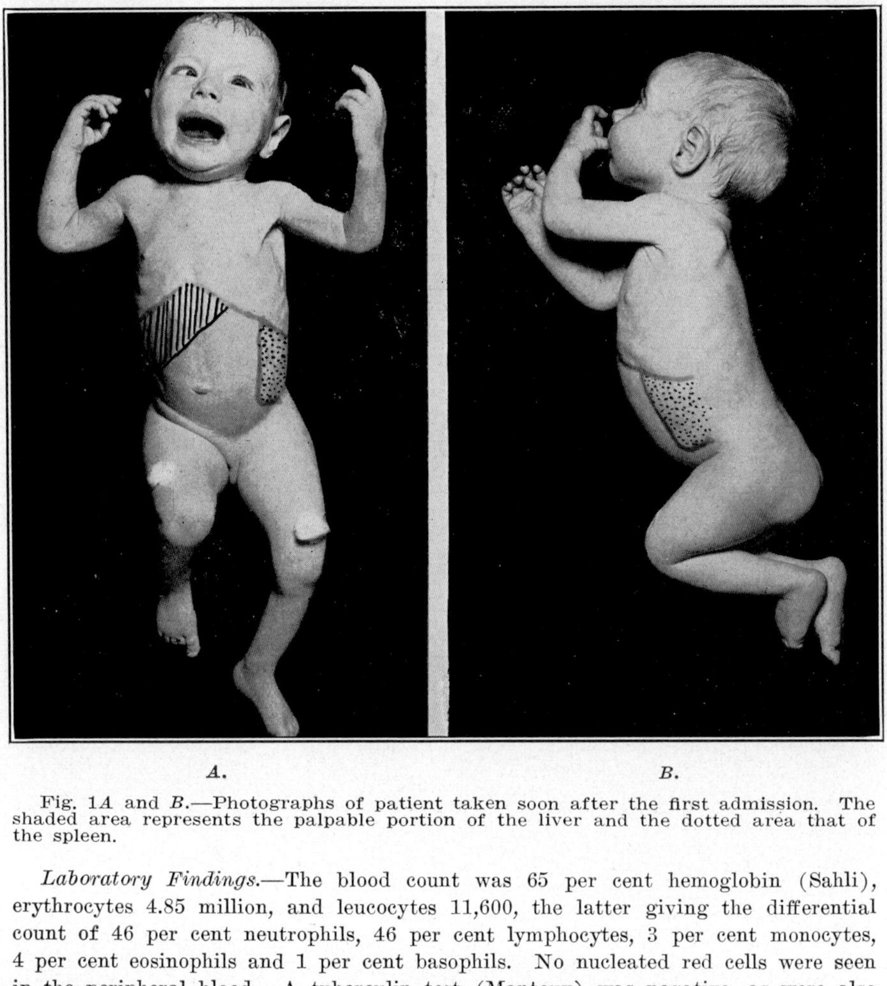

A. *B.*

Fig. 1*A* and *B*.—Photographs of patient taken soon after the first admission. The shaded area represents the palpable portion of the liver and the dotted area that of the spleen.

Laboratory Findings.—The blood count was 65 per cent hemoglobin (Sahli), erythrocytes 4.85 million, and leucocytes 11,600, the latter giving the differential count of 46 per cent neutrophils, 46 per cent lymphocytes, 3 per cent monocytes, 4 per cent eosinophils and 1 per cent basophils. No nucleated red cells were seen in the peripheral blood. A tuberculin test (Mantoux) was negative, as were also the Kahn and Wassermann tests. The spinal fluid, containing two to three cells (lymphocytes) per cubic millimeter, was clear, under no increased pressure, and there was no increase in globulin content. The urinalysis was negative. Roentgenography of the long bones revealed no abnormalities.

At this stage of observation it occurred to the authors that the case probably belonged to one of the groups of lipoidosis. While in the hospital the patient was unable to swallow food properly, taking no more than 2.5 oz. of formula at one feeding (a total of 500 c.c. daily). On April 15, 1937, a slight dullness was noted with diminished breath sounds over a portion of the right lower lung, and a roentgenogram of the chest taken at this time revealed a pneumonic infiltration extending outward from the right hilum. The following morning the patient developed a fever of 39° C. Daily hypodermoclysis was then instituted, and with the aid of two blood transfusions the temperature dropped to the normal level within ten days. During this period of febrile attack the patient had occasional spells of transient cyanosis. Blood cholesterol was then determined and showed to be 129 mg. per cent, which argued against the possibility of Niemann-Pick's disease. A sternal marrow puncture (Kato[20]) was performed on April 26, 1937, and the smears made from the aspirated material contained characteristic Gaucher cells (Fig. 2) which constituted conclusive proof of Gaucher's disease (infantile type).

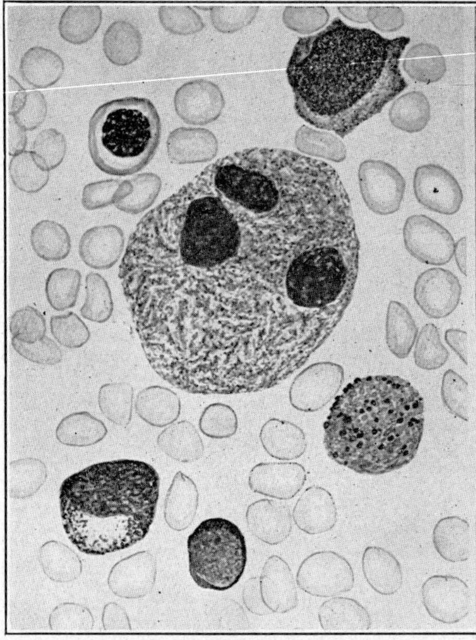

Fig. 2.

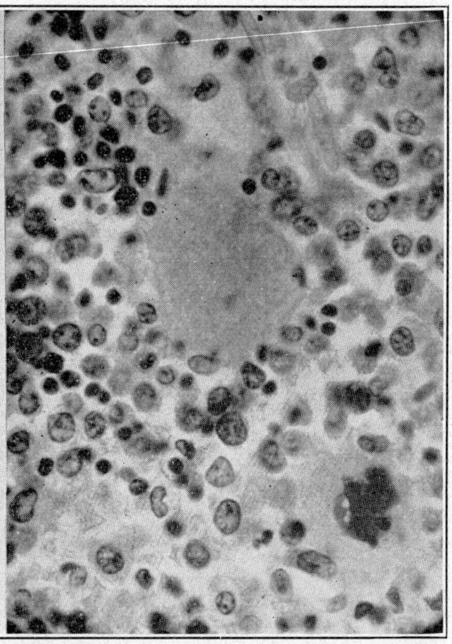

Fig. 3.

Fig. 2.—Camera lucida drawing of a Gaucher cell seen in the smear made from sternal marrow puncture material. Reduced from magnification of 1300 diameter. May-Grünwald-Giemsa stain.

Fig. 3.—Photomicrograph of a section of bone marrow showing a Gaucher cell and a megakaryocyte.

At the request of the parents the patient was taken home on April 28. Her weight was then 3,900 gm. While at home the baby took hardly any food or fluids, had a few attacks of laryngeal spasm, and was extremely restless. Two days later, cyanotic and pale, she was brought back to the hospital in a precarious condition. Her tissue turgor was very poor, the fontanel was sunken, and the respiration, labored. The weight decreased to 3,500 gm., but with daily hypodermoclysis and repeated intravenous administration of fluids her condition considerably improved. Gastric gavage had to be resorted to because of her inability to take food, after which the body weight increased to 4,305 gm. in six days. The blood count at this time was 59 per cent hemoglobin (Sahli), erythrocytes 4.84 million, and leucocytes 5,600, with a differential count of 26 per cent neutrophils, 66 per cent lymphocytes, 2 per cent monocytes, and 1 per cent each of eosinophils and basophils. The urinalysis was completely negative. On the seventh day, after an attack of diarrhea and an elevation of temperature up to 39.8° C., the infant, while being fed, suddenly became cyanotic and her respiration stopped abruptly (May 7, 1937).

Autopsy Protocol.—Autopsy, which was restricted to inspection of organs and removal of only necessary tissues through an abdominal incision, was performed by Dr. Humphreys and Dr. Steiner about seven hours after death and resulted in the following anatomic diagnosis:

(1) Lipoid histiocytosis, Gaucher type, with extreme splenomegaly and moderate enlargement of the liver; (2) lipoid storage in the lungs, lymph nodes, thymus, adrenal glands, bone marrow, and lymphoid tissue of the intestine; (3) acute bronchopneumonia; (4) hemorrhages in serous membranes; (5) emaciation; (6) excoriations on the buttocks and scalp.

The gross appearance of the liver and spleen was most remarkable. The liver (not removed) was estimated to weigh at least twice the normal for a child of this age. The capsule showed much irregular purple-red and yellow-gray mottling, coarser than normal lobular markings. The margins were strikingly rounded. Upon incision

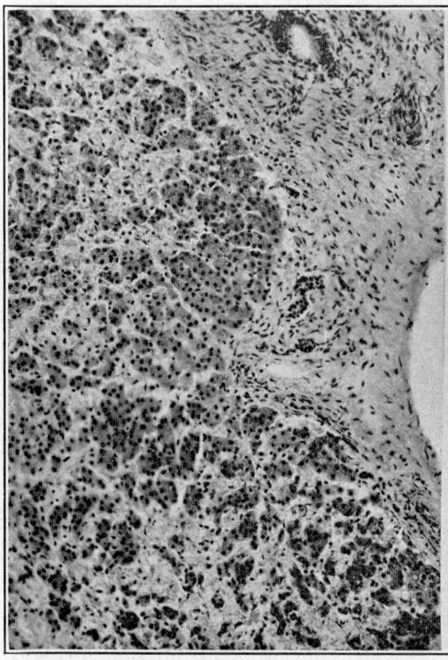

Fig. 4.

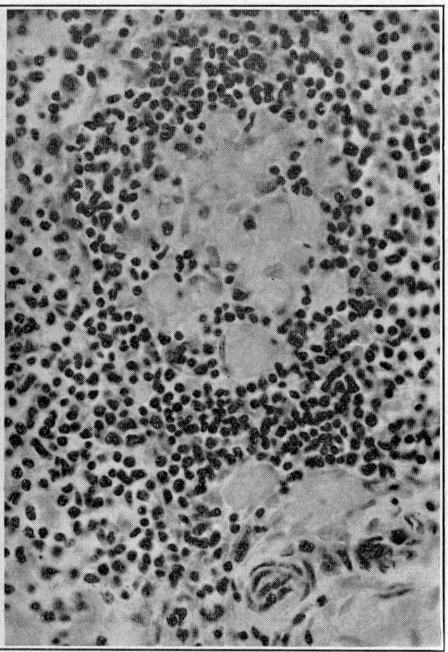

Fig. 5.

Fig. 4.—Photomicrograph of a section of liver, showing atrophy of liver cells due to accumulation of Gaucher cells.

Fig. 5.—Photomicrograph of a section of spleen, showing accumulation of Gaucher cells in the center of a small Malpighian corpuscle.

of the organ, bulging and very friable liver tissue protruded, to the extent that the organ was practically diffluent.

The spleen was an enormous soft organ weighing 110 gm. (seven times the normal), with delicate capsule. The splenic pulp which bulged forth upon incision of the capsule was uniformly pale purple red with no recognizable lymphoid bodies.

The most characteristic feature of the case was the histologic demonstration of ubiquitous presence of Gaucher cells, which were found in great abundance in the spleen, liver, thymus, lungs, lymph nodes, and in the lymphoid tissue of the intestines (Peyer's patches) and appendix, bone marrow, adrenal glands, and in moderate abundance in the kidneys (Figs. 3 to 7).

Histologic Characteristics of Gaucher Cells.—The Gaucher cells seen in this case were typical of those described in the literature: huge, pale cells, sometimes multinucleate and only occasionally definitely vacuolated. More frequent was the appearance of wrinkling or striping of the cytoplasm, well brought out by the Maximow and Mallory stains. Here too the cytoplasm was of a dingy grayish or brownish cast, quite in contrast to the other mononuclears. Foot silver stains failed to demonstrate any increase of reticulum. Scharlach R brought out no evidence of neutral fat or lipoid in any section, except in the adipose tissue cells (liver, spleen, kidney, lung, lymph node, bone marrow). With modified Weigert stains (Lorrain Smith-Dietrich) the only tissue in which lipoids could be unequivocally demonstrated was in the adrenal cortex; here Gaucher type cells, free from granules, surrounded by adrenal cortical cells packed with blue and blue-black coarse and fine granules, were definitely identified. Thus the fat stains strikingly demonstrated the absence of any chemically

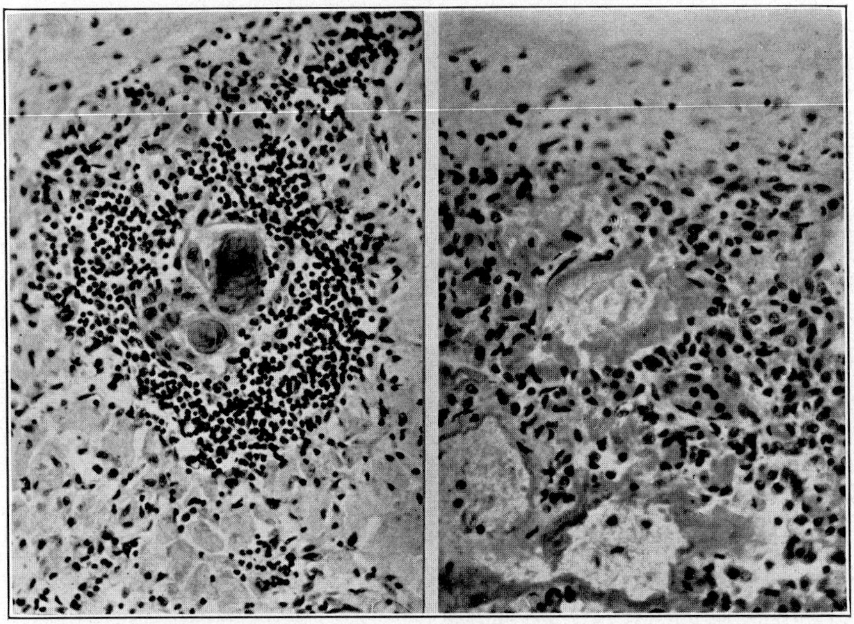

Fig. 6. Fig. 7.

Fig. 6.—Photomicrograph of a section of thymus, showing dense accumulation of Gaucher cells around a lymphoid follicle.

Fig. 7.—Photomicrograph of a section of lung, showing accummulation of Gaucher cells beneath the visceral pleura.

active lipoids (found in abundance in Niemann-Pick's disease where phospholipins abound), as well as the scarcity of sudanophilic fat and lipoid.* No granular iron was recognizable in the hematoxylin-eosin sections.

*Chemical analysis of the liver and spleen (Dr. Marberg) revealed the following values for various lipoids:

	LIVER	SPLEEN
Weight of sample used	81.0 gm.	72.0 gm.
Weight lipoidal extract	4.57 gm.	4.84 gm.
Weight of extracted dry residue	12.2 gm.	9.4 gm.
Total solids	16.6 gm.	14.2 gm.
Ratio total lip. total sol.	27.2%	34.0%
Free cholesterol		
Total cholesterol	66.0%	85.5%
Percentage of total lipoids		
Free cholesterol	4.5%	5.6%
Cholesterol ester	1.2%	1.6%
Phosphatides (as lecithin)	44.9%	30.6%
Cerebroside (as kerasin)	43.6%	36.6%
Balance, neutral fat plus fatty acid	5.8%	25.6%

ETIOLOGY

Cases of Gaucher's disease have been reported in every age period from infancy to old age. Attention has already been directed to the relatively large percentage of cases (more than one-sixth) in which the disease took its onset during the first year of life. In some instances evidence of its onset was even noted very shortly after birth. Kohn,[22] for example, found an infant during its first week of life to have an enlarged spleen, and in the case presented here the parents first noticed retraction of the head and strabismus on the ninth day of the child's life. Inasmuch as it seems logical to infer that before the typical symptoms appear, there must be a relatively extensive infiltration of organs by the pathologic cells, these cases bespeak a congenital origin.

The positive familial tendency of this illness has long been recognized. Rettig[38] and Bychowski[8] have reported cases in children and in the parents of one of them. Anderson[2] observed the disease in the first and third generations. Upon these grounds Bloem, Groen and Postma[5] suggest the recessive characteristic of the disease to be hereditary.

At one time it was supposed that females were affected more frequently than males. But in the infantile cases, summarized in Table I, the distribution as to sexes is about equal, in conformity with which the majority of authors consider there to be no significant sex predisposition. As to race there seems to be a much greater incidence in the white race; but contrary to the commonly accepted belief, the Jewish race shows a special predilection to Gaucher's disease. Cases have been reported in practically every race. The disease is also said to be very common in India, as observed by Spackman and Mackie.[43]

Along with most diseases of obscure origin, tuberculosis and syphilis have been regarded by some as etiologically related to Gaucher's disease. But the majority of cases on record have manifested no evidence of Koch's infection, and tuberculin and Wassermann tests have usually been negative.

PATHOGENESIS

The nature of the disease is still imperfectly understood. Gaucher,[15] in describing the first such case, regarded the condition as neoplastic, but Bovaird[7] denied such a possibility. Schlagenhaufer[42] based the disease on a systemic affection of the reticulum cells of the lymphatic and hematopoietic organs. Simultaneously, Marchand[28] stressed the significance of deposits of foreign material commonly found in the histogenesis of the Gaucher cell. In 1915 Mandelbaum and Downey[27] traced the origin of this cell to the reticulum of the lympho-hemopoietic organs. Later Pick[34] showed that they originate as well from the histiocytes of the arterioles of Glisson's capsule and from the periadventitial cells of the capsular vessels and central veins. With the aid of silver stains Pittaluga and Goyanes[35] uncovered further evidence of such sites being the origin of the Gaucher cell.

In infants Gaucher cells occur in unusual locations, a deviation partly explained by the differences between the development of the reticuloendothelial system of infants and that of adults. Epstein[13] and Lieb[24] were the first to identify the substance accumulated in the Gaucher cell as a complex cerebroside kerasin, an observation later verified by numerous other workers. Chemical determinations of the spleen have given variable results. Bloom and Kern[6] found no changes in nitrogen, phosphorus, cholesterol and fatty acids, but low values for these substances were reported by other workers. Metabolic studies in patients of various ages have also been inconclusive. Cholesterol, fatty acids, and phospholipids in the blood have been found by some to be low in values, and by others, normal. In infants, few of these substances have been determined except cholesterol, and that has been found to be consistently low in value. Phosphorus and calcium estimations, carbohydrate, and nonprotein nitrogen have all been invariably normal, and the spinal fluid uniformly negative.

Attempts to produce the disease experimentally have not as yet been successful, but the work of Beumer and Gruber[4] may lead to profitable findings in this field; these authors have reproduced the changes characteristic of Niemann-Pick's disease by injections of large amounts of sphingomyelin, the substance specifically concerned in this disease. When Beumer and Gruber used lecithin-cephalin, in place of sphingomyelin, no results were obtained. It is significant to mention that kerasin is chemically related to sphingomyelin, both containing sphingosine in their nucleus. The changes in the spleen observed by Babes,[3] after continued coal tar painting of rabbit's skin, closely simulate the essential pathology seen in Gaucher's disease, but a chemical confirmation of the storage substance is lacking.

As concerns the cause of Gaucher's disease the theory most widely accepted at present, and one upheld by Pick, is that the condition arises from an overloading of certain active elements of the reticulo-endothelial system with large quantities of kerasin, which in turn accumulates because of an abnormality of lipoid metabolism. Thannhauser[45] goes one step further and suggests that kerasin is produced at the expense either of sphingomyelin or of sphingosine normally present in the body.

PATHOLOGY

Pick outlined the major pathologic features of Gaucher's disease and clearly distinguished it from Niemann-Pick type of lipoidosis. In infants the spleen, liver, lymph nodes, and bone marrow undergo the chief outstanding gross changes. But the distinctive feature of the disease is the Gaucher cells, large (20 to 80 microns in diameter), pale polygonal cells with a homogeneous and opaque cytoplasm when observed in the fresh state. The nuclei are relatively small, hyperchromatic, and eccentrically placed; occasionally they are multinuclear.

With Mallory's stain a delicate network of dark blue wavy or straight lines can be observed, accentuating the wrinkled appearance of the cell; between these wrinkles the protoplasm appears pale blue. In Gaucher cells from adult patients Turnbull's reagent sometimes gives a faintly positive reaction for iron in the cells, and one of the striking features of these cells is their failure to give the usual reactions for fats and lipoids. In contrast to the orange coloration assumed by the Niemann-Pick cells, after mordanting with potassium bichromate, Gaucher cells stain very pale yellow with sudan III. Similarly, with nile blue sulfate only a light blue color is obtained. Anisotropic bodies rarely appear.

In the spleen and in lymph nodes Gaucher cells tend to collect in clusters presenting typically alveolar arrangement of cell nests, a phenomenon not observed in all organs. True to type they are most numerous in the spleen, lymph nodes, bone marrow, and liver, in which latter location they are found in the capillaries; in the marrow, compressed by the neighboring cells, they tend to be elongated and spindle-shaped. In addition to the above locations Gaucher cells have been found in the lungs, the suprarenals, and in the lymphatic reticulum of the intestines and tonsils. In infants these cells are less abundant and more widely scattered than in adults. These findings have been verified in the present case.

In the central nervous system the findings are unique, as pointed out by Jenny[19] and by Oberling and Woringer.[33] No typical Gaucher cells have ever been found here. Except for scattered gliosis under the ependyma of the third ventricle, the pathology is restricted to the pyramidal (large and small) cells of the cerebral cortex. The lesions are the most widespread in the occipital and parietal regions but are found throughout the cortical substance. With ordinary stains the pyramidal cells are sharp of outline. The ganglion cells are so retracted as to appear ''densified'' or ''mummified,'' and the contours are angular. With Nissl's stain the cytoplasm is seen to be modified by a conglomeration of the tigroid substance in a chromophilic mass filling a large portion of the cell body and involving a part of the processes. This almost conceals the nucleus. Many of these cells contain vacuoles of variable sizes, some large enough to distend the cell bodies. There is no neuronophagia, and no pathologic changes have been found in the brain stem.

SYMPTOMATOLOGY AND DIAGNOSIS

From the summary of symptoms observed in various cases of Gaucher's disease (Tables I and II) it is readily evident that when this disease sets in before the age of 6 months, neurological findings are likely to be the outstanding factor. These cases set in, for the most part, with dyspeptic manifestations and failure to gain in weight, together with more or less indefinite additional symptoms indicative of generally failing health. By the time this stage is reached, the spleen is usually moderately enlarged, and as this organ then progressively increases in size, hepatomegaly gradually becomes apparent. The neurological syndrome usually appears after the onset of the splenic enlargement. Retraction of the head, opisthotonus, and strabismus are the earliest signs of the neurological syndrome, followed by the development of laryngeal spasms, dysphagia, and spastic extremities with changes in the reflexes. The limbs are often maintained in the same position for prolonged periods, commonly referred to as catatonia. The patient assumes the characteristic position of elbows flexed, forearms adducted and slightly pronated, and hands held in front of the face. In most cases the legs are kept in flexion (Figs. 1*A* and *B*). The expression on the baby's face is one of peculiar sadness, and the infant rarely shows any awareness of its surroundings. In some cases, in a later stage of the disease, complete loss of sensation and even idiocy may ensue.

The course of the disease is accompanied by a gradual but steady loss of weight and arrest of physical and mental development. A slight anemia with leucopenia is frequently observed. The blood cholesterol is likely to be diminished. Off and on the temperature is elevated, the cause being undetermined except possibly in one case in which the fever appeared to coincide with low fluid intake. Finally within a few months' time the infant reaches a marantic stage, in the course of which he succumbs either to an intercurrent infection or as a result of the cachexia itself. In some instances death has occurred during a laryngeal spasm at any stage of the disease.

In cases in which the disease process begins after six months of age, neurological manifestations as a rule do not develop, the first evidence of the disease being only the definite symptoms of generally failing health. But soon thereafter the abdomen noticeably and rapidly enlarges; the spleen increases in size, followed by hypertrophy of the liver. A moderately severe anemia produces pallor. The course, although not as acute as in the younger group, is rapid and the immediate cause of death is most likely to be cachexia and intercurrent infection. Splenectomy may precipitate the termination.

It is noteworthy that in Gaucher's disease of infancy certain of the symptoms so frequently found at a more advanced age are rarely encountered. Pinguecula-like deposits on the conjunctivae and large brownish pigmentations of the skin have never been reported in infants suffering with the disease, although an ocher cutaneous discoloration may be seen. Hemorrhagic tendencies may become manifest during the second half of the first year, but bone involvement, at least as far as roentgenographic evidence is concerned, practically never occurs.

It must be added that neurological manifestations in Gaucher's disease are not wholly confined to infantile cases; they have also been observed in some older patients with Gaucher's disease, such as the case reported by Hoffman and Makler and those observed by Reiss and Kato. In the patients reported by the latter authors, neurological symptoms appeared long after the onset of the disease, at a time when hemorrhagic manifestations were prominent. In the absence of postmortem studies the plausible assumption is that the symptoms referable to the nervous system in these cases have been produced by hemorrhages, as at the time diagnosed, rather than being the result of the pathologic background of the nervous symptoms in the infantile form of Gaucher's disease.

DIFFERENTIAL DIAGNOSIS

If the neurological symptoms are pronounced and typical, the diagnosis of Gaucher's disease is not difficult to make on clinical basis alone. But in all other cases the proof of positive diagnosis must be derived from laboratory procedures (sternal and splenic punctures). The neurological form has to be differentiated from: (1) congenital syphilis, (2) cerebral agenesis, (3) erythroblastosis neonatorum, (4) Wilson's disease, and (5) Niemann-Pick's disease, including amaurotic family idiocy.

Congenital syphilis is ruled out by the absence of the usual symptoms and indications of syphilis, and by negative serology. The diagnosis of cerebral agenesis should be made only on the basis of elimination of other diseases. Even though an infant with glaring congenital defects in the brain is likely to be more predisposed to secondary anemias than is a normal baby, the enlargement of the spleen and liver is a signal conspicuous enough to arouse suspicion and, unless satisfactorily explained otherwise, diagnostic punctures should be performed. Erythroblastosis of the newborn infant may also cause an enlargement of the liver and spleen, attended by neurological findings, but the latter symptoms are usually in the nature of true paralysis or of generalized convulsions; moreover, erythroblastosis is frequently accompanied by jaundice, hydrops, and hemorrhagic tendencies, which do not occur in the neurological form of infantile Gaucher's disease. The blood study would settle the diagnosis beyond any doubt. Wilson's disease practically never occurs at this early age. But the greatest difficulty encountered in the differential diagnosis of Gaucher's disease is in distinguishing it from Niemann-Pick's lipoidosis. The more important points of contrast between these two diseases may best be tabulated in Table II.

In cases free of a neurological syndrome, the positive diagnosis can be made only from the characteristic cytology of the biopsy tissues, such as the sternal marrow, spleen and lymph node punctures. This group of Gaucher's disease has to be differentiated from: (1) syphilis, (2) Niemann-Pick's disease, (3) hemolytic icterus, (4) erythroblastic anemia of Cooley, (5) anemia pseudoleucemia infantum of von Jaksch, (6) adrenal neuroblastoma of Pepper type, (7) Letterer-Siwe's disease,

TABLE II

	GAUCHER'S DISEASE (NEUROLOGICAL FORM)	NIEMANN-PICK'S DISEASE
1. Age of onset	First six months	May begin after six months
2. Race	No special predisposition	Jewish race (50%)
3. General appearance	Usually no discoloration of skin; expression of sadness	Mongoloid facies frequent; discloration of skin usually
4. Neurological	Hypertonia; strabismus; laryngeal spasm; dysphagia; catatonia	Usually hypotonia; no pseudobulbar syndrome
5. Liver and spleen	Splenomegaly usually precedes hepatomegaly	The opposite may be found
6. Fundi	Negative; occasionally temporal pallor	Cherry red spot or pigmentation at macula lutea frequent
7. Blood	Slight anemia and leucopenia; no morphologic changes	More severe anemia with leucocytosis; vacuoles in the cytoplasm of lymphocytes frequent
8. Chemistry	Normal or low blood cholesterol and fatty acids	All these are definitely elevated
9. Biopsy	Relatively scarce presence of Gaucher cells in the sternal marrow, but numerous in splenic tissue	Relatively numerous Niemann-Pick cells in all aspirated tissues

(8) Banti's syndrome and, in tropical countries, (9) malaria, and (10) kala-azar.

But in each of the above conditions the characteristic Gaucher laboratory findings, particularly the absence of the Gaucher cells in the biopsy materials, are consistently missing.

COMMENT

A review of the literature on infantile Gaucher's disease discloses unmistakable evidence of a definite relationship between the age of onset of the disease and its clinical manifestations. As Reuben and Rowland emphasized, when the condition sets in during the first year of life, the course is almost always very rapid. It is furthermore to be noted that in cases of infantile Gaucher's disease developing before 6 months of age, as in the present case, a striking neurological syndrome is encountered, as well as pathologic changes in the cerebral cortex of a nature different from the usual findings of the disease (absence of true Gaucher cells). In addition the Gaucher cells themselves seem to overflow the usual boundaries and permeate the thymus, tonsils, suprarenal medulla, the lymphoid tissues of the intestinal tract, and even the lungs. In contrast to this, in cases beginning in the second half of the first year, the morbid anatomy is limited to the usual organs (spleen, liver, bone marrow, and lymph nodes), and the resultant clinical picture is merely characterized by enlargement of the liver and spleen and a moderately severe anemia. But in either instance the disease proceeds rapidly to fatal termination.

This swift course no doubt accounts for the absence of such chronic manifestations as pingueculae and bone changes, as well as for the diminished incidence of hemorrhagic tendencies. As there is but a slight variance in the acuteness of the process in both groups, it seems unlikely that the severity of the disease would in itself account for the great differences in the extent of the pathologic involvement. As Pick[34] suggests, it is more likely the particular stage of development of the reticuloendothelial system, in the individual case, which is responsible for these variations in pathologic picture among the numerous cases of Gaucher's disease. With the exception of the cerebral changes this statement is strongly supported by the work of Lubarsch,[25] whose investigations on the phagocytosis of iron pigment and fat in infants have shown that the phagocytic tendency undergoes a definite change towards the end of the first year of life. By that time cells hitherto capable of storage lose their capacity of phagocytosis. Among these cells Lubarsch included the reticulum cells of the thymus and the perivascular cells of the suprarenals and tonsils. Significantly enough, these are practically the same groups of cells that are specifically affected in the Gaucher's disease of early infancy.

Regarding the central nervous system no satisfactory explanation of the atypical pathology can be offered. But, in harmony with the view advanced by Meyer,[29] it may be assumed that the factor determining the pathologic changes is the peculiar substratum of the developing infantile cerebral cortex. It is universally accepted that active development of this portion of the nervous system takes place during the first year of life. Further studies in this field need to be undertaken with a view to uncovering important information on the relationship of different brain cell groups to the reticuloendothelial system.

SUMMARY AND CONCLUSIONS

The literature on Gaucher's disease in infancy has been reviewed, and a new case reported.

The cases reviewed fall into two rather sharply distinguishable groups: (1) those in which the disease begins before 6 months of age, and (2) those in which it begins after 6 months of age.

In the first group of cases, of which the present case is an example, neurological manifestations are frequently observed, while in the second group they are rarely encountered.

In view of the fact that in both forms the disease follows a rapidly fatal course, the differences between them in clinical manifestations and in pathologic findings can be explained only by the difference in distribution, and perhaps by functional variations, of the reticuloendothelial elements at different periods of infancy.

REFERENCES

1. Acuna, M., and De Filippi, F.: Arch. argent. de pediat. **5**: 489, 1934.
2. Anderson, J. P.: J. A. M. A. **101**: 979, 1933.
3. Babes, A.: Virchows Arch. f. path. Anat. **272**: 411, 1929.
4. Beumer, H. von, and Gruber, G. B.: Jahrb. f. Kinderh. **146-147**: 125, 1935.
5. Bloem, T. F., Groen, J., and Postma, C.: Quart. J. Med. **5**: 517, 1936.
6. Bloom, W., and Kern, R.: Arch. Int. Med. **39**: 456, 1927.
7. Bovaird, D.: Am. J. M. Sc. **120**: 377, 1900.
8. Bychowski, Z.: Wien. med. Wchnschr. **24**: 1519, 1911.
9. Davison, C., and Jacobson, S. A.: Am. J. Dis. Child. **52**: 345, 1936.
10. Di Guglielmo, G.: Haematologica (I. Arch.) **12**: 615, 1931.
11. Dienst, N., and Hamperl, H.: Wien. med. Wchnschr. **77**: 1597, 1927.
12. Donovan, E. J.: S. Clin. North America **11**: 517, 1931.
13. Epstein, E.: Biochem. Ztschr. **145**: 398, 1924; Zentralbl. f. allg. Path. u. path. Anat. **35**: 257, 1924-25.
14. Ewing, J.: Neoplastic Diseases, p. 313, Philadelphia, 1922, W. B. Saunders Company.
15. Gaucher, P. C. E.: De l'epitheliome primitif de la rate, These de Paris, 1882.
16. Graham, S., and Blacklock, J. W. S.: Arch. Dis. Childhood **2**: 267, 1927.
17. Hess, J.: Not published (cited by Hoffman and Makler).
18. Hoffman, S. J., and Makler, M. I.: Am. J. Dis. Child. **38**: 775, 1929.
19. Jenny, E.: Beitrag zur Kenntnis der Varianten der Gaucherschen und Niemann-Pickschen Krankheit, Thèse de Bale, 1930.
20. Kato, K.: Am. J. Dis. Child. **54**: 209, 1937.
21. Klenk, E.: Ztschr. f. physiol. Chem. **229**: 151, 1934; **235**: 24, 1935.
22. Kohn: Cited by Oberling and Woringer.
23. Kraus, E. J.: Ztschr. f. ang. Anat. **7**: 186, 1921.
24. Lieb, H.: Ztschr. f. physiol. Chem. **140**: 305, 1924.
25. Lubarsch, O.: Verhandl. Deutsch. Path. Gesellsch., Jena **18**: 63, 1921-22.
26. Macera, J. M., and Brachetto-Brian, D.: Arch. argent. de pediat. **7**: 11, 1936.
27. Mandelbaum, F. S., and Downey, H.: Folia haemat. **20**: 139, 1915-16.
28. Marchand, F.: München. med. Wchnschr. **54**: 1102, 1907.
29. Meyer, R.: Rev. franç. de pédiat. **8**: 559, 1932; Rev. neurol. **2**: 612, 1934.
30. Moncrief, A.: Arch. Dis. Childhood **5**: 265, 1930.
31. Nagao, N.: Trans. Soc. path. jap. **24**: 464, 1934 (Abst., Zentralbl. f. d. ges. Kinderh. **30**: 154, 1934).
32. Nauwerck: Cited by Pick: Med. Klin. **18**: 1408, 1922.
33. Oberling, C., and Woringer, P.: Rev. franç. de pédiat. **3**: 475, 1927.
34. Pick, L.: Med. Klin. **20**: 1399, 1924; Virchows Arch. f. path. Anat. **254**: 782, 1925; Ergebn. d. inn. Med. u. Kinderh. **29**: 519, 1926; Am. J. M. Sc. **185**: 453 and 601, 1933.
35. Pittaluga, G., and Goyanes, J.: Arch. d. mal. du coeur **26**: 65, 1933.
36. Reber, M.: Jahrb. f. Kinderh. **105**: 277, 1924.
37. Reiss, O., and Kato, K.: Am. J. Dis. Child. **43**: 365, 1932.
38. Rettig, P.: Berlin. klin. Wchnschr. **156**: 2047, 1908.
39. Reuben, M. S.: New York Med. J. **107**: 118, 1918; Arch. Ped. **41**: 456, 1924.
40. Rowland, R. S.: Brennemann's Practice of Pediatrics, Hagerstown, Md., Prior, 1936, Vol. 3, Ch. 23, p. 77.
41. Rusca, C. L.: Haematologica, I. Arch. **2**: 441, 1921.
42. Schlagenhaufer, F.: Virchows Arch. f. path. Anat. **87**: 124, 1906-07.
43. Spackman, W. C., and Mackie, F. P.: Indian Med. Gaz. **60**: 69, 1925.
44. Stransky, E.: Jahrb. f. Kinderh. **126**: 204, 1930.
45. Thannhauser, S. J.: Klin. Wchnschr. **12**: 49, 1933.
46. Vickery, D.: M. J. Australia **2**: 546, 1934.
47. Winter, S. J.: Am. J. Dis. Child. **43**: 1150, 1932.

THE TREATMENT OF GONORRHEAL VAGINITIS WITH CORBUS-FERRY GONOCOCCUS FILTRATE

LOUIS E. GOLDBERG, M.D., NEWARK, N. J., AND
KENNETH BLANCHARD, M.D., EAST ORANGE, N. J.

DESPITE a wide variety of empiric methods and new suggestions of treatment we are still struggling with gonococcus infections, one of the most resistant and age-old affections afflicting humans. Stockwell[1] holds that gonorrhea existed thirty-six centuries before Christ and was observed by Juvenal, Persius, and Galen. Efforts at cure still continue by new and old methods. While recent research devoted to the treatment of gonorrheal vaginitis with estrogenic substances is in process of development, the use of gonococcus filtrate for the condition has come to the fore. Controversial evidence seems to indicate that evaluation of these newer therapeutic agents awaits further corroboration in order to be established as superior to the local remedies. This study on treatment by Corbus-Ferry filtrate* was undertaken to determine the efficacy of the method in a group of twenty-four children with gonorrheal vaginitis.

In order to appreciate the variety of approaches to combat the disease it is necessary to recall that gonococci can be acted upon in two ways, as pointed out by Ernest Finger,[2] either directly by destroying them or indirectly by producing a change in their soil, that is, rendering the mucous membrane unfavorable to their proliferation. Treatment by filtrate is an example of the first method, that by estrogenic substances, of the second method. Chemical destruction of the gonococcus has yielded uncertain results because no chemical agent as yet available kills the submucosal bacteria.

The beginning of the method of producing counteraction to overcome the inroad of the gonococcus is traceable to the middle of the nineteenth century. It was Pasteur who laid the foundation of the present activities, the principal factor being the production in bouillon filtrate of a substance called the antivirus. As early as 1897 the first attempts at dealing with a gonococcus toxin were reported by de Christmas.[3] The opinion is that he used autolyzed cultures containing appreciable amounts of endotoxin. Herrold,[4] in 1925, did some important experimental work, obtaining a filtrate from cultures of the gonococcus.

Since we are concerned with the effectiveness of a bouillon filtrate containing antivirus it would be well to define the meaning of this

*We are indebted to Parke, Davis & Company for supplying us with the material for the treatment of these patients.

term. An antivirus, as described by Corbus and O'Conor[5] is an atoxic, nonantigenic, thermostable substance, formed in culture media, which is easily detached from the body of the bacterial cells and is antagonistic to them. It is more abundant in the liquid media when all the bacterial cells are dead or incapable of continued proliferation. The antivirus is said to cause the death of the bacteria in the culture medium. Besredka found that the action in vitro could be produced in vivo. To exert its specific activity the antivirus must come in contact with the bacteria.

Corbus, stimulated by the work of Besredka in specific immunization by antivirus, directed his attention to the possibility of producing a gonococcal antigen solution. After prolonged experimental work he and O'Conor[6] succeeded in producing a bouillon filtrate of the organism. The bouillon developed by them at this time was toxic and antigenic. After a thorough trial of intra-urethral injections in eighteen cases by Corbus and O'Conor, the results proved discouraging. The assistance of Dr. N. S. Ferry was requested by Corbus in making a new preparation. In the fall of 1929, Clark, Ferry, and Steele,[3] using a hormone broth, produced a gonococcus bouillon filtrate and discovered that it contained a soluble toxin and was not an antivirus. This gonococcus filtrate proved a difficult problem in analysis because of lack of adaptability to artificial conditions of culture and the inherent tendency of cultures of gonococcus to autolyze. In dilutions of 1:1,000 and 1:1,500 the toxin was found capable of causing skin effects similar to the Dick reaction. In experimenting with animals it was further revealed that this toxin stimulated the formation of an antitoxin which neutralized in vitro as well as in vivo. Using this new preparation by Ferry, Corbus and O'Conor injected it intradermally in two patients. Their results encouraged them to believe that intradermal injections of gonococcus bouillon filtrate, properly controlled, brought about specific immunizing effects destructive to the organism in most instances.[7]

In vivo bacteria are lodged in certain tissues or cells. In the application of the antivirus-containing filtrates the biologic fact that skin cells are capable of producing immunity has been utilized. In other words, they found that the antigenetic response from some toxins, if given intradermally, seems to have the power of inducing general immunity for their respective bacteria. It is generally believed that every virus has its cell and every cell its immunity. But such local immunity forms only a part of the general immunity which can be stimulated by intradermal injections introduced anywhere in the body.[8]

Corbus and O'Conor[7] later observed that by withholding all other therapeutic methods they could influence the course of the disease favorably in acute cases but that the rapidity of the cure did not always exceed that attained by means of medicaments. Treatment of eight women with gonorrheal endocervicitis yielded most encouraging results. In three young girls with vulvovaginitis of specific origin the outcome was equally promising. They felt that in some persons at least the gonococcus was eliminated permanently by these injections alone.

In 1932 Corbus again reported on the results of treatment with filtrate in a series of 151 male patients with gonorrheal infection.[9] Other investigators (McKay, Storts, Stockwell, Townsend, and Spence)[10] also sought to determine the effectiveness of this type of therapy. The Council of Pharmacy and Chemistry of the American Medical Association made two preliminary reports,[11] both times awaiting further evidence of the clinical value of the Corbus-Ferry filtrate. A recent survey of a number of urologists regarding their opinion of this product, based on actual trial, showed that with but few exceptions, its use has been discontinued either because of lack of therapeutic results or the too common precipitation of serious complications after its administration.[12]

Experimental observations, however, continued, with both favorable and unfavorable results (Jamieson, Deakin, Gardner, Whitehouse, and Anwyl-Davies).[13] After further consideration the Council of Pharmacy and Chemistry made its final report,[14] declaring that the Corbus-Ferry gonococcus filtrate is not acceptable for new and nonofficial remedies. In the meanwhile we had undertaken our investigation.

PRESENT CLINICAL STUDY

A series of twenty-four consecutive cases of gonorrheal vaginitis in children at the Essex County Hospital for Contagious Diseases, at Belleville, New Jersey, was made the subject of intensive study. Each child had a history of vaginal infection, associated with a purulent discharge, burning, and itching. The clinical experiment to determine the therapeutic value of Corbus-Ferry gonococcus filtrate in the treatment of this disease was begun on June 9, 1936, and terminated on July 13, 1937. The ages of the children ranged from 2 to 10 years. The duration of the gonorrheal infection in these patients before institution of the new form of therapy varied from eleven to seventy-nine days.

Previous treatment by local antiseptics had been given over a period varying from one to fifty-four days. In most of the cases it consisted of argyrol, 10 and 20 per cent twice a day, instilled locally, followed by a potassium permanganate douche of 1:8,000 twice a day. Some of the children were given a 2 per cent boric acid douche, followed by application of metaphen ointment ($\frac{1}{5}$ of 1 per cent) tri-weekly.

In all cases the employment of local medicaments was supplemented by hygienic measures.

For the purpose of ascertaining if the results in the types of gonorrhea would differ, the cases were divided into two groups: acute and chronic. This classification was made arbitrarily, the disease of a duration of forty days or less being considered acute and over forty days, chronic. The entire number consisted of fifteen acute cases and nine chronic cases. All patients originally showed positive gonococcus smears, that is, the presence of gram-negative intracellular diplococci of morphologic resemblance to gonococci, which is the criterion for the diagnosis of gonorrheal infection. In all but two cases the smears were positive for gonococcus at the beginning of the experimental therapy with the filtrate. These two patients, in whom the discharge had not cleared up by previous local treatment, were included in the series to determine the effect, if any, of the new treatment on the presence of the discharge. Their smears contained pus, but no microorganisms could be isolated.

The children were given varied dosages of the Corbus-Ferry gonococcus filtrate intracutaneously with the purpose of determining the optimum dosage. In eight cases the dosages given twice weekly ranged as follows: 0.0083⅓, 0.1, 0.075, 0.1, 0.125, 0.15, 0.175, and 0.2 c.c. In fourteen cases, from 0.01 to 0.02 c.c. of the filtrate were given twice weekly. Two patients received a bi-weekly constant dosage of 0.01 c.c. Judging from the response to the varied dosages we found that the smaller the dosage the better was the result. Probably a dosage in the neighborhood of 0.01 c.c. of Corbus-Ferry gonococcus filtrate given intracutaneously twice weekly is the optimum for use in children with gonorrheal vaginitis.

Regarding local reactions from filtrate injections, these varied from none whatsoever, which happened in a few instances, to cutaneous wheals of 50 to 75 mm. in twenty-four hours. In rare instances, in which there was an absence of any local reactions, they occurred in the latter part of the disease. These reactions did not tend to disappear as the patients became cured of the disease. In other words, there was no relationship between the presence or absence of a local reaction and the progress of the disease. In some instances (seven) a rise in temperature to a maximum of 101.6° F. was observed. These constitutional reactions appearing in variable periods of the disease showed no dependence on the strength of the dosage.

In a few cases, after the filtrate was given intracutaneously it caused an increased vaginal discharge. This was such an inconstant factor that no definite statement can be made in regard to it.

Previous to the institution of filtrate therapy the following diseases were present in association with the gonorrheal vaginitis: gonococcic pelvic peritonitis (two cases), congenital syphilis (one case), chronic rheumatic endocarditis (one case), scabies (one case), ringworm of the scalp (one case), and scarlet fever (one case). During treatment with filtrate therapy two complications occurred, namely, cellulitis of the left leg (one case), and acute tonsillitis (one case).

Three postulates governed the clinical results of treatment, namely: (1) the cessation of vaginal discharge, (2) absence of pus cells, and (3) the disappearance of gonococci in the smears. Before the children were dismissed as cured we had evidence of 22 to 44 consecutive negative vaginal smears. The number of days before the vaginal discharge ceased varied from 22 to 149 days. Before consecutive negative smears were obtained the children were under treatment from 6 to 119 days.

In the eighteen cases in which the patients were considered cured at the hospital the duration of treatment with filtrate ranged from the shortest of 28 days to the longest of 165 days, before dismissal and commitment to follow-up at the Health Department centers. These cases were checked periodically up to Jan. 7, 1938. The average length of treatment resulting in cure was 73.44 days. It was found that of the eighteen patients cured by filtrate therapy, five had recurrences. The length of time after dismissal from the hospital without a recurrence varied from 180 to 508 days. Thirteen, or 54.17 per cent, of the twenty-four patients in the series have continued without trace of the disease.

Six patients, representing 25 per cent, whom we were unable to cure by means of this form of therapy, were treated over a period ranging from 93 to 165 days, with varied dosages twice weekly, without apparent improvement.

In the two cases in which the patients had a vaginal discharge but did not show a positive smear, the infection cleared up in one and recurred in the other.

It may be definitely stated that no complication followed as the result of treatment by gonococcus filtrate in any case under observation.

COMMENT

We realize that twenty-four cases do not comprise a large number on which to pass judgment concerning the value of any therapeutic agent. But the fact should be stressed that these patients were under close observation at all times, data were accurately recorded, and smears were taken and examined daily.

The question arises whether the duration of the infection or the type of case was a factor in the cure. Of our thirteen patients who continue to be without trace of the disease, six were acute cases, and seven, chronic cases. Of the five recurrences three were acute and two, chronic cases. Obviously the difference is not sufficient to war-

TABLE I

SUMMARY OF PATIENTS TREATED WITH CORBUS-FERRY FILTRATE

PATIENTS	AGE IN YEARS	DURATION OF DISEASE BEFORE NEW TREATMENT (DAYS)	DURATION OF OLD TREATMENT (DAYS)	TYPE OF OLD TREATMENT	DURATION OF NEW TREATMENT (DAYS)	DURATION OF TREATMENT BEFORE CONSECUTIVE NEG. SMEARS STARTED (DAYS)	DURATION OF TREATMENT BEFORE VAGINAL DISCHARGE CEASED (DAYS)	NO. OF CONSECUTIVE NEGATIVE SMEARS BEFORE DISCHARGE FROM HOSPITAL	TIME SINCE DISCHARGE FROM HOSPITAL WITHOUT RECURRENCE (DAYS)
H. W.	9	36	29	Argyrol, 20%, B.i.d.* KMnO$_4$ douche, 1:8,000, B.i.d.	165	Not cured; treatment stopped 11/20/36			
J. M.	4	26	1	KMnO$_4$ douche, 1:8,000, daily	165	102	92	28	R†
C. M.	2	48	24	Argyrol, 25%, B.i.d. KMnO$_4$ douche, 1:8,000, B.i.d.	151	119	149	33	427
O. S.	6	22	12	Argyrol, 10% and 20%, B.i.d. KMnO$_4$ douche, 1:5,000 B.i.d.	95	66	77	32	481
M. T.	3	48	38	Argyrol 10% and 20%, B.i.d. KMnO$_4$ douche, 1:8,000, B.i.d.	70	39	64	32	508
A. H.	7	38	33	Argyrol, 20%, B.i.d. KMnO$_4$ douche, 1:8,000, B.i.d.	108	77	96	33	R
J. M.	10	15	1	KMnO$_4$ douche, 1:8,000, daily	130	Not cured; treatment stopped 11/20/36			
M. G.	7	13	3	Argyrol, 10%, B.i.d. KMnO$_4$ douche, 1:8,000, B.i.d.	71	40	67	31	508
G. B.	4	76	24	Argyrol, 20%, B.i.d. KMnO$_4$ douche, 1:8,000, B.i.d.	18	11	22	37	390

*B.i.d.: twice daily.

†R: recurrence.

‡These patients previously showed vaginal smears positive for gram-negative intracellular diplococci

TABLE I—CONT'D.

L. W.‡	4	69	27	Argyrol, 20%, B.i.d. $KMnO_4$ douche, 1:8,000, B.i.d. Boric acid douche, 2%, followed by metaphen ointment, 1/5 of 1 %, tri-weekly	28	Last positive vaginal smear 11/12/37	22	32	387
Ma. W.‡	7	68	54	Argyrol, 20%, B.i.d. $KMnO_4$ douche, 1:8,000, B.i.d.	28	Last positive vaginal smear 11/18/37	23	25	R
My. W.	7	79	38	Argyrol, 10% and 20%, B.i.d. $KMnO_4$ douche, 1:8,000, B.i.d. Boric acid douche, 2%, followed by metaphen ointment, 1/5 of 1%, tri-weekly	89	72	90	24	318
A. T.	10	40	34	Argyrol, 20%, B.i.d. $KMnO_4$ douche, 1:8,000, B.i.d. Boric acid douche, 2%, followed by metaphen ointment, 1/5 of 1%, one day	126	Not cured; treatment stopped 3/22/37			
M. S.	9	48	26	Argyrol, 20%, B.i.d. $KMnO_4$ douche, 1:8,000, B.i.d.	44	60	89	39	R
E. W.	3	35	29	Argyrol, 20%, B.i.d. $KMnO_4$ douche, 1:8,000, B.i.d.	114	Not cured; treatment stopped 3/22/37			
L. D.	9	38	29	Argyrol, 20%, B.i.d. $KMnO_4$ douche, 1:8,000, B.i.d.	62	45	71	30	340
E. F.	7	31	51	Argyrol, 20%, B.i.d. $KMnO_4$ douche, 1:8,000, B.i.d.	106	87	108	22	R
J. V.	3	39	33	Argyrol, 20%, B.i.d. $KMnO_4$ douche, 1:8,000, B.i.d.	93	Not cured; treatment stopped 5/18/37			
L. F.	5	41	33	Argyrol, 20%, B.i.d. $KMnO_4$ douche, 1:8,000, B.i.d.	132	88	134	47	196
M. H.	3	24	2	$KMnO_4$ douche, 1:8,000, B.i.d.	99	Not cured; treatment stopped 5/25/37			
W. M. M.	4	41	7	Boric acid douche, 2%, followed by metaphen ointment, 1/5 of 1%, tri-weekly	85	40	77	40	196
F. B.	7	19	1	Argyrol, 20%, B.i.d. $KMnO_4$ douche, 1:8,000, B.i.d.	38	6	22	31	245
E. McG.	3	11	3	Argyrol, 20%, B.i.d. $KMnO_4$ douche, 1:8,000, B.i.d.	91	51	70	43	180
M. K.	3	36	32	Argyrol, 10% and 20%, B.i.d. $KMnO_4$ douche, 1:8,000, B.i.d.	41	13	34	34	204

rant any other conclusion except that the effect of treatment by gonococcus filtrate is the same in acute as in chronic cases.

In the opinion of some investigators the filtrate is a means of reducing the possibility of complications and attaining a safe postinfectious period. Our study permits us only to point out that there were no complications following treatment by filtrate therapy in our cases of children with gonorrheal vaginitis.

In reviewing the literature on the use of gonococcus filtrate one is impressed by conflicting evidence in regard to its value. We can discern belief in the product as a worth-while discovery on a sound biologic basis and the hope of progress along this line. Others have expressed doubt and condemnation of its use. It is our opinion based on our experience that Corbus-Ferry gonococcus filtrate has some value, for 54.17 per cent of cures cannot plausibly be considered by us as accidental. But we hold that more scientific work is necessary and should be done before definite and absolute judgment is passed on the therapeutic value of the filtrate.

SUMMARY

Review of the literature on the treatment of gonorrheal infection by Corbus-Ferry gonococcus filtrate shows diverse and conflicting evidence of its therapeutic value.

The present study on the use of this therapeutic agent was undertaken in an attempt to determine the efficacy of the method in a group of twenty-four children with gonorrheal vaginitis.

Varied dosages of the filtrate, ranging from 0.0083⅓ c.c., initially, to 0.01 and 0.2 c.c. were given bi-weekly over a period of 28 to 165 days.

There appeared to be no difference in the results between the chronic and acute cases. Of the eighteen patients cured by Corbus-Ferry gonococcus filtrate, five had recurrences. Thirteen, or 54.17 per cent, of the twenty-four patients in the series continue to be without trace of the disease.

From our experience we are inclined to believe that further experimental work scientifically carried out is indicated before the value of gonococcus filtrate as a cure for gonorrheal infection can be definitely determined.

We wish to acknowledge our indebtedness to Dr. Rose Bass and Dr. Frank Giuffra for their assistance in checking the cases following the dismissal of the patients from the hospital.

REFERENCES

1. Stockwell, A. L.: J. Missouri M. A. **32**: 387, 1935.
2. Ref. 1, p. 388.
3. De Christmas: Quoted by Clark, L. T., Ferry, N. S., and Steele, A. H.: J. Immunol. **21**: 233, 1931.

4. Herrold, R. D.: J. A. M. A. **84**: 391, 1925.
5. Corbus, B. C., and O'Conor, V. J.: J. Urol. **24**: 336, 1930.
6. Ref. 5, pp. 336, 338.
7. Ref. 5, p. 340.
8. Corbus, B. C.: J. Urol. **26**: 730, 1931.
9. Corbus, B. C.: J. A. M. A. **98**: 532, 1932.
10. McKay, R. W.: South. M. J. **97**: 152, 1935; Storts, B. P.: Arch. Pediat. **52**: 567, 1935; Stockwell: Idem, Footnote 1, p. 389; Townsend, J. M.: Kentucky M. J. **33**: 463, 1935; Spence, H. M.: J. Oklahoma M. A. **28**: 443, 1935.
11. Report of the Council of Pharmacy and Chemistry: J. A. M. A. **98**: 554, 1932; Ibid. **104**: 1825, 1935.
12. Queries and Minor Notes: J. A. M. A. **107**: 302, 1936.
13. Jamieson, W. R.: Southwestern Med. **20**: 251, 1936; Deakin, R.: J. A. M. A. **107**: 956, 1936; Gardner, M. E.: J. Med. **17**: 488, 1936; Whitehouse, A. J.: Am. J. Obst. & Gynec. **33**: 523, 1937; Anwyl-Davies, T.: Brit. M. J. **1**: 321, 1937.
14. Report of the Council of Pharmacy and Chemistry: J. A. M. A. **110**: 47, 1938.

CELIAC DISEASE AND ITS ULTIMATE PROGNOSIS

SIDNEY V. HAAS, M.D.
NEW YORK, N. Y.

MORE than 150 articles on celiac disease have appeared in the literature during the past five years, but its etiology remains unknown. Thaysen[1] believes that tropical sprue, nontropical sprue, and celiac disease are identical, Parsons[2] believes otherwise. Some hold that carbohydrates are at fault,[6, 11] and some that it is the fats,[2a, 29] others believe it to be an avitaminosis,[38] and still others, an endocrine[3] disturbance.

In such a conflict of opinions the only criterion which can be satisfactorily applied is the result of therapy. Following, an attempt will be made to show there is no symptom pathognomonic of the disease, that the symptoms of celiac disease depend upon an intolerance of carbohydrates, that the fatty stools which are regularly present may be due to this fault, that it can be readily cured by a strict high protein-banana diet, from which other carbohydrates and plain milk have been excluded, and that the exclusion of fats[29] does not accomplish this.

Celiac disease, although first brought to attention by Gee[4] in 1888, was not known to the average physician until recent years.

Herter[5] in 1908 published a monograph on intestinal infantilism. His conclusions were that the tolerance for protein is excellent, for fats, variable, and for carbohydrates poor. This was the first step toward a correct understanding of the therapy necessary for the treatment of celiac disease. He also found a changed intestinal flora, the importance of which later investigators have minimized.

These observations were not given practical application until Howland,[6] in 1920, in a paper entitled "The Treatment of Prolonged Intolerance to Carbohydrate," advocated the use of a high protein, carbohydrate-free diet with limitation of the fats. His good results were later duplicated.[7]

At about this time I was fortunate enough to discover that ripe bananas, rich in carbohydrates, could be used in celiac disease with benefit, would supply all the carbohydrates required, and when added to a high protein diet regularly produced a cure.[8]

Although this treatment has proven successful in the hands of physicians in all parts of the world, there are still large numbers, especially among the English, who persist that the fats are at fault in celiac disease.

In 1931 Parsons,[9] in the opening remarks of his Ratchford Memorial Lectures, stated that "the outstanding feature in celiac disease is the inability of the child suffering from it, properly to absorb fat from the intestine," and ended with the statement[10] that "the treatment of celiac disease is very tedious and full of anxiety because it is so prolonged, lasting sometimes for years, and progress is so slow; at times there are bad, even catastrophic setbacks, hence, unless there is hearty cooperation and the will to conquer on the parts of the parents and the doctor, success will never be achieved.''

Thus, despite an unknown etiology, the difference in the results of treatment based on these hypotheses is striking and would seem to indicate that the symptoms depend upon an inability of the patient to utilize the usual carbohydrates.

Whenever a disease is described for the first time, it is natural that the severe cases which are outstanding should be the only ones recognized. This is what happened in the description of celiac disease, in which the anemic, irritable, stunted child with large abdomen, flat buttocks, large foul fatty stools, and symptoms of avitaminosis, first attracted attention.

Greater knowledge and experience have taught that there are all degrees of the disease which can be recognized. Early diagnosis and correct treatment have made the severe cases comparatively infrequent in this country.

DESCRIPTION

Two types must be considered in a description of celiac disease: The severe cases of long standing, due to neglect or unsatisfactory treatment, and the mild cases which may present only one or more of the usual symptoms. The former has been described so often that it is only necessary to recapitulate. It is rarely seen in a child under 1 year of age, for it takes time for the symptoms to be produced. There is a history of extreme irritability, profuse sweating, sleeplessness, marked asthenia, anorexia, rarely a voracious appetite, a prolonged diarrhea, continuous or intermittent, and occasionally vomiting and abdominal pain. None of the usual changes of diet seem to help. Examination shows marked pallor, a characteristic facies, and emaciation, best exemplified by the flattened pendulous buttocks. There is definite stunting in growth, a large abdomen, thin bones, and where the avitaminosis is great, glossitis, ecchymotic spots, and edema. The child lies quiet, whimpering, and cries when touched; he is unable to move the extremities because of a paresis of the parts. In some cases there is increased cardiac dullness.

The milder cases may arise so insidiously that there is no suspicion of their true nature. The most frequent symptoms calling attention to the possible existence of the disease are anorexia and diarrhea, and large stools, pale and foul, although in some cases there may be constipation. There is usually a history of failure to gain in weight, and growth is slow or entirely interrupted. The child may show no signs of unhappiness although inclined to be irritable. The abdomen is not enlarged, and there is absence of flattened buttocks. Emaciation is usually slight, and there are no definite symptoms of avitaminosis.

INCIDENCE

Celiac disease may begin at any age, often in the first months of life, but heretofore unrecognized in its early stages; symptoms of carbohydrate intolerance may appear even in the first weeks of life, i.e., frequent loose stools, and failure to gain in weight.

The disease is by no means as uncommon as was formerly believed, owing to the recognition of the milder cases. It would appear to occur more frequently among the poor and middle classes than among the well-to-do, and in this country is seen less frequently in hospitals than in private practice, which is contrary to the English experience.

It is likely to occur in several members of a family, in near or remote relatives.[11] Sauer[12] believes the disease may be transmitted, but I have never seen this nor am I familiar with other reports in the literature supporting this view.

COURSE

The course of the disease under correct treatment is very satisfactory; progress is regular and usually rapid, improvement sets in almost immediately, weight increases, the irritability and querulousness lessen, appetite improves, the stools become normal in appearance and less frequent, and after six to eight weeks the child acts normally and begins to grow in length. From the very beginning of the treatment there is no relapse from the disease itself. Relapses occur only as the result of an acute infection or a departure from a strict celiac diet. The tendency to relapse from infection diminishes as the celiac disease improves, but may occur from this cause until the disease is cured, after which there is no relapse from any cause.

Although all the active symptoms of the disease disappear early in the treatment, a strict diet must be maintained for at least a year and occasionally for as long as three years; failure to follow this rule may result in a relapse long after apparent cure.

DIAGNOSIS

Severe cases form a typical unforgettable picture which can hardly be mistaken for any other condition, although there is no individual symptom pathognomonic of the disease. In the milder cases anorexia and history of repeated attacks of diarrhea make the diagnosis probable, and the use of a strict carbohydrate-free diet, which I have termed a ''celiac diet,'' will prove or disprove the diagnosis depending on the therapeutic response.

Substantiation of the diagnosis in either the mild or severe types may be aided by the presence of a low blood sugar curve[13] which is flat in the active stage and approaches normal during convalescence. Although characteristic of and usually found in celiac disease, it is not pathognomonic,[14] since the low blood sugar curve, one in which the rise does not exceed 40 mg. per cent, is an inconstant phenomenon in about 5 per cent of normal individuals and is present in about 50 per cent of the cases of idiopathic steatorrhea.[15] It is also said to be found in marasmus, in any prolonged intestinal disturbance, and in cretinism.

There has been some work to show that the vitamin A absorption curve is low in celiac disease[16] but normal in some other types of steatorrhea. This may perhaps be of value in diagnosis.

Steatorrhea, although fairly characteristic of celiac disease, is not pathognomonic, for it is found in: congenital steatorrhea (fibrosis of pancreas),[17] tropical sprue,[16a] intestinal tuberculosis, excessive fat feeding, acholia,[18] severe diarrhea,[19] duodenal fistula,[20] pancreatic disease, and obstruction of the pancreatic duct.[21]

The avitaminosis may occur in any other disease where there is a lack of accessory food factors from any cause.

It is well known that infantilism occurs in many conditions, and although a striking and regular manifestation of severe celiac disease, it is in no sense pathognomonic unless it can be shown to be related to the intestinal disturbance.

Achylia is not found in celiac disease, and the blood picture is variable.

PROGNOSIS

The prognosis of celiac disease under the high protein banana diet is excellent. Of more than 200 patients seen in hospitals, consultation, and private practice, 134 consecutive patients were treated by me. The only therapy used was diet plus vitamin D and sometimes iron. One patient died of influenzal bronchopneumonia in the second week of treatment. One died of essential nephrosis, long after a cure had been effected. One, although recovered from the celiac condition, at 15 years of age is underweight and undersize, equaling a 10-year-old boy; he is scoliatic, with absent knee jerks, somewhat ataxic, and is believed to have suffered an attack of poliomyelitis. This is the only failure in the series, if it can be so considered. One proved to be a diabetic, probably a fibrosis of the pancreas. One, an adult, although generally well, is sensitive to carbohydrates and has an occasional loose stool. This is probably a case of sprue and is certainly benefited by injections of liver extract. The remainder are alive and well; seventeen cases are too recent to be of value in this analysis, although all of the patients are progressing satisfactorily. The eight patients for whom the diet was first used, after fifteen years are healthy, normal individuals. All are of normal height or above, five are of normal weight or above, three are underweight. All are on a full diet. There have been no relapses, and this small group can in no way be distinguished from any similar group in which celiac disease had never existed.

Among the remaining cases there have been no relapses so far as known.

In the entire series, of which forty-nine were males and sixty-six females, all are normal or above normal in height, eighty-six are normal or above normal in weight, nineteen (20 per cent) are below normal in weight. Of the underweights, 73 per cent are females.

TREATMENT

The treatment of celiac disease is one of diet alone, and this has held for the adult as well as the child. Failure to respond to the so-called celiac diet means that the patient has not celiac disease.

The correct treatment is exceedingly simple. A few principles must be borne in mind: first, no milk as such may be used; second, no sugar or starch in any form, excepting as it occurs in bananas and oranges and in protein milk or calcium caseinate milk or cottage cheese, may be used; third, protein may be used in any form as meat, egg white, gelatin, protein milk, calcium caseinate milk, cottage cheese.

This is the basic diet.

When the diagnosis is made or a suspicion of celiac disease exists the following diet is prescribed:

Breakfast.—Orange juice, cottage cheese, bananas, protein milk for children less than 2 years of age, and calcium caseinate milk for older children and adults, in any quantity desired by the patient.

Lunch.—Meat, liberal portion, preferably broiled or roasted, bananas, protein or calicum caseinate milk, and sugar-free gelatin.

Supper.—The same as breakfast; or egg white and bacon, may replace the cheese. Saccharin to be used for all sweetening.

Between Meals.—The permitted milk preparations and bananas may be used as desired.

Much Later.—Vegetables, except potato, and other fruits may be tried very carefully, one at a time. As a rule vegetables are not very well tolerated early in the treatment.

This diet, even in the face of apparent normality, should be continued for at least a year, when starch in the form of toast or cereal may be tried in addition, with the understanding that upon the reappearance of any symptom such as diarrhea, anorexia, or irritability it should be at once discontinued, to be tested again after three months.

If no ill results have followed by the end of three months, plain milk may be added with the same precautions and strictures.

If there have been no ill results at the end of another three months, then a full diet may be used and it will be found well tolerated. Sugar should be restricted in quantity for a long time.

During the course of the disease there is a variation in the tolerance for fats; some are more easily digested than others. Butter, as a rule, can be used early and freely, and sour cream is better tolerated than fresh cream; but cod-liver oil is not tolerated at all, although it has occasionally been reported as resulting in benefit. In my experience, egg yolk is frequently the cause of trouble.

The only vitamin required is vitamin D in concentrated, preferably dry form. This should be started after the diet is well initiated, early in the treatment.

The anemia is sometimes stubborn, and iron taken early in some form is advisable early.

Change of climate, massage, transfusion, etc., may be used, but are unnecessary, and hospitalization is necessary only when complications exist.

DISCUSSION

The value of banana in the treatment of celiac disease may depend upon one or more of the folllowing factors: First, it is rich in levulose. Mason and Sly[22] have shown that levulose or galactose can act differently from dextrose in the body, perhaps opening a new vista to the action of carbohydrates; however, the case upon which this observation was made was one of celiac disease, which may account for the better utilization of levulose, if not for galactose.

Mann[23] finds that levulose can be well utilized by hepatectomized animals for the formation of muscle glycogen, "although an apparently contrary opinion is expressed in that the tolerance for levulose is more often disturbed in clinical and experimental hepatic disorders than is that for glucose."

It has been found that sucrose and fructose, which make up a large part of bananas, raise the respiratory quotient to a greater extent than other sugars do, probably due to the large amount of lactic acid formed as the immediate intermediary product of these sugars.[24]

In healthy children, bananas as compared with glucose show a blood sugar curve only slightly higher, 9.1 mg. per cent; but in children suffering from celiac disease, bananas increase the blood sugar curve 50.2 mg. per cent and glucose only 22.9 mg. per cent.

The rise after equal amounts of levulose and dextrose is much less than the rise after an equal amount of banana.

It would appear, therefore, that the carbohydrate contained in banana is capable of raising the blood sugar to a normal height, which neither glucose nor levulose is able to do.[25]

In celiac disease dextrose produces a very flat curve; the curve obtained after the ingestion of a mixture of equal proportions of levulose and dextrose is similar to that found in normal children after the ingestion of dextrose.[26]

There also are certain enzymes in banana capable of converting starch into sugar.[27]

Kahn has said: "It is possible to convert the stool of a normal infant from an almost complete gram-negative to an almost complete gram-positive state by the use of 5 per cent of banana powder in the formula. The same effect was produced by 5 per cent of an equal amount of sucrose and fructose. A possible explanation is that fructose is the least well absorbed of the monosaccharides and offers an exceedingly favorable medium for the growth of the *Micrococcus ovis* and the gram-positive anaerobic intestinal bacteria.''[28]

In other fruits and vegetables there exists carbohydrate in some degree, the action of which in celiac disease is similar to that contained in banana. Many of these fruits and vegetables unfortunately are laxative in themselves, thereby limiting their use; apple alone of the common fruits seems to be an exception.

Unfortunately, the idea arose among many that bananas were specific in celiac disease and that it was only necessary to add them to any diet to obtain a good result; it was not realized that as long as other carbohydrates were being used the banana was valueless.

Celiac disease, tropical sprue and nontropical sprue are believed to be identical conditions by some, especially Dr. Hess Thaysen,[1] whose excellent monograph, ''Non Tropical Sprue, a Study in Idiopathic Steatorrhoea,'' would seem to prove beyond doubt that tropical and nontropical sprue are identical diseases, the only difference being that the patients in the one instance were never in the tropics.

Consideration of the subject would be simplified if in the future the term tropical sprue were used to include both types of the disease, for I believe that a given case of nontropical sprue is either definitely tropical sprue or it is definitely celiac disease.

Thaysen believes that celiac disease is only tropical sprue occurring in early life. This viewpoint is not entirely acceptable as it is insufficiently supported by the available evidence, although when the etiology is understood it may prove to have been correct.

It is the marked similarity in symptomatology between tropical sprue and celiac disease which has created confusion; for the presence in both conditions of steatorrhea, a low blood sugar curve, infantilism, and avitaminosis, tend toward mistaken interpretation. Steatorrhea is common to both but in the case of celiac disease this is the result of the absence of available carbohydrate necessary for the metabolism of the fats.

In the case of tropical sprue, as has been so splendidly demonstrated by Rhoads[30] and his collaborators, steatorrhea is due to the absence or imperfect interaction of certain gastric intrinsic and extrinsic factors.

The presence of large fatty stools, together with the use of the term steatorrhea in this relation, has fostered the idea that the fats are at fault. Although it is true that the stools in celiac disease contain an excess of fat, the same patient on a fat-free diet may present an equally fatty stool; ''the fats in this instance are believed to come from the epithelium of the intestinal wall and the intestinal bacteria.''[31]

The steatorrhea in celiac disease is apparently connected with the carbohydrate metabolism; clinically it is known that the tolerance for fats improves as the tolerance for carbohydrate increases. In a given case, a minute amount of carbohydrate will produce a steatorrhea even on a low fat intake, while with a high carbohydrate intake in the form of banana, the same case will not develop steatorrhea, even though a much larger amount of fat is ingested.

This can be shown by the simple test of putting the patient on a strict celiac diet, and when the symptoms are under control, if sugar, bread, cereal, cake, or even potato is added, the symptoms of the disease will return, to be again controlled by the omission of the offending carbohydrate from the diet.

Studies in metabolism have revealed an interdependence of carbohydrates and fats. The influence of carbohydrates in facilitating the combustion of fats is well known. It has been shown that the amount of fat which can be satisfactorily used by the organism holds a definite relation to the amount of carbohydrate introduced into the body, and the human organism appears to be incapable of oxidizing the common fatty acids unless a certain amount of carbohydrate or materials capable of forming glucose is burned simultaneously.[31]

It is now known that the fecal lipids may consist largely of fatty material secreted into the bowels rather than unabsorbed food lipids; and in the human subject on the exclusion of bile from the intestine, the fatty acids of the feces were found to equal or exceed the intake, and yet 65 to 75 per cent of the labeled ingested fats was absorbed.[32]

According to present day belief the fatty acids liberated by enzymic action in the small intestine are absorbed into the epithelial cells and then resynthesized to neutral fat.[33]

There can be no question that fats are poorly borne in celiac disease; but this depends chiefly upon the poor utilization of the carbohydrates, for from the beginning of treatment a certain amount of fat can be tolerated, an amount which increases rapidly with the improved utilization of the carbohydrates.

That the fats per se are not at fault in celiac disease is demonstrated by the use of protein milk, each quart of which contains 4 oz. of 20 per cent cream.

At the beginning of treatment I have used with excellent results, in this form, as much as 70 gm. of fat every twenty-four hours over an extended period. Only once was it necessary to avoid cream in making the protein milk. In this instance its replacement by an equal amount of butter was successful.

That the fats are of great importance in the celiac diet is well illustrated by the following report:

A girl 3¼ years of age, suffering from a severe case of the disease, was placed upon the ideal celiac diet, except that it was made as nearly fat-free as possible. With this diet she made a good symptomatic recovery. In nine months she gained 13¾ pounds but grew only ¾ of an inch. The fat was then returned to the diet, and during the following seven months she grew 3 inches and gained 7 pounds, and in the next eight months, another 3 inches, a rate five times as rapid as that of the fat-free period. In the next year there was a high normal gain of 3 inches, so that at 5¼ years of age her height was 42⅛ inches and her weight was 44¾ pounds, normal for the age.

This is in line with experimental work which has been done on rats by Mendel and others.[34]

Neither skimmed milk, nor lactic acid nor buttermilk can be successfully used, although in a few cases fermented milks have proved satisfactory late in the treatment.

The good results in celiac disease of an exclusive high protein diet may be accounted for by the conversion of approximately one-half the protein into carbohydrate, thus supplying the body's need for carbohydrate.

According to many, especially Parsons,[2] many cases of celiac disease show low calcium levels, often low phosphorus levels, thin brittle bones, and osteoporosis; tetany is common. Parsons has gone into this phase of the subject thoroughly and his work is detailed and authoritative; consequently, it has been a surprise that among all the cases of celiac disease which I have seen, the only clinical manifestation of tetany has been perhaps the abdominal colic. The cases are usually flaccid, and perhaps fail to show the usual symptoms because they are fed fat from the beginning and receive vitamin D early.

It has been found[35] that there is a marked reduction in the production of glycero- and hexosediphosphatase in the intestines of all patients with celiac disease, a finding which may prove to be of importance in its pathogenesis.

Herter's findings that there is an absence of the colon group and that the bacteria in the stools of patients with celiac disease are predominently gram-positive aciduric organisms which retain their infantile characteristics, particularly B. bifidus and B. infantilis, whose numbers rise and fall with the fluctuations in the course of the disease, have not been accepted as an explanation for its etiology, although Brown[36] and his collaborators "in its principal point have confirmed Herter's work."

Compatible with the theory of a bacterial background for the etiology of celiac disease is the experience that in treatment including a rigid celiac diet, relapse may occur from the addition of carbohydrate up to a certain time, after which relapses cannot be induced by any measure. The whole proceeding gives the impression that some organism requiring carbohydrate for its propagation continues to grow until deprived of its proper medium for a sufficient period, when it disappears from the intestinal tract, not to appear even though the carbohydrate which previously continued the disease may be fed in large amount. Experimentally[37] it has been shown that upon the addition of starch to the medium, bacteria can produce enterotoxic substances and can restore these substances after their exhaustion, when starch is again added. Although lack of evidence makes a bacterial etiology highly speculative, the idea is certainly worth continued consideration.

From this conflicting mass of evidence and theory there arise certain facts which have the appearance of truths and which can be used as a basis for further investigation and treatment.

CONCLUSIONS

Celiac disease is due primarily to a carbohydrate intolerance. It can be cured by a celiac diet. The differential diagnosis between celiac disease and the other steatorrheas can be made by the response to the celiac diet. The prognosis under correct treatment is excellent as to life and immediate and future health.

REFERENCES

1. Thaysen, T. E. Hess: Non Tropical Sprue. A Study in Idiopathic Steatorrhoea, p. 111, London, 1932, Oxford University Press.
2. Parsons, L. G.: Am. J. Dis. Child. 43: 1293, 1932.
2[a]. Miller, Reginald: Arch. Pediat. 40: 88, 1923.
3. Schick, B., and Wagner, R.: Ztschr. f. Kinderh. 35: 263, June, 1923.
4. Gee, S.: St. Barth. Hosp. Rep. 24: 17, 1888.
5. Herter, C. A.: Infantilism From Chronic Intestinal Infection, New York, 1908, The Macmillan Company.
6. Howland, John: Trans. Am. Pediat. Soc. 11: 15, 1921.
7. Sauer, L. W.: Am. J. Dis. Child. 29: 155, 1925.
8. Haas, S. V.: Am. J. Dis. Child. 24: 421, 1924.
9. Parsons, L. G.: See reference 2.
10. Parsons, L. G.: See reference 2, p. 1346.
11. Haas, S. V.: J. A. M. A. 99: 448, 1932.
12. Sauer, L. W.: Am. J. Dis. Child. 34: 936, 1927.
13. First Suggested by Thaysen, and First Carried Out in Celiac Disease by Elizabeth Svensgaard, Acta Pediatric Vol. 7, Suppl. 4, 1931.
14. Thaysen, T. E. H.: See reference 1, p. 94.
15. Curor, B. S.: Celiac Disease Dept. Pediatrics Glasgow University & BioChemical Lab., Royal Hospital for Sick Children.
16. Chesney, J., and McCoord, A. B.: Proc. Soc. Exper. Biol. & Med. 31: 887, 1934.
16[a]. Thaysen, T. E. H.: See reference 1, p. 32.
17. Parmelee, A. H.: Am. J. Dis. Child. 50: 1418, 1935.
18. Peters, John P., and Van Slyke, D. D.: Quantitative Clinical Chemistry, p. 235, Baltimore, 1931, Williams & Wilkins Company.
19. Foweather, F. S.: Brit. J. Exper. Path. 7: 7, 1936.
20. Mindline, J., and Rosenheim, M. L.: Lancet 2: 764, 1935.
21. Greenberg, J.: Yale J. of Biol. and Med. 6: 121, 1933.
22. Mason, H. H., and Sly, Grace E.: J. A. M. A. 108: 2016, 1937.
23. Mann, F. C., and Magath, T. B.: Quoted by Peters and Van Slyke in ''Quantitative Clinical Chemistry,'' p. 190, Baltimore, 1931, Williams & Wilkins Company.
24. Higgins, H. L.: Am. J. Physiol. 41: 258, 1916.
25. Badenoch, E., and Morris, N.: Quart. J. Med. 5: 227, 1936.
26. McClean, A. B., and Sullivan, K. C.: Am. J. Dis. Child. 38: 16, 1929.
27. Northcutt, R. T., and Haas, S. V.: Unpublished.
28. Kahn, B. S.: Arch. Pediat. 1: 330, 1933.
29. Neale, A. V., Smallwood, E. C., and Shippam, F.: Am. J. Dis. Child. 50: p. 1502, 1935.
30. Rhoads, C. P., and Miller, D. K.: J. A. M. A. 103: 387, 1934.
31. Peters, John P., and Van Slyke, D. D.: ibid. p. 33.
31[a]. Hill, E., and Bloor, W. R.: J. Biol. Chem. 53: 171, 1922.
32. Shapiro, A., Koster, H., Rittenberg, K., and Schoenheimer, R.: Am. J. Physiol. 117: 525, 1936.
33. Sinclair, R. G.: Am. Rev. Biol. Chem. 6: 245, 1937.
34. McAmis, A. J., Anderson, W. E., and Mendel, L. B.: J. Biol. Chem. 82: 247, 1929.
35. Heymann, Walter: Ztschr. f. Kinderh. 55: 92, 1933.
36. Brown, A.: Courtney, A. M., Davis, G. A., and MacLachlan, I. F.: Am. J. Dis. Child. 30: 603, 1925.
37. Jordan, Edward O., and Burrows, Wm.: J. Infect. Dis. 57: 1928-1935.
38. Rice, C. V.: Arch. Pediat. 50: 358, 1933.

Special Article

THE NATIONAL HEALTH CONFERENCE

HOW the Conference Came to Be Called.—At the time the Social Security Act of 1935 was being prepared and discussed, an attempt was made to include a number of ''health'' provisions. So much controversy developed about the question of health insurance and other matters, and there were so few factual data upon which to inaugurate legislation, that the subject was largely omitted from the provisions of the Act. Certain sections relating to the ''Public Health Service'' and ''Maternal and Child Welfare'' were, however, included.

In August, 1935, following the passage of the Act, President Roosevelt appointed an ''Interdepartmental Committee to Coordinate Health and Welfare Activities,'' consisting of Assistant Secretaries of four governmental departments (Treasury, Interior, Labor and Agriculture) and the Chairman of the Social Security Board, in order that the full benefits of the various federal programs under the provision of the Act might be carried on with minimum delay and maximum effectiveness.

This Interdepartmental Committee in turn appointed a ''Technical Committee on Medical Care'' to study the subject and formulate a program. The Technical Committee consists of Dr. Martha Eliot of the Children's Bureau, Dr. Falk of the Social Security Board and Drs. Mountin, Perrott, and Waller of the United States Public Health Service. The report and national health program recommended by the Technical Committee to the Interdepartmental Committee was presented to the President on February 14, 1938. At the suggestion of the President a ''National Conference on Health and Medical Care'' was called by the Interdepartmental Committee in Washington on July 18, 19, and 20, at which the recommendations of the Technical Committee were presented for discussion.

Invitations to attend the Conference were extended through the Chairman of the Interdepartmental Committee, Miss Josephine Roche, to men and women from the medical profession, from agencies actively interested in health and medical services, and from labor, agriculture, and other groups of citizens.

The purposes of the Conferences as stated by the Chairman were:

(1) To present and discuss the needs of the people of this country for preventive and curative service in illness and for the reduction of the economic burdens caused by illness, as revealed by governmental and other studies.

(2) To discuss steps which may be taken to meet these needs, as proposed by representatives of the government and by members of the conference.

It was distinctly understood and clearly stated that it was not the purpose of the Conference to take action on the recommendations as presented by the Technical Committee. Members of the Conference, however, were invited to present any program they had in mind.

A mimeographed report on ''The Need for a National Health Program'' was made available some time ago and has had a limited discussion in medical journals. Part of the information forming the basis of the report was obtained from the ''National Health Survey'' made by the United States Public Health Service in the winter of 1935-36, in which, for example, three-quarters of a million families in 84 urban centers of different sizes were canvassed and detailed information was obtained as to income, illnesses, and the extent of medical care.

The program recommended by the Technical Committee, in the form of five resolutions, was not available, as a whole at least, to the members of the Conference before the time of the meeting. Certain parts were sent a few days before the meeting to certain members selected for their interest in some particular phase, with the request that they take part in the discussion.

Composition of the Conference.—The nature of the conference is well pictured by a glance at its composition. In all there were 171 members, of whom about 80 took part in the discussions. In addition there were almost an equal number admitted as "observers" who were seated in the balcony, but took no part in the proceedings. A break-up of the membership shows the broad character of the interests represented. Somewhat less than a third were physicians. Resolving this group into parts, 6 were representatives of the American Medical Association although it was stated that in the entire membership there were 10 members of the House of Delegates present. There were 10 representatives of special fields, as tuberculosis, mental hygiene, obstetrics, etc. Nine were heads of city and state departments of health, and in addition several represented voluntary health organizations. About 10 belonged to specific hospital and industrial groups. A few represented organizations such as the Red Cross and College of Surgeons. Some 7 or 8 represented no particular category or organization, but were present as individuals. Several of these were members of the "liberal" group which has banded itself together loosely as the "Committee of Physicians." Many as a matter of fact represented several phases of interest or activities.

Over two-thirds of the members were "lay" and these may again be divided up into several groups. There was a large professional group made up of social workers, nurses, dentists, hospital executives, etc., who are working directly in the field of health. A smaller group was made up of board members, community workers, officers of women's organizations, and the like. A third large division was made up of representatives of what was referred to many times as the "consumer," viz., public welfare agencies, labor, and agriculture. There were over twenty representatives of labor, including the President of the A. F. L. and the Chief Counsel of both the A. F. L. and the C. I. O. For the purpose of the conference the labor group stood closely together. Some 10 representatives of agriculture and farm organizations were included. Nearly 15 journalists including members of the editorial staff of such magazines as *Time, Good Housekeeping, Survey, Liberty,* and *New Republic,* formed another distinct group.

That the membership was carefully picked to represent all phases of the question of medical care there was not the slightest doubt. The intermingling of the "technical" group with the "consumer" group marked a new phase of health conferences. The intermingling was further marked by seating the members alphabetically rather than by group interest or personal choice.

Program

The first day was given over to introductory remarks and scheduled discussions. On the second day there were three sessions at which the five recommendations for a program, which are discussed below, were presented. The third day was entirely given over to discussion by the members of the Conference, although considerable open discussion took place on both the first and second days. Members of the Interdepartmental Committee, Messrs. Altmeyer, Wilson and Chapman, presided at the various sessions.

Session I, Monday Morning, July 18, 1938.—The conference was opened by Miss Roche, who presented a message from the President which ended with the statement, "I hope that at the National Health Conference a chart for continuing concerted action will begin to take form."

Miss Roche then welcomed the members and began the theme of the first day's session, which was the ''Need for Medical Care.'' The viewpoint of the present government was summed up in the remark, ''We have established the principle that certain insecurities which individuals alone are powerless to withstand must be met through public action, that human conservation is an obligation of government.'' She then in a general way outlined the Committee's findings on needs. Stress was placed on economic differences. Among families on relief acute illness is 47% more prevalent and chronic illness 87% more prevalent than among families with incomes of $3000 or over. ''No physician's care is received in 30 per cent of serious disabling illnesses among relief families, and in 28 per cent of such families just above the relief level.'' ''. . . the death rate among infants in families with incomes of $500 was more than five times the death rate among families with incomes of $3000 or more.'' ''Half of the two million babies born each year—a million babies—are born to families either on relief or with less than $1000 annual income.'' ''Fifty million Americans are in families receiving less than $1000 income a year.'' ''On the average day of the year, four million or more persons in the United States are disabled by illness.'' ''The total cost of illness and premature death in this country is approximately ten billion dollars a year. This estimate includes only those factors which can be expressed in dollar values—the cost of health service and medical care, the loss of wages through unemployment resulting from disability and the loss of potential future earnings through death.'' The speaker pointed out that everything proposed could not be put into effect at once and that time would be required to put a full program into operation.

Miss Katherine Lenroot, Chief of the Children's Bureau of the Department of Labor, then spoke on the subject of ''Health Needs of Mothers and Children,'' discussing the problems of income and food for the family, the question of the infant mortality rate, the lack of medical care for the mothers and children in many areas, the lack of hospital facilities and medical care for children. ''A total loss of maternal and early infant life amounting to 160,000 a year, at least half of which is preventable.'' Forty of 49 State Health Officers declared that facilities for maternal care in their states are definitely inadequate. ''. . . as in meeting mass disaster, the needs of mothers and children require that they be among the first to be cared for.''

Dr. Thomas Parran, Surgeon General of the United States Public Health Service, concluded the brief program of the first session. He spoke of the necessity for increased emphasis upon the prevention of disease and the vital function of research. ''It is my firm belief that this Conference marks the ridge of the hill between the old indifference to health as a matter of national concern and a new understanding that health is the first and most appropriate object for national action.'' ''The significance of this meeting does not lie in the fact that it involves contemplation and discussion of health needs . . . discussion is requested of you as a preliminary to practical action by responsible government agencies.'' ''It is not unlikely that public health may be the next great social issue in this country.'' ''You are here to suggest the best, most practical and most profitable ways and means of putting medical science to work.'' ''. . . we should not continue to think in terms of the separateness of public, private and voluntary efforts or of the separateness of preventive or curative efforts to reduce death and disease . . . all are parts of the same entity.''

The inability for economists to solve our problems was pointed out and that medicine and public health should lead economics rather than follow it, as our proved ability to prevent disease exceeds greatly our proved ability to control other causes of poverty. ''Medical education and practice must keep pace with advances in science and with changing social concepts.''

"This Conference may reveal differences of opinion concerning the role of the federal government in putting medical knowledge to work for the benefit of all citizens. There can be no disagreement, however, with the principle that the federal government must increasingly assume leadership in the study of those great causes of disease and death before which we are now helpless." The coordination of investigative efforts and aid to scientific institutions were cited as examples of this government leadership.

Second Session. Monday Afternoon.—The second session started with a group of seven scheduled discussions. Dr. Irvin Abell, President of the American Medical Association, was the first speaker, and his address covered in general the same grounds as his address at San Francisco in June, which has been published in the *Journal of the American Medical Association.* He spoke in general of the work of the A. M. A.; the necessity of a plan under medical control. He felt it was impossible to isolate medical care from other unfulfilled needs, as food, clothing and housing. Dr. Abell stated that there could be little disagreement on certain fundamental objectives in regard to medical care, which were the provision of good medical care for all the people, the development of public health problems, and an improvement in the distribution of medical services and hospital facilities by geographic and economic division.

He was followed by Dorothy Kahn, Director of the Philadelphia County Relief Board, who spoke of the problem in obtaining good medical service for families on relief. The speaker felt it was difficult to obtain an idea of medical needs by a survey, but that when medical relief was given it brought out the needs.

The next two speakers, William Green, President of the A. F. L., and Dorothy J. Bellanca, Vice President of the Amalgamated Clothing Workers of America, discussed the problem in a broad way calling attention to the social and economic disintegration that results from sickness not only to the bread winner but to the children. The expansion of public health and maternal and child welfare services, the use of government funds to provide medical care for the needy, and the application of the insurance principle were urged by "labor." Mr. Green demanded compulsory insurance under government supervision for the low income group (under $3000) which he stated made up 87 per cent of the population even in the best times.

Next, two "Farm" representatives spoke, Benjamin Kilgore, Executive Secretary of the Kentucky Farm Bureau Federation, and Mrs. H. W. Ahart, President, Associated Women, American Farm Bureau. Both stated the farm people wanted better medical service and hospitals—medical service comparable to that obtainable in the urban districts which at the present time was not available for the farmer. Resolutions of the American Farm Bureau Federation were presented calling for the establishment of rural hospitals where they are needed and could be maintained on a good professional and financial standard, acknowledging the advantages of health insurance and pledging itself to work for such laws, and third the extension of all forms of preventive medicine throughout the country. Mrs. Ahart stated they had no quarrel with the American Medical Association but insisted the medical fraternity had a grave responsibility to the public and asked for greater cooperation between the medical profession and the lay public. "The demand for health insurance and for adequate medical care for our entire population, both urban and rural, is a force that must be recognized, despite any objections expressed by individuals within the medical profession."

The last scheduled speaker was Dr. Hugh Cabot. After referring to the rising tide of the "consumer," he stated he thought the fact of need was quite beyond discussion. He felt that further surveys to determine if needs existed were superfluous, and, referring to the survey now being carried on by the American Medical Association, that physicians were poorly qualified to carry out a survey. He felt further discussion of the need of improvement in medical care was futile and our attention should be turned to methods of improving care.

Several members were then called upon to speak whose remarks are included under the heading "Discussion" below.

Sessions III, IV and V. Tuesday, July 19.—At the three sessions on Tuesday, the five programs and recommendations of the Technical Committee were presented. "Maternal and Child Health" and "Public Health Service" in the morning, "Medical Care for the Medically Indigent" and "Hospitals" in the afternoon, and at the evening session (a) "A General Program for Medical Care" and (b) "Insurance against Loss of Wages During Sickness." All of the presentations followed the general plan of a brief summary of the needs, followed by the recommendations of the Committee, and ending with a brief discussion of plans and estimates of cost.

Program and Recommendations for Maternal and Child Health. Presented by Dr. Martha Elliot, Assistant Chief of the Children's Bureau.

This was presented first as the Committee was of the opinion that in any plan for a national health program primary consideration must be given to the subject of maternal and child health.

Attention was called to the high maternal death rate in the United States, to the 75,000 stillbirths each year, and to the death of 70,000 infants in the first month of life. Over 1,100,000 births occur in families on relief or with an income of less than $1,000 a year. Physicians estimate that from one-half to two-thirds of the maternal deaths are preventable, that the stillbirth rate can be reduced by two-fifths, and that the newborn infant deaths can be reduced by one-third to one-half. The total extent of dental defects, rheumatic disease, visual defects, crippling, etc., among children was pointed out, and the place of infectious diseases as a cause of illness and death in childhood. The need for consultation services in obstetrics and pediatrics was mentioned, and the national character of the problem with its economic and geographic differences was stressed. For example, 11 states in the Southeast, caring for 25 per cent of the children, receive only 12 per cent of the national income, while 12 states in the Northeast, caring for 29 per cent of the nation's children, receive 41 per cent of the income.

The Committee recommended expansion of the existing Federal-State cooperative program for Maternal and Child Welfare services under Title V of the Social Security Act, over and above the $3,800,000 now available. The program should provide facilities for (a) medical and nursing care for mothers throughout maternity, and (b) health supervision and medical care for children. The plan for extension under (a) called for the medical care of mothers and newborn infants, including delivery, by qualified local physicians assisted by nurses, facilities for expert diagnosis and consultation in centers and in the home, and hospital care when necessary for medical or economic reasons; under (b) health supervision and medical care by local physicians, the aid of specialized consultants and hospitalization when necessary. Increased opportunities for post graduate training of professional personnel were considered as essential in carrying out the program.

It was estimated that the cost to the federal, state and local governments of a program for the maternity and newborn services for families with an income level of $1000 or under, would be $95,000,000 a year, with a maximum federal participation of approximately one-half of this amount. It was recommended that for the first year the present federal appropriation should be increased by $4,500,000, and that the annual appropriation be gradually increased until it reached $35,000,000 by five years, and the total amount in not less than 10 years.

It was estimated that medical care for the 13,000,000 children under 15 years of age in the medically indigent group would cost $130,000,000 a year. Part of this would be carried by the provisions of Recommendations II and III (''Hospitals'' and ''Medical Care for the Indigent''). The Committee recommended that a sum beginning with $3,000,000 a year and increasing gradually to $30,000,000 by the tenth year should be provided for the medical care of children by the Children's Bureau under Title V, part 1, of the Social Security Act.

Under Title V, part 2, of the Act, an additional appropriation over and above the $2,850,000 now available was recommended for services for crippled children.

The Committee felt that the part played by the federal government in the early years, when the program was developing, should be relatively large, supplementing present expenditures by the state and local communities. In apportioning money to states such factors as the ability of the state to provide support, and the need for maternal and child health care as shown by the mortality and morbidity rates, should be taken into consideration.

In recapitulation the program recommended increased appropriations above amounts now available for expenditure under Title V of the Social Security Act, for Federal grants-in-aid to the states of $9,500,000 the first year, increasing gradually to a total of $82,500,000 by the tenth year.

Program for Public Health Services. Presented by Dr. Clifford E. Waller, United States Public Health Service.

The need for an increase in full time health administration, particularly in rural areas and smaller cities, and in inadequate state organizations was first pointed out, and the work of the United States Public Health Service under the provisions of the Social Security Act in the last few years.

Certain problems were discussed specifically. Tuberculosis with its spread from active cases. Venereal disease, in which early and adequate treatment is the only possible method of cutting down the incidence. Increased laboratory facilities and better treatment facilities are urgently needed. Some 60,000 cases of congenital syphilis occur yearly. By the development of serum treatment for pneumonia, which implies increased diagnostic laboratory facilities, the gross death rate of 150,000 annually could be reduced 25 per cent. Only eight states have active programs for typing and distribution of serum. Cancer with its high death rate is an active program in only seven states. Malaria control in the southern states is essential. Institutional care for the mentally ill is but part of the mental hygiene problem. Preventive facilities and services should be extended. Laboratory and field research is needed in the field of industrial hygiene as 15,000,000 people are engaged in productive occupations.

The Committee recommended the expansion of the existing Federal-State Cooperative Program under Title VI (Public Health Work) of the Social Security Act. Federal participation in state and local health services to be extended through increased authorization for grants-in-aid to the states.

Primary consideration under the program would be given to the development of local health organizations on a full time basis. The tuberculosis campaign would be carried on through case finding and isolation of active cases. Venereal disease would be attacked along the lines now being carried out. The pneumonia campaign would be to increase laboratory facilities and the free distribution of serum for the medically indigent. For cancer the setting up of diagnostic and treatment centers is required. An extension of the work of present hospitals or new centers might both be used. An adequate staff and therapeutic apparatus, as radium and deep x-ray therapy, are essential. The program for mental hygiene involves assistance to existing institutions and improved diagnostic and treatment facilities. Mental hygiene centers for the early preventive treatment of maladjustments must be provided. An industrial hygiene unit should be developed in every state with adequate laboratory and field workers. Prior to 1936 only 3 states and 1 city had programs for industrial health. Since 1936, under Title VI of the Social Security Act, units have been organized by federal assistance in 21 additional state departments of health. Departments should be developed in all states.

The total estimated maximum annual cost for all services would be $200,000,000. This includes federal, state and local expenditures combined.

Public health organization	$23,000,000
Tuberculosis	43,000,000
Venereal disease	47,000,000
Pneumonia	22,000,000
Cancer	25,000,000
Malaria	10,000,000
Mental Hygiene	10,000,000
Industrial Hygiene	20,000,000
	$200,000,000

It is not assumed that all items would remain at these maximum figures. It is considered proper that the federal government should contribute half of the amount. The Committee recommends that the initial federal appropriation should be $10,000,000 the first year, with a gradual annual increase to the maximum of $100,000,000 by the seventh year.

Hospital Facilities. Presented by Joseph W. Mountin of the United States Public Health Service.

The extent and control of existing hospitals was discussed. General hospitals by number are one-half nonprofit organizations, one-third proprietary, and 15 per cent operated by state and local governments. By beds, 27 per cent are governmental, 62 per cent nonprofit, and about 11 per cent are proprietarily owned. Fees collected from patients form 70 per cent of the income of nonprofit hospitals and 6 per cent of the income comes from endowment. Over 40 per cent of the counties in the United States do not contain a registered general hospital—the population of these counties amounts to 17,000,000. The ratio of beds per 1000 population exceeds 5.2 in 23 large cities of 200,000 or more inhabitants.

Hospital facilities exceed 4.7 per 1000 of population in 25 per cent of the states. Beyond the metropolitan counties 3.1 beds are found in 25 per cent of the states. On combining location with ownership, general hospital service is not available to a large segment of the population either through faulty location or inability to purchase care. Average occupancy is about 70 per cent of capacity, but in hospitals depending on revenue from patients it is 50 per cent. In tuberculosis sanitaria the bed occupancy amounts to 92 per cent of capacity where less than 10 per cent of the cost is paid by patients, and falls to 67 per cent when the revenue from patients amounts to 90 per cent or more. State and local governments have a practical monopoly (92 per cent) of institutions for the insane. Out patient services are most important in caring for the medically indigent. Each city over 250,000 has one or more such department, while only 2 per cent of cities under 10,000 have such resources. About half of the cities of 50,000 have outpatient services.

The Committee recommended federal grants-in-aid for the construction of needed hospitals and related facilities, and special grants on a diminishing basis toward defraying the operating costs of these new institutions in the first three years of their existence.

To bring all state averages for general hospitals up to 4.5 would require 180,000 additional beds. Some should be added to existing units and some would call for new units. The Committee estimates a need for 500 new hospitals, in areas largely rural in character, of a 30 to 60 bed capacity. There should be 2 sanitaria beds for tuberculosis for each death. This would call for an addition of 50,000 beds. Many of these should be incorporated into existing institutions, but in several states new institutions should be established. Mental institutions call for a capacity of 4.8 beds for 1000 population. This would call for 130,000 additional beds.

The estimated cost of such construction would be

General Hospitals	$ 630,000,000
Tuberculosis Hospitals	150,000,000
Mental Hospitals	325,000,000
	$1,105,000,000

For the construction program the Committee recommends federal government grants-in-aid equivalent to 50 per cent of the cost, or $552,250,000. Temporary maintenance grants over a period of three years were calculated at a total of $177,000,000. This construction program would extend through several years.

Medical Care for the Medically Needy. Presented by George St. John Perrot of the United States Public Health Service.

The formulation of a national health program implies acceptance of the principle that the maintenance of the health of its citizens is a responsibility of government. Government has assumed responsibility for the provisions of preventive health services on a community-wide basis, but wide variations exist throughout the country in the practical application of this policy. A more serious situation arises from the inertia of governmental bodies in the field of medical care of the needy sick. With some important exceptions medical care is ''an economic commodity'' purchased and paid for directly by the individual who needs it. The fact that it is chiefly a professional service does not alter the basic fact.

In the United States there are today probably 40,000,000 persons—almost one-third of the population—living in families with an income of less than $800. This sum supports the family at an emergency level. In this group are 11,000,000 in families on work relief, 6,000,000 in families on general relief and 3,000,000 wards of the government under the Social Security Act (dependent children, old age, dependent blind). This group of 20,000,000 is dependent on government for food, shelter and medical care. In the emergency of sickness 20 million more in the marginal income class become dependent on public aid for medical care.

In the 40 million there will be 20 million cases annually of disabling illness of which 8 million will be of at least a week's duration. Two million of the disabling illnesses will receive no medical care and the 6 million medically attended cases will include 2 million patients in general hospitals. It will include 250,000 cases of pneumonia, 190,000 cases of appendicitis, 425,000 cases of tonsillitis, etc.

There is an uneven distribution of our resources for the maintenance of health. A large population of the medically needy are found in small cities and rural areas in which facilities for care are limited.

The medical needs of this low income group exceed those of families at higher economic levels as demonstrated by numerous surveys. Among children in relief families the annual days of disability was 17 per cent higher per capita than the average for families of higher economic levels.

One in every 20 family heads in the relief population was unable to work on account of illness, contrasted with 1 in 250 in families with an income of $3000 or more. The tuberculosis case rate is 10 times as high under similar income conditions.

Despite this greater need, studies ''before depression'' showed well-to-do sick persons received 3 times as much medical service as the poor.

In 1935 the survey of the Public Health Service showed hospitalization was about the same for the rich and poor in the large cities, but the proportion of poor hospitalized in small cities and rural areas declined rapidly. In discussing the present financial basis of public medical care it was stated that in 1935 governmental expenditures for health and medical care amounted to one-sixth of the total medical bill for that year, or $520,000,000. After deducting expenditures for patients in federal hospitals, public health services, etc., a sum remains of roughly $130,000,000 which was spent for tax supported medical care for the needy. It is estimated that the cost of essential medical services at the emergency level for the medical needy would amount to about $400,000,000 annually.

The Committee recommended Federal grants-in-aid to the states toward the costs of a medical care program for recipients of public assistance and other medically needy persons.

Two broad groups of the population would be included (a) those for whom government has already accepted some responsibility through public assistance, and (b) those who, able to obtain food, clothing and shelter, are unable to obtain necessary medical care.

The program would be developed around existing preventive health services. It would provide minimum essential needs, including medical and surgical care, hospitalization, care of the tuberculous and mentally ill, bedside nursing and emergency dental care. It would extend to 40,000,000 persons in families under the $800 income level group. The total figure is based on an estimate of $10 per person. The proposed federal contribution might amount on the average to 50 per cent, or $200,000,000 annually. It is suggested that a start should be made in the first year of $50,000,000 increasing annually to the maximal expenditure at 10 years. This sum is over and above the recommendation for public health services.

A. *''A General Program of Medical Care.''* B. *''Insurance Against Loss of Wages During Sickness.''* Presented by Dr. I. S. Falk, Social Security Board.

Medical facilities are of no direct benefit to persons who do not use them. The most important barrier between individuals or institutions equipped to serve the sick, and the millions of people in need of this service is an economic wall. The cost of medical care must be brought within the means of the public.

The total expenditures in 1929 for all kinds of health and sickness services were about $3,700,000,000, of which patients paid 79 per cent, government 14 per cent and philanthropy and industry the remaining 7 per cent. In 1936 the total expenditures had declined to $3,200,000,000 of which patients paid 80 per cent and government 16 per cent.

Medical services to be effective must be geared to need. All studies and surveys show sickness is more prevalent among people of the low income groups. The well-to-do do not receive too much care—the poor receive too little. The large majority of people receive medical care not according to their needs but according to their income.

The average family with an income up to $5000 spends 4 to 5 per cent of the income for medical care. Average figures do not give a realistic picture, as the need by a specific family is uneven and unpredictable. Serious illness may be a catastrophe to the family budget. The burden is not due to the average expenditure, but to the unevenness. The savings of a lifetime are at times wiped out and the whole level of family life and security lowered by the economic loss of sickness. The adjustment of fees operates in only a limited way.

Adequate medical care purchased on an individual basis is estimated to cost $76 per year per person. On a group basis it can be purchased for $25 a year. Expenditures on this basis would mean doubling the amount now spent by families in the $1000 level, adding one-fifth to the $2000 level (60-80 per cent of the nation).

Families with incomes of $3000 or more spend more than $100 per year. "If medical care is to be made available to all families with small or modest incomes at costs they can afford, the costs must be spread among groups of people over periods of time."

The inadequate income of physicians deserves careful consideration. In 1929 for every physician who earned $10,000 there were two who earned less than $2,500. Since 1929 the economic status of doctors has become worse. While doctors are only partially occupied, millions of people in need of service do not receive it. Every sound arrangement to reduce the burdens created by sickness costs operates to increase and stabilize the incomes of those who furnish the services.

Voluntary insurance efforts, in the opinion of the Committee, is not the answer to the nation's needs. Many of the devices practiced to meet the burdens and distribute the costs, as organized charity, sliding scale of medical fees and commercial insurance, have long been in use and are inadequate to meet the needs.

Group payment in various forms has become more important, especially group hospitalization; while commendable, the proof of their value lies in their actual accomplishment. Voluntary sickness insurance, with or without subsidy, may be important as a method of experimentation, but it has nowhere shown the possibility of reaching more than a small fraction of those who need its protection.

The Committee recommended federal grants-in-aid to the states toward the costs of a more general medical program.

The wide variations in existing personnel, institutions, and economic conditions require that a national program must be flexible and adopted to the diverse conditions existing in different parts of the country. Hence effective operating programs should be designed and administered on a statewide basis. The role of the federal government should be principally to give financial and technical aid to the development of state programs.

There are two methods of expanding public health services. By one the government can make particular kinds of services available, by the other a general program can be developed. The second has fewer drawbacks of an administrative nature and is not complicated by economic groups. A general program would cost about $2,750,000,000. New tax funds for public medical services would not represent a new kind of expenditure, as most of these sums are now being spent from private funds. A general program can be financed through insurance contributions. It might be limited to specified income levels. A general program should include the medically indigent, through maintenance by public funds, combined with the insured groups.

A choice between public medical services (tax supported) and health insurance involves many considerations. It may be best, according to type of the population of a given area, to develop both methods. This is a choice to be made by the states rather than the federal government. Federal grants-in-aid should within reasonable limits be available whatever procedure or method the states decide to follow. The eventual federal support would amount to between one-fifth and one-third of the $2,600,000,000 overall cost.

B. *Insurance Against Loss of Wages by Sickness.—*

There are probably 7 to 10 days of disability per person a year among the gainfully employed, with a range of from 3 to 4 days up to 15 or more a year per person. The total wage loss by disability in 1929 amounted to nearly two billion dollars. The average loss of time is relatively unimportant, but the incidence is uneven, extending up to a year, or permanent disability in many cases.

Under the present Social Security laws workers are assured of partial income when unemployed, and most are protected by workingmen's compensation from accident or injury arising from employment. There is no protection from non-industrial accident or sickness, except in a very few instances where there is voluntary insurance.

The Committee recommended federal action toward the development of programs of disability compensation.

Two coordinated systems would probably be better than a single insurance system. A system for temporary disability is best patterned after unemployment compensation. For permanent disability the system should be patterned after old age retirement. The first would cost approximately 1 per cent of wages, the second 0.1 to 0.2 per cent at the start with a gradually increasing cost to 1 to 2 per cent of wages in 20 years.

A disability program is not primarily part of a medical care program, but there are important interrelationships.

Discussion

Nearly 80 members of the Conference took part in the discussion. There was, however, very little specific discussion of the recommendations, nor was there any continuity to the discussion. It was obvious that most members who spoke came prepared to say some specific thing, and most frequently read from a prepared manuscript. This was presented whenever the member got the chance to take the floor. Thus a member discussed ''insurance'' before the insurance report had been presented Tuesday night. It has seemed best to present the discussion by groups and topics, therefore, rather than the order in which it came. Many members had the opportunity to speak Tuesday and the entire sixth and seventh sessions on Wednesday were given over to the members of the Conference.

Discussion by Medical Members.—Unfortunately a certain element of discord and personal feeling entered into the discussion by the physicians, which was ''news'' and hence featured in the newspapers, and which gave a somewhat false impression of the attitude of the medical members of the Conference as a whole.

After Dr. Abell and Dr. Cabot had spoken on the scheduled program of the second session as noted above, Dr. West, Secretary of the American Medical Association, took the floor on Monday afternoon and pitched into Dr. Cabot whose remarks he considered as a criticism of the American Medical Association. He then continued with a defensive discussion of the American Medical Association and the medical profession, which was a tactical error, as it opened the way for future discussion on this point. It gave a number of speakers the opportunity to attack the American Medical Association while praising the medical profession. To quote Mr. Lee Pressman, Counsel for the C. I. O.: ''I do not criticize the individual doctors. I direct my attack specifically at the upper hierarchy of these medical associations that simply refuse to give adequate health to the people of this country.'' This is not quoted in support of Mr. Pressman's views but to illustrate the attitude taken by a member who spoke. There was no disagreement among the physicians present on Monday night, no matter what they represented or what their personal feelings or interests might be, that the medical profession as ''organized medicine'' had made a bad impression. The situation was so obvious that at his request Dr. Abell of the A. M. A. was given the floor the first thing on Tuesday morning and made some excellent conciliatory remarks, expressing the intention of organized medicine to cooperate. On Tuesday and Wednesday a number of physicians spoke in a general way, including Drs. Kerr, Peters, Veeder, Myers, Osgood, Hamilton, Grulee and Baehr. In general all expressed the attitude that they recognized medical needs were not being adequately met at the present time due to changing conditions, the increase in the load of the medically indigent, and the rapid technical development of medical science with its corresponding increase in the cost of good medical care. The importance of providing for the maintenance and development of the highest medical standards in any program was stressed in one way or another by all. Dr. Osgood spoke of the necessity of independence of action of physicians as is dictated by their consciences. He threw out the suggestion of the possibility of a National Health Council, without executive power, to act in an advisory capacity in matters of health. The importance of medical education and training in any program was stressed by several. Dr. Alice Hamilton, who was called upon impromptu, gave one of the finest talks at the Conference. She stated while in some particulars the figures presented might be wrong, the aggregate picture was correct. Her impressions of the Conference were first of the very great need and secondly of a ''body of people, the physicians, who have striven hard to meet the need, but who are suddenly faced with an increased demand which they themselves cannot meet.'' The ''federal government is not an invading hostile power . . . it is ourselves—ourselves organized.'' She felt there would be certain losses in this new approach to the medical problem, but that every advance has been accompanied by the loss of something precious. She felt we must go forward and meet this new need and did not agree with those who think the need is temporary.

Dr. Fishbein, Editor of the *Journal of the American Medical Association,* spoke Wednesday morning and his remarks were widely quoted in the lay press which was playing up opposition to the program by the American Medical Association. Dr. Fishbein did not attack the program from the standpoint of socialized medicine, but rather that it was based on a temporary need and that he considered other needs as more important. ''The fundamental needs of mankind are food, fuel, clothing, shelter and a job, and medical care and dental care must always be subservient to those main human needs.'' ''Let us concern ourselves with that question of food, fuel, clothing, shelter and a job with adequate wages.'' The importance of these factors was denied by no one and was brought out as related to health several times in the Conference; the Conference, however, was called to discuss a program for medical care not basic economic problems.

Dr. George Baehr, Chairman, Committee on Public Relations of the New York Academy of Medicine, was the last medical speaker. He stated he spoke ''as the average American physician who has been stood up before you throughout this Conference and buffeted about only to be stood up again by the next speaker in time to receive the next blow.'' ''I feel that the medical profession has, partly because of the manner in which it has presented its case, left you with a wrong impression. The average American physician . . . is deeply in sympathy with improving the adequacy of medical care and is ready to agree with you as far as you wish to go, that medical care in many fields of medical activity is not adequate.'' ''. . . you should be sure that we are really making progress forward and not backward.'' He spoke of how private enterprise had pointed the way to government in public health and considered some of the needs due to the failure of government support, and said that the responsibility must be laid at the door of government, not of the medical profession. He spoke of the vast number of communities served by political appointees. ''. . . you are responsible for keeping in office the political administrations which are responsible for this, and therefore to lay these evils at the door of American medicine, to make a scapegoat of the medical profession and not to acknowledge your own responsibility humbly and join with us in making such progress as can be made, is entirely wrong.''

Discussion by Labor.—One of the most interesting parts of the Conference was the discussion of the labor representatives. We have referred to the two scheduled discussions in the second session. Several of the union executives presented detailed medical programs for their groups, which were of significance only as it showed they were thinking of and considering a health program in detail. Several of the speakers dramatically described the conditions of medical care under which the workers were existing. The demand for better medical care was clear and distinct, and the point was made that regardless of what the medical profession thought, they were not satisfied with the medical services available to them, and accused the organized medical profession of blocking progress toward better medical care. Some labor members stated they did not want insurance under state control, as recommended by the technical committee, but would only be satisfied with a federal controlled system. There was some difference of opinion among them as to whether the entire cost should be borne by the employer, or whether a part of the cost of insurance should be borne by the employee. Mr. Green of the A. F. L. suggested that disability compensation be combined administratively with workmen's compensation. Mr. Padway, General Counsel of the A. F. L., believed, as did nearly all labor representatives, in a compulsory system of insurance. He stated the physicians had been criticized too much, and that much was unfounded. The physician has and is rendering excellent service to the community. He must realize that there is some place where he stops, a point beyond which he cannot advance. Beyond that line the government must take up the work. The physician is part of the problem. He must be consulted and have something to say of the plan. He must be an integral part. They must not oppose the plan, because it is coming. He (the physician) must see the handwriting on the wall. He must help devise the plan which will function best.

Specific Recommendations.—Turning to the discussion of specific points. As stated before, the discussion was general as a rule, rather than specific.

Maternal and Child Health. This was apparently accepted as of ''primary importance'' as stated by the Committee. No definite opposition to the expansion of Public Health Services was presented. Several warned of the necessity of going slow, as success would depend on the development and training of personnel.

Some criticism was directed to the hospital recommendations. Father Schwitala and one or two others questioned the factual data, and he stated he feared it would lead to the replacement by government institutions of the voluntary organizations which had given so much service. Dr. Goldwater thought that the program submitted arrives at its results by methods of calculation that are too simple to be reliable. He stated that thousands of hospital beds are now vacant and that efforts for a more complete utilization of existing resources would materially reduce estimates of need. Experience has shown that generous federal hand-outs almost invariably result in political log-rolling and wasteful expenditures.

Medical Care for the Medically Indigent: The question of ''needs'' was not as a whole challenged. There seemed to be a general acceptance of the fact that good medical care was not being received by many who could not afford to pay for it.

The subject of insurance perhaps provoked the most disagreement as to methods, but with few exceptions not as to its place in a national program. Thus labor on one extreme wanted a federally controlled compulsory insurance system. The Committee recommended a state plan. A number of representatives of existing voluntary associations thought the solution lay in the extension of voluntary group insurance plans. ''Group hospitalization'' came in for much favorable discussion, with the suggestion of its extension to include prepayment for medical services.

Capital and Industry: The lack of representatives of capital and industry in the Conference was striking. Huge sums of money were glibly talked about in a casual way that was rather staggering to the medical members of the conference at least. Except for a statement of one labor member that as far as insurance was concerned the ''employer'' must pay the bill, the problem of where the money was coming from was not mentioned. The idea seemed to be that it was for the technical interests and consumer to plan the program and Congress to find the means. The only representative of capital who spoke, Mr. Charles Taussig, President of the American Molasses Company, stated "Progressive business will regard an adequate health service as a subsidy to industry, not a burden."

Perhaps the best summing up of the discussion was that of Prof. Winslow of the Yale University School of Medicine near the close of the final session. We quote from his remarks taken from stenographic notes, and uncorrected by the speaker.

"I have met with groups, a good many of them in this very room or part of it, for ten or twenty years, discussing these problems, and I think in the back of our minds all that time was the dream and the hope that something might happen like this Conference.

"Dr. Grulee suggested that we were dealing here with a premature infant. It would be very presumptuous for me to differ on the point of diagnosis with a professor of pediatrics, but I hope he will take the subject back to his clinic and consider very carefully whether it may not be malnutrition, instead of prematurity. (Laughter.)

"I think this infant is older than he thinks, and I suspect that all it needs is a little administration of vitamins CIO and AFL and whatever kind of vitamin they make in the Farm Bureau, to make it a pretty husky child. (Applause.)

"Now I am going to break all precedents of this Conference by talking about the subject in hand, and the report that has been presented (laughter), and I think this Conference has been of extraordinary significance for three major reasons. In the first place, we have had presented to us here a report which is the work of five independent government departments working in cooperation. Now those of you who remember the one-time relations between the Children's Bureau and the Public Health Service will realize that that is nothing short of a miracle. Nearly half the President's Cabinet is represented in these proposals that have come to us, and for that type of coordinative action, as for so many other things, we owe a tremendous debt to Miss Roche. (Applause.)

"The second reason for which this conference seems to me significant is the excellence of the program that has been presented by the staff that has been working for so long upon it.

"This report is notable for the care with which it has been prepared, for its soundness and particularly for its balance. I think it is possible that in the discussions of yesterday and this morning, devoted largely to one or the other of the particular phases, we may tend to lose sight of the interrelationship which is so skillfully woven into that report. This is not a program of health insurance, it is not a program for the extension of medical service, it is not a program for hospital construction; it is a coordinated, complete, interlocking, dove-tailing health program for the nation in which all these things have their just and proper part.

"In the perfection of that program the members of this conference have brought incalculable aid. I am sure that as we read the printed report, even more than in listening to the speeches, we shall find innumerable instances in which practical, important difficulties have been pointed out and in which happier solutions of certain aspects of the problem have been suggested.

"Yet on the whole I think the most extraordinary thing about this Conference is the overwhelming preponderance of opinion in favor of the general objectives and general methods of the report. So far as I can recall, and I have sat here all through the Conference, partly because of the interest of the speeches and partly, like some of you, I think, because this room is air-cooled and the corridor is not air-cooled—a great addition to the success of any meeting—and I have listened to every paper, only one apparent criticism of the data presented has been made, and that criticism is only apparent. Father Schwitala referred to the study that has been made by the American Medical Association indicating that only a small number of counties in the United States were in all parts more than thirty miles from a hospital. Now that apparently is in conflict with the figures of the Committee, but it isn't in the least because the Committee based its judgment of hospital needs upon the number of beds available per thousand population, and people use beds in hospitals, not hospitals as a whole, and the American Medical Association study simply gives you the number of people within a certain distance of a hospital. On that basis, if there were one 10-bed hospital in the City of New York or the City of Chicago, it would be classified as adequately cared for. Now I don't think even Dr. Goldwater would be inclined to accept that as reasonable or important.

''There have been other suggestions which differed from the general tenor of the report from the standpoint of haste and the rate at which we want to move. Mr. Lee Pressman wants to move much faster and he wants to move more toward federal or centralized control than others. I presume that is because that is the characteristic way in which his temperament works. Dr. Goldwater and Dr. Olin West want to move more slowly, and with less centralization. That probably is the way their temperaments work, and both those points of view are helpful in arriving at exactly the proper pace that is desirable under given circumstances.

''I would like to say just one word about this question of federalization, though it was admirably treated by an earlier speaker today. I am a little troubled sometimes at the assumption that a Federal Government is a peculiar, strange kind of foreign body intruded into these United States by some mistake. I have never been able to regard it that way. I regard the Federal Government like the State government and the city government, and like my Community Chest of which I have for two years been president, as an organ through which I and my fellow citizens can function, and I don't think there is any particular spiritual or moral value about a voluntary or an official agency or a state or a federal agency. The problem is, how can a particular end best be achieved?

''I am an individualist, because I am a New Englander. I like to do things when I can on my own steam. If I can't, I like to do things as a member of my family, or as a member of a voluntary agency in the community, or as a citizen of my city or my state or my nation, and I quite agree that the simplest and most direct way of solving a particular problem should be sought, but I think the evidence presented here has been absolutely overwhelming that individual and voluntary and city and state agencies are inadequate to meet this situation without the help and the stimulus that this federal plan will give to them.

''Mr. Weiss in discussing his attitude about the matter said that he was one of those people who wanted to have his doctor. Judging by the success of *Time Magazine,* I suppose he can (laughter), but the reason why this conference is called is that there are a great many million American citizens who can't have their doctor, and the whole purpose of these projects that have been put before you is to give them somewhat similar opportunities to those enjoyed by Mr. Weiss. (Applause.)

''Now the further reason why this congress is significant is the astounding and thrilling support that has come to its main objectives from the groups that have been represented here. I have, as I say, discussed this thing in this room and in other rooms, but never before has it been discussed face to face with those great agencies that really represent the American people, and when this health program has received, as it has received in general principle and in broad method, the support of both the great labor organizations of the country, of the agriculture of the country, of the business of the country with that splendid phrase, which we never want to forget, of Mr. Taussig's, that 'tax-supported health program was not a tax burden but a subsidy to industry,' and with that other magnificent phrase of his, that 'democracy should be a sword as well as a shield'; when we have the support of the women of the country, and the parents of the country, and the youth of the country, and the press, that is a fact of the most profound and momentous significance.

''We have, I think, in the course of this discussion made it fairly clear that criticism of the existing situation is not criticism of the medical profession, any more than Dr. Baehr's admirable, just, and sound criticisms of our political force was a criticism of us as individuals. There are in my part of the country many people who don't like anything that is going on today in Washington, but because they do not like the acts of the present administration that happens to be in power, it doesn't mean that they are making an assault on the American home and on George Washington and the Constitution.

''On the contrary, I see in the discussions of this Conference, particularly on Monday, an extraordinarily touching appeal to the medical profession. It has been the boast of the medical profession, and the just boast, and the source of proper pride, that if a woman came with a sick child to an individual physician and said, 'My child is suffering and we want you to care for it,' that he never failed to respond. Now what has happened here this week is that the representatives of millions of men and women in the United States have come to the medical profession as a group and said, 'Our members are sick and suffering and we want medical care for them, and we want means provided by which we can pay.' Is it possible, is it conceivable that that appeal is going to be rejected? I think not. (Applause.)

''I was reading a rather poorly typed manuscript a day or two ago and I came to the title of a reference which I thought read, 'Medical Care Not Now.' I looked more carefully and saw it was in the *Survey* and realized that title couldn't be right (it might have been in some other magazines), and I found the title really was, 'Medical Care But How.' And I thought my mistake rather symbolized our situation. I think with this Conference the whole problem has shifted from medical care not now to medical care but how.

''Now I, like Dr. Davis, do not minimize the difficulties. There are many practical difficulties. I would like to point out that running through all these proposals that have been made, there are as it seems to me two fundamental problems. One is the problem of organizing the medical profession for effective service. It is not now organized effectively for physicians, because physicians are in large measure not where they are needed and it is not now organized in such a way as to give the maximum possible guarantees of quality. That is a professional question. It is a question which must be solved by the medical profession through their medical societies, and perhaps better through their hospital staffs, and by the health officers of the community, but underlying all these problems is that basic problem, that one basic problem of organizing the profession so as to make their services available where they are needed and to keep those services at the highest possible level of quality.

''The other problem, of course, is the question of organizing the profession properly for effective service and to organize the financial resources in the community to make the maximum possible and maximum reasonable payment for that service.

''It is quite clear, I think, that effective methods of organizing the community's contribution to payment can be made without any interference with the standards of the profession and without any interference with the principle of freedom of choice.

''I have great sympathy with the principle of freedom of choice of physician, but I should like to point out that any acceptable definition of freedom of choice of physicians must include the right of a group of patients to choose a group of physicians for their service. (Applause.)

''Any artificial attempts to interfere with that freedom cannot stand.

''Mr. Kellogg in his excellent address yesterday introduced the fable of King Canute. He did not make any application of it; he is much too diplomatic; nor will I. I do not know who he thought was attempting to hold the tide back, but I do know that I am not of that kind, and that as I think over these three days and the great wave of enthusiasm and devotion to the promotion of national health that has been manifest here, I say, thank God, at last the tide is coming in!'' (Applause.)

In closing the Conference Miss Roche stated that in light of the discussion and suggestions, the Technical and Interdepartmental Committees would move forward to a plan of action. She felt the discussion revealed substantial agreement on fundamental points, and many of the principles set forth in the recommendations. In preparing proposals for legislative action, the Interdepartmental Committee hopes to have the benefit of further counsel from those present as well as others who have not been present. ''I think it should be unnecessary to specify that among those from whom we expect to receive constructive suggestions and aid are the members of the medical profession.''

Borden Veeder.

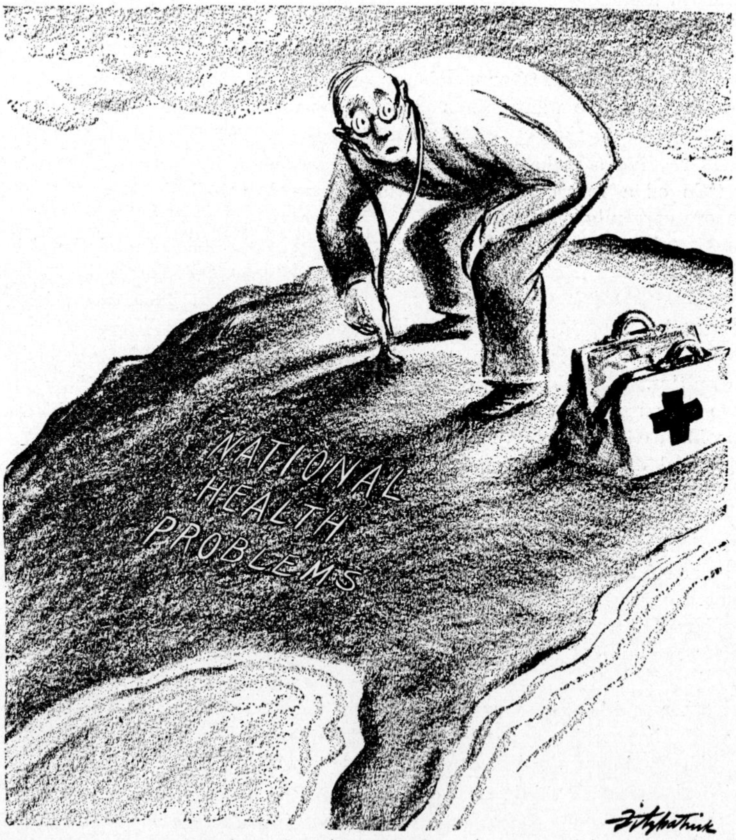

THE DOCTOR HEARS STRANGE RUMBLINGS.

—By permission of the St. Louis Post-Dispatch.

Critical Review

SOME PEDIATRIC PROBLEMS OF BEHAVIOR IN INFANCY AND EARLY CHILDHOOD

LEO KANNER, M.D.
BALTIMORE, MD.

INFANCY and early childhood have for a long time been the no man's land of child psychiatry. The personality and behavior problems of older children have for the past two to three decades been studied and treated in mental hygiene and child guidance clinics, psychiatric out-patient departments of some of our large hospitals, and by psychiatrists connected with schools, camps, placement agencies, juvenile courts, and correctional institutions. The developmental and training difficulties of infants, however, did not come to the attention of any of those groups. Valuable contributions were made by psychologists about the normal evolution of early functions and some of their fluctuations but usually not in a manner that would make those observations serve as immediate practical aids to parents and nurses. The few articles on disturbing behavior of infants, however meritorious, were almost lost like drops in the ocean of literature concerning behavior, training, socialization, and parent-child relationship after the third year of life. The psychoanalysts, through retrospective deductions from interpreted material obtained from adults, have built into the infant's, the newborn infant's, and even embryo's "unconscious" a wealth of mechanisms and experiences which have been substantiated about as convincingly as the reports of life after death.

And yet, "life," "behavior," "interpersonal relationship," all that goes gradually into the making of a person, certainly is present from birth. Maternal perplexities, uncertainties, apprehensions may be present then and may have existed even before then. The parents cannot, and should not, turn for advice about their infants' behavior to psychiatrists, most of whom will honestly admit that they have had no experience whatever with infants. The parents expect that advice to come from their pediatricians. For this reason, a review of the work with problems of behavior in infancy and early childhood has its proper place in a pediatric journal.

PROBLEMS OF FEEDING BEHAVIOR

Infant nutrition has rightly been a major issue of pediatrics. The factors of growth, health, and general development are closely interwoven with the adequacy of food and digestion. The process of establishing usable principles of feeding has been accompanied by much controversy, by rigidity and relaxation of rules, by an assortment of dogma, heresy, and skepticism. Attention was so thoroughly focused on *giving* food to infants, that the infants' *taking* of food, or feeding behavior, had little opportunity left for consideration. Refusal and fussiness that were not directly attributable to physical illness were labeled as nervous anorexia, which in turn was usually treated with more concentration on the food to be given and little, if any, regard for the child to be fed. This neglect of the eating habits of infants eventually came back as a boomerang when psychologists, pediatricians, and parents began to become person-conscious and look in the individual child for explanations of his acceptance or rejection of food. Anorexia, the dreaded *crux paediatrica,* came to be viewed not merely as a pseudodiagnostic alibi but as a definite therapeutic and prophylactic challenge. The last fifteen years have seen a wholesome and, as events have shown, practically helpful shift in the attitude towards eating difficulties of infants and children. Attention to food substances was supplemented by attention to feeding behavior. "Feeding behavior," as Gesell[17] has recently said, "is chiefly concerned with the intake of food rather than with food assimilation. Assimilation, however, may be indirectly affected by the mode of intake, so unified is the personality of the infant and so pervasive is the psychobiology of the alimentary tract. . . . Each child presents an individual pattern of growth and an individual pattern of personality. Although the feeding behavior of infants develops in accordance with certain laws, the expression of these laws takes on unique features in the individual. Therein lies the necessity of individualization in the supervision of feeding behavior. . . . In the diagnosis and supervision of feeding behavior we have an approach to a developmental hygiene which embraces at once the growing body and mind."

Important contributions to this change of front have come both from pediatricians and psychologists. Among the former group, Aldrich[1-3] and Brennemann[6-8] deserve a great deal of credit for doing pioneer work in this direction. Aldrich has had the courage to present his insights to the lay public in a readable and informative book which manages to steer clear of the pitfalls of overpopularization and unnecessary alarm. (Alarm is always unnecessary.) The incidence of anorexia in private pediatric practice has been variously estimated at from 50 to 85 per cent.[21] Brennemann stated: "Anorexia is not an occasional occurrence, an isolated phenomenon in childhood; it is the rule in that very stratum of society in which mothers are lying awake nights planning a gospel diet and the most effective way of administering it. . . . It has been stated that this condition exists only among the well-to-do—that a poor appetite is rare among the poor. My experience does not quite confirm this observation." As a matter of fact, in our own work at the Harriet Lane Home children with feeding difficulties have been referred with about equal relative frequency from the dispensary and the private consultation service, a total of not less than one-fourth of all cases sent for psychiatric advice. "This truly amazing phenomenon, the majority of the young of any animal refusing to eat a diet that is not only scientifically optimum, but as appetizing as culinary ingenuity can make it, can be explained only on a psychologic basis. It is, a priori, unthinkable that it is on a physical basis."[6] Brennemann found the psychologic feature to consist of two principal interrelated components, one to be sought in the environment and the other in the child himself. Obsession with the dangers of overfeeding, undernutrition, and deviation from rigid rules about quantities, percentages, calories, intervals, and stools, and a campaign of frequent weighing and measuring to attain narrowly delimited standards of "perfection" have tried to make of the infant something of a machine to be oiled with certain kinds of oil only, at certain times only, in a certain manner only, with just so much oil only, and according to specifications provided for all machines, regardless of their special makes and performances. Many infants, not being machines, rebel against this standardizing, "extraneously, arbitrarily imposed authority," inflicted dutifully and carried out to the letter by anxious mothers; the adults' emphasis on eating furthermore supplies the child with an effective tool for his desire for the spotlight and domination of the home.

How imperative and indispensable are those exacting diet prescriptions imposed upon mothers and infants? Clara Davis[10-13] approached this question in a very original way. She subjected three infants of weaning age to a self-selected diet experiment, two for periods of six months each, and one for a period of a year. Having previously had no other nourishment than breast milk, they were allowed to choose without any kind of restriction from a large assortment of ordinary foodstuffs. They were able from the first to select their own diets in quantities sufficient to maintain themselves with apparently optimal digestive and good nutritional results as far as immediate effects could be judged. They were omnivorous and in eating were governed not only by their caloric needs, but showed definite preferences which, however, changed from time to time and were unpredictable. These studies, carried out at the Children's Memorial Hospital in Chicago, were extended to include fifteen children. Cooked and raw, uncombined, unseasoned, and unsophisticated foods were served according to an unvarying schedule of three meals a day, and no food was given between meals. Each child had his own small table and the foods for the meal were set before him on a tray. Children ate with spoons or fingers, depending on ability or preference, and empty dishes were promptly refilled to make sure that the children got all they wanted of everything. Food and eating were never discussed by the attendants in the presence of the children. In this setting, "anorexia, other than as a transient loss of appetite with acute parenteral infection, was unknown among them, all eating heartily with keen appetite day in, day out. It was not unusual for children to eat three or four bananas at a meal or five to seven servings of potatoes or meat. One child a year old frequently drank a quart of milk at his noon meal besides eating other food. Yet none were fat, and all were solid well-built children, healthy and vigorous, presenting no problems in behavior. A few instances of vomiting or diarrhea occurred with an acute parenteral infection, but otherwise there were no digestive disturbances and never any constipation, laxatives never being needed or given to any. The study demonstrated that under the conditions of the experiment and with such natural foodstuffs young children could choose their diets and thrive without adult direction of eating."

In another equally fascinating study, Dr. Davis[12] allowed three infants their choice of four formulas from the end of the first week of life throughout the nursing period. The formulas consisted of (1) a proprietary "reconstructed" cow's milk (Similac), in which there was some readjustment of the fat and salt content and addition of lactose to approximate woman's milk as much as possible; (2) fermented lactic acid milk with 5 per cent of Blue Label Karo corn syrup; (3) a simple milk dilution formula (whole milk, boiled ten minutes, 20 ounces; water, 10 ounces; lactose, 1.5 ounces); (4) an orange juice, egg yolk, sugar, milk, and water formula. One of four bottles of equal make and size, with nipples of the same brand and shape, was offered; when the infant stopped sucking or did not suck, a second bottle was substituted, until all four had been proffered. A bottle emptied during the feeding was refilled to insure that the infant had all he wanted of that formula. The total quantity was left entirely to the infant. Undiluted orange juice was given twice daily. The infants showed individual differences in taste, though the preferences shown were moderate in degree. The most striking feature of their performance, however, was the wide variation in the quantities taken at a feeding. "This pattern of eating behavior, i.e., occasional 'stuffing' and meals of widely varying quantities, is, of course, the natural one not only of mammalian young in general, but also of the breast-fed baby. Furthermore, it is not only an infantile pattern but one that continues to a greater or less degree throughout life. Artificially fed infants appear to be the only large group on whom identical quantities for successive meals are meticulously imposed, and one cannot but wonder whether the comfort of these infants who exercised choice not only of formulas but of quantities and their complete freedom from digestive discomforts and symptoms of any sort were not due rather to the following of this natural eating pattern than to the combinations made by their choices of formulas."

I have reported the Davis experiments in some detail because I consider them as being of fundamental significance. They give scientific backing to the present trend of refusing to sacrifice regard for children's personal needs and domestic tranquillity on the altar of nutritional dogmatism. They make allowance for individual preferences, with strikingly satisfactory results. Confirmation of the early existence of personal differences with regard to food intake and feeding behavior has come from nursery observations made by reliable psychologists and published, among others, by Eliot,[15] Ripin,[22] and Dockeray.[14] An important recent contribution has come from Gesell and Ilg,[17] who reported their work comprehensively last year in a book entitled, *Feeding Behavior of Infants.* The authors made minute studies of infants' eating from the first day of life until the second year and recorded carefully the "foundational patterns" of feeding and related behavior, the motor mechanisms of feeding (basic adjustment, suckling, mastication, swallowing, from hand to mouth), behavior towards nursing utensils (breast, bottle, cup, spoon), reaction to different types and consistency of food, acceptance and rejection, food-sleep relationship, and the interplay between infant and adults in connection with eating. This book is a veritable storehouse of well-rounded information and renders a real service to pediatricians.

Attempts have been made to show how early feeding behavior may affect the development of character and conduct. The use of statistical correlations between feeding methods and later behavior problems or personality traits seems to this reviewer to be of questionable value in situations in which numerous other factors are variously and potently at play. It may be in order to correlate more specific items, such as satiation from breast feeding and finger-sucking, as Levy[32] has done (reported under the caption of thumb-sucking). Beyond that, however, one wonders how many errors are introduced by the neglect of many significant features in the life of the child. Childers and Hamil[9] studied the emotional problems of 469 children less than 13 years of age "as related to the duration of breast feeding in infancy." Their tabulations seemed to show that undesirable behavior manifestations (of patients referred to the Neuro-Psychiatric Clinic of Harper Hospital, Detroit) were greatest among those who had been weaned between the first and sixth months of life; next in frequency were those who had never been breast-fed; then came the group in which breast feeding had been continued into the "normal" period for weaning; the children in whom breast feeding had been prolonged beyond the eleventh month showed the smallest percentages of undesirable traits. The authors concluded honestly: "The statistical fallacies of this study are recognized, but the comparisons illustrated in the graphs of the four groups are quite interesting." Hill[18] selected from more than 500 consecutive admissions to a psychiatric clinic 172 children and adults (!) "because of the available detailed information regarding early childhood development for special study of the relation of infant feeding, digestive disturbances, and personality disorders." The group was composed of cases in which the breast feeding was inadequate, excessive, or adequate. Hill reached the following conclusions: "Inadequate or excessive breast feeding is undesirable both from the physiological and psychological viewpoints. Both of these extremes in infant feeding are common. It was inadequate in 49 per cent of the cases and excessive in 9 per cent. A strong familial interest in the upper alimentary tract and a faulty maternal emotional reaction to the child are most important factors in functional gastrointestinal and emotional disorders." The thirteen examples cited, of whom three only are children, are so heterogeneous and offer such extremes of schizophrenic, manic depressive, alcoholic and psychoneurotic conditions, that the jump from infant feeding to personality disorders appears to have skipped all sorts of biographic data certainly not less life-shaping than the feeding in infancy.

Mohr's study[20] keeps itself on much firmer ground. In an investigation of sixty-six children presenting problems of eating behavior, he stressed the importance of the emotional relationship between mother and child and advocated early instruction of the family on the part of physicians, for "failure to cope adequately with this problem implies a likelihood of similar unsatisfactory modes of behavior in other fields of activity." R. M. and H. Bakwin,[4] in a recent discussion of the prevention of anorexia, stated: "Anorexia during the first months of life, though usually organic in origin, often has a basis in the psychologic environment. The most potent psychologic factor at this early age is an agitated, uncertain parent or nurse. Young infants appear to be particularly susceptible to this attitude and react with restlessness, disturbed sleep, excessive crying, anorexia, and often vomiting."

Summary.—During approximately the past ten years, attention to the average and the undesirable feeding behavior of infants and children has been added to the interest in the foodstuffs to be given. Anorexia which is not solely due to physical illness is now recognized as the result of the combined behavior of the infant who is fed and the person or persons feeding him. The Davis self-selection experiments have tended to do away with nutritional obsessiveness, at the same time without losing sight of the sound basic principles arrived at in many years of patient pediatric work in laboratories as well as in the nursery. The pediatricians, encouraged by their personal experiences, the insight of leaders in their own ranks, studies made by psychologists and the fundamental work of Gesell, have come to include in their practice the prevention and treatment of faulty feeding behavior as part of the physical and mental hygiene of infancy and childhood. Education of the parents in matters of early feeding behavior is becoming in an increasing degree a part of the pediatrician's task.

THUMB-SUCKING

The great concern of present-day mothers over the thumb-sucking of their offspring is largely due to the warnings of alarmists in the ranks of dentists and psychologists. Prior to those scares, the habit received but scant notice from parents, pediatricians, or anyone else. Even folklore, seizing so promptly upon every portion and function of the human body, attributing great significance to such things as sneezing and yawning and firmly believing in the worm etiology of nose picking or grinding of teeth, has failed to consider finger-sucking as worthy of its attention. Several famous artists depicted children with thumbs in their mouths to give them an expression of serene tranquillity. Mazzini[38] and Bragman,[26] who compiled notes on thumb-sucking in productions of art, saw it presented in paintings and sculptures of Ghirlandajo (*Adoration of the Magi,* 1488), della Robbia, Borgognone, Credi, Lippi, and other Italian masters of the early Renaissance. The notion that it is bad or harmful did not arise until the end of the last century.

Since that time, dentists and especially orthodontists asserted that thumb-sucking results in malformations of the jaws and palate. Parents were therefore admonished to do everything within their power to curb a child's performance so injurious to his future mastication and physiognomy. All sorts of mechanical devices were invented, publicized, and marketed to keep the little thumbs from reaching the mouth. Illustrated articles in dental and pediatric journals[23, 25, 28, 40] described ever new varieties of cuffs, muffs, Elizabethan collars, and modified strait jackets. People who refrained from hampering children's movements took refuge to ill-tasting substances which were smeared on the fingers in order to preclude sucking and subsequent damage to the configuration of the jaws. Later investigations tended to show that the shape of the palate does not become affected by thumb-sucking. Temporary malocclusion may occur but does not become permanent. Lewis,[37] in 1930, concluding the observation of 170 children over a five-year period, found some degree of malocclusion of the deciduous teeth in twenty-four out of thirty thumb-suckers; if the habit had been stopped before 6 years of age, the deformity corrected itself spontaneously. Hence, early sucking certainly did not produce serious or lasting disfigurements. Yet it is mostly the wailings alone that reach anxious mothers, and not the calming reassurances. Popular books on the care of infants continue to discuss the harmful results of thumb-sucking.

Parents are also besought to beware of the germ danger. Says a famous psychologist who has become a very widely read mentor for mothers:[41] "From the standpoint of the child the matter is serious. Physicians tell us that some 90 per cent of diseases due to germs find their way into the body through the mouth. The child with its mobile hands gathers germs everywhere. Next it puts the hands into the warm, moist mouth. The germs are thus given an ideal breeding place." If a mother is not duly scared by that, she may read on as the text continues:

"If persisted in for long at an early age before the bony, tendinous, and muscular tissues harden, the mouth becomes misshapen and the fingers and hands are changed in their contours. There are many other bodily changes which may occur, such as interference with the proper growth and position of the teeth." You can see a frightened mother, after the perusal of this or similar bits of information, run to her physician, imploring him to save her thumb-sucking infant from a life of disease and ugliness, with misshapen mouth and teeth and fingers and hands, with his mouth a culture medium for germs introduced by the thumb! The mother does not have a chance to read statements in scientific journals, such as this:[4] "There is no evidence to indicate that thumb-suckers are more susceptible than other children to gastrointestinal disturbances, infection, or stomatitis."

As if the overemphasis on physical effects were not enough, parents have been harassed by psychologists. Said Watson:[41] "The effect of thumb-sucking upon the child's personality is the most serious aspect of all." According to him, "millions of mothers who are almost criminally careless" use a pacifier to keep the child quiet and, if they let their offspring suck the thumb (a "highly unsocial act"), they are "condemned in progressive communities." And, of course, he did not forget to tell mothers that thumb-sucking is "in part a sex response closely akin to masturbation." This wisdom had come to him from psychoanalysis. Freud,[27] in the second of his *Three Contributions to the Theory of Sex,* chose thumb-sucking "as a model of the infantile sexual manifestations." He believed that "association of the manifestations into which we have gained an insight through psychoanalytic investigation justifies us in claiming thumb-sucking as a sexual activity." Since not all children suck their thumbs, he assumed that "it is found only in children in whom the erogenous significance of the lip zone is constitutionally reinforced. If the latter is retained in some children they develop into kissing epicures with a tendency to perverse kissing, or as men, they show a strong desire for drinking and smoking. But should repression come into play, they then show disgust for eating and evince hysterical vomiting. By virtue of the community of the lip zone, the repression encroaches upon the instinct of nourishment." Thumb-sucking is viewed as a form of autoerotism, the sexual aim being under the control of an erogenous zone. If "autoerotism" simply means derivation of pleasure from certain sensations of the body, then the pleasure derived from sucking is autoerotic by definition. The hedonic component of many of the manipulations of the body cannot be denied or minimized. Nor does one wish to deny that some degree of lack of self-control is common to all of them. Homburger[29] has referred to the sensations which accompany them as "perverse pleasure sensations." But this is something altogether different from attributing sexual significance to the habit and even identifying it with "larvated masturbation." Psychoanalysis, though, is probably not to be blamed directly for the extent to which some of its adherents have gone in analyzing the habit of thumb-sucking. Melanie Klein,[31] reporting the case of six-year-old Erna, told a listening world that the little girl's thumb-sucking "was caused by phantasies of sucking, biting, and devouring her father's penis and her mother's breasts. The penis represented the whole father and the breasts the whole mother."

The etiology of thumb-sucking has been approached from still another angle. Levy[32, 35] has in an interesting study come to the conclusion that in a majority of instances it is due to insufficient lip movements or incompleteness of the sucking phase of the feeding act, regardless of the type of feeding (breast, bottle, or mixed). He named as the most frequent causative factors: (1) spontaneous withdrawal from a too rapidly flowing breast or bottle; (2) forced withdrawal from sucking at the termination of too short a period of time; (3) changing feeding schedules with increasing intervals between feedings and diminished duration of the feeding time. Each nursing period, according to Levy, begins with the child tense and restless because of hunger. As the feeding continues, he becomes relaxed, and after a fully satisfying meal he is sufficiently relaxed to fall asleep. If, however, he is not fully satiated, he may suck his thumb or fingers, thus maintaining something of the pleasures of nursing until he falls asleep. There can be nothing seriously undesirable about this form of behavior, provided it does not become chronic. But if the feeding is not entirely satisfactory, there is danger that each meal will so frequently be followed by thumb-sucking that the act will become thoroughly habitual. Levy[33, 34, 36] subsequently extended his investigations to dogs, calves, and chickens. If the feeding act was disrupted before the point of satiety was reached, a sucking habit resulted in dogs in the form of licking of the paw or the body of another dog, besides sucking of various inanimate objects. In calves, the licking habits concerned the ears of other calves, painted boards, clothes, anything suitable for licking. The pecking behavior of chickens raised on a platform of wire mesh (and that of turkeys) was found to follow the same law of instinct satiation as in the studies of sucking behavior. Levy stated that the percentage of finger-suckers was highest in infants fed every four hours, less in a group fed every three hours, and least in a group fed irregularly. On the other hand, Gesell[17] was led by his own observations to remark that "there are so many exceptions to this relationship that it cannot be set down as a general factor."

Gesell[17] found finger-sucking to be associated with hunger during the first few weeks of life, but then receding at the time when the postural development does not permit the hands to be readily brought to the mouth. By the third month, this movement becomes easier again, and the fists are sucked prior to and later also after feeding. In the fourth month, the sucking in many cases appears throughout the day. The infant "probably relieves the pain" from local irritations that may be present weeks or months before actual eruption of the teeth "and possibly aids dentition by mouthing his fist." The successive teething episodes seem to exacerbate the hand-to-mouth response. "With those who later become persistent thumb-suckers, the degree of the sucking may markedly lessen or even vanish between the teething periods. All of this behavior suggests that mouthing may play a part in the developmental economy of teething." Fatigue and frustration are other inciting factors. Gesell reported a most interesting observation. When an overzealous mother, in her efforts to train her child in toilet habits, places him on the toilet many times when he has no occasion to use it, the thumb-sucking child usually does not resist the procedure but promptly begins to suck his thumb and keeps it up contentedly for the duration of the séance. However, if he spontaneously asks for the toilet, he will not bring his thumb to his mouth.

Summary.—Thumb-sucking in infancy has been made the object of parental scare by insistence on its damaging effect on dental occlusion, the infectiousness of the sucked finger, and its identification with autoerotism. Sober observation has tended to remove these scares and thus free infants from all sorts of frantic attempts to break them from the habit. Pediatricians can help frightened mothers by explaining to them the relative harmlessness of a short period of indulgence. Reasonably well-fed and well-occupied children will sooner or later give up the habit without the much more harmful battle introduced by the application of devices which hamper their movements. Calm removal of the thumb from the mouth, substitution of play interests for the pleasure derived from sucking and absence of unwarranted alarm constitute the best method of treatment of thumb-sucking in infancy.

THE SO-CALLED AGE OF RESISTANCE

The earliest expressions of anger, resentment, remonstrance, disobedience, spitefulness, stubbornness, and destructiveness, the first refusals to conform to feeding, sleeping, and elimination routine, and the beginnings of any kind of willful resistance to adult direction and training have been said by many investigators to appear during the third year of life. This type of behavior, succeeding a biennium of relative submissiveness, has been frequently referred to in the literature as a characteristic manifestation of the "age of resistance" or "period of negativism"; German authors speak of it as the "spite period of childhood." It is generally stated that it lasts several months sometimes between the ages of 2 and 4 years. Thom[54] spoke of a group of children who develop what may be termed "contra-suggestibility" from 3 to 5 years of age. Many psychologists became first aware of this contrariness by the observation of the frequency of children's refusals to cooperate in mental test situations. Binet[44] mentioned the difficulties encountered in trying to obtain the cooperation of normal 3-year-old children, attributing them either to timidity or to "bad mood" and "bad will." Gesell[17] remarked that "the 2-year-old child is considered to be the most resistant to psychological examination." Reynolds[52] found in a study of 229 preschool children that the peak of negativism was at or below 2 years of age, with a gradual decrease from then on. The mean of the negativistic scores of the 2-year-old group was 6.44 and that of the 4½-year-old group was 2.26. The correlations between life age and negativistic score were higher than those between mental age and the score. There was no special difference shown in the reaction patterns of the refusals made by the different age groups, the distinction being one of frequency rather than of degree or kind. The 2-year-old child was more apt to refuse to cooperate on a situation but when he did refuse he showed the same kind of behavior as the older children. The 4-year-old subject was less likely to refuse, but when he did his behavior pattern was similar to that of the younger children.

Levy and Tulchin,[50, 51] who observed 983 infants and children during testing, found the manifestation of resistance to be typically pronounced at 18 to 23 months in girls and at 30 to 35 months in boys, yielding gradually with age in both sexes. They tabulated the resistance patterns during mental tests of 110 children ranging in age between 6 and 54 months. The earliest resistances noted, at 6 to 7 months, were crying and clinging to the mother. All reactions recorded before the fourteenth month were crying and withdrawal movements denoting some relation with the mother. At 16 to 17 months, assault reactions directed towards toys or the examiner and head shaking and verbal objections made their first appearance. Latest to arrive were more complex modes of behavior, such as slapping movements without slapping or walking back to the mother in the midst of the test. Crying, most frequent in the first year, gradually diminished in frequency with increasing age. Simple crying after two years and withdrawal reactions (looking away, covering the face, hand movements) occurred oftener in girls, clinging to the mother oftener in boys.

The majority of authors consider the resistant behavior of preschool children as a normal feature of child development. Thom[54] said: "The negativistic phase of the child's life is recognized as being a normal reaction occurring in the process of growing up. It is the period when the child begins to assert his own personality, when he resents domination by others. This is a natural and healthy reaction." According to Helen Woolley,[55] "negativism constitutes a very frequent stage of development in very young children. It seems to be a natural step in the development of personality. When a child begins to get a feeling of himself as an independent agency, he enjoys trying out his powers." Some attempts at accounting for the resistance have led the authors far afield into theoretical realms. Haeberlin (quoted by Benjamin[42]) was probably the first to compare the infantile remonstrances to the sulkiness and sullenness observed in the early part of the second decade. He was apparently so struck by certain resemblances that he spoke of this phase as the "first puberty." Charlotte Buehler[45] also found analogies between puberty and the so-called age of resistance, consisting chiefly of hostility to the environment and at the same time the formation of strong attachments. She concluded that the similarity indicates the presence from 2 to 4 years of age of a first spurt of sexual development, which then subsides to be resumed at the time of pubescence. A strange interpretation came from Busemann.[47, 48] He began with the assertion that the existence of the "spite period," which according to him begins at about 27 months of age, is an indisputable biologic fact. Like the sucking mechanisms and the instincts related to them, it is anchored genetically and provided for in the anlage. As a matter of fact, Busemann counted five different stages of resistance in the course of childhood and adolescence, the first between 2 and 4 years, the second at about 6, the third between 8 and 9, the fourth between 12 and 14, and the fifth from 16 to 17 years. Nature, he argued, has intended for women a birth rhythm with about three-year intervals between the arrivals of new offspring. If, contrary to this prescription, the next child fails to appear on schedule, the existing youngster suffers from a "luxuriant educational activity" on the part of his mother. She has enough time on her hand to will and act for the child, who in turn having developed his own volition and sense of power rebels against this with stubbornness and spite. Hence the only child is especially likely to go through the five "cycles of excitability," the tempo and course of which are said to be the "biological functions of the maternal birth rhythm."

The infantile period of resistance has been accorded particular significance by Benjamin,[42, 43] who saw in its manifestations and management a most important factor in the development of childhood neuroses and the determination of a child's personality formation. Mention of a connection with future character traits had been made previously by Hetzer,[49] who stated that the absence of any negativism in a 2- to 4-year-old child may result in weak-willed meekness. Benjamin, like others (Busemann, Levy, and Tulchin), felt that the display of resistance is evidence of an inherent behavior pattern: "Anlage is one of the most essential genetic factors. Differences of reaction forms are based on variations rooted in the anlage." Benjamin took the spite period most seriously as a phenomenon very closely related to morbidity. He wanted a sharp line drawn between normal behavior during that age, about which he had a very little to say, and psychopathologic conditions, to which he assigned the role of a distinct nosologic entity. The basic disturbance lies in the child's failure of adaptation to his environment, due to insecurity and anxiety. His difficulty of adjusting to the task of growing into relationships with other people and the acceptance of values determined by them leads to a state of disorientation, hostile refusals, and isolation, with aversion to cleanliness and to the acquisition of functions commensurate with his age. Hence, for example, come the persistence of enuresis and disorders of speech. This failure of adaptation leaves three possible avenues open to the child: developmental standstill, even to the point of regression to a previous stage of existence in which there was a greater feeling of security; introversive turning away from reality to find consolation in thumb-sucking, masturbation, and rhythmic body movements (such as rocking, head rolling, jactatio capitis nocturna); and spiteful rebellion, resembling the fluttering of a caged bird or the bewildered agitation of an adult in a panic situation. Out of the latter mode of reaction arise feeding problems, vomiting, rebellious wetting and soiling, destructiveness, breath-holding spells, and temper tantrums. A neurosis is characterized by the unnaturally protracted duration of the spite period and has its origin in a combination of social contact disturbances, partial inhibition of psychic development, inner insecurity, and faulty training. Although the rebellion seems to come as a sudden change, two-thirds of Benjamin's 205 cases presented difficulties from the first few months of life, expressed through restlessness, abundant crying, vomiting, constipation, pylorospasm, and stereotyped movements. Because of the etiological significance of the spite period as the basis for later neurotic conditions, Benjamin urged early prophylaxis and treatment not of the symptoms alone but of the total person. His case illustrations depict various problems of preschool children, which are much too readily interpreted as outgrowths of the spite reaction, though they contain ample evidence that many other factors are at play.

Those who believe in the existence of a circumscribed period of resistance have adduced support from some observations made by child psychologists. William Stern[53] and Karl Buehler[46] have noticed independently that a child's first "No" has a volitional meaning and that the significance as a simple denial of fact appears several months afterwards. The nearly uses of "No" mean: "No, I won't do that," "No, that is not to be." A child may have learned to scream "No, no" very energetically when a toy is taken away from him. But for another two or three months, although he can quite correctly show his hands and eyes, he is unable to say "No" when his hand is touched and he is asked, "Is this your little eye?'' Similarly, the volitional ''I'' precedes its intellectualized use even by a longer time, approximately five or six months. Stern's two eldest children said ''I'' for the first time at 24 months of age. When one was given a ball, the other said, ''I look for ball, me too.'' But not until 30 months of age was ''I'' employed in connection with a statement of fact, such as ''I am small.''

Whether a child's first remonstrances be regarded as an exquisitely specific, anlage-determined, circumscribed phase of infantile development or as the beginnings of self-awareness and self-assertiveness, much will be gained if parents could be prepared for those early negations and refusal practices as something to be looked forward to as signs of normal healthy evolution. They are useful functions of the growing individual that contain the nucleus for sound criticism, competition, and the preservation of self-dependence and self-respect. This attitude would help to remove from children trying to orient themselves in interpersonal relationships the odium of disobedience and contrariness and emphasize the constructive socializing value of self-assertion. The practice of meeting resistance with counterresistance only tends to make of the home a field of battle between the youngster and his elders. A child needs the same good-natured aid and encouragement in finding his place in the family group as he needs in his first attempts at walking, self-feeding, going up the stairs, or climbing on a chair. No harm is done if the petty and irrelevant ''No, no'' and ''I won't'' replies are disregarded, if at the same time the more important matters of daily routine and habit regularity are insisted upon with gentle firmness. A child's right to resist unreasonable demands should be acknowledged. Parental domination that wishes to break a child's will and keep him turned on like a mechanical toy, parental indulgence that shrinks from crossing a child's will with the excuse of his frail, delicate, nervous condition, or, out of sheer convenience, the extremes of tyranny and excessive leniency, should be equally discouraged.

Summary.—At the end of the second or at the beginning of the third year of life, children acquire the meaning and application of negation, which is added to their reactive equipment. This acquisition is a normal feature of infantile development. Much of the parent-child relationship for years to come, much of the child's contributions to the family life, much of his character formation depends on the adults' attitude to, and management of, those early negations, refusals, remonstrances, and resistances. Impatient adult counterresistance is apt to bring about an exaggeration and perpetuation in the child of a type of behavior which is a natural and desirable phenomenon to begin with. The one extreme of uncomprehending insistence on strict immediate obedience with harshness and violence often brings on spite and a long war, in which the child uses temper tantrums, refusal to eat and go to bed, and elimination caprices as handy weapons. The other extreme of ready ''giving in'' provides the child with a means of domination of the family, making use of the same symptoms as ''spoiled child reactions.'' Recognition of this natural phase of child development will help pediatricians to prepare mothers for its appearance, explain to them the early negations and refusals and introduce a type of management that would avoid parental despotism on the one hand and parental submission on the other.

THE MENTAL HYGIENE OF INFANCY

The mental hygiene of infancy lies entirely in the hands of pediatricians, who are the parents' first advisers in matters of child health and behavior. Yet the literature, which is so rich in suggestions with regard to older children, offers almost nothing that could serve the pediatricians as a practical guide. The article by R. M. and H. Bakwin[4] offers a helpful departure. Kanner,[56] in a recent article, tried to present to physicians the principles of mental hygiene during the first 2 years of life. The following passages are quoted from this article.

The interrelationship between an individual and his surroundings begins on the very first day of life and keeps increasing in variety and complexity. During the first two years the progressive unfolding of the inherent potentialities of the species transforms the infant from a passive, helpless, inarticulate being into a more and more differentiated little participant who walks, feeds himself, controls his eliminative functions, comprehends gestures and spoken language, forms words and short sentences, and becomes an active somebody to be reckoned with. Some of this unfolding comes from within; growth, locomotion, the formation of vowels and consonants are in the main independent of educational efforts. The chief danger to the normal progress of these functions lies in hazards to bodily health. The ancient adage, *Mens sana in corpore sano,* still holds true. Attention to physical well-being is therefore one of the principal pillars of mental hygiene. The direction taken by the development of many other functions depends to a much larger extent on the molding forces of the infant's environment, that is, the influences of his home. Hence the considerations implied in the slogan, *Mens sana in domo sana,* constitute the second pillar of the mental hygiene of infancy and childhood.

Child training works towards socialization, for which the groundwork is laid at the beginning of life. Adequate socialization hinges on the establishment of relative self-dependence, security, and conformity. The family physician, through his knowledge of the home and the confidence invested in him, can contribute a lion's share to the smooth introduction and maintenance of these features. As the parents' natural adviser consulted in all matters pertaining to the infant's health, he is in a strategic position that allows him to guard somatic developments, supervise home training, and inculcate sound attitudes.

The development of *self-dependence* is hampered by parental overindulgence and oversolicitude, the behavior commonly alluded to as "spoiling." Spoiling is made up of feelings and actions representing parental needs that may arise from various sources, such as the preceding death of a child, economic, marital, or health features precluding the birth of other children, the void created by the substitution of unsatisfying housework for the richness of a previous social or vocational life, overcompensation for the displeasure accompanying the arrival of an unwanted child, or memories of an unhappy childhood resulting in a desire to smother the child with excessive coddling and protection. A mixture of anxiety, puzzlement, impatience, and inexperience centers the family's attention on the infant's nutrition, sleep, and elimination. Weaning from the breast and the bottle is delayed. The child is not given an opportunity to learn how to feed himself. The meals become tragicomic events with coaxing, cajoling, threatening, and bribing by the adults, and refusal, gagging, and even vomiting on the part of the child.

Learning how to sleep through a whole night is made impossible by the parents' habit of jumping up at the infant's slightest whimpering, carrying him about the room or rocking his cradle. Bowel overconcern resorts to purgatives, suppositories, and enemas. The child, not left alone for a minute of his waking time, fondled and handled and shown off incessantly, does not have a chance to develop the socializing responsibilities commensurate with his age and remains physically and emotionally overdependent on his elders. The well-known spoiled infant syndrome of anorexia, insomnia, constipation, and attention-getting intrenches itself more and more firmly. This failure to establish a reasonable degree of self-dependence, if continued unabated, may lead in preschool age, during the school years, and even later to disturbing difficulties of adjustment.

The development of *security* may at an early age be interfered with by inconsistencies in the display of affection and recognition of achievement, emphasis on real or anticipated shortcomings, instillation of fear and confusion regarding authority. The average sensibly managed infant is happy and secure and as yet untroubled by "the slings and arrows of outrageous fortune." As the temperature of his baths should be neither too hot nor too cold, so should parental affection normally steer clear of the extremes of explosive demonstrativeness and chilly rebuff. Approval of success and encouragement in the face of occasional failure during the first attempts at walking, talking, self-feeding, handling breakable objects, meeting strangers, etc., help to impart to the infant a sense of progress and self-confidence when confronted with ever new tasks. But sometimes parental frustrations, overambition, overconscientiousness, or resentment of the child-training duties as annoying inconvenience lead to sternness, perfectionism, fault-finding, undeserved punishments, and nagging which make the child uncertain of himself and instill timidity, dread of his elders, and lack of self-assertion. The infant is being lectured to and reasoned with in terms which he does not and cannot comprehend and is then reprimanded for disobedience if the sermon has had no results. Constant corrections of initial hesitation in reporting his experiences with an as yet inadequate vocabulary may cause him to become speech conscious and start him on the road to stuttering. The parents' dissatisfaction with his left-handedness may make him miserable by their methods of enforcing a change of handedness. Their agitations about his thumb-sucking or touching his genitals may fetter him with all sorts of mechanical devices. Beating, bogey man threats, and the custom of locking him in a dark closet for punishment may introduce strong and disturbing fears. Under such conditions an infant cannot possibly be expected to develop a healthy sense of security. This is made even more difficult by the frequent inconsistency with which the same act, dependent on the mood of the moment, is tolerated at one time and severely rebuked at another. Besides, differences in the temperaments and attitudes of the parents and other adults in the household often create in the child a confusion of authority when the same behavior is condoned by some and turned into a great issue and censured by others.

The development of *conformity* depends mainly on the introduction of conventional manners, emotional control, and a give-and-take attitude. The first two years are the best time to train ("condition," if you wish) a child for habit regularity. Setting certain times for the meals and, in the second year, naps and night rest, and the use of the toilet offer the earliest opportunities for the establishment of routine, which is often hindered by parental overindulgence, laissez-faire negligence, or peculiar pseudomedical notions that turn an infant into the central object of his mother's hypochondriasis. The latter is often fostered by fear of inheritance of some relative's disease, superstitions about prenatal marking of the baby, difficult labor or birth or some early illness. The child, branded as sickly, frail, and delicate, receives a considerable amount of overprotection and is suspended from all reciprocal obligations. On the theory that sickly children should never be crossed, he is suffered to dominate the family, take toys away from his siblings and playmates, provided that he is allowed to have playmates, refuse violently to let them play with his own toys, eat, sleep, and soil himself whenever he pleases and destroy anything he wishes to destroy. Improper adult example renders him even more unmanaged and unmanageable. It is a fact that infantile breath-holding spells and temper tantrums are staged mostly in homes where unchecked emotional outbursts are common occurrences and the infants' own upheavals are met with yelling, hitting, and the dreadful habit of emptying a pitcher of cold water over him. The strange combination of giving in, screaming, spanking, and faulty habit training prevents the establishment in the infant of conformity, that is, good manners, sensible use of his emotional equipment and sharing.

Summary.—The family physician can help parents considerably in the mental hygiene of their children by trying to understand, inform and reassure them. He will not attain this purpose by blaming and scolding them and telling them in a general way not to pamper, worry about, or be impatient with their offspring. The desire to understand implies listening to what the parents have to say. An attentive ear will not fail to get the preoccupations, concerns, solicitudes, frustrations, and erroneous beliefs underlying unhealthy management and training. The average mother wants and needs enlightenment about the child's state of health, about what to expect and not to expect of him at a given age.

Herein lies a great challenge to the modern physician who is the only person privileged to administer mental hygiene during the first two years of life and steer the child in the direction of self-dependence, security, and conformity, in other words, in the direction of adequate socialization and good mental health.

REFERENCES

Problems of Feeding Behavior

1. Aldrich, C. A.: The Prevention of Poor Appetite in Children, Ment. Hyg. **10**: 701, 1926.
2. Aldrich, C. A.: Cultivating the Child's Appetite, New York, 1927; Ed. 2, 1932; reprinted 1936; The Macmillan Company.
3. Aldrich, C. A.: Science and Art in Child Nourishment, J. PEDIAT. **1**: 413, 1932.
4. Bakwin, R. M., and Bakwin, H.: Psychologic Care During Infancy, J. PEDIAT. **12**: 71, 1938.
5. Blatz, W. E.: A Study of Eating Habits in a Nursery School, Genetic Psychol. Monogr. **4**: 89, 1928.
6. Brennemann, J.: Vis Medicatrix Naturae in Pediatrics, Am. J. Dis. Child. **40**: 1, 1930.
7. Brennemann, J.: Psychologic Aspects of Nutrition in Childhood, J. PEDIAT. **1**: 145, 1932.

8. Brennemann, J.: Pediatric Psychology and the Child Guidance Movement, J. PEDIAT. **2**: 1, 1933.
9. Childers, A. T., and Hamil, B. M.: Emotional Problems in Children as Related to Duration of Breast Feeding in Infancy, Am. J. Orthopsychiat. **2**: 134, 1932.
10. Davis, C. M.: Self Selection of Diet by Newly Weaned Infants, Am. J. Dis. Child. **36**: 651, 1928.
11. Davis, C. M.: Self Selection of Food by Children, Am. J. Nursing **35**: 403, 1935.
12. Davis, C. M.: Choice of Formulas Made by Three Infants Throughout the Nursing Period, Am. J. Dis. Child. **50**: 385, 1935.
13. Davis, C. M.: Feeding After the First Year: In Brennemann's Practice of Pediatrics, Vol. I, Chapter 30, Hagerstown, 1937, W. F. Prior Company.
14. Dockeray, G. C.: Differential Feeding Reactions of Newborn Infants, Psychol. Bull. **31**: 747, 1934.
15. Eliot, A. A.: Eating Habits in Relation to Personality Development in Two- and Three-Year-Old Children, Genetic Psychol. Mongr. **13**: 399, 1933.
16. Gesell, A.: The Psychological Hygiene of Infant Feeding, Ment. Hyg. **22**: 216, 1938.
17. Gesell, A., and Ilg, F. L.: Feeding Behavior of Infants, Philadelphia, 1937, J. B. Lippincott Company.
18. Hill, A. B., and van Alstyne, D.: Learning Levels of Children in the Nursery School, With Reference to the Eating Situation, New York, 1930, Bureau of Publications, Teachers College, Columbia University.
19. Hill, J.: Infant Feeding and Personality Disorders; Study of Early Feeding in Its Relation to Emotional and Digestive Disorders, Psychiatric Quart. **11**: 356, 1937.
20. Mohr, G. J.: Emotional Factors in Nutrition Work With Children, Ment. Hyg. **12**: 366, 1928.
21. Moseley, M. R.: Reactions to Food of Children of Preschool Age, With Special Consideration of Management as a Conditioning Factor, 1926, M. A. Thesis, University of Chicago.
22. Ripin, R.: A Study of the Infant's Feeding Reactions During the First Six Months of Life, Arch. Psychol. **18**: 1, 1930.

Thumb-Sucking

23. Anderson, W. W.: Thumbsucking Apparatus, Am. J. Dis. Child. **39**: 70, 1930; **46**: 90, 1933.
24. Barton, E. A.: Relative Septicity of Dummy Teat and Thumb, Lancet **1**: 348, 1930.
25. Bonney, T. C.: Facial Deformities; Results of Thumbsucking, Mouth Health Quart. **4**: 12, 1935.
26. Bragman, L. J.: Thumbsucking and Other Auto-Erotic Tendencies in Children, As Portrayed in Art, J. Nerv. & Ment. Dis. **74**: 708, 1931.
27. Freud, S.: Three Contributions to the Theory of Sex. In: The Basic Writings of Sigmund Freud. Translation by A. A. Brill, pp. 585 ff., New York, 1938, The Modern Library.
28. Heimlish, A. F.: Correction for Thumb- and Fingersucking Habits (Description of Device), Internat. J. Orthodontia **21**: 1138, 1935.
29. Homburger, A.: Vorlesungen ueber die Psychopathologie des Kindesalters, Berlin, 1926, Julius Springer.
30. Kiernan, J. G.: Thumbsucking an Auto-Erotic Phenomenon, Pediatrics **23**: 197, 1911.
31. Klein, M.: The Psycho-Analysis of Children. Translation by A. Strachey, London, 1932; ed. 2, 1937, p. 84; Hogarth Press.
32. Levy, D. M.: Fingersucking and Accessory Movements in Early Infancy: An Etiological Study, Am. J. Psychiat. **7**: 881, 1928.
33. Levy, D. M.: Experiments on Sucking Reflex and Social Behavior of Dogs, Am. J. Orthopsychiat. **4**: 203, 1934.
34. Levy, D. M.: A Note on Pecking in Chickens, Psychoanalyt. Quart. **4**: 612, 1935.
35. Levy, D. M.: Thumb or Fingersucking From Psychiatric Angle, Angle Orthodontist **7**: 100, 1937.
36. Levy, D. M.: On Instinct-Satiation: An Experiment on the Pecking Behavior of Chickens, J. Gen. Psychol. **18**: 327, 1938.

37. Lewis, S. J.: Thumbsucking; Cause of Malocclusion in Deciduous Teeth, J. Am. Dent. A. **17**: 1060, 1930.
38. Mazzini, G.: Il bambino nell'arte, Rassegna di studi psichiat. **16**: 468, 1927.
39. Thom, D. A.: Everyday Problems of the Everyday Child, p. 104, New York, 1934, D. Appleton-Century Company.
40. Van der Bogert, F.: Device for Control of Hands in Facial Eczema and Thumbsucking, Arch. Pediat. **51**: 810, 1934.
41. Watson, J. B.: Psychological Care of Infant and Child, p. 133, New York, 1928, W. W. Norton & Company, Inc.

Age of Resistance

42. Benjamin, E.: Grundlagen und Entwicklungsgeschichte der kindlichen Neurose, Leipzig, 1930, Georg Thieme.
43. Benjamin, E.: Die Krankheit der Zivilisation, Munich, 1934, Rudolph Müller & Steinicke.
44. Binet, A., and Simon, T.: Méthodes nouvelles pour le diagnostic du niveau intellectuel des anormaux, Année psychol. **11**: 191, 1905.
45. Buehler, C.: Kindheit und Jugend, Leipzig, 1928, S. Hirzel.
46. Beuhler, K.: Die geistige Entwicklung des Kindes, p. 223, Ed. 2, Jena, 1921, Gustav Fischer.
47. Busemann, A.: Ueber das sogenannte ''erste Trotzalter'' des Kindes, Ztschr. f. pädagog. Psychol. **29**: 42, 1928.
48. Busemann, A.: Ueber die Urschen des ''ersten Trotzalters'' und der Erregungsphasen ueberhaupt, Ibid. **30**: 276, 1929.
49. Hetzer, H.: Entwicklungsbedingte Erziehungsschwierigkeiten, Ztschr. f. pädagog. Psychol. **30**: 77, 1929.
50. Levy, D. M., and Tulchin, S. H.: The Resistance of Infants and Children During Mental Tests, J. Exper. Psychol. **6**: 304, 1923.
51. Levy, D. M., and Tulchin, S. H.: The Resistant Behavior of Infants and Children, Ibid.: **8**: 209, 1925.
52. Reynolds, M. M.: Negativism of Pre-School Children, Contribution to Education, No. 288, New York, 1928, Bureau of Publications, Teachers College, Columbia University.
53. Stern, W.: Psychology of Early Childhood, p. 376, New York, 1924, Henry Holt & Company, Inc.
54. Thom, D. A.: Everyday Problems of the Everyday Child, p. 118, New York, 1934, D. Appleton-Century Company.
55. Woolley, H. T.: Enuresis as a Psychological Problem, Ment. Hyg. **10**: 42, 1926.

The Mental Hygiene of Infancy

56. Kanner, L.: Mental Hygiene During the First Two Years of Life, Preventive Medicine **7**: 233, 1938.

American Academy of Pediatrics

Proceedings

EIGHTH ANNUAL MEETING OF THE AMERICAN ACADEMY OF PEDIATRICS

DEL MONTE, CALIF., JUNE 10 AND 11, 1938

Round Table Discussion of Nursing Care in the Newborn Infant

Chairman: Dr. Jay I. Durand, Seattle, Wash.
Assistant: Dr. Amos U. Christie, San Francisco, Calif.

CHAIRMAN DURAND.—The probable reason for the choice of this subject for a round table discussion this year was the epidemics of diarrheas which have broken out in the nurseries of lying-in hospitals in various parts of the world. With this fact in mind, Dr. Christie and I have decided not to consider many conditions such as asphyxia, hemorrhagic diseases, and prematurity, in which the nursing care has been well covered in pediatric literature and shall confine our discussion largely to nursery technique in the newborn infant.

Beginning with the surgery, it should be noted that there has been great improvement in hospitals, but I believe that the last department of the hospital to receive attention has been the newborn nursery. The patients are inarticulate and defenseless or they would not tolerate the crowding, lack of proper heat regulation, rough garments, and shortage of nurses which so often occurs there.

There is a general awakening to the conditions and more has appeared on the subject of nursery technique in the medical and nursing journals during the past two years than during the preceding ten.

There has been a very definite reduction during two decades in the incidence of mouth, skin, umbilical, and intestinal infections, perhaps some reduction in respiratory infections. While there still were too many hospital acquired infections and deaths, we seem to be progressing. Then an acute communicable disease of the newborn infant made his appearance in the nurseries of many of our well-conducted hospitals. Since this infectious enteritis affects only the newborn patient, it seems an astonishing fact that outbreaks have been reported from such widely separated points as New York, Chicago, Buffalo, Memphis, and Seattle. The etiological agent is so far undetermined, but the symptomatology, progress of the individual case, course of the epidemic, the 50 per cent mortality, and post-mortem findings leave little doubt that it is the same disease. The New York Board of Health has investigated twenty-seven outbreaks in three years up to December, 1937. It has been made a reportable disease, and stringent measures for its control and prevention have been put into effect.

When a case is discovered there is no temporizing. The obstetrical ward of that hospital is closed, all suspected cases isolated, and as soon as the newborn infant can be discharged, the nursery is thoroughly renovated.

Regulations covering all lying-in institutions and newborn nurseries have been put into effect.

These regulations which were published in an article by Dr. William H. Best, Deputy Commissioner of Health in the *Journal of the American Medical Associa-*

tion, April 9, 1938, seem very exacting and perhaps unnecessary in some of their provisions, except in the presence of an epidemic.

They show much thought and painstaking care in their preparation, cover every point in the conduct of the nursery, but, to me, seem to be rather a guide to perfection than an enforceable set of health regulations to control all nurseries.

These regulations and the technique set up by Gladys Dick at the Cradle, as described by Louis Sauer in the JOURNAL OF PEDIATRICS, 1935, furnish the best texts I have found for the conduct of the newborn wards of an obstetric hospital or the teaching of their nursery technique.

Care of the Skin in the Newborn Infant.—The skin of the newborn baby is an extremely delicate and sensitive tissue. Very slight irritation will produce an erythema, and infections are extremely common unless great care is exercised.

Drugs administered to the mother and toxins in the maternal circulation are the cause of some of the irritations. The clothing often roughened and hardened by prolonged use and laundering is responsible for some cases. Washing in solutions, either alkaline or acid, will lead to irritations. Water, oil, and ointments are irritating to some skins. Such erythemas are short-lived and comparatively unimportant except for the concern they give the mothers and because infections are more frequent in infants in which they occur. These infections vary from an occasional bleb or pustule to the large multiple blebs of a virulent impetigo or pemphigus neonatorum.

Some of the more severe conditions are the following:

Intertrigo.—This occurs where skin surfaces are in opposition, especially in the presence of moisture and excessive heat. Air conditioning and heat control of the nurseries, avoidance of excess in clothing but care that a layer of nonirritating clothing is up under the arms, avoidance of excessive zeal in washing, wiping, and rubbing these surfaces, and supervision of the solutions used in the laundry will go far toward prevention.

The Circumcision Rashes.—An infant's skin is sensitive to the attendant trauma, to antiseptic solutions, vaseline and oil, and the secretions which result from the operation, and a fine papular rash with minute vesicles occurs quite regularly on the surrounding parts. In the absence of secondary infection, this heals quite promptly with a variety of treatments. Exposure to the air with heat from an incandescent bulb at a safe distance works very well, as it does also for irritation of the buttocks. A dry dusting powder composed of calomel, talcum, and zinc in proportions of parts 3, 2, and 1, is an assistance in preventing and curing mild infections.

The infections in the newborn skin may be acquired in the passage through the birth canal but are generally due to the hands of nurses, physicians, and mother. Washing the hands before touching any infant should be enforced in every nursery, and the actual skin-to-skin contact between these hands and the skin of the infant should and can be reduced to a minimum. The dry technique later to be described is of great assistance.

The occasional small isolated bleb or pustule is the mildest of these infections. It occurs occasionally in every nursery and in many cases will not spread on the child or to other infants if reasonable care is exercised. Breaking the top and touching with gentian violet or mercresin and applying the dusting powder will heal most of them in two days. Whether isolation of this infant is necessary, I do not know, but it is generally done.

Outbreaks of virulent pemphigus neonatorum have greatly reduced in recent years, but I have vivid recollections of several severe outbreaks. In these epidemics blebs up to two or three inches in diameter raised the superficial layer of the skin, often a considerable portion of the body was involved, and deaths occasionally occurred.

The worst and most obstinate epidemic which I remember occurred when a nurse from a neighboring city came to take care of a sister who was confined in one of our hospitals. About the third day a severe pemphigus appeared on the baby and rapidly spread in the nursery. The nurse told me that the last two babies she had cared for developed the infection and that in consequence she had taken no obstetric cases for the preceding four months. The infection had evidently persisted in her clothing or possibly in an infected sinus during this interval. This epidemic proved extremely obstinate, and in spite of opening three new nurseries while old ones were renovated and painted, sporadic cases appeared, though growing less virulent for weeks.

For the ordinary pyodermias ultraviolet irradiations are very useful in preventing the extension to new areas of the skin and in treatment. They may be a helpful prophylactic measure in sterilizing the skin of babies which may have been exposed to the infection.

In connection with the care of the skin I should like to discuss the ''dry technique.'' In 1931 this practice was instituted by Dr. W. F. Patrick in the White Shield Home of Portland, where approximately 100 babies are born annually, and it has been continued since that time. During the past few months I have visited hospitals in Portland, Seattle, and Vancouver where this technique has been established from one to seven years and I am convinced of its value.

Two reports describing this procedure and the results have been published during the past year. One is by Dr. Heyworth N. Sanford of Chicago. Covering a six-year study of 3,500 infants born in the Presbyterian Hospital, it gives the incidence of skin troubles during the years from 1930 to 1936, inclusive. A certain regime was followed: For two years 2 per cent ammoniated mercury inunctions were first given, followed by daily baths with castile soap and water; for one year, ammoniated mercury at birth followed with subsequent olive oil baths; one year, no antiseptic at birth and only olive oil baths; one year, a commercial antiseptic baby oil used exclusively; one year, only olive and mineral oil used; and one year in which the skin was untouched for nine days except to wipe off any excessive blood. The largest number of infections occurred during the period when ammoniated mercury was used, the largest number of skin irritations during the year of commercial oil application, and the best results of all during the past year when the skin was left practically untouched.

The second report is by Dr. L. Howard Smith of Portland, Ore., and covers the experience during two and a half years in nonbathing and nonoiling newborn infants at the Multnomah County Hospital of Portland, Ore. During this period only two of 1,734 babies developed pustules. These were single lesions and were treated with the calomel dusting powder and healed within thirty-six hours.

The procedure is simplicity itself. Excess of blood is gently wiped from the infant's head and meconium from the buttocks with sterile cotton balls, when the baby is brought from the delivery room. Care is taken not to remove the vernix. If the blood has dried, a little warm water may be necessary. The child is clothed and placed in the crib. Warm water is used to clean the buttocks following stools. The clothing is changed daily, but there is no bathing or oiling.

I quote Dr. Smith: ''Within twelve hours after birth the infant's skin is clean, and the vernix has disappeared. Unless one has witnessed the phenomenon, this miracle does not seem possible. It would appear that if this greasy, slimy newborn infant, who looks as if he had been rescued from a sewer pit, were not immediately cleaned up, he would smell like a dead fish in twenty-four hours. What a contrast to behold him a few hours later looking so fresh and clean.''

Sanford agrees that the skin is a better color and smoother if not washed or oiled. This is due to two causes. First, soap, oils, and even water are irritating to some skins; and second, freedom from handling and rubbing. What becomes of the vernix? It almost seems to evaporate. It absorbs into the clothing. It drops off, at any rate, it disappears very rapidly. If the hair is thick and the family will be shocked by seeing vernix there, a sterile fine comb is sometimes employed.

Care must be taken that the shirt comes up into the axilla for moisture and skin surfaces in apposition may lead to irritation. The groins are the only other area to be watched. The excretions on the skin at birth seem to have a role in protecting this delicate organ against irritation and infection. Furthermore, when babies are not bathed, the common bathing and diapering table can be eliminated.

Another point in favor of the dry technique is the nursing time saved. A study of this at the Multnomah County Hospital showed a saving of five minutes on the initial care and three minutes for the subsequent daily care of each infant. This saving in a nursery with an average population of thirty amounts to an hour and a half each day, and three to four weeks of nursing time during the year.

Mouth Infections.—Thrush may be acquired during birth. The same monilium has been found in the mother's vagina in many instances. It can live, as Faber has shown, in dust collections in the nursery.

It should not spread in the modern nursery from the sporadic case, as no dust collections will be permitted and nothing that is not surgically aseptic will touch the baby's mouth.

An epidemic of an apparently new mouth infection has been reported from Baltimore. So little is known about it that I shall only mention it. The commoner mouth infections will be taken care of, I am sure, by a better aseptic technique which Dr. Christie will discuss.

Conclusion.—The large nurseries commonly found in our hospitals with bassinets touching one another, and through whose narrow passages nurses and doctors and hospital employees travel back and forth all day long, is an ideal place for the spread of infection. I doubt whether any aseptic technique can be developed which can be effective in such quarters. Small units of four to eight cribs, far enough apart to make it possible to care for a child in one without contaminating those on either side will help. A technique which will insure surgical asepsis of anything touching the baby's nose and mouth will help. The dry technique is a real help. None of these will control air-borne infections. Should the menace of an infectious enteritis continue or perhaps extend, the suggestion made by Dr. Mandel Spivek in a paper to be read before the Pediatric Section in San Francisco, of giving up the nursery entirely and putting the baby in the mother's room, may prove to be the easiest and best solution.

DR. CHRISTIE.—Dr. Durand has already indicated the reasons for calling this round table. It is unnecessary to stress further the multiple problems involved in such a discussion, but I think I can best serve my purpose here by immediately arriving at some rather definite affirmative and negative conclusions which I hope will bring out a deluge of really critical and pertinent discussion.

I am not one who would return to the days of the horse and buggy or the coal oil lamp, and I would admit that renewing the discussion of home versus hospital delivery will serve no purpose. Still I wish to point out again the distinctly abnormal conditions under which we herd together from ten to thirty newborn infants in crowded quarters which will shock the housing experts of the future. All our problems in nursery technique seem to be due to this crowding, and the solution of them inevitably entails an analysis of cost and practicability of the remedy.

The development of nursery technique is like choosing a serologic test for syphilis. It must be sufficiently sensitive to exclude all possibility of infection, it must be specific, and finally it must be adaptable to the hospital, to the patient, and to the doctor.

We must also be practical regarding aseptic technique. Isolation technique has not been devised as yet that is foolproof and entirely consistent. This immediately brings up the question of masks. In the nursery these are worn, obviously not to protect ourselves, as in isolation technique, but as a protection to the infant. If the nurses working in a nursery are to wear masks, then the mother should also wear a mask when nursing the baby. Furthermore, I am reliably informed by nursery supervisors that the wearing of a gauze mask over the nose for even a few hours will bring undesirable symptoms such as headache and nausea which soon initiate a desire on the part of the nurse to return to private duty on a surgical ward. Finally, the wearing of a mask over the nose during an entire summer day in Baltimore is a very different matter than the same procedure in cooler San Francisco. It has been shown by McKhann that the usual gauze mask is not adequate to prevent cross-infection. I do not know the answer to this question but I would like to suggest here that the new types of masks, such as the plastic or deflecting mask which is impervious to air, prevents direct infection, and allows ventilation for the wearer, may be the solution of our problem as this type of mask approaches a 75 per cent effectiveness.

Recent observations on the sterilization of air by ultraviolet light by Wells and Hart, applied by McKhann to a children's ward, revealed the inadequacy of this method for the complete sterilization of air in a ward or room. Ultraviolet light will sterilize air, but all that can be hoped for at present is a dilution of contaminated air with the ultraviolet sterilized air.

At the University of California Hospital, where the nurseries are under the supervision of the Pediatric Department, many of our past difficulties have been traced to the private service where, for one reason or another (often because of special privilege), the aseptic technique has not been as stringent as for the clinic service. We have partially, and I hope permanently, remedied this situation by breaking the active nursery group into four separate units, each infant in each unit being on individual techniques. The units are: the premature unit separated by double doors from the rest of the nursery, a clinic nursery, a private nursery, and an isolation unit for babies whose mothers have rashes, sepsis, colds, pneumonia, syphilis, gonorrhea, or are suspected of harboring other communicable diseases. If the baby should develop any abnormality needing special observation or treatment he is likewise removed to the isolation unit, where he is cared for by nurses who never enter the other nursery units. Likewise, nurses assigned to any nursery unit are never allowed to care for infants in other units.

All cleaning is done while the infants are at the breast. No visitors are ever allowed in the nursery, and the babies are shown only through glass partitions at very limited hours to a limited group. This showing of infants to visitors as well as to the mothers, is further limited during the height of the season of respiratory infections.

The supervising nurse is held strictly responsible for all aseptic technique. No one may enter the nursery in street clothes but must wear sterile mask, cap, and gown at all times. Hands must be scrubbed with soap and water before touching an infant or any of the nursery supplies. All linen, blankets, diapers, and smocks used in the nursery are sterilized. All solutions, oils, and ointments are sterilized, and only sterile garments are put on the babies.

The nursing personnel should be adequately trained and instructed to recognize and record any suspected abnormality of the infant. Various methods may be advocated for this, and I have taken the opportunity of this meeting to collect several forms from leading medical centers throughout the eastern and middle western United States. They are not presented for critical comparison but rather as an interesting exhibit of how the same information can be efficiently recorded in many different ways.

It may be noted that in one form or another there should be room for recording all instances of injury at birth, congenital abnormalities, cyanosis, fever, convulsions, pallor, jaundice, rashes, weight gains out of proportion to normal (edema), snuffles, hemorrhage, etc., and the supervising nurse should see that any such instances are reported to the attending pediatrician. Adequate room should be available in the nursing notes for all abnormalities in the gastrointestinal system, such as failure to nurse, to take breast, or artificial feeding, character of stools, etc.

The care of the skin and mouth infections has been adequately covered by Dr. Durand. To go further giving details of my own experience would be like the doctor who reported a certain type of treatment which prevented hemorrhagic disease in 200 consecutive newborn infants. The point I am trying to make is that we lack definite scientific information to evaluate properly some of the methods we use in the care of the newborn infant. As for the evaluation of the pertussis vaccine, we need more fundamental understanding of the underlying immunology of newborn patients. If oiling the infant's skin raises the skin temperature, then we are increasing the possibility of infection by promoting a better culture medium.

In this regard I wish to add a word about nursery policy determined by weight and physical condition at birth. Dr. Durand tells me that in only about 50 per cent of hospitals he has visited do they have any means of placing the infant in a specially heated crib following delivery. I wish to make a point regarding this as I feel that every hospital should have a Nobel box or heated crib to receive infants who have just been delivered.

The greatest value for arbitrary standards to indicate prematurity is that below certain levels of weight these infants need special medical as well as nursing care. This arbitrary level for prematurity is 2500 gm., and without going into a discussion of premature care I would like to indicate the extreme importance to the infant of not allowing the body temperature to fall after delivery. In a preliminary analysis of premature mortality in those infants born at home and taken to the hospital, I have observed that the gross mortality was approximately doubled when the admission temperature was below 37° F. By use of heated premature ambulances (plus other means) Hess in Chicago has been able to reduce the inevitable premature mortality of over 50 per cent to approximately 34 per cent. This can be compared with the expected 25 per cent mortality for premature infants born in and cared for in hospital nurseries.

And so it would appear that the first duty of the delivery room nursing staff is to keep the infants warm, for some of the factors which add to premature mortality must also operate in other congenitally immature or possibly some full-term infants. Any attempt to remove vernix caseosa or to examine or measure the infants should be reserved for a time when the temperature is normal (at least 37° F.).

We do not have time nor is it within the scope of this round table on nursery technique to go into a discussion of air-conditioned nurseries. The work of Blackfan and Vaglou suggests the benefits of certain air conditions to premature infants. It has been my clinical observation and that of others that there are marked changes in the hydration of normal full-term infants when the relative humidity is very low. I believe also that we keep the temperature of our nurseries too high, which contributes to a lower humidity, subsequent dehydration, and dryness of the skin.

The nursery temperature for full-term infants should be 68° to 70° F., and the relative humidity should be between 50 and 55. I would also like to state that the production of these conditions is within the means of any institution considering a renovation or especially for those building a new nursery.

Before concluding and without meaning to appear too critical I must call your attention to the most complete and recent set of suggestions governing nursery technique which has appeared in the pediatric literature. I refer to the article of Frant and Abramson in the December, 1937, issue of the JOURNAL OF PEDIATRICS. It is entitled "Control and Prevention of Outbreaks in Hospital Nurseries." It was designed to control and prevent such disastrous epidemics as Dr. Durand has discussed and which unfortunately are spreading throughout the country with case fatality rates approaching 50 per cent.

These suggested regulations approach the ideal but do not seem always to be practical. For instance, the ratio of one nurse to two infants, as suggested by the authors quoting Brenneman, both day and night is undoubtedly a very good idea, but in dollars and cents there are few hospitals which are able financially to assume responsibility for meeting this suggestion. This recommendation is further complicated by a statement that ''no nurse who dresses, bathes, or diapers the babies should feed any newborn baby.'' Let us take a moment to analyze these suggestions. They must mean literally that in a small private hospital where twelve infants are cared for, there would be three nurses bathing and diapering and three nurses for feeding. For three eight-hour shifts this would entail the employment of eighteen nurses to supply adequate care for the newborn infants during the twenty-four-hour period.

The routine daily inspection of nursing personnel by a regularly assigned physician and the monthly stool culture likewise seem impractical for most private and teaching hospitals. From the standpoint of hospital administration it is out of the question, and our efforts can be better directed to developing a more efficient aseptic technique for which the supervising nurse should be held strictly accountable.

Under a discussion of nursery personnel the authors suggest that ''the nursing staff should be a constant one and not ever changing.'' In a hospital where nurses are in training, this suggestion is obviously most difficult to attain.

Now in conclusion I would like to make a plea for improvement in maternal education. This inevitably devolves upon the nursing personnel. Every mother should have not one but several demonstrations of modern methods of feeding, clothing, airing, and bathing her baby. She is an unusual patient in that she is intimately under the care of her physician for approximately a year, if we include her prenatal and post-partum care. It is possible by collaborative effort with our existing knowledge, hospital, and clinic facilities, to do a much more complete and better job in this regard, giving the mother a lasting impression of the advantages of modern obstetrics and pediatrics for herself and for her baby. The advantages of such a program in timesaving and services rendered are obvious.

DISCUSSION

DR. CHRISTIE.—I observed an epidemic of diarrhea at Johns Hopkins Hospital which began very much like a thrush. The children lost much weight, were greatly dehydrated, and had an explosive type of diarrhea. Venoclysis seemed to help more than anything else, but the mortality was 50 per cent.

CHAIRMAN DURAND.—Every delivery room should have a heated crib ready before every birth.

DR. H. K. FABER (SAN FRANCISCO).—We had a series of skin infections which lasted a period of months. We looked everywhere for the source of infection and found that it was a common bathing table. We prepared separate units and had the nurse scrub her hands and change her gown before bathing each baby. With this technique we got rid of the skin infection. We use glass caps for all nursing bottles and keep the babies separated.

DR. R. G. FLOOD (SAN FRANCISCO).—In our old hospital we were crowded but had very few skin infections. When we moved into our new hospital we began to get an increase in the number of skin infections, and had periodic outbreaks of impetigo. We looked everywhere for the source of infection and took swabs from the nurses' hands after they had scrubbed. The first swab would be negative, the second still negative, and the third swab from the same place would show staphylococcus. We decided that the soap formed a filament which covered the skin and when the filament was rubbed off, the skin still carried micro-organisms. We tried having the nurses wash their hands with Lugol's solution, and this dry technique appeals to me.

CHAIRMAN DURAND.—Tell us how you use Lugol's.

DR. FLOOD.—We have the nurse keep her hands in 3 per cent Lugol's solution until the hands are colored, and then decolorize with hyposulfite.

DR. R. P. SEITZ (San Francisco).—I believe that many of these infections originate in the mother's room.

DR. CHRISTIE.—That is the weak point in the whole thing. We autoclave everything around the nursery and then take the baby to the mother's room where nothing is autoclaved.

DR. SEITZ.—Do not carriers serve as a menace?

DR. FLOOD.—We have abandoned carriers. The nurse has a gown for each crib and puts it on to take the baby to the mother. We tried gloves, but when gloves are wet they slip, and the nurses let a few babies fall so we quit gloves.

DR. FABER.—If nipples are not covered they become contaminated.

CHAIRMAN DURAND.—We had the nipples autoclaved, milk and all, but the babies developed a diarrhea and we quit the autoclaving.

DR. CHRISTIE.—We had an epidemic of diarrhea in the University Hospital which we thought was due to irradiated milk.

CHAIRMAN DURAND.—At the hospital in Portland no babies are bathed until they are fourteen days old. The blood is wiped off, and they sometimes use oil on genitals of girl babies.

DR. E. P. COOK (San Jose, Calif.).—Is it not true that the baby's skin is much tougher at two weeks of age?

DR. CHRISTIE.—There is no question in my mind but what that is true. I believe that oil irritates the skin. We use one-half strength tincture of green soap.

DR. G. B. KRYDER (Glendale, Calif.).—How long do you leave the baby in the heated crib?

CHAIRMAN DURAND.—That depends on conditions. If there is any repair work for the mother (or trouble with the baby), the baby may be there for some time.

DR. J. M. RECTOR (San Francisco).—Why show the baby to the mother?

DR. CHRISTIE.—When a baby's temperature goes up to normal and it begins breathing all right, it usually stays all right.

DR. R. L. PORTER (San Francisco).—What about the obstetrician as the source of infection? I heard of one who left one hospital where he got impetigo. He went to another hospital and it happened again, and then he went to a third hospital and the impetigo still followed him. It developed that he had a streptococcic sinusitis and was probably infecting his own babies.

DR. P. J. HOWARD (Detroit).—At the Ford Hospital, when the dry technique came out, some of our men tried it, but others refused; so we had two classes, one dry and the other, the old regime. The skin infections of the babies handled with the dry technique ran about 5 per cent, and of the babies handled with the old regime about 10 per cent. In the Women's Hospital in Detroit I have observed that their methods are about the same as ours, but their results were better.

DR. SEITZ.—At the County Hospital in San Francisco they have less skin infection than any other hospital in the city. I think this is because they have the same set of nurses year in and year out.

DR. RENA CRAWFORD (New Orleans).—At the county hospital in New Orleans they have practically no cases, but they have lots of them in the private hospitals.

DR. PORTER.—I dropped in to listen to the dermatologists yesterday afternoon and someone was telling them that negro sweat was antiseptic and, therefore, negroes did not get fungous infections that white folks do. I wonder if the negro babies have as much impetigo as the white babies?

DR. FLOOD.—Watch a nurse who is wearing a mask. She is constantly pulling at it and changing its position. You cannot wear them all day in comfort.

DR. CHRISTIE.—I have here a transparent mask which is much easier to wear. It is called the Penn mask and is made in Germany.

DR. FLOOD.—I would like to hear a discussion on incubators.

DR. CHRISTIE.—I believe that in ten years we will have air-conditioned nurseries. They are much nearer ideal than any incubator now in use.

CHAIRMAN DURAND.—Air conditioning is a thing which we should consider.

DR. FABER.—Can anyone here tell us anything about the new incubator of Dr. Chappell of Philadelphia?

DR. CHRISTIE.—This incubator controls humidity. The nurse puts her arm into the incubator through a sleeve when she wishes to care for the baby or do anything for it.

DR. SEITZ.—This incubator almost requires an engineer to run it. You could spend the same amount of money and air condition the room and take care of several babies.

DR. HOWARD.—We made a glass box, equipped it with an electric pad, and we have a tank of oxygen and a tank of carbon dioxide and oxygen connected. We have one side open so we can get to the baby easily.

DR. L. E. RECTOR (BOSTON).—At the Boston Children's Hospital a combination respirator and incubator heated with bulbs works beautifully.

CHAIRMAN CHRISTIE.—There have been recent reports in the literature throughout the country in the past few years on diarrhea in the newborn infant. I think it well to discuss this quite fully.

DR. M. L. BLATT (CHICAGO).—The diarrheas in the newborn infant which have occurred under my observation have been cases of sepsis; they do not begin with diarrhea. Many of the patients died of bronchopneumonia. We were unable to isolate any definite organisms, and in many instances more than one organism was found in similar cases throughout the nursery. A source of infection may be from the milk supply, from the nursery, and, I think, it may probably be air borne.

DR. DURAND.—Looking for sepsis is probably right. It is interesting that not many cases occur at one time; there will be three or four cases and then a lull, to be followed by three or four cases later on. In some instances we found on examination of the stool fat droplets which were first thought to be Monilia. In these epidemic diarrheas the stools are acid, fermented, yellow, watery consistency, and practically no blood. It is the same picture seen the country over. At autopsy there is no ulceration found in the intestinal tract but marked hyperemia with terminal bronchopneumonia. Definite pathogens are not known; it may be virus.

DR. V. CULLOTA (BALTIMORE).—Are cases ever seen in older children?

DR. DURAND.—None.

DR. BLATT.—We have had patients return to the hospital twenty-one days after being discharged. These cases, like the ones occurring in the hospital, did not begin with diarrhea. There was a gradual onset, first of anorexia, fever, progressing gradually to diarrhea, etc.

CHAIRMAN CHRISTIE.—Have any breast-fed babies developed the disease?

DR. BLATT.—Some few. The feedings of breast milk, which introduce into the gastrointestinal tract *Bacillus bifidus,* seem to be of help.

DR. A. F. ABT (CHICAGO).—I am not quite so certain concerning the portal of entry in these cases. In the Michael Reese hospital in Chicago, in 1931, cases occurred until the culture from the nose and throat of two nurses revealed *B. mucosus capsulatus*. The same organism was recovered from the stool. The nurses were removed, and the epidemic stopped. Tonsillectomy and adenoidectomy were performed on the nurses; they returned to the nursery, and no further cases developed. It appears from this that the portal of entry may be from the air and not through the gastrointestinal tract. I have noticed too that in the beginning the infections of these babies did not act primarily as gastrointestinal infections; more, they resemble sepsis.

DR. DURAND.—There has been some question as to whether this is a new form of disease. I think it certainly must be; it has never been seen before in epidemic form and it has occurred in forty-odd places throughout the country in the past few years. All the cases seem to be the same. There is approximately a 50 per cent mortality, so that it must be a new disease. It resembles influenza in many instances.

We might discuss somewhat the question of nursery technique and personnel. It seems that unless something is done along developing a definite technique we will be forced to give up the nurseries.

CHAIRMAN CHRISTIE.—The temperature of the nursery is usually kept at 68° to 70° F., the humidity 50 to 55 per cent. Under conditions of this sort very little clothing is put on the babies. A baby wears a shirt and diaper. If the buttocks become excoriated, the diaper is removed, and the buttocks are exposed to the sun and air. Babies never seem to be chilled or affected by this routine. The temperatures, when taken, are always normal. In the care of the skin, ammoniated mercury inunctions produce a high amount of skin irritation, but very little impetigo occurs. The dry technique is quite satisfactory. It is surprising that no irritation of the skin results as well as that the babies are devoid of odor. At the University Hospital half strength tincture of green soap bath is used.

DR. J. B. BILDERBACK (PORTLAND, ORE.).—The nurse with a cold should be removed from the nursery.

CHAIRMAN CHRISTIE.—The nurses' supervisor is invaluable and is of great help. There should be a medical examination of the nurses daily, and a monthly throat and stool culture should be made.

DR. E. G. SCHWARTZ (FORT WORTH, TEXAS).—It seems to me the question of impetigo is a climatic one. We see a number of cases in Texas in the summer only. I might say that we have had no cases of diarrhea that have been discussed. I have seen an occasional baby with sporadic bleeding from the bowel but they all seem to act well, and many times the cause for this condition is not explained.

DR. W. A. REILEY (SAN FRANCISCO).—I have seen, during the winter in San Francisco, diarrheas occurring in older children. The stools are quite loose, some mucus and occasional blood, and they are negative to organisms. Do you think these cases are the same as those occurring in the newborn infant?

DR. DURAND.—A few epidemics of diarrhea have occurred in Portland but they are not similar to those that are seen in the newborn infants, and I do not believe these cases are of a similar nature. We are very seldom troubled with diarrhea in older children; because of the cool nights we have very little effect from the hot weather or changes in the milk from heat.

DR. CULLOTA.—I have noticed very definitely that evaporated milk is more laxative now than before the milk was irradiated. Do you suppose radiation accounts for this?

DR. SAMUEL HURWITZ (SAN FRANCISCO).—Is there any particular physiologic reason for not giving cold milk to a baby; which milk has a low bacterial count?

DR. DURAND.—It does not seem right to give cold milk to a young baby, and certainly heating the milk just before it is given should not affect the count.

DR. REILEY.—Do you remove nurses who show streptococci on culture?

DR. BLATT.—They are removed from the premature room, the milk laboratory, and the newborn nursery. As nothing used in the nose and throat will be of any advantage, it is necessary that the nurses be removed.

DR. HURWITZ.—We have followed a plan in Oakland which seems to offer some help in that the mothers are delivered at the hospital and discharged on the fourth day. These periods of short hospitalization seem to give a lessened amount of trouble with babies in the nursery. I should like to ask at what time infections occur and what time do skin infections develop as a rule in the newborn infant?

DR. DURAND.—They usually occur early, about the fourth day. They are acquired by passage through the birth canal.

DR. BLATT.—Making a smaller unit and more of them will remove a large incidence of infection.

CHAIRMAN CHRISTIE.—Has anyone any suggestion to make as to how to preserve technique during circumcision rituals?

DR. DURAND.—The separation of the patient and operator by glass partitions might help to solve the problem.

DR. BLATT.—Why is humidity of the nursery necessary?

CHAIRMAN CHRISTIE.—According to the report of Dr. Blackfan and clinical evidence, it is indicated.

DR. BLATT.—We have no humidification in the premature room. The humidity is 10 to 45 per cent, and no difference has been seen.

M. K. WYLDER, M.D., Albuquerque, N. M.
F. B. SMITH, M.D., Baltimore, Md.
Secretaries.

EIGHTH ANNUAL MEETING OF THE AMERICAN ACADEMY OF PEDIATRICS

DEL MONTE, CALIF., JUNE 10 AND 11, 1938

Round Table Discussion of Diabetes Mellitus

Chairman: Dr. H. Clare Shepardson, San Francisco, Calif.
Assistant: Dr. Howard F. West, Los Angeles, Calif.

CHAIRMAN SHEPARDSON.—In bringing before this group a subject which permits of such latitude in discussion as does that of diabetes mellitus, I realize that we may stray far afield. In the past two or three years, largely as a result of the impetus provided by the discovery of protamine insulin by Hagedorn, many investigations concerning this disease have been accelerated. Yet we find from practical experience that many doctors, including pediatricians, still do not fully appreciate the incidence and symptomatology, the diagnosis nor the prognosis of the juvenile diabetic. This largely results from the fact that emphasis in discussions and in the literature has been placed on problems of management, types of diet, and of more recent months, the several types of insulin, to the more or less exclusion of these various fundamentals. Even yet we see children who have been neglected during the first weeks of symptoms, and we see mothers who have been given inadequate or misleading information about their prognosis or proper management. Tragic examples could readily be cited, but for this representative group they would be superfluous. Nevertheless, it is felt that proper education of the physicians throughout the country is the only means of obviating this distressing state of affairs.

In order to properly open this discussion I have asked Dr. West to present to you a brief analysis of the information resulting from the study recently made by him of some 300 juvenile diabetics. Possibly these problems can be amplified later by a frank consideration of the mortality rates, the changed status of girls relative to menstrual development, and pregnancy, and the manner in which these youngsters, if adequately controlled, are able to meet the physical, economic, and sociologic complications to which they will later be subject. One problem of tremendous importance is the ability of the girl diabetic to subsequently overcome the difficulties of pregnancy, which may later ensue. This of course immediately suggests many other phases which are the result of the advent of long acting insulins. It seems obvious that the greatest accomplishment of protamine insulin has been the elimination of acidosis in childhood. Formerly it was not at all uncommon to see repeated attacks of coma in the child diabetic. These apparently will be almost entirely eliminated in the future. As a result of this improvement in the therapeutics of diabetes tremendous significance is added to the statement made by Joslin, several years ago, that "no longer is the child diabetic a dying child, but rather a living one."

Consequently we are now confronted with the fact that only rarely do children die of diabetes. It is to be expected, therefore, that the life expectancy of the child diabetic will increase immensely as a result of the use of these insulins with prolonged hypoglycemic effect.

There are other very interesting subjects concerning diabetes which, of late, have assumed considerable prominence. One of these particularly applicable to pediatricians is the association of diabetes with disturbances in function of various members of the endocrine system. Because of the increase in life expectancy of the child diabetic, and the consequent increase in the number of patients so afflicted, it seems obvious that the incidence of endocrine diseases in the juvenile diabetic population will be proportionately greater as time goes on. As you well know, there recently has been a great deal of investigative work done in several laboratories throughout the world on the relationship of various ductless glands, particularly the adenohypophysis and the adrenal cortex, to diabetes mellitus. From the relevant data available at the moment, it seems quite probable that alterations in function of either the anterior pituitary gland, or the suprarenal cortex, will profoundly effect carbohydrate metabolism. We are all aware of the effect of a hyperfunctioning thyroid on the general metabolism; consequently it is not surprising that the metabolism of carbohydrates is adversely affected in the presence of thyrotoxicosis. On the other hand, I cannot subscribe to the theory that disturbances in function of the pituitary or of the adrenal cortex, or of the thyroid gland, are causative factors in the development of diabetes. The incidence of a condition to all intents and purposes identical with diabetes mellitus is relatively high among the acromegalic population. The same statement can be made of that group of women inflicted with the suprarenogenital syndrome. It is felt that in all probability the abnormal effects evident from a hyperfunctioning acidophilic adenoma and the pituitary exercise their effect through the adrenal cortex. In order to produce diabetes under such conditions we must, for the present, hypothecate a functional disturbance of islet cell activity as a pre-existing factor in those patients afflicted with such diseases as acromegaly or the suprarenogenital syndrome and who subsequently develop an associated diabetes.

Of equal interest is the study of the reduced activity of the pituitary and the thyroid in the child diabetic. Priscilla White recently has been extremely interested in the incidence of dwarfism among her group of diabetic children. She has used growth hormone with very gratifying results in these youngsters. Unfortunately the determination of the cause of the dwarfism among diabetic children is sometimes extremely difficult to make. The diabetes itself when improperly treated can be responsible. Bone age studies should be made in each instance, and the results thus obtained should not be ignored. Dr. White is placed in the position of having to defend her results, which, in certain instances, are open to question because she has administered, simultaneously with growth hormone, thyroid substance. And in that group of children whose dwarfism results from thyroid deficiency, it seems unnecessary to employ growth hormone to enhance their growth, for we are all familiar with the extremely favorable effects resulting from the administration of thyroid substance alone. One other factor is of serious importance; these children have all been placed on protamine zinc insulin. As a consequence, their nutrition has undoubtedly improved. This alone may account in part, at least, for some of Dr. White's results.

As a concluding feeature of this very interesting round table discussion I should like to introduce the subject of long acting insulins, with their effect not only on the disease itself, but particularly on the patient's prognosis. There seems to be no question that Hagedorn's introduction of protamine insulin has greatly enhanced the comfort of the child diabetic. Diabetes in childhood is almost uniformly a severe disease. Prior to 1935 it was necessary to give these children multiple doses of insulin during twenty-four hours in order to even partially control the disease. As a matter of fact, it was not until protamine insulin came into use that we actually realized how inadequately treated and how poorly controlled, even under the most favorable conditions, had been the child diabetic in the past. Following the institution of protamine zinc insulin the number of daily injections was reduced 50 to 75 per cent, and the control of the diabetes greatly improved. As a result, the psychic status of the child diabetic under the present regime is far superior to that which existed three or four years ago. More recently Sahyun, of Detroit, has introduced a new crystalline insulin. This substance in the hands of many investigators has proved equally satisfactory and in some respects more so than have other so-called long acting insulins.

The advantage of the newer insulins with a prolonged hypoglycemic effect have been thoroughly established. They effect a more constant, hence, better physiologic control of diabetes, a reduction in the number of daily injections of insulin, and, incidentally, frequently a considerable reduction in the total daily insulin requirement. The various disadvantages accompanying the use of these substances have been emphasized by many investigators. Suffice it to say, however, that the magnitude of those disadvantages has steadily decreased with increasing knowledge and experience in the use of these preparations. Protamine zinc insulin has produced uniformly favorable results in the treatment of diabetes. Yet, it is by no means an ideal substance. The ideal insulin should promise a lowering of blood sugar throughout the digestive period. It should be so controllable that when adequate doses are given, a maximum sugar-lowering effect would be obtained without producing hypoglycemia and the accompanying reactions or shock. For the present there seems to be some disagreement as to whether the hypoglycemic effect of crystalline insulin is sufficiently different from that of unmodified insulin to warrant its inclusion in the therapeutic armamentarium of the diabetic specialist.

Juvenile Diabetes

DR. WEST.—Fifteen years after the introduction of so radical an improvement in therapy as insulin gave to the management of juvenile diabetes would seem to be an opportune time for a review of progress. This would seem to be indicated not only for the sake of gaining what satisfaction we may, but also because experience shows that many doctors do not as yet appreciate the changed status of the diabetic child. The extremely bad prognosis, an average expectation of life of about two years from onset of symptoms, of a decade and a half ago apparently remains fixed in many minds. This point of view is a decided handicap to the child, often delaying the institution of adequate treatment, and is especially disheartening to the anxious parents.

As an introduction to this discussion I would like to refer to the experience of my associates and myself with 328 juvenile diabetics (onset of symptoms before the age of 16 years) seen since 1917. We have included in this group children seen in private practice and in three charity hospitals and clinics. They have not all been continuously under our personal care. The results, good and bad, would, therefore, more nearly represent a cross section of community experience than individual attainment.

From the information obtained in a review of this group the following pertinent points are presented briefly:

Age of Onset.—While juvenile diabetes may become manifest at any age after birth, our patients conformed to the general experience that symptoms most frequently develop in the prepubescent years, 9 to 12 years among girls and 11 to 12 years for the boys. Onset during the first year is relatively rare (only three instances in this series). The youngest was only 8 weeks of age. No instance of congenital diabetes was seen. There is a sharp falling off in frequency during the fifteenth year.

Sex.—Also conforming to other experiences the sexes were almost equally divided with a slight preponderance of females, 174 girls and 154 boys.

Race.—Only 10.3 per cent of these children were of the Jewish race. This incidence is practically the same as found in all other series reported and is in sharp contrast to the high incidence among adult Jews. Among the non-Jews, the group included seven Mexicans, five colored persons, one Italian, one Assyrian, and one Portuguese.

Heredity.—Of all the known predisposing causes, heredity is preeminent. This information is available in 313 records, with a family history of diabetes recorded as positive in 32.8 per cent. For those with diabetes of a duration of ten or more years the family history has had time to reach 41.4 per cent. For the Jewish group it is 45.4 per cent.

Twins.—In a family under observation there is one pair of twins, each having diabetes. They are Jewish females, one having developed symptoms at 3 years and 2 months of age, the other at 3 years and 11 months. Both are living, six years and seven months and five years and ten months, respectively, since onset. Three other pairs of twins have been seen, but in only one of each pair has diabetes so far become evident. The others are under close observation.

Previous Illnesses.—H. J. John has been impressed with the importance of infections as predisposing factors in the diabetes of childhood. While acute illness and especially infections do lower carbohydrate tolerance and make existing diabetes more severe, in only about 24 per cent of the entire group did we obtain a history of an acute illness sufficiently close in time to the onset of recognizable symptoms to be considered as a possible factor in etiology or a precipitating event. As a group the records of preceding illness were little different from those obtainable from other children of similar ages. On the other hand, it must be remembered that acute symptoms of diabetes not infrequently follow immediately after one of the exanthemas or an acute respiratory infection, and even after tonsillectomy (four instances), other operations, or vaccination. In our group acute upper respiratory infections were the most common among what might be classed as precipitating events. The record shows thirty-four instances.

Presenting Symptoms and Diagnosis.—The symptoms of diabetes in the child tend to follow the classical pattern. From 316 records in which the original symptoms were adequately recorded we find that polyuria occurred in 91.4 per cent, polydipsia in 88.8 per cent, loss of weight and strength in 79.6 per cent, and polyphagia in 73.9 per cent. Nervous irritability and difficulty in school were not uncommon. The onset of symptoms was definitely acute in 83 per cent.

Yet, in spite of the typical nature of the symptoms and the acuteness of onset, diagnosis was much too often delayed. In 252 records sufficient data were recorded to permit the calculation of the number of days elapsing between the onset of symptoms and the discovery of glycosuria. The average delay was 55.3 days. In this the younger children fared better than those of the older age groups. The average time elapsing between onset of symptoms and diagnosis for those less than 5 years of age was 38.4 days, between 6 and 10 years, 49.2 days, while in the group more than 10 years of age symptoms had been present for an average of 77.1 days, over two and one-half months. The bathroom habits and general condition of younger children are obviously more closely observed than their older brothers and sisters. The failure to recognize the symptoms of diabetes reflects the utter astonishment of most parents when they are finally given the correct diagnosis. Doctors also are too often taken unaware and prescribe extra feedings, tonics, and vitamin concentrates or vacations before making an analysis of the urine.

The unhappy significance of this delay in diagnosis is illustrated by the fact that over 37 per cent of these children had developed a more or less severe ketosis, and an additional 21 per cent, one out of every five, were actually in coma when the diagnosis was first made. Of more particular importance is the revelation that 31.5 per cent of all deaths occurred within less than thirty days following the onset of symptoms. In the preinsulin period 50 per cent of the deaths occurred during the first month. It is obvious that the profession and also parents must be made more conscious of diabetes if these children are to be spared the hazards of delay.

Mortality.—Of 302 children whose present status is known, 248 are living and 54 or 17.9 per cent are dead, a regrettably high mortality. Insulin was first available to our group in November, 1922. Prior to this date twenty-five patients of our series had been diagnosed as diabetic. Of these twenty-five, fourteen died without benefit of insulin, a mortality of 56 per cent. Of these, eight died within a month of onset of symptoms, one lived for seven years, one for six years, and four from two years and one month to two years and eight months. Of the remaining eleven of the preinsulin group, two have died, each at five years and seven months from onset, and nine are still living. Of these nine, the onset of one was in 1920, of two in 1921, and of five in 1922. For those patients receiving no insulin, the mortality was 100 per cent. The outcome to date of 288 children for whom insulin has been available is known. Forty have died, a mortality of 13.8 per cent. If we subdivide the fifteen years of insulin experience into three five-year periods, the mortality experience is as shown in Table I.

TABLE I

PERIOD	PATIENTS			KNOWN DEATHS
	NEW PATIENTS	HELD OVER	TOTAL	
Jan. 1923—Jan. 1928	65	11	76	12 or 15.8%
Jan. 1928—Jan. 1933	122	64	186	17 or 9.1%
Jan. 1933—Aug. 1937	123	169	292	11 or 3.7%

For purposes of analysis computations have been made as of August 1, 1937. One death has occurred, however, since that date.

The steady improvement in the mortality rate is modified partly by the constant addition of new patients who have been exposed to the hazards of diabetes for a shorter period of time, but we also believe it reflects earlier diagnosis and more effective treatment.

Of particular interest is a group of eighty-three children with onset of diabetes prior to August 1, 1927, and for whom insulin has been available, in other words, those who have had an opportunity to live ten or more years. Twenty-one, or 25.3 per cent, have died. Only three of these deaths have occurred since 1930; two-thirds of the deaths of this group occurred during the first half of the period analyzed. For those exposed less than ten years the mortality has been 9.25 per cent.

Causes of Death.—Inquiry into the cause of death in this entire group shows that 60.1 per cent of the deaths must be attributed directly to diabetes. The highest incidence is naturally in the preinsulin group, 79 per cent, but even in the insulin period we must admit that for 55 per cent there is no other adequate cause. These figures are based on the total known causes of death, but the actual cause of death is unknown for five.

In the preinsulin period ten of the diabetic deaths were due to uncomplicated coma and one to a very severe ketosis complicated by gangrene of the nose and severe malnutrition.

In the insulin period twenty patients, or 50 per cent of the total deaths, died in coma. There was one death due to hypoglycemia during the early days of insulin and one with acute pancreatitis and ketosis. Twelve of the comas were uncomplicated, but in eight—two-thirds—of these insulin was stopped, refused, or the institution of treatment was too late, because of delay on the part of the parents, delay in diagnosis or, in some instances, because of both factors. Four charts gave indication of inadequate treatment; in one the treatment appeared to be adequate, but sudden death ensued, unexplained even at autopsy. In the other eight cases of coma there were severe complications, such as pneumonia, three cases; severe enteritis, one; lateral sinus thrombosis, one; otitis media, one; hyperpyrexia, one; gangrene of the bowel with peritonitis (possibly the result of huge doses of castor oil administered by the parents before admission), one.

What we may call nondiabetic deaths during the insulin period include pneumonia, three; myocardial failure after diphtheria (diabetes well controlled), one; lymphosarcoma, one; influenza, one; pertussis, one; cerebral embolism, one; drowning, one; lateral sinus thrombosis, one; pulmonary tuberculosis, one; head injury, one; and pneumococcic meningitis, one.

Duration of Life.—Prior to the use of insulin, as is well known, the average expectation of life for a diabetic child was but a little over two years from onset. Today no one knows with accuracy what it is or will be. A curve has been projected from data obtained by Dublin and Marks, of the Metropolitan Life Insurance Company, from the clinic of Dr. Joslin, indicating that the expectation is well over thirty years when onset occurs before 10 years of age.

Sixty-two, or 25 per cent, of our group have already lived ten years or more, the longest nearly eighteen years; while 156, or 62.5 per cent, have lived five years or more; and 87.8 per cent have passed the two-year mark. At least nine more patients would be added to the ten-year group if we were to carry our analysis to June, 1938, instead of closing it on August 1, 1937.

Nonfatal Complications.—There is perhaps no better way to evaluate both the hardihood of these modern diabetic youngsters and the efficacy of present-day treatment than to consider some of the many complications that have been successfully met during the course of their diabetes. The list is much too long for a detailed report at this time. Only some of the more severe tests are reported.

There are 71 individuals who have survived coma, 32 of them on more than one occasion. An additional 171 have experienced more or less severe ketosis. There have been 40 repeaters. Other complications met successfully were: measles, in 38 patients; mumps, 14; chicken pox, 25; pertussis, 19; pneumonia, 7; scarlet fever, 4; diphtheria, 3; tonsillitis, 46; appendicitis, 12; typhoid fever, 1; upper respiratory infections of note, 104; enteritis, 25; pulmonary tuberculosis, 1; poliomyelitis,

1; tonsillectomy, 42; appendectomy, 8; gangrene of the nose, 3; tracheotomy, 1; operation for squint, 1; extensive burns with skin grafting, 1; fracture of leg, 2; fracture of spine, 1; mastoidectomy, 1; removal of ovarian cyst, 1; herniotomy, 1; traumatic rupture of spleen with laparotomy, 1.

Retinitis has been observed in 2 patients and cataract in only one. In only 1 patient has there been detected any evidence of arteriosclerosis of clinical importance.

Of all the complications the most interesting and perhaps the most significant is pregnancy.

Prior to the insulin period girls developing diabetes before the sixteenth year did not live long enough, as a rule, to marry. Sexual development was delayed and total amenorrhea was the rule rather than the exception.

A new generation has been added to medical history. These girls are beginning to marry and to have children. In this group there have been at least thirteen pregnancies in eight individuals. There have been six cesarean sections for five mothers. One abortion was induced because of intractable ketosis and vomiting before the patient came under our observation. There has been no maternal mortality. (Two pregnancies have not reached term.)

The increasing frequency of pregnancy among diabetic women is adding new problems for the pediatrician.

The newborn infants of diabetic mothers may be oversized, fat, and flabby. Congenital anomalies are somewhat more frequent than the general average. The newborn infants of diabetic mothers are apparently somewhat more prone to develop hypoglycemia of clinical significance than other infants. However, the importance of spontaneous hypoglycemia among all newborn infants has but recently begun to be appreciated. Emergency treatment may be indicated to prevent deaths. To date we have not observed diabetes developing in the offspring of a mother diabetic at the time of delivery. One parent of each of three of the children in this series has developed diabetes since the onset in the child.

DISCUSSION

DR. A. E. FISCHER (NEW YORK CITY).—Were the twins identical?

DR. WEST.—They were; however, in many cases reported, twins were not identical

CHAIRMAN SHEPARDSON.—The factor of heredity is much higher than heretofore. Dr. West shows a present incidence of 32.8 per cent.

DR. LEE COHN (SAN FRANCISCO).—What is the attitude toward pregnancy for a woman having diabetes since childhood?

CHAIRMAN SHEPARDSON.—If there is no diabetic history in the paternal family, we advise pregnancy. If the history is positive in the paternal family, we advise against pregnancy. Diabetes is a recessive Mendelian character. If limited to one side of the family, the recessive will not become dominant. The mother could not reasonably be sterilized.

DR. WEST.—Joslin states that if the mother is prohibited from becoming pregnant, then all of her brothers and sisters should not have children.

DR. COHN.—This is a great economic problem.

CHAIRMAN SHEPARDSON.—Also it is a great social problem. The diabetic child's life is pathetic, and probably no child would want to come into life under such conditions.

DR. WEST.—If the diabetic mother has one normal child sterilization could be advised.

CHAIRMAN SHEPARDSON.—Dr. West has significantly pointed out the results of a delayed diagnosis. The adult internist sees more sick children than the pediatrician; he should keep diabetes of childhood in mind in diagnosis. He is often at fault for the delay in diagnosis.

On the other hand, many parents are at fault in withholding insulin therapy. Death in coma is due to carelessness. Sixty per cent of Dr. West's fatal cases were patients with coma, and this should never occur. Severe acidosis also is inexcusable.

DR. COHN.—The coma cases were under your care, were they not?

DR. WEST.—Not always. This one 15-year-old boy was operated for hernia by another physician who failed to care for the diabetes.

DR. P. J. HOWARD (DETROIT).—Did you note any relation between enuresis and diabetes?

DR. WEST.—We have seen a few diabetics with enuresis but without glycosuria at the time. Occasionally other enuretics have had mild glycosuria but not true diabetes.

DR. HOWARD.—Is there any contraindication to general anesthesia for surgery?

DR. WEST.—No. Surgery, if it helps elimination of infection, should be done.

CHAIRMAN SHEPARDSON.—Any necessary surgery can be done if the diabetes is under good control. Anesthesia is not a major question.

DR. COHN.—What are your criteria for good control?

CHAIRMAN SHEPARDSON.—Blood sugar determination is not absolutely essential. If there is no glycosuria the patient is burning his blood sugar efficiently.

DR. COHN.—Does diabetes occur without glycosuria?

CHAIRMAN SHEPARDSON.—Probably not in childhood. If so, it is very rare. The symptoms will help in diagnosis.

DR. HOWARD.—Is glucose tolerance essential in every diabetic suspect?

CHAIRMAN SHEPARDSON.—No. But a fasting test and one after a high carbohydrate meal could be done first. If the fasting test is high the glucose tolerance need not be done.

DR. W. A. REILLY (SAN FRANCISCO).—What is your preparation for surgery?

DR. WEST.—Emergency surgery can be done immediately. In the meantime, we give enough carbohydrate and adequate insulin to control ketosis. Urinalysis is important. A blood sugar can be done but it is not absolutely necessary. The important thing is sufficient fluid and a good storage of glucose in the liver. For elective cases, store carbohydrate ahead of time in liver and have diabetes under control.

CHAIRMAN SHEPARDSON.—Often in comatose diabetics the abdomen (rigid abdomen, 100,000 white blood count, acidosis with vomiting and pains) may simulate surgical abdomen. These patients can be treated medically from three to five hours and then operated if doubt still exists. The mortality is less if the infection can be relieved surgically.

DR. R. S. LEET (OAKLAND, CALIF.).—What do you think of the substitutes for insulin?

CHAIRMAN SHEPARDSON.—There are none. Hexylresorcinol and inulin are no good. Synthaline causes liver diseases. Myrtillin is not at all reliable. Mehlitol is a fraud.

DR. COHN.—Are pathologic changes definite in infancy?

CHAIRMAN SHEPARDSON.—Very often they are not.

DR. REILLY.—Do diabetic children later develop polyglandular syndromes?

DR. WEST.—Some adolescent girls become obese and develop amenorrhea. Thus other glands can become hypofunctional as well as the pancreas.

DR. REILLY.—Do these girls grow normally?

DR. WEST.—A few fail to grow well. This is probably a question of undernutrition, even though they are obese. Since diabetic children have been fed more liberally, the dwarfism has disappeared. Adequate growth and weight (short of obesity) is the desideratum. The skeletal dwarfism was fundamentally a nutritional deficiency.

DR. J. W. BRUCE (LOUISVILLE, KY.).—What do you think of free choice of diet and control with protamine insulinate?

CHAIRMAN SHEPARDSON.—All diets should include adequate calories for occupation or growth. Secondly, there must be an adequate amount of protein. Before insulin was introduced sugar and carbohydrate were taken out of the diet; the diet was mainly high in protein and fat. In 1914 Frederick Allen postulated that total calories should be lessened. In 1922, when insulin was first in use, carbohydrate was put into the diet to the extent of about 50 gm. daily.

There are three schemes of diet. Newburgh raised the fat to 100 gm. daily. He and Gellan, in New York, suggested a high fat diet because they thought blood sugar would be more stable, and complications like arteriosclerosis would be less frequent. Rabinowitch, Allen, Bast, Joslin, etc., all have used variable diets, and their patients do quite well. I have stuck to an intermediate course and use about 150 gm. of carbohydrate. One can use whatever satisfies the patients and keeps them happy. Of course the blood sugar and urine have to stay within normal limits. Any diet which does not violate the ketogenic-antiketogenic ratio is satisfactory if palatable. It probably matters little if a high fat, low carbohydrate diet or the reverse is used. Much depends on the patient and the physician.

DR. WEST.—What is a diabetic diet? It is only a quantitative diet, which free choice of diet is not. Insulin dosage always has to be anticipated. This cannot be done with the free choice diet if the insulin is used before meals, as it usually has to be. If the patient would take the same amount of protein, carbohydrate, and fat on a free choice diet every day, then the insulin dosage could be satisfactorily anticipated.

CHAIRMAN SHEPARDSON.—All diabetic diets are weighed diets. There is normally a 10 per cent variation with weighing. Too many variables already exist in diabetic therapy without using the free choice diet. Blood sugar will vary greatly. The hypoglycemia is far more dangerous than hyperglycemia.

We will learn much from the use of insulin for dementia precox.

DR. BRUCE.—Is protamine insulin better than insulin for children?

CHAIRMAN SHEPARDSON.—This is hard to answer. Neither one is adequate. I would stay with regular insulin; also it acts more quickly. I have to use the same number of injections with protamine as with old insulin. Few children can get along with a single injection; if so, old insulin is still adequate.

DR. BRUCE.—How do you counteract protamine reactions in early morning?

CHAIRMAN SHEPARDSON.—I would try diet as 1/5, 2/5, and 2/5 at night. At 6:00 P.M. give 60 per cent of the 2/5 and 40 per cent at 10:00 P.M. Extra crackers can be given at early morning if reactions occur. Give less of protamine before breakfast and give some regular insulin after breakfast for short immediate use. Crystalline insulin is very good and possibly superior to protamine insulin in that less injections are required.

DR. BRUCE.—How much exercise do you recommend?

CHAIRMAN SHEPARDSON.—It depends on the child. Some children may develop hypoglycemia in the morning if overexercised. However, exercise in general should not be restricted.

DR. P. F. DWAN (MINNEAPOLIS).—What percentage of your cases were treated with protamine insulin?

DR. WEST.—The majority have had it during the last two years. There are very few who are on one dose of protamine alone. We do not share the enthusiasm which prevailed several years ago, but we do feel that protamine has definite advantages.

DR. S. R. KALISKI (SAN ANTONIO).—Can you follow a case to your own satisfaction solely by the micromethod of sugar determination?

CHAIRMAN SHEPARDSON.—Yes.

DR. KALISKI.—At what time of day do you give protamine insulin?

CHAIRMAN SHEPARDSON.—Almost uniformly before breakfast.

DR. C. A. BOST (SAN FRANCISCO).—How do you handle new patients in the office?

CHAIRMAN SHEPARDSON.—If marked ketosis is present, they are better off in the hospital. I put them on reduced diets and small doses of regular insulin as required. If definite coma or drowsiness exists, plenty of fluid and saline solution should be used. Insulin is given in amounts depending on the glycosuria.

DR. A. A. WALKER (BIRMINGHAM, ALA.).—How much?

CHAIRMAN SHEPARDSON.—In general about 25 units for a brick red reduction, 20 for orange, 15 for yellow, 10 for green reduction. This can be varied depending on the child's weight.

DR. REILLY.—Do you recommend alkali for coma?

CHAIRMAN SHEPARDSON.—I do not use it. Those who do, use so little that it is not effective. Salt solution does well; alkali may produce anuria. Water and sodium chloride are very important and almost equal to insulin.

DR. REILLY.—How do you manage diabetic coma?

CHAIRMAN SHEPARDSON.—The patient in uncomplicated coma is a patient in shock. It is essential that this be combated immediately by warmth, administration of fluids, and the use of drugs, such as caffeine, to support the failing circulation. Insulin can be immediately started in small doses, i.e., 25 units every half hour until the glycosuria begins to diminish. The small insulin doses are then rapidly reduced. The previously mentioned doses, of course, will be reduced depending on the ratio of the child's weight to a normal adult weight.

The two important procedures following the institution of shock therapy are the administration of adequate amounts of fluid in the form of normal salt solution in the use of unmodified insulin in frequently repeated relatively small doses. It is difficult to tell which of these two is the more important. As soon as the patient is sufficiently conscious to swallow, carbohydrate fluids are given by mouth. Early in the course of treatment the stomach should be washed.

The dosage of insulin can be regulated quite safely by observing the urine. Of course a blood sugar determination is very helpful when available.

DR. REILLY.—Do you use glucose infusions during coma?

CHAIRMAN SHEPARDSON.—No. Given a patient with high blood sugar, the intravenous injection of glucose may produce anuria; also one does not know exactly how the insulin will act. If too effective the best indicator, glycosuria, is not available. The clinician should never think first of glucose administration in diabetic coma; only very rarely is it needed, and its use may produce untoward and extremely undesirable effects. Likewise alkalies are not used.

WILLIAM ANTHONY REILLY, M.D., San Francisco, Calif.
SIDNEY R. KALISKI, M.D., San Antonio, Texas.
Secretaries.

Comments

THE National Health Conference may well be the greatest event in medical science which has happened in our time.'' Even if this statement of Dr. Parran, Surgeon General of the United States Public Health Service, in a network broadcast during the Conference held in Washington, July 18, 19 and 20, should prove to be a marked exaggeration, nevertheless its significance to American medicine is beyond question. For the first time the medical profession met face to face with the specific demands of the public. And these demands were put forward in no pleading, hesitant way.

Although some of the discussion of the Conference was carried as news in the press, and will be featured in a number of journals, of both a medical and social nature, it is the feeling of some of the Editorial Board and officers of the Academy that a report of the Conference in THE JOURNAL OF PEDIATRICS might help for a better, unprejudiced understanding of what took place and is taking place. Three Fellows of the Academy were present as ''Members of the Conference,'' Allan Butler, Clifford Grulee and Borden Veeder. A report written by Veeder of the Editorial Board appears as a special article on page 400 of this issue. The report attempts to present what took place, what was said and done, and to avoid any critical analysis or expression of personal viewpoint. The report is based on notes taken at the Conference and on stenographic copies of the remarks of a number who took part in the discussion. Many exact quotations have been used and care has been taken that in no instance the quotations give a false interpretation or meaning by removing them from the context.

The pediatricians have been the outstanding group in the medical profession who have recognized ''medical needs,'' and who have whole-heartedly recognized their responsibility in the inauguration and support of measures aimed for the betterment of the health of American children, and thus in turn for the nation as a whole.

The planned extension of the work for children under the direction of the Children's Bureau has been approved by the Academy, and there is no question but that the Fellowship will continue to cooperate as they have done in the past and are now doing.

The Journal of Pediatrics

Vol. 13 | October, 1938 | No. 4

Original Communications

THE TONIC NECK REFLEX IN THE HUMAN INFANT

Morphogenetic and Clinical Significance

Arnold Gesell, M.D.
New Haven, Conn.

THE tonic neck reflex is an asymmetric pattern of behavior, common to man and beast. Magnus, in his classic work on *Körperstellung,* reported an analysis of the postural reaction of decerebrate quadrupeds when their heads were experimentally turned to an extreme right or left position. He found a characteristic response: (a) extension of the forelimb on the side toward which the head was turned; (b) flexion of the opposite forelimb. The reflex occurred in pure form when the labyrinths were extirpated, and it was ascribed to proprioceptive impulses arising in the neck from torsion.

Magnus demonstrated the existence of the tonic neck reflex in idiots and patients suffering from extrapyramidal tract lesions; he was unable to induce the reflex in some twenty-six normal infants from a few hours to 16 weeks of age. He came to the conclusion that in man the tonic neck reflex is a pathologic phenomenon.[1]

This conclusion is somewhat amazing because we have found the tonic neck response a ubiquitous, indeed, a dominating characteristic of normal infancy in the first 3 months of life. In a clinical sense the response should be regarded as abnormal only when it occurs in children of more advanced age who are suffering from arrest or damage of the central nervous system.

The accompanying illustrations show that this attitudinal pattern is clearly evident in the spontaneous waking postures of the normal infant, whether he lies quiescent or active. We shall use the convenient symbol T.N.R. to designate the general pattern, both in its quiescent and activated forms.

From the Yale Clinic of Child Development, Yale University.

Fig. 1 illustrates T.N.R. in a rabbit and in a normal infant. The rabbit is adapted from Magnus; the infant is a healthy 8-week-old subject basking in the photographic dome of our clinic at Yale. Both are in the right T.N.R. attitude.

A.

B.

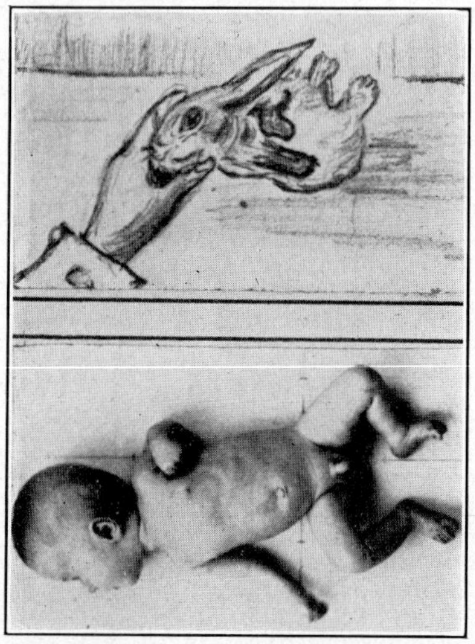

Fig. 1.—*A*, Right T.N.R. in rabbit induced by head torsion. (Adapted from Magnus.) *B*, Right T.N.R. in normal human infant (aged 8 weeks), spontaneously assumed.

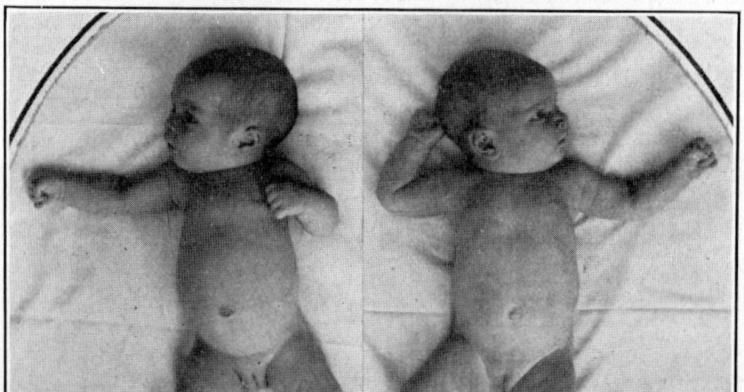

A. *B.*

Fig. 2.—*A*, Right T.N.R. in a normal 6-week-old infant. *B*, Left T.N.R. in another normal infant of the same age.

Fig. 2 pictures two normal infants, both 6 weeks of age. One is in right T.N.R., and the other in left T.N.R. In each instance the face-arm and face-leg are in extension, the contralateral extremities in flexion. Note the striking semblance to a fencing stance.

Fig. 3 shows a normal infant who at 1, 6, 8, and 12 weeks of age spontaneously and consistently exhibited a right T.N.R.

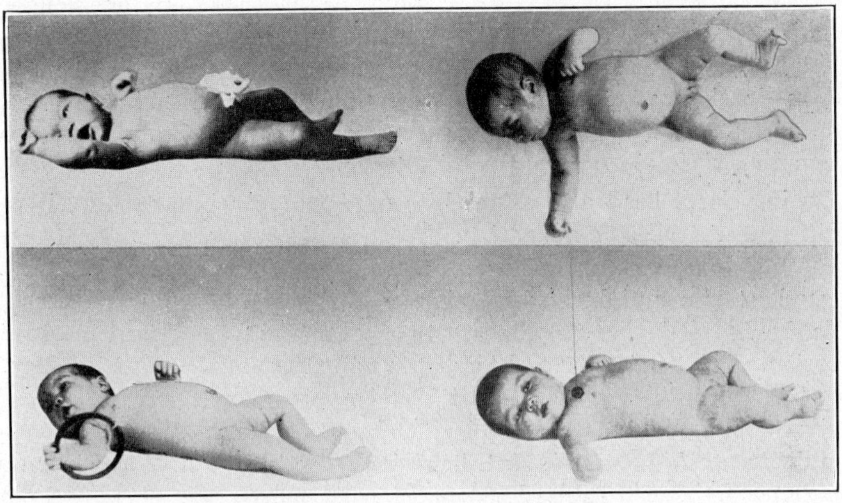

Fig. 3.—Right T.N.R. spontaneously and consistently exhibited in infant V. W. at 1, 6, 8, and 12 weeks of age.

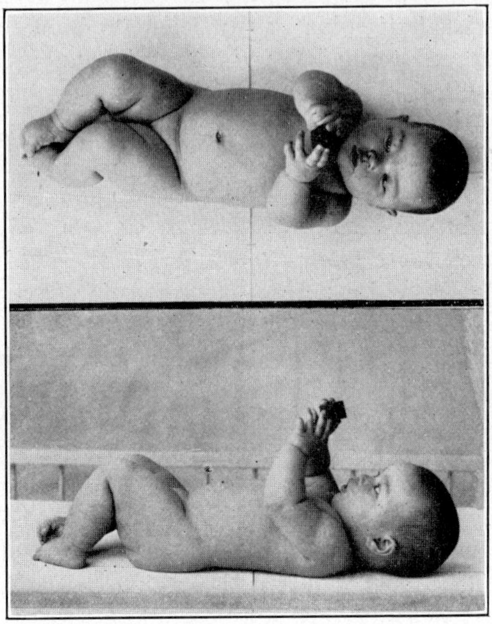

Fig. 4.—Symmetric prehensory and postural patterns in infant V. W., aged 24 weeks. Simultaneous photographs taken with one camera at the zenith and the other at the horizon of the photographic dome.

Fig. 4 pictures the same infant at 24 weeks of age. The spontaneous postural asymmetry of the earlier ages has been superseded by a symmetric attitude in which both arms flex and the hands engage above the chest at the midline. This is a lawful, developmental sequence. The

T.N.R. mechanisms are not extinguished at 24 weeks; they are simply submerged by symmetric, bilateral patterns. In another month the bilateral in turn give way to new unilateral patterns: one-handed reaching, one-handed manipulation and hand-to-hand transfer, and ultimately to well-defined dextrality or sinistrality. Throughout early human development there is an almost periodic, interweaving maturation, now of symmetric and then asymmetric behavior forms, with corresponding shifts in postural manifestations.

During sleep, head and extremities tend to lapse into symmetric or indifferent attitudes of relaxation. Whether drowsing, asleep, or awake the infant's posture may burst into momentary general symmetry, through startle and body jerk reflexes. The prevailing waking attitude, however, during the first three months is characterized by head aversion. The head seeks and holds the mid-position for relatively brief and infrequent intervals. Round heads rotate more freely than long heads in the early weeks, and since head posture initiates arm postures, this difference influences T.N.R. behavior. By 16 weeks of age infants usually show considerable freedom of head movement. I have been able to induce alternating right and left T.N.R. responses in a supine 16 weeks old infant simply by passing an object slowly across the field of vision. This visual stimulus was sufficient to induce a right T.N.R. when my hand moved toward the right, and a left T.N.R. when my hand moved to the left. The infant responded almost like an automaton under photoelectric control. These responses and other manifestations of the tonic neck reflex are delineated in a motion picture film.*[5]

Morphogenetically the human T.N.R. should not be envisaged as a stereotyped reflex but as a growing pattern, changing with the maturity and the economy of the organism. Torsion of the head to one side in a living fetus 20 weeks old arouses a movement of the arm on that side. This is a rudimentary T.N.R. which becomes better defined and elaborated in the latter half of the prenatal period. Fifteen minutes after the birth of a normal infant, I recently detected a greater tonicity in the right as opposed to the left arm (the legs were in equal relaxation). This discrepancy was predictive of a left T.N.R. in which the right, or occiput arm tends to show the greater tonus. The infant was kept under continuous observation for fourteen days and nights, and although he was placed in varying postures, he consistently displayed a waxing left T.N.R. Another infant, belonging to the right wing, was photographed daily in a standard supine position, from the fifteenth day

*This film is based on normative, experimental, and clinical cinema records as follows: (1) Reactions of a supine infant (age 20 weeks) to a dangling ring. Shows symmetry of postural and prehensory approach. (2) Overhead view of infant M. H., consistently showing right T.N.R. at 64, 65, 66, 67, 68 days of age, based on daily cinema records under experimentally repeated conditions. (3) Microphotographic section of a birth lesion of the basal ganglia (status marmoratus). (4) Active T.N.R. of boy A. C., aged 7 years, associated with a basal brain lesion. (5) Active T.N.R. of normal infant G60, similar in pattern to that of A. C. (6) Persisting T.N.R. in presence of distracting visual stimulus in infant G. 47, age 12 weeks. (7) Alternating T.N.R. in infant A. R., age 16 weeks, induced by visual stimulus. (8) Postural bilateral symmetry in infant G48, age 20 weeks, superseding T.N.R.

throughout most of the first year of life.* This infant spent approximately one-half of the 834 seconds of cinematically recorded behavior up to the eighty-second day in T.N.R. Sixty-five separate T.N.R.'s were observed; only one of these was leftward.

Fig. 5 graphs the incidence of these T.N.R.'s which fell to zero on the nineteenth day, when the head preferred a mid-position and the arms assumed more symmetric and versatile attitudes.

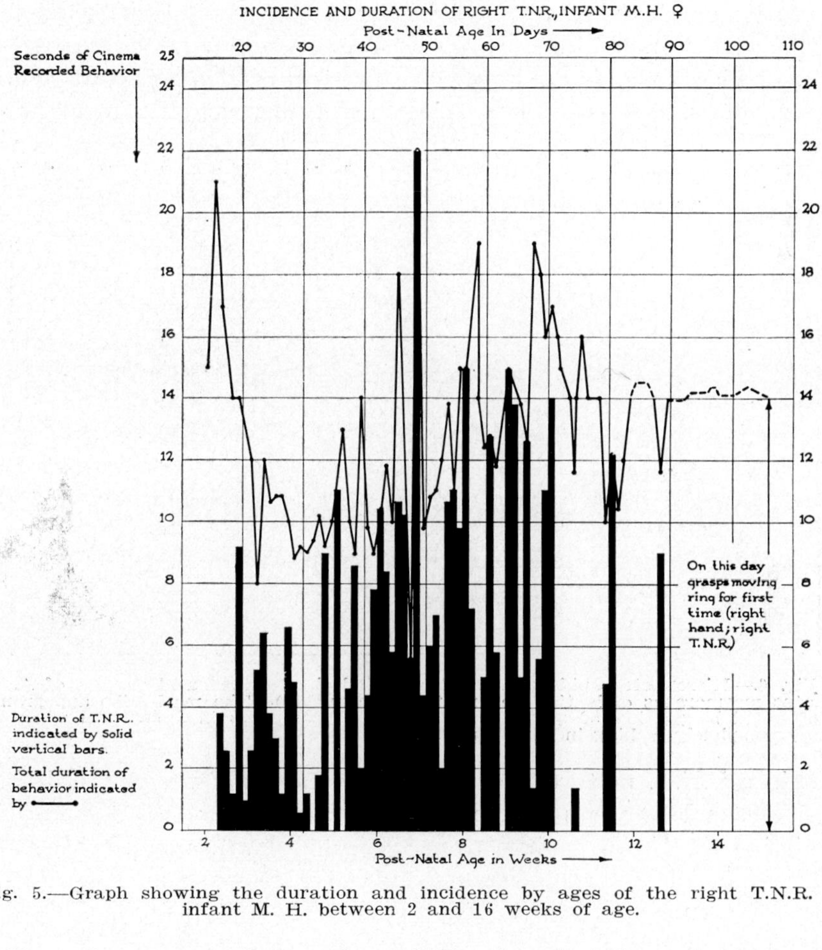

Fig. 5.—Graph showing the duration and incidence by ages of the right T.N.R. in infant M. H. between 2 and 16 weeks of age.

The submergence of the naïve T.N.R. of early infancy is the result of the ascendancy of cortical controls, probably in the motor and premotor regions, if Bieber and Fulton's data, regarding ablation, for monkeys and baboons apply to man.[2] This probability is strengthened by our findings in a case of cerebral palsy, in which necropsy (at the

*These observations were incidental to a study, with H. M. Halverson, of the visual and postural reactions of an infant to three interlocked rings, red, white, and blue, 4 cm. in diameter. The infant (M. H.) lay supine in a small photographic cubicle. The rings within easy reach were suspended on a horizontal string above her head and slowly moved left and right across the field of vision.

age of 14 years) revealed a severe but uncomplicated birth lesion of the basal ganglia (status marmoratus) (Fig. 6).[3] The boy in question, A. C. was afflicted with extreme double athetosis and, although intelligent, could not sit, walk, talk, grasp, or even hold up his head sustainedly. Cinema records of his spontaneous behavior in the supine position were made at the age of 7 years. Subjected to frame-by-frame analysis, these records revealed temporal and spatial patterns remarkably similar to those of the activated T.N.R. of normal infancy. Fig. 7 portrays eleven comparable phases in the arm and head movements of the palsied boy, aged 7 years, and of a normal infant, 4 weeks old.

These phases may be envisaged as a slashing windmill reaction emerging out of and returning to a basic T.N.R. attitude. The presence of the T.N.R. was obscured by lively athetotic movements, but when the cinema films were quantitatively studied, it was found that this boy

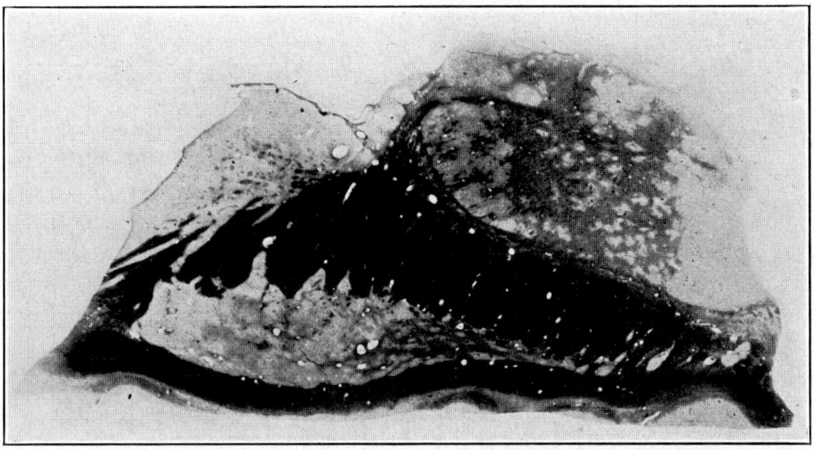

Fig. 6.—Microphotographic section of a birth lesion of the basal ganglia of A. C. (Status marmoratus of lenticulate and thalamic nuclei.) The marblelike appearance is produced by patches of gliosis and delicate myelin fibers in a striation which is nearly completely lacking in ganglion cells.[3]

was in a T.N.R. posture from 41 to 56 per cent of the recorded time at 7, 10, and 13 years of age. The head generally took the lead in initiating the T.N.R. attitude. In no instance was a reversed T.N.R. attitude (head averted to one side with the arm of that side flexed) assumed even momentarily. All this suggests that the proprioceptive stimulus in the neck was operating to bring about the natural reflex.

Although the T.N.R. is a normal and prominent feature of early infant behavior, it becomes a pathologic symptom if it persists with undue dominance beyond the age of 6 months. In cases of cerebral palsy such persistence may usually, if not always, be taken as a prognostic sign that the child will never acquire the ability to walk. In primary and secondary amentia the T.N.R. may persist for many months as an evidence of slowed down or arrested development. We refer here to spontaneous manifestations of the T.N.R. which may be naturalistically observed while the child lies supine, either quiescent or in general postural activity. In some instances, as already suggested, it is possible to induce the T.N.R. indirectly by slowly moving a stimulus across the field of vision, thereby inducing head rotation. In aments of lower grade, and in certain neurological conditions, the examiner is able to elicit the T.N.R. response by forcible or passive rotation of the head. In normal infants, however, such attempted manipulation by the examiner arouses resistance reactions. This is probably the reason Magnus failed to find the T.N.R. in the absence of abnormality.

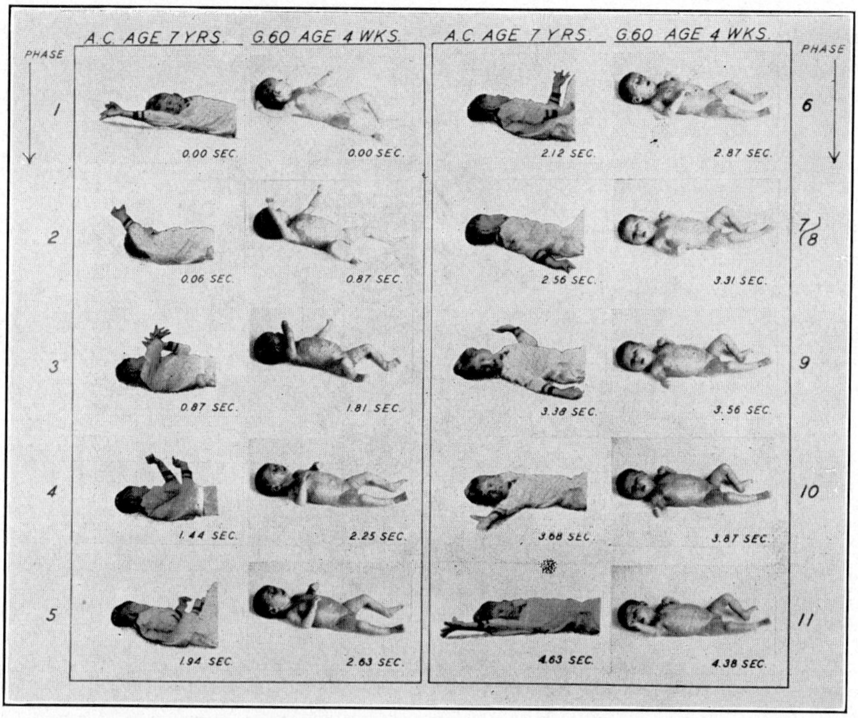

Fig. 7.—Comparative consecutive phases of the athetotic action pattern of A. C., aged 7 years, and of the spontaneous supine action pattern of a normal infant, G60, aged 4 weeks. Eleven phases, with the elapsed time indicated in seconds, are shown side by side in vertical columns. These phases may be envisaged as a slashing windmill reaction emerging out of and returning to a basic T.N.R. attitude.

When a large number of normal infants are examined at intervals during the first three months, we find that at least one-third consistently assume a right T.N.R.; possibly a third, the left T.N.R.; and the remainder adopt either right or left in a somewhat ambivalent manner. These figures are crude (the problem needs refined study), but they suggest important trends and individual differences in the genesis of laterality. Handedness is a partial and sometimes a misleading index of physiologic unilaterality. It is probable, however, that emphatic, constitutional left handedness is correlated with a strong infantile left T.N.R.

In our normative survey of the ontogenetic sequences of behavior pattern, from twenty-six to forty-nine infants were examined at lunar month intervals up to the age of 56 weeks.[4] It is a remarkable fact that 100 per cent of the infants at 4 weeks of age, when observed in a free supine posture, spontaneously maintained the head predominantly rotated to one side; 100 per cent likewise held their arms in characteristic T.N.R. attitudes. We conclude that the T.N.R. is a normal and virtually universal feature of neonatal infancy. Indeed, for 8 weeks the T.N.R. holds strong sway; at 12 weeks it is less conspicuous; at 16 weeks it is in transition; at 20 weeks, in eclipse, for at 20 weeks 100 per cent of our normative infants maintained the head in mid-position. And when the head is predominantly held in mid-position, at least one-half of each

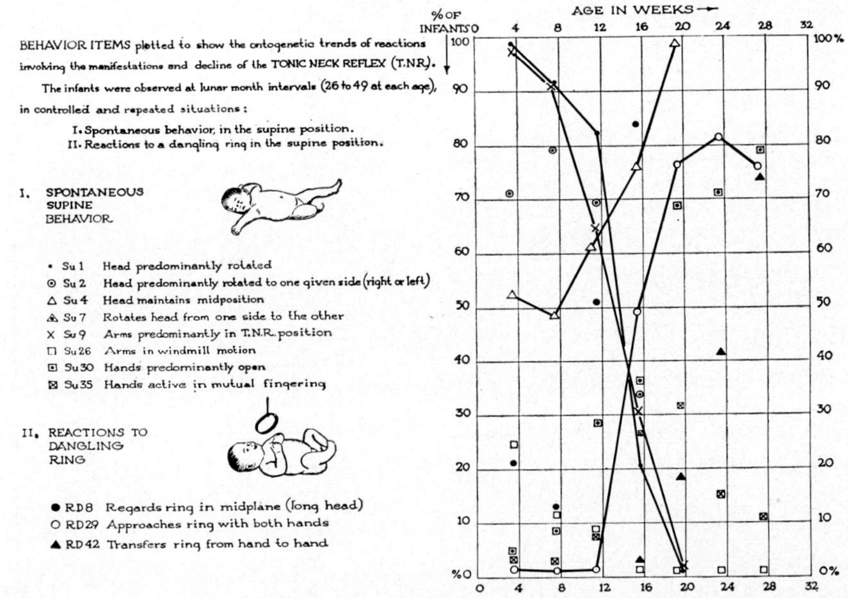

Fig. 8.—Graph showing the ontogenetic trends of the components of the tonic neck reflex.[4]

T.N.R. subsides, and tonic symmetry displaces tonic neck asymmetry. The ontogenetic trends which underlie these transformations of postural pattern are plotted in Fig. 8.

The process of transformation is extremely complex. It is not a process of simple substitution but one of progressive interlocking, so that neither symmetry nor asymmetry gains permanent or complete ascendancy. It implies an intricate neurological cross-stitching which organizes antagonistic muscles and unilateral functions into reciprocal relationships. The addiction of the young infant to T.N.R. postures is both a symptom and a condition of his behavior growth. The infantile T.N.R. represents a morphogenetic stage in which fundamental neurological coordinations are laid down to form the framework for later postural, manual, locomotor, and psychomotor reactions. Indeed, the T.N.R. is part of the ground plan of the organism pervasively identified with its unitary, total action system.

The T.N.R. accordingly has an ecology. More or less directly it subserves adaptations to the environment, prior to birth as well as later. The T.N.R. helps the fetus to accommodate to the conformation of the uterine cavity; and it may even facilitate the longitudinal presentation and orientation of the fetus at the entrance of the birth canal. The T.N.R. of the neonatal infant is well suited to postural attitudes which the child needs to assume when suckled at the breast. The activated windmill T.N.R. of the early weeks with its intensification of grasp responses suggests vestiges of arboreal groping and clinging. But the future and formative references of the T.N.R. are more significant. The T.N.R. attitude promotes and channelizes visual fixation by the infant on his extended hand; it leads to hand inspection, to eye-hand coordinations, to prehensory approach, and eventually to unidextrality. It contributes to the organization of the diagonal reflexes of prone locomotion. It reduces the hazard of suffocation to the infant and is well adapted to acts of rejection and withdrawal. Elaborated and inflected, it finally figures in innumerable adult acts of skill, aggression, and extrication. Attitudinal asymmetry always remains in reflex reserve, as well as subject to voluntary mobilization.

Man does not face the world on a frontal plane of symmetry, but at an angle, and he makes his escapes obliquely! This orientation is prefigured in the T.N.R. attitude of infancy. The bias is grounded in the primitive anatomy of the nervous system and entails such elaborate present and future ramifications that much developmental time is needed to mature the neuromotor structure. For such morphogenetic reasons the T.N.R. is a prolonged and conspicuous feature of the early patterning of human behavior. For the same reasons the T.N.R. is a diagnostic indicator of development status and a clinical sign of neurological defects.

SUMMARY

1. The tonic neck reflex (T.N.R.) is an asymmetric postural attitude, so basic that it is found in lower animals as well as in man. It involves the total action system, but particularly arms and head.

2. It is a normal characteristic of the human infant during the first 12 weeks of waking life, spontaneously manifested in the supine position. At 20 weeks it is normally supplanted by symmetric head and arm postures.

3. Marked persistence of the T.N.R. beyond the first half year is indicative of retarded, arrested, or defective development.

4. In association with basal ganglion lesions it is a prognostic indication that the child will not "learn" to walk.

5. The T.N.R. is a natural but not a stereotyped reflex. It undergoes progressive growth changes. It serves useful adjustments in the fetus as well as the infant in neonatal life. It is morphogenetically so fundamental that it has clinical value both as an index of maturity and as a symptom of neurological abnormalities.

REFERENCES

1. Magnus, R.: Körperstellung, pp. xiii, 740, Berlin, 1924, Julius Springer, Animal Posture, Croonian Lecture, Proc. Roy. Soc., Series B., Vol. 98, No. B 690, pp. 339-353.
2. Bieber, I., and Fulton, J. F.: Arch. Neurol. & Psychiat. **39**: 433, 1938.
3. Gesell, A., and Zimmerman, H. M.: Am. J. Psychiat. **94**: 507, 1937.
4. Gesell, A., and Thompson, H., assisted by Amatruda, C. S.: Infant Behavior: Its Genesis and Growth. New York, 1934, McGraw-Hill Book Company, pp. viii, 343.
   An Atlas of Infant Behavior: A Systematic Delineation of the Forms and Early Growth of Human Behavior Patterns, Vol. 1, p. 523, New Haven, 1934, Yale University Press.
   The Psychology of Early Growth, Including Norms of Infant Behavior and a Method of Genetic Analysis, pp. ix, 290, New York, 1938, The Macmillan Company.
5. Gesell, A., et al.: The Tonic Neck Reflex (T.N.R.) in the Human Infant. From the Photographic Library of the Yale Clinic of Child Development, 16 mm., 130 feet, 1938.

THE USE OF HONEY AS A CARBOHYDRATE IN INFANT FEEDING

F. W. Schlutz, M.D., and Elizabeth M. Knott, Ph.D.
Chicago, Ill.

Although honey has been known as a food from the earliest days of which we have historical record, its importance to man seems to have decreased as civilization has advanced. In view of the fact that honey is a product occurring free in nature ready for use without artificial treatment and that it is composed of two monosaccharides most acceptable to the organism, it is strange that honey has not enjoyed wider use, especially in the feeding of infants and children.

The composition of honey has been reported by Browne, in 1908, as follows: water, 17.70 per cent; sucrose, 1.90 per cent; levulose, 40.50 per cent; glucose, 34.02 per cent; dextrin, 1.51 per cent; ash, 0.18 per cent.

Luttinger, in 1922, published values for honey constituents comparable to the figures quoted from Browne except for a slightly higher ash content. Luttinger also included figures for acetic, malic, and formic acids, the content of these being 0.2, 0.3 and 1.1 per cent, respectively.

The mineral value of honey has been studied more in detail by Schuette and Remy (1932). They found dark honeys to be superior and reported the following results in milligrams of mineral per kilogram of honey:

Table I

	Light Honeys			Dark Honeys		
	Min.	Max.	Av.	Min.	Max.	Av.
Iron	1.20	4.80	2.40	0.70	33.50	9.40
Copper	0.14	0.70	0.29	0.35	1.04	0.56
Manganese	0.17	0.44	0.30	0.52	9.53	4.09

Thus honey is seen to contain valuable minerals in amounts large enough to be significant in infant feeding.

In addition to the carbohydrates, acids, and minerals, Luttinger believed vitamins A, B, C, and D also to be present in honey in appreciable amounts. Other workers (notably Dutcher, 1918; Hawk, Smith, and Bergeim, 1921; Scheunert, Schlieblich, and Schwanebeck, 1923; and Hoyle, 1929) have not been able to confirm the presence of these vitamins in honey except in perhaps negligible quantities. It may be

From the Department of Pediatrics, University of Chicago.

that different sources for honey affect its composition sufficiently to account for the different results reported by these workers.

The best reports in the literature regarding the use of honey come chiefly from European sources, although Luttinger, in 1922, had advocated its use in the United States. Luttinger summarized historical and literary references to honey and commented upon its ease of digestion, good utilization, and valuable mineral and vitamin content. His conclusion that honey was an excellent source of carbohydrate for infants was based on 419 feeding cases, but he did not report any details for his work. Comby in 1926 gave a brief review and praised the use of honey for infants because its aseptic nature made it an excellent and safe source of minerals and vitamins for addition to pasteurized milk. Comby, however, like Luttinger, included no experimental data in his paper.

In 1931 two papers based on carefully controlled experiments were presented by Lahdensuu and Muniagurria. Lahdensuu reported twenty cases in which honey had been alternated with saccharose as a supplement to milk. The honey feedings gave better weight gains than did the saccharose, although they contained fewer calories per unit amount of feeding. Lahdensuu believed the natural form of the sugars in honey somehow enabled the body cells to bind water to better advantage and thus facilitate gain in weight. Lahdensuu commented on the good digestion which accompanied the feeding of honey. Diarrhea and vomiting were decreased, presumably because the natural sugars of honey were easily and quickly digested and the natural acids aided the digestion of milk. Lahdensuu also made blood sugar tolerance studies comparing saccharose with honey and found the blood sugar rose more rapidly and to higher levels following honey administration than after saccharose. No glycosuria, however, occurred as a result of the higher levels of blood sugar, nor was acidosis observed in the urine.

Muniagurria, in the introduction to his paper on honey, discussed the conditions required for a carbohydrate to be suitable for infant feeding. He evaluated honey and compared it with other common sources of carbohydrates, using case reports to illustrate his various points. His major conclusion was that honey was not laxative per se, but because of the completeness and ease with which it was digested it corrected conditions which had caused constipation when other less easily digested carbohydrates had been fed. He found honey especially suited to cases of dystrophy and also obtained good results with honey therapy for enterocolitis. Muniagurria stated that honey, by improving digestion, could correct dyspeptic states as effectively as did Finkelstein's protein milk. He tested his hypothesis by feeding relatively large quantities of honey, adapting the treatment to individual needs and increasing honey feedings from low initial amounts up to 40 or 50 gm. per kilogram of body weight.

Stancanelli (1933), following the suggestions of Muniagurria, also used honey successfully in the treatment of dystrophy. He reported fourteen cases in which favorable clinical effects had resulted from the substitution of honey for dextrimaltose. The infants made regular gains in weight following the introduction of honey into their formulas.

Following the work of Emrich who had increased the rate of growth of older children by means of honey administration, Rolleder (1934) gave two tablespoons of honey daily, in addition to the regular diet, to a group of twenty-nine school boys. His control group of twenty-nine was carefully paired for both age and weight with the individuals in the honey group. The boys receiving honey were superior at the end of six weeks not only because of greater weight gains but also because of increases in hemoglobin.

Farioli (1936) has made the most thorough recent study in regard to the use of honey for infants. The eighteen infants in his case reports ranged in age from 10 days to 16 months, and suffered from a variety of disorders, such as rickets, enteritis, malnourishment, and prematurity. He was able to confirm the opinions of former observers since he found excellent tolerance for honey as demonstrated by the good weight gains and well-being of his infants. Farioli studied particularly the fecal flora and observed a shift during honey administration from gram-negative to gram-positive bacteria. In blood sugar tolerance tests he found no excessive elevation of the blood sugar following honey ingestion.

From the above review of the literature it would appear that honey, because of its ease of digestion, its ability to control diarrhea, its favorable effect upon weight gains, and its normal intermediary metabolism, might have special advantages as a carbohydrate for use in infant feeding.

EXPERIMENTAL PROCEDURE AND DISCUSSION

In order to investigate the suitability of honey for infant feeding it was used under controlled conditions for ten healthy male infants who had been admitted to the hospital for various metabolism studies. Most of the infants were about 1 month of age or less on admission, and all were normal in every respect. Seven of the ten infants were studied until they were about 6 months old. Throughout the study the infants were fed either evaporated milk, one-half skimmed dried milk, or one-half skimmed lactic acid powdered milk* The source of carbohydrate was either honey† or karo corn syrup. In addition, solutions of ferric pyrophosphate, copper sulphate, thiamin, cevitamic acid, and crystalline vitamin D were used in the formulas at different levels. Table II

*These milks were furnished through the courtesy of Irradiated Evaporated Milk Association, The Borden Company, and Mead Johnson & Company.

†Honey, carefully selected as to source, purity, and uniformity, was supplied by the Lake Shore Honey Company, Chicago.

TABLE II

NAME	BIRTH	AGE DURING HOSPITALIZATION	MILK	CARBOHYDRATE	WEIGHT	
					INITIAL	FINAL
John	8/31/36	4 wk.—5½ mo.	Evaporated	Karo-honey	3650	7325
Hal	10/7/36	7 wk.—6 mo.	Evap.-Dryco	Honey	3535	7030
Rob	1/18/37	18 da.—7 wk.	Evaporated	Honey	3660	4515
Bart	2/17/37	18 da.—5 mo.	Dryco	Honey-karo-honey	3365	6770
Myles	8/19/37	19 da.—6½ mo.	Dryco	Honey-karo-honey	3170	7320
Ned	9/3/37	14 da.—6½ mo.	Dryco	Honey-karo-honey	3170	6770
Kermit	11/5/37	6 wk.—2½ mo.	Skim lactic acid powdered (½)	Karo	3850	4600
Ray	12/1/37	7 wk.—3½ mo.	Dryco	Karo	4180	5810
Noel	12/19/37	4 wk.—5½ mo.	Dryco	Honey	2895	7710
Jack	2/18/38	4 wk.—3¼ mo.	Dryco	Honey	3004	5680

gives the birth dates, the duration of hospitalization, the type of formula, and the initial and final weights for each infant.

Since the number of stools per day is one indication of an infant's well-being, careful records were kept by the nurses in charge of the infants. To facilitate analysis and charting of results the average number of stools per day was calculated for each period during which no changes were made in an infant's formula. These data are presented in Fig. 1. It will be observed that in general all of the infants maintained an average of less than two stools per day. The chief exceptions

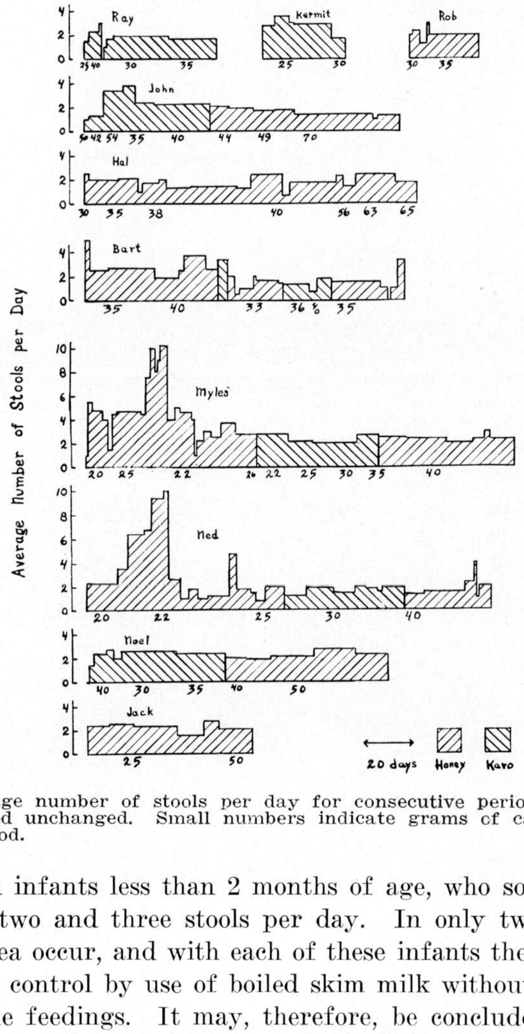

Fig. 1.—Average number of stools per day for consecutive periods during which formulas remained unchanged. Small numbers indicate grams of carbohydrates per day for each period.

to this were in infants less than 2 months of age, who sometimes averaged between two and three stools per day. In only two cases did a definite diarrhea occur, and with each of these infants the diarrhea was brought under control by use of boiled skim milk without omitting the honey from the feedings. It may, therefore, be concluded that honey was well tolerated by these infants.

In addition to the average number of stools per day recorded in Fig. 1, the type of carbohydrate for each period is included in the graph, together with the number of grams of carbohydrate in the formula per day. When results with karo corn syrup and honey were compared for infants of similar ages, or for older infants who received first one and then the other of these two carbohydrates, but little difference in number of stools per day was noted. The level of carbohydrate was altered from time to time in order to maintain a proper soft consistency for the stools. Individual infants varied in this respect, some requiring more and some less of the karo or honey. The role of the carbohydrate ap-

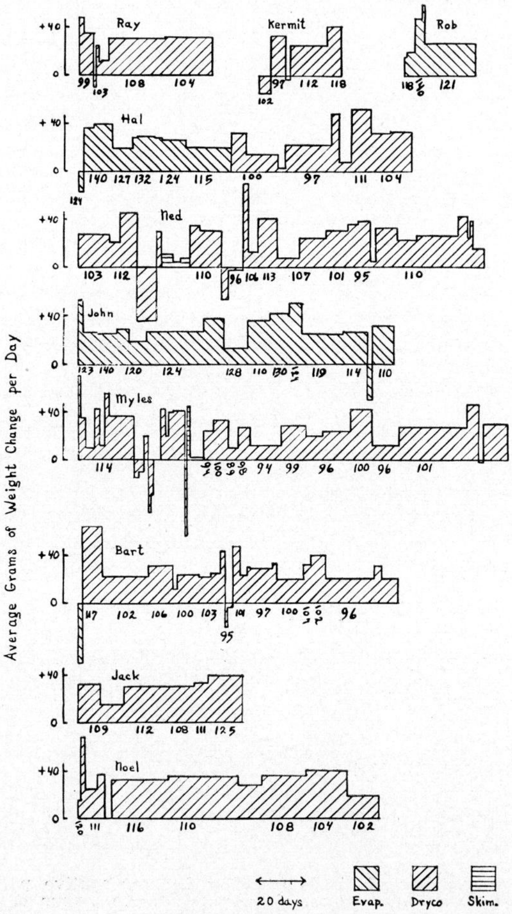

Fig. 2.—Average weight changes per day for consecutive periods during which formulas remained unchanged. Small numbers indicate calories per kilogram per day for each period.

peared to be that described by Muniagurria, since increases of honey apparently relieved constipation by improving digestion without causing a diarrhea. Honey may thus have a distinct advantage in infant feeding over those carbohydrates which have a tendency to be laxative.

Another means of evaluating the utilization of honey by the infants was found in the daily weight records. In order to show the regularity with which weight gains were maintained, the average gain or loss per day has been calculated for each period of days during which the infant's formula remained unchanged. These weight changes are plotted in Fig. 2. The only weight losses of consequence occurred with the two infants who each had a short period of diarrhea. Other than these two periods, during which an infection may have caused the digestive disturbance, weight gains were quite consistently maintained at about 20 to 30 gm. per day.

Since weight gains are, to a large extent, controlled by the energy value of the ingested food, the average caloric intake per kilogram of body weight has been calculated for each period for each infant and is included in Fig. 2. In Fig. 3 these caloric intakes have been plotted

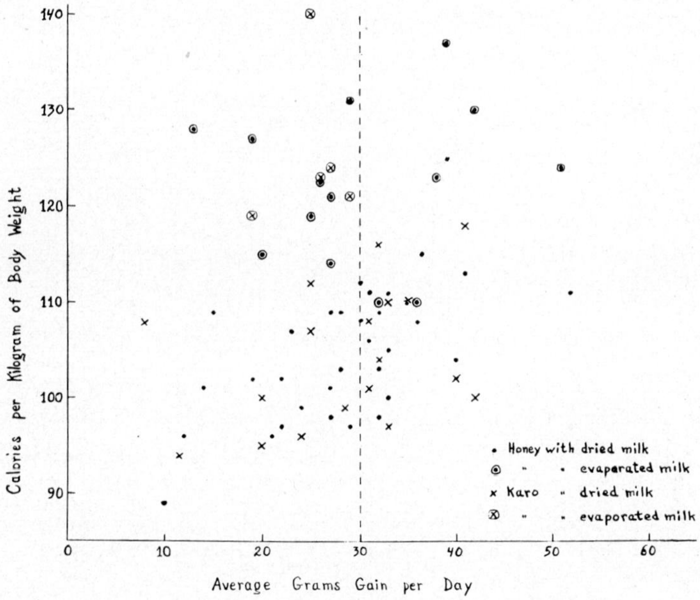

Fig. 3.—Relation of calorie intake and type of milk and carbohydrate to gain in weight.

against the average weight gains for all periods during which an infant's formula had remained unchanged for at least a week.

Although weight gains are always under the influence of a number of related factors besides the caloric intake, there was a tendency for slightly greater weight gains to occur with those infants receiving honey instead of karo. This was most noticeable when these two carbohydrates were contrasted as supplements to evaporated milk. Out of a total of thirty-seven periods during which the infants averaged less than 30 gm. gain per day, honey had been fed in 65 per cent of the cases. On the other hand, with average weight gains above 30 gm. per day, honey had been fed in 71 per cent of the thirty-four cases. When just the evaporated milk feedings were considered, honey had been fed in 62 per cent of the cases gaining less than 30 gm., while it had been used for 100 per cent of the cases gaining more than 30 gm. It would seem that honey, at least to a moderate extent, had facilitated higher weight gains.

Another means of evaluating the utilization of honey by infants has been a series of blood sugar tolerance tests which have been conducted on these infants. In these tests, the details of which are being published in another paper (Schlutz and co-workers, 1938), various sugars which are commonly used in infant feeding were administered in 20 per cent solutions and blood sugar determinations made at the end of 15, 30, 60, 90, and 120 minutes. Honey appeared to have special advantages for infants because, with the exception of dextrose, it was absorbed most quickly of all the sugars tested during the first fifteen minutes following ingestion, yet did not flood the blood stream with exogenous sugar. It also maintained both a steady and a slow decrease in blood sugar until the fasting level was again reached. This response of honey is presumably due to the unique combination of the two easily digested monosaccharides, dextrose and levulose. Honey is quickly digested and absorbed into the body because if its dextrose content, while the levulose, being somewhat more slowly absorbed, is able to maintain the blood sugar. Honey has an advantage over sugars which contain higher levels of dextrose since it does not cause the blood sugar to rise to higher levels than can be easily cared for by the body.

SUMMARY

Ten healthy male infants have been studied during the first 6 months of their lives for a total of 151 weeks. Formulas for all infants were restricted to either evaporated or dried milk and carbohydrate, with additional supplements of pure vitamin or mineral solutions. The response of the infants to honey as a source of carbohydrate has been contrasted with their response when receiving karo corn syrup.

The general well-being of the infant, the number of stools per day, and weight gains have been used to determine the value of honey in regular feedings. Besides these criteria, blood sugar tolerance studies have been employed to contrast the response to honey with that resulting from administration of other common sources of carbohydrate.

From these studies it is concluded that honey is easily digested, being absorbed more rapidly than most sugars during the first fifteen minutes after ingestion. It is well tolerated by the infant and does not cause diarrhea. It may facilitate weight gains, since there was a slight tendency for greater average gains per day to occur on lower calorie intakes when honey was included in the formulas.

It would seem, therefore, that honey is a type of carbohydrate which is well suited to the infant's needs and probably should be recommended for wider use in infant dietaries.

The authors wish to acknowledge the courtesy and suggestions of Dr. M. C. Tanquary, Professor of Apiculture, University of Minnesota, and Mr. W. F. Straub, Director, Wieboldt Foundation.

REFERENCES

Browne, C. A.: U. S. Dept. Ag. Bur. Chem. Bull. **110**: 1908.
Comby, J.: Arch. de méd. d. enf. **29**: 46, 1926.
Dutcher, R. A.: J. Biol. Chem. **36**: 551, 1918.
Farioli, A.: Riv. di clin. pediat. **34**: 337, 1936.
Hawk, P. B., Smith, C. A., and Bergeim, O.: Am. J. Physiol. **55**: 339, 1921.
Hoyle, E.: Biochem. J. **23**: 54, 1929.
Lahdensuu, S.: Acta Soc. med. fenn. duodecim. **15**: 1, 1931.
Luttinger, P.: New York M. J. **116**: 153, 1922.
Muniagurria, C.: Bull. Soc. de pédiat. de Paris **29**: 227, 1931.
Rolleder, A.: Arch. f. Kinderh. **101**: 244, 1934.
Scheunert, A., Schieblich, M., and Schwanebeck, E.: Biochem. Z., **139**: 47, 1923.
Schlutz, F. W., Knott, E. M., Gedgoud, J. L., and Loewenstamm, I.: J. PEDIAT. **12**: 716, 1938.
Schuette, H. A., and Remy, K.: J. Am. Chem. Soc. **54**: 2909, 1932.
Stancanelli, G.: Pediatria **41**: 524, 1933.

STATISTICAL STUDIES ON PREMATURITY

I. The Incidence of Prematurity and the Effect of Certain Obstetric Factors

C. H. Peckham, M.D.
Baltimore, Md.

In 1932 during the course of an analysis, "The age distribution of 15,370 obstetric patients and its effect upon the type of delivery," the author recorded the births of 974 infants who had been classified as premature. This study included only patients delivered of viable babies, while all those having abortions, i.e., fetuses less than 1500 gm. in weight and less than 35 cm. in length, were omitted from the series. The infants termed premature had reached the above standards either in weight or length or both but weighed less than 2500 gm. and were less than 45 cm. long. All others were classed as "full term." This arbitrary standard for abortion and prematurity has long been used in the Obstetrical Department of the Johns Hopkins Hospital, whence came the above series of cases. The 974 premature infants made up 6.34 per cent of the total cases, and the incidence in white and colored women was 4.75 and 7.97 per cent, respectively.

It has frequently been noted in the clinic that whereas almost all infants whose length is less than 45 cm. are less than 2500 gm. in weight, a considerable number are seen with a birth weight between 2000 and 2500 gm. but measuring 45 to 47 cm. in crown-heel length. It was decided to examine the punch card abstracts of the case records for the clinic, both hospital and outside services, in order to determine how many babies there were who, while above the standards for abortion, were below the individual weight and length criteria for full term. Such a series of cases would enable the derivation of both weight and length incidences of prematurity for contrast with the previously mentioned one. Also it would be possible to determine the effect of certain obstetric factors such as race, age, and parity of the mother upon these incidences.

Gross Incidence.—A total of 39,394 deliveries of theoretically viable children occurred in the hospital and outside obstetric services from the beginning of the department in 1896 to Jan. 1, 1936. Among these there were 4,055 infants weighing less than 2500 gm., yet at least 35 cm. in length. This number includes certain very small children weighing less than 1500 gm., yet 35 cm. or more in length and hence technically classified as "premature." It does not include fetuses below the premature

From the Department of Obstetrics, Johns Hopkins University and Hospital.

standard in both weight and length. Also included in the series are a considerable number of infants whose birth weight was below 2500 gm. yet whose length was 45 cm. and over, hence, who had been catalogued as full term. In other words, excluding abortions, this series includes all infants premature according to weight alone at birth.

In a similar fashion a second series of babies was accumulated, including all whose length at birth was less than 45 cm., but excluding fetuses below the premature standard in both length and weight. This series corresponds in all respects to the former except that here the prematurity is decided according to length instead of weight. It was of interest and, in our opinion, of considerable significance that while 4,055 infants were found whose weight at birth was less than 2500 gm., only 2,415 were delivered who were less than 45 cm. in length. The make-up of these series, subdivided according to race, together with the incidences for prematurity derived, are shown in Table I. Since small babies

TABLE I

THE INCIDENCE OF PREMATURITY, ACCORDING TO VARIOUS WEIGHTS AND LENGTHS

	NUMBER OF INFANTS			PER CENT OF TOTAL DELIVERIES		
	WHITE	BLACK	TOTAL	WHITE	BLACK	TOTAL
Single Births						
Total viable deliveries	18,375	20,569	38,944	100.00	100.00	100.00
Less than 2500 gm.	1,120	2,458	3,578	6.10	11.95	9.19
Less than 2400 gm.	929	2,048	2,977	5.06	9.96	7.64
Less than 2300 gm.	781	1,692	2,473	4.25	8.23	6.35
Less than 2200 gm.	637	1,348	1,985	3.47	6.55	5.10
Less than 2100 gm.	525	1,134	1,659	2.86	5.51	4.26
Less than 2000 gm.	429	902	1,331	2.33	4.39	3.42
Less than 1500 gm.	148	315	463	0.81	1.52	1.19
Less than 1000 gm.	26	33	59	0.14	0.16	0.15
Less than 45 cm.	666	1,496	2,162	3.62	7.27	5.55
Less than 44 cm.	447	1,033	1,480	2.43	5.02	3.80
Less than 43 cm.	316	752	1,068	1.72	3.66	2.74
Less than 42 cm.	238	527	765	1.30	2.56	1.96
Less than 41 cm.	183	386	569	1.00	1.88	1.46
Less than 40 cm.	129	259	388	0.70	1.26	1.00
Less than 35 cm.	12	13	25	0.07	0.06	0.06
Multiple Births						
Total viable twins	426	474	900	100.00	100.00	100.00
Less than 2500 gm.	190	287	477	44.60	60.55	53.00
Less than 2000 gm.	82	137	219	19.25	28.90	24.33
Less than 1500 gm.	27	59	86	6.34	12.45	9.56
Less than 1000 gm.	7	11	18	1.64	2.32	2.00
Less than 45 cm.	86	167	253	20.19	35.23	28.11
Less than 40 cm.	18	42	60	4.23	8.86	6.67
Less than 35 cm.	3	8	11	0.70	0.17	1.22

occur much more frequently in multiple than in single births these have been analyzed separately in order to determine a more exact incidence. Omitting twins from consideration it will be noted that the delivery of infants weighing less than 2500 gm. occurred 3,578 times, while only 2,162 were found who were less than 45 cm. in length. Moreover, there were 463 premature infants weighing less than 1500 gm. and 59 less than 1000 gm., but all at least 35 cm. in length. In contrast, however, only twenty-five children were found less than below 35 cm. but weighing at least 1500 gm. The total incidence of prematurity according to weight was 9.19 per cent, while for length it was only 5.55 per cent. A weight incidence comparable to 45 cm. length fell between 2200 and 2300 gm. An interesting feature of Table I is the racial disparity which was noted, showing that the incidence for the various weights and lengths in colored infants was almost twice as great as for white. Of all white infants delivered 6.1 per cent weighed less than 2500 gm., while a similar incidence for blacks fell between 2100 and 2200 gm. Similarly, 3.62 per cent of white children were less than 45 cm. long and the corresponding black rate was approximately at 43 cm. Whether these figures indicate a true racial difference in incidence of prematurity or whether different criteria are necessary for the two races will be discussed in a subsequent paragraph.

That portion of Table I dealing with multiple births was computed according to the same weight and length specifications as was used in the analysis of deliveries of single children. It will be noted that over one-half of all viable twin infants weighed less than 2500 gm. and more than a quarter were under 45 cm. in length. A similar racial difference in incidence was found as has been described for single births. Judging by weight alone prematurity occurred almost six times as often in twin deliveries, while for length a five to one ratio was observed. It is of interest in this connection to note the disparity between the numbers of first and second twins upon such division of the total premature multiple births. A definite tendency for the heavier child to be born before the lighter one was indicated by the following number of infants under 2500 gm. in birth weight: 219 (first born) and 258 (second born). No similar difference was noted, however, in the comparative series selected according to total length.

Age.—It is generally stated that the likelihood of premature delivery is increased by excessive multiparity, as well as through too closely spaced childbearing. If this is so, one would expect the incidence of prematurity to increase with advancing age of the mother. Table II indicates the proportion of those small infants under analysis (both weight and length series) according to several age groups for the mothers, and for comparison there is submitted the age distribution of the patients making up the general clinic population. No significant difference in incidence was found for the three groups, although certain rather suggestive discrepancies were noted. First, 33.66 per cent of the total deliveries occurring on the service were in women less than 20 years old, while 37.70 per cent of the infants weighing less than 2500 gm. and 30.04 per cent of those less than 45 cm. in length fell in the same cate-

TABLE II

THE EFFECT OF AGE OF MOTHER UPON THE INCIDENCE OF PREMATURITY

AGE	PER CENT OF TOTAL					
	WEIGHT				LENGTH UNDER 45 CM.	GENERAL CLINIC POPULATION
	–1499 GM.	1500-1999 GM.	2000-2499 GM.	TOTAL		
16 and under	7.43	9.82	9.39	9.26		7.41
17 to 19	21.67	23.87	31.39	28.44		26.25
20 to 24	32.20	29.00	29.24	29.53		33.08
25 to 29	18.27	13.60	13.18	13.88		16.49
30 to 34	10.84	10.27	8.65	9.30		9.23
35 to 39	5.88	10.27	6.56	7.37		5.53
40 and over	3.72	3.17	1.58	2.22		2.01
19 and under	29.10	33.69	40.78	37.70	30.04	33.66
20 to 34	61.31	52.87	51.07	52.71	59.54	58.80
35 and over	9.60	13.44	8.14	9.59	10.41	7.53

gory. We would interpret this to indicate that early childbearing does not increase the incidence of true premature birth, but rather that the young woman at term gives birth to an infant smaller in weight but equal in length to that of the more mature individual. Furthermore, it would seem that this small child is more vigorous and stands a better chance of survival than does one of the same weight born to an older woman. Further analysis would seem to substantiate these statements, as the percentage of infants 2000 to 2499 gm. to the total number of infants less than 2500 gm. was found to decrease with advancing age of the mother. Thus for the age group 17 to 19, 68.22 per cent of the total number of infants less than 2500 gm. weighed between 2000 and 2499 gm., while for the group aged 40 years and over a similarly calculated rate of 47.62 per cent was obtained. Finally, from Table II we obtained suggestive evidence of an increased incidence of prematurity in women aged 35 years and older, and found in this age group 7.53 per cent of the patients comprising the general clinic population as contrasted with 9.59 and 10.41 per cent of the total prematures as determined by weight and length, respectively.

Parity.—In view of what has been said concerning the effect of age of mother upon the incidence of small infants, it was not surprising to find that primiparous births made up a larger proportion of the total in both the weight and length (premature) series as contrasted with the general clinic population. This is illustrated by Table III. Furthermore, the comparative incidence of premature births was less for each group with parity more than one, except for the group para x and over, for weight, and the group para viii and over for length, where practically identical incidences obtained. As was stated under the discussion of age, we do not believe that the large number of small children born to primiparas represents a true index of prematurity, but rather that this group, particularly if young, tends to give birth to relatively undersized but essentially mature infants. Moreover, it is known that each successive child tends to be larger than the one before. This may explain the low incidence of infants weighing less than 2500 gm. found in our series as contrasted with the general clinic population for the higher para groups. This had been a somewhat surprising finding, since it is in this type of patient that certain obstetric complications predisposing to premature delivery, such as placenta previa, premature separation, chronic nephritis, etc., are most likely to occur. Moreover, the incidence of twins increases with the parity of the mother. In this bracket no figures are available for the effect of increasing weight or length as analyzed under the heading "age."

TABLE III

THE EFFECT OF PARITY OF MOTHER UPON THE INCIDENCE OF PREMATURITY

PARITY OF MOTHER	PER CENT OF TOTAL								
	WHITE			BLACK			TOTAL		
	GENERAL CLINIC POPULATION	WEIGHT LESS THAN 2500 GM.	LENGTH LESS THAN 45 CM.	GENERAL CLINIC POPULATION	WEIGHT LESS THAN 2500 GM.	LENGTH LESS THAN 45 CM.	GENERAL CLINIC POPULATION	WEIGHT LESS THAN 2500 GM.	LENGTH LESS THAN 45 CM.
1	36.64	46.28	41.44	35.16	43.89	37.32	35.87	44.65	38.60
2	18.67	13.95	13.44	21.24	20.56	21.46	20.01	18.47	18.97
3	11.55	9.77	10.89	12.34	8.89	10.51	11.96	9.17	10.63
4	8.54	7.69	9.34	8.32	6.84	7.90	8.43	7.11	8.34
5	6.16	5.93	6.36	5.91	5.02	5.80	6.03	5.31	5.97
6	4.95	3.84	3.82	4.60	3.79	4.01	4.77	3.80	3.95
7	4.21	3.34	3.11	3.26	2.94	3.31	3.72	3.06	3.25
8	2.93	2.09	2.69	2.53	2.43	2.99	2.72	2.32	2.90
9	2.06	1.75	2.40	1.81	1.47	1.97	1.93	1.56	2.11
10 and over	4.27	5.34	6.51	4.82	4.17	4.71	4.56	4.54	5.27

Rupture of Membranes.—Labor before term is preceded often by premature rupture of the membranes, and accordingly the series under discussion was analyzed in order to determine how often this accident occurred and to contrast its frequency with that pertaining for the general clinic population of term deliveries. The results of this analysis are shown in Table IV. It will be seen from this table that rupture before the onset of labor was observed somewhat more frequently with prematurity than at term, but the difference amounted to only 3 per cent and was considered insignificant. It is interesting to note, furthermore, that the time of rupture was almost identical in the two series analyzed according to weight and length, respectively.

TABLE IV

THE TIME OF RUPTURE OF MEMBRANES IN PREMATURE LABOR

	PER CENT OF TOTAL		
	GENERAL CLINIC POPULATION	WEIGHT LESS THAN 2500 GM.	LENGTH LESS THAN 45 CM.
Before onset of labor	17.14	20.22	18.73
First stage	32.66	17.61	17.70
Second stage	50.20	62.17	63.58

Maternal Complications.—The incidence of certain maternal complications predisposing to premature labor, either spontaneous or induced, is shown in Table V. A positive Wassermann was noted four and one-

TABLE V

THE INCIDENCE OF SOME MATERNAL COMPLICATIONS PREDISPOSING TO PREMATURE DELIVERY

COMPLICATION	PER CENT OF TOTAL			
	WEIGHT LESS THAN 2500 GM.			GENERAL CLINIC POPULATION
	WHITE	BLACK	TOTAL	
Syphilis	4.66	21.35	16.07	2.55—White 20.76—Black
Heart disease	3.33	1.58	2.13	0.57
Eclampsia	4.91	2.43	3.21	0.70
Other toxemia	18.06	10.75	13.06	14.01
Placenta previa	4.49	1.58	2.50	0.76
Premature separation	2.91	1.62	2.03	0.52
Prolapse of cord	1.33	1.00	1.11	—
Total	39.69	40.31	40.11	

half times as often in the colored as in the white patient. As contrasted with the general clinic population, syphilis was found more frequently in the white, but about equally often in the colored woman delivering prematurely. Heart lesions, eclampsia, premature separation, and placenta previa had a much higher incidence in the premature series. In about 40 per cent of the cases some maternal complication was found which might possibly have contributed to the early termination of the pregnancy. It is interesting to note that the incidence of total complications was approximately the same in the black and white, the high rate of syphilis in the former group being compensated for by a disparate number of other complicating factors in the latter. In other words, omitting cases with maternal complications, there remained the same preponderance of colored over white infants in the series.

The figures given in Table V were obtained from the series of infants analyzed according to weight. Similar statistics derived according to length of child have been omitted since the totals as well as the incidence of each individual maternal complication were almost identical with the ones shown here. It is of interest to note that on detailed examination of this portion of our material, it was found that the total incidence of maternal complications decreased significantly with increasing weight and length of the child. Thus a maternal abnormality was found in 46.81 per cent of those infants weighing less than 1500 gm., a figure which fell to 32.89 per cent in the group 2000 gm. and more. Similar analysis revealed percentages of 59.99 and 38.11 with lengths of less than 35 cm. and 40 cm. and more, respectively.

Sex.—Investigators have repeatedly noted that the sex ratio of newborn infants shows a preponderance of males. Thus Crews estimated a conception ratio of 170 males to 100 females, Schultz, 110 to 100 during the abortion stage, and Rauber, 106 to 100 at full term. In view of this, it was surprising to note in this series of infants weighing less than 2500 gm., a reversal of this ratio in both white and black infants, with females outnumbering males 110 to 100, and 107 to 100 for the two races, respectively. Moreover, a similar reversal was found in infants whose length

TABLE VI

THE SEX OF PREMATURELY BORN INFANTS

	PER CENT					
	WHITE		BLACK		TOTAL	
	WEIGHT LESS THAN 2500 GM.	LENGTH LESS THAN 45 CM.	WEIGHT LESS THAN 2500 GM.	LENGTH LESS THAN 45 CM.	WEIGHT LESS THAN 2500 GM.	LENGTH LESS THAN 45 CM.
Males	47.55	46.33	48.35	48.25	48.09	47.65
Females	52.45	53.67	51.65	51.75	51.91	52.35

TABLE VII

SEX RATIOS

	WHITE	BLACK	TOTAL
	MALES TO FEMALES	MALES TO FEMALES	MALES TO FEMALES
Weight less than 2500 gm.	100-110	100-107	100-108
Length less than 45 cm.	100-116	100-107	100-110

at birth was less than 45 cm., with ratios existing of 116 to 100 (white) and 107 to 100 (black). It is our belief, however, that these findings do not indicate a true preponderance of females in prematurely born infants but are to be explained by the normally lower weight and length at birth of this sex, as contrasted with the male. Thus we have found the average birth weight in a series of term infants to be, male and female, respectively: white primiparas, 3270 and 3165 gm.; white multiparas, 3441 and 3313 gm.; black primiparas, 3034 and 2947 gm.; and black multiparas, 3162 and 3027 gm. It would seem plausible to assume that a disproportionate number of females over males are born at full term with weights of less than 2500 gm. and lengths under 45 cm. Further proof of this will be adduced subsequently by the significantly lower stillborn and neonatal mortality rates found for the female infants in the series. In passing, attention is drawn to the unequal ratios found in white infants analyzed by weight and length (110 to 100 and 116 to 100, respectively) although for the black race identical figures were obtained.

Type of Delivery.—Premature labor which begins accidentally and spontaneously will, in the vast majority of cases, terminate without instrumental or manual aid, breech extraction being the only general exception to this. Other types of operative delivery are occasioned chiefly by some obstetric complication which has necessitated premature termination of the pregnancy or ensue in the desire to immediately deliver a second twin. In other words, we believe that Table VIII reflects

TABLE VIII

INCIDENCE OF CERTAIN OPERATIONS—PER CENT OF TOTAL DELIVERIES

OPERATION	PREMATURE	GENERAL CLINIC POPULATION
Cesarean section	3.45	4.61
Breech extraction	6.78	4.35
Forceps	3.94	13.54
Version	4.35	1.62
Destructive operations	0.67	0.41

the incidence of the causative complications rather than the incidence of various types of delivery deliberately selected as the safest obstetric procedures for the undersized infant. It will be noted that in our series one out of five babies weighing less than 2500 gm. and roughly one out of six less than 45 cm. in length were delivered by operative means. These rates are only slightly below that found for the general clinic population of term infants provided the material is divided according to race of mother as shown in the footnote to Table IX. However, the

TABLE IX

THE OPERATIVE INCIDENCE WITH PREMATURE DELIVERY

	DELIVERY		PER CENT OPERATIVE
	SPONT.	OPER.	
Weight of infant in gm.			
1499 and under	399	119	22.97
1500 to 1999	743	216	22.52
2000 to 2499	1962	442	18.39
Total	3104	777	20.02
Length of infant in cm.			
34 and under	20	11	35.48
35 to 39	309	82	20.97
40 to 44	1584	319	16.76
Total	1913	412	17.72

Operative Incidence: Premature—white 28.09 per cent; black 16.24 per cent. Clinic—white 29.64 per cent; black 19.88 per cent.

type of operation selected to effect delivery of the premature infant as contrasted with the full-term infant varies considerably. Thus, breech extraction and podalic version were necessary more frequently with immature babies, while forceps and cesarean section were employed more often at full term. Attention is drawn to the marked difference in operative incidence for the two races. This is probably explained to a considerable extent by the fact that those maternal complications predisposing to operative delivery (those previously listed with the exception of syphilis) occurred more frequently in white women than in black, 35.03 and 18.96 per cent of total patients, respectively. Finally, it seems significant that the operative rate fell with increasing weight and length of the child, which is graphically illustrated in Table IX.

DISCUSSION

Little discussion seems necessary in addition to that given with each individual analysis. It would, however, seem worthy of emphasis at this point that any attempt at a single standard of prematurity, whether based on weight or length, or both, would result in inaccuracies due to differences according to race, age, parity, and sex. Furthermore, separate criteria would seem necessary in single as contrasted with multiple births. Speculation concerning an accurate weight-length standard, with corrections for the above factors, and particularly with reference to mortality rates, would seem of considerable interest from a practical standpoint as well as contributing to our knowledge of constitution. Such a study, however, to be valuable, should include term as well as premature infants and is not within the province of this article. It is proposed to examine our complete material from the above points of view in the near future.

It is, consequently, our opinion that the figures presented here do not offer a true picture of the incidence of prematurity and that the following rates offer only an indication of the frequency of the birth of infants theoretically viable but below average in weight or length and not necessarily truly premature: less than 2500 gm., 9.19 per cent; and less than 45 cm., 5.55 per cent.

The marked racial differences noted throughout the study are of interest. It would not appear that the increased number of small infants born to colored women is to be explained solely by the fact that this average weight at birth is several ounces below that found for white patients. Syphilis occurred approximately four times as often in the colored as in the white portion of the series, yet this factor also does not afford a complete explanation of the disparity. The negresses making up this clinic population are for the most part second- or third-generation tenement dwellers in a large city. They show evidences generally of physical degeneration, and it seems possible that this might result in an increased number of prematurely born children, as well as a decreased birth weight or length at term. It would be of interest to learn if a similar racial difference would be found in rural areas.

CONCLUSIONS

1. In a large series of consecutively delivered infants, 9.19 per cent weighed less than 2500 gm. at birth, while only 5.55 per cent were under 45 cm. in length. For multiple births similar incidences of 53.00 and 28.11 per cent, respectively, were obtained.

2. The number of second born twins weighing below 2500 gm. was significantly greater than that of first born, indicating a tendency for the heavier child to pass through the birth canal first.

3. Judged by either weight or length the incidence of small infants was almost twice as great in the black as in the white race.

4. Although the obstetrically youthful woman relatively frequently gives birth to a child below the average in size, no definite correlation was determined between maternal age and the true incidence of premature births. A possible exception to this was found in the groups aged 35 years and over where some increase in the number of very small and undoubtedly premature infants was noted.

5. Small infants were born to primiparas more frequently than to any other parous group.

6. No significant increase in the frequency of premature rupture of the membranes was noted in the groups under discussion, as contrasted with a series of deliveries at term.

7. As was to be expected, certain maternal complications, in themselves resulting in premature delivery, either spontaneous or induced, were observed more frequently in this series of cases than in the general clinic population.

8. The sex ratio of the infants comprising this series showed a predominance of females, probably due to the normally smaller birth weight and birth length of the female child.

9. The percentage of premature babies delivered by operative means was essentially that of the general clinic population. Breech extraction and version occurred more frequently and forceps and cesarean section less often in the premature groups.

10. It is our belief that present methods of establishing prematurity on the basis of weight, or length, or both, are grossly inaccurate. Allowances must be made for race, age, and parity of mother, as well as sex of infant. Separate standards are necessary for single and multiple births. Further investigation is necessary to definitely establish these points.

STATISTICAL STUDIES ON PREMATURITY

II. The Mortality of Prematurity and the Effect of Certain Obstetric Factors

C. H. Peckham, M.D.
Baltimore, Md.

In a preceding communication a statistical analysis was made on a series of prematurely delivered infants from the point of view of the incidence of early birth and the effect upon the incidence of certain obstetric factors. In the present study it is proposed to reinvestigate the same group of cases in order to derive certain rates of mortality, both stillborn and neonatal, according to varying weights and lengths of the infants at birth. Furthermore, it is desired to ascertain the effects, if any, of such factors as the race, age, and parity of the mother, the type of delivery, etc., upon mortality rates. The series is composed of 4,055 infants weighing less than 2500 gm. at birth and 2,415 measuring less than 45 cm. in length, the two groups comprising 10.29 per cent and 6.13 per cent respectively of 39,394 consecutive viable deliveries occurring on the Obstetrical Service of the Johns Hopkins Hospital.

Gross Mortality Rates.—The general mortality figures obtained from the study are shown in Tables I and I *A* and certain trends are further illustrated in Figs. 1 to 4. Divisions by 100 and 500 gm. and 1 and 5 cm. are noted, together with differences occurring between single and twin births, and white and colored infants. Upon reaching 2500 gm. and 45 cm., mortality rates were found to be still decreasing. Since it was desired to ascertain at what level of weight and length a stationary death rate began, small series of infants between 2500 and 3000 gm. and 45 and 49 cm. were selected at random and the data incorporated into the tables. For the sake of clarity the findings according to weight and length will be discussed separately. For premature infants, recorded in the three brackets under 1200 gm., a falling stillborn rate was compensated for by an increasing neonatal mortality percentage, so that the total mortality remained relatively stationary and at about 90 per cent. From 1200 gm. on there was a steady mortality decrease for each 100 gm. division, becoming relatively rapid in the brackets between 1800 and 2400 gm., then slowing and finally becoming stationary at 2700 gm. and more (Fig. 1). The total mortality fell below 50 per cent in the bracket 1800 to 1900 gm. Deaths per 100 live births also declined steadily above 1200 gm. and became stationary at less than one per cent from 2700 gm. on. This rate fell below 50 per cent between 1600 and 1700 gm. (Fig. 2).

From the Department of Obstetrics, Johns Hopkins University and Hospital.

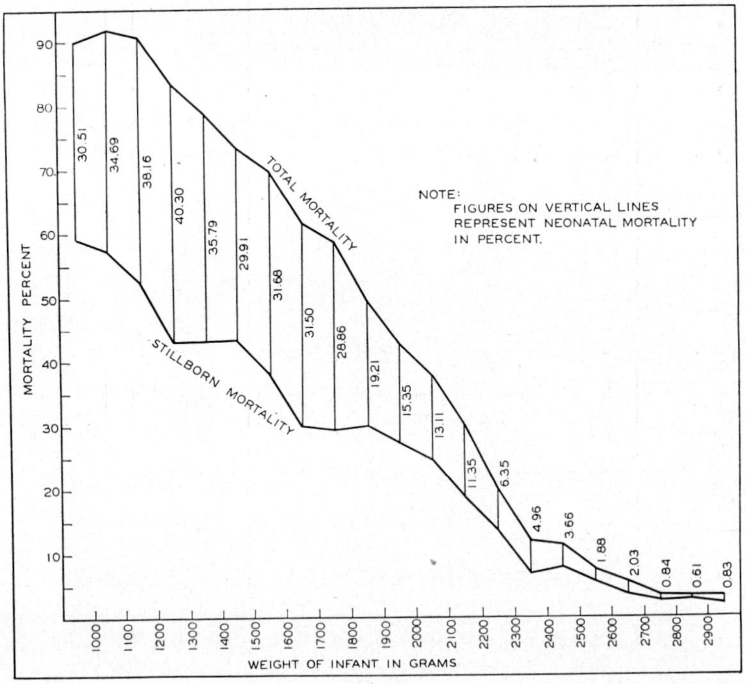

Fig. 1.—Total, neonatal, and stillborn mortality according to weight of infant (single births only).

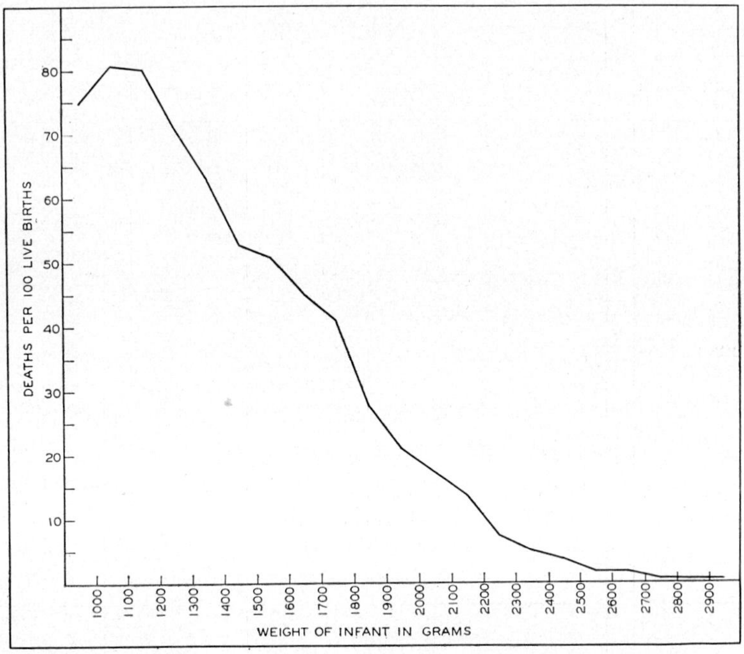

Fig. 2.—Deaths per 100 live births according to weight of infant (single births only).

TABLE I

WEIGHT OF CHILD (GM.)	WHITE								BLACK								BOTH RACES							
	TOTAL BIRTHS	STILLBIRTHS	LIVE BIRTHS	NEONATAL DEATHS	% STILLBORN	% NEONATAL DEATHS	% TOTAL MORTALITY	% NEONATAL DEATHS TO LIVE BIRTHS	TOTAL BIRTHS	STILLBIRTHS	LIVE BIRTHS	NEONATAL DEATHS	% STILLBORN	% NEONATAL DEATHS	% TOTAL MORTALITY	% NEONATAL DEATHS TO LIVE BIRTHS	TOTAL BIRTHS	STILLBIRTHS	LIVE BIRTHS	NEONATAL DEATHS	% STILLBORN	% NEONATAL DEATHS	% TOTAL MORTALITY	% NEONATAL DEATHS TO LIVE BIRTHS
Mortality Rates: Single Births (By 100 Gm.)																								
Less than 1000	26	14	12	11	53.85	42.31	96.16	91.67	33	21	12	7	63.64	21.21	84.85	58.33	59	35	24	18	59.32	30.51	89.83	75.00
1000-1099	15	10	5	3	66.67	20.00	86.67	60.00	34	18	16	14	52.94	41.18	94.12	87.50	49	28	21	17	57.14	34.69	91.83	80.95
1100-1199	25	13	12	10	52.00	40.00	92.00	83.33	51	27	24	19	52.94	37.25	90.19	79.17	76	40	36	29	52.63	38.16	90.79	80.56
1200-1299	18	11	7	6	61.11	33.33	94.44	85.71	49	18	31	21	36.73	42.86	79.59	67.74	67	29	38	27	43.28	40.30	83.58	71.05
1300-1399	25	10	15	10	40.00	40.00	80.00	66.67	70	31	39	24	44.29	34.29	78.58	61.54	95	41	54	34	43.16	35.79	78.95	62.96
1400-1499	39	17	22	15	43.59	38.46	82.05	68.18	78	34	44	20	43.59	25.64	62.23	45.45	117	51	66	35	43.59	29.91	73.50	53.03
1500-1599	48	11	37	23	22.92	47.92	70.84	62.16	113	50	63	28	44.24	24.78	69.02	44.44	161	61	100	51	37.89	31.68	69.57	51.00
1600-1699	50	10	40	16	20.00	32.00	52.00	40.00	77	28	49	24	36.36	31.17	67.53	48.98	127	38	89	40	29.92	31.50	61.42	44.94
1700-1799	61	19	42	19	31.15	31.15	62.30	45.24	88	25	63	24	28.41	27.27	55.68	38.10	149	44	105	43	29.53	28.86	58.39	40.95
1800-1899	69	23	46	14	33.33	20.29	53.62	30.43	160	46	114	30	28.75	18.75	47.50	26.32	229	69	160	44	30.13	19.21	49.34	27.50
1900-1999	53	16	37	7	30.19	13.21	43.40	18.91	149	39	110	24	26.17	16.11	42.28	21.82	202	55	147	31	27.23	15.35	42.58	21.09
2000-2099	96	16	80	13	16.67	13.54	30.21	16.25	232	65	167	30	28.02	12.93	40.95	17.96	328	81	247	43	24.70	13.11	37.81	17.41
2100-2199	112	13	99	12	11.61	10.71	22.32	12.12	214	48	166	25	22.43	11.68	34.11	15.06	326	61	265	37	18.71	11.35	30.06	13.96
2200-2299	144	20	124	10	13.89	6.94	20.83	8.06	344	47	297	21	13.66	6.10	19.76	7.07	488	67	421	31	13.73	6.35	20.08	7.36
2300-2399	148	13	135	13	8.78	8.78	17.56	9.63	356	22	334	12	6.18	3.37	9.55	3.59	504	35	469	25	6.94	4.96	11.90	5.33
2400-2499	191	15	176	10	7.85	5.24	13.09	5.68	410	33	377	12	8.05	2.93	10.98	3.18	601	48	553	22	7.99	3.66	11.65	3.98
2500-2599	165	7	158	6	4.24	3.64	7.88	3.80	366	23	343	4	6.28	1.09	7.37	1.17	531	30	501	10	5.65	1.88	7.53	2.00
2600-2699	203	7	196	5	3.45	2.46	5.91	2.55	389	15	374	7	3.86	1.80	5.66	1.87	592	22	570	12	3.72	2.03	5.75	2.11
2700-2799	277	3	274	1	1.08	0.36	1.44	0.36	557	19	538	6	3.41	1.08	4.49	1.12	834	22	812	7	2.64	0.84	3.48	0.86
2800-2899	346	10	336	3	2.89	0.87	3.76	0.89	630	19	611	3	3.02	0.48	3.50	0.49	976	29	947	6	2.97	0.61	3.58	0.63
2900-2999	442	10	432	4	2.26	0.90	3.16	0.93	760	21	739	6	2.76	0.79	3.55	0.81	1202	31	1171	10	2.58	0.83	3.41	0.85
Mortality Rates: Single Births (By 500 Gm.)																								
Less than 1000	26	14	12	11	53.85	42.31	96.15	91.67	33	21	12	7	63.64	21.21	84.85	58.33	59	35	24	18	59.32	30.51	89.83	75.00
1000-1499	122	61	61	44	50.00	36.07	86.07	72.13	282	128	154	98	45.39	34.75	80.14	63.64	404	189	215	142	46.78	35.15	81.93	66.05
1500-1999	281	79	202	79	28.11	28.11	56.22	39.11	587	188	399	130	32.03	22.15	54.18	32.58	868	267	601	209	30.76	24.08	54.84	34.78
2000-2499	691	77	614	58	11.14	8.39	19.53	9.45	1556	215	1341	100	13.82	6.43	20.25	7.46	2247	292	1955	158	13.00	7.03	20.03	8.08
2500-2999	1433	37	1396	19	2.58	1.33	3.91	1.36	2702	97	2605	26	3.59	0.96	4.55	1.00	4135	134	4001	45	3.24	1.09	4.33	1.12
Mortality Rates: Twin Births (By 500 Gm.)																								
Less than 1000	7	1	6	5	14.29	71.43	85.71	83.33	11	7	4	4	63.64	36.36	100.00	100.00	18	8	10	9	44.44	50.00	94.44	90.00
1000-1499	20	6	14	11	30.00	55.00	85.00	78.57	48	5	43	23	10.42	47.92	58.34	53.49	68	11	57	34	16.18	50.00	66.18	59.65
1500-1999	55	4	51	11	7.27	20.00	27.27	21.57	78	11	67	15	14.10	19.23	33.33	22.39	133	15	118	26	11.28	19.55	30.83	22.03
2000-2499	108	1	107	2	0.93	1.85	2.78	1.87	150	7	143	6	4.67	4.00	8.67	4.20	258	8	250	8	3.10	3.10	6.20	3.29

TABLE I *A*

LENGTH OF CHILD (CM.)	WHITE								BLACK								BOTH RACES							
	TOTAL BIRTHS	STILLBIRTHS	LIVE BIRTHS	NEONATAL DEATHS	% STILLBORN	% NEONATAL DEATHS	% TOTAL MORTALITY	% NEONATAL DEATHS TO LIVE BIRTHS	TOTAL BIRTHS	STILLBIRTHS	LIVE BIRTHS	NEONATAL DEATHS	% STILLBORN	% NEONATAL DEATHS	% TOTAL MORTALITY	% NEONATAL DEATHS TO LIVE BIRTHS	TOTAL BIRTHS	STILLBIRTHS	LIVE BIRTHS	NEONATAL DEATHS	% STILLBORN	% NEONATAL DEATHS	% TOTAL MORTALITY	% NEONATAL DEATHS TO LIVE BIRTHS
Mortality Rates: Single Births (By 1 cm.)																								
Less than 34	12	9	3	1	75.00	8.33	83.33	33.33	13	8	5	3	61.54	23.08	84.62	60.00	25	17	8	4	68.00	16.00	84.00	50.00
35	23	10	13	8	43.48	34.78	78.26	61.54	28	21	7	6	75.00	21.43	96.43	85.71	51	31	20	14	60.78	27.45	88.23	70.00
36	19	9	10	8	47.37	42.11	89.48	80.00	41	25	16	11	60.98	26.83	87.81	68.75	60	34	26	19	56.67	31.67	88.34	73.08
37	25	14	11	9	56.00	36.00	92.00	81.82	48	26	22	15	54.17	31.25	85.42	68.18	73	40	33	24	54.79	32.88	87.67	72.73
38	23	14	9	3	60.87	13.04	73.91	33.33	64	31	33	26	48.44	40.63	89.07	78.79	87	45	42	29	51.72	33.33	85.05	69.05
39	27	11	16	7	40.74	25.93	66.67	43.75	65	22	43	28	33.85	43.08	76.93	65.12	92	33	59	35	35.87	38.04	73.91	59.32
40	54	18	36	21	33.33	38.89	72.22	58.33	127	51	76	31	40.16	24.41	64.57	40.79	181	69	112	52	38.12	28.73	66.85	46.43
41	55	19	36	14	34.55	25.45	60.00	38.89	141	45	96	39	31.91	27.66	59.57	40.63	196	64	132	53	32.65	27.04	59.69	40.15
42	78	15	63	15	19.23	19.23	38.46	23.81	225	64	161	38	28.44	16.89	45.33	23.60	303	79	224	53	26.07	17.49	43.56	23.66
43	131	20	111	30	15.27	22.90	38.17	27.03	281	57	224	34	20.28	12.10	32.38	15.18	412	77	335	64	18.69	15.53	34.22	19.10
44	219	38	181	34	17.35	15.53	32.88	18.78	463	76	387	47	16.41	10.15	26.56	12.14	682	114	568	81	16.72	11.88	28.60	14.26
45	95	8	87	6	8.42	6.32	14.74	6.90	236	15	221	4	6.36	1.69	8.05	1.81	331	23	308	10	6.95	3.02	9.97	3.25
46	204	12	192	2	5.88	0.98	6.86	1.04	419	20	399	12	4.77	2.86	7.64	3.01	623	32	591	14	5.14	2.25	7.39	2.37
47	357	6	351	8	1.68	2.24	3.92	2.28	725	18	707	7	2.48	0.97	3.45	0.99	1082	24	1058	15	2.22	1.39	3.61	1.42
48	601	12	589	7	2.00	1.16	3.16	1.19	1034	36	998	11	3.48	1.06	3.55	1.10	1635	48	1587	18	2.94	1.10	4.04	1.13
49	907	13	894	9	1.43	0.99	2.42	1.01	1417	31	1386	9	2.19	0.64	2.83	0.65	2324	44	2280	18	1.89	0.77	2.66	0.79
Mortality Rates: Single Births (By 5 cm.)																								
Less than 34	12	9	3	1	75.00	8.33	83.33	33.33	13	8	5	3	61.54	23.08	84.62	60.00	25	17	8	4	68.00	16.00	84.00	50.00
35-39	117	58	59	35	49.57	29.91	79.48	59.32	246	125	121	86	50.81	34.96	85.77	71.07	363	183	180	121	50.41	33.33	83.74	67.22
40-44	537	110	427	114	20.48	21.23	41.71	26.70	1237	293	944	189	23.69	15.28	38.97	20.02	1774	403	1371	303	22.72	17.08	39.80	22.10
45-49	2164	51	2113	32	2.36	1.48	3.84	1.51	3831	120	3711	43	3.13	1.12	4.25	1.16	5995	171	5824	75	2.85	1.25	4.10	1.29
Mortality Rates: Twin Births (By 5 cm.)																								
Less than 34	3	0	3	2	0.00	66.67	66.67	66.67	8	4	4	3	50.00	37.50	87.50	75.00	11	4	7	5	36.36	45.45	81.81	71.43
35-39	15	3	12	9	20.00	60.00	80.00	75.00	34	6	28	18	17.65	52.94	70.59	64.29	49	9	40	27	18.37	55.10	73.47	67.50
40-44	68	5	63	15	7.35	22.06	29.41	23.81	125	11	114	18	8.80	14.40	23.20	15.79	193	16	177	33	8.29	17.10	25.39	18.64

In the series analyzed according to length at birth (Table I *A*) the total cases in the lower centimeter brackets were so few as to permit the chance of a considerable sampling error. A steady and relatively consistent fall in stillborn mortality occurred with each added centimeter, an essentially level rate being reached at 47 cm. and above. The total mortality remained fairly constant between 84 and 88 per cent through the length 38 cm., following which a steady fall occurred, this rate also becoming stationary at 47 cm. The total mortality fell below 50 per cent at 42 cm. Deaths per 100 live births declined steadily after 36 cm., the fall becoming very slow from 45 cm. on. This rate fell below 50 per cent at 40 cm.

From the foregoing discussion the following comparative rates may be derived:

1. A steady total mortality was reached at 2700 gm. and 47 cm.

2. The total mortality became less than 50 per cent at 1800 gm. and 42 cm.

3. Deaths per 100 live births fell below 50 per cent at 1600 gm. and 40 cm.

The determination of racial differences in mortality rates was difficult since the probability of sampling errors due to insufficient figures in each individual rubric was great. Generally speaking, stillbirth rates were greater and deaths per 100 live births less in colored infants judged both by weight and length standards. The lower neonatal mortality was particularly evident in the groups 2300 to 2399 and 2400 to 2499 gm., when rates of 9.63 and 5.68 per cent were found for white prematures as contrasted with 3.59 and 3.18 for black. These black percentages correspond roughly with the figure of 3.8 obtained for white babies weighing 2500 to 2599 gm., and it seems probable that the latter weight range in the white race is about the equivalent in maturity to the 2300 to 2400 range level in the black. A finding of considerable interest was the marked difference in death rates for single as contrasted with twin births, as is illustrated in Fig. 4. With the exception of extremely immature infants of less than 1000 gm., the chances of live birth and of survival were much greater for all weights in the twin series, and in the group 2000 gm. and over the ratio was almost three to one. A similar tendency, but by no means as marked, was observed for various lengths. This is taken as confirmation of the closer approach to maturity, at any given weight, of twin infants as contrasted with single born children, whereas the length of the former tends to correspond more closely to the true gestational age.

Attention is drawn at this time to two items illustrated in Tables I and I *A*. Many more infants were found whose weight at birth was under 2500 gm. than whose length was below 45 cm., 3,578 and 2,162, respectively. The stillborn, neonatal, and total mortality rates in the

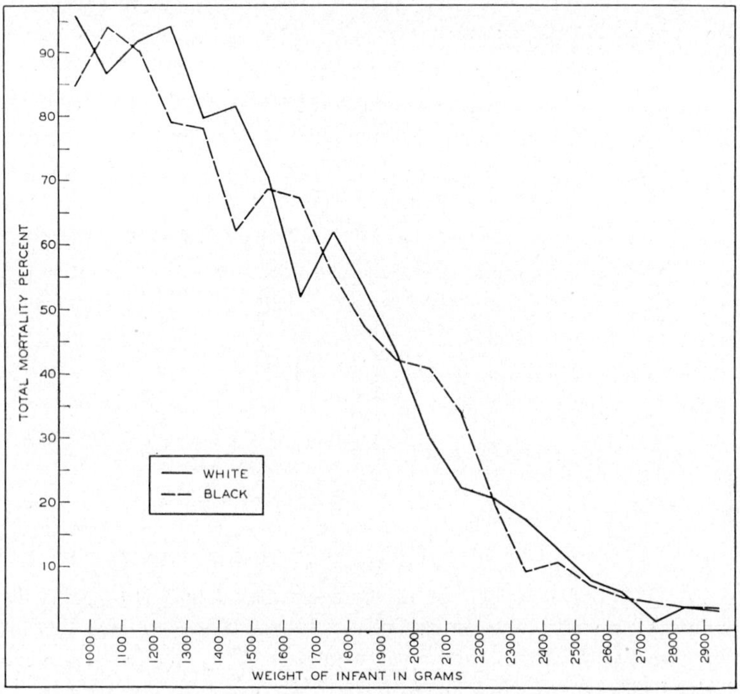

Fig. 3.—Total mortality according to race and weight of infant (single births only).

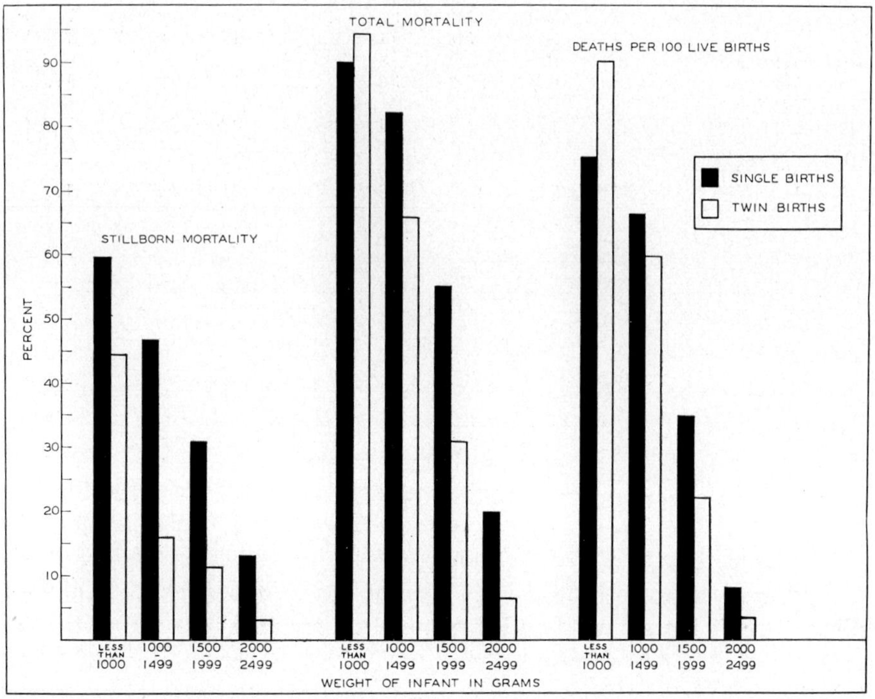

Fig. 4.—Stillborn mortality, total mortality, and deaths per 100 live births according to weight of infant (single versus twin births).

smaller series (length) were considerably higher than in the larger (weight). It is our opinion that these findings indicate the inaccuracy of criteria for prematurity which now link a weight of 2500 gm. and 45 cm. together. If the weight is accepted the length must be increased, and if the length is correct a decrease in the weight criterion must follow. Or, and this has seemed the more logical to us, both of the commonly accepted weight and length standards should be discarded and new ones derived, the accuracy of which would be subject to less criticism.

Mortality Rates: First Versus Second Twin.—In the remaining analyses of this series of prematurly born infants it is planned to group together the single and twin births. First, however, it is desired to present mortality rates for the first born, as contrasted with the second born in twin pregnancies, the prediction having been made that since the former theoretically received the greater trauma during labor (dilatation of cervix, perineum, etc.) its risk should be higher. Table II shows

TABLE II

MORTALITY RATES: FIRST VERSUS SECOND TWIN

WEIGHT	TOTAL BIRTHS	STILL-BIRTHS	LIVE BIRTHS	NEO-NATAL DEATHS	PER CENT STILL-BORN	PER CENT NEONA-TAL DEATHS	PER CENT TOTAL MOR-TALITY	PER CENT NEONATAL DEATHS TO LIVE BIRTHS
First twin:								
1499 and under	39	9	30	22	23.08	56.41	79.49	73.33
1500 to 1999	65	6	59	11	9.23	16.92	25.15	18.64
2000 to 2499	115	2	113	3	1.74	2.61	4.35	2.65
Total	219	17	202	36	7.76	16.44	24.20	17.82
Second twin:								
1499 and under	47	10	37	21	21.28	44.68	65.96	56.76
1500 to 1999	68	9	59	15	13.24	22.06	35.29	25.42
2000 to 2499	143	6	137	5	4.20	3.50	7.69	3.65
Total	258	25	233	41	9.69	15.89	25.58	17.60

the results of this analysis and, although not conclusive, apparently indicates that the risk is about equal for the two infants. Indeed, most of the rates derived according to weight were slightly lower for the first born, but the margin of difference was so small that it could easily be accounted for by a sampling error. On the other hand the chances of the second twin were somewhat better, both for live birth and survival in the series analyzed according to length.

Age.—Table III indicates that whether judged by weight or length at birth, the risk to the prematurely born child increased materially with advancing age of the mother in the series under discussion. This discrepancy would seem to permit explanation in two ways. In the first place, there is both clinical and statistical evidence that the young woman tends to give birth to an infant relatively below average in weight and length. This infant, however, is vigorous and stands a better chance of survival than a similar one born to an older woman and one more premature in its essential reactions. Secondly, advancing parity accompanies advancing age and it is in these higher parous groups that certain maternal complications, adding materially to the risk of prematurity and infant death, are most commonly found.

TABLE III

MORTALITY RATES ACCORDING TO THE AGE OF THE MOTHER

AGE OF MOTHER	TOTAL BIRTHS	STILL-BIRTHS	LIVE BIRTHS	NEO-NATAL DEATHS	PER CENT STILL-BORN	PER CENT NEO-NATAL DEATHS	PER CENT TOTAL MOR-TALITY	PER CENT NEONATAL DEATHS TO LIVE BIRTHS
			Weight					
19 and under	1272	195	1077	177	15.33	13.92	29.25	16.43
20 to 29	1749	395	1354	253	22.58	14.47	37.05	18.69
30 and over	759	205	554	128	27.01	16.86	43.87	23.10
			Length					
19 and under	781	140	541	144	17.93	18.44	36.37	26.62
20 to 29	1096	309	787	210	28.19	19.16	47.35	26.68
30 and over	490	159	331	104	32.45	21.22	53.67	31.42

Parity.—In view of what has been said regarding age of mothers, rising mortality rates with increasing parity were probably to be expected. The extent to which multiparity adds to the risk of the child is shown in Table IV. The growing stillborn rate was explainable in terms of the previously mentioned maternal complications. However, the increased number of neonatal deaths in parous women did not lend itself to immediate interpretation. Although not shown in the table it is of interest that both the stillborn rate and that for deaths per 100 live births were twice as great in the group para x and more as in the primiparous division.

TABLE IV

MORTALITY RATES ACCORDING TO THE PARITY OF THE MOTHER

PARA	TOTAL BIRTHS	STILL-BIRTHS	LIVE BIRTHS	NEO-NATAL DEATHS	PER CENT STILL-BORN	PER CENT NEO-NATAL DEATHS	PER CENT TOTAL MOR-TALITY	PER CENT NEONATAL DEATHS TO LIVE BIRTHS
			Weight					
1	1690	270	1420	208	15.98	12.31	28.29	14.65
2 to 4	1315	308	1007	215	23.42	16.35	39.77	21.35
5 and more	780	219	561	137	28.08	17.56	45.64	24.42
			Length					
1	879	196	683	171	22.30	19.45	41.75	25.04
2 to 4	864	242	622	175	28.01	20.25	48.26	28.14
5 and more	534	173	361	116	32.40	21.72	54.12	32.13

Rupture of Membranes.—Table V indicates the mortality rates derived by both weight and length according to the time of rupture of the membranes. Little discussion seems necessary except to note that the lowest rates found were in the group with rupture occurring before the onset of labor. This may be taken as additional evidence that this accident, formerly considered of grave import, is essentially harmless, even to the premature child.

TABLE V

MORTALITY RATES AS AFFECTED BY TIME OF RUPTURE OF MEMBRANES

TIME OF RUPTURE	TOTAL BIRTHS	STILL-BIRTHS	LIVE BIRTHS	NEO-NATAL DEATHS	PER CENT STILL-BORN	PER CENT NEO-NATAL DEATHS	PER CENT TOTAL MOR-TALITY	PER CENT NEONATAL DEATHS TO LIVE BIRTHS
			Weight					
Before onset of labor	582	83	499	77	14.26	13.23	27.49	15.43
First stage	507	121	386	55	23.87	10.85	34.72	14.25
Second stage	1790	365	1425	280	20.39	15.64	36.03	19.65
			Length					
Before onset of labor	309	66	243	64	21.36	20.71	42.07	26.34
First stage	292	80	212	45	27.40	15.41	42.81	21.23
Second stage	1049	271	778	224	25.83	21.35	47.18	28.79

Sex.—In a previous communication attention has been drawn to the interesting finding that the normal preponderance of males at birth was reversed in this series of prematurely born children. In Table VI we

TABLE VI

MORTALITY RATES AS AFFECTED BY THE SEX OF CHILD

RACE AND SEX	TOTAL BIRTHS	STILL-BIRTHS	LIVE BIRTHS	NEO-NATAL DEATHS	PER CENT STILL-BORN	PER CENT NEO-NATAL DEATHS	PER CENT TOTAL MOR-TALITY	PER CENT NEONATAL DEATHS PER 100 LIVE BIRTHS
			Weight less than 2500 gm.					
White, male	620	125	495	124	20.16	20.06	40.16	25.05
White, female	684	116	568	95	16.96	13.89	30.85	16.73
Black, male	1321	327	994	212	24.75	16.05	40.80	21.33
Black, female	1411	248	1163	170	17.58	12.05	29.62	14.62
Total, male	1941	452	1489	336	23.29	17.31	40.60	22.57
Total, female	2095	364	1731	265	17.37	12.65	30.02	15.31
			Length less than 45 cm.					
White, male	347	93	254	97	26.80	27.95	54.75	38.19
White, female	402	92	310	78	22.89	19.40	42.29	25.16
Black, male	799	261	538	174	32.67	21.78	54.45	32.34
Black, female	857	181	676	143	21.12	16.69	37.81	21.15
Total, male	1146	354	792	271	30.89	23.65	54.54	34.22
Total, female	1259	273	986	221	21.68	17.55	39.23	22.41

record the significantly higher mortality rates, both stillborn and neonatal, found throughout in the males as contrasted with the females. It is our opinion that the normally smaller weight and length at birth of the female infant only partly accounts for the observed discrepancy. It is probable that a true sexual difference in ability to survive is presented here.

Effect of Type of Delivery.—In recent years a number of articles have appeared dealing with the effect of the type of delivery upon the mortality rate of prematurely born infants. In order that our figures may be contrasted with those already published by others, Table VII, dealing

TABLE VII

MORTALITY RATES ACCORDING TO TYPE OF DELIVERY

WEIGHT OF CHILD (GM.)	TOTAL BIRTHS	STILL-BIRTHS	LIVE BIRTHS	NEO-NATAL DEATHS	PER CENT STILL-BORN	PER CENT NEO-NATAL DEATHS	PER CENT TOTAL MOR-TALITY	PER CENT NEONATAL DEATHS TO LIVE BIRTHS
Spontaneous Delivery								
1499 and under	399	178	221	152	44.61	38.10	82.71	68.78
1500 to 1999	743	195	548	169	26.24	22.75	48.99	30.84
2000 to 2499	1962	206	1756	135	10.50	6.89	17.38	7.69
Total	3104	579	2525	456	18.65	14.69	33.33	18.06
Operative Delivery								
1499 and under	119	58	61	36	48.74	30.25	78.99	59.02
1500 to 1999	216	81	135	57	37.50	26.39	63.89	42.22
2000 to 2499	442	86	356	27	19.46	6.11	25.57	7.58
Total	777	225	552	120	28.96	15.44	44.40	21.74
Cesarean Section								
1499 and under	22	9	13	11	40.91	50.00	90.91	84.62
1500 to 1999	31	9	22	7	29.03	22.58	51.61	31.82
2000 to 2499	81	12	69	9	14.81	11.11	25.92	13.04
Total	134	30	104	27	22.39	20.15	42.54	25.96
Breech Extraction								
1499 and under	38	18	20	7	47.37	18.42	65.79	35.00
1500 to 1999	88	24	64	29	27.27	32.95	60.22	45.31
2000 to 2499	137	20	117	5	14.60	3.65	18.25	4.27
Total	263	62	201	41	23.57	15.59	39.16	20.40
Forceps								
1499 and under	13	2	11	5	15.38	38.46	53.84	45.45
1500 to 1999	17	3	14	3	17.65	17.65	35.30	21.43
2000 to 2499	123	14	109	5	11.38	4.07	15.45	4.59
Total	153	19	134	13	12.42	8.50	20.92	9.70
Version and Extraction								
1499 and under	28	12	16	13	42.86	46.43	89.29	81.25
1500 to 1999	58	30	28	15	51.72	25.86	77.58	53.57
2000 to 2499	83	30	53	5	36.14	6.02	42.16	9.43
Total	169	72	97	33	42.60	19.53	62.13	34.02

TABLE VIII

MORTALITY RATES

STILLBIRTHS, NEONATAL DEATHS, AND DEATHS DURING FIRST YEAR

WEIGHT	WHITE				BLACK				TOTAL			
	PER CENT STILL-BORN	PER CENT NEONATAL DEATHS	PER CENT DIED FIRST YEAR	TOTAL	PER CENT STILL-BORN	PER CENT NEONATAL DEATHS	PER CENT DIED FIRST YEAR	TOTAL	PER CENT STILL-BORN	PER CENT NEONATAL DEATHS	PER CENT DIED FIRST YEAR	TOTAL
1499 and under	46.86	40.57	4.00	91.43	43.05	35.29	8.56	86.90	44.26	36.98	7.29	88.53
1500 to 1999	24.70	26.79	9.52	61.01	29.92	21.80	13.38	65.10	28.17	23.48	11.99	63.64
2000 to 2499	9.76	7.51	8.26	25.53	13.01	6.21	10.14	29.36	11.98	6.63	9.66	28.27
G. C. P.*	4.43	2.60	3.76	10.79	6.47	3.08	5.09	14.64	5.75	2.91	4.61	13.27

*General clinic population.

with this item, is included. It is not our belief that this table shows in any way the comparative risk rate to the infant according to the method of delivery, per se. In the vast majority of those cases delivered by operative means, breech extraction alone excluded, the choice was dictated by some maternal complication such as heart disease or placenta previa rather than through conscientious effort to produce a living infant. Consequently, the rates appearing in Table VII would seem to reflect the mortality from the maternal abnormality rather than that associated with any given type of delivery. Mortality rates according to type of delivery but derived according to length of child were so similar to those shown here that they have not been included in the table.

Mortality During the First Year of Life.—A relatively large number of the mothers of the infants under analysis returned to the dispensary for examination one year after delivery, and at this time information was obtained concerning the course during the first year of those children discharged alive. This mortality during this period, coupled with the stillborn and neonatal rates, is shown in Table VIII, which further includes similar figures obtained from the general clinic population on children normal in weight at birth. No similar figures are available according to length. It has been the policy of the clinic to discharge the small baby from the hospital only when it has attained a minimum weight of 5½ pounds, presents no abnormality, and is gaining satisfactorily. Despite apparent normality at this time, the death rate of these infants during the first year of life was high, and even in the theoretically most hardy group, with a birth weight between 2000 and 2499 gm., was 8.26 and 10.14 per cent for the white and colored races, respectively. As contrasted with a normal series of term infants, stillbirths, neonatal deaths, and deaths during the first year of life occurred at least twice as often in both black and white children weighing between 4.4 and 5.5 pounds at birth.

DISCUSSION

In the foregoing paragraphs data have been presented on two series of infants below average in weight or length at birth. Little discussion seems necessary in addition to that noted under each individual topic. The purpose of this article has been to present facts obtained from statistical data. Accordingly no positive statements on the prevention of premature birth seem warranted or desirable. Moreover, the care of the prematurely liveborn infant is deemed a problem for the pediatrician rather than the obstetrician. It is of interest to note, however, that the babies making up this series have been born over a period of the past forty years and have been cared for under the rapidly changing regimes of that time. Despite radical alterations in care and feeding, attempts on our part to adduce changes developing in neonatal mortality rates from decade to decade have not met with any significant findings.

A number of articles have appeared recently dealing with the effect of the type of delivery and anesthetic upon the prematurely born infant. We are unable to agree with the rather optimistic findings of some of these. A relatively high stillborn mortality rate seems unavoidable, since the premature labor and birth so often is the result of fetal death in utero, which in turn has been caused by some maternal complication such as nephritis or syphilis. Furthermore, the premature baby, although born alive, often succumbs in the first few hours of life as the result, apparently, of prolonged partial asphyxia from such conditions as placenta previa or premature separation of the placenta. It would seem that when the early birth is due to maternal complications, high mortality rates are unavoidable and that only when the premature labor is apparently accidental may reasonably low results be expected. Obviously the immature fetus cannot withstand the stresses and strains of labor and delivery with such impunity as does the term one. Consequently, whatever course will subject it to the least number of uterine contractions during labor, and the least trauma at birth, would seem to offer the best results. Each case must then be individualized, and as a guide one can only suggest conservatism. Forceps, version, etc., may occasionally be warranted because of maternal conditions, but should rarely be indicated by the prematurity of the infant. Furthermore, it is well to remember that even cesarean section does not guarantee a live baby and that stillbirths and neonatal deaths will occasionally follow this procedure. Finally, it seems evident that anesthesia and analgesia are to be avoided in this type of case in so far as is possible and that the former, when necessary, be of the saturation rather than the asphyxiation type.

CONCLUSIONS

1. In two large series of premature infants, decreasing stillborn and neonatal mortality rates were noted with increasing weight and length. This decrease was slow in the lower weight brackets (under 1200 gm.), became particularly rapid with weights between 1800 and 2400 gm., and reached a relatively stationary low level at 2700 gm. With increasing length the fall was steady, and a level rate was reached at 47 cm.

2. In general, stillborn rates were higher and deaths per 100 live births lower in black than in white infants.

3. Stillborn and neonatal rates were definitely lower in multiple than in single births. No significant difference was noted in the mortalities of first versus second twins.

4. Judged by either weight or length standards mortality rates increased significantly with advancing age of the mother.

5. A rising mortality was observed with increasing parity of the mother and was twice as great in the group para x and more as in the primiparous portion of the series.

6. No significant effect on mortality was found according to time of rupture of membranes.

7. A much higher stillborn and neonatal death rate was noted in male as contrasted with female infants.

8. An analysis of mortality rates according to type of delivery permitted no definite statement as to the most favorable procedure for the immature infant.

9. A high mortality during the first year was found in those premature infants who survived the first weeks of life.

THE INFLUENCE OF METABOLISM ON TEETH

JOHN OPPIE MCCALL, D.D.S., AND FRANCES KRASNOW, PH.D.
NEW YORK, N. Y.

THE medical profession no less than the dental profession has reason to be interested in the welfare of the human dentition, and signs are not lacking that this interest is becoming articulate, as indicated by the appearance in medical journals of articles dealing with teeth and the causes and prevention of dental caries. Under the circumstances we feel that it may be appropriate to present briefly various causal factors influencing the caries syndrome in the light of newer data.

Miller[1] in 1883 focussed the attention of the dental profession on local causes of dental caries by his demonstration that this process is inaugurated by chemicoparasitic activity in carbohydrate material retained on the tooth surface either in crevices or on areas not readily cleansed by food scouring or other methods. Miller's theory failed to explain completely all clinical facts, hence there has been a more or less continuous search through the intervening years for an explanation of discrepancies as well as a means for control of the carious process itself.

Recently conviction has been gaining strength that metabolic factors have much to do with the etiology and also the control of dental caries. These may influence the incidence of caries in one of two ways: (1) the tooth structure may be defective (shown chiefly as enamel hypoplasia) because of abnormal metabolism during the period of tooth formation, making it susceptible to what may be called amelolytic influences; (2) current metabolic influences expressing themselves (a) as functions of the saliva, which controls largely the environment of the tooth, and (b) possibly through nutrient channels (as yet little understood) within the tooth. Most recent researches in dental caries tend to be directed toward the solution of the problem by means of efforts to influence metabolism in one or the other of the senses just stated by regulation of the diet and other physiologic factors.

ENAMEL HYPOPLASIA

There are several important differences between formative enamel defects (hypoplastic enamel) of the deciduous and permanent teeth. In the deciduous dentition the crowns are fully formed and very largely calcified in utero, hence hypoplastic enamel in these teeth is chargeable to prenatal systemic disturbance. The hypoplastic deciduous tooth is smooth when erupted but lacks density. Jones[2] has stated that in severe

From The Murry and Leonie Guggenheim Dental Clinic, New York.

hypoplasia the enamel may be soft and chalky at the time of tooth eruption. Caries attacks large areas of the hypoplastic deciduous tooth which may decay with rapid loss of enamel en masse (Figs. 1 and 2).

In the permanent dentition, crown formation and calcification of even the first teeth to erupt, the central incisors and first molars, begins at about the time of birth, hence hypoplasia of enamel is traced to

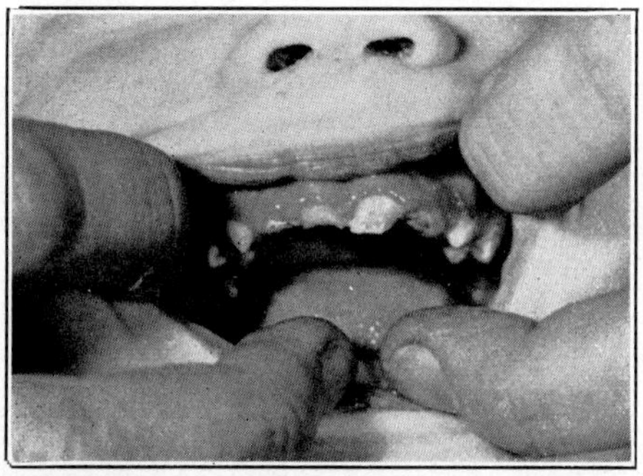

Fig. 1.—Photograph of girl, 21 months of age, showing extensive decay due to deficient enamel formation. The mother's diet during the pregnancy was extremely deficient in calcium and vitamins.

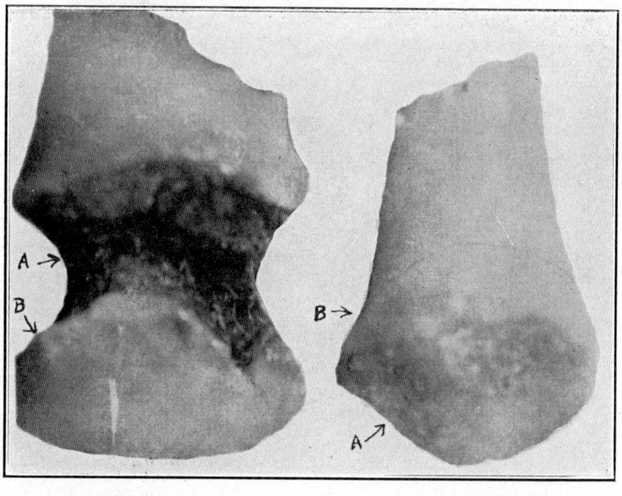

Fig. 2.—Photomicrograph (×6) of upper central and lateral incisor from the same mouth. Caries has attacked areas *A,A* of hypoplastic enamel but has not attacked areas *B,B* where enamel was well formed and well calcified. The crowns of the deciduous teeth are formed in utero, hence the enamel defect and subsequent decay are chargeable to prenatal conditions. What apparently occurred was an illness causing deranged metabolism at the time when areas *A,A* were being formed, preceded and followed by good health with normal metabolic status as evidenced by the good enamel found at *B,B*. (The central incisor [left] begins to form before the lateral incisor.)

systemic disturbance at and following birth. Hypoplastic enamel is pitted and may present grooves, but calcification of the deformed structure is usually normal in its density. It is not prone to decay unless the grooves and pits are of such a depth as to make self-cleansing and cleansing by the tooth brush difficult (Figs. 3 and 4).

In this connection it should be mentioned that Mellanby[3] has claimed that enamel structure is the chief factor in caries resistance and that hypoplastic enamel is likely to decay because of inferior resistance. Clinical evidence does not corroborate this view as regards the permanent teeth, and it seems more likely, in view of other evidence, to be mentioned later, that the same metabolic influences that caused the enamel hypoplasia produce also influences favoring dental caries. However, decay may occur in enamel through environmental or metabolic influences, no matter how perfectly it is formed and calcified.

Fig. 3.

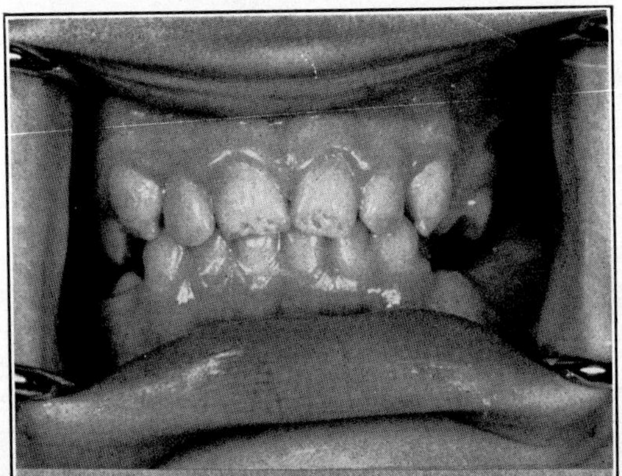

Fig. 4.

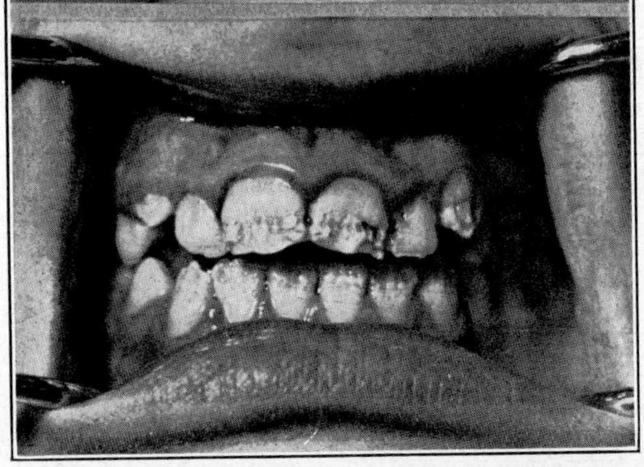

Fig. 3.—Photograph of teeth of boy, aged 10 years, showing mild enamel hypoplasia of the upper central incisors. These teeth usually are not susceptible to caries.

Fig. 4.—Photograph of teeth of girl, aged 10 years, showing marked enamel hypoplasia of all incisors and cuspids. Because of the depth of some of the pits, decay will occur unless protective fillings are placed.

PREGNANCY AND DENTAL CARIES

Tooth structure in relation to caries has received attention from a different viewpoint, viz., the influence of pregnancy on caries. There has been a rather general assumption (1) that women are more susceptible to caries during pregnancy than at other times, and (2) that this assumed special susceptibility is due to withdrawal of calcium salts from the teeth to meet fetal needs. This would imply that tooth structure could be altered after eruption.

Schour[4] has recently presented certain phases of the pathology of the dental tissues, also evidence that teeth are not a storehouse for calcium. He then infers that pregnancy does not influence caries. Review of other evidence seems to indicate that this viewpoint is not conclusive. He derives support for this hypothesis largely from a research by Ziskin,[5] which consists of observations made primarily from the dental standpoint. Because of inherent difficulty in an investigation of this type, little evidence was brought forward as to the metabolic status of the women examined. Indications of this might be obtained by one of several methods. Jay, Hadley, and Bunting[6] have shown a relationship between presence or absence of *Lactobacillus acidophilus* in the mouth and caries immunity or susceptibility. Fosdick and Hatton[7] have announced a test, based on solution of tooth shavings by the saliva as a criterion of caries immunity or susceptibility. Krasnow, Oblatt, and Hirschfeld,[8] through salivary analysis, have suggested a double correlation between certain elements in the saliva and tendency to caries and other dental disease. Still others might be enumerated.

The metabolic state would have to be determined by some reliable method in a study of caries in pregnancy, since it could easily happen that many of the nonpregnant women examined would be caries susceptible and the pregnant women nonsusceptible. Also, pregnant women, except in the lowest economic strata, have prenatal care involving not only diet recommendation, but also instructions tending to bring the physiologic plane to the optimum level. Even in earlier generations, metabolism (hence tooth metabolism) during pregnancy might have been better because of the belief that the expectant mother should have sufficient rest and should eat for two. This would tend to provide good caries resistance in the average case.

GENERAL HEALTH: DENTAL HEALTH

Until more evidence is forthcoming it is safer to assume that dental health is no less a resultant of those conditions which make for the health and life of the body as a whole than that it is itself one of these factors. The teeth have their specific function and in all probability are associated with specific metabolisms. Dental disease, caries, erosion, etc., therefore, may be interpreted as the effect of specific syndromes.

Jones,[9] from her work with dogs at the University of California as well as with children in Honolulu, concludes a relationship between food and teeth. Similar interdependence is implied by Hawkins.[10] Boyd, Drain, and Stearns[11] hypothesize a close correlation between metabolic efficiency and resistance of the tooth to decay. In order to reduce substantially the incidence of dental disease, especially in temperate zones, Mellanby[12] believes that it is necessary to introduce large changes in the diet and habits of pregnant and lactating women, of

TABLE I

ANALYSES ON TOTAL UNSTIMULATED SALIVA[8]

SUMMARY OF RESULTS OBTAINED BY THREE COMMON STATISTICAL METHODS FOR EVALUATING PROBABLE SIGNIFICANCE OF FIGURES

ANALYSES	EROSION*									CARIES†								
	AVERAGE RANGE NOT OVERLAPPING NORMAL‡			DISTRIBUTION MORE THAN 50% ABOVE AVERAGE NORMAL RANGE			ODDS AGAINST RANDOM DEVIATIONS[6]			AVERAGE RANGE NOT OVERLAPPING NORMAL‡			DISTRIBUTION MORE THAN 50% ABOVE AVERAGE NORMAL RANGE			ODDS AGAINST RANDOM DEVIATIONS[6]		
	TOTAL	ALK.	ACID	TOTAL	ALK.	ACID	TOTAL	ALK.	ACID	TOTAL	ALK.	ACID	TOTAL	ALK.	ACID	TOTAL	ALK.	ACID
H^+, pH	6.83 ±0.05	7.19 ±0.07	6.73 ±0.04	89	–	–	1341.0	1.0	15×10^6	6.92 ±0.06	7.21 ±0.04	6.71 ±0.04	62	–	–	26.4	1.9	4×10^5
Calcium	7.6 ±0.5	5.5 ±0.5	8.2 ±0.5	74	25	87	6.3	1.6	13.6	6.2 ±0.2	6.0 ±0.25	6.4 ±0.19	22	11	33	–	1.0	–
Magnesium	0.75 ±0.10	0.41 ±0.04	0.84 ±0.12	68	0	87	8.5	1.0	13.6	0.65 ±0.06	0.63 ±0.06	0.73 ±0.08	65	67	75	5.4	2.2	9.9
Inorganic phosphate	18.0 ±1.4	12.2 ±1.6	19.7 ±1.5	53	25	60	2.6	2.6	9.9	14.4 ±0.6	12.6 ±0.7	15.2 ±0.7	39	11	50	1.0	6.3	–
Protein	446.0 ±46.0	284.0 ±33.0	489.0 ±53.0	68	25	80	22.2	–	44.8	346.0 ±24.0	315.0 ±33.0	359.0 ±39.0	54	33	67	3.0	1.0	2.2
Lipid phosphorus	0.52 ±0.11	0.26 ±0.11	0.60 ±0.14	78	50	86	37.4	1.4	44.8	0.20 ±0.03	0.19 ±0.02	0.22 ±0.04	63	78	50	7.3	4.6	3.5
Cholesterol	11.2 ±2.0	5.3 ±2.1	12.9 ±2.5	57	25	65	3.5	1.0	7.3	10.7 ±0.77	9.2 ±0.7	11.9 ±1.2	82	67	92	31.4	3.0	26.4

*Erosion refers to subjects suffering from wastings: erosions or abrasions.

†Caries refers to subjects with active decay processes only.

‡Normal values obtained from analyses on subjects who as far as medicodental clinical and laboratory tests could discern had no ailments. Hydrogen-ion concentration: 7.14±.04; calcium: 6.3±.4; magnesium: 0.46±.07; inorganic phosphate: 15.2±1; protein: 298±17; lipid phosphorus: 0.13±.02; cholesterol: 7.5±.7.

infants, and of children during the whole period of dental development, and, indeed, during the whole lifetime.

RECENT DATA ON SALIVA

Researches by Krasnow et al.[8] on the quantitative salivary analysis of individuals suffering from caries or erosion and also of those who are caries-free indicate characteristically different chemical pictures of saliva for different dental conditions. Table I summarizes some recent data. From this it will be seen that in erosion the average range of hydrogen-ion concentration, calcium, magnesium, inorganic phosphate, protein, lipid phosphorus, and cholesterol lies entirely beyond that for the same constituents in saliva of normal individuals. The standard deviations are relatively small, and none of the average ranges overlap, hence variations from the normal are probably significant. In caries-active individuals variations from the normal are fewer, nonoverlapping figures appearing only for hydrogen-ion concentration, magnesium, lipid phosphorus, and cholesterol.

It seems plausible to assume a common mechanism at work. The results imply a tendency to that type of derangement often associated with acidic states in the body,[13] notwithstanding that the subjects, for the most part, had no other pathologic involvement as far as the usual medicodental clinical and laboratory tests could discern. Detailed perusal of accumulated data, coordinated with the fact that the organism makes every effort to rid itself of acid ions in salt form, led to the examination of the dietary acid-base potentialities in addition to the usual orthodox factors.[9, 10]

In the plan adopted[14, 15] the chief criteria of physiologic response are subjective guides, clinical manifestations (roentgenograms), weight changes, and variation in the chemical composition of saliva. To insure saliva samples which are duplicable and representative of an individual, conditions are set for a definite metabolic plane over a period of at least one week preceding any analyses.

The variations noted in the saliva in different oral conditions, especially as regards the number of constituents in which variations are found, furnish the basis for the view indicated earlier, that the teeth are associated not with calcium metabolism alone, but with several specific metabolisms upon which general metabolism depends, and that dental health is closely related to the health and life of the body as a whole. It is interesting and perhaps significant that aberrant salivary values can be brought within the normal range by nutritional regulation (Table II). Furthermore, clinical evidence is accumulating which points to the lessening of susceptibility to erosion and caries under such a regime. Indications are that while calcium values in the saliva may not, under certain conditions, vary markedly from the normal, other constituents do, and calcium intake should receive consideration along

TABLE II[14]

CASE REPORT

Patient 16 C, 15 years old, healthy, from excellent home of good economic status.

DEC. 6, 1935	APRIL 1, 1936	OCT. 10, 1936
I. Findings:	I. Findings:	I. Findings:
A. *Saliva*	A. *Saliva*	
pH 7.1	pH 7.0	
Calcium mg % 5.3	Calcium mg % 5.0	
Phosphorus mg % 13.2 Tending low	Phosphorus mg % 15.5 Increased	
Magnesium mg % 0.62 High	Magnesium mg % 0.41 Decreased	
Protein mg % 300	Protein mg % 306	
Cholesterol mg % 10.9 High	Cholesterol mg % 6.5 Decreased	
Lecithin mg % 0.18 Tending high	Lecithin mg % 0.14 Decreased	
B. *Diet*	B. *Diet*	
Water, milk low.	Milk increased, water low.	
Calories somewhat low.	Calories increased.	
Acid:base 61:45.	Acid:base 41:55.	
High bread, cake, cereal.	Decrease in bread, cereal.	
C. *Dental Report*	C. *Dental Report*	C. *Dental Report*
Caries extremely rampant occlusally and interproximally.	Apparently no noticeable change.	Interproximal decalcification arrested.
		No new cavities.
		Enamel texture improved.
II. Recommendations:	II. Recommendations:	II. Recommendations:
Increase milk to 3 glasses.	Increase water intake.	Continue with previous advice.
Slowly increase water to 8 glasses.	Use pablum instead of other cereal.	
Slowly increase vegetables } especially	Substitute fruit for cake dessert.	
Slowly increase fruits } raw	Use irradiated milk instead of cod-liver oil.	
Take 2 teaspoonfuls cod-liver oil.		
Decrease slowly bread, cake, etc.		
Keep caloric intake at 1,800.		

with other factors in dietary correction. It should apparently be, and can well be, gained from natural food sources.

We hope that with the presentation of this evidence the medical profession will defer acceptance of theories founded on limited investigation, pending the inauguration of a much needed and really comprehensive research.

CONCLUSIONS

Hypoplastic enamel of the permanent teeth is no more subject to caries than normal enamel unless structural defects are severe. In the deciduous teeth hypoplastic enamel is much more susceptible to caries than normal enamel; a governing factor in the incidence of caries in these teeth seems to be environmental influence, which is, in its turn, apparently related to the metabolic status of the body.

Calcium may not be withdrawn from the teeth through the blood stream during pregnancy, but there exists the possibility that the caries process may be accelerated as a result of unfavorable metabolic conditions, which in turn may also result in unfavorable environmental conditions.

Calcium therapy per se (administration of calcium salts) has not been proved to be beneficial to the teeth. At the same time adequate intake of calcium-containing foods cannot be overlooked in its relationship to normal tooth formation.

Stress laid on one need must always be coordinated with all other physiologic needs directly or indirectly associated with the situation at hand.

REFERENCES

1. Miller, W. D.: Am. J. Dental Science. Third Series **17**: 83, 126, 525, 1883.
2. Jones, M. R.: J. A. M. A. **99**: 1849, 1932.
3. Mellanby, M.: Influence of Diet on Caries in Children's Teeth. Medical Research Council, Special Report, Series No. 221, London, 1936.
4. Schour, Isaac: J. A. M. A. **110**: 870, 1938.
5. Ziskin, D. E.: Am. J. Obst. & Gynec. **12**: 710, 1926.
   Ziskin, D. E., and Hotelling, H.: J. Dent. Research **16**: 507, 1937.
6. Jay, P., Hadley, F. P., and Bunting, R. W.: J. Am. Dent. A. **23**: 846, 1936.
7. Fosdick, L. S., and Hatton, E. H.: Northwestern University Bulletin **37**: No. 47, 1937.
   Hansen, H. L., Fosdick, L. S., and Epple, C. F.: J. Am. Dent. A. and Dental Cosmos **24**: 1611, 1937.
8. Krasnow, F., Oblatt, E. B., and Hirschfeld, I.: Salivary Analysis of Patients Subject to Wastings: Abrasions and Erosions, J. Periodontology **9**: 42, 1938.
9. Jones, M. R.: Dental Cosmos **77**: 535, 651, 747, 1935.
10. Hawkins, H.: J. Am. Dent. A. **16**: 781, 1929.
11. Boyd, J. D., Drain, C. L., and Stearns, G.: J. Biol. Chem. **103**: 327, 1933.
12. Mellanby, M.: Brit. Dent. J. **62**: 241, 1937.
13. Hawk, P. B., and Bergeim, O.: Practical Physiological Chemistry. Ed. 11, Philadelphia, 1937, p. 407, P. Blakiston's Son & Co.
14. Krasnow, F.: J. Am. Dental Assoc. and Dental Cosmos **25**: 216, 1938.
15. Krasnow, F.: Nutritional Influence on Teeth, Am. J. Public Health **28**: 325, 1938; J. Canadian Dental Assoc. **4**: 135, 1938.
16. Pearl, R.: Introduction to Medical Biometry and Statistics. Ed. 2, p. 438, Philadelphia, 1930, W. B. Saunders Company.

THE BIOPHOTOMETER AS A TEST FOR VITAMIN A DEFICIENCY

Charles E. Snelling, M.B.
Toronto, Ontario

METHODS for the detection of subclinical avitaminosis are being sought for all the vitamins. Considerable investigation has been carried out with regard to vitamin A.

One of the conditions resulting from vitamin A deficiency is night blindness. It is caused by a failure in the regeneration of visual purple after a bleaching by strong light. Administration of cod-liver oil, butter, or milk results in improvement by the third to fifth day, and vision becomes practically normal by the seventh to fourteenth day. Night blindness may be caused by other conditions than vitamin A deficiency.

Using the fact that night blindness is caused by lack of vitamin A, Jeans and Zentmire,[2, 3] with a Birch-Hirschfeld photometer, studied the dark adaptation of a group of children. As a result of this study they found that 26 per cent of the children from rural districts, 53 per cent of children from villages, and no less than 56 to 79 per cent of urban children showed decreased dark adaptations. In a group of eighty-seven children with decreased dark adaptation, eighty-four or 95 per cent returned to normal with the administration of vitamin A. Similar results have been reported by others. Using the same type of instrument and technique, we were unable to obtain satisfactory and consistent results.[5] We concluded, "In our hands the Birch-Hirschfeld photometer was unsatisfactory for the estimation of small variations in dark adaptation such as might be produced by vitamin A deficiency."

Subsequently, Jeans et al.[6] in a later report stated, "This instrument (Birch-Hirschfeld) is not adapted for the satisfactory use in the manner employed," and they described a new instrument devised for this particular test called the biophotometer. Using the latter instrument on a group of thirty-seven children, they obtained results which indicated that 19 per cent were suffering from vitamin A deficiency.

Jeghers,[7] with a group of adults, reports that vitamin A deficiency was common and could be photometrically detected. In a group of medical students 35 per cent were low, and 12 per cent had clinical manifestations of the deficiency. There was complete recovery in three days after an experimentally produced vitamin A deficiency.

From the wards and laboratories of the Hospital for Sick Children and the Department of Paediatrics, University of Toronto, under the direction of Alan Brown, M.D., F.R.C.P. (C).

Read at the Tenth Annual Meeting of the Society for Pediatric Research, Great Barrington, Mass., May 4, 1938, and at the Sixteenth Annual Meeting of the Canadian Society for the Study of Diseases of Children, Kingston, Ont., June 3 and 4, 1938.

Palmer and Blumberg[8] recently have reported that "the biophotometer test does not appear to constitute an accurate or reliable technique for detecting mild degrees of vitamin A deficiency in the routine survey of school children." Palmer[9] further reported an investigation of the effect of vitamin A administration on the biophotometer dark adaptation measurements in school children. He states "The results showed no significant difference in the improvement in biophotometer measurements between a group of children whose diet was supplemented and a control group whose diet was not supplemented with vitamin A."

These reports were of extreme interest to us. We have subsequently obtained a biophotometer* as described by Jeans et al. and have made tests according to the technique and standards given in their report.

PROCEDURE

A group of average Toronto school children were tested on repeated occasions during the past year. They were tested on Saturday mornings so as to not interfere with school attendance. They came from all parts of the city with no special selection. The first test was made and it was repeated within three weeks, with no addition to the diet. The children were then given 13,000 units of 50 per cent oleum percomorphum† daily for three weeks, and then a third test was done. The oil was continued for a second three-week period, and a fourth test was made. As far as could be ascertained the children all took the oil.

RESULTS

Table I shows the comparison of the dark adaptation in the first test with the second test. Theoretically these two tests should show a marked degree of correlation as there was no change in the feeding routine in

TABLE I

A COMPARISON OF DARK ADAPTATION AS SHOWN BY THE FIRST TEST WITH THE SECOND TEST: NO CHANGE IN VITAMIN A INGESTION

	FIRST TEST	SECOND TEST		
		UNCHANGED	IMPROVED	DECREASED
Abnormal	17	11	6	–
Borderline	14	5	3	6
Normal	3	2	–	1
Total	34	18	9	7

the interval. Of 34 children, 18 gave readings in the same range on the second test, and 16 were different. Of those that changed, 9 improved and 7 decreased in dark adaptation.

Table II shows the comparison in 34 subjects of the dark adaptation in the second test which was made prior to the administration of vitamin A, with the third test made after three weeks of administration of

*Frober-Faybor Company.

†Kindly supplied by Mead Johnson & Company.

at least 13,000 international units of vitamin A. Theoretically one would expect the abnormal and borderline subjects to improve. Eight of 17 abnormal subjects and 3 of 8 borderline improved; one borderline decreased, and no less than 4 of 9 normal range subjects became borderline or abnormal.

TABLE II

A COMPARISON OF DARK ADAPTATION AS SHOWN BY THE SECOND TEST WITH THE THIRD TEST, MADE AFTER THREE WEEKS OF DAILY INGESTION OF VITAMIN A*

	SECOND TEST	THIRD TEST		
		UNCHANGED	IMPROVED	DECREASED
Abnormal	17	9	8	–
Borderline	8	4	3	1
Normal	9	5	–	4
Total	34	18	11	5

*At least 13,000 international units were used.

Table III shows the comparison in 24 subjects between the third test which was made after three weeks of vitamin A administration with the fourth test after six weeks of vitamin A administration. Three of 10 abnormal subjects improved and none of 6 borderline improved; 3 of 6 borderline subjects decreased, and 3 of 8 normal became borderline or abnormal subjects.

TABLE III

A COMPARISON OF DARK ADAPTATION AS SHOWN BY THE THIRD TEST, MADE AFTER THREE WEEKS OF INGESTION OF ADDITIONAL VITAMIN A, WITH THE FOURTH TEST, MADE AFTER INGESTION OF ADDITIONAL VITAMIN A FOR SIX WEEKS

	THIRD TEST	FOURTH TEST		
		UNCHANGED	IMPROVED	DECREASED
Abnormal	10	7	3	–
Borderline	6	3	–	3
Normal	8	5	–	3
Total	24	15	3	6

Table IV shows the comparison in 24 subjects between the second test and the fourth test, or before and after six weeks of vitamin A administration, during which time 13,000 international units of vitamin A were administered daily. Three of 13 abnormal subjects and 2 of 6 borderline improved; 1 borderline and 2 of 5 normal range subjects decreased.

TABLE IV

A COMPARISON OF DARK ADAPTATION OF THE SECOND TEST, MADE PRIOR TO ADMINISTRATION OF ADDITIONAL VITAMIN A, WITH THE FOURTH TEST, MADE AFTER A PERIOD OF SIX WEEKS*

	SECOND TEST	FOURTH TEST		
		UNCHANGED	IMPROVED	DECREASED
Abnormal	13	10	3	–
Borderline	6	3	2	1
Normal	5	3	–	2
Total	24	16	5	3

*Thirteen thousand units of vitamin A were administered daily during this period.

DISCUSSION

The results shown above are variable and have very little consistency. Hecht et al.,[10] in investigating dark adaptation, have shown that certain factors play a part which may explain the inconsistencies observed with the use of the Birch-Hirschfeld instrument and biophotometer. They pointed out that dark adaptation to ordinary bright light was a factor of both rods and cones. The cones adapted very rapidly, approximately ten times as fast as the rods, and had completely recovered in three to five minutes. Adaptation to red light was mainly by the cones. Adaptation to violet light corresponded to the usual cone adaptation seen with ordinary bright light, after which it followed the curve of rod adaptation, but the subject stated that the light appeared colorless during this latter period. These observers showed that the time of complete cone adaptation and appearance of rod adaptation varied with normal individuals to quite a large degree, but the shape of the curves was similar. They found that the shape of curve for adaptation could not be drawn from the average of a number of individuals because this flattened out the dividing portion between cone and rod adaptation. They also found a rapid and a delayed type of rod adaptation. The former was thought to be due to regeneration of the visual purple that had been changed by exposure to bright light, and the latter, due to a new formation from fresh substances in retina and blood stream; this formation is only called into play when there is extreme destruction of visual purple following exposure to very bright light. In the method used by these observers the test light entered the eye from an angle, and also it was intermittent. This would be difficult to manage with young children. Obviously from the report of the above authors the measurement of dark adaptation is a complicated process and requires a much more difficult technique than is at present used with the biophotometer.

CONCLUSIONS

We have found the biophotometer unsatisfactory as a method of estimation in children of the variations in dark adaptation such as might be produced by vitamin A deficiency.

REFERENCES

1. Tisdall, F. F.: Practice of Pediatrics, Brenneman, vol. 1, chapter xxxii, 1937, W. E. Prior, Inc.
2. Jeans, P. C., and Zentmire, Z.: J. A. M. A. **102**: 892, 1934.
3. Jeans, P. C., and Zentmire, Z.: J. A. M. A. **106**: 996, 1936.
4. Maitra, M. K., and Harris, L. J.: Lancet **2**: 1009, 1937.
5. Snelling, C. E.: J. Pediat. **9**: 655, 1936.
6. Jeans, P. C., Blanchard, E., and Zentmire, Z.: J. A. M. A. **108**: 451, 1937.
7. Jeghers, H.: J. A. M. A. **109**: 756, 1937.
8. Palmer, C. E., and Blumberg, H.: Reprint No. 1866 from the Pub. Health Rep. **52**: 1403, 1936.
9. Palmer, C. E.: Am. J. Pub. Health **28**: 309, 1938.
10. Hecht, S., Haig, C., and Chase, A. M.: J. Gen. Physiol. **20**: 831, 1937.

THE NEW TUBERCULIN PATCH TEST

W. DEAN STEWARD, M.D.
CHATTANOOGA, TENN.

THE object of this paper is to discuss the tuberculin patch test recently described by Vollmer and Goldberger,* and to point out its ease of application and its reliability. Although previous attempts have been made to produce a successful patch or plaster test for tuberculosis, none have been satisfactory. It is not within the scope of this paper to discuss these reasons, nor to discuss the history of the tuberculin test in its various forms.

At the Pine Breeze Sanatorium patch tests† were run on ninety-one tuberculous children in the institution, and on five normal adults. In all but two instances, coincidental Mantoux tests (dilution 1:1000 O. T.‡) were performed. On these two patients recent Mantoux tests had been strongly positive.

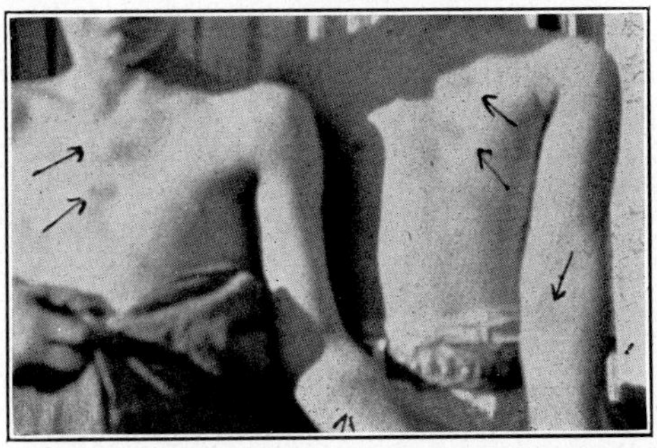

Fig. 1.—Mantoux test and patch test.

Half of the patch tests were prepared from old beef extract medium, and the remaining half were prepared with the use of a synthetic medium made after Siebert's formula. No discrimination was made between the two types. They were applied in rotation—first one, then the other, etc.

The results of this series show the reliability of the patch test as compared with the Mantoux test. Ninety (93.75 per cent) of the persons

TABLE I

	CASES	PERCENTAGE
Conformity between Mantoux and patch tests	90	93.75%
Positive patch test—negative Mantoux test	6	6.25%
Negative patch test—positive Mantoux test	0	0%

*Vollmer, H., and Goldberger, E. W.: Am. J. Dis. Child. 54: 1019, 1937.
†Furnished for this study by The Lederle Laboratories, Inc.
‡Furnished by City Health Department. Made from Lot No. 491, Parke, Davis & Company.

tested gave parallel results between the patch test and the Mantoux test. All of the remaining six (6.25 per cent) showed a positive patch test and a negative Mantoux. There was only a slight difference recorded with the two types of patch tests.

TABLE II

COMPARISON BETWEEN (1) BEEF EXTRACT MEDIUM AND (2) SYNTHETIC MEDIUM MADE ACCORDING TO SIEBERT'S FORMULA

	TOTAL CASES		CASES	PERCENTAGE
(1)	48	Conformity of patch and Mantoux*	46	95.83%
		Positive patch and negative Mantoux	2	4.17%
(2)	48	Conformity of patch and Mantoux*	44	91.66%
		Positive patch and negative Mantoux	4	8.33%

*Including one case each in which recent Mantoux was positive.

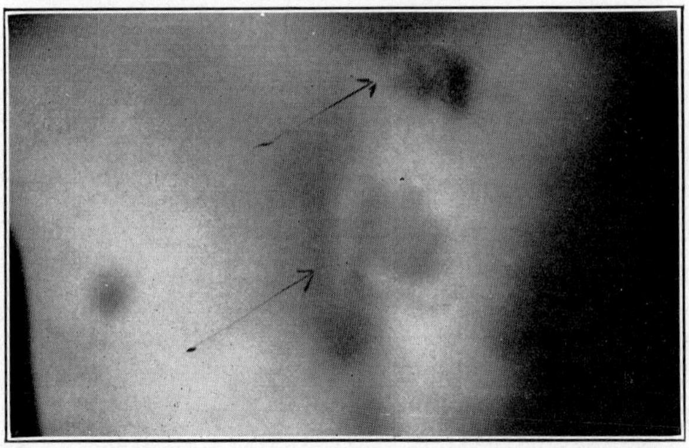

Fig. 2.—Close-up of patch test.

In twenty-four cases (25 per cent of entire group) there was some reaction in the skin, due either to the control patch or to the adhesive plaster. In no instance was it marked enough to interfere with the reading and reliability of the test.

The above figures would lead one to believe that the patch test, as described by Vollmer and Goldberger, is at least as efficient as the Mantoux test when used for routine testing purposes.

In performing and recording a series like the above, several interesting and worth-while facts are noted. In the first place, many children feared the needle, but none feared the ether cleansing and adhesive tape. Secondly, numerous severe local reactions occurred following the Mantoux test. These included several cases with adenitis and occasional ones with lymphangitis. None of the patch tests produced more than transitory itching. Thirdly, the ease of application is important. The patch test can be applied rapidly, even by an inexperienced person. Contact is always obtained. There is no chance of misplacing the tuberculin as occurs in the Mantoux test when the needle is accidentally introduced subcutaneously because of movement on the part of the child.

A factor equally as important as the above is the availability of the patch test to the general practitioner and pediatrician. It removes the necessity of keeping O. T. in stock and also the trouble of preparing dilutions from the stock mixture. Since it comes in a dried form, it should keep indefinitely.

CONCLUSIONS

1. The tuberculin patch test of Vollmer was tried on ninety-six persons, ninety-one of whom were children in a tuberculosis sanatorium. 90 (93.75 per cent) showed conformity between the patch test and the Mantoux test in a 1:1000 dilution. The remaining 6 (6.25 per cent) showed positive patch test and negative Mantoux test.

2. The patch test was found to be as reliable as the Mantoux test.

3. Equally good results were obtained with patch tests prepared from old beef extract medium and with synthetic medium from Siebert's formula.

4. The test is painless and children do not fear it because no instruments are required.

5. Severe local and constitutional reactions do not occur, and there is no danger of infection.

6. It should prove of great service to the general practitioner and the pediatrician in the diagnosis of tuberculosis during childhood.

RELATION OF INTESTINAL BLEEDING TO HETEROTOPIC GASTRIC MUCOSA AND ULCERATION IN MECKEL'S DIVERTICULUM

ALFRED L. ABRAMS, M.D.
NEW YORK, N. Y.

IN ORDER to elucidate the relationship of intestinal bleeding from a Meckel's diverticulum to the type of mucosa existing in the diverticulum and to the occurrence of ulceration in the mucosa, the series of surgical and autopsy cases at the Babies Hospital has been reviewed along the following lines. First, on the pathologic side, the incidence of heterotopic gastric mucosa and of mucosal ulceration, gross and microscopic, was determined in all the cases of Meckel's diverticulum in which this question had been investigated histologically or in which material was still available for suitable study. Second, on the clinical side, the occurrence of intestinal bleeding in these cases was determined from the history by checking the progress notes for hematemesis, melena, and tarry stools, from the laboratory reports by reviewing the chemical tests for blood, and from the nurses' notes by evaluating descriptions of vomitus and stools. Since this is presented as the experience of one hospital rather than as a compilation, no other reference will be made to the literature except to the work of Schullinger and Stout,[1] which carries an extensive bibliography.

Of a total of eighty-eight cases of Meckel's diverticulum in our files, nine were surgical, and seventy-nine (or an incidence of 1.3 per cent in all our autopsies) were post-mortem specimens. Clinical reports were lacking on one case in each group, leaving a total of eighty-six. Of these eighty-six cases we have complete data—clinical, gross, and microscopic pathology—in seventeen cases (nine autopsy and eight surgical). These seventeen cases form the chief basis for this report, and the findings in the remaining sixty-nine will be summarized briefly.

Of the nine autopsy cases, in all of which Meckel's diverticulum was an adventitious finding unrelated to cause of death, two contained heterotopic gastric mucosa, none exhibited mucosal ulceration, and in only one was there evidence of intestinal bleeding. In the latter case the terminal coffee ground vomitus was ascribed to uremia.

Of the eight surgical cases, five exhibited intestinal bleeding, seven contained gastric mucosa, and two were ulcerated, one grossly in the intestinal type mucosa, the other microscopically in the heterotopic gastric mucosa. There seemed a definite relationship between intestinal bleeding and heterotopic gastric mucosa, since all five bleeding cases exhibited gastric mucosa. However, two of the three nonbleeding patients also exhibited gastric mucosa. There was no definite relation of intestinal bleeding to ulceration, since of the five bleeders only one exhibited ulcera-

From the Babies Hospital and Department of Diseases of Children, Columbia University Medical School, New York.

tion, whereas of the three nonbleeding patients, one was also ulcerated. The one case showing ulceration of heterotopic gastric mucosa was not associated with intestinal bleeding. Thus, in the combined surgical and autopsy series of seventeen cases, ulceration was present in no case without heterotopic gastric mucosa, and of the nine cases containing heterotopic gastric mucosa, ulceration occurred in only two. In one of these latter two cases ulceration was located in the heterotopic gastric mucosa, and in the other in the intestinal type mucosa.

Thus, five of the seventeen cases exhibited intestinal bleeding attributable to no other cause than coexisting Meckel's diverticulum; nine contained heterotopic gastric mucosa; two were ulcerated. All five of the bleeders contained heterotopic gastric mucosa, but in none was it ulcerated; four of the twelve nonbleeding patients also contained gastric mucosa, which was ulcerated in one. It might be derived tentatively that if intestinal bleeding is encountered with Meckel's diverticulum, the presence of heterotopic gastric mucosa is likely.

In the sixty-nine additional autopsy cases we are justified in the main, for lack of more specific gross description and microscopic sections, only in correlating intestinal bleeding with the presence of a Meckel's diverticulum, and this only when other sources of intestinal bleeding have been ruled out. In three cases of the sixty-nine such intestinal bleeding was detected.

In summary, Table I expresses the relationship of ulceration and of heterotopic gastric mucosa to the bleeding syndrome, as shown in this series of cases.

Table I

Histologic Picture in Meckel's Diverticulum, With Relation to the Bleeding Syndrome

	Surgical Cases		Autopsy Cases		Total
	With Bleeding	Without Bleeding	With Bleeding	Without Bleeding	
Heterotopic gastric mucosa	5	2	0	2	9
Ulceration in heterotopic gastric mucosa	0	1	0	0	1
Ulceration in intestinal type of mucosa	1	0	0	0	1
No bleeding source discovered	4	–	–	–	4
Total cases examined histologically	8		9		17

CONCLUSION

The conclusions drawn from the material available for this survey are:

1. Intestinal bleeding in the clinical syndrome Meckel's diverticulum indicated the presence of heterotopic gastric mucosa, but in our series ulceration was rarely found.

2. Heterotopic gastric mucosa was present in many cases and in a fair number occurred without intestinal bleeding.

REFERENCE

1. Schullinger and Stout: Arch. Surg. 28: 440, 1934.

THE NERVOUS SYSTEM IN ACRODYNIA

Review of the Literature and Report of a Case

Albert J. Lubin and Harold K. Faber, M.D.
San Francisco, Calif.

ALTHOUGH acrodynia has become a well-defined and fairly common clinical entity, reported examinations of the nervous system are not only somewhat meager but are conflicting. The confusion is evident not only in locating the site of the lesion, but also in the type of cellular response noted. This great variance in findings is demonstrated in the accompanying tabulation, which includes all of the available pathologic descriptions.

The original description of acrodynia was published by O. Selter[1] in 1903. In 1914 Swift[2] reported a series of cases in Australia. Since that time it has gone under a variety of names: "Selter-Swift-Feer's Disease," "pink disease," "erythroedema," "dermatopolyneuritis," "trophodermatoneurosis," and "vegetative neurosis." It appears in young children, chiefly "toddlers," and has been said to have occurred in epidemics. The onset is usually insidious. Changes in the disposition, such as apathy, may appear first. The extremities become swollen and podgy, and erythematous rashes appear on the skin. Hyperesthesias and pruritis are common. Signs of dysfunction of the autonomic nervous system include profuse sweating, digestive disorders, tachycardia and hypertension, dilatation of the pupils and photophobia, increased metabolic rate, alopecia neurotica, rhinorrhea, sialorrhea, vasomotor disturbances in the extremities, and trophic ulcers. Occasionally muscular weakness is the first symptom, and the deep reflexes often disappear. In severe cases this weakness is followed by paralysis. Pleocytosis and increase of spinal fluid protein have been noted. The prognosis is usually good, and complete recovery occurs in three to nine months. Emaciation or intercurrent infection is the cause of death in a few cases.

SUMMARY OF NEUROPATHOLOGIC CHANGES REPORTED

Spinal Cord.—Of the total of thirty-seven cases reported, nothing abnormal was noted in eighteen. Four cases showed only a slight diffuse increase of small round cells. Edema without inflammatory infiltration was observed in two cases. One case contained inflammatory nodules, consisting mostly of lymphocytes, near the entrance of the dorsal roots. Involvement of nerve cells was described in twelve cases. One of these consisted of vacuolar degeneration of posterior horn cells, one of poorly stained anterior horn cells, and one of a few swollen anterior horn cells. Distinct chromatolysis of nerve cells was cited in nine cases; in seven of these it was confined to anterior horn cells, in one to cells of the anterior horns, lateral horns, and Clarke's column, and in another to cells of the lateral horns, with lesser changes in the anterior horns.

From the Division of Neuropsychiatry (Neuropathology Laboratory) and the Department of Pediatrics, Stanford University School of Medicine.

In eleven cases a diffuse increase of small round cells was noted, Willie and Stern reporting seven of these. Myelin sheath abnormalities were observed in only three instances, and in two of these it was mild.

No abnormalities noted		18
Slight increase of small round cells		4
Edema without inflammatory reaction		2
Inflammatory nodules		1
Nerve cell involvement		12
posterior horn cells	1	
anterior horn cells alone	9	
anterior and lateral horn cells	1	
anterior and lateral horn cells and cells of Clarke's column	1	
Total		37

Brain.—No pathologic manifestations were noted in eighteen cases. In another ten the changes were nonspecific, consisting of generalized congestion, edema, hyperemia, anemia, or slight increase of small round cells. In seven cases there was involvement of the region adjacent to the third ventricle, postulated as the site of the diencephalic sympathetic center. In two cases the lesions were widely scattered throughout various portions of the brain.

No abnormalities noted	18
Nonspecific changes, as edema and congestion	10
Involvement of sympathetic center in diencephalon	7
Scattered lesions	2
Total	37

Peripheral Nerves.—Involvement of peripheral nerves was described in twelve instances. Actual degeneration of myelin sheaths or axis cylinders was present in seven of these. Chromatolysis of cells in the gasserian ganglion was noted in two cases. In nine cases there was specific mention that no abnormalities were found in the peripheral nerves.

Sympathetic Nervous System.—The peripheral sympathetic system was involved in eight cases. In one case many nerve cells with two nuclei were found; lymphocytic infiltration was described in three cases; in two cases there was neuronophagia in addition to the lymphocytic infiltration; in another two cases there was marked neuronophagia and cellular degeneration. There is specific mention that no abnormalities were found in eight cases. There were few cases, however, in which adequate examination was made of the paravertebral chain ganglia and their peripheral connections.

Vagus Nerve.—Some degeneration was noted in one instance.

Peripheral nerve involvement	12
Sympathetic nerve involvement	8
Gasserian ganglion, chromatolysis	2
Vagus degeneration, mild	1
Dorsal root involvement	9

Table I

Neuropathologic Changes Described in Acrodynia

AUTHOR	SPINAL CORD AND ROOTS	BRAIN	PERIPHERAL AND SYMPATHETIC NERVES
Byfield (1920)	A few anterior horn cells stained poorly; gliosis around central canal; some variation in fiber size in lumbar posterior roots with edema and swelling of myelin sheaths.		Edema of myelin sheaths and connective tissue about nerve fibers in sciatic nerve.
Paterson and Greenfield (1923) 2 cases	Slight diffuse increase of small cells, apparently glial, in cervical and lumbosacral enlargements and in roots (especially dorsal roots).	Cortex, thalamus, and pons negative.	Vagus and cervical sympathetic nerves negative; nuclei appeared to be more numerous in brachial plexus but median nerve was negative.
	Capillary congestion and diffuse increase of small cells in cord and roots; swelling, eccentric nuclei, and chromatolysis of anterior horn cells, most marked in lumbosacral region.	Negative.	Myelin degeneration in internal and external popliteal nerves; most marked distally; some changes in lumbar nerve.
Helmholz (1925)		Negative.	Definite nerve changes.
Howland (1925)	Cord negative	Negative.	Few changes but not enough to warrant diagnosis of peripheral neuritis.
Warthin (1926) 2 cases	Cord and roots negative except for edema of meninges.	Marked congestion and edema of meninges with proliferation of reticulo - endothelial cells.	
	Perivascular edema; no degenerative or inflammatory changes.	Marked congestion and edema of brain and meninges and marked proliferation of reticulo-endothelial cells.	
Feer (Vetter) (1925)	Cord negative		Sympathetic nerves negative.
Woringer (1926)		Brain edematous; some macrophagic foci at posterior commissure of third ventricle.	Many cells in sympathetic ganglion with two nuclei, some with chromaffin granules.
Kernohan and Kennedy (1928)	Chromatolysis of anterior horn cells, especially in ventrolateral group in sacral region; lateral horn cells and cells of Clarke's column involved in thoracic region; apparent increase in glia; no one cell group completely involved; chromatolysis in posterior root ganglia, especially at lumbar level.	Advanced chromatolysis in floor of fourth ventricle, locus caeruleus, mesencephalic root of fifth nerve, lenticular nucleus, anterior nucleus of thalamus.	Myelin sheath disintegration and swollen, nodular axis cylinders, especially in sciatic and femoral nerves; marked chromatolysis in gasserian ganglia.

TABLE I—CONT'D

AUTHOR	SPINAL CORD AND ROOTS	BRAIN	PERIPHERAL AND SYMPATHETIC NERVES
Francioni and Vigi (1928) (developed after epidemic encephalitis)		Chromatolysis, eccentric nuclei, and some shadow cells in infundibulum and tuber cinereum; dissipation of lesions toward hypothalamus.	Perivascular collars of small round cells in cervical sympathetic ganglia.
Findlay and Stern (1929)	Small round cell infiltration in cord and along posterior roots; early anterior horn cell changes.	Small round cell infiltration in medulla; negative above medulla.	Cervical and abdominal sympathetic ganglia negative.
Orton and Bender (1931) (review of Byfield's case)	Chromatolysis, sclerosis, and destruction of many lateral horn cells; loss of myelin sheaths, glial increase, small hemorrhages in lateral horns; chromatolysis of anterior horn cells without glial reaction.		
Willie and Stern (1931) 7 cases	Slight anterior horn cell chromatolysis with some satellitosis in seventh cervical segment; advanced changes in anterior horn cells in fourth and fifth lumbar; slight round cell infiltration; some myelin degeneration.	Negative.	Beading and fragmentation in sciatic nerve and brachial plexus.
	Few swollen anterior horn cells; diffuse infiltration of small round cells; fat droplets in dorsal roots.	Increased vascularity of cortex; slight small cell infiltration in cortex and medulla.	Negative.
	Some anterior horn cell chromatolysis in lumbar region; small cell infiltration, especially in dorsal horns.	Small round cell infiltration in cortex and basal ganglia.	Negative.
	Slight excess of small cells.	Negative.	Negative.
	Few rounded anterior horn cells in cervical enlargement; slight chromatolysis in anteromedial group in third and fourth lumbar; small round cell infiltration.	Negative.	Fat globules along course of all peripheral nerves, especially median.
	Chromatolysis and few eccentric nuclei in anterior horn cells of lumbar enlargement; small cell infiltration.	Negative.	Early degeneration of peripheral nerves, especially near Ranvier's nodes.
	Slight increase of round cells.	Negative.	Some degeneration of vagus fibers.

TABLE I—CONT'D

AUTHOR	SPINAL CORD AND ROOTS	BRAIN	PERIPHERAL AND SYMPATHETIC NERVES
Soós (1931)		Brain substance soft, doughy, and anemic.	Marked differences in size, pyknotic and absent nuclei, poorly stained tigroid substance, and marked neuronophagia in cells of solar and paravertebral chain ganglia.
de Lange (1932)	Spinal cord negative; chromatolysis and eccentric nuclei in posterior root ganglia.	Circumscribed frontal meningitis, perivascular infiltration in pia-arachnoid; increase of glia (especially microglia) without neuronophagia in infundibulotuberous region and "gliaknötchen"; less marked glial increase in midbrain, locus caeruleus, putamen, globus pallidus, and right dentate nucleus; changes not found in controls.	Chromatolysis and eccentric nuclei in gasserian ganglion.
Bellocq and Meyer (1932)	Some degeneration and vacuolization of posterior horn cells.	Cellular lesions and neuronophagia in the infundibulotuberous region and along the walls of the third ventricle.	Numerous foci of neuronophagia and cellular degeneration in sympathetic chain ganglia; myelin degeneration in crural and intraspinal nerves.
Blackfan and McKhann (1933) 5 cases	Examination of the central nervous system, peripheral nerves, and sympathetic nervous system failed to disclose changes which could not be related to the terminal infection.		
Braithwaite (1933) 2 cases	Cord negative.	Brain injected; increase in cerebrospinal fluid; apparent increase in neuroglial cells of white matter.	
	Cord negative.	Brain congested and edematous; glia slightly edematous.	
Wolf and Davison (1934)	Chromatolysis and vacuolization in nucleus ventralis of eleventh nerve and anterior horn cells; mild disintegration of single fibers in spino-olivary, spinocerebellar, and lateral pyramidal tracts.	Slight disarrangement of all layers of cortex, especially third; some chromatolysis and falling out of cells, slight increase in glia in cortex; swelling of ganglion cells in basal ganglia; severe cell changes in locus caeruleus; absence of fibrillary processes, lack of chromatin, and swelling of Purkinje cells in cerebellum; some swelling of ganglion cells about fourth ventricle and pons.	Early disintegration and swelling of myelin, early axis cylinder changes in peripheral nerves, more advanced in lower extremities.

TABLE I—CONT'D

AUTHOR	SPINAL CORD AND ROOTS	BRAIN	PERIPHERAL AND SYMPATHETIC NERVES
Deamer and Biskind (1934)	Spinal cord negative; chromatolysis and neuronophagia in thoracic posterior roots.	Negative.	Chromatolysis and neuronophagia in sympathetic chain ganglia with phagocytic cell infiltration resembling tubercle of rabies; sympathetic ganglia of thoracic aorta negative; slight spreading of bundles of vagus and sciatic nerves.
Fessler (1935)		Hyperemia and edema of brain; internal hydrocephalus.	
Mouriquand, Dechaume, Bernheim, and Weill (1935)	Inflammatory nodules, consisting mostly of lymphocytes, in thoracic region near entry of dorsal roots; lymphocytic infiltration and satellitosis of ganglion cells in dorsal root ganglion.	Brain congested; slight inflammation, perivascular cuffing of lymphocytes and plasma cells in meninges; nodules of lymphocytes or glia in supraoptic nuclei; vascular congestion and distention of perivascular sheaths around third ventricle.	Lymphocytic masses, perivascular cuffing, lymphocytic invasion of stroma, satellitosis and pseudoneuronophagia, and some neuronophagia in coeliac and cervical sympathetic ganglia; peripheral nerves negative.
Pehu, Dechaume, and Boucomont (1936)	Cord and roots negative.	Perivascular cuffing and lymphocytic infiltration in meninges; marked congestion, and engorgement of vessels, leucocytic thrombi in region of third ventricle; lymphoplasmocytic infiltration, as partial perivascular cuffs, near vegetative nuclei in walls of third ventricle.	Increase of lymphocytes, perivascularly and in stroma, and of satellite cells in sympathetic ganglia.
Mouriquand, Dechaume, and Sédallian (1936)	Cord negative.	Congestion of small vessels with hemorrhages in perivascular spaces in walls of third ventricle; similar changes in cerebral cortex.	Perivascular lymphocytic infiltration in coeliac ganglion.
Harris (1935)	Small round cell infiltration and well-marked chromatolysis of anterior horn cells in spinal cord.	Congestion of cortical vessels; small round cell infiltration; but no degeneration.	Patchy demyelinization in most peripheral nerves, especially in left phrenic and left sciatic nerves and in right brachial plexus; both vagi negative.

Dorsal Roots and Ganglia.—Abnormalities in the dorsal roots were present in nine cases. In four this consisted of an increase or infiltration of small round cells, in three there was chromatolysis of ganglion cells, in one fat droplets were noted, and in one there was edema.

CASE REPORT

P. R., a boy, 2 years and 10 months old, entered the hospital May 25, 1935, with bronchopneumonia. He had had a previous attack of pneumonia in December, 1934, accompanied by otorrhea and tonsillitis.

In February, 1935, he became listless, his legs became weak, and all of his extremities cold and pink, turning definitely red in a few days. His temperature was slightly elevated. There was profuse sweating. When he was placed on his feet, he showed evidence of discomfort. Later in the month his feet scaled, and the distal phalanges of the fingers became swollen and puffy. He slept in grotesque positions and was very irritable. His appetite was poor, and he lost a slight amount of weight. During March he became somewhat worse. In April an abscess developed in the right ear and was drained. Swelling of the hands increased and also appeared in the feet. The child was unable to walk. During the next month the paralysis increased and involved both arms and legs. The pink color disappeared. On May 23 a cough developed, he became prostrated, breathing became difficult, and the temperature rose to 102.2° F., dropping to 101.6° F. the next day when he entered the hospital.

Physical Examination.—He was a well-developed but malnourished boy, breathing rapidly and coughing frequently. There was marked scaling and thickening of the epidermis of the extremities. The tonsils were reddened but not enlarged. The percussion note was dull over the entire right side of the chest; the breath sounds were diminished and were bronchial in character posteriorly. X-ray films revealed collapse of the right middle and upper lobes.

The neurological examination showed a flaccid paralysis of both legs with absent knee and ankle jerks. No pathologic reflexes were elicited. Both biceps and triceps reflexes on the right were not obtained. There was marked weakness of both upper extremities. The electrical reactions of the muscles were not impaired. The abdominal and cremasteric reflexes were absent. There was marked hyperalgesia.

Blood Count.—5,300,000 red cells; 95 per cent hemoglobin; 47,800 white cells, with 85 per cent polymorphonuclears, of which 29 per cent were banded.

Course.—During the next few days he improved; the right lung expanded, and the white count decreased to 26,000 on May 29. But on June 1 the respiratory rate increased, the right lower lobe collapsed, and a mucous rattle was audible. Carbogen was given, but on the morning of June 2 the patient suddenly died. No cyanosis was present.

Autopsy.—Sections of skeletal muscle from the back, pectoral muscles, and diaphragm were normal. There was a slight fatty infiltration of the heart, but the muscle fibers were normal. Sections through the aorta were negative. Hassall corpuscles were quite numerous in the thymus; the cellular elements were normal. The lungs were moderately congested, and there were a few areas of collapse. In places the alveoli were filled with fluid and contained large mononuclears, lymphocytes, and polymorphonuclear leucocytes. The bronchi contained desquamated epithelial cells, a few lymphocytes and polymorphonuclears, and red cells; the mucosa was moderately infiltrated. Smears from the right middle lobe contained gram-positive cocci in pairs and short chains; no acid-fast bacilli were seen. A peribronchial lymph node was moderately congested and contained many leucocytes; the germinal centers were large and several mitotic figures were present.

Nothing abnormal was present in the gastrointestinal tract. The capsule and trabeculae of the spleen were normal; some large phagocytic cells in the pulp contained a small amount of brown pigment. Adrenal cortical cells contained moderate amounts of lipoid material.

Examination of the Nervous System.—Examination of the coeliac ganglion revealed nothing abnormal. Unfortunately no other part of the sympathetic nervous system and none of the peripheral nerves were available for examination.

Macroscopically there were no abnormalities in either the brain or spinal cord.

Celloidin sections were made from various portions of the brain and spinal cord. Nothing abnormal was found in the cortex, mesencephalon, pons, cerebellum, or medulla. Serial sections of the diencephalon from the level of the subthalamic nucleus through the tuber cinereum were studied. Careful examination was made of the paraventricular nucleus, the supraoptic nucleus, the nucleus of the tuber cinereum, the mammillary body, and the subthalamic nucleus (corpus luysi). There was no perivascular infiltration or increase of glia. Many of the cells contained eccentric nuclei and only small amounts of Nissl substance; pseudoneuronophagia was present in places. Such findings, however, were interpreted as normal in this portion of the brain. There was no true neuronophagia. The nuclei were of regular contour, the nuclear membranes were intact, and the nucleoli were not pyknotic. The cells were neither swollen nor shrunken, and no shadow forms were present.

In the spinal cord, sections through the cervical region were normal. The intermediolateral cell column in the thoracic region contained many degenerating cells. Extrusion of the nucleus, folding of the nuclear membrane, absence of Nissl bodies, vacuole formation, and occasional shadow forms were observed (Fig. 1). The cells of Clarke's column were larger than the anterior horn cells at the same level, and degenerative changes were seen in a few of them. Anterior horn cells in the cervical, thoracic, and upper lumbar segments were normal. The most striking changes were present in the lower lumbar and upper sacral regions, involving the anterior horn cells of the posterolateral cell column (Fig. 2). There were many round and swollen cells, marked central chromatolysis, eccentric nuclei, and vacuole formation. The nuclear membranes were often hyperchromatic and folded and the nucleoli pyknotic. In some cells the nuclei were missing or protruding. Shadow forms indicated advanced degeneration. Compared with the amount of cellular involvement, there was but little glial response. Satellitosis and neuronophagia were seen only in a few places. Frozen sections stained with the Cajal gold-sublimate method revealed no increase in neuroglia. No myelin sheath abnormalities were present with the Weigert stain.

DISCUSSION

The clinical picture of acrodynia clearly points in all cases to an involvement of the sympathetic nervous system. The symptomatology is so widespread that this involvement must necessarily be either localized in a center of sympathetic activity, as in the diencephalon, or diffuse throughout more peripheral portions of the sympathetic system. Pathologic changes have been located by various authors in the following places: (1) the diencephalic sympathetic centers, (2) the intermediolateral cell column in the spinal cord, (3) the paravertebral chain ganglia and the other peripheral sympathetic nervous pathways, and (4) the peripheral nerve trunks and posterior roots.

Francioni and Vigi,[10] de Lange,[15] and Bellocq and Meyer[16] described lesions in the region of the tuber cinereum and infundibulum; Mouriquand, et al,[22] noted inflammatory lesions in the region adjacent to the third ventricle. Orton and Bender[12] found the most marked changes in the intermediolateral cell column, in which sympathetic motor cells

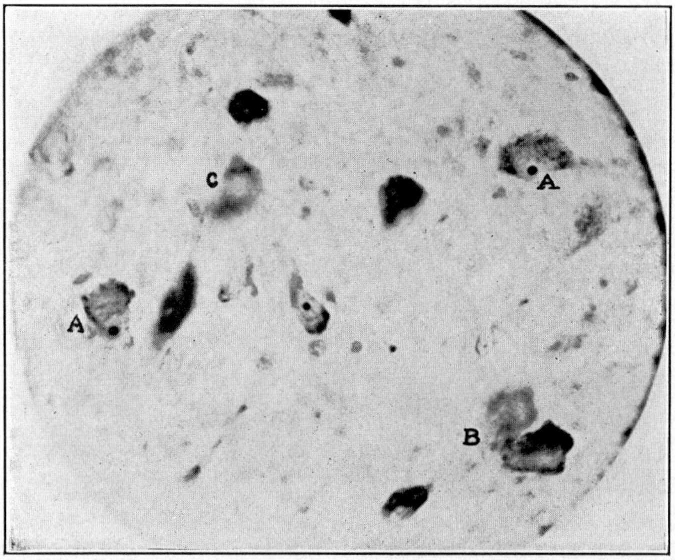

Fig. 1.—Extruding nuclei (A) and degenerated cells with absent nuclei (B) in intermediolateral cell column. A cell which is not in focus (C) contains a large vacuole. Cresyl violet stain.

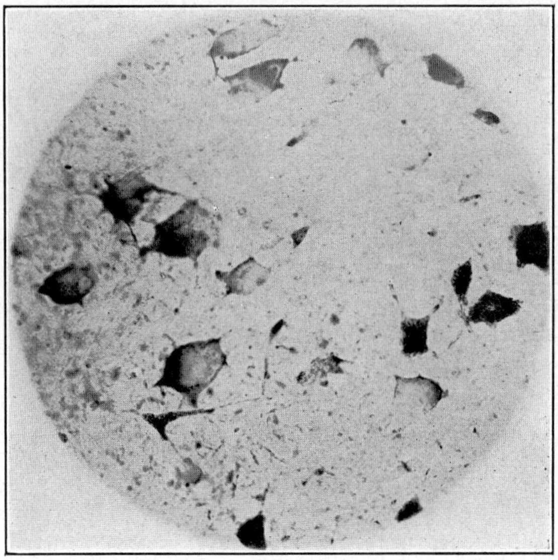

Fig. 2.—Anterior horn cells of the posterolateral cell column in the upper sacral region, showing marked swelling, chromatolysis, eccentric nuclei, and shadow forms. Cresyl violet stain.

form synapses with descending sympathetic pathways in the spinal cord and give off sympathetic neurones to the peripheral sympathetic ganglia. Kernohan and Kennedy[9] also noted involvement of this region, although merely as part of widespread damage. Soós[14] and others described neuronophagia in paravertebral and other sympathetic ganglia. Paterson and Greenfield[4] believed that the disease was a polyneuritis. Varying degrees of posterior root involvement were mentioned in nine cases.

Those findings in the diencephalon particularly warrant skepticism. Schwarz, Goolker, and Globus[24] have pointed out normal findings in infants' brains that are frequently misinterpreted as pathologic. This was in an attempt to disprove Goldzieher's theory that intestinal intoxication of infants (Goldzieher's ''diencephalitis dehydrans'') was due to cellular infiltration of the region adjacent to the walls of the third ventricle. They observed that discrete cellular aggregations, often perivascular, in this region were but normal manifestations of a ripening brain.

In the case described here interest was particularly focused on the diencephalic sympathetic nuclei. Serial sections through this region, including the subthalamic nucleus, the periventricular nuclei, and the tuber cinereum, failed to reveal anything which could be interpreted as pathologic. Eccentricity of nuclei and lack of centrally placed Nissl bodies were considered as normal in this area. Pathologic findings were all confined to the spinal cord. Involvement of anterior horn cells in the lumbosacral region and of cells of the intermediolateral cell column in the thoracic region were noted, the changes being especially striking in the anterior horn cells. These changes consisted of swelling and central chromatolysis, folding of the nuclear membrane, nuclear displacement, and shadow forms, but there was no marked glial reaction. Changes in the anterior horn cells explain the flaccid paralysis found in this case. The changes in the intermediolateral cell column, in which are located sympathetic motor cells, seem significant. In only two other cases (Kernohan and Kennedy[9] and Orton and Bender[12]), however, have similar changes been noted, so that it is difficult to evaluate whether they are of fundamental importance.

A review of the literature shows that reported changes in the nervous system are inconstant. Degenerative changes in anterior horn cells, as noted in this case, were lacking in many reports. For example, in Willie and Stern's series[13] of seven cases chromatolysis was not noted in two, was mild in four, and was advanced in only one case. In the same series varying degrees of peripheral nerve involvement were found in four cases, and there were no changes in three; in two of the cases small cell infiltration in the cerebrum was mentioned and was not found in five.

Failure in finding constant and fundamental pathologic changes, however, is not without precedent in diseases of the nervous system. Honeyman[25] has reported four fatal cases of acute febrile polyneuritis (or neuronitis) in which a detailed and systematic histopathologic examination failed to reveal any significant changes. The etiology of this condition, as is the case with acrodynia, is not known. There is evidence indicating that infections or toxins may ascend in the perineural lymph spaces and pass through large areas of the nervous system without leaving behind evidence that is demonstrable by modern methods.

A glance at the summary of the pathologic studies will make it clear that many of them have not been systematic or thorough. The vascular changes, forming so constant and characteristic a feature of the clinical picture, suggest that alterations in the sympathetic fibers of the peripheral blood vessels might be found, but they apparently have not been sought. Detailed studies of all of the sympathetic ganglia have rarely been made. This is, of course, the more surprising since the constant and characteristic features of the disease are those of disturbed sympathetic function. The present study will best serve its purpose if it encourages more detailed examinations of the entire nervous system, with special emphasis on its autonomic components. While previous studies and the present one have failed to show any constant lesions, either in occurrence, character, or distribution, nevertheless nervous lesions have been noted frequently enough to indicate quite strongly that a specific etiologic agent with special effects on the nervous tissues actually exists. Since clinically the disease appears to be of an infectious nature, further search is certainly desirable for a specific virus or perhaps a bacterial agent with toxic properties.

SUMMARY

1. The findings in the nervous system in a case of acrodynia are reported.

2. No pathologic changes were found in serial sections through the diencephalic sympathetic nuclei. This fails to support the belief that this region is the primary focus of involvement.

3. Degenerative changes were present in the anterior horn cells of the lumbosacral region and in the intermediolateral cell column of the spinal cord.

4. A review of the literature and the data supplied by the present case show that while alterations in the nervous system are not infrequently observed, they are not constant in occurrence, kind, or localization and hence do not offer a satisfactory explanation of the clinical picture.

5. Since the latter, nevertheless, quite consistently points to a disturbance in the sympathetic nervous system, it is desirable that further and more systematic search for lesions in this system be made.

REFERENCES

1. Selter, P.: Arch. f. Kinderh. **80**: 244, 1927.
2. Wood, A. J.: M. J. Australia **1**: 145, 1921.
3. Byfield, A. H.: Am. J. Dis. Child. **20**: 347, 1920.
4. Paterson, D., and Greenfield, J. G.: Quart. J. Med. **17**: 6, 1923.
5. Helmholz and Howland, in Discussion of Rodda, F. C.: Am. J. Dis. Child. **30**: 597, 1925.
6. Warthin, A. S.: Arch. Path. & Lab. Med. **1**: 64, 1926.
7. Feer, E.: Jahrb. f. Kinderh. **108**: 267, 1925.
8. Woringer, P.: Rev. franç. de pédiat. **2**: 440, 1926.
9. Kernohan, J. W., and Kennedy, R. L. J.: Am. J. Dis. Child. **36**: 341, 1928.
10. Francioni, C., and Vigi, F.: Bull. d. sc. med. Bologna **6**: 66, 1928; Riv. sper. di freniat. **52**: 307, 1928.
11. Findlay, G. M., and Stern, R. O.: Arch. Dis. Childhood **4**: 1, 1929.
12. Orton, S. T., and Bender, L.: Bull. Neurol. Inst. New York **1**: 506, 1931.
13. Willie, W. G., and Stern, R. O.: Arch. Dis. Childhood **6**: 137, 1931.
14. Soós, J.: Centralb. f. allg. Path. u. path. Anat. **53**: 211, 1931.
15. de Lange, C.: Jahrb. f. Kinderh. **136**: 193, 1932.
16. Bellocq, G. Ph., and Meyer, R.: Rev. franç. de pédiat. **8**: 495, 1932.
17. Blackfan, K., and McKhann, C. F.: J. Pediat. **3**: 45, 1933.
18. Braithwaite, J. V.: Arch. Dis. Childhood **8**: 1, 1933.
19. Wolf, I. J., and Davison, C.: J. Pediat. **4**: 498, 1934.
20. Deamer, W. C., and Biskind, G. R.: Am. J. Dis. Child. **48**: 1326, 1934.
21. Fessler, A.: Arch. f. Dermat. u. Syph. **173**: 283, 1935.
22. Mouriquand, G., Dechaume, J., Bernheim, and Weill, L.: Lyon méd. **156**: 203, 1935; Pehu, M., Dechaume, J., and Boucomont, J.: Lyon méd. **157**: 301, 1936; Mouriquand, G., Dechaume, J., and Sédallian, P.: Lyon méd. **158**: 210, 1936; Pehu, M., Dechaume, J., and Boucomont, J.: Rev. franç. de pédiat. **12**: 239, 1936.
23. Harris, C. F.: St. Barth. Hosp. Rep. **68**: 137, 1935.
24. Schwarz, H., Goolker, P., and Globus, J. H.: Am. J. Dis. Child. **43**: 889, 1932.
25. Honeyman, W. M.: Bull. Neurol. Inst. New York **6**: 519, 1937.

SULFANILAMIDE IN THE TREATMENT OF GONORRHEAL OPHTHALMIA IN CHILDREN

Merrill W. Michels, M.D.
Detroit, Mich.

SINCE the introduction of the Credé method of prophylaxis, the incidence of ophthalmia neonatorum has not diminished to the extent that many anticipated. Ernst Fuchs, in 1884,[1] reported the statistics of Credé to the effect that the incidence of this disease had diminished from 10.8 per cent to 0.1 to 0.2 per cent following the introduction of the use of silver nitrate. More recent information has shown that ophthalmia neonatorum is responsible for more cases of blindness today than from any other affection. McKee[2] states that 10 per cent of the 300,000 blind persons in Europe and 30 to 60 per cent of all those in asylums were rendered so by this disease. Surveys by Mayou[3] in London have shown that the number of cases has not materially decreased in a fifteen-year period. Lehrfeld[1] found a similar situation in Philadelphia; the Department of Public Health records investigated showed no diminution despite the generalized application of the Credé method of antisepsis. In those hospitals in which ante-partum antisepsis of the expectant mother known to have gonorrhea was carried out, there was not a single case of ophthalmia. Hospitals using no prenatal antisepsis showed 43.7 failures per 1,000 births, with a total of 535 cases. The inference is that the Credé method of prophylaxis is not being carried out as originally described and is in need of revision to include antisepsis of the Neisserian-infected mother.

Ophthalmia occurs more frequently in infants than in adults, probably on the basis of the less effective mechanical barrier that is present. The cornea of the infant is only three cells in thickness, the ocular conjunctiva is much thinner than in adults, and with the mucoid changes occurring as a result of infection, the basement membrane is bared, allowing a ready entrance of organisms to the subconjunctival tissues. At birth there is little or no lymphoid tissue in the conjunctiva. There is a gradual increase in this type of tissue, but the rapidity with which it forms is dependent upon the amount of irritation present. This explains the thickened conjunctiva which occurs in the chronic state of ophthalmia.

Stephenson[4] reviewed the subject of ophthalmia thirty years ago and concluded after a thorough study of the literature that two-thirds

From the Department of Ophthalmology and Otolaryngology, Children's Hospital of Michigan, Detroit.
I wish to acknowledge the suggestions of Dr. H. L. Begle.

of all cases in the newborn infant were due to the gonococcus. May[5] agrees with these figures. In Bellows' series[6] of 188 cases, 45 per cent were due to the gonococcus. Thygeson,[7] however, found an incidence of less than 0.03 per cent in a series of 261 cases of ophthalmia neonatorum. He points out the common diagnostic error of confusing staphylococcus conjunctivitis and inclusion blenorrhea with gonorrheal ophthalmia. *Staphylococcus aureus* is the most frequent cause of abundant purulent secretion and mild conjunctival infiltration. This condition responds rapidly to treatment, in contradistinction to inclusion blenorrhea and gonorrheal ophthalmia. Thomas[8] reports 100 consecutive cases of purulent conjunctivitis in the newborn infant caused by a single strain of *Staphylococcus aureus,* probably transmitted by contamination.

During the last few years there has been nothing significant reported in the treatment of gonorrheal ophthalmia. Many of the commonly employed antiseptics are of little or no value in shortening the duration of the disease. Bellows has shown that argyrol, mercuric oxycyanide, and metaphen are without great beneficial effect in shortening the course of the disease. He found acriflavine 1:1,500 the most efficacious of the antiseptics tried.

Opinion varies concerning the value of gonococcal vaccines. Many writers, as McKee, state that vaccines are equal but in no way superior to whole milk. Mayou concludes that such vaccines are without any influence in shortening the duration of the disease.

There is also a divergent view concerning the value of foreign protein in the treatment of the ophthalmias. Brewster[9] has found them efficacious in the treatment of corneal ulcers. Hektoen[10] objects to the widespread and indiscriminate use of nonspecific foreign protein therapy as whole milk on the grounds that it may give rise to more or less permanent sensitizations. Bernstein[11] reports specific sensitization following the use of milk and advocates instead the use of a protein not closely related to the dietary or environmental proteins. It would seem wise to reduce all foreign protein administrations to a practical minimum.

In view of the numerous inadequacies of our present forms of therapy, any treatment which will reduce the length of hospitalization and decrease complications is acceptable. Following the accounts of Domagk[12] and later of Long,[13] Dees and Colston[14] were the first in this country to report on the use of sulfanilamide in the treatment of gonococcic infections. Marshall[15] showed that sulfanilamide is rapidly absorbed from the gastrointestinal tract, entering practically all the body fluids, and is excreted almost entirely in the urinary tract. Concerning its mode of action, Long[16] concluded that bacteriostasis occurs with sulfanilamide. Mellon[17] found no indication that phagocytosis is a factor in the mechanism of the drug.

Following favorable isolated reports and realizing the close relationship of the gonococcus to the meningococcus, we started the use of sulfanilamide in cases of gonorrheal ophthalmia. We have included in this series only cases of proved gonorrheal origin, determined by direct smear of the conjunctival scrapings or by culture on chocolate agar medium.

We have taken cases treated in the two-year period prior to the use of sulfanilamide as a control. These cases had repeated positive smears and were treated as follows:

1. Warm boric irrigations sufficient to keep the eyes free of discharge; irrigations were carried out every thirty minutes or more often as needed and decreased as the discharge diminished.

2. Instillation of antiseptics: argyrol, 20 to 25 per cent, was used every three to four hours after the irrigation.

3. Ice compresses were used only in cases with marked swelling and tumefaction of the lids. Care was used to avoid corneal maceration that accompanies the prolonged use of cold. Premature infants did not receive such treatment.

4. Silver nitrate, 1 per cent, was used in the more chronic cases with papillary thickening of the palpebral conjunctiva. Applications were made to the everted lids once daily.

5. Atropine sulfate, ½ to 1 per cent, was used in patients with marked spasm or corneal involvement.

6. Special measures, as external canthotomy and conjunctival flaps, were carried out as the case demanded. One group of four patients received foreign protein therapy in the form of sterile milk.

7. Daily eye smears were taken, and when three consecutive negative smears were obtained, the clinical examination giving support, the patient was removed from the isolation of the ophthalmia ward.

The control group consisted of thirty-two patients with an average hospital duration of 28.5 days. Four patients had corneal involvement, two going on to perforation. Eighteen patients had involvement of both eyes. There were twenty white patients and twelve negroes. Of the entire group, there were seven illegitimate children. There were no positive serologic findings in the entire group (many of the Kahn tests, however, were taken in children prior to the third month of life). Of eighteen females, six had positive vaginal smears. The ages of the patients varied from 1 day to 10 years.

Four additional patients were treated by sterile milk with an average hospital duration of 16.5 days; of these, none showed corneal involvement.

The children treated with sulfanilamide had an identical local care as outlined above, except that silver nitrate was not used. Sulfanilamide was given on the approximate dosage basis of one grain per

Table I

Controls

Average Hospitalization: 28.5 Days

CASE NO.	AGE	RACE, SEX	HISTORY	ADMITTED	DISCHARGED	DURATION	OD	OS	CORNEA	NOTES
1. 120873	2 D.	W-F	1 day	12/ 4/34	1/10/35	8 days	+	–		Premat-Credé
2. 120915	2 D.	W-M	1 day	12/12/34	2/ 2/35	33 days	–	+		
3. 121384	7 D.	C-F	5 days	12/21/34	2/ 7/35	32 days	+	+		Credé Proph.
4. A-776	6 D.	W-M	?	2/ 1/35	3/21/35	31 days	+	+	+ O.U.	Illegitimate
5. A-1485	5 D.	W-F	2 days	3/ 3/35	4/ 5/35	29 days	+	+		Credé Proph.
6. A-1699	9 Yr.	W-F	8 days	3/13/35	4/ 2/35	18 days	–	+		Vaginitis
7. A-2191	14 D.	W-M	14 days	3/21/35	4/24/35	29 days	+	+		Mother's smear positive
8. A-3397	2 Yr.	W-F	14 days	5/ 4/35	6/17/35	39 days	+	+		for gonococcus
9. A-3407	6 D.	C-F	?	5/ 6/35	5/29/35	20 days	–	+		Canthotomy vaginitis
10. A-4973	16 D.	W-F	10 days	6/24/35	7/ 2/35	7 days	+	–		Illegitimate
11. A-6593	2 Yr.	W-M	3 days	8/16/35	9/ 6/35	21 days	+	+		Vaginitis
12. 88882	10 Yr.	W-F	2 days	8/16/35	9/19/35	34 days	+	+		Vaginitis
13. A-7194	9 D.	W-M	7 days	9/14/35	10/11/35	27 days	+	+		
14. B-6527	3 W.	C-M	?	9/21/35	10/ 9/35	11 days	+	–		Illegitimate
15. A-7262	3 D.	W-F	?	9/26/35	10/16/35	21 days	+	+		Illegitimate
16. A-7842	4 D.	W-M	2 days	10/16/35	12/ 1/35	30 days	+	+	+	
17. 109028	2 Yr.	C-F	21 days	10/24/35	11/28/35	15 days	–	+		Vaginitis
18. A-8296	4 D.	W-M	3 days	10/26/35	12/13/35	47 days	+	–		
19. A-8307	17 Mo.	C-M	2 days	10/28/35	11/21/35	25 days	+	–		
20. A-8856	7 D.	W-M	7 days	11/12/35	1/ 5/36	32 days	–	+		Strep. otitis media
21. B-17	8 D.	W-F	3 days	1/ 4/36	3/11/36	65 days	+	+		
22. B-308	5 D.	C-M	2 days	1/23/36	2/ 2/36	10 days	+	+		Illegitimate
23. B-400	4 D.	W-M	1 day	1/31/36	4/ 8/36	64 days	+	+	+ perf.	
24. 115608	2 Yr.	C-F	5 days	3/25/36	4/ 9/36	15 days	+	+		Vaginitis
25. B-2698	1 D.	C-F	1 day	4/ 3/36	6/18/36	61 days	–	+		Premature
26. B-3435	8 Mo.	C-F	2 days	5/11/36	6/11/36	16 days	+	+		
27. B-3162	4 Mo.	W-F	1 day	7/ 9/36	8/20/36	41 days	+	+		
28. B-5130	1 D.	W-F	1 day	7/17/36	10/15/36	34 days	+	+		Premature
29. C-6836	1 Mo.	C-M	?	10/22/37	11/ 3/37	13 days	+	–	+ perf.	
30. C-986	4 D.	W-F	?	2/ 7/37	4/ 6/37	26 days	+	+		
31. C-2101	1 Mo.	C-M	14 days	3/16/37	4/22/37	37 days	+	+		Illegitimate
32. C-3007	1 D.	C-F	1 day	4/28/37	6/ 3/37	23 days	+	–		Illegitimate

D: days
Mo: months

Yr: year
OD: right eye

OS: left eye
Perf: perforation

W: white
C: colored

M: male
F: female

TABLE II

SULFANILAMIDE

Average Hospitalization After Sulfanilamide Started: 5.8 Days

CASE NO.	AGE	RACE, SEX	HISTORY	ADMITTED	DISCHARGED	DURATION	OD	OS	CORNEA	NOTES
1. C-3583	23 Mo.	C-F	1 day	5/28/37	6/10/37	11 days	+	−		Rickets
2. C-4292	1 Mo.	W-M	1 mo.	6/28/37	7/10/37	6 days	+	+		
3. C-4445	21 D.	C-F	10 days	7/ 6/37	7/10/37	4 days	+	+		
4. C-4799	6 D.	C-M	3 days	7/20/37	7/25/37	5 days	+	−		
5. C-5258	9 D.	W-F	5 days	8/ 9/37	9/ 9/37	7 days	−	+		Premature
6. C-5265	3 Yr.	W-F	9 days	8/10/37	8/22/37	11 days	−	+	+	Vaginitis
7. C-6368	1 Mo.	W-M	1 mo.	9/25/37	10/19/37	5 days	+	−	+	
8. C-7450	11 Mo.	C-M	3 days	11/ 8/37	11/16/37	5 days	+	+		
9. C-7465	3 Yr.	C-M	1 day	11/11/37	11/19/37	7 days	−	+		
10. C-7548	10 D.	W-M	6 days	11/14/37	11/19/37	4 days	−	+		
11. C-7817	7 D.	C-M	1 day	11/18/37	12/ 8/37	4 days	+	+		Premature
12. C-7972	5 D.	W-M	3 days	11/30/37	12/ 7/37	5 days	−	+		
13. C-8385	12 D.	C-F	3 days	12/15/37	1/10/38	5 days	+	+		Premature
14. C-8425	12 D.	W-F	4 days	12/21/37	12/25/37	4 days	−	+		
15. A-3537	21 D.	C-F	10 days	1/ 1/38	1/ 5/38	4 days	+	+		

See footnote at bottom of Table I.

pound body weight daily, combining it with equal amounts of sodium bicarbonate. The drug was incorporated in karo water feedings with smaller infants, with no difficulty encountered by this mode of administration. Older children were given oral administration; one resistant child was gavaged. In no instance was parenteral administration found necessary. Sulfanilamide blood level determinations were made according to the method described by Marshall.[18] The levels found were much lower as a group than with older children on a similar dosage basis. Blood levels taken in the morning after a nocturnal period with no drug administration were uniformly low. Levels taken during or within a few hours after a day's administration were higher.

Fifteen patients were treated with sulfanilamide with an average hospital duration of 5.8 days. The ages of the patients varied from 5 days to 3 years. Of these, two showed corneal involvement; perforation did not result after sulfanilamide was started. Six of the group showed bilateral involvement. There were seven white and eight negro patients, seven females and eight males. One had vaginal involvement.

None of the complications attributed to sulfanilamide were observed in this group; no appreciable acidosis or cyanosis was observed. No cases showed a morbilliform rash; no nausea or vomiting was encountered.

TABLE III

SUMMARY OF TREATMENT

NO. OF CASES	TREATMENT	AVERAGE DURATION
32	Routine	28.5 days
4	Routine + milk	16.5 days
15	Routine + sulfanilamide	5.8 days*

*After sulfanilamide was started.

PRESENTATION OF CASES

CASE 1.—P. F., C-3853, colored female, aged 23 months, weight, 16½ pounds, was admitted May 28, 1937, and discharged June 10, 1937. Pain, swelling, and discharge developed in the right eye two weeks prior to admission. No home treatment was given. There was no definite history of contact.

On admission examination showed that there was massive chemosis of the right eye, with a thick, yellow, purulent discharge. The palpebral conjunctiva was edematous and injected; the cornea was clear. The left eye was apparently uninvolved. Examination revealed a malnourished, colored female child, not acutely ill. Clinical signs of active rickets were present. Direct smears of both eyes showed gram-negative intracellular and extracellular diplococci. The patient was isolated and the usual treatment instigated. In addition sulfanilamide and sodium bicarbonate were given in equal amounts. There was a rapid subsidence of symptoms, and three consecutive negative smears were obtained by the eleventh day (Table IV). On June 15, 1937, the patient had a recurrence of symptoms in the right eye, but three smears were negative. She was seen one week later with no involvement or discharge. Tuberculin test (1:5000) was negative, as well as Kahn test and vaginal smears.

TABLE IV

DAYS	SMEARS		DISCHARGE		SULF.	SULF. LEVEL
	RIGHT EYE	LEFT EYE	RIGHT EYE	LEFT EYE		
5/28	+	+	++++	–	0	
5/29	+	+	+++	–	15 gr.	
5/30	–	–	++	–	15 gr.	
5/31	–	–	+	–	15 gr.	
6/1	–	–	–	–	15 gr.	4.5 mg.
6/2	–	–	–	–	15 gr.	
6/3*	–	–	–	–	15 gr.	
6/4	+	+	–	–	15 gr.	
6/5	–	–	–	–	10 gr.	
6/6	–	–	–	–	10 gr.	
6/7	–	–	–	–	0	
6/8	–	–	–	–	0	

*Blood count: Hb. 12 gm.; R.B.C. 4,000,000; W.B.C. 9,400; polymorphonuclears, 62 per cent; small lymphocytes, 23 per cent; large lymphocytes, 15 per cent.

CASE 2.—S. W., C-4292, white male, aged 4 weeks, weight 5½ pounds, was admitted June 28, 1937 and discharged July 10, 1937 (Table V).

This child was born at the Armour Hospital, Ferndale, premature seven months. Discharge was noted in both eyes on the third day. On admission to the hospital, the patient showed swollen lids; palpebral conjunctivae, thickened and beefy with a copious, thick, yellow purulent discharge present in both eyes. The mother had a vaginal discharge during the last four months of pregnancy. Sulfanilamide was started on the sixth day after repeated positive smears. Discharge rapidly ceased, and smears were negative on the third day. A checkup two weeks after discharge from the hospital showed no recurrence, and the palpebral conjunctivae had lost all thickening. Kahn test was negative.

TABLE V

DAYS	SMEARS		DISCHARGE		SULF.	SULF. LEVEL
	RIGHT EYE	LEFT EYE	RIGHT EYE	LEFT EYE		
6/28	–	+	++	++		
6/29	+	–	++	++		
6/30	+	+	+	+		
7/1	+	+	+	+		
7/2	+	+	+	+		
7/3	+	+	+	+	5 gr.	
7/4	–	–	–	–	5 gr.	
7/5	+	+	–	–	5 gr.	
7/6	–	–	–	–	5 gr.	
7/7	–	–	–	–	5 gr.	
7/8	–	–	–	–	5 gr.	Trace*
7/9	–	–	–	–	5 gr.	
7/10	–	–	–	–	0	

*Blood level taken in the morning after a night with no administration.

CASE 3.—C. J., C-4445, colored female, aged 3 weeks, weight 7½ pounds, was admitted July 6, 1937 and discharged July 12, 1937 (Table VI).

The child was born at home; no prophylaxis was used. At 1 week of age, the right eye began to discharge; three days later the left eye became involved. On admission both lids were swollen. The conjunctivae were reddened and the corneas were clear. Marked photophobia and lacrimation was present. Smears taken were positive. Sulfanilamide was started on the second day following admission. Discharge ceased, and smears promptly became negative. Patient was discharged on the seventh day with complete subsidence of involvement. Kahn test was negative.

TABLE VI

DAYS	SMEARS		DISCHARGE		SULF.	SULF. LEVEL
	LEFT EYE	RIGHT EYE	RIGHT EYE	LEFT EYE		
7/6	+	+	++	++		
7/7	+	+	+	–	5 gr.	
7/8*	–	–	–	–	5 gr.	
7/9	–	–	–	–	5 gr.	1.5 mg.†
7/10	–	–	–	–	5 gr.	
7/11	–	–	–	–		
7/12	–	–	–	–		

*Blood count: Hb. 13 gm.; R.B.C. 3,930,000; W.B.C. 5,500; polymorphonuclears, 60 per cent; small lymphocytes 36 per cent; large lymphocytes, 4 per cent.
†Blood level taken in the morning.

CASE 4.—C. D., C-4799, colored male, aged 6 days, weight 5 pounds, was admitted July 20, 1937 and discharged July 25, 1937 (Table VII).

The child was born at home, attended by a midwife, and was referred by the Board of Health with a history of purulent discharge from one eye for three days. Patient showed an edematous right eye, swollen lids, and purulent discharge. Palpebral conjunctiva was injected; cornea was clear. Left eye was apparently not involved. Smears were positive, and sulfanilamide was started on the second day with rapid clearing of the discharge and subsidence of all conjunctival involvement. The child was seen on July 27, 1937, and on Aug. 2, 1937, at which times there was no involvement. Kahn test was negative.

TABLE VII

DAYS	SMEARS		DISCHARGED		SULF.	SULF. LEVEL
	RIGHT EYE	LEFT EYE	RIGHT EYE	LEFT EYE		
7/20	+	–	+++	–	5 gr.	
7/21	+	–	++	–	5 gr.	5.3 mg.
7/22	–	–	+	–	5 gr.	2.5 mg.
7/23*	–	–	–	–	5 gr.	
7/24	–	–	–	–	0	
7/25	–	–	–	–	0	trace

*Blood count: Hb. 14 gm.; R.B.C. 4,800,000; W.B.C. 12,000; polymorphonuclear, 70 per cent; small lymphocytes, 28 per cent; large lymphocytes, 2 per cent.

CASE 5.—G. G., C-5258, white female, aged 9 days, weight 4½ pounds, was admitted Aug. 9, 1937 and discharged Sept. 9, 1937 (Table VIII).

The patient was born in a Dearborn hospital, seven months premature. Credé prophylaxis was used. On the fourth day discharge started in the left eye and continued to discharge in increasing amounts since then. The patient was admitted with a copious, yellow discharge, with moderate edema and papillary swelling. The child, otherwise, was a normal, well-developed, premature baby with no significant physical findings. Smears were positive for gram-negative diplococci. On the third day after admission sulfanilamide was started. Negative smears were obtained five days later and remained negative. The child was transferred to the Medical Service and remained in the hospital until it reached the weight of 5 pounds. On final discharge the eyes showed no recurrence of symptoms. Vaginal smears and Kahn tests were negative.

TABLE VIII

DAYS	SMEARS		DISCHARGE		SULF.	SULF. LEVEL
	RIGHT EYE	LEFT EYE	RIGHT EYE	LEFT EYE		
8/9	–	+	–	++		
8/10	–	+	–	++		
8/11*	–	+	–	++	5 gr.	0
8/12	–	+	–	++	7½ gr.	
8/13	–	+	–	+	7½ gr.	4.3 mg.
8/14	–	+	–	+	7½ gr.	
8/15	–	–	–	–	7½ gr.	
8/16	–	–	–	–	7½ gr.	
8/17	–	–	–	–	7½ gr.	

*Blood count: Hb. 14.6 gm.; R.B.C. 4,300,000; W.B.C. 9,400; polymorphonuclears, 65 per cent; lymphocytes, 34 per cent; basophiles, 1 per cent.

CASE 6.—R. M. W., C-5265, white female, aged 3 years, weight 22 pounds, was admitted Aug. 10, 1937 and discharged Aug. 22, 1937 (Table IX). This patient was the daughter of circus performers. The mother, an acromegalic dwarf of 41 inches, was delivered by cesarean section. Three weeks prior to admission the patient developed a profuse vaginal discharge and was treated at St. Luke's Hospital, Milwaukee, Wis. When the parents changed location the patient was seen in the outpatient department. At this time there had been a discharge from the left eye for at least twelve days. Both eyes had swelling of the lids with a purulent discharge present. The corneas were uninvolved. Physical examination showed nothing remarkable save the eye involvement and a vaginal discharge. The patient was started on sulfanilamide. On the fourth day, despite the clearance of much of the injection and edema, the left cornea showed ulcerative changes. Atropine, 1 per cent, was started, and sterile milk was also given in doses of 2 and 3 c.c. on Aug. 14, 1937, and Aug. 16, 1937. Sulfanilamide was continued at the initial dosage of 30 grains daily. Owing to the lack of cooperation, gavage feedings became necessary. She had an excellent febrile reaction to the foreign protein and a rapid clearing of the corneal ulcer by the seventh day. Daily vaginal smears throughout her entire course failed to show gram-negative cocci. Kahn test was negative.

TABLE IX

DAYS	SMEARS		DISCHARGE		SULF.	SULF. LEVEL
	RIGHT EYE	LEFT EYE	RIGHT EYE	LEFT EYE		
8/10*	–	+	–	++++	30 gr.	
8/11	–	+	–	+++	15 gr.	
8/12	–	+	–	ulcer	30 gr.	
8/13	–	+	–	++	30 gr.	11.2 mg.
8/14	–	+	–	+	30 gr.	
8/15	–	–	–	+	30 gr.	
8/16	–	–	–	+	30 gr.	7.2 mg.
8/17	–	+	–	–	30 gr.	
8/18	–	–	–	–		
8/19	–	–	–	–		
8/20†	–	–	–	–		
8/21	–	–	–	–		
8/22	–	–	–	–		

*Blood count: Hb. 11 gm.; R.B.C. 4,240,000; W.B.C. 9,600; polymorphonuclears, 74 per cent; lymphocytes, 24 per cent; eosinophiles, 2 per cent.

†Blood count: Hb. 11.5 gm.; R.B.C. 4,000,000; W.B.C. 12,400; polymorphonuclears, 66 per cent; lymphocytes, 30 per cent; monocytes, 4 per cent.

CASE 7.—R. B., C-6368, white male, aged 4 weeks, weight 5¾ pounds, was admitted Sept. 25, 1937 and discharged Oct. 19, 1937 (Table X). The child was born at the Florence Crittenden Hospital, seven months premature, and received Credé prophylaxis. Shortly after birth the eyes began to discharge, and despite routine treatment discharge continued with no abatement. Smears taken prior to admission were positive on several occasions. On the fifth day after admission corneal ulceration was noted and 1 c.c. of sterile milk was given, with no subsequent improvement. On the fifteenth day sulfanilamide was started, with a rapid cessation of discharge and a healing of the ulcer. Patient was seen one week and three weeks after discharge, with normal conjunctiva and a leucomatous patch at the site of the ulcer. Kahn test was negative.

TABLE X

DAYS	SMEARS		DISCHARGE		SULF.	SULF. LEVEL
	RIGHT EYE	LEFT EYE	RIGHT EYE	LEFT EYE		
9/26	+	–	+	–		
9/27	+	–	+	–		
9/28	+	–	+	–		
9/29*	+	–	+	–		
9/30	+	–	ulcer	–		
10/1	+	–	+	–		
10/2	+	–	+	–		
10/3	+	–	+	–		
10/4	+	–	+	–		
10/5	+	–	–	–		
10/6	+	–	–	–		
10/7	+	–	–	–		
10/8	+	–	–	–		
10/9	+	–	–	–		
10/10	+	+	–	+		
10/11	+	+	–	+	5 gr.	
10/12	+	–	–	–	5 gr.	
10/13	–	–	–	–	5 gr.	
10/14	–	–	–	–	5 gr.	4.6 mg.
10/15	–	–	–	–	5 gr.	
10/16	–	–	–	–		

*Blood count: Hb. 12.5 gm.; R.B.C. 5,200,000; W.B.C. 11,300; polymorphonuclears, 72 per cent; lymphocytes, 28 per cent.

TABLE XI

DAYS	SMEARS		DISCHARGE		SULF.	SULF. LEVEL
	RIGHT EYE	LEFT EYE	RIGHT EYE	LEFT EYE		
11/8	+	+	++	++++	20 gr.	
11/9*	+	+	+	++	30 gr.	
11/10	–	–	+	+	30 gr.	
11/11	–	–	–	–	30 gr.	5.0 mg.
11/12	–	–	–	–	30 gr.	
11/13	–	–	–	–	30 gr.	
11/14	–	–	–	–	10 gr.	
11/15	–	–	–	–		
11/16†	–	–	–	–		

*Blood count: Hb. 12 gm.; R.B.C. 3,900,000; W.B.C. 11,600; polymorphonuclears, 63 per cent; small lymphocytes, 20 per cent; large lymphocytes, 14 per cent; monocytes, 3 per cent.

†Blood count: Hb. 12 gm.; R.B.C. 4,100,000; W.B.C. 8,000; polymorphonuclears, 54 per cent; lymphocytes, 46 per cent.

CASE 8.—N. J., C-7450, colored male, aged 11 months, weight nineteen pounds, was admitted Nov. 8, 1937 and discharged Nov. 16, 1937 (Table XI). The child's mother had a discharging eye two weeks before the patient was infected. The child had a very profuse discharge from both eyes which started three days prior to admission, with the lids markedly swollen and the conjunctivae chemotic. The cornea was negative. Smears were positive. Sulfanilamide was started promptly on admission. On the second day scanty discharge was present; on the fifth day both eyes were opened and the discharge had ceased; the conjunctivae approached a normal state. On the seventh day three negative smears were obtained, and sulfanilamide was discontinued. The patient was seen on Nov. 19, 1937, and on Nov. 26, 1937, with no recurrence; Kahn test, negative.

CASE 9.—A. J., C-7465, colored male, aged 3 years, weight 44 pounds, was admitted Nov. 11, 1937 and discharged Nov. 19, 1937 (Table XII). (This patient is a brother of No. C-7450.) On the evening prior to admission reddening of the left eye was noted. By morning the eye was swollen shut and pus was oozing between the lids. On admission chemosis was marked and symptoms of general constitutional involvement were present. Sulfanilamide was started promptly, and within two days there was considerable reduction in the local reaction and the discharge. Discharge continued, however, until the sixth day, at which time the left eye was open. By the ninth day all conjunctival involvement had subsided; Kahn test, negative.

TABLE XII

DAYS	SMEARS		DISCHARGE		SULF.	SULF. LEVEL
	RIGHT EYE	LEFT EYE	RIGHT EYE	LEFT EYE		
11/11*	–	+	–	++++	20 gr.	
11/12	–	–	–	+++	40 gr.	
11/13	–	–	–	+++	40 gr.	3.5 mg.
11/14	–	–	–	+	40 gr.	
11/15	–	–	–	+	40 gr.	
11/16	–	–	–	–	40 gr.	
11/17	–	–	–	–	40 gr.	5.8 mg.
11/18	–	–	–	–	40 gr.	
11/19†	–	–	–	–	40 gr.	

*Blood count: Hb. 13 gm.; R.B.C. 3,620,000; W.B.C. 15,700; polymorphonuclears, 84 per cent; lymphocytes, 12 per cent; monocytes, 3 per cent; eosinophiles, 1 per cent.

†Blood count: Hb. 13.2 gm.; R.B.C. 4,350,000; W.B.C. 7,900; polymorphonuclears, 55 per cent; small lymphocytes, 26 per cent; large lymphocytes, 18 per cent; eosinophiles, 1 per cent.

CASE 10.—D. B., C-7548, white male, aged 10 days, weight 4¾ pounds, was admitted Nov. 14, 1937 and discharged Nov. 19, 1937 (Table XIII). Discharge was noted on the fourth day after birth, involving the left eye. The mother had a profuse, purulent discharge during the last few months of pregnancy. She was treated by the family physician, and at delivery Credé prophylaxis was used. Two smears taken at home were positive for Neisserian infection. The child was admitted to the hospital showing puffy edematous lids of the left eye with a moderate yellow, purulent discharge. The conjunctiva was thickened and injected; no corneal involvement was noted. The right eye appeared negative. After obtaining positive smears, sulfanilamide was started. By the fifth day the discharge had entirely ceased. The eyes were opened and the conjunctiva appeared normal. The child was seen subsequent to discharge on March 2, 1938, and March 5, 1938, and smears taken at that time were negative; Kahn test, negative.

TABLE XIII

DAYS	SMEARS		DISCHARGE		SULF.	SULF. LEVEL
	RIGHT EYE	LEFT EYE	RIGHT EYE	LEFT EYE		
11/14*	–	+	–	++	5 gr.	
11/15	–	+	–	++	5 gr.	
11/16	–	–	–	++	5 gr.	
11/17	–	–	–	+	5 gr.	3.2 mg.
11/18	–	–	–	–	5 gr.	
11/19†	–	–	–	–	5 gr.	

*Blood count: Hb. 14 gm.; R.B.C. 4,800,000; W.B.C. 17,000; polymorphonuclears, 42 per cent; lymphocytes, 58 per cent.

†Blood count: Hb. 12 gm.; R.B.C. 4,530,000; W.B.C. 9,900; polymorphonuclears, 57 per cent; lymphocytes, 42 per cent; eosinophiles, 1 per cent.

CASE 11.—W. H., C-7817, colored male, aged 7 days, weight 3¾ pounds, was admitted Nov. 18, 1937 and discharged Dec. 4, 1937 (Table XIV). This child was a seven-month premature baby, born at home; Credé prophylaxis was used. Discharge started on the second day after birth with considerable chemosis of both eyes. The mother gave a history of a vaginal discharge during the last four months of pregnancy. Eye smears were positive, and the patient was admitted to the hospital. Hemolytic jaundice of the newborn infant was present. The child was placed on sulfanilamide, and by the third day discharge had become scanty. On the fifth day both eyes were open, discharge had ceased, and the smears were negative. The child was transferred to the premature ward and kept in the hospital until he had attained a weight of 5 pounds. He was seen in the out-patient department on Feb. 14, 1938, and Feb. 16, 1938, at which time the eyes appeared normal. Kahn test was negative.

TABLE XIV

DAYS	SMEARS		DISCHARGE		SULF.	SULF. LEVEL
	RIGHT EYE	LEFT EYE	RIGHT EYE	LEFT EYE		
11/18*	+	+	+++	++	2½ gr.	
11/19	–	–	+	+	5 gr.	
11/20	–	–	–	–	5 gr.	3.5 mg.
11/21	–	–	–	–	5 gr.	
11/22	–	–	–	–	5 gr.	
11/23	–	–	–	–		
11/24†	–	–	–	–		

*Blood count: Hb. 16.7 gm.; R.B.C. 3,800,000; W.B.C. 7,600; polymorphonuclears, 60 per cent; lymphocytes, 38 per cent; eosinophiles, 2 per cent.

†Blood count: Hb. 15.8 gm.; R.B.C. 3,600,000; W.B.C. 7,500; polymorphonuclears, 61 per cent; lymphocytes, 36 per cent; monocytes, 2 per cent; eosinophiles, 1 per cent.

CASE 12.—W. T., C-7972, white male, aged 5 days, weight 5 pounds, was admitted Nov. 30, 1937 and discharged Dec. 7, 1937 (Table XV). This child's left eye became involved on the third day after birth, with discharge and swelling of the lids. Credé prophylaxis was used at birth. The father had been treated at Receiving Hospital six months previously for a urethral stricture. On admission there was a thick, yellow discharge from the left eye; the conjunctiva was involved, the cornea was clear. Sulfanilamide was started promptly, and by the fourth day discharge had ceased. Conjunctival thickening had resolved. The smears were negative. The child was seen one week after discharge from the hospital, at which time the eyes were clear; Kahn, negative.

TABLE XV

DAYS	SMEARS		DISCHARGE		SULF.	SULF. LEVEL
	RIGHT EYE	LEFT EYE	RIGHT EYE	LEFT EYE		
11/30	–	+	–	++	5 gr.	
12/1	–	+	–	++	5 gr.	
12/2	–	–	–	+	5 gr.	
12/3	–	–	–	–	5 gr.	3.1 mg.
12/4	–	–	–	–	5 gr.	
12/5	–	–	–	–	5 gr.	
12/6*	–	–	–	–	5 gr.	
12/7	–	–	–	–		

*Blood count: Hb. 17.5 gm.; R.B.C. 4,200,000; W.B.C. 10,100; polymorphonuclears, 42 per cent; lymphocytes, 52 per cent; monocytes, 1 per cent; eosinophiles, 5 per cent.

Blood count, Dec. 21, 1937: Hb. 17.6 gm.; R.B.C. 4,560,000; W.B.C. 13,100; polymorphonuclears, 49 per cent; lymphocytes, 41 per cent; monocytes, 2 per cent; eosinophiles, 7 per cent; basophiles, 1 per cent.

CASE 13.—J. D., C-8385, colored female, aged 12 days, weight 4 pounds, was admitted Dec. 15, 1937 and was discharged Jan. 10, 1938 (Table XVI). The child was born at home, 7 months premature; Credé prophylaxis used: mother had a positive Neisserian history and had received prenatal care. Both eyes were involved three days prior to admission. Smears were positive. Lids were edematous and tumefied; the conjunctivae were thickened and protruded through the lids. The corneas were clear. Sulfanilamide was started, and by the fourth day both eyes were open, discharge had ceased, and the smears were negative. The child was kept in the hospital until it had reached the weight of 5 pounds. She was seen in the out-patient department, at which time the eyes were negative. Kahn test was negative.

TABLE XVI

DAYS	SMEARS		DISCHARGE		SULF.	SULF. LEVEL
	RIGHT EYE	LEFT EYE	RIGHT EYE	LEFT EYE		
12/15	+	+	+	++	2½ gr.	
12/16*	–	–	–	+	5 gr.	
12/17	–	–	–	+	5 gr.	3.6 mg.
12/18	–	–	–	–	5 gr.	
12/19	–	–	–	–	5 gr.	
12/20	–	–	–	–	5 gr.	

*Blood count: Hb. 15 gm.; R.B.C. 5,390,000; W.B.C. 13,400; polymorphonuclears, 60 per cent; small lymphocytes, 36 per cent; large lymphocytes, 4 per cent.

Blood count, Dec. 27, 1937: Hb. 15.5 gm.; R.B.C. 5,000,000; W.B.C. 16,800; polymorphonuclears, 54 per cent; lymphocytes, 44 per cent; basophiles, 1 per cent; eosinophiles, 1 per cent.

Blood count, Feb. 7, 1938: Hb. 7.5 gm.; R.B.C. 2,600,000; W.B.C. 5,500; polymorphonuclears, 52 per cent; small lymphocytes, 20 per cent; large lymphocytes, 20 per cent; eosinophiles, 8 per cent.

CASE 14.—M. W., C-8425, white female, aged 12 days, weight 6½ pounds, was admitted Dec. 21, 1937 and was discharged Dec. 25, 1937 (Table XVII). The child was born at Grace Hospital and received Credé prophylaxis. She was discharged for home on the fifth day. The following day the left eye began to swell and a copious, yellow discharge began and persisted until admission to the hospital. There was no corneal involvement on examination; there was moderate swelling of the lids of the left eye, and tumefied, moderate involvement of the conjunctiva was noted. Smears were positive, and sulfanilamide was started. By the fifth day the discharge had ceased entirely. The eye was open and the conjunctiva less involved. Patient was seen on Jan. 1, 1938, at which time there was no involvement noted. Kahn test was negative.

TABLE XVII

DAYS	SMEARS		DISCHARGE		SULF.	SULF. LEVEL
	RIGHT EYE	LEFT EYE	RIGHT EYE	LEFT EYE		
12/21	–	+	–	++	$2\frac{1}{2}$ gr.	
12/22*	–	–	–	+	5 gr.	
12/23	–	–	–	–	5 gr.	2.5 mg.
12/24	–	–	–	–	5 gr.	
12/25	–	–	–	–	$2\frac{1}{2}$ gr.	

*Blood count: Hb. 17 gm.; R.B.C. 4,500,000; W.B.C. 18,200; polymorphonuclears, 44 per cent; lymphocytes, 56 per cent.

CASE 15.—A. B., A-3537, colored female, aged 3 weeks, weight 9 pounds, was admitted Jan. 1, 1938 and discharged Jan. 5, 1938 (Table XVIII). This child was born at home and was referred by the Board of Health with a discharging right eye which began shortly after birth. On admission smears were positive from both eyes, and moderate palpebral conjunctival involvement was present. There was slight discharge from both eyes. No corneal ulceration was present. Sulfanilamide was started, and by the fourth day complete resolution with negative smears and normal appearing conjunctivae were present. Patient was seen on Jan. 25, 1938, and the eyes were negative; Kahn, negative.

TABLE XVIII

DAYS	SMEARS		DISCHARGE		SULF.	SULF. LEVEL
	RIGHT EYE	LEFT EYE	RIGHT EYE	LEFT EYE		
1/1	+	+	+	+	$2\frac{1}{2}$ gr.	
1/2*	–	–	–	–	5 gr.	
1/3	–	–	–	–	5 gr.	
1/4	–	–	–	–	5 gr.	2.1 mg.
1/5	–	–	–	–		

*Blood count: Hb. 13 gm.; R.B.C. 4,600,000; W.B.C. 7,600; polymorphonuclears, 67 per cent; small lymphocytes, 28 per cent; large lymphocytes, 5 per cent.

SUMMARY

The most satisfying observation in the use of sulfanilamide in the treatment of gonococcic ophthalmia was the rapid decrease in the swelling and discharge. Patients with red, chemotic, bulbar conjunctivae, with swollen retrotarsal folds and tumefied lids showed a uniformly prompt subsidence. Since this type of case is more apt to have implication of the cornea, if untreated, the rapid arrest noted with sulfanilamide is responsible, we believe, for a much better prognosis.

In conclusion, we have observed a reduction of hospitalization of from 28.5 days for a control series of thirty-two patients with gonorrheal ophthalmia to 5.8 days for a series of fifteen patients treated with sulfanilamide. We believe the use of sulfanilamide is warranted in the treatment of gonorrheal ophthalmia for the following reasons: (1) economic importance, sharply reducing the length of hospitalization; (2) the ease of administration; (3) the apparent lack of complications; (4) the rapid improvement found; and (5) the general increase in the comfort of the patient.

REFERENCES

1. Quoted from Lehrfeld, Louis: J. A. M. A. **104**: 1468, 1935.
2. McKee, S. H.: The Eye and Its Diseases. Edited by Berens, C., p. 368. Philadelphia, 1936, W. B. Saunders Company.
3. Mayou, M. S.: Brit. M. J. **2**: 973, 1931.
4. Stephenson, Sydney: Practitioner **93**: 374, 1914.
5. May, Charles H.: Diseases of the Eye, p. 103, Philadelphia, 1924, William Wood & Company.
6. Bellows, J. G.: Illinois M. J. **70**: 154, 1936.
7. Thygeson, Phillip: Tr. Am. Ophth. Soc. **34**: 340, 1936.
8. Thomas, A. B.: J. Infect. Dis. **43**: 306, 1928.
9. Brewster, N. F.: New Orleans M. & S. J. **88**: 508, 1936.
10. Hektoen, Ludwig: J. A. M. A. **105**: 1765, 1935.
11. Bernstein, C., Jr., and Ginsberg, J. E.: J. A. M. A. **108**: 193, 1937.
12. Domagk, Gerhard: Deutsche med. Wchnschr. **61**: 250, 1935.
13. Long, P. H., and Bliss, Eleanor A.: J. A. M. A. **108**: 32, 1937.
14. Dees, J. E., and Colston, J. A. C.: J. A. M. A. **108**: 1855, 1937.
15. Marshall, E. K., et al.: J. A. M. A. **110**: 252, 1938.
16. Long, P. H., and Bliss, Eleanor A.: J. A. M. A. **108**: 1524, 1937.
17. Mellon, R. R., Gross, P., and Cooper, F. B.: J. A. M. A. **108**: 1858, 1937.
18. Marshall, E. K., Jr., Emerson, Kendall, Jr., and Cutting, W. C.: J. A. M. A. **108**: 953, 1937.

RUPTURE OF THE LIVER IN THE NEWBORN INFANT

Harry B. Silver, M.D.
Newark, N. J.

ALTHOUGH vascular abnormalities of the liver are by no means rare, rupture of the liver with resulting death in the newborn infant is seldom reported. Hemangiomas, either small or of the large cavernous type, are very frequently described, although they rarely give rise to any symptoms in the newborn period. Small subcapsular hemorrhages are frequently met with on the autopsy table, but actual damage to the liver structure is very rarely seen. Apart from the rare reports of cases of liver rupture due to direct trauma, rupture of the liver occurs as a cause of death in a small group of the newborn infants. The etiology of this condition is inadequately explained.

Before 1917, when Hedren compiled the literature, it was felt that rupture of the liver was not possible in spontaneous labor. Since that time, however, Pim and Barlow described one case in 1932, and McNitt described two cases in the same year. In 1933 Henry S. Meyer described another case. In 1936 Schmitt described three cases, only one of which, however, occurred in spontaneous delivery. Although in stillbirths injury to the liver is very frequently demonstrated, it is rare in children born alive. All of these cases reported were in living children.

The liver of the newborn child averages about 4 per cent of the total body weight of the newborn child. It is normally palpable, about 2 to 3 cm. below the free costal margin. As the child lies in the uterus in the fetal position, the liver is at what may readily be conceived of as a point of maximum pressure. It is the keystone of an arch, formed by the back of a child, against which the legs and feet are pressed when the tremendous forces incident to active labor occur. When it is remembered how forcible the uterine contraction is and how exposed to injury this large, soft organ seems to be, it is surprising that injury occurs as infrequently as it does. Due to the protective capsule about the liver, unless the lacerations are extreme, immediate severe bleeding does not occur. What actually happens is that a slow, continuous hemorrhage from the lacerated liver tissue lifts the capsule and causes a subcapsular hematoma. Ordinarily the pressure upon this hematoma within the capsule controls the bleeding. In occasional cases, however, where the injury is severe enough, the bleeding continues until the pressure within the hematoma has risen to a point where the capsule is ruptured and free blood is poured into the abdomen. This produces the characteristic clinical history of the condition.

From the Beth Israel Hospital, Newark, N. J.

The child is born apparently normal and with only moderate evidence of birth shock. It seems perfectly well until about the third or fourth day, when it suddenly goes into collapse and dies. Occasionally, as occurred in our case, some of the characteristic symptoms of free intra-abdominal bleeding are present. There is a doughy feel of the abdomen and a discoloration either about the umbilicus or along the inguinal gutter and the scrotum. Aspiration of the abdomen may reveal free blood. On the autopsy table the tear in a capsule is readily seen. There is ordinarily no definite tear of the liver structure, although the adherent blood clot of the subcapsular hematoma gives direct evidence of the injury to the liver itself.

In going over the literature I have been able to find four other cases reported that appear in their clinical manifestations to be of the same type as the case that we are reporting.

Pim and Barlow[1] report the following case:

A primipara was delivered of a male infant weighing 10 pounds 14 ounces. The labor lasted about twenty-three hours, the presentation being left occipitoanterior, and terminated naturally, but with considerable laceration of the perineum. The infant started to breathe shortly after the head was born. There was a good deal of delay in the birth of the shoulders, and toward the latter part of this delay breathing ceased, and some cyanosis became apparent. After the birth of the shoulders, breathing restarted with slight stimulation. Neither Schultze swinging nor compression of the chest was used.

The child was well-formed and apparently quite healthy. On the second and third days it seemed quite well and was fed from the breast. On the fourth morning it was observed that it was slightly jaundiced, but otherwise well. In the afternoon the nurse noticed that the child seemed weak and listless, and from that time the weakness increased, until at 6 A.M. on the fifth day the baby collapsed and died.

Post-Mortem Examination.—When the peritoneum was opened, it was found to be full of dark liquid blood. All the organs appeared normal except the liver. On the outer surface of the right lobe was a hematoma, the size of half a billiard ball, full of diffluent blood, and about the center of the hematoma there was a linear tear ½ inch long in the capsule of the liver, through which blood was leaking. Around the edges of the tear was a small, soft clot.

McNitt[2] reported the following two cases:

A multipara, aged 29 years, had three previous full-term labors with two forceps deliveries. One day before the estimated date of confinement the patient went into labor. At this time the position was R.O.P., and the fetal heart was strong. After six hours of hard labor with the cervix practically dilated, the position was still R.O.P. The abdomen was manipulated between pains, with the end in view of turning the fetus. This was accomplished quite easily, and about twenty minutes later a baby boy, weighing 8 pounds, was born.

The child took the breast well and appeared perfectly normal. Two days later the baby suddenly vomited, its respiration became more rapid, and its skin became anemic in appearance. One hour later it died. Artificial respiration failed, as did intracardiac injections of adrenalin.

Autopsy Report.—On opening the abdomen many large clots of blood were seen. A large clot was noted more firmly attached to the under surface of the liver. On close examination, a rent in Glisson's capsule, approximately 1 inch in length, was found, and beneath this, a corresponding laceration of the liver substance. This tear extended from a point on the inferior surface of the right lobe near the vertebrae, laterally, and forward for the distance of 1 inch. A clot was firmly attached to the bed of the laceration. All organs were anemic in appearance. The tentorium cerebelli showed no laceration or hemorrhage.

A white multipara, aged 23 years, in a previous pregnancy had twins who died when 3 days old. The cause was unknown, and there was no autopsy. On Oct. 31, 1930, the patient went into labor at 4:30 A.M.; the membranes ruptured at 4:00 P.M., and birth of a male infant weighing 9 pounds 3 ounces took place at 7:35 P.M. on the same day. The position was L.O.A. Ether anesthesia was used and there was a loop of cord around the infant's neck. Three days later, on November 3 at 4:30 P.M., the baby apparently became very hungry (thirsty?), regurgitated, grew pale, defied all attempts at resuscitation, and died at 12:30 A.M. The child's temperature ranged from 99° F. to 101.8° F.

At the end of the second stage of labor, mild pressure was exerted on the abdomen during pains in order to assist the slow descent of the large child through the birth canal. This was the only antepartum manipulation made.

Autopsy Report.—There was an intra-abdominal hemorrhage of dark thick blood. A large clot was found toward the posterior inferior aspect of the right lobe beneath the capsule of Glisson, filling the proximal portion of the right lateral gutter. Dissecting the capsule of Glisson, almost over the entire postinferior aspect of the right lobe, the subcapsular hemorrhage measured 2½ inches by 1½ inches. On removal of the liver, a more or less elliptical slit or rupture was noted in the capsule, extending toward the lateral aspect of liver margin.

In both of these cases, extra-abdominal manipulation of the uterus was attempted, and the author felt that possibly this manipulation was the cause of the rupture.

In 1933 Henry S. Meyer[3] reported the following case:

L. S., a white male, was delivered July 8, 1933. The labor was hard and of eight hours' duration. The child was delivered by low forceps. A median episiotomy was done. The position was occipitoanterior. The child weighed 10 pounds at birth. There were no cyanosis, convulsions, paralysis, or malformations. The child apparently nursed well but continued to lose weight very rapidly during the first five days. On July 13 there was a sudden collapse, and a diagnosis was made of collapse, due to hemorrhage into one of the viscera.

Autopsy Report.—The abdomen, when opened, revealed about 500 c.c. of sanguineous fluid. The capsule of the liver showed a rent about 3 cm. long. It had been dissected from the anteroinferior surface of the right lobe and part of the left lobe. The liver was spongy over the entire area.

Author's case:

The mother was a 24-year-old primipara. The entire pregnancy had been normal. She entered the hospital in labor at 4:15 P.M., on Jan. 11, 1936, and delivered spontaneously at 8:28 the same day. Labor was short, no medication was used; episiotomy was done, and gas-oxygen anesthesia was employed. The mother's condition was normal and remained so throughout the post-mortem period. Kahn and Wassermann tests were all negative for father, mother, and child.

The child, born at 8:28 P.M., Jan. 11, 1936, weighed 7 pounds 2 ounces. There was normal spontaneous delivery. No anomalies or cyanosis were noted. The child began to cry immediately and for the first twenty-four hours seemed to be perfectly normal. At 9:15 P.M. on the following day, Jan. 12, the nurse noted that the scrotum and right inguinal region were edematous and cyanotic. The extremities were cold, and the baby appeared to be in shock. At 1:10 A.M., Jan. 13, the baby was seen. The right inguinal region and right scrotum were definitely ecchymotic, and the baby still appeared to be in shock. Temperature was subnormal, pulse very rapid, and abdomen weak. Paracentesis was done, and 5 c.c. of liquid blood was obtained. Diagnosis of a ruptured viscus was made, and the child was treated for shock. By 10:30 A.M., Jan. 13, there was marked edema of the scrotum with increasing ecchymosis. The discoloration was sharply defined and extended upward along the right inguinal region. The abdomen was distended and had a doughy feel. There was no blood in the stools or vomit. The child died within about three hours.

Autopsy Report.—The body was that of a 2-day-old white, male infant. Rigor mortis was absent. There was no jaundice, edema, or petechiae. The abdomen appeared unusually distended. Just below and to the left of the umbilical scar, which was well-healed, there was a pinhead-sized dark red zone, the site of a recent paracentesis. The right scrotal sac appeared purple in color and felt tense on palpation. The left scrotal sac was less markedly discolored. Both testes were in the scrotum. There was no external anomaly.

Internal Examination.—On opening into the abdominal cavity, a gush of fluid blood resulted. The whole abdominal cavity was filled to distention with a considerable quantity of dark red fluid blood, which enveloped all the intra-abdominal viscera, but was most pronounced in the right lumbar gutter. The under surface of the right lobe of the liver presented a circumscribed area about 2 cm. in diameter consisting of a collection of semifluid and coagulated blood lying beneath the capsule. The latter was intact except at one point where a ragged rent was visible, from which a moderately firm, grayish-red, friable cylindric blood clot extended down into the right lumbar gutter. The remainder of the liver appeared intact.

The lungs were pinkish in color, soft, and crepitant.

The heart presented no abnormalities. The foramen ovale was represented by a crescentic opening. The kidneys showed fetal lobulations. The capsules stripped readily, leaving a smooth surface. Cut section showed the usual cortical and medullary structure. Pelves, ureters, and bladder were negative.

The scrotal sac was distended and discolored to a dark red color. The right processus vaginalis was found to contain a large collection of fluid and partially coagulated blood which surrounded and compressed the testis, which appeared normal.

The diagnosis was subcapsular hematoma of under surface of the right lobe of the liver, with rupture into peritoneal cavity and resultant hemoperitoneum.

DISCUSSION

The etiology of the rupture of the liver in the newborn infant is difficult to explain. A number of theories have been advanced. McNitt felt that the possibility of abdominal ante-partum manipulations, utilized in attempting to change the position of the fetus before delivery, may have been the distinctive factor in his cases. It is conceivable that with the application of pressure binders the normal forces of the uterine contractions may be so distorted that forcible pains acting against a brace, supplied by the abdominal binding, might conceivably injure the liver. However, there is really no direct evidence for this. In our own case, no such ante-partum manipulation was done.

In a case of Pim and Barlow, the difficulties of the labor itself may have been a factor in the injury. The twisting of the body, incidental to the difficult delivery of the shoulders, could possibly have put the liver in a more exposed position. In the other cases, however, those of Meyer and our own, labor was practically normal. It would seem that some abnormality of either the position of the fetus or of the stresses of labor would be necessary to cause the rupture. In addition, it may also be essential that some underlying congenital anomaly exists.

Another possibility has been discussed at some length by Schmitt, who believes that mechanic-traumatic asphyxia should be considered as one of the etiological factors. The abnormally increased tendency to hemorrhage, the so-called pseudohemophilia, indicates a constitutional cause. The inability to demonstrate on the autopsy table actual laceration of the liver structure is in all probability dependent on the structure of the liver itself. Injuries of sufficient magnitude to cause tremendous bleeding in such a spongy organ may still present disintegration of the liver structure rather than definite tearing.

REFERENCES

1. Pim, H. A., and Barlow, Cecil H.: Brit. M. J. **1**: 887, 1932.
2. McNitt, Russell H. J.: Am. J. Obst. & Gynec. **23**: 431, 1932.
3. Meyer, Henry S.: Arch. Pediat. **50**: 814, 1933.

CONGENITAL ABSENCE OF TEETH

Absent Deciduous and Permanent Right and Left Central and Lateral Incisors and the Canines of the Lower Jaw

Jacob L. Stein, M.D., and Alexander Gerber, M.D.
Brooklyn, N. Y.

The congenital absence of teeth is an uncommon occurrence as judged from experience both in the dispensary and in private practice. It is for this reason that we are reporting a case of this type. The medical literature on this subject is very small. Only occasionally does one find a reference in the orthodontic literature.

The etiology must be sought in the embryologic development of the teeth. The endocrines, whose importance in development is appreciated, have also been incriminated. Syphilis is known to interfere with normal development often involving the teeth. In this condition absence of teeth is uncommon. Dwarfism and changes in contour of the teeth are the usual picture in syphilis.

The teeth are derived from both ectoderm and mesoderm. In human embryos, before the lip groove is formed, a thickening of surface ectoderm takes place along the edges of the processes that bound the slitlike entrance to the mouth. When the lip groove appears, the epithelial thickening comes to lie along the edge of the jaw, i.e., along the edge of the gums. This ridge grows into the mesoderm of the jaw, toward the lingual surface, and is now known as the dental shelf. This shelf is at first of uniform thickness throughout, but soon five enlargements appear in it in each upper and lower jaw, indicating the beginnings of the milk teeth. At the 40 mm. stage (eleven weeks), a condensation of mesenchymal tissue beside the deciduous teeth pushes its way into the enlargements of the dental shelf. These ingrowths are called dental papillae. The epithelium gives rise to the enamel organ and the dental papillae (mesoderm) give rise to the dentine and the pulp. These anlagen are connected to each other by dental shelf and to the surface by original ingrowth of ectoderm. Part of the dental shelf grows even further lingually, in which portion the beginnings of the permanent teeth arise. From the foregoing description, it is obvious that any interference with the surface ectoderm in this region, or the region of the dental shelf, may produce either partial or complete edentia.

Congenital absence of teeth may be familial, as pointed out by Pitts,[1] who reports the absence of both deciduous and permanent central incisors with absence of the permanent lateral incisors in two members of a family. The same author reports another case in which there was congenital absence of all teeth but two molars in the lone survivor of pre-

From the Pediatric Department, Jewish Hospital.

mature twins. This patient had coarse, dry hair, suggesting also a faulty primitive ectoderm.

Bray,[2] in 1934, reported a case of complete edentia in an otherwise normal child. Another child in the same family had normal development in every respect. Gardner and Dillery[3] report a case in which twenty-three of the permanent teeth failed to develop.

The description of our case follows:

M. B., aged 4½ years, has been under the care of one of us (J. L. S.) since birth. The birth weight was 5 pounds and 6 ounces. The child was fed a modified cow's milk formula with the usual additions in the later months. Cod-liver oil and orange juice were given in sufficient quantity.

At birth the patient presented a right inguinal hernia. This had incarcerated on several occasions and required surgical intervention at the age of 3 months. Development was normal in all respects, with exception of the teeth. The mother's Wassermann test was negative, and there were no stigmas of congenital syphilis in the child. There were no other evidences of ectodermal or endocrinal defect.

The patient was referred to Dr. Glen H. Whitson for orthodontic examination and treatment. The following is his report:

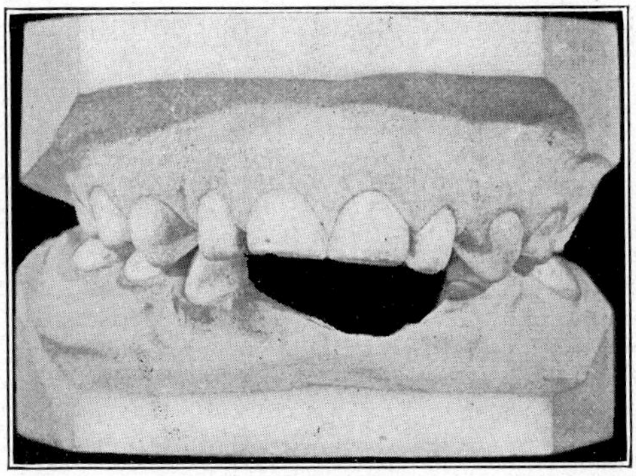

Fig. 1.

"Normal mesiodistal relationship of the upper and lower dental arches one to the other and to the cranium. The intercuspal relationship of the canine, first and second deciduous molars is normal. The upper deciduous incisors are protruding labially due to a tongue thrust habit. The lower left deciduous central and lateral incisors and the canine and the lower right deciduous central and lateral incisors and canine, six teeth in all, are missing. No history of a fall or blow which might account for the absence of these deciduous teeth.

"*Radiographic examination.*—The lower permanent right and left central and lateral incisors and the canines, six teeth in all, are apparently not present as there is no sign of their development. In the upper jaw all the permanent teeth are apparent, though the presence of the upper permanent canines at this age has not been definitely determined. In my personal experience, extending over twenty-five years, this is the first instance where the entire lower anterior deciduous dentition from left canine to right incisor is congenitally missing."

Treatment as suggested by Dr. Whitson is as follows:

"The all important objective right now for this boy is incisor function. This I believe can be established by making hard gold alloy cast overlay anchorage in combination for the first and second deciduous molars on the left side and cast overlays in combination for the deciduous canine and first molar on the right side.

Connect these anchorages with a heavy triangular shaped clasp metal bar so placed that it will function with the maxillary deciduous incisors. I feel justified in saying that such an appliance could remain in place until the four first permanent molars and maxillary central incisors are fully erupted. In addition to this, I would place an orthodontic appliance upon the upper teeth to restore the incisors in that jaw to their normal axial inclination and function."

A perusal of the scanty literature on this subject reveals no figures as to the frequency of this condition. The significance of absent teeth is obvious from both an esthetic and a nutritional viewpoint. Etiologically, the condition is related to developmental defect involving the primitive ectoderm of the oral region. A further possibility to be considered is

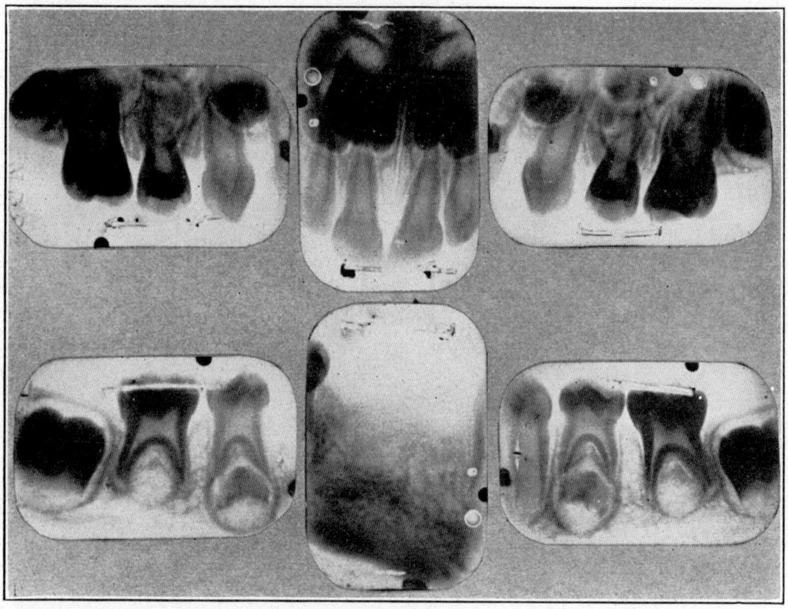

Fig. 2.

that of multiple defects in the ectodermal tissues related to defects in the primitive streak. Endocrinal disfunction and syphilis have been mentioned.

SUMMARY

The rarity of congenitally missing deciduous and permanent teeth is emphasized. A case is presented, a plan of treatment outlined, and the possible etiology suggested.

REFERENCES

1. Pitts, A. T.: Proc. Roy. Soc. Med. **16**: 44, 1922-1923.
2. Bray, Charles H.: Internat. J. Orthodontia **20**: 602, 1934.
3. Gardner, B. S., and Dillery, J. L.: J. Am. Dent. A. **21**: 2032, 1934.
4. Porter, C. G., and Edwards, R. W.: J. Am. Dent. A. **24**: 1852, 1936.
5. Schreiber, G.: Bull. méd., Paris **51**: 124, 1937.

135 Eastern Parkway, Brooklyn, N. Y.
61 Eastern Parkway, Brooklyn, N. Y.

METHYL SALICYLATE POISONING IN AN INFANT

Report of a Patient with Partial Necropsy

Aaron Eimas, M.D.
Bridgeport, Conn.

Although methyl salicylate poisoning is a comparatively rare occurrence, especially in infancy, steps should be taken toward its prevention. When taken internally for therapeutic purposes symptoms of intoxication may occur; but the accidental or intentional taking of an overdose has been followed by a mortality in 59 per cent of the cases. Forty-one[1] per cent of the cases of poisonings occurred in infants. A review of the literature, from the case reported by Gallaher[2] in 1852 to the one reported by Stevenson in 1937, reveals a total of 47 cases.

The following case is of interest because of the severe intoxication and death that was produced from a dose of only one teaspoonful of synthetic oil of wintergreen, and because of the normal carbon-dioxide tension with clinical symptoms of a severe acidosis.

Case Report.—D. C., a boy aged 22 months, was sent into the Park City Hospital on the evening of Oct. 25, 1937, having swallowed one teaspoonful of oil of wintergreen at 8 o'clock that morning. Soon after, the child began to vomit, but the mother thought nothing of it. Vomiting increased and the child began to breathe rapidly and appeared quite drowsy. A physician was called and advised immediate hospitalization. At time of entrance the child had not retained any food or fluids for twelve hours and had become quite stuporous.

Physical Examination.—On admission the child appeared very ill; breathing was rapid and slightly labored. Soon after admission the respirations took on the Kussmaul type of breathing. The pupils were equal and regular but slightly contracted. The skin, lips, and tongue showed evidence of marked dehydration. The child was restless and craved for water, which was immediately vomited. The abdomen was soft. There were no abnormal neurological signs. The temperature on admission was 99° F., pulse rate, 110, and respiration rate 40. Blood pressure was 95 systolic, with a diastolic pressure of 60. The respirations became deeper and more labored, and there was an odor of oil of wintergreen on the breath, but no acetone could be detected. Immediate urinalysis showed only a slight trace of albumin and acetone. Microscopic examinations were negative. The Benedict reaction was negative.

Course in Hospital.—Shortly after admission the child was given an intravenous injection of 350 c.c. of 5 per cent glucose in a normal saline solution. Blood was taken for a carbon-dioxide tension and sugar determination. During the night the child had several clyses which were immediately absorbed because of the severe dehydration present. Since the carbon-dioxide tension was 57 volume per cent, and the blood sugar was normal, 112 mg. per 100 c.c., alkali treatment was not given, but a continuous intravenous infusion of 5 per cent glucose in a normal saline solution was started the following morning. The patient showed no response to these therapeutic measures, and his condition became steadily worse. A transfusion of 200 c.c. of whole blood was given by direct method. That evening the child became cyanotic and was placed in an oxygen tent. During the day several urine specimens were obtained, which gave a positive Gerhardt test of a violet color for salicylates. Tests for acetone and diacetic acid were only slightly positive. Early the following morning the patient developed generalized convulsions. A lumbar puncture was performed, and the spinal fluid was normal in pressure and cell count. The spinal fluid gave a negative Gerhardt test for salicylates. Thirty-six hours after admission the child's condition became very poor, signs of pneumonia appeared, the temperature rose to 105° F., and pulse rate increased to 160. The child died.

Additional Laboratory Examinations.—The admission specimen of urine showed only slight trace of albumin and acetone, but no sugar. Subsequent urine examination showed traces of acetone and diacetic acid. Sugar continued to be negative. Microscopic examination of the urine was negative. A blood count taken on admission showed: red blood cells, 4,300,000; hemoglobin, 65 per cent (Sahli); white blood cells 18,500; polymorphonuclears, 47 per cent; lymphocytes, 53 per cent. The red cells appeared normal on the smear.

Autopsy.—There were no scars or deformities present. Rigor mortis was weak, and post-mortem settling was slight. The eyes were sunken and the pupils moderately dilated and equal.

On section, the body showed the following:

Abdomen: no abnormalities.
Right and left pleural cavities: no abnormalities.
Pericardial sac: no abnormalities.
Heart: the myocardium was friable and pale; the endocardium and its valvular leaflets were normal.
Lungs: slight pulmonary edema.
Liver: the capsule was smooth; the parenchyma on section showed considerable fatty infiltration.
Gall bladder and bile ducts: normal.
Spleen: normal.
Pancreas: normal.
Gastrointestinal tract: normal.
Kidneys: the capsule stripped readily; the parenchyma was pale and bulged from beneath the capsule.
Pelvis, ureters, and bladder: normal.

Anatomic Findings:

Pulmonary edema.
Cloudy swelling of all the parenchymatous organs.
Fatty infiltration of the liver.

Microscopic Examination:

Liver: marked fatty degeneration of the liver cells.
Spleen: no changes.
Kidney: marked congestion with a swollen granulated appearance of the convoluted tubules; there was marked irregularity in the size of the glomeruli.
Lungs: moderate degree of congestion of the septal vessels.

Heart muscle: cells had cross striations and presented a hyaline appearance.

Histological findings:

Nephrosis, of kidney.

Cloudy swelling and albuminous degeneration of the heart muscle.

Fatty degeneration of the liver.

Congestion of the lungs.

DISCUSSION

In reviewing the literature on methyl salicylate poisoning, the amount of methyl salicylate swallowed in the fatal cases varied from 4 c.c. to 15 c.c. The smallest recorded lethal dose was reported by Hughes,[3] in a male infant who was given 4 c.c. of synthetic oil of wintergreen by mistake. However, recovery has occurred in cases in which the dose was considerably in excess of this. Meyers[4] reported a case in a child, 2 years of age, who swallowed 30 c.c. and recovered.

The intimate relationship of the salicylates to the phenols and their possible toxic properties was stated by Wetzel and Nourse[5] in 1926. Of the salicylates, the methyl ester is much more respected, therefore, the sodium salt is more frequently used in treatment. The toxicity of methyl salicylate, according to Hanzlik and Wetzel,[6] is said to be due, in part, to the greater lipoidal solubility and, in part, to the fact that it suffers less destruction within the body after absorption.

The symptomatology and physical observations in the cases previously reported are similar in many respects. My case presents many of the clinical features reported in those cases. The symptoms can be grouped under three classes, namely: gastrointestinal, respiratory, and central. The gastrointestinal symptoms are due to the direct irritant action of the drug on the mucosa of the stomach and intestines. Some cases presented few, if any, outstanding symptoms. Vomiting and diarrhea are constant features. Woodbury and Nicholls[7] reported two cases: in one, the only symptom was vomiting; in the other, there were vomiting and convulsions. In my case, the vomiting occurred early and persisted for twenty hours, although it was never bloody. The cerebral symptoms are prominent in the severe cases. These symptoms such as marked irritability, increasing stuporousness, mental dullness, and generalized convulsions were very prominent in my case. The causation of the cerebral symptoms is less obvious, and some of the symptoms such as deafness and disturbance of vision are known to accompany salicylate poisoning.[8] The most spectacular symptom, the hyperpnea, seen also in my case, seems to be the most widely discussed. Because of the Kussmaul type of breathing, it was thought to be caused by an acidosis, since most investigators agree that there is some reduction in the carbon-dioxide capacity of the blood plasma in salicylate poisoning. Johnson[9] found that in four of his eight experimental cats which had received the equivalent of a full therapeutic dose of sodium salicylate there was a significant decrease on the alkali reserve and that in these four there was an increase in blood lactates. Hanzlik,[10] on the other hand, does not consider the reaction of air hunger in salicylate poisoning to be of the nature of an acidosis because he did not find any shift in the hydrogen-ion concentration. Veil and Graubner,[11] Gebert,[12] and Odin[13] suggest that the salicylates have an irritative action on the respiratory center, which produces hyperventilation. This in turn causes a decreased carbon-dioxide content of alveolar air and blood and a reduction of fixed alkali in the blood by excretion of an alkaline urine. For this reason they believe alkali treatment is contraindicated in salicylate poisoning. Morris and Graham,[14] on the other hand, state that the air hunger in salicylate poisoning cases was due to a nongaseous acidosis, and because of the acidosis and impairment of renal function, they believe the only form of treatment is by alkalies and not glucose.

Although many cases of salicylate poisoning have been reported and their similarity to diabetic coma noted, few authors have determined the actual existence of a severe acidosis by means of a carbon-dioxide combining power of the blood plasma. Longmead[15] in 1906 reported eight cases of salicylate poisoning in children and called attention to the similarity of these cases to diabetic acidosis. In 1936, Bowen, Roufa and Clinger[16] reported a case of methyl salicylate poisoning in a child eighteen months of age and noted in their patient the similarity of salicylate poisoning to diabetic coma. The carbon-dioxide capacity was found to be 50 volumes per cent. These authors believe the symptoms resembling diabetic coma to be one of an irritative action on the respiratory center, rather than a true acidosis. Pincus and Handley,[17] on the other hand, in their case found the carbon-dioxide combining power to be 36 volumes per cent. Olmstead and Aldrich[18] reported two cases, and their determinations were 33.5 per cent and 37.6 per cent. Dwyer,[19] in 1933, reported one case of 36.5 per cent. In my case the findings of the carbon-dioxide combining power were 57 volumes per cent. Because of this normal value, the child was treated with intravenous saline solutions and 5 per cent glucose. Most investigators agree that the ideal treatment of salicylate poisoning is large amounts of alkalies, both by mouth and rectum, and intravenously in the more severe cases. Nevertheless, every patient suspected of any salicylate poisoning should have a carbon-dioxide combining power done before alkali therapy is started.

While a number of cases were studied at necropsy, the pathologic conditions described seem to show certain changes which were found in my case. In 1928 Woodbury and Nicholls described an acute gastritis, congestion and edema of the lungs, and acute degenerative parenchymatous nephritis. Wetzel and Nourse found hemorrhagic areas in the lungs; the liver showed generalized fatty changes and cloudy swelling; with cloudy swelling and fatty degeneration of tubular portion of the renal cortex. Meyerhoff[20] reported changes of an early glomerular nephritis; cloudy swelling and fatty degeneration of the liver.

SUMMARY

1. Four cubic centimeters of methyl salicylate can produce death in infants. Methyl salicylate should be dispensed with proper warning as to its possible dangers when taken internally, and since the drug is used so freely, steps should be taken toward its prevention.

2. The clinical and pathologic findings in this case are similar to those previously reported.

3. When dealing with a case of coma, salicylate poisoning should be considered, and if possible a carbon-dioxide combining power should be done so as to determine whether to give alkali therapy or not.

4. Since most cases that have been reported show a low carbon-dioxide combining power, the therapy of choice would be some form of alkalies, either by mouth or intravenously if the case is severe.

REFERENCES

1. Stevenson, C. S.: Am. J. M. Sc. **193**: 772, 1937.
2. Gallaher, T. J.: Philadelphia Med. Exam. **16**: 347, 1852.
3. Hughes, R. F.: Canadian M. A. J. **27**: 417, 1932.
4. Meyers, H. B.: J. A. M. A. **75**: 1783, 1920.
5. Wetzel, N. C., and Nourse, J. D.: Arch. Path. & Lab. Med. **1**: 182, 1926.
6. Hanzlik, P. J., and Wetzel, N. C.: J. Pharmacol. & Exper. Therap. **14**: 43, 1920
7. Woodbury, F. V., and Nicholls, A. G.: Canadian M. A. J. **18**: 167, 1928.
8. Cushney, A. G.: Pharmacology and Therapy, Philadelphia, 1911, Lea & Febiger.
9. Johnson, C. C.: J. A. M. A. **94**: 784, 1930.
10. Hanzlik, P. J., Scott, R. W., and Thorburn, T. W.: J. Pharmacol. & Exper. Therap. **9**: 247, 1917.
11. Veil, W. H., and Graubner, W.: Arch. f. exper. Path. u Pharmakol. **117**: 208, 1926.
12. Gebert, K.: Ztschr. f. klin. Med. **117**: 147, 1931.
13. Odin, M.: Acta med. Scandinav. **50**: 177, 1932.
14. Morris, N., and Graham, S.: Arch. Dis. Childhood **6**: 273, 1931.
15. Longmead, F.: Lancet **1**: 1822, 1906.
16. Bowen, B. D., Roufa, J. F., and Clinger, O. W.: J. A. M. A. **107**: 276, 1936.
17. Pincus, J. B., and Handley, H. E.: Bull. Johns Hopkins Hosp. **41**: 163, 1927.
18. Olmstead, J. G. M., and Aldrich, C. A.: J. A. M. A. **90**: 1438, 1928.
19. Dwyer, H. L.: J. Kansas M. Soc. **34**: 166, 1933.
20. Meyerhoff, I. S.: J. A. M. A. **94**: 1751, 1930.

Critical Review

HEREDITY IN DISEASE

A Review of the Recent Literature

David Beres, M.D., and Viva Schatia, M.D.
New York, N. Y.

THE increasing recognition of the importance of genetic factors in disease warrants a detailed study of the recent literature on this subject. There are available several reviews of heredity which give general summaries of the subject.[1, 2] The purpose of this article is not merely to catalogue the work done by various authors, but rather to present a critical survey of the past year in order to emphasize the recent trends in this field.

There are three important fields in which genetic data find application. There is, first, the immediate clinical significance to the physician in the care of a given case. Second, there is the application of the data of human heredity to eugenic problems. This is a very controversial field which we shall touch upon but briefly. Third, there is the application of the data to political and economic problems about which, unfortunately, a great deal of harmful and vicious misinformation has been promulgated. We shall not touch upon this interesting aspect of the subject, which includes the consideration of race biology, but refer the reader to a recent book by J. B. S. Haldane.[3] This review will be limited for the most part to articles of clinical significance.

Material for the study of human heredity is so scarce that in this more than any other field of medicine are communal interests of different workers indicated. The isolated case reported by one author assumes increased significance when similar observations by another worker add to the statistical validity of the material.

It will not be possible in this review to consider the basic biologic material, the understanding of which is essential for any discussion on heredity. Such material, written especially with the view to its application to human problems, is available in a number of excellent books on the subject.[4]

The authors of this review have attempted as thorough a search of the literature as possible within the limits discussed above. There is no doubt, however, that a considerable number of articles have been missed, especially because so often genetic data are buried in articles in which the whole emphasis is either clinical or pathologic.

INTERNAL MEDICINE AND PEDIATRICS

Allergy.—The importance of heredity in development of allergic diseases has long been recognized and accepted. The questioning of this conclusion by Ratner[5] is surprising. His report, unfortunately, is in abstract form and the author himself apologizes for the generalities

From the Pediatric Service of Dr. Bela Schick and the Department of Laboratories, Mount Sinai Hospital.

of his data. Ratner analyzes the family background of 250 allergic children and finds among them an incidence of allergy no greater than that in the general population. Wiener[6] and his colleagues present a more valid study of inheritance in allergic disease. They sought also for evidence of linkage with eye color and the blood group properties A, B, M, and N.[7] They distinguish, among patients with asthma, two types: the one with onset before puberty, the other with onset in the third decade of life. They postulate, instead of the accepted Mendelian mechanism which is that of simple dominant heredity, the existence of two allelomorphs, H and h. Individuals having the genetic composition HH are normal. Those with hh are asthmatics presenting the early type of the disease, while those with the heterozygous composition Hh either have the disease late in life or not at all. The authors did not find any evidence of linkage between allergic diseases and genes determining the blood group properties and eye color.

Digestive Diseases.—Körner[8] studied fifty-seven families of individuals who had been operated upon for gall bladder disease. He found an increased incidence of gall bladder disease in the families of 47.3 per cent of the patients. In these families there was also an increased incidence of diseases, considered by the author to be related to gall bladder disease, such as appendicitis, peptic ulcer, adiposity, and gout. In fifty-seven control families only two presented an increased incidence of the disease itself, and thirty-three families in this group had members who suffered from the so-called associated diseases. The author emphasizes that increased frequency of incidence of disease in a family is not necessarily the same as heredity, and the extrinsic factors in the causation of gall bladder disease must not be minimized.

Necheles and Levitsky,[9] in a study of the relation of constitution to peptic ulcer, conclude that ulcer patients secrete less saliva following pilocarpine than do normal individuals. In a previous article the same authors concluded that the apparently healthy members of the families of ulcer patients suffered from a similar type of pharmacodynamic abnormality.

The incidence of appendicitis in two families was compared with that computed for the general population by Baker.[10] Although the pedigrees are interesting and suggestive, the statistical work-up does not appear to be very reliable.

Sheldon[11] reports a case of hypertrophic pyloric stenosis in one of a set of uniovular twins. He reviews the literature on the subject, emphasizing that his experience is different from that of most other reports, in which usually both of the twins, when identical, are afflicted.

Cardiac Diseases.—Hecht and Gupta[12] studied the electrocardiograms of twins and concluded that the similarity of the tracings in identical twins is striking as compared to the lesser degree of similarity in ordinary twins.

A paper of unusual excellence is one by Wilson and Schweitzer[13] on rheumatic fever. This paper is important not alone for the material presented and the conclusions drawn, but also as an example of a careful, valid, statistical analysis. The authors emphasize the increased familial incidence of rheumatic fever, which is reported to be from 15 to 58 per cent. They consider three factors to be responsible. First, home environmental conditions; second, communicability; and third, susceptibility, probably on a hereditary basis. By an analysis of the relative significance of these factors, the authors believe that hereditary susceptibility would seem to determine the familial incidence of rheumatic fever. They conclude: "It is reasonable to suppose that the acquisition of rheumatic fever may be dependent on the exposure of the susceptible individual to an etiological agent that is widespread in this geographical environment."

Ayman,[14] in a study of 1,524 persons in 277 families, ascribes a tendency to hypertension in early life to a hereditary basis. He states that so-called emotional hypertension occurs almost wholly in the young members of hypertensive families. However, he carries his conclusions too far in assuming the existence of a "special personality" in these hypertensive individuals, and the assumption that there is a heredity of personality demonstrable in his data.

Ullrich[15] describes a most unusual study of a set of triplets, all boys, two of whom were identical. These two presented congenital cardiac hypertrophy with fibrosis of the endocardium. The pathologic studies of the two abnormal children are included.

Infectious Diseases.—The study of heredity in relation to infectious diseases presents many difficult problems. Lehmann,[16] in a brief general discussion, assumes the existence of hereditary differences determining susceptibility to infectious diseases in human beings. An excellent summary of experimental studies of this subject on animals is presented by Hill[17] in which the available literature is subjected to a critical survey. The author points out the difficulty of eliminating the environmental factors concerned, particularly that of acquired immunity transmitted from infected ancestors. It was demonstrable, however, that between strains of the same species, differences in mortality from specific infections existed, which could be ascribed to differences in genetic composition.

Hofmeier[18] summarizes recent literature on the relation of heredity to immunity in human beings. He emphasizes the importance of studies in twins.

Metabolic Diseases.—Two papers on heredity of brittle bones and blue sclerae describe the usual dominant type of heredity that has previously been worked out in this disease. Burch and Sodeman[19] found forty-one afflicted individuals among seventy-six persons in five generations. Hills and McLanahan[20] found the condition in twenty-seven out of fifty-one persons in five generations.

Harnapp[21] describes the occurrence of a form of osteosclerosis in a father, two brothers, and three sisters. This condition is usually considered to be nonhereditary.

HEMATOLOGY

Hemophilia.—The heredity of hemophilia has long served as an exquisite example of heredity in the human being, demonstrating the Mendelian mechanism of recessive sex-linkage. Fonio,[22] who has reviewed the entire subject of hemophilia in an extensive monograph, has another long article[23] on the hemophiliacs of Bern. He lists several new family pedigrees which do not deviate from the recognized form of recessive sex-linked inheritance. He discusses the hematologic findings in so-called female carriers and claims to have demonstrated changes in the functions of the platelets and increased bleeding time in several such individuals. He includes in his pedigree a child 3 years of age as a female hemophiliac, but unfortunately there were no clinical studies on this case.

The question of female hemophiliacs is creating increased interest. Rosenthal, Vogel, and Beres[24] present a detailed hematologic study of a female with the classical features of hemophilia. There were no other cases in the family of this patient, whose symptoms developed at the age of 28 years. The patient had a son who was entirely normal and the authors conclude that this case of hemophilia in a female was therefore genetically of different character from the hemophilia ordinarily seen in the male. The authors state that a careful search of the literature prior to the case reported has not yielded a single case of hemophilia in a female in which the hematologic criteria could be accepted.

Bauer and Meller[25] describe five cases in females who showed prolonged coagulation time and a familial incidence of the disease. Their data include a family in which the father and the mother were both hemophiliacs, and only one of their two daughters was a hemophiliac. They also report abnormalities in the bleeding time and platelet counts. The accuracy of this entire report is to be most seriously questioned. Studt[26] also believes that there is a quantitative abnormality in coagulation time demonstrable in female conductors. Birch[27] has prepared a monograph on hemophilia and includes a consideration of its genetic aspects.

Hereditary Pseudohemophilia.—This disease is to be sharply differentiated from hemophilia, both on clinical grounds and on those of genetic behavior. Clinically these cases present normal coagulation time. Handley and Nussbrecher[28] describe the occurrence of this disease in both male and female. Debré et al.,[29] in a study of seven families, confirmed the accepted hereditary pattern of dominant Mendelian heredity.

Other Hematologic Diseases.—Brockmann,[30] in a very careful study of seventeen families of individuals with polycythemia, found no increased frequency of the disease in these families and concludes that there is no relation to any constitutional disease entity. He believes, however, that a complex polyfactorial heredity is most probable. Wiskott[31] presents three cases of purpura hemorrhagica in three brothers. Four sisters were normal. Ardashnikov[32] describes a family pedigree of four generations with cases involving both sexes and transmitted directly from parent to child. The patients had increased bleeding time, normal platelets, and normal coagulation time. The hemorrhages were usually localized to the throat.

Macklin,[33] in a statistical analysis of cases of erythroblastosis foetalis reported in the literature, considers the relationship of this disease to icterus neonatorum and congenital anemia. She believes that the genetic behavior of these three diseases is sufficiently different to indicate a different genetic basis for each one. Pache[34] describes three families with severe jaundice of the newborn infant. He demonstrates that the percentage of diseased children is greater in later births.

Cardozo[35] attempts an immunologic study of sickling and blood groups and finds no definite relationship. Haden and Evans[36] studied a family of five white children, two of whom suffered from sickle-cell anemia, one with sickling but no anemia, and the other two with no blood dyscrasia. Bauer[37] studied a pair of 7-month-old identical twins, both of whom presented, on sternal puncture, a picture which the author considers characteristic of von Jaksch-Hayem's anemia. Only one of the children had clinical symptoms of this disease.

Schemensky[38] describes a rare anomaly of the red blood cells characterized by an oval shape which is present under all circumstances. The condition was present in a mother and daughter. It has no clinical significance. Sternal puncture revealed a normal bone marrow. Strauss and Daland[39] describe a family with a similar condition in which ten individuals were involved. Heredity was typically dominant in character.

Gunn[40] reports the presence of hereditary acholuric jaundice in a strain of rats. This condition appeared by mutation in a laboratory strain of the animal. The author indicates the close similarity to the disease as it appears in human beings. Especially interesting is the fact that 50 per cent of normal-appearing hybrid rats showed increased fragility of the red blood cells and increased reticulocytosis, indicating that the condition is inherited as an incomplete dominant factor.

SKIN

The striking manifestations of hereditary skin conditions have given reports in this field a prominent place in the literature. An excellent summary of the available material up to 1933 has been prepared by Cockayne.[41] Munro[42] describes twenty persons with sebaceous cysts in four generations of a family and concludes that the disease is determined by a dominant gene subject to modification. West[43] describes a case of congenital ichthyosis in a mother and three sons. He concludes that the disease is determined by a dominant gene. He discusses Cockayne's analysis of heredity in this disease and dismisses that author's theory that it may be transmitted as a sex-linked recessive trait. West makes the error of assuming that the heredity of a disease must be explained by only one Mendelian mechanism. This is contrary to experience in both human and animal genetic material. Beres and Messeloff[44] describe a family in which ichthyosis vulgaris is inherited as a sex-linked recessive character. Idelberger and Haberler[45] describe a family in which the disease appears as a dominant character. Gilch,[46] in an exhaustive analysis of ichthyosis, describes several types of hereditary mechanism and attempts a clinical distinction on the basis of the different forms of heredity behavior.

Gillespie[47] describes four children in one family presenting total alopecia. The parents were related to each other but the author could not determine the exact relationship. A boy, 9 years old, presenting an ectodermal dysplasia is reported by Kerley.[48] Fitch[49] presents photographic evidence of the dominant inheritance of white forelock in four generations of one family. The abnormality was associated in some cases with white spots on the skin, while the latter occurred in one member without the hair anomaly. Anderson[50] describes an interesting family studied for four generations, presenting wooly hair in both male and female. The disease is transmitted only through affected individuals in direct line from parent to child.

McCrackin[51] describes a family of seven negro children, five of whom (three boys and two identical twin girls) suffer from albinism. In an elaborate summary article, Sanders[52] analyzes 140 families with 216 cases of albinism, gathered from the literature and his own experience. The heredity is typically recessive in character.

TEETH

Hyde,[53] in a general article directed to the dental profession, emphasizes the importance of heredity in various dental conditions, including double deciduous teeth, transparent dentine and enamel, congenital missing teeth, and hereditary hypoplasia.

Haldane[54] publishes a pedigree presented by C. H. Bampton to the Sixth International Dental Congress in 1914 in which the appearance of brown teeth was studied in five successive generations, and concludes that this anomaly follows a dominant sex-linked pattern, a type of heredity which is very rare.

The relationship of dental abnormalities to cleidocranial dysostosis is emphasized by Rushton.[55] The dental abnormalities he finds in the latter disease include supernumerary teeth, failure of eruption, deformities of the teeth, abnormalities of the jaw, and the formation of cysts.

EAR

Studies of the hereditary factors in diseases of the ear have been limited within the past year to congenital abnormalities of the external ear. Potter[56] presents a pedigree of a family followed for five generations in which a bilateral external ear malformation appeared to be transmitted as a dominant characteristic. Powell and Whitney,[57] who describe pedigrees of two families, conclude that free ear lobes are dominant, whereas adherent ones are recessive. They are criticized by Wiener[58] who believes that, although there is a correlation between types of ear lobes in parents and children, no definite genetic mechanism has been determined as yet.

EYE

A most unusual series of articles by Hamilton[59] undertakes the analysis of the entire population of Tasmania, with special reference to the incidence of hereditary eye diseases. He considers the problem from all angles, including social and economic significance of the various factors involved. The different hereditary eye conditions which have been found are described and analyzed from a genetic point of view. This study is of importance, not alone for the ophthalmologic material which it presents, but also as an example of a genetic study of the highest order.

Vogt and Meyer[60] present two families with angiomatosis retinae of the type associated with von Hipple-Lindau's disease. In one family father and daughter were affected; in the other, uncle and nephew. In the second case, there were two other uncles who had cerebellar tumors. The article is illustrated by beautifully colored plates demonstrating the lesions in the fundi. Walsh and Wegman[61] present a pedigree of hereditary cataract affecting the males more severely than the females. The data were submitted to Dr. C. W. Metz of the Carnegie Institute of Washington for an opinion of the genetic mechanisms involved. He made the suggestion: "Rather than speculate on the possible genetic basis of the cataract at present, it seems desirable to await the appearance of another generation which ought to provide significant information." Allan[62] presents a number of pedigrees of retinitis pigmentosa with several different forms of genetic behavior. This study suffers from the fact that of the fifty-nine patients, only fifteen were personally examined by the author. Two of the pedigrees were developed entirely on the basis of hearsay information, and not a single individual in these families was examined. Bonnet and Paufique[63] described a father and three children presenting bilateral ophthalmoplegia. The father was the only affected member of eleven siblings.

White and Fulton[64] describe an unusual pupillary anomaly in monozygotic female twins. The anomaly consists of large, irregular pupils incapable of responding to constricting stimuli except in certain quadrants, which were the same in both subjects. The mother was reported to have the same condition. The father, five siblings, and five offspring were free of the abnormality.

Lisch[65] describes a family in which twelve members in three generations were afflicted with keratoconjunctivitis sicca. The author states that this is the first description of the familial incidence of this disease. Mann[66] describes three cases of congenital vascular veils in the vitreous, all in males, two in brothers. The author emphasizes the embryologic basis of this condition.

ORTHOPEDICS

The appearance of skeletal anomalies presents a complex problem which has been handled by two types of articles; broad surveys, in which an attempt is made to discuss congenital anomalies in general, and reports of the familial incidence of a given anomaly. Streeter,[67] in a Harvey lecture, discusses the general problem of congenital abnormalities, emphasizing their dependence on genetic factors. Macklin[68] offers a general statistical study of the relation of external factors, such as barometric pressure, to the etiology of malformation. She concludes that external factors are of little or no importance, heredity being the chief etiological factor. Müller,[69] in a monograph on the congenital abnormalities of the hand, discusses especially the developmental bases of the various abnormalities. He considers in detail the genetic factors involved.

Weidenmüller,[70] in a discussion of the heredity of spina bifida, emphasizes the importance of a careful search for mild atypical forms of the disease in supposedly normal members of the family. He describes a family with syndactylia in two generations and syndactylia and spina bifida in the third.

Schwarzweller[71] describes cases of congenital winged scapula and emphasizes the existence of associated anomalies such as fusion of vertebral arches, defects in the vertebral column, and scoliosis.

Pfeiffer[72] describes a variety of anomalies of the femur and concludes that in his cases the basic etiology is a genetic one. Schwarzweller,[73] in a discussion of acrocephalosyndactylia, emphasizes the presence in siblings of portions of this syndrome and its appearance with other hereditary anomalies. Hangarter and Dieker,[74] in a discussion of the Klipple-Feil syndrome, also emphasize the presence of minor abnormalities in other members of the family.

Jarcho and Levin[75] report a brother and sister with a form of the Klipple-Feil syndrome. They postulate the existence of a general dysplastic tendency, which is evidenced in these cases and in other members of the family by the existence of minor abnormalities, such as accessory nipple, anomalies of the heart, and undescended testicle. A second specific dysplastic factor is considered to be responsible for the deformity itself. An interesting observation which the authors made was that corresponding to the reduced number of vertebrae in the thoracic region there was also a reduction in the number of thoracic spinal roots. They conclude, therefore, that the so-called "segmentation of the spinal roots really depends upon extrinsic structures rather than upon a fundamental pattern within the nervous system."

Bakwin and Krida[76] present a brother and sister with x-ray evidence of metaphyseal dysplasia. Fused fingers were present as a dominant hereditary characteristic in a family studied by Wightman,[77] with data for seven generations. Jackson[78] describes a family in which six digits appeared as an irregular dominant factor for four generations. Duncan,[79] in an article written from a therapeutic point of view, presents a pair of identical twins with coxa vara, the deformity in one being the mirror image of that in the other.

Achondroplastic nanism, associated with musical ability, appeared as a dominant nonsex-linked characteristic in a family known personally to Capinpin.[80] Volhard and Drigalski[81] describe a family in which three brothers present a peculiar deformity of the spine. They mention a family with a similar picture described by Nilsonne in which also only males were affected. Gaugele[82] discusses congenital dislocation of the hip. Though he recognizes its increased familial incidence, he doubts that it is a hereditary disease.

GENITOURINARY DISEASE AND SURGERY

Gruber[83] presents a detailed analysis of a variety of congenital anomalies of the genitourinary system. He discusses especially pedigrees of families with cystic kidney. He describes the relationship of this anomaly with other anomalies, especially those involving the skeletal system. There is an extensive bibliography. Gordon and Trasoff[84] describe a family in which five children out of seven have polycystic kidney. The parents of these children were related as uncle and niece. The author stresses the importance of examining all members of a family in which polycystic kidney occurs.

West[85] presents two pedigrees illustrating the familial incidence of hernia. His data do not allow a definite conclusion as to the Mendelian mechanism involved.

A case of unusual interest is described by Pettersson and Bonnier.[86] The patient was a girl, apparently normal, who was operated upon for double inguinal hernia and was found to have testes and other internal male structures but no internal female structures. Examination of the family revealed similar sex mosaic inheritance among other individuals. The authors discuss possible genetic explanations of this inherited anomaly but do not arrive at a final conclusion. They consider it most probable that the individuals begin as normal males but that a sex-linked recessive gene inhibits the development of the external male genitals.

CANCER

In the articles so far discussed several cases have arisen in which a hereditary factor has been pointed out as of significance in the development of an individual type of tumor growth. Examples of this are von Hipple-Lindau's disease and sebaceous cysts.

One must, however, make a sharp distinction between heredity as regards a specific type of unusual growth and the heredity of cancer in general. With regard to the former, a great deal of information is available. With regard to the latter, there is little convincing material to be found in human studies. Little and Reimann,[87] in an unusual paper, present a discussion on the subject of heredity in relation to neoplastic disease, which is valuable as an indication of the problems which are being emphasized in studies of this subject.

Bell and Rothnem[88] describe two cases in brothers aged 16 and 13 years who had xeroderma pigmentosum with carcinoma. The parents were second cousins. Hauser and Weller[89] describe additional cases in the so-called cancer family of Warthin, in which forty-one individuals out of a total of 174 over 25 years of age have some form of neoplasm. Twenty-six of these were carcinoma of the intestinal tract, and fifteen were of the uterus. No definite Mendelian mechanism was indicated. Martynova[90] studied the families of 201 women who had carcinoma of the breast. Seven hundred and ninety-six patients from a dental clinic were used as controls. In the families of the cancer patients there was an incidence of carcinoma, in general, of 12.08 per cent and of cancer of the breast of 2.65 per cent. Among the controls the general incidence of cancer was 2.96 per cent and cancer of the breast 0.17 per cent. This study would seem to indicate the operation of a very definite hereditary factor. Körbler,[91] in his presentation of several cases of familial incidence of cancer, poses the problem of the basis of this increased incidence. He considers heredity and contagiousness to be possible factors but he leaves the problem unanswered because of insufficient available data.

In the consideration of cancer heredity, animal experiments are of interest. Stark[92] describes an interesting study in the Drosophila melanogaster, which has been the animal most used in genetic studies. He describes several different hereditary tumors presenting a variety of hereditary mechanisms. One was sex-linked, never being seen in the male because all males who were afflicted died before reaching maturity. Another type due to multiple genes in several chromosomes is described. Some of the tumors arise from embryonic rests in the walls of the larval digestive tract. Another form resembles lymphosarcoma, another melanoepithelioma. The importance of this study is that it allows detailed genetic investigation of definite neoplasms presenting certain histologic similarities to human material. Murray[93] describes the relation of genetics to transplantation of neoplastic tissue and emphasizes the importance of genetic factors in the success of transplantation experiments in animals.

Bittner,[94] in a review of the genetics of cancer in mice, warns against the application of findings in animal experimentation work to the human problem. He says: "The impossibility of securing human data to compare with inbred strains of animals where controlled matings may be made needs little comment. The reliability of considerable of the human data is questionable and leaves much to be desired."

ENDOCRINE DISEASES

Two papers of extreme interest have been published in which endocrine disturbances in one of a set of identical twins have resulted in gross dissimilarity in the individuals. In all the cases the identity of the twins was established by the usual biologic criteria. Lüth[95] describes three sets of identical twins with differences in growth and development in one individual of each set. Lewis[96] describes in detail two brothers who until puberty were always mistaken for each other. After that, one grew larger than the other and developed acromegalic features.

He grew to a height of 6 feet, 4 inches, while his brother was 5 feet, 8 inches. The only etiological clue in the former was a head injury sustained at the age of 12 years.

Munro[97] describes two cases in brother and sister with a similar atypical and uncommon psychosis associated with endocrine malfunction suggestive of the hyperactivity of the adrenals or of the anterior pituitary. The parents were first cousins.

Warkany and Mitchell,[98] in a discussion of heredodegenerative diseases, warn against the tendency to assume a relationship to endocrine disease, even when both may be present in the same patient. Goldman and Smith[99] describe several cases of hyperparathyroidism occurring in siblings.

Laurence-Moon-Biedl Syndrome.—A great deal of interest has been manifested in this disease. The syndrome contains in its complete form the following manifestations: mental defect, retinitis pigmentosa, adiposogenital dystrophy, syndactylia, polydactylia, microglossia, and various skull defects. The disease has a definite familial incidence, though any one individual may have varying degrees of the affliction, from the disease in its entirety to the appearance of isolated features. Warkany and Frauenberger,[100] in a detailed study of the literature, emphasized the fact that the syndrome rarely appears in its full form. They conclude that the syndrome does not represent a disease entity but is rather a combination of more or less frequent heredofamilial symptoms.

Van Bogaert[101] describes a family in which two brothers have the disease in its classic form, while the mother had only retinitis pigmentosa and two aunts had obesity, hypogenitalism, and mental disturbances. Panse[102] also discusses the hereditary basis of this disease. Cooperstock[103] accepts the explanation of two recessive linked genes to account for a large family he studied, the various members of which had one or more stigmas of the syndrome.

NEUROLOGY AND PSYCHIATRY

The problem of hereditary factors in nervous and mental diseases has aroused the interest of physicians, sociologists, and geneticists for practical as well as theoretical reasons. Much data have been accumulated, particularly by German authors, and many conclusions, both correct and erroneous, have been drawn. An excellent critical analysis of the entire subject has been prepared by a special committee appointed by the American Neurological Association to investigate the problem of eugenic sterilization. This committee, consisting of Drs. Abraham Myerson, James B. Ayer, Tracy J. Putnam, Clyde E. Keeler, and Leo Alexander, have presented the results of their studies in a book entitled *Eugenical Sterilization,*[104] to which repeated references will be made in this review. Additional sources of critical evaluation of the data relating to heredity of mental and neurological disorders is to be found in the publications of the English scientists, who have given to this subject a series of brilliant and basic works, those of Hogben,[105] Haldane,[3] and Penrose[106] being especially valuable.

Huntington's Chorea.—Huntington's chorea, which is a classical example of dominant heredity in the human being, has been reported by a number of different authors. Spillane and Phillips[107] describe twenty-four cases with typical dominant heredity, and explain those instances in which both parents of afflicted individuals were normal by the assumption that the affected parent died before he was old enough to manifest the disease. Hempel[108] describes several cases with typical heredity but with atypical clinical pictures that created considerable difficulty in diagnosis. Meierhofer[109] in his paper stresses the appearance of atypical psychoses in a family afflicted with Huntington's chorea. Stone and Falstein[110] describe a group of cases with atypical heredity.

Minski and Guttmann[111] offer a detailed analysis of thirty-four families, considering also the clinical manifestations of the disease in its usual and unusual forms. Their data confirm the accepted mechanism of dominant heredity.

Familial Ataxia, Multiple Sclerosis, and Related Diseases.—Hall and MacKay,[112] in an excellent paper, describe two forms of familial ataxia and emphasize the diagnostic difficulties involved in differentiating this disease from multiple sclerosis. This point is very important in the evaluation of several articles which have appeared in the German literature in which multiple sclerosis is described as a hereditary disease. Curschmann[113] describes three brothers afflicted with a disease diagnosed as multiple sclerosis. Jentsch[114] describes two sets of identical twins with a disease diagnosed as multiple sclerosis. He considers it to be an infectious disease with a hereditary predisposition. Curtius and Speer,[115] in a general analysis of the subject, consider multiple sclerosis to be forty times as frequent among the relatives of patients affected as in the general population.

Schröder[116] describes a family in which two brothers, one sister, the mother, and the maternal grandmother had Friedreich's ataxia. Lux[117] considers hereditary ataxia as an hereditary disease in which the clinical course is profoundly affected by external factors, such as intercurrent infections. In a paper on hereditary cerebellar ataxia by Waggoner, Löwenberg and Speicher,[118] the difficulties of diagnosis and classification are strongly brought out. The report includes the pathologic study of a patient and genetic study of five generations of the patient's family, which included twenty-seven cases of ataxia. The pathologic study showed abnormalities in the pons, olivary bodies, and the cerebellum. The authors, however, refuse to consider this a case of olivo-ponto-cerebellar atrophy, and on the basis of the heredity, classify this as an example of the heredocerebellar ataxia of Pierre Marie.

Two papers on familial spinal spastic paralysis describing a familial incidence interpreted as due to a dominant hereditary factor are presented by Röhricht[119] and Kahlstorf.[120] The fact that the authors describe the same disease under different names is an indication of the difficulties that beset analysis in this field. Turner and Roberts[121] describe a sex-linked heredity in a condition resembling Friedreich's ataxia. This has never before been reported in this disease.

The myelopathies, of which there are so many types, present striking examples of heredity in organic neurological disorders. Two general reviews on the subject are available, one by Aring and Cobb[122] in English, and one by Sjövall[123] in German. The diagnostic difficulties in differentiating the various types of this disease must be taken into consideration in evaluating the reports which follow. Boeters[124] describes a large series of cases involving the various forms of myelopathies. Cooper[125] presents a history of a 55-year-old man and three sons, ages 28, 24, and 21 years, who had Dejerine-Sottos disease. In addition, one other member of the family had muscular atrophy, and a maternal grandmother presented wasting of peripheral portions of all limbs. Rütenik[126] describes a case of amyotrophic lateral sclerosis (confirmed at autopsy) with a family history including a sister who had had the same symptoms and a brother with early symptoms which were discovered by routine examination of the family. Schneider and Abeles[127] present clinical histories of two brothers with a Charcot-Marie-Tooth syndrome associated with primary optic atrophy. The parents were first cousins. A case of myotonia congenita in a boy 9 years of age is described by Breitfort.[128] There was no other case in the family.

Rothbart[129] describes the occurrence of myasthenia gravis in four brothers. This disease is not usually considered to be a hereditary one, the only evidence heretofore having been the occasional coexistence of myasthenia and congenital anomalies. This report therefore assumes increased importance.

Heredodegenerative Diseases.—An interesting report of Niemann-Pick's disease in a set of identical twins is described by Freudenberg.[130] He emphasizes the "Aryan" descent of these patients. There were no reports this year of heredity in amaurotic family idiocy of the infantile type which is pathologically and clinically closely related to Niemann-Pick's disease. In the former there is strong evidence that heredity is determined by a single recessive gene. Van Bogaert and Borremans[131] present a series of cases which they consider to be an adult form of amaurotic family idiocy. The clinical details make very questionable the accuracy of their diagnosis and further observation is necessary. Jakobsen[132] describes a case of juvenile amaurotic family idiocy in which the patient was the only afflicted member of a family in which four generations were studied.

Two papers on Wilson's disease have appeared. Schwyn[133] describes two cases occurring in brother and sister, and includes a detailed pathologic report. Müller[134] describes a case in a boy with a suggestive family history. The father had pernicious anemia and combined sclerosis, and a sister died of a disease manifesting extrapyramidal symptoms. He considers the disease to be determined by a metabolic anomaly that may affect different organs.

Forsberg and Stromme[135] describe a family in which a brother and three sisters had dysarthria, spastic phenomena, cerebellar ataxia, and nystagmus. The grandparents were cousins. The authors have diagnosed these cases as Pelizaeus-Merzbacher disease but offer no anatomic confirmation.

The pathogenesis of congenital diplegia has caused considerable discussion. Alpers[136] in a recent review of the subject agrees with the prevailing general opinion that it is a degenerative disease, probably due to the effect of prenatal factors. The theory of birth injury as a causative factor has steadily lost in acceptance in the years that the subject has been studied. In an important paper by Thums[137] there is an analysis of a series of twins in which one or both members were afflicted with Little's disease. His findings are very striking. Among nine pairs of identical twins only one pair presented the appearance of the disease in both individuals. Among ten sets of nonidentical twins there is no case in which both had the disease. In a group of ten sets of twins of different sex and therefore biovular, one set presented the disease in both individuals. Lisch and Thums[138] analyze a pair of identical twins, one of whom was entirely normal, whereas the other suffered with congenital spastic diplegia and mental deficiency. The diagnosis of identity was made on the basis of the accepted biologic criteria. This paper apparently proves that the disease is not determined on a purely hereditary basis.

Van Bogaert and de Savitsch[139] describe a group of cases which they cannot classify exactly, in which rhythmic tremor of the head, eyes, and upper extremities presents the outstanding clinical features. Forty members of a family of 109 individuals were afflicted. The data were interpreted as presenting evidence of a dominant type of heredity.

Russell and Tallerman[140] describe the occurrence (confirmed by autopsy) of familial progressive diffuse cerebral sclerosis in two Jewish children whose parents were first cousins and whose two siblings were normal.

Other Conditions.—Allan[141] studied seventy-two consecutive cases of parkinsonism. In forty-five he found a positive family history, of which he presents forty-three complete pedigrees. He considers the genetic mechanism to be that of an autosomal gene acting as dominant. The author indicates the incompleteness of his study, emphasizing the need for observation by other workers, and claims only that he has demonstrated beyond doubt the importance of heredity in shaking palsy.

Menninger and Grotjahn[142] studied a group of cases of juvenile dementia paralytica and conclude that the tendency for neurosyphilis to appear with increased frequency in a family is due to the existence of a neurotropic strain of *Spirochaeta pallida* rather than to familial predisposition to cerebrospinal syphilis.

Laubenthal[143] describes a family presenting several individuals with congenital word blindness.

Craig[144] describes the interesting occurrence of intracranial tumors in two sisters. The symptoms developed in both patients at approximately the same age. One of the patients had a craniopharyngioma and died postoperatively; the other had a primary glioma of the optic chiasm and recovered following surgical intervention. The case of a boy 19 years of age with intraocular neuroma of the optic nerve head is described by Stollard.[145] The patient subsequently developed signs of increased intracranial pressure. There were in the family of the patient several cases of multiple neurofibromas of the central nervous system and cranial nerves, in two generations.

In a study of sciatica, involving seven sets of identical twins and eight sets of fraternal twins, Becker[146] postulates the existence of a hereditary predisposition to this disease which is, however, brought out by various environmental factors.

The Epilepsies.—It must be recognized that in using this term one includes a heterogeneous group of diseases which are better described under the general heading of convulsive disorders. The reports which have appeared on the hereditary basis of this disease have almost universally indicated an increased incidence in the families of afflicted individuals, the conclusion being that in epilepsy one is dealing with a disease which is basically hereditary in character. Conrad[147] has published an elaborate series of articles consisting of a study of twins and of the familial incidence of the disease as compared with that in the general population. His general conclusion has been that the disease is basically a hereditary one, and he has pointed out that the incidence is twenty to thirty times as great in families of epileptics as in the general population. Paskind and Brown[148] attempted to differentiate the so-called institutional deteriorated type of epileptic from the nondeteriorated, well-adjusted, ambulatory patient. They find a smaller incidence of so-called neuropathic taints in the families of nondeteriorated patients than in the families of deteriorated patients. This search for neuropathic taints, which characterizes the paper of Paskind and Brown, is to be found in most studies of the heredity of mental disorders. It raises the general question of so-called polymorphism, under which term one makes the assumption that a poor hereditary constitution may manifest itself in one of several abnormal traits. This conception is subjected to severe criticism by the Committee of the American Neurological Association. In this work the opinion is stated that so far no conclusive studies have appeared which justify this lumping together of a variety of abnormalities under the one general group. It must be remembered that no advance in knowledge is achieved by giving to an unknown entity a new and longer name.

Franke[149] studied the children of epileptics, distinguishing between so-called true epilepsy and symptomatic epilepsy. He found a lower incidence of epilepsy and other mental defects among the children of the symptomatic group. The Committee of the American Neurological Association devotes considerable space to the subject of heredity in epilepsy and concludes that epilepsy occurs more frequently in the descendants of the epileptic than in the descendants of the nonepileptic, and also agrees that the vast bulk of epileptics arise from families having a low incidence of epilepsy and who, in the main, are indistinguishable from the mass of the population. They hold forward little hope at present for the effective eradication of epilepsy on the basis of its eugenic control.

Latham and Munro[150] describe a family in which the parents were first cousins and in which five out of eight siblings present myoclonic epilepsy and deaf-mutism. Other members of the family showed what the authors call psychosis of the affective type. This is the first recorded example of the coexistence of these anomalies. Minkowska[151] also emphasizes the coexistence of epilepsy and psychosis in a very long report attempting to establish a basic relationship between these two conditions. Keschner[152] presents the clinical history of an unusual case of myoclonic epilepsy in a 46-year-old man whose maternal aunt had a similar disease; one second cousin was epileptic, and one third cousin had a myoclonic convulsive condition. The patient's brother suffered from multiple sclerosis and ataxia and was feeble-minded, but never had convulsive seizures.

Mental Deficiency.—Under the general heading of mental deficiency, Mongolian idiocy is the one clear-cut entity. Doxiades and Portius[153] present an elaborate study of mongolism, from which they conclude that the condition is twenty times as frequent in families presenting the disease as in the general population. They find also the presence in mentally normal relatives of single anatomic characteristics usually associated with the disease. They recognize the well-established fact that the disease is more common among the children of older mothers. Schröder[154] considers that the hereditary basis of this disease is highly suggestive but not proved. Bleyer[155] presents an interesting analysis of the relation of maternal age to the incidence of mongolism, based on

2,822 cases, and presents very strong evidence that the age of the mother is an important factor, the disease being far more common among the offspring of older mothers. It appears that mongolism is a disease in which two important factors operate: heredity and prenatal environment. On this basis, the various apparently conflicting theories can be reconciled. This interpretation is developed in detail by Penrose.[106]

Lahdensuu[156] in a study of Mongolian idiocy in Finland, collected 250 cases. He considers heredity to be the basic factor and does not believe the age of the mother to be of importance. In this regard his experience is contrary to that of most other observers. An unusual case report of paraplegia and mongolism occurring in twins is offered by Gordon and Roberts.[157] The twins, both girls, were considered to be fraternal in type. One had only moderate manifestations of both the paraplegia and mongolism. The intelligence quotient of one twin was 59; the other 89.

An interesting animal experiment presenting a similar genetic relationship to that found in mongolism is described by Haldane,[3] in discussing a paper by Wright on heredity of polydactylia in the guinea pig. In a given strain, in which polydactylia is present, it was found that the percentage of newborn infants presenting this condition varied according to the age of the mother, younger mothers having over 80 per cent polydactylic offspring, while older mothers had 30 per cent polydactylic offspring. This illustrates the coexistent effect of hereditary and environmental factors in the development of a characteristic, the essential basis of which is hereditary, and the environmental factor prenatal.

In considering other types of mental deficiency, one is faced with enormous difficulties which are basically due to the lumping together of all forms of mental deficiency with scarcely any knowledge of the underlying pathology or basic etiology of the condition. Hogben[105] in a discussion of human inheritance has most eloquently indicated the danger of applying elaborate mathematical analysis to data which are basically inadequate when he says: "There is the danger of concealing assumptions which have no factual basis behind an impressive façade of flawless algebra."

Rosanoff, Handy, and Plesset,[158] in an elaborate monograph, analyze 336 pairs of twins with mental deficiency in one or both of the pair. They conclude that the hereditary factors play an important part but are not the only ones involved. They conclude from their data that sex-linked genetic factors also operate in the manifestation of this condition on the basis of the greater incidence of mental deficiency among males.

A special committee appointed by the British Research Council has prepared a study of 1,280 cases of mental defects in which the existence of hereditary factors is emphasized.[159]

The Mental Deficiency Committee of the Royal Medico-Psychological Association[160] in an analysis of the relatives of normal individuals found an incidence of mental defect and psychologic abnormality, including psychosis, in 57 per cent of the families of these normal persons. This figure is compared with the usually quoted one, that 80 per cent of mental defectives have positive family histories. This article is of basic importance as an indication of the difficulty of determining hereditary significance in a disease by the method of studying the general familial incidence.

Jervis[161] presents a preliminary study of fifty cases of mental deficiency associated with urinary excretion of phenyl pyruvic acid and concludes that both the involvement of the nervous system and the metabolic error in these patients are an expression of the same degenerative processes, genetic in character.

Schwesinger,[162] in an exhaustive analysis, indicates that the degree of intelligence of a given individual is in large part determined by hereditary factors. However, the mechanism of this heredity is most complex and no detailed knowledge is available at present. Environmental factors too are of vast importance in the development of the inherent intellectual capacities of the individual. This would indicate the caution with which one should approach this problem. It is doubtful whether, in the present state of knowledge, any effect on the incidence of mental deficiency would be achieved by eugenic measures.

One may also bring up at this time the question which has frequently been raised as to whether or not feeble-minded and other mentally defective individuals are propagating at a rate which threatens the survival of our civilization. The Committee of the American Neurological Association, in analyzing this point, brings out quite clearly that statistical data show that there is no indication of increased fertility among feeble-minded or other mental defectives and that actually their rate of reproduction is lower than that of the general population.

A book by Dubitscher[163] on mental deficiency has just appeared. It assumes unusual importance because it is an official publication appearing under the direction of Dr. A. Gütt, who carries the title "Ministerialdirektor im Reichs- u. Preuss. Ministerium des Innern. Prasident des Preuss. Landesgesundheitzrates." The book is the first in a series which will cover other diseases in which heredity is considered to be important. The expressed purpose of the work is to justify the sterilization laws which have been put into effect by the German government. This volume includes a detailed summary of the clinical and pathologic aspects of feeble-mindedness and on this account is of great value. It presents no new data with regard to the genetic aspect of the problem.

Psychosis and Neurosis.—It is a truism that among the many schools of psychiatry there is the greatest divergence of opinion regarding all matters concerning mental diseases. This lack of agreement is manifest in considering etiology, pathogenesis, clinical manifestations, psychodynamics and prognosis.

It was pointed out in the beginning of this review that one of the basic elements for a valid study in heredity is the diagnostic accuracy of the clinical material. Certainly in a subject as complicated as that of the mental diseases, the clarity of clinical thought which would allow an author unquestioned confidence in his material is not possible. Unfortunately, most papers on heredity in psychoses and neuroses are concerned more with statistical acrobatics and conclusions concerning the fate of the human race than with a clinical evaluation of the material presented.

An example of an elaborate study in which the author goes so far with his genetic formulas as to diagram the position of the genes for schizophrenia in the chromosomes is found in a paper by Ziehen.[164] Schnitzenberger,[165] in a study of the incidence of mental disease among the relatives of thirty patients with involution melancholia, found among the parents of the patients 5.31 per cent of affective psychoses. In 138 siblings there was no other case of involution melancholia, but there were 3.3 per cent of affective psychoses. These figures indicate no greater incidence than in the general population. In this regard one may recall the findings of the Mental Deficiency Committee of the Royal Medico-Psychological Association in which the incidence of psychoses and neuroses among the relatives of normal persons was studied and found to be 23 per cent.

McInnes[166] studies the comparative incidence of neuroses in the families of fifty patients with anxiety neurosis and thirty with hysteria. He had seventy-five control families. Among the controls the parents were normal in 72 per cent of the cases and siblings in 70.6 per cent of the cases. In the families of his patients only 46 per cent of the parents and of the siblings were normal. Among the patients with hysteria, on the contrary, the percentage of normal parents was higher than in the controls; that is, 93.4 per cent. Among the siblings 16.6 per cent of the cases presented symptoms of hysteria. The study was conducted by the questionnaire method. There is no discussion of possible environmental factors in these cases. An important paper bearing on this point is one by Powdermaker,[167] presented by the author at the Third International Congress of Eugenics in 1932, in which an attempt is made to weigh the relative importance of nature and nurture in mental disease. The author emphasizes the unusual abnormal environment that is created for a child when one or both parents are suffering from a mental illness.

The Committee of the American Neurological Association gives considerable space to the problem of heredity of mental disease. They emphasize the point that the various conditions being discussed, such as schizophrenia, manic-depressive psychosis, feeble-mindedness, and epilepsy are probably each of heterogeneous composition and that all considerations of this problem must keep in mind this limitation. They consider unfounded the tendency to lump together various mental illnesses as indicative of a so-called neuropathic trend, a subject discussed above when considering polymorphism. They state that most of the early conclusions which are extensively quoted to prove the heredity in these various diseases were "merely statistical illusions due to the artificial elements of selection." They emphasize also the lack of adequate control studies in most cases. They conclude, however, that "in spite of criticism we have made of the above material, it is probable that there is some hereditary factor operating in dementia praecox, although it cannot be stated that this has been satisfactorily demonstrated in a clear-cut, inconvertible way." Their discussion of manic-depressive psychosis too is most surprising. They say: "It is curious to note that while the literature is quite unanimous as to the hereditary character of manic-depressive psychosis, very little valuble statistical material is available." They believe that the studies presented indicate an increased incidence of the disease among siblings of patients as compared with the general population. They conclude as follows: ". . . fewer cases than in schizophrenia have been studied, and the statistical value of most of the publications is not high. It is safe to say that manic-depressive psychosis is inheritable."

It is our opinion that this conclusion is not warranted either by the original data under review or by the arguments presented by the Committee. We believe the facts indicate an increased familial incidence of mental illness, still to be adequately measured and due to unknown factors. Future study should demonstrate the relative importance of heredity and environment in these diseases. At present there is no reason to venture any conclusion beyond the facts, especially because of the tendency in some places to apply drastic sterilization laws, not alone to patients with mental illness but also to their relatives.

Kretschmer,[168] in a general article, summarizes his well-known theory of the relation of heredity and constitution to mental disease. He assumes that there is a hereditary basis for schizophrenia and manic-depressive psychosis. He describes certain physical types which present a definite tendency to develop in each case a specific variety of mental illness. The basic types he considers "radical forms of personality." He emphasizes, however, that the psychosis is subject to environmental factors. He says: "Often external experience is not so much the real cause of a neurosis; it is rather a flame which ignites the inner typologically determined mass of conflicts within the personality."

HEREDITY AND EUGENICS

There are a number of reports which are directed mainly toward the general problem of heredity, using human material only as the means of establishing some basic genetic point. These papers are, however, of no less interest to the clinician and usually are of greater value as careful genetic studies than the more definitely clinical papers.

The study of twins has afforded an approach to the study of human genetics, the full benefit of which is still to be realized. Newman, Freeman, and Holzinger[169] have published in a book the results of many years of study. The book presents the product of collaboration of a biologist, a psychologist, and a statistician. It is a careful critical analysis which warrants careful reading by any student of the subject. Their conclusions are drawn with great caution. It is not practical to present a summary of this book at this point.

Schiller[170] describes an extensive study of 214 pairs of twins, of which eighty were identical twins. She studied a variety of characteristics and confirms the accepted findings with regard to similarity of body size, pigmentation, and other bodily characteristics in identical twins. She adds considerable data regarding similarities in capillary patterns in identical twns. The greatest difference in identical twins was in their characters and emotional expressions. Lehmann[171] also emphasized the importance of capillary studies as a means of establishing identity in twin sets. A monograph by Brander[172] discusses the study of twins with special emphasis on its relation to pediatrics.

Studies regarding Mendelian mechanisms in human material are obviously difficult to carry out, but the recent literature has been unusually rich in this regard. Several papers have been published on linkage, evidence of mutation, and other genetic manifestations previously studied only in animal material. Haldane,[173] in a study of hemophilia, points out that hemophiliacs die young and have a low fertility rate, despite which the percentage of hemophilia in the population has remained constant. The assumption is that the loss of genes by the early death of hemophiliacs is replaced by mutation. In this way are explained the not infrequent cases of hemophilia in which no family history is obtained.

Riddell[174] describes a family in which hemophilia and color blindness, both of which are sex-linked characters, are present in the expected linked relationship. Bell and Haldane[175] discuss in detail the mathematical implications of this relationship. Csik and Mather[176] describe a group of cases including oligophrenia, Laurence-Moon-Biedl syndrome, harelip, cleft palate, and allergy, in all of which there has been described an excess of affected males. This has usually been ascribed to sex linkage of some of the genes concerned in their inheritance. The authors consider the data insufficient to explain adequately what is the mechanism behind the difference in incidence of these diseases in the sexes.

The hereditary blood groups have afforded an opportunity for genetic study in human beings unequaled by any other character, due to the universal appearance of blood groups in all individuals. Friedenreich[177] presents a general summary of the subject. Hogben and Pollack,[178] in a study of several cases of Friedreich's ataxia, emphasize the value of carrying out with all genetic studies a detailed investigation of the blood groups and taste deficiency. The aim of such studies is the accumulation of data regarding linkage relationships in human material. In recent years it has been established that taste deficiency to a variety of substances is an inherited characteristic. All individuals present either the ability to taste these substances or the inability to taste them. The evidence indicates that deficiency of taste is a recessive factor. Studies of taste deficiency are indicated in all genetic human studies.

Snyder and Davidson[179] describe the inheritance of taste deficiency to diphenylguanidine as a recessive factor. Gottschick[180] obtains a similar result in a study of p-athoxyphenylthio acid. Boyd and Boyd[181] carried out an extensive study of taste deficiency and pointed out certain complexities in the problem due to differences in distribution of tasters and nontasters in different anthropologic groups. Studies were carried out in Dublin, Wales, Russia, and Egypt. They emphasized that there are fewer tasters in the males than in females. The significance of this finding is not yet clearly understood.

Herman and Derby[182] studied the relation of the blood group properties A, B, M, and N to mental disease. They found no significant distribution of the blood group properties to exist in mental disease.

Faust[183] presents a theoretical, statistical analysis of the probability that a given individual is the carrier of a defective gene. This is based on incidence of the disease in the relatives, its frequency in the general population, and the mechanism of its heredity. The weakest link in this elaborate statistical structure is that the method is applied to such diseases as schizophrenia, in which not only is there no adequate proof of a mechanism of heredity but even the degree of significance of hereditary factors is not entirely established.

One should mention at this point a new journal[184] which has made its first appearance this year, devoted to review articles on heredity, race hygiene, and related subjects. Verschuer[185] has put out a book on human heredity in which he describes the indications for sterilization, listing as the diseases in which this procedure is most frequently carried out the following conditions: congenital feeble-mindedness, schizophrenia, manic-depressive psychosis, hereditary epilepsy, Huntington's chorea, hereditary blindness, hereditary deafness, serious hereditary bodily malformation, and serious alcoholism.

Summary.—There exists in the literature on human heredity a tendency for the selection of cases presenting a positive hereditary history. This would result in overemphasis on the whole of the importance of heredity as a factor in the pathogenesis of disease. There is also the mistaken impression that when a disease is proved to be hereditary nothing can be done for the patient. It is perhaps for this reason that in most discussions of the subject by clinicians there enters a feeling of futility regarding the therapeutic approach to the cases under consideration.

Actually, one must realize that in the development of any clinical syndrome there are always the two factors, variously termed intrinsic and extrinsic, hereditary and environmental, or nature and nurture. The significance of this is that no discussion of the cause of a disease is complete which assumes only a hereditary basis or only an environmental basis. The task is to weigh the proportionate importance of each. Stated practically, this means the need of determining what environmental factors the physician can bring into operation to overcome the hereditary factors which are obviously beyond his control. For example, in such a disease as hemophilia it is apparent that the hereditary factors are the predominating ones. The physician may, by repeated blood transfusions (an environmental factor), modify the course of the disease. His therapy is at best most unsatisfactory. The correct procedure in the broad sense is to avoid the birth of hemophiliac individuals, which calls for eugenic measures. In cases such as this there is no disagreement.

An example of a disease in which heredity is an unquestionable fact, yet one in which the environment is of striking importance, is the group of allergic diseases. Here heredity determines that an individual can become allergic and so develop asthma, hay fever, and other allergic manifestations. However, in order for the disease to appear certain environmental factors are necessary as, in the case of an individual susceptible to ragweed, the presence of ragweed pollen in the atmosphere. Furthermore, it is possible for the physician to modify the clinical course of this hereditary disease by a variety of therapeutic measures. Certainly in this disease the therapeutists have not taken a fatalistic attitude.

At the other extreme are a group of diseases in which heredity may play a part but in which at the present time no conclusive evidence for this has been presented. The mental diseases present the most striking examples of this group. Here the proved genetic data are so scarce that no practicable eugenic plan can be presented for the elimination of these diseases. The optimistic claims of eugenicists, as exemplified especially in the noncritical enthsiasm of certain authors abroad, is not justified by careful and sober study. It would seem that with the present state of knowledge the wiser approach both therapeutically and as a preventive measure would be the environmental aspect, namely a psychotherapeutic and socio-economic one.

REFERENCES

1. Macklin, M. T.: The Rôle of Heredity in Disease, Medicine 14: 1, 1935.
2. Hofmeier, K.: Die Bedeutung der Erbanlagen für die Kinderheilkunde, Beihefte zum Arch. f. Kinderh., 14. Heft, 1938.
3. Haldane, J. B. S.: Heredity and Politics, New York, 1938.

4. Blacker, C. P.: ed., The Chances of Morbid Inheritance, Baltimore, 1934.
Mohr, O. L.: Heredity and Disease, New York, 1934.
Hogben, L.: Genetic Principles in Medicine and Social Sciences, London, 1931.
Baur, E., Fischer, E., and Lenz, E.: Human Heredity, New York, 1931.
5. Ratner, B.: Does Heredity Play a Rôle in the Pathogenesis of Allergy? (abstr.), J. Allergy **8**: 273, 1937.
6. Wiener, A. S., Zieve, I., and Fries, J. H.: The Inheritance of Allergic Disease, Ann. Eugenics **7**: 141, 1936-37.
7. Zieve, I., Wiener, A. S., and Fries, J. H.: On the Linkage Relations of the Genes for Allergic Disease and the Genes Determining the Blood Groups, MN Types and Eye Colour in Man, Ann. Eugenics **7**: 163, 1936-37.
8. Körner, G.: Über die familiäre Häufung der Gallenblasenkrankheiten, Ztschr. f. menschl. Vererb.- u. Konstitutionslehre **20**: 526, 1936-1937.
9. Necheles, H., and Levitsky, P.: Studies on Constitution and Peptic Ulcer. IV. Salivary Secretion Test in Peptic Ulcer Patients and Normal Subjects, J. Lab. & Clin. Med. **22**: 624, 1937.
10. Baker, E. G. S.: A Family Pedigree for Appendicitis, J. Hered. **28**: 187, 1937.
11. Sheldon, W.: Hypertrophic Pyloric Stenosis in One of Uniovular Twins, Lancet **1**: 1048, 1938.
12. Hecht, H., and Gupta, I. C.: Elektrokardiogramm und Vererbung, Deutsches Arch. f. klin.Med. **181**: 160, 1937.
13. Wilson, M. G., and Schweitzer, M. D.: Rheumatic Fever as a Familial Disease. Environment, Communicability and Heredity in Their Relation to the Observed Familial Incidence of the Disease, J. Clin. Investigation **16**: 555, 1937.
14. Ayman, D.: Added Evidence of Heredity in Arteriolar Essential Hypertension: Medical Papers Dedicated to H. A. Christian, Baltimore, 1936.
15. Ullrich, O.: Angeborene Herzhypertrophie mit Endokardfibrose bei zwei eineiigen Partnern von männlichen Drillingen, Ztschr. f. menschl. Vererb.- u. Konstitutionslehre **21**: 585, 1938.
16. Lehmann, W.: Die Vererbung der Immunität, Med. Klin. **33**: 444, 1937.
17. Hill, A. B.: The Inheritance of Resistance to Bacterial Infection in Animal Species, London, 1934. Great Britain Medical Research Council, Special Report Series 196.
18. Hofmeier, K.: Vererbung und Immunität, Klin. Wchnschr. **16**: 329, 1937.
19. Burch, G. E., and Sodeman, W. A.: Hereditary Hypoplasia of the Mesenchyme (Blue Sclerotics and Brittle Bones), Am. J. M. Sc. **194**: 844, 1937.
20. Hills, R. G., and McLanahan, S.: Brittle Bones and Blue Sclerae in Five Generations, Arch. Int. Med. **59**: 41, 1937.
21. Harnapp, G. O.: Zum Bilde der Marmorknochenkrankheit. Die familiäre, gutartige Form der diffusen Osteosklerose, Monatschr. f. Kinderh. **69**: 1, 1937.
22. Fonio, A.: Die Hämophilie, Ergebn. d. inn. Med. u. Kinderh. **51**: 443, 1936.
23. Fonio, A., Lang, E., and Tillmann, A.: Die Bluterkrankheit im Kanton Bern, Arch. d. Julius Klaus-Stiftg. f. Vererbungsforschg. **12**: 495, 1937.
24. Rosenthal, N., Vogel, P., and Beres, D.: Acquired Hemophilia in a Female: Festschrift Dedicated to Robert T. Frank, 1937.
25. Bauer, H., and Meller, J.: Zur Frage der weiblichen Hämophilie, Ztschr. f. klin. Med. **130**: 445, 1936.
26. Studt, H.: Die Bluter von Calmbach, Arch. f. Rassen- u. Gesellsch.-Biol. **31**: 214, 1937.
27. Birch, C. L.: Haemophilia: Clinical and Genetic Aspects, Illinois Medical and Dental Monographs **1**: No. 4, 1937.
28. Handley, R. S., and Nussbrecher, A. M.: Hereditary Pseudo-Haemophilia, Quart. J. Med. **4**: 165, 1935.
29. Debré, R., Lamy, M., See, G., and Schrameck, S.: La maladie hémolytique, Ann. de méd. **40**: 251, 1936.
30. Brockmann, H.: Untersuchungen über die Erblichkeit der Polycythaemia vera rubra, Ztschr. f. menschl. Vererb.- u. Konstitutionslehre **20**: 380, 1936-1937.
31. Wiskott, A.: Familiärer angeborener Morbus Werlhoffii? Monatschr. f. Kinderh. **68**: 212, 1937.

32. Ardashnikov, S. N.: A Hereditary Case of a Peculiar Hemorrhagic Diathesis, J. Hered. **29**: 14, 1938.
33. Macklin, M. T.: Erythroblastosis Foetalis: A Study of Its Mode of Inheritance, Am. J. Dis. Child. **53**: 1245, 1937.
34. Pache, H. D.: Die Erythroblastose der Neugeborenen als Familienkrankheit, Ztschr. f. Kinderh. **59**: 73, 1937-38.
35. Cardozo, W. W.: Immunologic Studies of Sickle-Cell Anemia, Arch. Int. Med. **60**: 623, 1937.
36. Haden, R. L., and Evans, F. D.: Sickle-Cell Anemia in the White Race, Arch. Int. Med. **60**: 133, 1937.
37. Bauer, E.: Latente und manifeste Anämie bei eineiigen Zwillingen, Deutsche med. Wchnschr. **63**: 776, 1937.
38. Schemensky, W.: Die Ovalocytose, eine vererbbare Anomalie der Erythrocyten, Med. Welt **10**: 1686, 1936.
39. Strauss, M. B., and Daland, G. A.: Hereditary Ovalocytosis (Human Elliptical Erythrocytes); Observations on Ten Cases in One Family, New England J. Med. **217**: 100, 1937.
40. Gunn, C. H. Hereditary Acholuric Jaundice in a New Mutant Strain of Rats, J. Hered. **29**: 137, 1938.
41. Cockayne, E. A.: Inherited Abnormalities of the Skin, London, 1933.
42. Munro, T. A.: Hereditary Sebaceous Cysts, J. Genetics **35**: 61, 1937.
43. West, L. S.: Observations on a Family Manifesting Congenital Ichthyosis, Eugenical News **22**: 77, 1937.
44. Beres, D., and Messeloff, C. R.: Ichthyosis Vulgaris. Report of a Case Illustrating Sex-Linked Inheritance, J. Mt. Sinai Hosp. **1**: 181, 1934.
45. Idelberger, K., and Haberler, G.: Kasuistische Beiträge zur Erbbiologie der Ichthyosis vulgaris, Dermat. Wchnschr. **104**: 374, 1937.
46. Gilch, T.: Über die Verbreitung und Vererbung der familiären Hornhautentartung in Württemberg, Ztschr. f. menschl. Vererb.- u. Konstitutionslehre **21**: 1, 1937-1938.
47. Gillespie, J. B.: Congenital and Familial Alopecia Totalis, Am. J. Dis. Child. **53**: 132, 1937.
48. Kerley, C. G.: Hereditary Ectodermal Dysplasia: Anhidrotic, Non-Sex-Linked Type, Arch. Pediat. **55**: 211, 1938.
49. Fitch, L.: Inheritance of a White Forelock, J. Hered. **28**: 413, 1937.
50. Anderson, E. An American Pedigree for Woolly Hair, J. Hered. **27**: 444, 1936.
51. McCrackin, R. H.: Albinism: Albinism and Unialbinism in Twin African Negroes, Am. J. Dis. Child. **54**: 786, 1937.
52. Sanders, J.: Die Heredität des Albinismus, Genetica **20**: 97, 1938.
53. Hyde, W.: Heredity in Relation to Malocclusion, J. A. D. A. **25**: 88, 1938.
54. Haldane, J. B. S.: A Probable New Sex-Linked Dominant in Man, J. Hered. **28**: 58, 1937.
55. Rushton, M. A.: Dental Abnormalities in Cleido-Cranial Dysostosis, J. Hered. **29**: 129, 1938.
56. Potter, E. L.: A Hereditary Ear Malformation Transmitted Through Five Generations, J. Hered. **28**: 255, 1937.
57. Powell, E. F., and Whitney, D. D.: Ear Lobe Inheritance, J. Hered. **28**: 185, 1937.
58. Wiener, A. S.: Complications in Ear Genetics, J. Hered. **28**: 425, 1937.
59. Hamilton, J. B. The Significance of Heredity in Ophthalmology. Preliminary Survey of Hereditary Eye Diseases in Tasmania, Brit. J. Ophth. **22**: 19, 83, 129, 1938.
60. Vogt, A., and Meyer, G.: Aufdeckung eines Stammbaumes von E. von Hippel'scher Angiomatosis retinae in der Schweiz, Arch. d. Julius Klaus-Stiftg. f. Vererbungsforschg. **12**: 575, 1937.
61. Walsh, F. B., and Wegman, M. E.: A Pedigree of Hereditary Cataract Illustrating Sex-Limited Type, Bull. Johns Hopkins Hosp. **61**: 125, 1937.
62. Allan, W.: Eugenic Significance of Retinitis Pigmentosa, Arch. Ophth. **18**: 938, 1937.
63. Bonnet, P., and Paufique, L.: Ophthalmoplégie congénitale à caractère familial, Ann. d'ocul. **173**: 135, 1936.
64. White, B. V., and Fulton, M. N.: A Rare Pupillary Defect Inherited by Identical Twins, J. Hered. **28**: 177, 1937.

65. Lisch, K.: Über hereditäres Vorkommen des mit Kerato-Conjunctivitis sicca verbundenen Sjögren'schen Symptomenkomplexes, Arch. f. Augenh. **110**: 357, 1937.
66. Mann, I., and Macrae, H.: Congenital Vascular Veils in the Vitreous, Brit. J. Ophth. **22**: 1, 1938.
67. Streeter, G. L.: The Significance of Morbid Processes in the Fetus, Harvey Lectures, ser. XXIX, 1933-34.
68. Macklin, M. T.: Heredity as the Cause of Congenital Malformations, Am. J. Obst. & Gynec. **32**: 258, 1936.
69. Müller, W.: Die angeborenen Fehlbildungen der menschlichen Hand, Leipzig, 1937.
70. Weidenmüller, K.: Beitrag zur Frage der Erbbedingtheit der Spina bifida, Ztschr. f. menschl. Vererb.- u. Konstitutionslehre **20**: 42, 1936-1937.
71. Schwarzweller, R.: Der angeborene Schulterblatthochstand und seine Beziehungen zu den Missbildungen der Wirbelsäule, Ztschr. f. menschl. Vererb.- u. Konstitutionslehre **20**: 350, 1937.
72. Pfeiffer, R.: Die Variabilität der angeborenen Femurhypoplasie (sog. kongenitaler Oberschenkeldefekt), Ztschr. f. menschl. Vererb.- u. Konstitutionslehre **20**: 493, 1937.
73. Schwarzweller, F.: Die Akrocephalosyndaktylie (Ein Beitrag zur Ätiologie dieser Missbildung), Ztschr. f. menschl. Vererb.- u. Konstitutionslehre **20**: 341, 1936-1937.
74. Hangarter, W., and Dieker, W.: Die Erbgenese des Klippel-Feilschen Syndroms, Ztschr. f. menschl. Vererb. u. Konstitutionslehre **21**: 236, 1937-1938.
75. Jarcho, S., and Levin, P. M.: Hereditary Malformation of the Vertebral Bodies, Bull. Johns Hopkins Hosp. **62**: 216, 1938.
76. Bakwin, H., and Krida, A.: Familial Metaphysial Dysplasia, Am. J. Dis. Child. **53**: 1521, 1937.
77. Wightman, J. C.: A Pedigree of Syndactyly, J. Hered. **28**: 421, 1937.
78. Jackson, V. W.: Four Generations of Polydactyly, J. Hered. **28**: 267, 1937.
79. Duncan, G. A.: Congenital Coxa Vara Occurring in Identical Twins, Am. J. Surg. **37**: 112, 1937.
80. Capinpin, J. M.: Inheritance of Nanism in Man, J. Hered. **28**: 361, 1937.
81. Volhard, E., and Drigalski, W.: Über eine eigenartige familiäre Entwicklungsstörung des Rumpfskeletts, Zentralbl. f. inn. Med. **58**: 243, 1937.
82. Gaugele, K.: Die Hüftgelenksverrenkung, Zentralbl. f. Chir. **64**: 983, 1937.
83. Gruber, G. B.: Entwicklungsstörungen im Rahmen der Urologie und Vererbungsfragen, Ztschr. f. Urol. **31**: 9, 1937.
84. Gordon, G. R., and Trasoff, A.: A Congenital Polycystic Kidney with Report of Its Occurrence in Several Members of One Family, Am. J. M. Sc. **194**: 112, 1937.
85. West, L.: Two Pedigrees Showing Inherited Predisposition to Hernia, J. Hered. **27**: 449, 1936.
86. Pettersson, G., and Bonnier, G.: Inherited Sex-Mosaic in Man, Hereditas **23**: 49, 1937.
87. Little, C. C., and Reimann, S. P.: Dialogue on the Relations of Genetics and Experimental Embryology to Neoplasia, Am. J. Clin. Path. **8**: 109, 1938.
88. Bell, E. T., and Rothnem, T. P.: Xeroderma Pigmentosum with Carcinoma of the Lower Lip in Two Brothers Aged Sixteen and Thirteen Years, Am. J. Cancer **30**: 574, 1937.
89. Hauser, I. J., and Weller, C. V.: A Further Report on the Cancer Family of Warthin, Am. J. Cancer **27**: 434, 1936.
90. Martynova, R. P.: Studies in Genetics of Human Neoplasms, Cancer of the Breast Based Upon 201 Family Histories, Am. J. Cancer **29**: 530, 1937.
91. Körbler, J.: Zur Frage der Vererbung und der Kontagiosität bei Krebs, Ztschr. f. Krebsforsch. **47**: 84, 1937.
92. Stark, M. B.: The Origin of Certain Hereditary Tumors in Drosophila, Am. J. Cancer **31**: 253, 1937.
93. Murray, W. S.: The Genetic Theory of Transplanted Neoplasms, M. Times **66**: 32, 1938.
94. Bittner, J. J.: The Genetics of Cancer in Mice, Quart. Rev. Biology **13**: 51, 1938.
95. Lüth, K. F.: Endokrine Störungen bei eineiigen Zwillingen, Ztschr. f. menschl. Vererb.- u. Konstitutionslehre **21**: 55, 1937-1938.

96. Lewis, A. A.: A Case of Apparent Dissimilarity of Monozygotic Twins, Ann. Eugenics **7**: 58, 1936-1937.
97. Munro, T. A.: Familial Psychosis Associated with Endocrine Disorder, J. Ment. Sc. **83**: 707, 1937.
98. Warkany, J., and Mitchell, A. G.: Relation of Endocrine Disturbances to Certain Heredodegenerative Symptoms, Am. J. Dis. Child. **55**: 231, 1938.
99. Goldman, L., and Smyth, F. S.: Hyperparathyroidism in Siblings, Ann. Surg. **104**: 971, 1936.
100. Warkany, J., Frauenberger, G. S., and Mitchell, A. G.: Heredofamilial Deviations. I. The Laurence-Moon-Biedl Syndrome, Am. J. Dis. Child. **53**: 455, 1937.
101. Van Bogaert, L.: Ein Stammbaum einer Familie mit Laurence-Moon-Bardetscher Krankheit, Ztschr. f. menschl. Vererb.- u. Konstitutionslehre **21**: 314, 1937-1938.
102. Panse, F.: Über erbliche Zwischenhirnsyndrome und ihre entwicklungsphysiologischen Grundlagen (Dargestellt am Modell des Bardet-Biedlschen Syndroms), Ztschr. f. d. ges. Neurol. u. Psychia. **160**: 1, 1938.
103. Cooperstock, M.: Laurence-Moon-Biedl Syndrome, Am. J. Dis. Child. **54**: 334, 1937.
104. Committee of the American Neurological Association for the Investigation of Eugenical Sterilization: Eugenical Sterilization: A Reorientation of the Problem, New York, 1936.
105. Hogben, L.: Nature and Nurture, New York, 1933.
106. Penrose, L. S.: The Influence of Heredity on Disease, London, 1934.
107. Spillane, J., and Phillips, R.: Huntington's Chorea in South Wales, Quart. J. Med. **6**: 403, 1937.
108. Hempel, H. C.: Ein Beitrag zur Huntingtonschen Erkrankung, Ztschr. f. d. ges. Neurol. u. Psychiat. **160**: 563, 1937-38.
109. Meierhofer, M.: Atypische Psychosen in einer Chorea-Huntington-Familie, Monatschr. f. Psychiat. u. Neurol. **97**: 13, 1937.
110. Stone, T. T., and Falstein, E. I.: Huntington's Chorea: A Genealogical Study, Arch. Neurol. & Psychiat. **38**: 910, 1937.
111. Minski, L., and Guttmann, E.: Huntington's Chorea: a Study of Thirty-Four Families, J. Ment. Sc. **84**: 21, 1938.
112. Hall, G. W., and MacKay, R. P.: Forms of Familial Ataxia Resembling Multiple Sclerosis, Arch. Neurol. & Psychiat. **37**: 19, 1937.
113. Curschmann, H.: Über multiple Sklerose bei drei Brudern, Deutsche Ztschr. f. Nervenh. **145**: 225, 1937-38.
114. Jentsch, F.: Zur Erblichkeit der multiplen Sklerose (Konkordantes Vorkommen der multiplen Sklerose bei eineiigen Zwillingen), Deutsche Ztschr. f. Nervenh. **145**: 144, 1937-38.
115. Curtius, F., and Speer, H.: Multiple Sklerose und Erbanlage, Ztschr. f. d. ges. Neurol. u. Psychiat. **160**: 226, 1937-1938.
116. Schröder, W.: Zur Vererbung der Friedreichschen Krankheit, Deutsche Ztschr. f. Nervenh. **142**: 221, 1937.
117. Lux, E.: Die hereditäre Ataxie, eine erbbiologische Studie, Monatschr. f. Psychiat. u. Neurol. **96**: 211, 1937.
118. Waggoner, R. W., Löwenberg, K., and Speicher, K. G.: Hereditary Cerebellar Ataxia, Arch. Neurol. & Psychiat. **39**: 570, 1938.
119. Röhricht, W.: Familiäre spastische Spinalparalyse. Ein Beitrag zur Lehre von der Heredodegeneration, Monatschr. f. Psychiat. u. Neurol. **96**: 268, 1937.
120. Kahlstorf, A.: Klinischer und histopathologischer Beitrag zur hereditären spastischen Spinalparalyse, Ztschr. f. d. ges. Neurol. u. Psychiat. **159**: 774, 1937.
121. Turner, E. V., and Roberts, E.: A Family with a Sex-Linked Hereditary Ataxia, J. Nerv. & Ment. Dis. **87**: 74, 1938.
122. Aring, C. D., and Cobb, S.: The Muscular Atrophies and Allied Disorders, Medicine **14**: 77, 1935.
123. Sjövall, B.: Dystrophia musculorum progressiva: eine erblichkeitsmedizinische und klinische Studie, Lund, 1936. (Supplement X of Acta psychiat. et neurol.)
124. Boeters, H.: Der erbliche Muskelschwund. Genealogische Untersuchungen bei neurospinaler Muskelatrophie, Ztschr. f. d. ges. Neurol. u. Psychiat. **160**: 455, 1937-38.

125. Cooper, E. L.: Progressive Familial Hypertrophic Neuritis (Dejerine-Sottas), Brit. M. J. 1: 793, 1936.
126. Rütenik, G.: Familiäre amyotrophische Lateralsklerose, Arch. f. Psychiat. 107: 248, 1937.
127. Schneider, D., and Abeles, M. M.: Charcot-Marie-Tooth Disease with Primary Optic Atrophy. Report of Two Cases Occurring in Brothers, J. Nerv. & Ment. Dis. 85: 541, 1937.
128. Breitfort, K.: Über Myotonia congenita (Thomsensche Krankheit), Arch. f. Kinderh. 113: 110, 1938.
129. Rothbart, H. B.: Myasthenia Gravis in Children. Its Familial Incidence, J. A. M. A. 108: 715, 1937.
130. Freudenberg, E.: Klinische Beobachtungen und Untersuchungen an einem Zwillingspaar mit Niemann-Pickscher Krankheit, Ztschr. f. Kinderh. 59: 313, 1937.
131. Van Bogaert, L., and Borremans, P.: Über eine adulte, sich bis ins Präsenium hinziehende Form der familiären amaurotischen Idiotie, Ztschr. f. d. ges. Neurol. u. Psychiat. 159: 136, 1937.
132. Jakobsen, J.: Un cas solitaire d'idiotie amaurotique juvénile familiale de Spielmeyer-Stock, Encéphale 32: 266, 1937.
133. Schwyn, H.: Über zwei Fälle von Wilson'scher Krankheit bei einem Geschwisterpaar, Schweiz. Arch. f. Neurol. u. Psychiat. 40: 221, 1937.
134. Müller, W.: Zur Pathologie und Erbbiologie der Wilson-Pseudosklerose, Deutsche Ztschr. f. Nervenh. 145: 234, 1938.
135. Forsberg, R., and Stromme, R.: On Four Cases of Leucodystrophia Cerebri Hereditaria Progressiva (Merzbacher-Pelizaeus), Acta psychiat. et neurol. 12: 639, 1937.
136. Alpers, B. J., and Marcovitz, E.: Pathologic Background of Cerebral Diplegia, Am. J. Dis. Child. 55: 356, 1938.
137. Thums, K.: Zwillingsuntersuchung bei cerebraler Kinderlähmung (Littlescher Krankheit, angeborener spastischer Hemi-, Di-, und Tetraplegie). Ztschr. f. d. ges. Neurol. u. Psychiat. 158: 151, 1937.
138. Lisch, K., and Thums, K.: Diskordantes Vorkommen von Mikrophakie mit Schichstar und Littlescher Krankheit bei einem eineiigen Zwillingspaar mit Zeichen des Status dysraphicus, Ztschr. f. menschl. Vererb.- u. Konstitutionslehre 21: 220, 1937-38.
139. Van Bogaert, L., and de Savitsch, E.: Sur une maladie congénitale et hérédofamiliale comportant un tremblement rythmique de la tête, des globes oculaires et des membres supérieurs, Encéphale 32: 113, 1937.
140. Russell, D. S., and Tallerman, K. H.: Familial Progressive Diffuse Cerebral Sclerosis of Infants, Arch. Dis. Childhood 12: 71, 1937.
141. Allan, W.: Inheritance of the Shaking Palsy, Arch. Int. Med. 60: 424, 1937.
142. Menninger, W. C., and Grotjahn, M.: Familial Neurosyphilis of the Dementia Paralytica Type, Arch. Neurol. & Psychiat. 39: 343, 1938.
143. Laubenthal, F.: Sippe mit kongenitaler Wortblindheit, Ztschr. f. d. ges. Neurol. u. Psychiat. 158: 321, 1937.
144. Craig, W. M.: Intracranial Tumors of Sisters Occurring at Approximately the Same Age and Presenting Similar Syndromes, Proc. Staff Meet., Mayo Clinic 12: 798, 1937.
145. Stollard, H. B.: A Case of Intra-Ocular Neuroma (von Recklinghausen's Disease) of the Left Optic Nerve Head, Brit. J. Ophth. 22: 11, 1938.
146. Becker, P. E.: Zur Erblichkeit der Ischias (Zwillingsstudien über die Erbanlage bei der Neuritis lumbosacralis), Ztschr. f. d. ges. Neurol. u. Psychiat. 162: 183, 1938.
147. Conrad, K.: Erbanlage und Epilepsie. I. Untersuchungen an einer Serie von 253 Zwillingspaaren. Ztschr. f. d. ges. Neurol. u. Psychiat. 153: 271, 1935; II. Ein Beitrag zur Zwillingskasuistik. Die konkordanten Eineiigen, Ibid. 155: 254, 1936; III. Ein Beitrag zur Zwillingskasuistik. Die diskordanten Eineiigen, Ibid. 155: 509, 1936; IV. Ergebnisse einer Nachkommenschaftsuntersuchung an Epileptikern, Ibid. 159: 521, 1937.
148. Paskind, H., and Brown, M.: Hereditary Factors in Epilepsy, J. A. M. A. 108: 1599, 1937.
149. Franke, G.: Erbbiologische Untersuchungen an Kindern von Epileptikern, Ztschr. f. d. ges. Neurol. u. Psychiat. 160: 381, 1937.

150. Latham, A. D., and Munro, T. A.: Familial Myoclonus Epilepsy Associated with Deaf-Mutism in a Family Showing Other Psychobiological Abnormalities, Ann. Eugenics **8:** 166, 1938.
151. Minkowska, F.: Epilepsie und Schizophrenie im Erbgang mit besonderer Berücksichtigung der epileptoiden Konstitution und der epileptischen Struktur, Arch. d. Julius Klaus-Stiftg. f. Vererbungsforschg. **12:** 33, 1937.
152. Keschner, M.: Unusual Case of Myoclonic Epilepsy, Arch. Neurol. & Psychiat. **38:** 896, 1937.
153. Doxiades, L., and Portius, W.: Zur Ätiologie des Mongolismus unter besonderer Berücksichtigung der Sippenbefunde, Ztschr. f. menschl. Vererb.- u. Konstitutionslehre **21:** 384, 1937-38.
154. Schröder, H.: Die Sippschaftder mongoloiden Idiotie, Ztschr. f. d. ges. Neurol. u. Psychiat. **160:** 73, 1937.
155. Bleyer, A.: Rôle of Advanced Maternal Age in Causing Mongolism, Am. J. Dis. Child. **55:** 79, 1938.
156. Lahdensuu, S.: Über Vorkommen und Ätiologie der Idiotia mongoloidea im Lichte des in Finnland gesammelten Materials, Acta paediat. **21:** 256, 1937.
157. Gordon, R. G., and Roberts, J. A.: Paraplegia and Mongolism in Twins, Arch. Dis. Childhood **13:** 79, 1938.
158. Rosanoff, A. J., Handy, L. M., and Plesset, I. R.: The Etiology of Mental Deficiency with Special Reference to Its Occurrence in Twins: A Chapter in the Genetic History of Human Intelligence, Psychol. Monog. **48:** 4, 1937.
159. Penrose, L. S.: A Clinical and Genetic Study of 1,280 Cases of Mental Defect, London, 1938. (Great Britain Medical Reserch Council, Special Report Series 229.)
160. Report by the Mental Deficiency Committee of the Royal Medico-Psychological Association: An Inquiry Into the Incidence of Neuropathic Conditions in the Relatives of Normal Persons, J. Ment. Sc. **83:** 247, 1937.
161. Jervis, G. A.: Phenylpyruvic Oligophrenia, Arch. Neurol. & Psychiat. **38:** 944, 1937.
162. Schwesinger, G. C.: Heredity and Environment: Studies in the Genesis of Psychological Characteristics, New York, 1933.
163. Dubitscher, F.: Der Schwachsinn, Leipzig, 1937.
164. Ziehen, V.: Manifestationswahrscheinlichkeit und Erbgang der Schizophrenie, Arch. f. Psychiat. **107:** 1, 1937.
165. Schnitzenberger, H.: Die Erblage in der nächsten Verwandschaft von 30 Fällen klimakterischer bzw. involutiver Melancholie, Ztschr. f. d. ges. Neurol. u. Psychiat. **159:** 11, 1937.
166. McInnes, R. G.: Heredity in Neurosis, Proc. Roy. Soc. Med. **30:** 895, 1937.
167. Powdermaker, F.: Considerations on the Social Factors in Mental Development; A Decade of Progress in Eugenics, Baltimore, 1934.
168. Kretschmer, E.: Heredity and Constitution in the Aetiology of Psychic Disorders, Brit. M. J. **2:** 403, 1937.
169. Newman, H. H., Freeman, F. N., and Holzinger, K. J.: Twins, a Study of Heredity and Environment, Chicago, 1937.
170. Schiller, M.: Zwillingsprobleme, dargestellt auf Grund von Untersuchungen an Stuttgarter Zwillingen, Ztschr. f. menschl. Vererb.- u. Konstitutionslehre **20:** 284, 1936-1937.
171. Lehmann, W., and Hartlieb, J. Capillaren bei Zwillingen, Ztschr. f. menschl. Vererb.- u. Konstitutionslehre **21:** 271, 1937-1938.
172. Brander, T.: Über die Zwillingsforschung und ihre Berührungspunkte mit der Kinderheilkunde, Acta paediat. **21:** 5, 1937.
173. Haldane, J. B. S.: The Rate of Spontaneous Mutation of a Human Gene, J. Genetics **31:** 317, 1935.
174. Riddell, W. J. B.: Haemophilia and Colour-Blindness Occurring in the Same Family, Brit. J. Ophth. **21:** 113, 1937.
175. Bell, J., and Haldane, J. B. S.: The Linkage Between the Genes for Colour-Blindness and Haemophilia in Man, Proc. Roy. Soc. London, Series B **123:** 119, 1937.
176. Csik, L., and Mather, K.: The Sex Incidence of Certain Hereditary Traits in Man, Ann. Eugenics **8:** 126, 1938.
177. Friedenreich, V.: Blood Groups and Genetics, Ann. Eugenics **8:** 152, 1938.

178. Hogben, L., and Pollack, R.: A Contribution to the Relation of the Gene Loci Involved in the Isoagglutination Reaction, Taste Blindness, Friedreich's Ataxia and Major Brachydactyly of Man, J. Genetics **31**: 353, 1935.
179. Snyder, L. H., and Davidson, D. F.: Studies in Human Inheritance. XVIII. The Inheritance of Taste Deficiency to Di-phenyl-guanidine, Eugenical News **22**: 1, 1937.
180. Gottschick, J.: Erbliche Unterschiede der Geschmacksempfindungen auf p-Äthoxyphenylthioharnstoff, Ztschr. f. menschl. Vererb.- u. Konstitutionslehre **21**: 254, 1937-1938.
181. Boyd, W. C., and Boyd, L. G.: Sexual and Racial Variations in Ability to Taste Phenyl-Thio-Carbamide, With Some Data on the Inheritance, Ann. Eugenics **8**: 46, 1937.
182. Herman, M., and Derby, I. M.: The Blood Groups and M-N Types in Mental Diseases, J. Immunol. **33**: 87, 1937.
183. Faust, H.: Die theoretische Erbvorhersage bei Erkrankung von Vettern, Neffen und Stiefverwandten, Ztschr. f. menschl. Vererb.- u. Konstitutionslehre **20**: 657, 1936-37.
184. Fortschritte der Erbpathologie, Rassenhygiene und ihrer Grenzgebiete.
185. Von Verschuer, O.: Erbpathologie, ein Lehrbuch für Ärzte, Ed. 2, Dresden, 1937.

American Academy of Pediatrics

Proceedings

EIGHTH ANNUAL MEETING OF THE AMERICAN ACADEMY OF PEDIATRICS

DEL MONTE, CALIF., JUNE 9, 1938

Panel Discussion on the Role of Allergy in Pediatric Practice

Chairman: Dr. Bret Ratner, New York.

Assistants: Dr. Francis Scott Smyth, San Francisco.
Dr. Albert H. Rowe, Oakland.
Dr. George Piness, Los Angeles.

PRESIDENT PHILIP VAN INGEN.—This panel discussion will be conducted by Dr. Bret Ratner; there will be no questions asked from the floor. Anybody who wishes a question will please write it, send it to the table. It will be answered during the evening as far as possible.

CHAIRMAN RATNER.—It is indeed a privilege to be invited to be chairman of this panel. My teacher, Dr. Schloss, told me that he had to decide soon after he started work in the allergy field, whether he was to become an allergist or remain a pediatrician. I have unwittingly been placed in the same dilemma and find to my disappointment and chagrin that the allergists insist that I am a pediatrician and the pediatricians make it known that I am an allergist.

My own feeling is that the time has arrived when allergy must become an integral part of pediatrics. You will hear Dr. Smyth, the other pediatrician on this panel, express the same idea.

The situation is not unique; the pediatrician finds that he must include within his province such fields as psychology and endocrinology. The purpose of this panel therefore is to show how important a role allergy plays in the practice of pediatrics.

Our knowledge of the basis of allergic diseases is incomplete. Problems we are unable to solve beset us. After most painstaking studies and treatment our patients may continue to scratch or wheeze unmercifully. At times when we are delighted with the remission of all symptoms for many months and when we feel that we have obtained a brilliant result, the child has a sudden return of symptoms, and we are confronted by a disappointed mother who in consternation declares that after all we have not cured her child. Nevertheless, it is gratifying to know that in a large number of cases the well-trained allergist obtains good results.

The men working with allergy in the adult have found that a large proportion of their patients date the onset of their symptoms from childhood. Those who have made observations on allergic children find that the onset of allergy often occurs very early in life. My own observations indicate that 50 per cent of our cases have had their onset of symptoms in the first year and that by the eighth year 80 per cent of our children have manifested their allergic symptoms; by the tenth year practically all of our patients have developed symptoms. It is apparent from this that the pediatrician must be ever watchful for early allergic symptoms.

There are many problems which we would like to clarify for you, but in the short time allotted we cannot hope to do more than present some of the phases which may confront you, and make suggestions which we believe may be helpful.

I am particularly fortunate in having associated with me men whose contributions in the field of allergy have been noteworthy and whose opinions are mellowed by broad experience.

The first problem with which we will concern ourselves will be the early manifestations of allergy in infants. Since I know of no one better qualified to speak on this topic than Dr. Smyth, I shall ask him to open our discussion.

DR. SMYTH.—I have been asked to speak on the sensitivities in childhood, their importance, early diagnosis, management and treatment.

Those of us dealing with the health of children have failed to be impressed by the frequency with which some problem related to sensitivity is encountered. Hardly a day goes by but some child is seen with a skin manifestation related to an obvious sensitivity, or as seems more likely a skin response in which the cause is not readily recognized. For this reason I believe it is the duty of pediatric departments to maintain allergy clinics in order to train properly the pediatricians of the future. This statement is not intended to invite controversy with those colleagues on this panel who are exclusively engaged in the study of allergy, but rather to state my position regarding educational policy. And, while I do not doubt that there are times when it is a relief to refer a troublesome patient to a specialist in the field of allergy, the fact remains that the pediatrician in intimate relation with his patients may have advantages and duties with respect to this frequently encountered complaint. In the matter of history alone the pediatrician is able to evaluate and clarify information which seldom is obtained from a limited number of interviews.

Besides its frequency, allergy in early childhood is important for the very reason of our rather limited understanding of it. In general it may be said that the disease entities in the adult are often confused by complications and that the pure entities seen in childhood give us the hope not only of earlier recognition, but also of preventive measures. This statement, however, implies an accuracy of diagnosis, which as yet I am unable to admit.

For clarity let us list the conditions encountered in young children: Urticaria, eczema, purpura, angioneurotic edema, asthma, and hay fever. First perhaps in frequency would come skin manifestations. More specifically I refer to the urticarias and the eczemas, or just eczema.

Regarding urticaria in young children, it is surprising how diverse the reports can be. Our experience has led us to suspect that a fairly large percentage of young children may have urticaria, but that this may be of a transitory nature and is perhaps less likely to be preceded or followed by any more serious allergic complaint. The large macular urticaria is usually transitory in that it disappears in the course of a few hours. Certain observations are, however, worth noting. First, the response is often obtained with the initial feeding of certain foods such as shellfish or strawberries and much of its history is often influenced by the nature of the offending fraction. In our experience shellfish as a causative agent is likely to become more fixed, while we have seen the urticaria from strawberries fade out if the patient continues eating them. There is then the greatest response at the onset of the season and minimal response or disappearance by the end of the season. There is also to be seen the contrast between these two foods, that while cooking will often reduce or prevent the response to the fresh strawberries, no such alteration is obtained with the fish. Another observation worth mentioning is the digestive cycle causing an apparent tidal appearance or disappearance of skin lesions. For example, initiated by the ingestion of shellfish, the urticaria reappeared though in decreasing severity with subsequent meals. This evanescence, somewhat like the course of serum sickness, is directly related to the absorption cycle in the digestive tract, and may point to methods by which it may be combated. The treatment and management of these types of urticaria differ accordingly, and our interest might well be directed toward the offender—not the patient.

I have implied without so stating that in recognition of the causal substance, this type of urticaria is understood best by history. This may be easily obtained by a diary and trial-and-error diet. As far as eosinophilia, leucopenic index, skin tests, etc., are concerned, I am not impressed.

I am willing to admit, however, that occasionally *Pulex San Francisco* has embarrassed me. I was much chagrined in the case of a doctor's child recently. The appearance of the lesion strongly suggested a food urticaria. However, the distribution was unusual, being peculiarly concentrated around the waist band. A few of the lesions had a central pinpoint hemorrhage. By that I mean the reaction was not confined to the immediate zone of the bite. By history the mother was also hypersensitive to fleas. Whether this is a case of placental transmission I would not attempt to answer. However, in the absence of major sensitivity the use of pyrethrum in calamine lotion was very effective.

Papular urticaria is the second type seen in children; here, too, I must confess that but for distribution and microscopic search for mites I have found scabies annoying in the differential diagnosis. And my most recent confusion in diagnosis was with regard to lesions—again in a physician's child—suggesting papular urticaria. Involvement of the mucous membranes suggested to others the diagnosis of chicken pox. A sister in the home and a ward in the hospital have to date shown no subsequent contagion, despite the usual ease of transmission of varicella.

The use of skin tests, eosinophile count, leucopenic index, etc., is of little value in this type of urticaria. It is a much more chronic condition and seems to have a slow appearance and disappearance time. As such even more careful sleuthing is required. Dietary trial and error should allow no changes in less than four days. Oats and orange pulp seem to be frequent offending foods. I have, however, seen some instances in which fats such as butter and bacon are apparently responsible; these latter foods are emphasized by Bray who goes further and mentions the seasonal summer occurrence, noted also in our clinic. Bray also reports eosinophilia which as yet we have not found characteristic.

Eczema of infants has been subject to repeated studies and various terminologies. As yet I am unable to be enthusiastic about the term neurodermatitis nor to predict with assurance those who will continue into adult life with involvement of the floor surfaces and those who will have a spectacular improvement toward the end of the second year. The skin of infants is notoriously tender. Eczema to me is a response to irritation; that irritation may be single or multiple. A peculiar number of instances are associated with sensitivity to foods in which eggs, milk, meat, or oranges are found by frequency likely offenders. However, few if any pediatricians would rely on dietary measures alone. We have all witnessed the remarkable amelioration in the condition when the use of ointments and restraint is not neglected. And I think we have also been parties to those trying cases which result in shopping for the final improvement, which brings gratification to the physician fortunate enough to see the baby at about 16 months or 2 years, when that certain spontaneous improvement occurs.

A few years ago I visited Scheer's clinic in Frankfort. He had a number of infants in the hospital with an eczematous appearing lesion involving the buttocks, which he said was eczema and his remarkable success was due to the use of Hydrochloric milk. To me the condition is none other than the ammoniacal diaper which we customarily treat by eradication of *B. ammoniagenes*, by bichloride and strong boric acid soaking of the diaper. Cooke showed very clearly that the bacillus could be influenced by acid feeding, hence Scheer's results. The point I would emphasize, however, was that Scheer was sure that the eczema in which I was interested was of a similar nature, even though distributed differently on the body. Dr. Hansen of Minneapolis has likewise suggested that unsaturated fatty acid content of the blood is diagnostic and gives an important clue in the therapy of eczema. Visiting Minneapolis I saw several infants so treated with considerable improvement, yet such improvement may occur after hospitalization alone. For a similar reason it is suggested that the rationale of sobee may be of value because of fatty acid content. The German program, however, is for lowering the fat content of the diet. To me the diagnosis and treatment, the classification and therapy of causation of infantile eczema are far from settled. Eczema is a response to irritation, and the more the infants scratch, the more they itch. The irritation may come from food, contact with wool or silk, exposure to light, sudden changes in temperature, excessive soap and water, etc. Its diagnosis is not absolute.

The purpuric type of reaction is in our experience rare in children. I can illustrate the difficulty in this diagnosis no better than to mention an instance when Dr. Piness, the mentor of our children's allergy clinic, was visiting us. A 4-year-old child was seen by us and discussed in relation to allergic purpura. All agreed allergy was unlikely, yet under study we were able to induce or alleviate the symptoms by administration of orange with or without pulp. The skin tests, while faint, were interpretable because repetition showed consistent erythema only to orange.

I have had little experience with angioneurotic edema. In the one recent study the paternal history of allergy was strong. Another instance shall we say of germ plasm transmission? In this patient there is no doubt that certain foods aggravate the condition, but contributing factors such as excitability and/or the combination of foods are important in the production of response. Both parents are physicians and we have observed responses which admit no other interpretation.

In the second classification of symptoms we see the respiratory tract manifest sensitivities. While it is true that asthma and hay fever are found in very young children, the majority of recognized sensitivities in the young are still associated with skin manifestations. On the other hand, it must be admitted that a certain habit of mind has perhaps neglected the possible role of sensitivity for respiratory responses casually considered of infectious origin. An increasing number of instances without the premonitory skin manifestations have on suspicion shown a probable allergic nature. It is perhaps too early to predict, but I am of the opinion that rhinitis which looms so large in pediatric practice will warrant suspicion which should be directed toward an allergic study.

Osler I believe was responsible for suspecting the bronchopneumonia seen in the eczematous infant, as the initial onset of asthma. Pertussis has likewise proved dangerous for the subsequent course of such infants; nevertheless many instances of asthma in the older child may have little on which to trace the course of sensitivity. It pays, I believe, to anticipate probable asthmatic tendency, when infancy has been marked by eczema and food sensitivity, removing possible contact not only of the known ingestant offenders, but also of inhalants which by frequency are likely to be offensive.

In spite of such precautions there remains the possibility of sensitization to pollens, it being impractical to eliminate contact with these. We have seen pollinosis with either hay fever or asthma, or on the other hand with seasonal colds for which the pollens were responsible. However, it has been our policy, right or wrong, not to give courses of pollen injection unless the symptoms were marked.

With regard to the intestinal tract—the abdominal pain or colic of certain infants was early suspected by Schloss as of allergic origin. Associated with purpura or eczema, the implication is obvious. Eczema or asthma having previously been seen to follow ingestion of egg, I am impressed with the cramps and diarrhea which may later characterize the response. Peanut which is less frequent in the diet may produce symptoms of this sort in the child otherwise without sensitivities. Will such a response persist into adult life? Who knows?

And another question. Is mesenteric adentitis allergic, rheumatic or both? We have seen relief with salicylates, none with epinephrine, but it has been present in several known hypersensitive children.

However, the lability of the intestinal tract in infants and young children is notorious. Colic, or bellyache, is far from rare and to suspect an allergic basis for symptoms readily produced by causes other than allergy, is I believe at this time dangerous. We have all seen the hypertonic infant with perfect nutrition screaming half the night spectacularly relieved with atropine or phenobarbital. We have also witnessed colic and diarrhea caused by an infection without a doubt. For this reason I am loath to suspect all instances of enterospasm or pyloric stenosis as allergic. With regard to its popular usage, I believe there is disrepute for the term, if we adopt it in lieu of the word ''toxic'' merely to screen our ignorance.

What is to be said concerning the initiation and the premonitory signs of allergy? Are we ready to grant Mayerhofer's contention that even in the neonatal period the transient rashes, etc., are allergic? If so, are we able to predict with some degree of accuracy the subsequent course the patient will follow? For my part I am unwilling to do so. There have been a few instances where as early as the first month I have told parents that I consider the rash suggestive of eczema, and have had the subsequent course typical of the milk-, egg-, and wheat-sensitive child, where eczema and later asthma have been related to these foods. However, not a little of my consideration was based on the family history, and, Dr. Ratner, in the instance that comes to my mind, the sensitivity was paternal. I inject this, not to disprove the possible placental transmission but to emphasize the hereditary factor, that is, the capacity to become sensitized.

I believe we are justified in guarding against likely offense in those children or infants suspected of sensitivity. On the other hand, I doubt if we are ready to advise against parenthood even where that hereditary strain is recognized. This you will recall was the suggestion of Glaser and Laudou.

We are still a long way from exact methods in allergy. I know of too few life histories to be assured that sensitivity in the young will be aggravated or alleviated by age. The marked lability of infants as a group affords no gauge for the reactions seen in older children or adults, and, while I think there is greater danger in the artful promise of outgrowing the disease, I have seen amelioration with adolescence far exceeding my hopes. All too frequently natural processes or at least factors beyond the knowledge or intent of medical treatment alter the nature and severity of the later manifestations. It would seem likely to me that, particularly with regard to skin responses, some tendency analogous perhaps to ''street immunity'' establishes some degree of protection. On the other hand, episodes such as infections may suddenly precipitate more violent responses than would have been predicted by the premonitory signs—a so-called minor allergy being followed by a major response. Perhaps the studies of Burky showing the ability of certain bacterial toxins to alter antigenicity will have more than casual bearing on the infection.

Now to summarize a few points concerning diagnosis, management, and treatment. So many of the symptoms we associate with allergy in infants may be produced by causes other than allergy that a diagnosis and the recognition of the causes are not easy.

The history of the family and a detailed account of the young child's responses are of the greatest value in the diagnosis of allergy. In very young infants direct skin tests are notoriously unreliable, tending to develop perhaps from delayed to marked tests at about 4 months of age. The skin tests are decidedly helpful in older children but are not absolute. Eosinophilia is likewise fallible as a guide, having significance when positive, but its absence does not rule out sensitivity. The leucopenic index would appear to be of least value because of the normal fluctuations in the young child. There remains the detective work with trial-and-error diets and detailed diary follow-up.

On treatment I believe we are justified in suspecting the rashes suggesting eczema and the colic which may be associated with them. However, the treatment of eczema by dietary means alone is likely to be disappointing. Avoidance of certain foods, contacts, and inhalants, which are found offensive for many of these patients, as well as those suffering with asthma, is logical and perhaps preventive. Urticaria may be a transitory or minor allergy but it is not always easy to differentiate. In many infants there remains the role of nervous disposition occasionally seen to a marked degree in angioneurotic edema.

The very symptomatic treatments such as ointments and lotions for eczema, epinephrine and neosynephrine for asthma and hay fever, air filtration, etc., are of great value. Quite apart from the immediate relief so essential to medical practice these measures are in the same category with the rest of the program. To borrow a psychiatric term every effort should be made to break the pattern of response.

CHAIRMAN RATNER.—I am sure you will all agree with me that Dr. Smyth's survey is highly philosophical and yet he has offered many practical points of value. It is a pity that time does not allow Dr. Smyth to tell us more of the complexities of the eczema problem. Chevalier Jackson once said that ''all is not asthma that wheezes,'' and after listening to Dr. Smyth's description of eczema we might apply this aphorism and say that ''all is not eczema that itches.'' Dr. Smyth, you've stated that eczema is a response to irritation which comes from many sources, and I am wondering what your opinion is about the metabolic causes for eczema, whether you believe that certain types of hypothyroidism influence eczema, particularly in cases with delayed ossification.

DR. SMYTH.—I don't believe, Dr. Ratner, I could answer that. I have not been impressed with the theory that the thyroid had a direct relation to those youthful types of infantile eczema which we find with definite skin tests and in relation to some foods by trial-and-error administration.

CHAIRMAN RATNER.—I am almost in total agreement with everything you have stated, but I cannot let the remark about the hereditary factor versus intrauterine sensitization pass without comment. I regret that because of my work on intrauterine sensitization, the general impression seems to be that I regard this as the sole mode of sensitization in the young infant. We have found only about 30 per cent of our children who gave adequate evidence of that type of sensitization. On the other hand, I do not think that the child necessarily requires a family history to develop allergy. I believe with others that allergy or the capacity to acquire allergy is a universal attribute of the animal kingdom. I think that heredity may play some role, but it influences a rather small percentage of the children who actually develop allergy.

DR. SMYTH.—Of course, Dr. Ratner, you take us again into a realm of philosophy rather than allergy. I think in one of the allergy reviews I quote the Quaker ''Everybody's allergic but me and thee, and thee is a little allergic.'' I think Vaughan's use of the term minor allergy also points to the fact that perhaps you are right; the animal kingdom has this general tendency, some in marked degree, some to a lesser degree; nevertheless, at least from a practical standpoint I would be unwilling to neglect the importance of family history. I rather think that while granting placental transmission, Woringer's criticism of the wholesale acceptance, in view of the instances where the paternal influence was so marked, prompts one to keep a rather liberal point of view. It is true, even with careful histories, that there are plenty of instances where one cannot obtain a story of hereditary. On the other hand, sometimes I feel the history on allergy is an open book because you begin, and sometimes parents will say, ''There was nothing like that in my family.'' At a later date when they understand it, they will come in with a history and you wonder why they held back because it is a beautiful story.

CHAIRMAN RATNER.—How do you explain, Dr. Smyth, those cases of individuals who react the first time they ingest milk or eggs? Do you have any explanation other than the congenital concept?

DR. SMYTH.—I grant you that this case may be due to a type of activity similar to serum sickness. I recall Dr. Piness' pointing out that some of the reactions that we get would be group reactions and that we might find some individuals reacting to pollens found only in the high Sierras, when you know very well they haven't been up there. In the matter of egg white there is something confusing in that to me. I have often wondered whether proteins of the larger molecular structure are multiples of albumin, and whether that accounts for the peculiar predominance of egg white which is something, I think, in a class by itself.

CHAIRMAN RATNER.—I am familiar with that viewpoint of yours, but after all egg white does have one of the smallest molecular weights of all the proteins. It is highly diffusible and it is an ubiquitous component of the average diet. For these reasons I believe that egg white is so common an offender. I do not think that we must put it in a class by itself, any more than any other albumin.

DR. SMYTH.—I still feel there is something peculiar about egg white in its activity, its frequency, and its violent peculiar actions, out of all proportion to the tests with other allergens. One of the earliest experiences that I have had (I think Dr. Piness remembers when I started with the intracutaneous testing) using in a known egg-sensitive child what I thought was a very weak solution of egg white; I injected the egg white solution intracutaneously and either hit a capillary or was, as Dr. Piness said, so unfortunate as to strike the one in twelve thousand, but at any rate that child had anaphylaxis; so did I.

CHAIRMAN RATNER.—Before proceeding with this discussion I want to remind the panel that we are to have a free, easy, and informal discussion, interrupting one another at any point; I hope that you will all join in that spirit. Those in the audience can write their questions and send them up to us, and we will try to answer them as time permits.

DR. PINESS.—Dr. Smyth, I want to ask you if there is such a thing as a minor allergy. If there is, what is it and how do you explain the cycle that follows?

DR. SMYTH.—In my experience a minor allergy as I see it is an urticarial response, for example, that is transitory, with no other developments—for example, transitory hives from strawberries. Patients may have them one year only, they may come up the first of the season, or they may have them for two or three years. I do not think that this type of patient develops asthma or of necessity has urticaria of the nature through life.

CHAIRMAN RATNER.—Do you believe that type of urticaria is allergic?

DR. SMYTH.—Well, it is an altered sensitivity which the majority of us do not show.

CHAIRMAN RATNER.—In what percentage of urticarias that you have seen in which you have been able to determine the etiology would you say that the etiology is determinable by skin testing? What percentage of this group do you believe is definitely of the so-called allergic type?

DR. SMYTH.—Of course, again you have raised the question of terminology. Let's forget terminology. I believe that the majority of these patients with urticaria have not skin tests which we can interpret, but I think that we have a cause and effect that are demonstrative by trial-and-error diet.

CHAIRMAN RATNER.—Do you believe that these patients do by trial-and-error diet bring out the etiology and that they are definitely food sensitive?

DR. SMYTH.—Some of them, yes.

DR. PINESS.—Would it be interesting for you to know that in a large series of urticaria patients, only 10 per cent were determined by specific tests or by guess, as it were, on the part of the patient and the family, due to some food, and that 90 per cent were due to drugs, the chief worry being aspirin and the second largest in the series being phenolphthalein. Has that been your experience?

DR. SMYTH.—We have some hypersensitive children, but I think, not so large a series as you may have, from which to draw conclusions. I still unfortunately remember certain ones in whom I think we have ruled out the possibility of drugs; now I would not leave you for a moment with a feeling of any satisfaction about our ability to diagnose and to understand these cases.

CHAIRMAN RATNER.—Dr. Piness, do you infer that drug sensitivity is not truly allergic?

DR. PINESS.—I believe it is a true allergic thing. I am not discussing the question of its being all allergic phenomena. I believe the drug sensitivities are definitely allergic, the best proof being the work of Landsteiner that it is possible to hook up body proteins with drugs, particularly the acting group and make them then result in drug allergy. Now it is very possible that is what happens in the aspirin group particularly, not impossible and probable with the phenolphthalein group. Many of the other drugs which produce these urticarial eruptions are, in the nature of, or are, alkaloids. But I am convinced that skin tests give very little information as far as urticaria is concerned, and I am certain that patch tests give no information because I have never seen as yet, a patch test with any drugs that are common, accepted causes of urticaria which has ever produced a similar lesion by their application to the skin. In the literature which has been reviewed by us recently, we found that of all of the men that have discussed drug allergies none ever reported a ways and means of discovering the etiology by these tests, or by any chemical tests of the excretions or the blood. So I say that we must assume that there is such a thing but we are not able to prove it by specific means.

CHAIRMAN RATNER.—I think we shall proceed with our discussion. Dr. Smyth has commented on the fact that the nature of the offending factor may differ in foods; thus, although heat may reduce the antigenicity of certain foods, among which are milk, eggs, fruit, berries and cereals, yet with others, such as fish, cooking actually enhances its antigenicity.

He has also indicated to you that while sensitivities may not be entirely limited to foods, even in the cases of infantile allergy, as has been the general impression, foods do play a major role. Hence I shall call upon Dr. Rowe, who has contributed so much to our better understanding of the food allergy problem, to discuss its many intricacies, especially as related to childhood.

DR. ROWE.—Dr. Ratner and members of the section, I am very glad to be able to take part in this discussion this evening and I will proceed to give you some of the ideas that I have gathered according to Dr. Ratner's suggestion.

Why should my baby or child, or why should I myself, above all others, develop an allergy is a question which greets all physicians today. The best answer is that everyone tends to become allergic, but the tendency is heightened by heredity, that allergies due to inhalants, ingestants and contactants may develop at any time of life.

Now how does our food allergy develop in infancy? This has already been discussed in part, but I am going to have my little expression at this time. Usually allergy arises after birth, to foods following their addition to the diet. Intermittent feeding of a food may at times be responsible. The former practice of feeding a little egg white during the first few days of life until the breast milk appeared may have initiated some allergy in susceptible babies.

The same result probably arose from the temporary feeding of milk at birth. Thus if cow's milk in any form must be given during the first days of life, even though plenty of breast milk is soon available, it would seem advisable, particularly in babies with a strong family history of allergy, to continue small amounts of cow's milk until weaning. This same precaution should be taken against occasional feeding of vegetables, fruits, and other foods to subjects predisposed to allergy.

Overfeeding, particularly of one food, is another likely factor in the production of food allergy. If one remembers that allergy is essentially a protective response of the tissues to foreign substances, the origin of sensitization to a food fed in excessive amounts is not surprising. Moreover, food allergy may arise during digestive upsets or during acute illnesses in susceptible children.

The emphasis must be on the degree of positivity of the family history, for comparatively only few children or adults exist whose family history fails to reveal some evidence of allergy in its various forms; with marked evidence of food allergy in the progenitors, therefore, infants and children will be more susceptible to various disturbances from food allergy.

A similar tendency to develop manifestations of pollen or other inhalant allergies exists in the progeny of inhalant-sensitive parents. Also there is an inherited predisposition, in my experience, to definite manifestations of food allergy, such as gastrointestinal, cutaneous, nasal or bronchial symptoms. Asthma, eczema, nasal allergy, or migraine, or recurrent headaches certainly tend to run in families, also the tendency to become allergic to a specific food such as egg, milk, or even individual vegetables or fruits at times seems to be determined in part by heredity. Many instances of milk or egg allergy in three or four generations are recorded in the literature. Such specific effect of heredity, however, is not the rule.

From the practical viewpoint, if a definite history of milk, egg, or wheat, or other food allergy exists in the family it might seem wise to be cautious in the addition of such foods to the infant's diet. In the case of milk, evaporated milk, which Ratner has shown to be less allergic than other milk products, might be utilized. Or if milk allergy has been a great problem in the progenitors, a milk substitute like sobee, could be used entirely, with the gradual addition of minute and increasing amounts of denaturized milk, hoping that hyposensitization would gradually arise. This procedure fortunately should be rarely necessary.

Where egg allergy exists in the family or marked sensitization to other foods in the family is evident, egg may be excluded for a varying number of years. This is especially true when skin reactions to egg are present. When egg is finally added, it should be given with minute amounts, gradually increasing it over a period of several months, according to evidences of any clinical reactivity.

Food allergy also develops from foods eaten by the mother during the uterine life, as demonstrated clinically and experimentally by Ratner. The one-cell membrane in the placenta is largely responsible for the passage of food allergy from the blood vessels of the mother to those of the child. If there is an inherited tendency to the development of a specific food allergy such as egg, the ordinary amount of such food eaten by the mother could lead to such allergy in the fetus. In cases in which such predisposition does not exist, overeating by the mother during pregnancy is probably responsible for the origin of specific food allergy in the fetus. One patient aged 20 years developed a marked allergic conjunctivitis whenever rice was eaten; her mother overate of rice given her by the Chinese cook during her pregnancy. The origin of such specific food allergies during fetal life as a result of chromosonal action, but not by food allergy transmitted through the placenta, must also be remembered.

How frequently it occurs, whether the actual sensitization is inherited or whether it is due to the predisposition to become sensitive to specific foods, is impossible to state with the present available knowledge. How much sensitization of the infant arises from food allergens in the mother's milk it is difficult to say. Food allergens in such milk, as demonstrated by Donnally, are present but in extremely small amounts; such small amounts of food allergens might lead to sensitization in an infant with a marked inherited predisposition to allergy to such food. If this tendency existed, however, it would seem that placental transmission of such food allergies would establish fetal sensitization. Moreover, before sensitization through breast milk is accepted, the possibility of previous feedings of small amounts of food, or the deposit of such food on the lips of the infant by kissing or by the infant's hands, which have touched that food, might in turn have to be considered.

We will now discuss some of the problems of food allergy after its establishment in the patient. After one sensitization to a food arises, allergies to biologically related foods frequently, though not necessarily, develop. One may be sensitive to all citrous fruits, or to orange and not to lemon and to grapefruit. Likewise allergy may be present to several or merely to one of the pit fruits. As marked fruit sensitizations continue, allergies to other unrelated foods may arise. In a few patients allergies to many or nearly all fruits unfortunately may occur.

Extensive sensitizations to practically all pollens are encountered, which indicates that allergy to a great number of foods of all types may also develop. Thus with the establishment of specific food sensitizations it would seem important to control them in order to prevent more extensive difficulty.

Food sensitizations vary in the degree of their resultant manifestations. There are many more mild indefinite results than severe marked disturbances and those mild effects may produce discomfort and inefficiency which need relief. The symptoms may arise rapidly after the ingestion of the food or may delay for a few hours or even a few days; they may appear only after repeated ingestion of the food for days or even weeks depending on the amount of tolerance existing to the food. Moreover, a refractory period in which desensitization is present often arises after a marked clinical reaction to a specific food has occurred. This explains recurrent attacks of asthma, every one to four weeks, or nasal allergy, headache, even though the food is eaten every day.

One food may produce asthma, other foods may produce hives, others may result in gastrointestinal symptoms in the same patients according to the location of the specific reacting bodies to the food allergens in the cells of the body. Manifestations of the food allergy tend to decrease or disappear during the summer months. Patients sensitive to wheat, milk, or eggs often can eat such foods from May until mid-August or September without the asthma, nasal allergy, or eczema which arises from them during the fall, winter, and spring. A history of lessening of allergic manifestations during the summer months therefore should suggest possible food allergy.

Of great interest also is the fact that manifestations of food allergy especially are decreased, or may disappear when the patients go ten to twenty miles away from the Bay or coast line. Such nasal or bronchial allergy may disappear in one to three days in such territory only to reappear in a day or so on returning to the maritime region. This favorable influence is especially noted in the foothills or mountains of the Sierras here in California, or in the desert. Altitude is not responsible, since the benefit occurs in Death Valley, 300 feet below the sea level. It has been suggested that the mineral content of the air, being greater near the ocean, or that ionization of the air may explain this effect, but no assured explanation is at hand.

Uncontrolled pollen or other inhalant allergy may enhance food sensitizations which exist.

The statement that food allergy must always be studied with the possibility of inhalant, contactant, and to a less extent bacterial allergy in mind is important to emphasize.

Manifestations of food allergy at times gradually diminish or disappear, giving place to another symptom complex. Thus allergic dermatitis in infancy may be superseded by allergic bronchitis, asthma, or nasal allergy at the end of the second year. Recurrent vomiting or bilious attacks in childhood may resolve into recurrent sick headaches or migraine in the teens. Food allergy, however, rarely if ever disappears entirely and may remain potentially present without manifestations all through life.

A few comments will now be made on the diagnosis of food allergy. A dietary history often offers important clues concerning active food sensitization; all histories, whether of infants, children, or adults, and I may say for any medical condition, should contain this dietary information. In infants foods which are regurgitated, produce erythema or rashes of the skin or gastrointestinal symptoms must come under suspicion. In them, as in children and adults, foods that are disliked or produce definite disturbances of skin, nasal, bronchial, or gastrointestinal tracts must be suspected.

Such history may be more important than skin testing, but skin testing should always be done. Skin reactions, especially by the scratch test, are often negative to foods causing definite allergy. Skin-reacting bodies to such foods are absent, the sensitization itself being confined to the cells of the shock tissues whether in the lung, the nose, or the gastrointestinal tract. Positive reactions may only indicate the potentiality or may be nonspecific in nature and must therefore be checked by clinical trial or by a definite history of allergy thereto. The patient may give a few skin reactions to foods some of which are productive of allergy and may fail to react to other foods which cause equal or greater difficulty.

More reactions are often obtained with the intradermal tests with food allergies than with scratch tests. Here, however, a greater number of nonspecific reactions tend to arise and negative reactions to allergy-producing foods still may occur. Thus for the diagnosis of food allergy in childhood, as well as in adult life, diet trial, at times with several types of elimination diets, often over a period of weeks must be utilized. Such diet trials, however, are absolutely contraindicated if any nutritional damage is likely.

Food allergy in infancy probably produces more manifestations in the gastrointestinal tract than in any other tissue. Regurgitation, colic, distention, diarrhea, and feeding difficulties often may be due to mild or more definite allergies; spasm of the pylorus has been reported as due to food allergy in certain instances, and it is possible with its continuance that actual stenosis might arise.

How many of these gastrointestinal symptoms are due to food allergies or how many arise from impaired digestive function is impossible to tell. Deficiencies in hydrochloric acid or digestive ferments or in the peristaltic action in the intestines themselves may account for a definite number of such symptoms. Food allergy is often responsible, however, and must be constantly in mind.

After infancy food allergy continues to affect the gastrointestinal tract. Canker sores so frequently due to food allergy are probably urticarial or small Arthus-like lesions. It is entirely possible that such cankerlike lesions may occur in the stomach or duodenum, and, when increased by the acid and digestive ferments, they may develop into peptic ulcer.

Localized allergy in the stomach, intestines, and colon in childhood producing disturbances in peristalsis and digestive function may result in coated tongue, belching, regurgitation, distention, nausea, vomiting, cramping, abdominal soreness, spasms, irritable bowel, mucous colitis, diarrhea, constipation, rectal spasm, and irritation. Pruritus ani at times is due to allergy and may result in a localized eczema.

Recurrent vomiting often producing acidosis should always suggest food allergy. A refractory period develops after such an attack with a gradual building up of the allergic reactivity over a period of days or weeks as an explanation of such interims of relief. Such vomiting occurred in a five-year-old boy whom I recently saw and resulted in acidosis associated with a high blood sugar. At first diabetes was suspected, but with the recurrence of vomiting three weeks later allergy was assumed; with the use of trial diets no difficulty occurred in the last seven months except on one occasion when milk was taken against orders.

Anorexia, especially when mild or severe gastrointestinal allergy is present, should suggest food allergy as one possible cause. It also occurs when food or another allergy productive of nasal, bronchial, and especially of toxic symptoms is present.

Perennial nasal allergy, allergic bronchitis, or recurrent asthma is frequently due to food sensitizations at all times of life especially in childhood. As noted above, such symptoms are helped by inland residence and by the summer months. Sneezing, nasal congestion, and watery discharge without definite itching of the nose should suggest food allergy. Inhalant allergy more often results in itching. Opaque antra often arise from sinusal allergy, especially to foods. Eosinophiles are usually found in the nasal secretion. Mucous membrane edema and at times polyps cause the opacities. Thorough allergic study and prolonged treatments are imperative; opaque antra in themselves are never an indication for surgery.

Bronchial asthma arising from food allergy in childhood is usually indicated by allergic reactivity in the nose and sinuses for one or two days, giving the impression that a cold produces the asthma. Such nasal symptoms, however, actually are not due to infection. The secretions contain eosinophiles and not pus cells. They are the result of allergic reactivity which starts in the upper part of the nasal bronchial mucosa and localizes in the bronchial tissues after the first day or two. Since more attention has been paid to food and associated inhalant allergy as a cause of such asthma, and bacterial allergy has been relegated to its rare and infrequent role, results have been most satisfactory.

In the skin, food allergy is a usual cause of urticaria and angioneurotic edema. Fruits should always be suspected in urticaria and if elimination diets are used to study such cases, fruit should be excluded. Eczema or allergic dermatitis in children, and especially in infants, demands consideration of food allergy. As age increases, the inhalants must receive increasing study, and contactants as a cause of sensitizations must be recognized. In allergic dermatoses information derived from history, skin reactions and the results of diet trial, environmental control, and hyposensitization therapy in varying degrees must be used to determine finally the etiological causes of the difficulty. Food allergy as one cause of allergic purpura and mucous membrane bleeding must also be mentioned at this place.

Other manifestations of food allergy alone or associated with inhalant allergy must be kept in mind. Allergic conjunctivitis, corneal ulcers, and other less frequent ocular disturbances occur. Genitourinary tissues are not exempt. Recurrent vulval edema, congestion, itching, eruption, associated with fever and vomiting occurred in two children in my experience. Enuresis from uncontrolled food allergy has been recorded and observed in my work. Frequent and urgent urination with negative findings in the urine may be due to bladder allergy, which occurs occasionally in adults. Fever arising from food allergy has been studied by several students, emphasizing the consideration of allergy as one cause of the so-called idiopathic fevers.

Finally, uncontrolled allergy, especially to foods, leads to irritability, nervousness, restlessness, incorrigibility, wakefulness, nightmares, and other associated evidences that allergy directly or indirectly may act detrimentally on the brain and the nervous structures of the body.

In considering food allergy and other types of allergies as a cause of any symptoms, it must be stressed and emphasized that most careful physical examinations, laboratory tests of all indicated types must be done to recognize and rule out any diseases or pathologic states other than allergy that might be causing the patient symptoms.

CHAIRMAN RATNER.—Dr. Rowe, your discussion was so thorough and complete that I am sure that your remarks will give rise to many questions. I know that your task was the discussion of food allergy, but I had the feeling as I listened to you that probably food allergy was stressed a little too forcibly. We have had a peculiar reaction recently in evaculating our cases and find that infants who had food sensitivity even with eczema, as Dr. Smyth has brought out, or urticaria or rhinitis, may actually be sensitive not only to food, but also to inhalants and contactants. It seems to me that undue stress laid on food alone might tend to give us the impression that the finding of the food factor may solve the problem, but I doubt it very much, although I realize that food is a very important factor.

DR. ROWE.—I thoroughly agree with you, Dr. Ratner, about that; I believe though that in infancy and in the first few years of life food sensitization probably is more frequent in relation to inhalants than it is as years progress, and I believe that the criticism of the emphasis on food during infancy and in the first year or two of life is possibly well taken.

I took the occasion, however, in my discussion—I might have made it a little more definite and I realize that I was talking about food allergy all through the paper—to point out the fact that food allergy should never be considered alone—that inhalant allergy should always be kept in mind. And as I go along with my work I am in full accord with you that inhalant and contact allergy must always be given due consideration.

CHAIRMAN RATNER.—Dr. Rowe, I realized that that was your opinion and I just wanted to emphasize it. You brought up a question that is of particular interest to pediatricians, namely, the dangers of giving raw egg white or raw milk during the neonatal period. You emphasize, however, that these infants should not get this type of food if they have a background strongly suggestive of hereditary allergy. I for one believe that no infant should get these highly allergenic foods, irrespective of their heredity because of Schloss's work which showed that in normal and athreptic infants unchanged proteins do pass the intestinal wall in the native state.

DR. ROWE.—I believe that that is a point which is well emphasized; however, I still feel that many of these food sensitivities develop in children who have a strong inherited tendency and that there is in certain of them an inherited tendency to develop specific sensitizations to definite foods. I believe though in pediatric practice, with which I am not acquainted to any degree, that the custom today in the early days of infancy is not to feed uninterruptedly these foods that Dr. Ratner spoke about.

DR. W. A. McGEE (RICHMOND, VA.).—Dr. Rowe, I should like to mention two or three things. Do you find with the feeding intervals at three days when you have a child that is apparently allergic you can often steer clear of that offending food? I am not talking of inhalants. Have you found when you put them on the milk substitute you mentioned, if you have used it, clinical evidences of olive oil sensitivity? I have recently run across three of them that could not take milk and could not take olive oil, ruling out one of the most available milk substitutes. The other is that in an allergic child I feel the use of multiple cereals, multiple fish oils, and vegetable soups is definitely contraindicated.

DR. ROWE.—I am not in a position to discuss the practical aspects in feeding in the early days or months of infancy because I do not do any of that at all; but it seems to me that if milk has to be given and breast milk is not available, it would be a great mistake to stop the milk—if it is decided later on to use breast milk for a period of time, and particularly if there is a marked history of allergy in the family. In other words, if the breast milk is to be given in place of cow's milk that has been given previously, I would suggest that small amounts of cow's milk be administered every day or two or every four or five days to possibly prevent any establishment of future milk sensitivity.

About these other suggestions that the doctor made, I believe that it is entirely possible when a complex food like sobee is used, it must be remembered that sensitization to any one of the ingredients might certainly exist. How often it occurs, of course, I think is uncertain. I believe it is rather rare.

CHAIRMAN RATNER.—Dr. McGee, with reference to your remark about the multiple foods of infancy I see no objection at all to giving multiple foods provided that those multiple foods are denatured by heat. For example pablum, which has a multiplicity of cereal ingredients, has been shown experimentally to be quite free of antigenicity, and there is no reason at all to eliminate the multiple foods so long as they are heated and not given in a raw state. I think this is a point that is important to pediatrics practice.

DR. McGEE.—Dr. Ratner, that might be true experimentally and may sound true, but practically, I have seen many an infant who could not take it. We are not talking of skin tests, and it comes home to my own child.

DR. SMYTH.—I do not know whether I am just timid or reactionary, but when I listen to Dr. Rowe, the list of complaints from which you get an allergy I think you are very enthusiastic. I think it is perhaps almost dangerous to leave the impression, for example, that migraine is solved on an allergic study. Migraine to me is a riddle. If you solve it—God be praised. I think of the vomitus; how do you account for the frequency with which we find ketonuria preceding the episode of vomiting? There surely is a metabolic picture at least in some of them which deserves recognition fully as much as an allergic study.

I noted you mention also the dislike of certain foods. Have you not encountered certain individuals who with known sensitivity, even adults, will partake of shrimps when they full well know the symptoms they will have; they do not get edema of the glottis, and they like the sensation of eating the forbidden food.

This is perhaps baiting you, among pediatricians. What would be your feeling about the eczema of the breast-fed infant? You mention Donnally's work, but it seems to me the technique that Donnally used is not above criticism. He was injecting curds of milk, and I think there is some real room for controversy about that. Dr. Ratner mentioned Schloss's thesis, which I think is a fine one; nevertheless, the work with intestinal absorption has shown that even the normal individual will absorb protein from the intestinal tract and show a positive skin test by the Prausnitz-Küstner technic, so that that may be a normal mechanism in part. In fact, I wonder if our physiology is not perhaps erroneously worded that it leaves us with the impression that even in the normal gut certain types of protein may be absorbed and altered.

CHAIRMAN RATNER.—Dr. Smyth, there has been a great deal of discussion about the factors which influence heredity. Your bringing up the point of the work of Schloss and calling it a normal phenomenon leads me to express the following idea. Do you not think that allergy is a normal physiologic type of reactivity? There is no reason to suspect that heightened reactivity is not a normal physiologic capacity of the animal kingdom.

DR. SMYTH.—It seems to me that that suggestion, as well as Lippard's work, more recently, which is certainly aiming in that direction, and also the statement that allergy may be a protective reaction, is today one of the controversies from a theoretical angle that is far from settled. I refer to Arnold Rich, particularly working with tuberculin, who challenges very definitely the idea that perhaps it is an awful price to pay for the protection that certain individuals have.

DR. PINESS.—Dr. Rowe, I should like to ask in your experience, which is long and very wide, how many cases did you actually see in children from the age of one year, or under one year, to ten years who have been actually sensitive to foods and foods alone?

DR. ROWE.—It is my impression that quite a number of patients have in childhood and in infancy food sensitizations without actual clinical manifestations of inhalant allergy. That is a statement, of course, which could be modified by reference to the records, but I think that there are a great many children who are sensitive to food alone.

DR. PINESS.—That statement, I take it, is based on both skin test and elimination diet. Well, on the basis of skin tests alone how many have you observed? Up to 1930—was that when elimination diets came up? No; 1927. Your reports were formerly on the basis of skin tests?

DR. ROWE.—Well yes. In 1925 I reported—

DR. PINESS.—Well up to 1925, if I remember correctly, you reported that some 95 per cent cases were skin sensitive; we are not speaking of clinical sensitivity for the moment. And in that 95 per cent how many were sensitive to foods and foods alone by skin tests? And since then, if you know that?

DR. ROWE.—I cannot remember.

DR. PINESS.—Well, would it not be interesting to you to know that in five thousand children alone, we found only 1 per cent were sensitive to foods and foods alone, and the others were divided up into groups sensitive to pollens alone, epidermals alone, and then the multiple group. You are, I think, in accord with most of us that multiple sensitivity is the common type of sensitivity, is not that right?

Well, under those circumstances which do you believe is the most common food that one is sensitive to?

DR. ROWE.—Well, I have never really gathered statistics which would give me any basis to discuss that, but I think that milk is unquestionably a very common one, and egg; I think many of the fruits are equally frequently causative. Of course, I believe that many of these food sensitizations as demonstrated by skin tests are not associated with clinical sensitivity. Just because a patient gives a positive skin test, particularly by the intradermal method, does not mean that the patient is clinically sensitive to that food.

DR. PINESS.—Anticipating that from you I brought with me some facts that I think are rather interesting. In a thousand children of consecutive cases at the Allergy Clinic, Children's Hospital at Los Angeles—these children are clinically sensitive and not skin sensitive cases, and in them we were able to reproduce the facts at will—we found the following: Wheat, which you take to be one of the chief offenders, was fifty-fifth in that list; milk was forty-second; orange was fourth and of the cereal group in which we are all interested, particularly the pediatrician, barley was the most common. The most common fruit was orange, and the most common vegetable was lettuce, which was fifteenth; egg white was fifth. Now the others—white potato, for example, which is commonly used, was fortieth; and an interesting fact was that cod-liver oil was sixty-second on the list. One hundred seventy-three in one thousand children were sensitive to cod-liver oil. I think that is rather interesting because I do not believe that skin tests should be minimized to the extent that you suggest. I believe that skin tests have a real value and that value is dependent upon the clinician's ability to correlate a skin test with the clinical history. I think that the advantages of that are much greater than one obtains from elimination diets. It was rather interesting too in this whole group of cases in Southern California, we were able to get a higher percentage of children with pollen reactions than we did with foods. Orris root, which we are all discussing, was eleventh in the list of inhalants, and it's rather interesting, too, from our observation and from asking the mothers bringing children to the clinic the type of powders they are using, that very few of the powders these days contain orris root. I should like to have you answer how you can reconcile yourself to the elimination diet, disposing of such a report as this one. It seems to me illogical on the basis of scientific studies to accept the elimination diet as a substitute for such work as this.

CHAIRMAN RATNER.—I knew that there would be a very lively discussion. I feel that Dr. Rowe has some justification for his stand and that Dr. Piness is somewhat justified in his assertions. It seems to me, however, that the most important thing to be gathered from this discussion should be the fact that foods and foods alone play a minor role in the sensitivities of childhood, even in the very earliest instances, as Dr. Smyth has brought out and Dr. Piness has emphasized. It seems to me that no method as important as the skin test should ever be discarded; it is entirely too important and we should use all the methods available.

DR. PINESS.—Dr. Ratner, I did not want to give the impression that Dr. Rowe advocates the discarding of skin tests because he emphatically states in his paper that both systems should be correlated. My experience has been, and I believe, that there is a greater specificity to skin tests than there is to the elimination diet.

I should like to ask Dr. Rowe just one other question and that is on what he bases his theory that cases of asthma, I take it they were inhalant allergy, were better in the summer and might be due chiefly to foods.

DR. ROWE.—That is largely true experience, Dr. Piness, experience that I have gathered through a period of fifteen years of study. I am absolutely confident that most—many of these patients who have asthma or nasal allergy due to specific food sensitizations—are better in the summer than they are in the winter, and they are also definitely better when they go inland away from the bay region. There is not any question about that from my clinical experience, and after all clinical experience, as you all know, is a great deal more valuable in many instances than laboratory tests. I am perfectly willing to recognize the value of the scratch test or the skin test for foods, but I feel that with the intradermal tests that Dr. Piness uses there are a great many nonspecific irritant reactions that may indicate potential allergy that is confusing. When Dr. Piness gets a positive reaction to a food, he certainly has to check it up with a clinical trial in order to prove its worth. I feel really that trial diet modified by such reactions that are definite by the scratch test is about the best method that I have been able to work out through a period of fifteen or twenty years' effort in the study of food sensitizations.

CHAIRMAN RATNER.—Well, I think we all realize that there is a difference of opinion. I am going to ask Dr. Rowe just one more question. Am I wrong in assuming that you would have us believe that food allergies rarely if ever disappear?

DR. ROWE.—I think that the potential food sensitizations may continue. You cannot be absolutely sure that they disappear entirely. They may be potentially present for a long period of time.

DR. PINESS.—Dr. Ratner, since you have asked another question I think it my privilege to ask one too. I would like to ask you, Dr. Rowe, how would you prevent a child from acquiring a new food sensitivity, assuming that he is food sensitive? Pediatricians would like to know.

DR. ROWE.—Well, I think that overfeeding is important, as I have stated in this paper. Overfeeding of foods is an important thing to guard against, and certainly you have to be very careful about the way foods are fed during a digestive upset, particularly those affecting the gastrointestinal tract. Those are I would say the main ways.

DR. PINESS.—I would like to suggest a better and more simple method, if it is in order, and that is this: I believe that the easiest way and the most efficient way to prevent food sensitivities, that is the acquisition of new sensitivities, is by diversifying the diets. That is a very simple and very pleasing way for the child. I have found in my experience that feeding a child the same thing all the time is a very easy way to acquire new sensitivities.

CHAIRMAN RATNER.—I believe the suggestions of Dr. Rowe and Dr. Piness for the prevention of food allergy are both good.

There have been some questions from the floor and we will attempt to answer some of them.

DR. SMYTH.—The question is: How early may raw egg-yolk be added to the diet? Well I shall answer it in part by saying that at the New York Orphanage a number of years ago they had this formula—which I think they included for infants as young as two months—raw egg-yolk, lemon juice, and milk. To my knowledge they did not encounter a very high percentage of unfortunate reactions, but I think that if you are dealing with a nonallergic infant I would still be inclined to use hard boiled egg yolk crushed with a fork and avoid the egg white. It is true, however, that in quite a number of instances egg yolk can be incorporated into a formula, especially in an anemic undernourished infant, and little or no difficulty will be encountered. I would be guided, I think, entirely by the patient, that is, if there is a marked allergy or sensitivity I would be inclined to avoid the raw egg yolk.

CHAIRMAN RATNER.—A question: Did Dr. Ratner say pablum does not cause allergic manifestations due to its having been heated? Is it not true that the individual sensitive to wheat is not able to eat cooked wheat bread? Now that's a very significant question. Pablum, as you know, has been heated to an extremely high temperature in the presence of moisture, about twenty-two pounds of pressure for quite a while. When proteins are heated in the presence of water at a high temperature they become denatured. The reason bread is not denatured is simply that bread is baked in an oven not in the presence of moisture —the outside of the bread comes in contact with about 500° F. and the inside of the bread with about 200° F. Experimentally we have found that guinea pigs sensitive to raw wheat can be killed by an extract made from wheat bread, but guinea pigs sensitized to raw wheat will survive an injection of pablum.

DR. SMYTH.—The statement: I use a great deal of powdered protein milk, due to its low albumin content. It is used successfully in milk-sensitive babies. What is your thought?

We have used the 2 per cent dried milk in the form of dryco which I think Dr. Ratner would tell us was equally altered in its reactivity along with evaporated milk.

CHAIRMAN RATNER.—Dr. Smyth, experimentally we did not find that dryco was altered. It is prepared by heating on a hot plate for a few seconds, and apparently this dry heat to which it is subjected does not change it antigenically. No protein is denatured by heat in the absence of water. On the other hand, evaporated milk is altered or denatured in the heating process to which it is subjected because of the presence of moisture.

DR. SMYTH.—Well then, Dr. Ratner, what is your opinion of this commercial protein milk? Have you any comment?

CHAIRMAN RATNER.—Lactalbumin is the most frequent offender in milk. I should say that powdered protein milk which has a much lower content of albumin than dryco might very well be used with good results in milk-sensitive children.

DR. ROWE.—The next question is: Did I understand you to say that you have observed all manifestations to food allergy to have a seasonal incidence?

It has been my experience that most of the manifestations of food allergy, as I have observed them, tend to be worse during the winter and particularly during the spring months of the year. That they seem to be better between April 15 or around there until about September 15.

DR. SMYTH.—The question: Please explain teething rash. It is a very convenient term. I do not know that it is always as easily explained. I think earlier in my discussion I said that the skin of infants was notoriously tender. We have seen instances in which about the time of teething a tendency for rash appears with increased tension. There seems to be an association, but that it is necessarily allergic I, for one, am not ready to state.

DR. PINESS.—Embarrassing question No. 1: If skin tests are valuable, how do you explain a child with no reaction to skin tests in whom symptoms to foods occur?

That is not very difficult to explain because after all no one contends that skin tests are 100 per cent; they are not infallible. On the other hand, skin tests that are negative may be due to certain other factors. One, the antigen may not be active; two, the child may be in an anti-anaphylactic state. I do not know what it means. It may be a period when the skin is not reactive. And those of you who have done skin tests have observed, no doubt, that a child who has been tested once and gives 100 per cent negative reactions may come back in a month and give a very specific reaction. I think skin tests cannot be condemned on the basis of one child, or even the 24 per cent of children who are not reactive to skin tests, but it is a fact that many of these children will react on second testing.

DR. SMYTH.—Question: If the thyroid has no place in eczemas how do you explain the disappearance of eczema following the administration of thyroid gland?

I have seen eczema disappear without thyroid gland. I have seen thyroid gland used in the process called the treatment of its edema, simulating thyroid myxedema. I have seen eczema disappear in a sort of a profound diarrhea, only to reappear again when the fluid was re-established. It seems to me that the question involves some discussion of thyroid and its place in our therapy. There are some of us who feel that perhaps it can be overdone.

The second part of the question: If eczemas are a reaction to irritation, how do you explain the metabolic or constitutional differences between susceptible allergic individuals and normal ones? I am still looking for an explanation myself. Another question: What food should be avoided with the infant, allergic or non-allergic? Well, that would be open to discussion. Perhaps it varies with the section of the country, but I think perhaps strongly spiced foods and excessive use of stimulants, pickles, and a lot of indigestibles.

In general, the question is too broad to be specifically answered. Do you think of any answer? How would you think of that question?

CHAIRMAN RATNER.—Well, I think the question of what food should be avoided might be answered by stating that it is my belief that we would not have much food allergy if infants were fed denatured foods, provided an adequate amount of vitamin C were incorporated into the diet. It seems to me, for example, that the advent of evaporated milk is fast destroying the need for our skill as expert infant feeders, because practically all infants do well on evaporated milk. The application of this principle of heat denaturation to other foods in the infant's diet is a reasonable prophylactic measure.

CHAIRMAN RATNER.—Dr. Shaw states, "All children are allergic, at least that is all when given antigen parenterally. Is not the capacity to absorb unchanged protein a fundamental defect, the capacity to react to protein so absorbed being relatively universal? This better explains the mass action effect of the ingestion of excess amounts of food."

The question is really a good one, and Dr. Shaw answers it. His first statement, I presume, means that most children will develop serum sickness if given horse serum. I agree with him that the mass action of proteins coming in contact with normal membrane barriers accounts largely for the inception of allergy in childhood. We must accept the fact that serum sickness is truly an allergic phenomenon and does not differ basically from any other allergic phenomena we have been discussing.

The next question: Is it your impression that the frequency of allergy in infancy is the price paid for artificial feeding instead of breast feeding? Is not allergy less frequent in European clinics with 100 per cent breast fed infants? I cannot answer that question categorically. We do see allergy in the breast-fed infant, and I imagine that, when things clear up in Europe and some of our American allergists go over there, they will find plenty of allergies.

The next question raised is a rather interesting one. The doctor proposes a change of cereals, vegetables, and fruits on alternate days, and he asks what we think of this as a practical manner of feeding a baby. A diet consisting of a great variety of foods in small quantities and partially denatured will to a large extent eradicate food allergy, I am convinced.

CHAIRMAN.—I knew that Dr. Rowe's paper would arouse a great deal of discussion but didn't think it would take up so much time. I am sorry, therefore, that I will have to ask Dr. Piness who will continue our discussion to try to shorten his remarks. There are few men who know as much about the problem of rhinitis or hay fever in childhood or who have had any more experience than Dr. Piness.

DR. PINESS.—I came prepared to make my discussion a very short one realizing that I was coming so late in the program. Very few disorders of infancy and childhood are observed so commonly by the pediatrician as is allergic rhinitis. The reason for this is not hard to see. Mothers are well aware of the fact that coryza is the most common harbinger of evil at this age, and at the first sign of a running nose the pediatrician is consulted. Since coryza is also the most common symptom of allergic rhinitis and is also the most persistent and most frequently recurrent, we find sufficient justification for the statement made that there are very few disorders of infancy in childhood which the pediatrician observes so commonly. Because allergic rhinitis often foretells future frank hay fever and bronchial asthma and because it is a means of identifying the allergic constitution, it is important that the pediatrician be prepared to recognize this condition early in life so that the proper measures may be instituted to prevent the characteristic complications, and sequelae that result from the untreated allergic constitution.

How common then is the allergic constitution? The final answer is not yet determinable. In this regard it is interesting to note the various studies made on the incidence of allergy by the various workers in different sections of this country. An analysis of all the reports indicates a considerable similarity in their findings. Rowe in the study of 2,000 students in the University of California reported 35 per cent gave a positive family history and 33 per cent gave a positive history of having had or having some form of allergy. That is rather high. Vaughan surveyed a community of 508 individuals in which 60 per cent had some minor form of allergy (I contend again that there is no such thing as minor allergy because it is a constitutional disease and it is quite the same). Service made such a survey in a city of 35,000 population, using the sampling method according to economic distribution. He studied 1,000 families, whose total comprised 3,500 persons of all ages. He reports 44.9 per cent of the families surveyed had some form of allergic disease, and that 19.68 per cent of individuals in the general population had some form of allergy.

A positive history of heredity was elicited in about 32 per cent of these cases. This is considerably less than had heretofore been found by other writers but is quite in line with our own observations, resulting from a study made in Arizona of two communities with a total population of 4,000 persons, of whom 30 per cent gave positive histories of heredity—which at the time we thought to be lower than was to be expected. It would seem that heredity does not play a great part in determining how long an individual must be exposed before developing allergic symptoms. The consensus is that allergy in its various forms has its onset most frequently during the first decade of life. In a study made by us of a series of about 4,500 individual cases, 1,489, or 32.4 per cent gave a history of onset in the first decade of life, which is quite in line with the findings of other writers.

Rowe is of the opinion that food is responsible for most allergy during the first two years of life, inhalant allergy gaining increasing importance after that first year. We agree to the importance of foods as a factor during this age but wish to emphasize the importance of inhalants, particularly the environmental group, as being equally important in that exposure to them is equally as great as that to foods, perhaps more so. A consideration of this fact will result in more etiological information and better results from treatment. Hill reports observations in accord with our own.

Allergic rhinitis may be acute or chronic, it may be seasonal or perennial. It is a recurrent and often constant disturbance, and it is not infrequently considered as a repeated or persistent acute upper respiratory infection. The symptoms are characteristic. The acute attacks have a sudden onset, intense itching in the nose, eyes, ears, and pharynx, sneezing with a profuse discharge of serous fluid which, if the attack continues, becomes mucoid. There may be lacrimation and photophobia. The nose becomes completely or partially obstructed and usually symptoms subside rather acutely. Examination of the nose reveals usually an edematous congested, turgescent, mucous membrane with hypertrophy and edema of the turbinates. All nasal membranes have a characteristic bluish-white to deep pink color. The conjunctiva is usually edematous and has a granular appearance. This type is usually due to inhalants, and when seasonal, particularly during the summer months, is invariably pollen sensitivity. On the other hand, acute attacks that are not related to season are usually traceable to some environmental factor, such as insecticides, cosmetics, animal epithelium, and occasionally foods of the seasonal type.

The chronic and perennial types are characterized by recurrent daily symptoms chiefly occurring in the morning upon arising or upon retiring at night. Frequently the mother will observe similar attacks occurring when the child is put down for the afternoon nap. Here the symptomatology differs somewhat from the acute types in that the patient is usually free of symptoms the greater part of the day, symptoms are not as severe, but nasal obstructions in varying degrees are more or less constant. Examination of the nasal mucous membrane reveals a pale, boggy, water-logged, chronically turgescent mucous membrane, the chronic edema resulting in polyp formation on the turbinates and in the sinuses. Removal of polypi is disappointing in that they recur almost as rapidly as removed. In the pharynx there is a marked redness with hyperplasia of much lymphoid tissue in the lateral and medial positions. When the tonsils have been removed, much lymphoid tissue is evident on the pillars and on the fossae. The latter may be mistaken for tonsil regrowth. The diagnosis of allergic rhinitis should not be difficult and must not be missed, particularly when the above facts as to clinical history, symptomatology and pathology are known. Additional aids in making the diagnosis are a study of the nasal cytology, making smears from the nasal secretions, staining with Giemsa stain and noting whether or not eosinophilia is present. I refer to the work of Hansel who through his studies of nasal cytology has given us much information on the subject.

While blood studies are helpful, the presence of eosinophilia is not conclusive evidence of allergy; but in the presence of a positive family history, a story of having some other form of allergy, and a clinical history suspicious of allergy or a history of known allergic sensitivities, should be considered seriously in helping to establish a diagnosis.

Etiology of allergic rhinitis regardless of the type must of necessity be due to allergens, the nature of which we believe to be protein, although substances nonprotein in nature are known to produce it, and by means of skin testing one may in the majority of cases determine it. Time and space do not permit, nor is it necessary because of your familiarity with the procedure, discussion of the various techniques and methods of skin testing.

Much valuable information and considerable help are obtainable by eliciting certain facts in the clinical history, particularly such information as time of onset, relation of season, duration of symptoms, frequency of attacks, environment, noticeable factors that precipitate attacks—such as foods, domestic animals, cosmetics, certain portions of the home, and hobbies that might be factors, too.

Foods alone as the cause of allergic rhinitis, in my experience, do not occur as the etiological factor as often as some writers would lead us to believe. Our observations, particularly in a child with chronic allergic rhinitis, show that there is usually multiple sensitivity. While on the other hand, in the seasonal type, particularly that occurring in the summer months, the symptoms are usually due to pollen. Those having their severest season during the cold months are usually due to environmental allergens, such as wool, feathers, etc., while the perennial types who find no relief either by moving from place to place, or through seasonal variations are most likely to be due to food or allergens from the environmental group.

I wish to stress the point that skin tests are not employed to make a diagnosis of allergy but merely to confirm the diagnosis made by assisting in determining the etiology. They are not infallible, and are only of value when they can be proved clinically as well.

Since we are dealing with a constitutional disease, possibly of hereditary nature, at least predisposition to acquiring sensitivity, one must not make unwarranted claims for cure but can assure the patient's family that relief from all symptoms is possible, the degree of freedom from symptoms depending upon the ability to eliminate from the diet or environment those substances to which the patient is clinically as well as skin sensitive and on the complete cooperation of the patient and parents. This cooperation is also necessary in the pollen-sensitive individual in whom relief may be obtained only by persistent treatment with specific pollen antigens over a long period of time.

One must not consider all positive reactions as being the cause of the present symptoms, but they must be considered as potential factors either in the past or perhaps in some future time.

The treatment of allergic rhinitis then resolves itself into the removal of the offending allergens by eliminating the offending food from the diet, by removing from the environment the offending substances, and, if this is impossible, to make and treat with an antigen prepared from those known offenders. In the pollen-sensitive patient, prepare antigens from pollen and treat with these, but only after a careful study is made of the patient's history and after it is considered with regard to the reacting pollens that the patient may contact. To be able to accomplish this, it is necessary for the clinician to familiarize himself with the flora in the vicinity in which he resides, as well as the pollinating seasons. We are of the opinion that the majority of children affected by this condition are relieved of their symptoms by specific therapy, particularly when the etiology has been determined, and we have found that nonspecific means, such as nasal surgery, certain drugs, and endocrine products have been most disappointing.

Surgery is indicated only when there are anatomical defects, polyps, and secondary infections of the sinuses. As a matter of fact, the latter will very often clear up if the allergic condition is controlled.

In closing may I state that the many refractory and repeated upper respiratory conditions will disappear if treated on an allergic basis, and many complicating conditions such as sinus disease, bronchial asthma, and its sequelae might be obviated, making for a healthier, happier and better child.

CHAIRMAN RATNER.—Dr. Piness, I do not think that there can be much discussion of your paper because you have covered the field so well and we all agree with practically everything you said.

There are just two points which you brought up that I must comment on. You say that minor allergy does not exist. This is surprising, for there are all degrees and kinds of reactivity, the same as there are all degrees and kinds of so-called normality. The next point which I would like to stress is that I believe that your work done in the Arizona valley with the development of hay fever in a group of individuals who never suffered from hay fever prior to entering this community is probably one of the most important contributions that I find in the literature to indicate that heredity plays a minor role in allergy, for those people without positive family histories developed hay fever before the others who had positive family histories.

DR. PINESS.—Regarding the question of minor and major allergies, I contend that any individual who has an allergy of any kind at all is suffering from a major effect, and, regardless of whether the symptoms be mild or severe, he still is potentially predisposed to having all of the severe types of allergy. I do not think we can measure allergy by degree since it is a constitutional disease.

CHAIRMAN RATNER.—It seems unnecessary to summarize this discussion at this late hour because I believe my collaborators have done such a thorough job. I want to leave you, however, with the feeling that we have made no attempt to cover the allergy problem in childhood. We merely wanted to suggest to the pediatrician that he must interest himself in this problem and include a consideration of the allergic phenomena in his everyday practice. No period from earliest infancy throughout childhood is devoid of the possibility of hypersensitive reactivity. The pediatrician, as Dr. Smyth has brought out, is in intimate relation with his patients and has the opportunity to see these phenomena from their beginnings—free from the complications so often encountered in adult life. Early recognition offers the hope of introducing prophylactic measures and I hope my colleagues will bear with me if I venture the following statement: Although there will always be the need for the highly trained allergist, the time must come when the facts gleaned from the maze of work that is now being carried on in this field will be formulated into broad principles which may be readily applied in general pediatric practice.

I trust that you have all derived as much profit from this discussion as my colleagues and I have in preparing for it. It was a pleasure to present some of our viewpoints to you.

Meeting adjourned at 10:45 P.M.

EIGHTH ANNUAL MEETING OF THE AMERICAN ACADEMY OF PEDIATRICS

Del Monte, Calif., June 10 and 11, 1938

Round Table Discussion of Sulfanilamide

Chairman, Dr. Paul M. Hamilton, Alhambra, Calif.

CHAIRMAN HAMILTON.—During its three and a half years in the limelight of American medicine, sulfanilamide has inspired more clinical and laboratory investigation than any other development of its generation. Medical and even lay literature has reached stupendous proportions as workers have attempted to evaluate the merits, the dangers, and the mode of action of this remarkable new healing agent. And yet many fundamental questions remain either partly or totally unanswered.

From this vast and in many respects still debatable field only a limited area can be surveyed in the present summary. We shall concern ourselves therefore only with those phases which have a clinical application, and only with those conditions which may be seen by the pediatrician. Most of the comments will be based upon cases we ourselves have treated, though in most instances similar observations are plentiful in the literature. For a concise summary and bibliography one may refer to Holman and Duff.[1]

Mode of Action

The mode of action of sulfanilamide is not yet fully established. It seems certain that the actual destruction of bacteria is accomplished by the natural defense mechanisms of the body, aided in some way by the drug. Sulfanilamide is only weakly bactericidal in vitro, and, contrary to experience with true germicides, its efficiency is enhanced when various body fluids are added to the media. When added to specific antibody, the increase in potency is greater than would be expected from a simple additive effect. Long and Bliss[2] believe that the action is one of bacteriostasis and that the leucocytes are an indispensable part of the process, even though it is not one of simple phagocytosis. Osgood[3] believes that the drug in some way neutralizes bacterial toxins, thus permitting free attack on the organisms by all the mechanisms of body defense. Response is regularly greater and more rapid during the stages of active tissue change than in the more chronic phases of infection, such as the formation of walled-off abscesses. Rather contradictory observations are made that while clinically recovered animals may harbor the infecting organism for a long time, other animals may die with sterile organs. At present we may only say that the drug is not in itself strongly bactericidal.

Toxic Effects and Complications

The mechanism behind its toxic effects and complications is likewise incompletely understood. These actions of the drug are so numerous and varied that they must be considered separately. Despite their imposing array, the drug is relatively innocuous provided it is properly used and the patient carefully watched for evidence of serious reactions.

Cyanosis occurs with such frequency as to make it appear almost a concomitant of intensive treatment. It has most often been ascribed to methemoglobinemia; sulphemoglobinemia has also been demonstrated repeatedly, sometimes when no other sulfur medication has been given; and in some instances it occurs without either of these conditions. To explain this, Marshall and Walzl[4] postulate a black oxidation product which stains the red cells without measurably affecting their functioning ability. Hartmann[5] feels that the cyanosis is nearly always due to methemoglobinemia, and cites good results in treatment and prevention by the use of methylene blue either by vein or by mouth. Thus it appears that the cause of cyanosis is not always the same, and that at least in some instances it is not clearly understood.

Only rarely does cyanosis embarrass respiration or otherwise distress the patient, so that its appearance need not necessarily interfere with treatment. When due to methemoglobin, it can be relieved by methylene blue or oxygen, and it tends to disappear rapidly with discontinuance of the drug. Sulphemoglobinemia tends to be more severe and may persist for days after the sulfanilamide is discontinued.

Acidosis has been anticipated as a frequent result of intensive treatment and has been demonstrated through reduced carbon dioxide combining power. Hartmann,[5] however, has recently presented evidence to show that alkalosis is the primary response, and that such degree of acidosis as may occur later is no more than an exaggerated compensatory reaction. It has also been observed that nonfebrile patients, such as those with gonorrheal infection, usually have an alkaline urine. This naturally raises the question whether acidosis (when observed) is perhaps due to the disease rather than the drug. Proceeding on the assumption that acidosis is liable to occur, it has been our custom to give ⅙ molar sodium lactate solution, 10 c.c. to each 100 c.c. of 1 per cent solution of sulfanilamide, when given subcutaneously, or sodium bicarbonate in equal amounts when given by mouth; with the added precaution of frequent urine tests to be sure that the pH does not fall below 5. Hartmann stresses the need for maintaining chlorides and suggests a mixture of sodium lactate and Ringer's solution as being superior to sodium bicarbonate.

Anemia of great severity may occur, though fortunately it is not common. It is of the hemolytic type and may occur with such rapidity following the first dose as to suggest sensitivity, or it may come later (three to seven days) as if due to a cumulative action of the drug. Keefer[6] states that the outcome in these cases is good if the drug is stopped and transfusions are given, but our own experience has not always been so fortunate. We have seen hemoglobin drop from 80 per cent to 40 per cent in two days, despite transfusions, and continue to drop until death occurred. The only safeguard against this type of reaction is repeated blood examinations, with cessation of treatment and immediate transfusion at the first evidence of anemia. In this connection it should be remembered that a slight drop of 5 per cent to 10 per cent in hemoglobin is common during the first day or two and need cause no alarm unless it continues or accelerates.

Agranulocytosis is rare, but it is of serious import when it occurs. It tends to occur when considerable amounts of sulfanilamide have been given, and like the anemia should be anticipated by frequent blood examinations. It is treated with pentnucleotide K19 and transfusions, but it is difficult to control and may cause a fatal outcome.

Skin reactions which tend to take the form of a morbilliform rash are not uncommon. Other types of rashes may also occur, sometimes to the extent of an exfoliative dermatitis. Photosensitivity is a possibility which calls for protection of the patient from unnecessary exposure to sunlight.

Fever appearing for a few days after the disappearance of all evidence of the disease may be due to the drug. This fever is usually not high and has little effect on the patient, but it may be confusing from a therapeutic standpoint.

Malaise is common, and especially in ambulatory patients it may be so severe as to lead them to refuse treatment. It is seldom extreme in bed patients.

Psychoses are reported, but are very rare unless one should include mild confusion, depression, and moroseness, which are common. Both excitement and semistupor have been seen.

Jaundice is a warning of possible liver damage, or of hemolytic anemia. It tends to disappear if dosage is stopped.

Nausea is rather frequent, especially when the drug is given by mouth; *diarrhea* occurs occasionally; *toxic neuritis* and *deafness* for a short period have been reported.

Indications

Indications for the use of sulfanilamide are in some respects still ill defined, though its chief uses are fairly well established. It was first used against the staphylococcus and brilliant results have been obtained with this organism, but, in general, results have been erratic and disappointing. Possibly its greatest application has been with the streptococci of the Lancefield group A, which includes most of the streptococci ordinarily pathogenic to man. The beta (or hemolytic) organism is especially susceptible; some strains of the anhemolytic variety almost equally so; while *Streptococcus viridans* is resistant. Both meningococcic and gonococcic infections are treated with great success, gonorrheal ophthalmia in particular showing dramatic improvement over previous methods. The usual organisms of urinary tract infection respond well, with the exception of *Streptococcus fecalis.* The pneumococcus is sometimes though not always susceptible, and there is some reason to believe that a combination with type-specific serum may prove superior to either alone. Undulant fever has been treated with apparently good results, and also malaria; and experimentally, at least, it seems effective in choriolymphocytic meningitis.[7]

Clinically it is of no value in typhoid fever, although in mice it does have a definite protective effect; poliomyelitis does not respond,[8] and neither does nonspecific laryngitis, although it is commonly considered a streptococcal infection (incidentally, we have had great difficulty in recovering the streptococcus from our cases).

Contraindications

Contraindications are relative only and may alter the method of treatment rather than preclude it entirely. Gross *kidney damage* is not likely to be aggravated, but blood concentration of sulfanilamide should be watched because of diminished excretion. Marked *anemia* indicates special vigilance in watching for possible hemolysis; and a *low leucocyte count* is similarly significant. In the presence of either of these, other treatment is preferable if available. *Sulfur* in any form taken concurrently predisposes to sulphemoglobinemia. *Jaundice* may sometimes have dangerous significance.

Precautions have already been indicated. They consist above all else in repeated and careful blood examinations. Urine examinations especially for acidity should not be omitted, and we have learned that a smoky appearance of urine often precedes a severe reaction. The possibility of idiosyncrasy to the drug should be borne in mind; and variations in blood concentration with identical doses in different individuals may make blood titration desirable at times.

Dosage

Dosage is tending toward standardization at 15 grains for each 20 pounds of body weight per day, sometimes with the entire first day's amount given at the first dose when the subcutaneous route is employed. It is usually stated that, provided vomiting does not occur, the oral route provides essentially the same speed and completeness of absorption as does the subcutaneous method. We have insufficient data to offer, but we have felt that the subcutaneous route is more uniform and certain and have found no reasons to avoid it. The solution for this purpose is made up with normal saline, and can be made in 1 per cent strength by heating. The sulfanilamide will then stay in solution at ordinary room temperature, if it has been stored in the refrigerator it can be redissolved by heating. We have found no deterioration in solutions stored as long as two months. When necessary, it may be sterilized in the autoclave at about one-half the usual pressure. Antacids have already been discussed.

Several factors indicate that the question of dosage should not be considered as arbitrarily settled in every instance. It is anticipated that the dosage indicated will produce a blood concentration of about 10 mg. per cent within about four hours, with only a slightly lower concentration in the spinal fluid. This concentration is assumed to be optimal for most cases, but we have found that some patients recover rapidly with a considerably lower concentration; in like manner, it seems possible that some failures might be avoided if a higher level were maintained, which apparently can often be done without serious effects. Thus it may be that further study may show that some diseases may be treated with much less intensity than others. Again, the recommended dosage may produce a blood concentration far below that expected of it, in our experience sometimes falling as low as 3 or 4 mg. per cent, presumably because of unusually rapid excretion. In such instances, in the absence of evidence of undue toxicity, the dose may be increased far beyond the usual amount until the desired concentration is finally reached. In one instance of a young adult with epidemic meningitis we finally gave 1,100 c.c. of 1 per cent solution in one day, with immediate sterilization of a hitherto intractable spinal fluid and complete recovery. With present methods of rapid blood titration we may expect light on some of these questions in the near future.

Sulfanilamide is excreted rather rapidly by the kidney through glomerular filtration, and appears in the urine partly unchanged and partly conjugated in the acetylated form. The blood concentration is insignificant twelve hours after it has reached its maximum.

Results

With these generalities in mind, it is desirable to consider individually the more important diseases in which sulfanilamide is indicated, and to attempt to estimate its value. Many factors inherent in the shortness of the period in which it has been used preclude exact conclusions, but when results differ markedly from those hitherto obtainable the underlying trend at least is indisputable. When figures are given, these limitations must be realized until further experience permits greater accuracy.

Erysipelas has been notably amenable to treatment. It may confidently be expected to respond definitely in the first twenty-four hours, and very commonly the skin is almost clear, and the temperature is normal during the second day. Treatment should be continued for several additional days or relapse is liable to occur.

Of our 105 treated cases, 73 were discharged from the hospital within seven days; 30 of the remaining 32 were discharged during the second week; and 2 died. These two deaths deserve special comment, as they illustrate some of the dangers of sulfanilamide.

The first was a man, aged 54 years, admitted with facial erysipelas of three days' duration, and classed as moderately severe. He was given sulfanilamide by mouth, and by the third day the disease had subsided; but on that day jaundice developed, the patient became confused, and hemoglobinuria appeared. His hemoglobin dropped from 88 to 71 per cent the first day, and continued to fall despite daily transfusions of 500 c.c. each until death occurred three days later. The white count was 28,000, with over 90 per cent granulocytes. Fragility tests showed hemolysis beginning at 0.5 and complete at 0.32, the control being 0.44 and 0.36. The blood serum was coffee colored; hemoglobinuria was constant; cyanosis began the second day. The total dosage of sulfanilamide was 255 grains over a period of four days, and the blood concentration the day symptoms began was 3.3 mg. This death is ascribed to acute hemolytic anemia due to sulfanilamide.

The second death was an infant of 22 days, admitted after one day's illness, with erysipelas over the abdomen and a temperature of 105° F. The child was slightly jaundiced, but because of his critical condition sulfanilamide was begun at once, the dose being 35 c.c., 40 c.c., and 20 c.c. of 1 per cent solution daily for the first three days. During this time the rash faded very rapidly, and on the third day the temperature was 98° F. The temperature rose to 102.6° F. on the fifth day without apparent reason other than a mild diarrhea. The hemoglobin was found to be 60 per cent as compared with 87 per cent the day of admission; the white cells numbered 32,650, of which 59 per cent were polymorphonuclears. From 10 to 15 c.c. of sulfanilamide solution had been given daily, but the blood showed only a trace of the drug. A transfusion was given and the sulfanilamide stopped, but it had to be started again on the eighth day because the erysipelas recurred. By the following day the jaundice had markedly increased; the icteric index was 40 units; the van den Bergh, prompt direct. The drug was again stopped and daily transfusions given, but the child died on the eleventh hospital day with acute hemolytic anemia, liver damage, and erysipelas. The total dose of sulfanilamide was 170 c.c.

Scarlet fever should a priori be most favorably influenced by sulfanilamide, but for some reason this logical expectation is not fulfilled. For some time we have given it to attempt a comparison of efficiency with convalescent pooled human serum, both as to the disease itself and also its complications. So far as immediate abatement of signs and symptoms of the disease is concerned, this comparison has given all the advantage to the serum. With the latter, both rash and fever were found to disappear almost miraculously in the first twenty-four to thirty-six hours, whereas under sulfanilamide treatment these persisted for some days and the patients seemed to have a dull malaise possibly even more marked than in the untreated cases. In the treatment of complications, however, sulfanilamide seemed to give quicker and more certain relief than did the serum.

The efficiency of serum in preventing complications has been so gratifying that for some time we made no attempt to evaluate sulfanilamide in this respect. Over the five-year period before we began to use serum, our complication rate had been between 35 per cent and 40 per cent, whereas with serum in 109 cases treated up to last October, there had been only 9 complications. When we began to compile the records of the sulfanilamide-treated patients we found that they too showed a decreased complication rate as compared with the previous figures, and as more cases have been treated we now find, somewhat to our surprise, that the sulfanilamide group shows a slightly better percentage than does the serum group.

Among 194 previously uncomplicated cases receiving serum, 25, or 13.4 per cent, developed complications; while among 113 such cases treated with sulfanilamide there were 13 complications, or 11.5 per cent. It should, of course, be emphasized that these figures are inconclusive, both because of the small number of cases and because of the lack of concurrent control cases; but even so, the disparity between cases treated by either method and those of past years with no specific treatment at all is at least suggestive.

Dosage in these groups was: sulfanilamide, full dose two days, ⅔ dose three days, ⅓ dose five days; serum, 40 to 60 c.c. intravenously on admission.

The complications in each group are listed below:

Complication	*Serum*	*Sulfanilamide*
Cervical adenitis	11	8
Peritonsillar abscess	1	1
Otitis media	4	2
Recurrent scarlet	0	2
Paronychia	4	0
Pyrexia undetermined	2	0
Nephritis	2	0
Chalazion	1	0
Cellulitis	1	0

Gonorrhea in its common forms of urethritis and vaginitis has been treated extensively with sulfanilamide. First reports were more enthusiastic than later ones, due to the discovery that some patients apparently cured showed relapses. There is rather frequently some difficulty in establishing criteria of cure, in that organisms may be found under the microscope which will not grow on culture. The acute case in the male may be expected to show about 75 per cent success within two weeks; if cure is not established within this time, other methods are likely to be needed. Female patients seem to respond less well, although many reports testify to the definite value of the drug; and evaluation is made more difficult by greater uncertainty in demonstrating cure. Chronic cases in both sexes show much poorer results.

A blood concentration of at least 10 mg. per cent must be maintained in these patients for good results, and medication should continue for two weeks after smear and culture are negative. Antacids are rarely necessary. Malaise under treatment may be so worked as to make the patient refuse to continue unless he can go to bed.

Gonorrheal ophthalmia responds to sulfanilamide phenomenally well, and, since to my knowledge no series so extensive as our own has been reported, it seems worth while to recount our experience in some detail.

Before the advent of sulfanilamide, using almost constant eye irrigations plus many combinations of local disinfectants of the silver group plus occasional nonspecific or ''shock'' therapy plus attempts at specific therapy in the form of gonococcus antigen and the like, it took us an average of almost three weeks to obtain our first negative eye smear and culture, and almost a month to discharge the patient. In addition, especially among adult patients, there was a most distressing toll of lost or impaired vision. Since beginning to use sulfanilamide, we have treated 21 cases with 18 cures and 3 failures; the first negative eye smear and culture has usually been obtained in less than forty-eight hours; and no eye has suffered any impairment if it was undamaged when treatment was begun.

Treatment at first consisted of the previous routine plus sulfanilamide in regular doses. Later local drug treatment was less rigorously performed, and in the last few cases has been omitted entirely without loss of efficiency; whether it can be permanently discarded is not yet certain. Irrigations were carried out with great care in every case as long as discharge appeared, regardless of whether the smear and culture had become negative, and often enough to keep the eye clean even though this might require almost constant irrigation. This seems an indispensable part of the program, as the pressure of exudate when allowed to accumulate tends to cause corneal ulceration even when infection is subsiding. If ulceration was already present, treatment was given with 1 per cent of silver nitrate in the usual way.

The patients successfully treated included 10 adults, 2 children aged 5 and 9 years, and 6 infants under 30 days of age. The failures were all in infants, two of them premature; these deserve special comment as they illustrate points in treatment which I believe are important.

The first was a 4 pound premature infant admitted the eleventh day of the disease. Under treatment, smear and culture became negative within thirty-six hours, and the baby was sent home after smear and culture had remained negative for five consecutive days. Five days therafter it was readmitted, and this time the organisms disappeared with two and one-half days of treatment. This patient may have relapsed because treatment was stopped too soon, or it may have been reinfected by its mother who was known to have gonorrhea.

The second case was also a premature infant weighing 4 pounds 2 ounces admitted after one day of illness. This child had negative eye smears and cultures after twenty-four hours and for the five succeeding days, when the drug was stopped because of vomiting. The same day there was a relapse in one eye and although sulfanilamide was resumed at once it appeared to have no effect whatever. The baby finally recovered, but only after seventy-seven days in the hospital under all the treatment of the old methods plus repeated attempts to get results with sulfanilamide. This case illustrates the possibility that organisms may become resistant to this drug if they are not promptly and completely eliminated by it and suggests that possibly treatment should not be stopped until at least a week after the organisms disappear.

The third case, a 6 pound 4 ounce baby admitted after seven days of illness, illustrates somewhat the same points. This child showed an immediate and marked decrease in discharge from the eyes, and the dose of sulfanilamide was decreased despite the fact that smears were still positive. The eyes became worse immediately. Dosage was increased at once, but cure was very slow; the child was in the hospital forty-seven days. Obviously treatment had been inadequate.

These cases are too few for statistical significance, but no one seeing them could question the dramatic effect of treatment, and as the discussion of the failures shows, one might possibly get even better results as the series progresses.

Meningitis is one of the more serious conditions in which sulfanilamide has been used with particularly good effect. Our own experience with the meningococcic variety has been limited to 20 cases treated with sulfanilamide alone, in addition to which there have been 25 others treated with this drug plus one or more other methods. These do not lend themselves well to a comparative analysis to determine the relative worth of the various mediums used, inasmuch as the number of patients is small and those who received more than one type of treatment may well have had more severe infections. However, out of 109 patients receiving sulfanilamide, antiserum, antitoxin, or combinations of these agents, the group treated with sulfanilamide alone showed a mortality of 10 per cent, which is much lower than that of any other method or combination of methods. A great deal more work will be needed to establish exactly the relative merit of these various preparations, as both therapeutic efficiency and therapeutic hazard must be determined; and it seems unlikely that any one of them will be able to supplant the others entirely. At present it would seem wiser to consider sulfanilamide as simply an extremely valuable aid in this serious disease and to attempt no accurate comparative evaluation.

We have had one patient with pneumococcus Type 32 meningitis, who recovered following drainage of a sinus plus sulfanilamide therapy. Several cases due to the streptococcus appear in the literature; we have had two, with one recovery. The drug has been ineffective against the influenza bacillus.

Pyelitis and allied urinary tract infections, when due to any of the common organisms except *Streptococcus fecalis,* have been shown to respond to sulfanilamide at least as well as to any of the other methods commonly used. As the drug is excreted through the glomerulus and partially reabsorbed through the tubule, it should be able to attack kidney infections from both the blood and urinary streams. Its effect is usually greater in alkaline urine and has been shown experimentally to be greater when urine is added to the ordinary culture media. Helmholz[9] in particular has studied this type of infection.

Undulant fever, which so far has resisted all efforts toward specific therapy, may prove at least to some extent to be amenable to treatment with sulfanilamide. We have had four cases in which the temperature has become normal within a week and has remained so, and I have learned of three similar cases within the past few months. This disease is so uncommon that final evidence may be slow in coming, but it would seem that an attempt at treatment with this drug is justified.

Minor conditions in which sulfanilamide may be indicated include simple *cervical adenitis,* in which it is strikingly effective in most instances; *otitis media,* which usually responds unless due to a resistant organism but which must be treated as long as there is any discharge if relapse is to be prevented; *mastoid infections,* in which it would appear that surgery is sometimes avoided; *streptococcal infections* of the *throat;* and countless others. At present it is considered wise not to treat mild infections which may be expected to resolve satisfactorily under other treatments because of the slight but definite hazard of the drug itself; and in no event should intensive therapy be attempted unless the patient can be properly watched and necessary laboratory data obtained.

This summary of a remarkable new drug is admittedly incomplete; even our total knowledge of it is incomplete. Enough is known, however, to establish its undoubted potency and wide application. There is reason to believe that it may usher in a series of advances in chemotherapy as the possibilities of other related compounds are discovered.

REFERENCES

1. Holman, W. L., and Duff, G. L.: Am. J. M. Sc. **195**: 379, 1938.
2. Long, P. H., and Bliss, E. A.: J. A. M. A. **109**: 1524, 1937.
3. Osgood, E. A.: J. A. M. A. **110**: 349, 1938.
4. Marshall, E. K., Jr., and Walzl, E. M.: Bull. Johns Hopkins Hosp. **61**: 140, 1937.
5. Hartmann, A. F.: (to be published in Calif. & W. Med.)
6. Keefer, C. S.: Am. J. M. Sc. **195**: 701, 1938.
7. Rosenthal, S. M., Wooley, J. G., and Bauer, H.: Pub. Health Rep. **52**: 1211, 1937.
8. Kelson, S. R.: Proc. Soc. Exper. Biol. & Med. **36**: 718, 1937.
9. Helmholz, H. F.: J. Pediat. **11**: 243, 1937; J. A. M. A. **109**: 1039, 1937.

DR. E. S. PLATOU (Minneapolis, Minn.).—We have attempted to compare a series of one hundred scarlet fever patients treated with sulfanilamide during 1937-1938 with an equal number of controls who did not receive the drug. The two series, although not comprised of alternate cases, ran concurrently and were comparable with respect to age, severity, and duration of disease prior to treatment. Although the criteria for evaluating our results may be subject to criticism, some observations have been made which we believe are significant and seem to suggest that sulfanilamide is of value in the treatment of scarlet fever.

The drug was administered orally except to patients with nausea or extreme toxemia. The latter were given an initial large dose subcutaneously in the form of 1 per cent solution in normal saline. The dosage used was that recommended by Long and Bliss for severe infections; an initial massive dose of 0.05 gram per pound of body weight and a maintenance dose of 0.03 gm. per pound per twenty-four hours. It is our impression that per unit of weight, children tolerate the drug better than adults. With the exception of the development of leucopenia in two cases, a fever and rash in two additional cases, in which we were compelled to discontinue therapy, no serious complications were encountered with the drug. Cyanosis without sulphemoglobinemia was observed in several instances but therapy was continued without any ill effects. The dosage was gradually decreased but was continued on an average of twelve days. Too early discontinuance of the drug was believed to be the cause of the appearance of mild complications in a few of our cases. The best results were obtained when sulfanilamide was continued during the entire convalescent period. The fever curve in the treated cases, once it became normal, remained so in practically all cases without complications, whereas the untreated cases showed irregular rises in temperature, often without demonstrable explanation for this rise.

In our treated cases the rate of recovery from the acute toxemic phase of the disease (6 days) was no more rapid than it was in the control cases (6 days). The sulfanilamide-treated cases did not show the prompt subsidence of toxic symptoms such as we have observed following the administration of serum. The incidence of complications was 41 per cent in the controls as compared to 8 per cent in the treated cases. There were nine suppurative conditions in the control cases as compared to one in the treated series. In a few septic cases recently treated by massive intravenous doses of serum combined with sulfanilamide, the results have been so striking as to suggest a synergistic effect.

DISCUSSION

CHAIRMAN HAMILTON.—Dr. Platou's figures are most impressive. It would be of interest to see what can be done with both treatments.

DR. PLATOU.—We had six cases by the combined treatment. The results were dramatic and the complications nil.

DR. S. H. NICHOLS (ASBURY PARK, N. J.).—What are your results in the treatment of throat conditions, for example, acute tonsillitis?

CHAIRMAN HAMILTON.—We have had some good results and some poor results. I have no controlled group to report and would use it only if the patient were very sick.

DR. NICHOLS.—I have used it in 25 cases with very poor results. In a few cases it seemed to help.

DR. R. P. SEITZ (SAN FRANCISCO).—Have you used sulfanilamide in pneumonia?

CHAIRMAN HAMILTON.—In pneumonia our results are discouraging. We have had better results with serum and are now attempting serum and sulfanilamide for additive effects. We have not used serum very often in children.

DR. FAIRFAX HALL (NEW ROCHELLE, N. Y.).—Sulfanilamide in rheumatic fever shows bad results.

CHAIRMAN HAMILTON.—It is useless.

DR. V. E. TAPPAN (TUCSON, ARIZ.).—Reports from the Rockefeller Institute show fair results.

DR. G. L. KAUFMAN (CHICAGO).—What results were obtained in combined treatment in meningococcic meningitis?

DR. PLATOU.—We used it concurrently in 22 cases with no deaths.

DR. G. J. LEVY (MEMPHIS, TENN.).—Can sulfanilamide be used intraspinally?

CHAIRMAN HAMILTON.—It can be done, and there are no contraindications. The spinal fluid concentration is only slightly less than the blood concentration when sulfanilamide is given by mouth. The only advantage of giving the drug intraspinally is the speed of administration, in that when given, it is there at once. Spinal punctures in meningitis are only for relief of pressure, cell counts, and criteria of prognosis.

DR. SEITZ.—What results have you had in influenzal meningitis? I know one patient it apparently cured.

CHAIRMAN HAMILTON.—We have had two patients die, and sulfanilamide failed to affect them in any way.

DR. R. G. SHARP (SAN DIEGO, CALIF.).—We had one patient in the San Diego Hospital who seemed to have been cured by sulfanilamide.

DR. E. J. LAMB (SANTA BARBARA, CALIF.).—We have treated four cases of spider bites (black widow?) with sulfanilamide. A one-month-old infant died after twenty-four hours and one four-year-old child died within twenty-six hours after being bitten. The patients who recovered showed immediate results.

DR. TAPPAN.—Sulfanilamide gives results in chronic brucella infections.

CHAIRMAN HAMILTON.—How definitely chronic?

DR. TAPPAN.—In four cases of unexplained fever of three to four months' duration.

DR. HALL.—In mastoid infections sulfanilamide may bring fever to normal, but there are still some streptococci present in the mastoid cells, and the treatment should be continued over a long period of time.

DR. TAPPAN.—It is very important to continue treatment even after improvement as some bacteria are left which are still active.

DR. HALL.—Is six weeks too long to continue treatment?

CHAIRMAN HAMILTON.—Not necessarily. Two weeks are necessary in gonorrhea cases beyond the time of a negative smear.

DR. TAPPAN.—The results in tuberculosis have been undesirable.

CHAIRMAN HAMILTON.—The results in laboratory animals are poor.

DR. TAPPAN.—It has rendered animals less susceptible.

DR. E. C. MITCHELL (MEMPHIS, TENN.).—Sulfanilamide is of no benefit in malaria. We have treated 75 cases of pyelitis in the last two years. Sulfanilamide will clear up streptococcal infections, usually clears colon infections, but in staphylococcal infections the results are not as good. In gonorrheal vaginitis it will clear up the discharge, but it often returns.

DR. S. C. HENN (CHICAGO).—This seems to be a common occurrence. We often find the bacteria under the microscope but the bacteria will not grow. We always try to check the patient by culture as well as smear.

DR. G. W. KUTSCHER, JR. (ASHEVILLE, N. C.).—The pneumococcus acts the same as the gonococcus on culture.

DR. H. F. DIETRICH (LOS ANGELES, CALIF.).—I would like to report two cases.

CASE 1.—A child whose appendix had ruptured six days before was treated by surgical drainage; large doses of sulfanilamide were started and thirty hours after admission there was noted a dramatic improvement.

CASE 2.—A seven-year-old girl was ill for four or five days with general peritonitis; culture of the abdominal fluid revealed pneumococcus and beta streptococcus. Large doses of sulfanilamide were started and within twenty-four hours the patient had a critical drop in her fever. She went home in two weeks.

QUESTION.—Can sulfanilamide be used to begin the treatment of pyelitis?

CHAIRMAN HAMILTON.—Sulfanilamide is rapidly superseding previous medications in pyelitis. Pediatricians rarely isolate the organism in private practice.

DR. DIETRICH.—The routine use of sulfanilamide in pyelitis should be discouraged; 80-90 per cent of the infections are self-limited, and we are inviting undue risk by using sulfanilamide routinely. If we segregate those with chronic or obstructive cases, sulfanilamide is indicated.

DR. NICHOLS.—When is pyelitis self-limited? What are the criteria?

DR. DIETRICH.—The great majority of cases become sterilized in eight days; the rest in five to six weeks. If it persists four weeks, then the infection is certainly refractile and suggests the use of sulfanilamide.

DR. HENN.—Twelve years ago one of my patients (a boy) had 600 white blood cells per cubic centimeter. He was operated on for diverticulum of the bladder, and he continued to have pus in the urine. After ten years one kidney was removed, and he still had pus. He was treated with all the antiseptics with no result. Eight months ago he was given sulfanilamide in ''tonic'' doses (5 gr. every 4 hours), and the urine was clear in one week. The pus recurred in ten days and sulfanilamide therapy was repeated for ten days. Since then the urine has been absolutely clear.

DR. SEITZ.—What about ''tonic'' doses?

CHAIRMAN HAMILTON.—I see no reason for ''tonic'' doses. If using sulfanilamide one should give enough to get a concentration of 10 mg. per cent.

DR. MITCHELL.—I believe the use of alkalies hinders the effectiveness of sulfanilamide and have observed no benefit from them. For malaise, cyanosis, and other distressing symptoms, I inject 10 per cent methylene blue solution (dosage 10 c.c. per 150 pounds of weight) intravenously, and it also clears up the patient's subjective symptoms.

CHAIRMAN HAMILTON.—We use methylene blue occasionally.

DR. S. G. HENRICKE (PORTLAND, ORE).—I find that in hemolytic streptococcal infections one-tenth the dosage is equally effective. In pneumococcus Type 3, full dosage, with the serum, gives good results.

DR. HALL.—Does toxicosis depend upon dosage?

CHAIRMAN HAMILTON.—Not always. It may be an idiosyncrasy. There are many reports of sulfanilamide causing anaphylactoid reactions.

DR. HALL.—Small doses may cause an hemolytic anemia with rash in twenty-four hours.

CHAIRMAN HAMILTON.—If a rash appears, one should stop treatment.

DR. MITCHELL.—At the university we give 3 grains per kilogram of body weight per twenty-four hours and find sometimes this is entirely inadequate.

CHAIRMAN HAMILTON.—Do you divide your doses?

DR. MITCHELL.—Yes, we divide the twenty-four-hour dose into six parts and give it every four hours.

DR. HENRICKE.—When is the ideal time to take pooled scarlet fever serum?

CHAIRMAN HAMILTON.—Twenty-one days up to three or four months.

DR. W. W. QUILLIAN (CORAL GABLES, FLA.).—I have seen two patients treated with sulfanilamide who developed unusual blood pictures; i.e., a marked leucocytosis (34,000 white blood cells) instead of leucopenia. There were many abnormal types including 28 per cent eosinophiles. Later the blood picture gradually returned to normal. The patients' color became cyanotic though the blood concentration was only 9 mg. per cent.

DR. LEVY.—We try to maintain a concentration of 20 mg. per cent unless unusual toxic symptoms appear; we also control our patients with daily blood counts. We give an initial dose of 150 grains and rarely use subcutaneous administration because we think the oral administration ideal. In newborn infants we use the nasal tube. We have had one failure in gonorrheal conjunctivitis. This was a 29-year-old negro who had an initial 150 grain dose then 30 gr. every four hours. He received 450 grains before a toxic condition of jaundice and anemia occurred. We gave him glucose intravenously and a blood transfusion of 600 c.c. The anemia and jaundice progressed, and he developed anuria in eight hours. There was no autopsy, but our diagnosis was acute hemolytic anemia from sulfanilamide.

CHAIRMAN HAMILTON.—The only psychic symptoms we have noticed are dullness and confusion.

DR. PLATOU.—We have treated 16 cases of serious nephritis and had the impression that sulfanilamide did some good. The local treatment of sulfanilamide injected into a body cavity (as the pleural cavity) had no results. In my experience with the pneumococcus Type 3 it was not effective. I believe the greatest need is a test for predetermination of allergy or idiosyncrasy.

CHAIRMAN HAMILTON.—The local use of this drug has not been shown to be effective. An ointment has been used locally but not much is known about it.

DR. TAPPAN.—In what type of nephritis and in what stage was sulfanilamide used?

DR. PLATOU.—Acute glomerular nephritis, and its use is purely experimental.

DR. TAPPAN.—Aspirin given at the same time with sulfanilamide will cause toxicity.

DR. M. SWIGART (MONTEREY, CALIF.).—How much is secreted in the breast milk?

CHAIRMAN HAMILTON.—I have no definite report, but I believe the same concentration is present as in the blood and that it may have a toxic effect on the baby.

DR. HALL.—How about magnesium sulfate?

CHAIRMAN HAMILTON.—I have had no personal experience, but it should not be used.

DR. TAPPAN.—We have seen patients whose skin is very sensitive to the sun after treatment with sulfanilamide.

DR. M. M. NICHOLSON (WASHINGTON, D. C.).—Does the vitamin and mineral content of the child as he becomes ill influence the prognosis when using sulfanilamide?

CHAIRMAN HAMILTON.—I do not know of any data on this subject.

QUESTION.—If amidopyrine is a cause of agranulocytosis, how does sulfanilamide compare?

CHAIRMAN HAMILTON.—To answer this one should have a comparison of the frequency of use of amidopyrine and sulfanilamide, and one cannot do this because amidopyrine is bought so frequently over the drug counter. There are three types of infections being treated with sulfanilamide:

1. Those which sulfanilamide will cure.
2. The in-between infections, i.e., questionable cures.
3. Those infections which the drug will not affect.

We are still groping for infections sulfanilamide will cure.

DR. R. N. ANDREWS (MANKATO, MINN.).—In medicine the pendulum swings one way or the other too far. Several years ago I reported the use of urea in the treatment of pneumonia with good results. Now the subject has been practically dropped. There is no question that sulfanilamide has proved its usefulness. However, when patients die of the effects of sulfanilamide therapy, it should not be used indiscriminately. Why use it in tonsillitis when the infection is self-limited?

CHAIRMAN HAMILTON.—That attitude cannot be stressed too much.

A. L. GLEASON, M.D.
Oakland, Calif.
Secretary.

Academy News

Region I of the Academy will meet on Nov. 11 and 12, 1938, at Rochester, N. Y. Details of the meeting have not yet been announced. Dr. Paul W. Beaven, state chairman for New York, is in charge of the committee on arrangements. Dr. Stanley H. Nichols has been chosen chairman of Region I to succeed Dr. Schroeder, who died.

Region II of the Academy will meet on Wednesday, Nov. 16, 1938, at the Skirvin Hotel, Oklahoma City, Okla. This meeting will be held at the time of the Southern Medical Association. There will be a scientific session on Wednesday morning followed by round table discussions in the afternoon by invited guests. The business meeting of this region will be held at 4:30 P.M. At 7:00 P.M. there will be a joint banquet of the section on pediatrics of the Southern Medical Association and members, and the Academy members who wish to attend the meeting should write to Dr. Ben H. Nicholson, 301 West Twelfth Street, Oklahoma City, for reservations at the Skirvin Hotel, which is headquarters for the Academy.

Final announcements have been made of arrangements for the meeting of Region III at Detroit, Michigan on Thursday, Friday, and Saturday, Oct. 27, 28, 29, 1938. Headquarters will be at Hotel Statler.

The November issue of the JOURNAL will be a memorial to the late Williams McKim Marriott, who died Nov. 12, 1936. It will consist of contributions from his associates at Johns Hopkins, where he started his pediatric training with Howland, and from those who were associated with him at Washington University. The list of contributors is as follows: Blackfan, Clausen, Cooke, Darrow, Elliott, Hartmann, Hempelmann, Jeans, McCulloch, Park, Powers, Smyth, Tallerman, Utheim-Toverud and Veeder. Any one desiring an extra copy of the issue should notify the publisher, The C. V. Mosby Company, 3525 Pine St., St. Louis, at once, so that they may be provided for at the time of printing.

Dr. Ruth M. Mahon, of Grand Forks, N. D., died August 31 at Livingston, Mont., of encephalitis contracted while touring Yellowstone Park.

M. G. Peterman, M.D. has announced his resignation from the faculty of the Marquette University School of Medicine, effective September 1, 1938.

Dr. Arch B. Chappell, of Middletown, N. Y., died August 28.

Erratum

In the account of the Eighth Annual Meeting of the American Academy of Pediatrics, which appeared in the August issue of the JOURNAL, page 263, line 31, the following quotation:

> "DR. ANDREW J. THORNTON (SAN DIEGO, CALIF.).—All the school children in San Diego have an examination every year, including a Wassermann test for $1.50."

is incorrect and should be changed to read:

> "DR. ANDREW J. THORNTON (SAN DIEGO, CALIF.).—All *food handlers* in San Diego have an examination every year, including a Wassermann test, for $1.50. A similar program for examining nursemaids and others in close contact with children might be arranged as a public health measure."

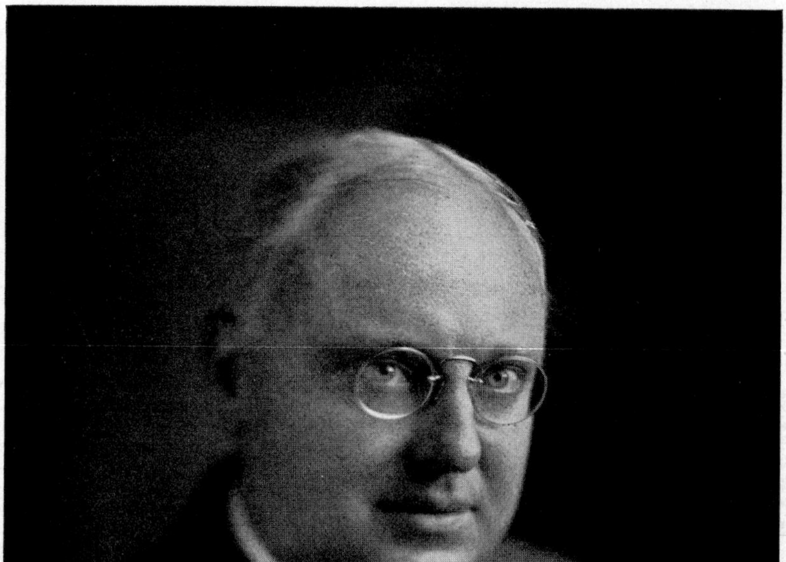

Williams McKim Marriott
1885-1936

WILLIAMS McKIM MARRIOTT was one of the most distinguished of the group responsible for the remarkable scientific advancement of American pediatrics in the quarter century 1910 to 1935. While it is true in general that time alone, with the historical perspective, fixes the exact place of an individual in the story of any advance or movement, nevertheless Marriott's contribution was of such decided influence upon, and of such importance to, his contemporaries, that as a mark of their appreciation and respect this number of THE JOURNAL OF PEDIATRICS is dedicated to his memory. Only pediatricians, and furthermore only those closely associated with him in Baltimore and St. Louis have been invited to contribute; for if all of his friends and associates in pediatrics and other fields were included, it would be necessary to devote many issues to their contributions. Dr. Blackfan, Dr. Park, and Dr. Powers represent Marriott's Baltimore years at Johns Hopkins; Dr. Tallerman and Dr. Utheim-Toverud, those who came from foreign countries to study under him; and the remainder, his associates during the years at Washington University in St. Louis. Dr. Eliot represents the large group who served as resident physicians on his service in the St. Louis Children's Hospital.

In its relationship to pediatrics it is convenient to look upon Marriott's life and work as divided into three periods. First, his background and early training and interests which led up to, and were in large part responsible for, the brilliant second phase of active pediatric work. The third period comes when his interests centered increasingly on administrative work, and pediatric interests diminished until he reached the decision he had had in mind for several years to leave this field, a change that was made only shortly before his early and untimely death. A study of his bibliography which is appended clearly reflects these three periods.

Marriott was graduated from the University of North Carolina with the B.S. degree in 1904, when he was only 19 years old. He had majored in chemistry and during the last year of his college course was an assistant in the chemical laboratory. In the fall of 1904 he became an assistant under Wolf in the Department of Biochemistry at Cornell Medical School in New York City, where he remained for six years, teaching and at the same time studying medicine, graduating with the M.D. degree in 1910. In the fall of that year he went to St. Louis with Shaffer as an assistant in the Department of Biochemistry of the newly reorganized School of Medicine of Washington University, where he remained for four years. He had no clinical medical training or hospital experience beyond that of the undergraduate course. Correspondingly one finds his publications during these years devoted to chemical research. It was a preparation with which few men have entered the field of clinical medicine, and naturally gave direction to the line of research and investigation which he later carried out.

It was in 1913 that I first heard him express the desire to take up problems more directly connected with clinical medicine. He had no particular interest in pediatrics and his entering the field was a matter of chance. He tried to obtain a position in a department of internal medicine, but, fortunately for pediatrics, was told they had no place for a "chemist." In 1913 an opportunity came to enter a department of pediatrics. Through unforeseen circumstances this fell through, and Howland, who was looking for a chemist in the pediatric department he was organizing in Baltimore, learning of the situation, offered him a place. As no opportunity to enter a department of internal medicine developed, he accepted and became a part of the pediatric department of Johns Hopkins in 1914. Marriott was never particularly interested in children as a problem or study, but rather in the study of disease. Once shortly before he left St. Louis, when discussing his future in San Francisco as dean and professor of research medicine, he remarked it would give him the opportunity to study some problems of adult medicine which he had in mind for many years.

He entered his pediatric years with an extraordinarily unusual technical training in chemistry, a keen, alert, analytical mind, and a scientific approach to the problems he was to undertake which foreshadowed the position he was later to hold. Furthermore he was entering at the opportune time on the special phase of pediatrics which he was to develop. Scientific progress in large part depends upon the development of methods of study, and it was just at this moment that methods of chemical research were being worked out, which to a large extent revolutionized our knowledge of metabolic processes and conditions. In this he played a prominent part. The remark of Pasteur that "chance favors the prepared mind," is eloquently exemplified in Marriott's career.

The association of Marriott and Howland from 1914 to 1917 was most fortunate and happy for both men and for pediatrics. Howland had an excellent clinical knowledge of pediatrics with an intense desire for scientific investigation, but with little technical training or knowledge of methods, while Marriott had no clinical knowledge or experience but splendid technical training. The results of their collaboration during these three years on the subjects of acidosis in alimentary intoxication and calcium metabolism in infancy are in some respects the finest work each produced. It can be said without exaggeration that with this work American pediatrics began to have a world-wide influence. Howland wished to keep Marriott in the laboratory and away from clinical medicine. Marriott, however, had different ideas and insisted after the first year upon spending part of his time in clinical work. According to his associates, with his brilliant mind he developed clinical experience with an uncanny ease.

In 1917 he was invited to become head of the Department of Pediatrics at Washington University which had recently been put on a full-time basis. Despite his limited clinical training and the advice of his friends, he accepted. As it turned out, he was right in his judgment.

His clinical training with Howland and his associates had given him the best in American pediatrics at that time. His short clinical training in a way was a decided advantage, as he was uninhibited by the traditional methods of infant feeding which were taught in American schools, and with which the average young man entering pediatrics at that time had been imbued by the authority of his elders. Nor had he come under the influence of the German school whose ideas were being handed out to the many pediatric neophytes studying abroad, for previous to Howland's clinic there was no place where training in this field could be obtained in America. He thus had little to unlearn and entered pediatrics with a free untrammeled approach to the subject. Nevertheless, it required courage to attempt what Marriott did, and only an unusually brilliant and sound mind could have made a success of his new responsibilities.

It is necessary only to go over his bibliography from 1919 to 1926 to note the spread of Marriott's interest and studies during his early years in St. Louis. During this time he did important work in the further study of diarrheal conditions and parenteral infections affecting metabolism, and he turned the weight of his rapidly growing influence toward simplified methods of infant feeding which were coming into use. But to realize fully the significance of his contribution, it is necessary to take into consideration the work of his associates, as Jeans, Hartmann, and Clausen, whose work was carried on with the stimulation of his interest and counsel.

In 1923 an event took place on which many of us look back as somewhat of a tragedy. He became dean of Washington University School of Medicine. This was the beginning of a steadily progressive decreasing interest in his scientific work and pediatrics, and a steadily increasing interest and engrossment in administrative details and problems. A glance at his bibliography shows this change. It is only fair to say that Marriott liked the administrative work, but at the same time was unwilling to give up his clinical work. For years he tried to carry the full-sized load of two men on his shoulders. He worked day and night. The tragedy lies not only in the effect it had on his health, but in that, while many men had as good or even better administrative ability, one does not need the fingers of a hand to count the men with his brilliant scientific mind and ability. His scientific output became trivial when compared with his earlier work. It was due only to the loyal support of his two associates, Hartmann and Cooke, that he was able to carry on his hospital and departmental work during his last few years in St. Louis. It is significant of the situation that in these later years there was no such development of younger men under him as had taken place earlier. This is not a criticism of Marriott—he liked the administrative work—but simply an explanation of the change which took place in his work and productivity which is obvious to any one who studies his career. He was conscious of it himself. Once when we were returning from a pediatric society meeting in the early thirties, he replied to a remark that he had not said a word at the meeting, that he felt "out of the pediatric picture."

In 1933 he had a serious illness which left its traces. In 1935 a streptococcus infection developed which in part led him to the decision to resign at St. Louis and accept the position of dean and professor of research medicine at the University of California Medical School. He felt this would allow him to take things easier, to carry on his educational interests, while the freedom from teaching and hospital responsibility would give him the opportunity to return to the laboratory. Those of us who knew him best feel that had he lived, his years at San Francisco would have been most fruitful.

This in brief, so far as pediatrics is concerned, is the story of the meteoric career of one of the most brilliant minds that has flashed across the field of pediatrics in America. His influence through his scientific work and writings, through the hundreds of students and practitioners who sat under his clear and forceful teaching, and particularly through the development of his associates who now hold places in many medical schools will last for many years.

It is not the place in a limited biographical note of this kind to discuss McKim Marriott as an individual, the concentration of his interest in his work, his simplicity of life, his interest in medical education, and his work as dean of the School of Medicine. In pediatrics he had the respect and loyalty of the men with whom he was associated, and this in itself speaks sufficiently for his character.

—*Borden Veeder.*

Bibliography

1904

(With R. Stevenson) An apparatus for the Continuous Preparation of Large Quantities of Gases for Laboratory Use, J. Am. Chem. Soc. **26**: 64, 1904.

1905

(With A. S. Wheeler) Strontium Malate, J. Am. Chem. Soc. **27**: 295, 1905.

(With C. G. L. Wolf) Contributions to the Study of Sulfur: 1. The Metabolism in Brombenzol Poisoning, Am. Med. **9**: 1026, 1905.

1906

(With C. G. L. Wolf) Cystinuria, Am. J. M. Sc. **131**: 197, 1906.

(With C. G. L. Wolf) The Composition of Cystin Calculi, Montreal M. J. **35**: 186, 1906.

The Determination of Ammonia and Urea in Blood (Abstr.), Proc. Soc. Exper. Biol. & Med. **4**: 89, 1906-07.

(With C. G. L. Wolf) The Determination of Small Quantities of Iron, J. Biol. Chem. **1**: 451, 1906.

1907

(With C. G. L. Wolf) The Colloidal Nitrogen in the Urine, Am. J. M. Sc. **133**: 404, 1907.

(With C. G. L. Wolf) Eiweiss Stoffwechsel bei Brombenzolvergiftung, Biochem. Ztschr. **7**: 213, 1907.

The Air They Breathe in New York Factories, Charities and the Commons, Vol. 17, No. 6.

1910

Bestimmung von Ammoniak und Harnstoff im Blut, Biochem. Ztschr. **26**: 165, 1910.

1913

The Determination of Acetone Bodies in Blood and Tissues by Micro Methods (Abstr.), Proc. Soc. Biol. Chem. **14**: 27, 1912-1913.

(With P. A. Shaffer) The Determination of Oxybutyric Acid, J. Biol. Chem. **16**: 265, 1913-1914.

The Determination of Acetone, J. Biol. Chem. **16**: 281, 1913-1914.

Nephelometric Determination of Minute Quantities of Acetone, J. Biol. Chem. **16**: 289, 1913-14.

The Determination of Oxybutyric Acid in Blood and Tissues, J. Biol. Chem. **16**: 293, 1913-14.

1914

The Metabolic Relationships of the Acetone Substances, J. Biol. Chem. **18**: 241, 1914.

The Blood in Acidosis From the Quantitative Point of View, J. A. M. A. **63**: 397, 1914. Also J. Biol. Chem. **18**: 507, 1914.

(With J. Howland) Observation Upon the So-Called Food Intoxication of Infants, With Especial Reference to the Alveolar Air, Proc. Soc. Exper. Biol. & Med. **12**: 51, 1914.

1915

(With J. Howland) The Indications for Treatment in Severe Diarrhea in Infancy, Arch. Pediat. **32**: 374, 1915. Also: Am. J. Obst. **72**: 544, 1915. Also: Pediatrics **27**: 592, 1915.

(With R. L. Levy and L. G. Rowntree) A Simple Method for Determining Variations in the Hydrogen-Ion Concentration of the Blood, Arch. Int. Med. **16**: 389, 1915. Also Tr. A. Am. Physicians **30**: 102, 1915.

A Study of the Acidosis Occurring in the Nutritional Diseases of Infancy, Tr. A. Am. Physicians **30**: 330, 1915.

1916

The Therapeutic Value of the Hypophosphites, J. A. M. A. **66**: 486, 1916.

A Simplified Procedure for the Determination of the Carbon Dioxide Tension in the Alveolar Air, Proc. Am. Soc. Biol. Chemists, 1916, p. 18. Also J. A. M. A. **66**: 1594, 1916.

A Method for the Determination of the Alkali Reserve of the Blood Plasma, Arch. Int. Med. **17**: 840, 1916.

(With J. Howland) Phosphate Retention as a Factor in the Production of Acidosis in Nephritis, Arch. Int. Med. **18**: 708, 1916.

(With J. Howland) A Discussion of Acidosis, With Special Reference to that Occurrence in the Diseases of Childhood, Med. Rec. **89**: 125, 1916. Also Johns Hopkins Bull. **27**: 63, 1916. Also Am. J. Obst. **72**: 556, 1916.

(With J. Howland) Use of a New Reagent for Microcolorimetric Analysis, as Applied to the Determination of Calcium and of Inorganic Phosphates in the Blood Serum, Proc. Am. Soc. Biol. Chemists, p. 18, 1916.

(With J. Howland) Acidosis Occurring With Diarrhea, Am. J. Dis. Child. **11**: 309, 1916.

(With J. Howland) The Calcium Content of Blood in Rachitis and Tetany, Am. J. Obst. **74**: 541, 1916. Also Tr. Am. Pediat. Soc. **28**: 202, 1916.

(With J. Howland) Acetone Body Production in Infancy and Childhood, Am. J. Dis. Child. **12**: 459, 1916.

(With J. Howland) Observations on Acid-Base Equilibrium in the Body, Am. J. Physiol. **42**: 587, 1916-17. Also Proc. Am. Soc. Biol. Chemists **5**: 11, 1916.

1917

(With H. L. Higgins) A Colorimetric Method for the Determination of the CO_2 Percentage in Air, J. Am. Chem. Soc. **39**: 68, 1917.

Case of Haematemesis and Melaena Neonatorum With Recovery, Brit. M. J. **2**: 516, 1917.

(With F. H. Haessler) A Micro Method for the Determination of Inorganic Phosphates in the Blood Serum, J. Biol. Chem. **32**: 241, 1917.

(With J. Howland) A Micro Method for the Determination of Calcium and Magnesium in Blood Serum, J. Biol. Chem. **32**: 233, 1917.

(With J. Howland) Observations Upon Calcium in Rickets and Tetany. Tr. A. Am. Physicians **32**: 307, 1917.

1918

(With W. R. Sisson) Variations in the Lipoid (Fat) Content of the Blood of Infants Under Certain Nutritional Conditions, Am. J. Dis. Child. **16**: 75, 1918.

(With W. R. Sisson) Variations in the Lipoid (Fat) Content of the Blood, New York Med. J. **108**: 531, 1918.

(With J. Howland) The Influence of Acid Phosphate on Elimination of Ammonia in the Urine, Arch. Int. Med. **22**: 477, 1918. Also Bull. Johns Hopkins Hosp. **29**: 264, 1918.

(With J. Howland) Acidosis, Pennsylvania M. J. **21**: 429, 1917-18.

(With J. Howland) Observations Upon the Calcium Content of the Blood in Infantile Tetany and Upon the Effect of Treatment by Calcium, Quart. J. Med. **11**: 289, 1917-18. Abstr., Bull. Johns Hopkins Hosp. **29**: 235, 1918.

1919

Mineral Equilibrium in the Blood Plasma and Its Relation to Certain Clinical Conditions, J. Missouri M. A. **16**: 99, 1919.

The Artificial Feeding of Athreptic Infants, J. A. M. A. **73**: 1173, 1919.

The Pathogenesis of Certain Nutritional Disorders, Tr. Am. Pediat. Soc. **31**: 34, 1919.

1920

Severe Diarrhea in Infancy, Med. Clin. North America **4**: 717, 1920.

Post-Diphtheritic Paralysis of the Respiratory Muscles, J. A. M. A. **75**: 668, 1920.

Some Phases of the Pathology of Nutrition in Infancy, Am. J. Dis. Child. **20**: 461, 1920.

1921

Abnormal Metabolism in Infancy and Its Relationship to Symptomatology, Brit. J. Dis. Child. **18**: 129, 1921.

1922

Digestive Insufficiency (Coeliac Disease), J. Missouri M. A. **19**: 90, 1922.

(With R. J. Terry) Congenital Malformation of the Auditory Organs, J. Missouri M. A. **19**: 196, 1922.

Nutritional Disorder, J. Missouri M. A. **19**: 196, 1922.

Pathology of Metabolism in Infancy and Early Childhood, Endocrinology and Metabolism, Appleton & Co., 1922. Vol. 41, pp. 781-811.

Chronic Digestive Insufficiency (Coeliac Disease), M. Clin. North America, pp. 91-96, 1922.

The Teaching of Infant Feeding, South. M. J. **15**: 530, 1922.

(With L. T. Davidson and L. P. Harshman) Studies on the Digestion in Infancy: Hydrogen-Ion Concentration of the Gastric Contents, Arch. Pediat. **39**: 361, 1922. Tr. Am. Pediat. Soc. **34**: 39, 1922.

1923

Anhydremia, Physiol. Rev. 3: 275, 1923.
Zur Kenntnis der Ernahrungsstörungen des Saüglingsalters, Monatschr. f. Kinderh. 25: 426, 1923.
(With L. T. Davidson) Acidified Whole Milk as a Routine Infant Food, J. A. M. A. 81: 2007, 1923.
Acidity of the Gastric Contents of the Gastric Contents of Infants, Am. J. Dis. Child. 26: 542, 1923.
(With S. W. Clausen) Intoxications Associated With Alterations in the Physico-Chemical Equilibria of the Body Cells and Fluids, Tr. Am. Pediat. Soc. 35: 205, 1923.
(With J. Howland) Acidosis. Vol. II, Chap. XXVII, p. 827, in "Pediatrics," edited by I. A. Abt, Philadelphia, W. B. Saunders Co.

1924

The Treatment of the Child, South. M. A. J. 17: 15, 1924.
Nephritis in Children, Acute Hemorrhagic Nephritis: Treatment, M. Clin. North America 7: 1417, 1923-24.
Nephritis in Children, Acute Parenchymatous Nephritis (Nephrosis); Treatment, M. Clin. North America 7: 1413, 1923-24.
Food Requirements of Malnourished Infants With a Note on the Use of Insulin, J. A. M. A. 83: 600, 1924.
Use of Bromin Sodiosalicylate (Diuretin) in Treatment of Hydrocephalus, Am. J. Dis. Child. 28: 479, 1924. Tr. Am. Pediat. Soc. 36: 30, 1924.
Celiac Disease, Vol. III, Chap. XLVII, p. 386 in "Pediatrics," edited by I. A. Abt, Philadelphia, W. B. Saunders Co.

1925

Broadening of the Medical Curriculum, South. M. J. 18: 147, 1925.
Hydrocephalus, M. Clin. North America 9: 45, 1925.
Further Observation Concerning Nature of Nutritional Disturbances, Laryngoscope 35: 592, 1925.
Nephritis; Newer Viewpoints Concerning Its Nature and Treatment, Northwest Med. 24: 472, 1925.
Application of Recent Studies on Nature of Nephritis, Proc. Inst. Med. Chicago, 5: 231, 1923-25.
Acute Nephritis in Children and Relation of Childhood Affections to Kidney in Adult Life, J. Michigan M. Soc. 24: 650, 1925.

1926

Remote Results of Certain Focal Infections Occurring During Infancy and Childhood, South. M. J. 19: 157, 1926.
(With B. Kramer and J. Howland) Inorganic Composition of Bones, J. Biol. Chem. 68: 721, 1926.

1927

Infant Feeding and Nutrition, South. M. J. 20: 352, 1927.
Newer Knowledge Concerning Nephritis, Illinois M. J. 51: 120, 1927.
Pediatric Aspects of Otolaryngology, Ann. Otol., Rhin. & Laryng. 36: 686, 1927. Ann. Otol., Rhin. & Laryng. 37: 71, 1928. Abstr. Tr. Ann. Laryng., Rhin. & Otol. Soc. 33: 470, 1927.
Relationship of Certain Focal Infections to General Disease in Infants and Young Children, Ann. Int. Med. 1: 1, 1927.
Practical Points in Feeding and Care of Infants, Kansas City Clin. Soc. Monthly Bull. 3: 15, 1927. J. Missouri M. A. 25: 411, 1928.
Preparation of Lactic Acid Milk Mixtures for Infant Feedings, J. A. M. A. 89: 826, 1927.

1928

Recent Advances in Chemistry in Relation to Medical Practice. St. Louis, 1928, The C. V. Mosby Company.
Lectures of the San Diego Academy of Medicine, December, 1927.
Infections in Infants, Proc. Inter-State Post.-Grad. M. Assemb., North America (1927) 3: 19, 1928.

Sequelae of Acute Infectious Diseases in Children, With Special Reference to Their Effect Upon Kidneys, Proc. Inter-State Post.-Grad. H. Assemb., North America (1927) **3**: 74, 1928.
Simplicity of Infant Feeding, J. Am. Dietet. A. **4**: 1, 1928.
(With A. F. Hartmann) Newer Aspects of Acidosis, J. A. M. A. **91**: 1675, 1928.

1929

(With L. Schoenthal) Experimental Study of Use of Unsweetened Evaporated Milk for Preparation of Infant Feeding Formulas, Arch. Pediat. **46**: 135, 1929.
Nutrition in Its Relation to Dentition and Bone Growth, Internat. J. Orthodontia **15**: 835, 1929.

1930

Infant Nutrition, St. Louis, 1930, The C. V. Mosby Company, ed. 2, St. Louis, 1935, The C. V. Mosby Company.
Uses of Proprietary and Medicinal Foods in Hospital, J. A. M. A. **94**: 1281, 1930.
Effects of Vomiting, Diarrhea and Water Loss on Body and Newer Methods of Treatment. Proc. Internat. Assemb. Inter-State Post.-Grad. M. A. North America (1929) **5**: 153, 1930.
Influence of Diet on Bones and Teeth, J. A. D. A. **17**: 1648, 1930.

1931

Enteral and Parenteral Factors in Causation of Diarrhea, South. M. J. **24**: 278, 1931.

1933

Diarrhea in Infants, Hygeia **11**: 503, 1933.
Recognition and Treatment of Certain Disturbances in Chemical Equilibrium of the Body. Proc. California Acad. Med. pp. 1-20, 1932-33.
(With A. F. Hartmann and M. J. E. Senn) Observations on Nature and Treatment of Diarrhea and Associated Systemic Disturbances, J. PEDIAT. **3**: 181, 1933.

1934

Some Therapeutic Procedures Based Upon Recent Advances in Biological Chemistry, South. M. J. **27**: 130, 1934.
The Feeding of Infants. McLester, ''Nutrition and Diet in Health and Disease,'' Philadelphia, 1934, pp. 270-287, W. B. Saunders.

1935

Graduate Teaching from Specialist's Standpoint, J. A. Am. Med. Coll. **10**: 129, 1935.

1936

Uses of Outpatient Department in Medical Education: Newer Points of View, J. A. M. A. **106**: 1442, 1936. Proc. Ann. Cong. M. Educ. pp. 52-56, 1936.
Unification of Medical Curriculum, South. M. J. **29**: 927, 1936.

1937

Serious Nutritional and Digestive Disturbances in Infancy, Vol. I, Chap. XXVIII, and Celiac Disease, Vol. I, Chap. XXIX, Practice of Pediatrics, edited by Joseph Brennermann, W. F. Prior Co.

The Journal of Pediatrics

Vol. 13 | November, 1938 | No. 5

Original Communications

INSPISSATION OF SECRETION, DILATATION OF THE DUCTS AND ACINI, ATROPHY AND FIBROSIS OF THE PANCREAS IN INFANTS

A Clinical Note

Kenneth D. Blackfan, M.D., and Charles D. May, M.D.
Boston, Mass.

During the past fifteen years examination of the pancreas in over 2,800 necropsies has disclosed thirty-five examples of a well-defined pathologic lesion, the existence of which was unsuspected during life. The patients in this series of cases, with the exception of five who died soon after birth, either failed to gain or lost in weight. Frequently episodes of diarrhea developed, and they finally died with a widespread pulmonary infection. Separate consideration will be given to seven patients who presented, in addition, wasting, especially apparent in the buttocks and thighs, distention of the abdomen, and "fatty" stools.

The lesion of the pancreas here under consideration was observed and its importance recognized by S. B. Wolbach many years ago. At necropsy, on gross examination, the transverse diameter of the pancreas is decreased. The organ is extremely firm in consistency so that considerable resistance to cutting is encountered. Microscopic examination reveals severe distortion of the architecture (Fig. 1). The acini and small ducts are greatly dilated, and their lining epithelium is flattened or occasionally obliterated. The lumina are filled with inspissated material laid down either in concentric rings or in homogenous masses. Extensive fibrosis is found. In many areas small islands of dilated acini and small ducts, separated from each other by delicate connective tissue, are surrounded by large amounts of coarse fibrous tissue. Atrophy of acini and ducts and replacement of large portions of the exocrine tissue of the pancreas by fibrous tissue marks the most advanced stage

From the Departments of Pediatrics and Pathology of the Harvard Medical School and the Infants' and the Children's Hospitals.

of the process (Fig. 2). Lymphoid and leucocytic infiltration of the interstitial tissue is often, but not always, present. The islet tissue does not partake actively in the pathologic process. No evidence of congenital anomalies or gross obstruction of the ducts could be found in those instances where it was possible to examine completely the duct system. In addition to the thirty-five patients with such advanced lesions in the pancreas, early stages of the process have been encountered in over two hundred patients at necropsy. Slight fibrosis is frequently encountered. The early changes are not recognizable on gross examination but microscopically there is dilatation of acini which contain inspissated secretion.

From a study of the development of the lesion in the large amount of material available, Blackfan and Wolbach, in 1933,[1] offered a provisional explanation in regard to pathogenesis. They stated, "Our preliminary studies indicate that the pathogenesis of this striking pancreatic affection resides in the production of an abnormal secretion which inspissates and leads to distention and atrophy of ducts and acini."

The lungs showed changes characteristic of the usual type of chronic pneumonia in infants and children. This type of pneumonia is primarily an interstitial one with secondary involvement of the alveoli and alveolar ducts. Characteristically the bronchioles and small bronchi are greatly dilated. Their walls are thickened and surrounded by collections of large mononuclear cells and lymphocytes. The dilated lumina of the bronchioles are filled with collections of polymorphonuclear cells. Frequently destruction of the walls of the bronchioles is encountered. Widespread replacement of lung parenchyma by connective tissue, and scattered manifestations of regeneration of alveolar epithelium are found in the more chronic examples of the condition.

The histologic change characteristic of vitamin A deficiency, namely metaplasia of lining epithelium in various parts of the body (trachea, bronchi, renal pelvis, or pancreas) to a stratified squamous type, was found in seven of the patients at necropsy.

From an analysis of the records of this series of patients it was found that the clinical manifestations begin very early in life. Five infants died within the first few days of life. In the remaining thirty patients the early signs of a disorder of nutrition developed before they were one year of age, the average age of onset of symptoms being about two months.

As to the family history, one patient was born of a mother who had an "intolerance" for fats and on this account had eliminated "fats" from her diet. The twin of this infant who died at another hospital is not included in this series, but both of these infants presented at necropsy histologic changes of vitamin A deficiency in addition to the pancreatic lesion. Another example of multiple occurrence in a family

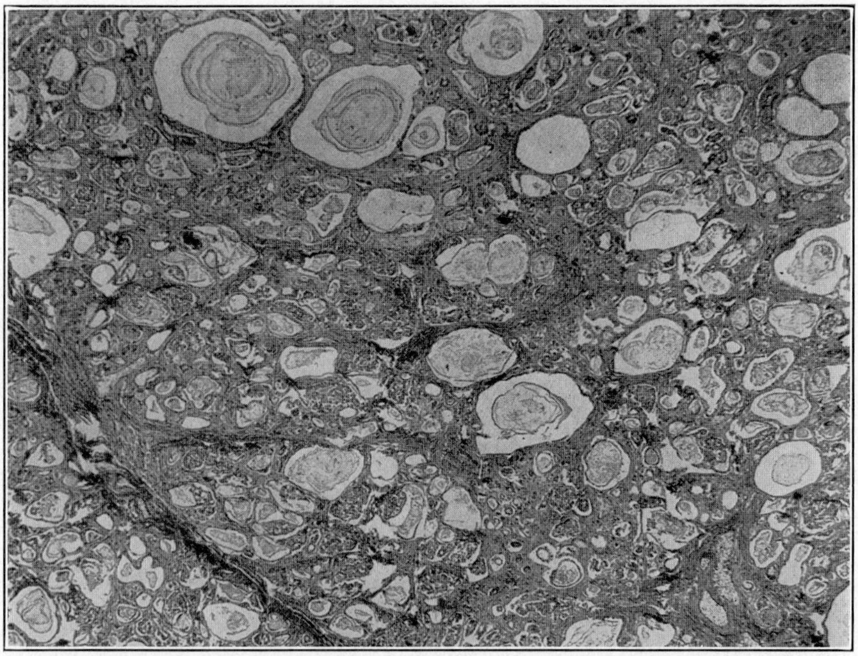

Fig. 1.—Pancreas of patient in Case A-34-21. (×33—aniline blue.) Symptoms from birth. Weight 12 pounds at 1 year of age. Developed "celiac disease" syndrome. Died at 2 years of age weighing 10 pounds. Chronic pulmonary infiltration was present but no pathologic evidence of vitamin A deficiency.

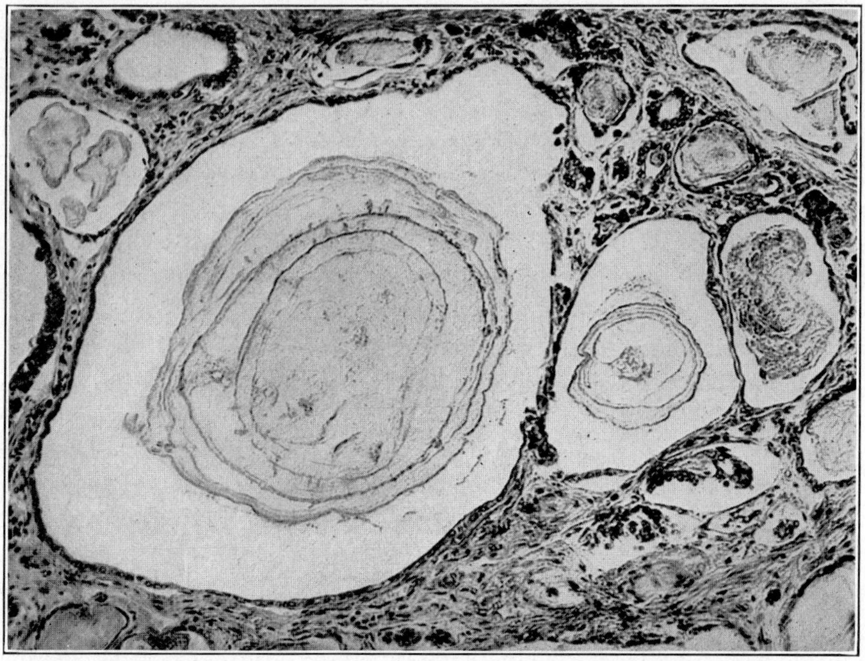

Fig. 2.—Pancreas of patient in Case A-34-21. (×233—aniline blue.) Detail of same section of pancreas shown in Fig. 1.

is that of twins who died a few days after birth. Both of these infants showed at necropsy a lesion of the pancreas as well as intestinal stenosis and meconium ileus. Mild episodes of vomiting, pyelitis, or eclamptic symptoms were reported during pregnancy by seven mothers. The mother's diet during pregnancy was restricted in only one case, that mentioned above where the "intolerance" for fats was claimed. In all but two cases, the infants were born at term by normal delivery.

Eighteen of the patients were breast-fed for from one to thirty-two weeks, the average being eight weeks. Those artificially fed were given modifications of cow's milk. The fat was markedly reduced in the food of five patients. Fifteen patients who lived more than one month had not received cod liver oil or vitamin A concentrates. Some infections, such as conjunctivitis, pyodermia, pyelitis, or frequent upper respiratory infections were conspicuous in the past history of twenty-five patients. So far as we were able to determine, there were no other specific incidents in the family or past history which might have a bearing on the production of the symptoms or the underlying associated lesion in the pancreas.

The clinical manifestations were limited in variety but were so common to many disorders in infancy that it has not been possible to determine accurately the dependable diagnostic features. However, there was an apparent uniformity in the onset and course of the illness which may be summarized as follows: In the usual course of events the patients developed symptoms of illness referable either to the gastrointestinal system or the respiratory system. In many instances such signs of ill health as vomiting and diarrhea, with failure to gain or loss of weight preceded the onset of signs of infection of the respiratory system, but in other instances a pronounced and unproductive cough was an early complaint. Sooner or later a productive cough and physical signs of pulmonary infiltration made their appearance. Vomiting as a rule was neither persistent nor frequent. Diarrhea was more significant, occasionally being severe, and often present for prolonged periods. The stools did not show pus or blood. The appearance of "fatty" stools was not observed except in seven patients who will be mentioned later.

With the persistence of these symptoms and with continuing loss of weight, the appearance of the infants was that of extreme emaciation with the attendant signs of a disorder of nutrition with or without the physical findings indicative of bronchopneumonia. Fever and dehydration did not become outstanding features until relatively late in the course of the illness. Roentgenograms showed generalized infiltration of the lungs in twenty-four patients. The tuberculin test and the Hinton test were negative.

The average duration of illness for the thirty patients who lived beyond the neonatal period was six months, and their average age at death was eight months. Several infants lived a year or more after the appearance of symptoms, but all died before the age of two years. The other five infants died, as mentioned above, within three weeks of birth—three of them with intestinal stenosis and meconium ileus, one with atresia of the ileum, and the other infant with cirrhosis of the liver.*

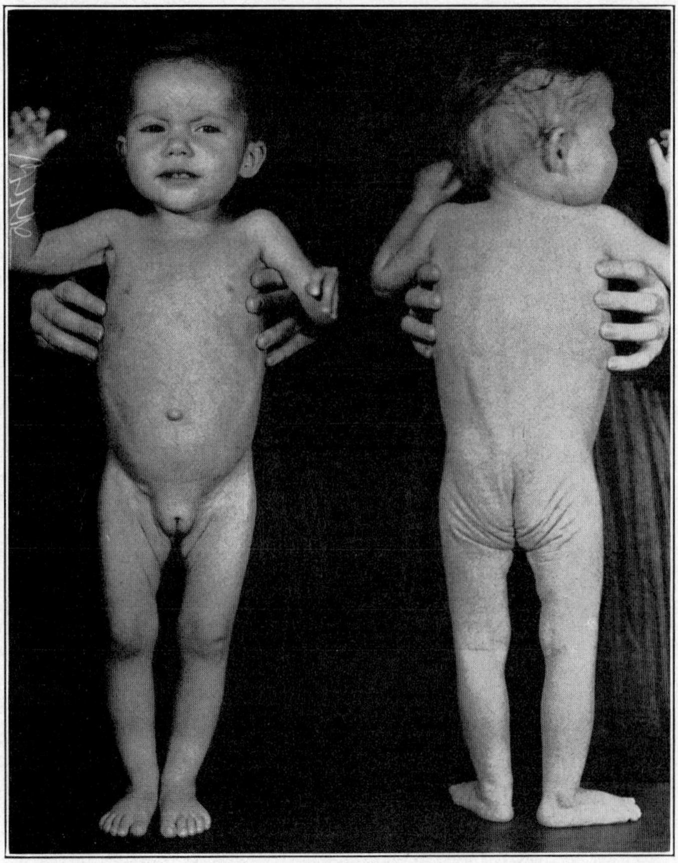

Fig. 3.—M.C. (Case 1, Table I.) at the age of 22 months. Died at 2 years.

Let us now consider the seven patients who presented such clinical features as emaciation, distention of the abdomen, and large, pale, putrefactive, "fatty" stools. While in general their illness and course were uniform with those of the other patients who lived beyond the

*Pathological examination revealed no evidence of defect in the biliary system. The bile capillaries were distended with bile and the liver cells laden with pigment. Small foci of necrosis were found in the portal areas, and a definite but slight increase in connective tissue was evident throughout the liver. The pathogenesis of the changes in the liver was obscure.

neonatal period, they stand out because in addition they developed these signs usually providing the basis for a tentative diagnosis of "celiac disease" (Fig. 3).

The ages of these seven patients at the onset of their symptoms were scattered from birth to one year. However, in this group the average duration of symptoms was sixteen months, which is much longer than the average of six months for the entire series of thirty patients who lived beyond the neonatal period. Thus their average age at death was twenty months in contrast to the average of eight months for the group of thirty patients.

While seven patients developed clinical symptoms suggesting "celiac disease," adequate data to determine the presence of all of the features of this syndrome* were obtained in only two patients because of limitations imposed by brief periods of observation or the severe illness of the patient. The clinical and laboratory data of these two patients whose symptoms dated from birth and continued with exacerbations and remissions until death occurred at twenty-four and thirteen months, respectively, are presented in Table I.

TABLE I

	CASE 1 M. C.	CASE 2 N. D.
Wasting	+	+
Abdomen	Distention	Distention
Diarrhea	+	+
Stools	"Fatty"	"Fatty"
Vomiting	0	0
Gastrointestinal roentgenograms	Clumping	Clumping
Chronic bronchopneumonia	+	+
Glucose tolerance curve	Flat	Flat
Stool analysis—Fat (% dry wt.)	58%	41%
Blood	Secondary anemia	Secondary anemia

It has been pointed out in this group of seven patients that the symtoms had existed for a much longer period than was true of the majority of the infants. That the "celiac disease" syndrome should develop when such severe lesions in the pancreas had existed so long is not too surprising, as similar manifestations have been reported in association with loss of pancreatic tissue in humans[4, 5] and in experimental animals.[6]

As to the occurrence of definite evidence of vitamin A deficiency on pathologic examination in seven of the patients in the entire series of thirty-five cases, it would be expected that any interference with the

*Until recently we have considered the "celiac disease" syndrome as including the characteristic wasting, distention of the abdomen, large, pale, putrefactive, "fatty" stools, excess fat in the feces by chemical analysis, clumping of barium in the small intestine, and "flat" glucose tolerance curve.

As mentioned by Fanconi,[2] Schiff,[3] and others, and as we have observed repeatedly, the features of the "celiac disease" syndrome may appear as a result of a variety of disorders which interfere with the proper utilization of food substances, particularly fat. Thus it would seem unwise to take these criteria as pathognomonic signs of a particular disease.

absorption of fat as a result of this lesion in the pancreas might affect the absorption of fat-soluble vitamin A.

Vitamin A absorption tests* were performed in the two patients whose clinical and laboratory data are summarized in Table I. When a single large dose of oleum percomorphum was given orally, the level of vitamin A in the blood did not rise during the following twenty-four hours as it usually does in normal children. But when thirty drops of oleum percomorphum were given daily, the vitamin A gradually rose to a normal level. After death the liver tissue was found to contain an abundance of vitamin A. The inference may be drawn that although vitamin A could be absorbed, the efficiency of absorption was probably diminished.

In the group of seven patients whose illness was of long duration and who finally developed the ''celiac disease'' syndrome, the only one who revealed pathologic evidence of vitamin A deficiency had not received accessory vitamin A in the diet. It is interesting to note that five of the total of seven patients who showed histologic evidences of vitamin A deficiency had not received accessory vitamin A in their diet. One may presume that the requirements of vitamin A for these patients may well have been greater than usual because of diminished absorption and infections. However, this should not be construed as indicating that vitamin A deficiency plays an important part in the production of the lesion, as we have seen an even greater number of patients with vitamin A deficiency in whom the pancreas was normal in every respect.

The clinical and laboratory manifestations herein reported together with so characteristic a lesion in the pancreas (dilatation of ducts, etc.) are similar in many respects to reports which have appeared in the literature for many years.[9-14] That an interrelationship exists between them certainly must be entertained, but further studies are needed before a clear understanding of any such interrelationship can be established.

While the possibility of a lesion of the pancreas should be considered in infants presenting the clinical and laboratory features which have been outlined, it is apparent that before a definite diagnosis can be established, investigation of the exocrine function of the pancreas will be needed. This would consist of indirect estimation through ''balance'' studies of fat and nitrogen absorption,[15] or direct estimation of the concentration of the pancreatic enzymes in the duodenum.[16]

SUMMARY

A note is presented on the clinical manifestations of thirty-five infants in whom an advanced lesion of the pancreas was found at necropsy. The

*Vitamin A analyses were performed by techniques based on those of Clausen[7] and Chesney and McCoord.[8]

lesion is characterized by inspissation of secretion, dilatation of the ducts and acini, atrophy and fibrosis. The need for further information concerning the absorption of fat and especially nitrogen, as well as pancreatic enzymes, as an aid to diagnosis, is suggested.

We are indebted to Dr. S. B. Wolbach and Dr. Sidney Farber for their assistance in describing the pathology of the pancreas and in the preparation of this communication.

REFERENCES

1. Blackfan, K. D., and Wolbach, S. B.: J. Pediat. **3**: 679, 1933.
2. Fanconi, G.: Der Intestinale Infantilismus, pp. 3-23, Berlin, 1928, S. Karger.
3. Schiff, E.: Klinische Fortbildung **2**: 81, 1934.
4. Clark, C., and Hadfield, G.: Quart. J. Med. **17**: 358, 1924.
5. Thomas, J., and Schlutz, F. W.: Am. J. Dis. Child. **56**: 336, 1938.
6. Greenberg, J.: Yale J. Biol. & Med. **6**: 121, 1933.
7. McCoord, A. B., and Luce-Clausen, E. M.: J. Nutrition **7**: 557, 1934.
8. Chesney, J., and McCoord, A. B.: Proc. Soc. Exper. Biol. & Med. **31**: 887, 1934.
9. Andersen, D. H.: Am. J. Dis. Child. **56**: 344, 1938. (Comprehensive bibliography.)
10. Garsche, R.: Ztschr. f. Kinderh. **58**: 434, 1937.
11. Harper, M. H.: Arch. Dis. Child. **13**: 45, 1938.
12. Hess, J. H., and Saphir, O.: J. Pediat. **6**: 1, 1935.
13. Parmelee, A. H.: Am. J. Dis. Child. **50**: 1418, 1935.
14. Kornblith, B. A., and Otani, S.: Am. J. Path. **5**: 249, 1929.
15. Pratt, J. H.: Am. J. M. Sc. **187**: 222, 1934.
16. McClure, C. W.: Functional Activities of the Pancreas and Liver. New York, 1937, Medical Authors' Publishing Company.

THE CAROTINOIDS AND VITAMIN A OF THE BLOOD

S. W. Clausen, M.D., and A. B. McCoord, Ph.D.
Rochester, N. Y.

THE proof that carotene is converted into vitamin A by the body[1] suggested that a study of the concentration of the carotinoid pigments and of vitamin A in the blood might be profitable. Such a study is obviously necessary for the elucidation of the problem of the intermediary metabolism of these substances. In this paper we shall call attention to the more important factors which affect the blood content of the carotinoids and of vitamin A, i.e., placental transmission, diet, infection, age and season, and we shall discuss the effect of chronic morbid states—diabetes, Bright's disease, celiac disease and hypothyroidism—on the concentration of carotinoids and vitamin A in the blood.

The carotinoid pigments are derived from plants and include isomeric carotenes ($C_{40}H_{56}$), of which those containing a β-ionone ring may serve as precursors of vitamin A, unsaturated hydrocarbons without rings of the same empirical formula (such as lycopin, the pigment of the tomato), and carotinoids containing oxygen, such as the xanthophylls, the function of which in the animal is not yet apparent.

The blood and tissues of man may contain appreciable amounts of several of these pigments.[2] So far as we know, the "lipochromes," or yellow fat-soluble pigments are carotinoids, possibly exclusively so.

METHODS

Since the blood cells contain little, if any, carotinoid, the analyses here reported have been made upon serum or plasma. For total carotinoids we have used a modification of the method of Connor.[3]

Method for Determining Total Carotinoids.—Three milliliters of plasma or serum are mixed with an equal volume of 95 per cent ethyl alcohol; 3 ml. of petroleum ether are added. The mixture is shaken at intervals for ten minutes and is centrifuged. The upper layer, containing all the carotinoids (and the vitamin A), is compared in the micro-Duboscq colorimeter with a standard of 0.02 per cent aqueous solution of potassium bichromate. The standard is prepared by dilution of a 0.2 per cent solution which keeps well for months. When the upper layer has exactly the same intensity of color as the dilute standard, the original plasma is said to contain 100 units of carotinoid per 100 ml. We have found that when solutions of pure carotene or xanthophyll are used, the relationship between colorimeter readings and concentration is linear

From the Department of Pediatrics, University of Rochester School of Medicine and Dentistry.

over a very considerable range. One hundred units of carotene are equal to 137 micrograms (γ); 100 units of xanthophyll are equal to 146 γ.

Method for Determining Carotene and Xanthophyll.—For carotene and xanthophyll analyses, we have used the method described by Clausen and McCoord.[4] We are aware of the fact that this method may give high results for carotene because lycopene and the esters of xanthophyll may be included with it; also, the results for xanthophyll may be low (*l.c.*). But the more important conclusions of the present study are not influenced by these facts because the factors investigated affect the carotene and the xanthophyll in a like manner.

Method for Determining Vitamin A.—The vitamin A content of the plasma (or serum) was estimated by a modification of the Price-Carr antimony trichloride reaction.[5] One milliliter of the petroleum ether extract of plasma already described is evaporated to dryness in a small test tube. One-tenth milliliter of chloroform is added; then 1 ml. of a 30 per cent solution of antimony trichloride in chloroform is added, and the mixture is rapidly transferred to the cup of the micro-Duboscq colorimeter with the plunger set at 10 mm. The other cup of the colorimeter contains an aqueous solution of 10 per cent copper sulfate ($CuSO_4 \cdot 5\,H_2O$). The comparison of the blue colors must be made within 30 seconds after mixing. When the color of the solution containing vitamin A is exactly matched by 10 mm. of copper sulfate, the original specimen is said to contain 100 units of vitamin A per 100 ml. Corrections are made for the carotene and xanthophyll content of the plasma by subtracting 3.7 blue units for each 100 γ carotene, and 4.1 blue units for each 100 γ xanthophyll or 2.7 blue units for each 100 units total carotinoid. Details will be published later. In many cases the analyses for total carotinoids *or* for carotene and xanthophyll were carried out on the same specimen as was the analysis for vitamin A. We are aware of the error which we tacitly make in identifying the "units" of blue color with "units of vitamin A" but feel that the average results to be presented may be a fairly accurate measure of vitamin A concentration.

CLINICAL MATERIAL

Early in this investigation it became evident that the concentration of carotinoid pigments and of vitamin A in the plasma varied considerably. A marked and prompt decrease in concentration accompanied infection and was proportional to the duration and severity of the infection. Consequently, some arbitrary classification of infections in the persons observed was necessary. We have considered as "severe" infections pneumonia, mastoiditis, meningitis, septicemia, and any fatal infection. All others were considered "mild or moderate" infections.

Since the carotinoid pigments of the blood are exogenous so far as we know and may enter the body through the placental circulation or from the food (colostrum, milk during the first few months, and pigmented vegetables later), we have presented separately the results of analysis (1) at birth, (2) in children under 6 months of age, (3) in those from 6 months to 24 months of age, and (4) in persons over 2 years of age. Each of these four age groups is divided into three subgroups: (a) those with no infection, those (b) with mild or moderate infection, and (c) those with severe infection. We have separated from all these groups for special consideration those metabolic disorders found to have a marked effect upon the level of plasma carotinoids and vitamin A—diabetes, Bright's disease, celiac disease, and hypothyroidism and hyperthyroidism. If the mean values in any group are to be of statistical significance, the groups must be fairly large, because the coefficients of variability are large. In several of the tables will be found the number of observations, the mean, the standard deviation (σ) and the probable error of the mean (P. E. M.). As a rule, the frequency distributions of the values are not normal, the mode being considerably below the mean. This is apparent in Tables V and VIII.

NEWBORN INFANTS AND THEIR MOTHERS

Blood was obtained from the umbilical artery and vein of the infant and from the mother's vein at delivery. The results of individual analyses permit the calculation of various correlations, as well as the calculation of means and standard deviations, which are presented in Table I. In a preliminary discussion of these results,[9] we have presented evidence that we are dealing with carotene and xanthophyll. If Table I is compared with Table III, containing the results in normal older children and adults, it will be evident that (1) the carotinoid pigments of the plasma at birth are lower than in later life, (2) the xanthophyll concentration at birth exceeds that of carotene, the reverse being true later, (3) vitamin A is relatively low in the blood at birth, and (4) the concentration of carotene and xanthophyll in the blood of parturient women is higher on the average than it is in other older persons. Table I also shows that the mean value of concentration of carotene and xanthophyll is significantly higher in the venous blood (that from the placenta) than it is in the arterial blood (that from the child). When the venous and arterial blood of the *same* individual were compared, it was found that the concentrations in the venous blood exceeds that in the arterial blood in *every case* (Table II). This fact is strong evidence that the carotinoids are passing by way of the placenta to the fetus at the time of birth. A very rough estimate shows that about 1 mg. of carotene per kilogram of fetus per day might be furnished to it in this way, provided the rate of transfer during life in utero is the same as that at

TABLE I*

CAROTINOID AND VITAMIN A OF FETAL AND MATERNAL BLOOD PLASMA AT BIRTH

	NUMBER	MEAN	σ	P.E.M.
Carotene				
Infant venous blood	63	16.60	5.73	0.49
Infant arterial blood	38	12.90	4.70	0.53
Maternal venous blood	32	114.0	40.6	4.94
Xanthophyll				
Infant venous blood	63	27.8	9.07	0.78
Infant arterial blood	38	21.3	8.20	0.91
Maternal venous blood	31	83.7	26.6	3.23
Vitamin A				
Infant venous blood	63	12.8	4.78	0.41
Infant arterial blood	37	13.1	4.80	0.54
Maternal venous blood	32	15.2	6.49	0.79

*In the tables, *N* designates number of observations; *M*, means; σ, standard deviation; *P.E.M.*, probable error of mean; *C*, carotene, γ per 100 ml.; *X*, xanthophyll, γ per 100 ml.; *Total C*, total carotinoid, units per 100 ml.; *A*, vitamin A, units per 100 ml.

TABLE II

DIFFERENCES BETWEEN CONCENTRATION OF CAROTINOIDS IN VENOUS AND IN ARTERIAL BLOOD OF THE NEWBORN CHILD

	NUMBER	MEAN	σ
Carotene	36	6.7	2.7
Xanthophyll	34	7.2	6.9

TABLE III

CAROTENE, XANTHOPHYLL AND VITAMIN A OF PLASMA AT VARIOUS AGES (INFLUENCE OF INFECTION)

	INFECTIONS								
	NONE			MILD OR MODERATE			SEVERE		
	N	M	σ	N	M	σ	N	M	σ
Carotene									
Birth	63	16.60	5.73	–	–	–	–	–	–
0-6 mo.	5	25.5	–	1	49.5	–	1	9.5	–
6-24 mo.	3	76.2	–	23	71.6	55.7	7	40.9	–
2 yr. +	108	94.1	42.6	61	70.8	32.6	19	50.6	7.25
Xanthophyll									
Birth	63	27.8	9.07	–	–	–	–	–	–
0-6 mo.	5	29.5	–	1	49.5	–	1	29.5	–
6-24 mo.	3	29.5	–	23	38.2	24.8	7	23.8	–
2 yr. +	108	53.0	25.2	61	38.4	16.4	19	37.9	15.0
Vitamin A									
Birth	63	12.8	4.78	–	–	–	–	–	–
0-6 mo.	14	23.8	10.7	20	15.0	7.1	14	9.1	5.2
6-24 mo.	12	19.9	5.2	75	12.9	7.05	24	9.5	6.9
2 yr. +	116	20.2	10.0	144	15.1	8.2	67	6.8	5.5

birth. The mean concentration of vitamin A in the venous blood plasma of the fetus is about equal to that in the arterial blood plasma. The variations in individual cases were found to take place in both directions. This may be due to errors of analysis, or, assuming that the analyses are correct, may be due to transfer of vitamin A by way of the placenta in some of the cases.

CAROTINOIDS AND VITAMIN A OF PLASMA AFTER BIRTH

The mean values for carotene, xanthophyll, and vitamin A are shown in Table III. In persons without infection the values for carotene rise after the sixth month, when, as a rule, green vegetables and carrots are added to the diet. The rise in xanthophyll occurs at about the second year. Vitamin A rises soon after birth to an approximately constant average level of about 20 units per 100 ml. Severe infections are accompanied by a marked fall in carotene and in vitamin A; after the second year, also by a fall in xanthophyll.

The mean value for vitamin A of the plasma in childhood does not vary greatly at different seasons of the year (Table IV), whereas in normal older children the plasma carotinoids are higher in the late summer (Table VII).

The distribution of values for vitamin A in the plasma in the group studied is very asymmetrical about the mean (Table V). For example, the vitamin A of plasma in normal persons most frequently lies between 10 and 20 units per 100 ml., whereas the mean is 20.5 units. For this reason, too much significance must not be placed upon a single low result. Either a series of analyses must be made upon one individual under controlled conditions, or the mean and the probable error of the mean must be determined in a sufficient number of different individuals

TABLE IV

SEASONAL VARIATIONS IN VITAMIN A OF PLASMA

MONTHS	INFECTIONS					
	NONE		MILD OR MODERATE		SEVERE	
	N	M	N	M	N	M
December, January, February	35	21.9	112	13.2	45	8.1
March, April, May	33	22.8	60	14.9	33	7.5
June, July, August	71	18.7	52	15.9	19	7.5
September, October, November	3	23.7	15	15.3	8	7.6

TABLE V

VITAMIN A OF PLASMA

UNITS A PER 100 ML.	INFECTIONS		
	NONE	MILD OR MODERATE	SEVERE
0- 4	2	13	29
5- 9	18	69	46
10-14	32	53	17
15-19	30	48	12
20-24	14	28	1
25-29	20	14	
30-34	6	10	
35-39	7	2	
40-44	4	2	
45-49	9		
N	142	239	105
M	20.5	14.4	7.72
σ	11.3	8.1	4.90

in whom one known factor is abnormal, and in whom the other variable factors do not affect the level of vitamin A.

A correlation exists between the levels of carotene and xanthophyll of the plasma. Considering only persons over 2 years of age, without infection, and without metabolic diseases which affect the levels of plasma carotinoids, we have estimated the coefficient of correlation and have calculated the mean, standard deviation and regression lines for 450 pairs of observations.

Coefficient of correlation	$r = 0.816$
Mean carotene concentration	$c = 90.52\ \gamma$ per 100 ml.; $\sigma = 45.3$
Mean xanthophyll concentration	$x = 53.9\ \gamma$ per 100 ml.; $\sigma = 28.7$

$$c = 1.29\ x + 2.07$$
$$x = 0.394\ c + 18.2$$

It follows that for certain statistical purposes, the total carotinoids may be used instead of carotene and xanthophyll. The high coefficient of correlation undoubtedly is due to the fact that the carotene and xanthophyll contents of the average diet are correlated.

TOTAL CAROTINOIDS OF THE PLASMA IN CHILDHOOD

The chief factors which affect the plasma concentration of carotinoids are the intake, infection, and certain metabolic disturbances.

The Effect of Intake.—It has been shown[6] that the level of plasma carotinoid rises slowly in young infants who are fed carrot puree, or solutions of carotene in oil, and that the presence of infection may interfere with the rise in level. If a large single dose (20 ml. 0.3 per cent carotene in oil) is administered to normal children, the increase in level appears to be influenced to some extent by the original level present (Table VI). With original levels below 150 units per 100 ml., a slow rise occurs which reaches a maximum in three days, and which is still apparent after seven days. With original levels above 150 units, the rise is greater, and the maximum is reached in twenty-four hours. The rate of absorption of carotene appears to be slower than the rate of absorption of vitamin A, for, when large doses of halibut liver oil are given, the maximum concentration of vitamin A in the plasma is found four hours afterwards.[6]

TABLE VI

MEAN INCREASE IN LEVEL OF PLASMA CAROTINOIDS FOLLOWING ADMINISTRATION OF SINGLE DOSE OF 20 ML. 0.3 PER CENT CAROTENE IN OIL

GROUP I—ORIGINAL PLASMA LEVEL BELOW 150 UNITS PER 100 ML.
GROUP II—ORIGINAL PLASMA LEVEL OVER 150 UNITS PER 100 ML.

(TEN OBSERVATIONS IN EACH GROUP)

	TIME UNITS PER 100 ML.								
	3 HR.	5 HR.	10 HR.	24 HR.	30 HR.	48 HR.	72 HR.	92 HR.	1 WK.
Group I	6.8	8.2	17.0	37.8	41.8	43.2	48.0	41.8	25.6
Group II	20.6	37.4	50.8	53.2	28.2	29.2	40.7	56.6	41.2

The average level of plasma carotinoids rises from about 20 units per 100 ml. at birth to about 100 units at 18 months, and falls to a constant level of about 90 units by the fifth year. The average level during the winter months is about 77; in late autumn about 100 (Table VII). These observations are readily explained by the varying intake of carotinoids which is low until infants receive vegetables, and which is lower in midwinter than in the spring and summer. When the intake of carotinoids is diminished by giving a diet free of pigmented vegetables, eggs, butter, and cream, the level of plasma carotinoids falls gradually from about 100 units to about 50 units in the course of a week (Fig. 1).

Correlation of Total Carotinoids With Vitamin A of Plasma.—Since both the carotinoids and vitamin A of the plasma fall during infection,

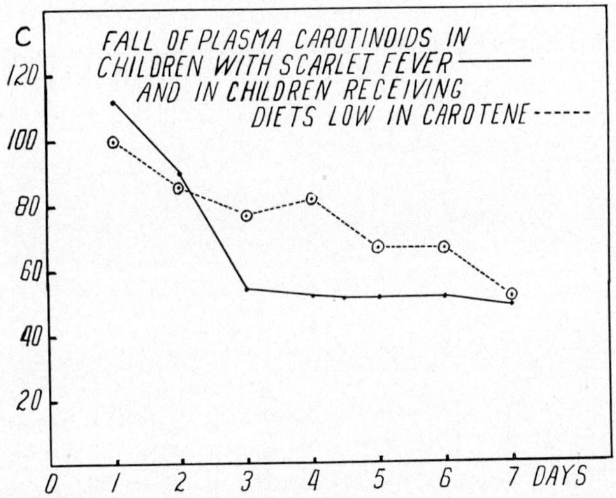

Fig. 1.—The fall in carotinoids of the plasma of children receiving diets low in carotinoids is gradual. The fall in carotinoids of the plasma of children with moderately severe scarlet fever is rapid.

it would seem natural to suppose that a correlation should exist between those substances in a large group of persons. In 1,414 pairs of observations we found that the coefficient of correlation was +0.305. When,

TABLE VII

SEASONAL VARIATION OF PLASMA CAROTINOIDS IN PERSONS OVER 2 YEARS OF AGE

MONTHS	INFECTIONS					
	NONE		MILD OR MODERATE		SEVERE	
	N	M	N	M	N	M
December, January, February	187	77.2	157	70.0	37	36.6
March, April, May	241	93.3	189	69.7	35	38.7
June, July, August	213	90.7	103	69.1	8	40.0
September, October, November	306	109.5	58	73.4	19	35.9

however, the groups were divided into subgroups (1) with no infection, (2) mild or moderate infection, and (3) severe infection; we found in the subgroups very low coefficients of correlation.

Correlation of Total Carotinoids With the Lipids of the Plasma.—In 84 children convalescent from rheumatic fever or from scarlet fever, the coefficient of correlation between total carotinoids and phospholipids or residual fat was too small to be of significance. The coefficient of correlation between total carotinoids and total cholesterol was +0.585.

The Effect of Infection.—The fall in level of plasma carotinoids during infection is also illustrated in Fig. 1 which shows that in 11 cases of mild scarlet fever the fall in plasma carotinoids to a low nearly constant level (about 50 units) may take place in 3 days. The frequency with which various levels of carotinoids are found in the plasma of children with no infections, mild or moderate infections, and severe infections, is shown in Table VIII. It will be observed that the distributions are not symmetrical about their means but that there is a marked tendency for the occurrence of instances with higher values than the mode, especially in persons without severe infection. The variability

TABLE VIII

FREQUENCY OF VARIOUS LEVELS OF THE CAROTINOIDS OF THE PLASMA IN CHILDREN OVER 2 YEARS OF AGE

UNITS PER 100 ML. PLASMA	INFECTIONS					
	NONE		MILD OR MODERATE		SEVERE	
	CASES	PER CENT	CASES	PER CENT	CASES	PER CENT
250-259	2	0.21	1	0.17		
240-249	1	0.11	0			
230-239	1	0.11	0			
220-229	2	0.21	0			
210-219	2	0.21	1	0.17		
200-209	7	0.74	3	0.52		
190-199	5	0.53	0			
180-189	11	1.16	4	0.69		
170-179	10	1.05	0			
160-169	12	1.27	3	0.52		
150-159	23	2.43	1	0.17		
140-149	27	2.85	2	0.34		
130-139	36	3.80	6	1.03		
120-129	45	4.75	20	3.43		
110-119	59	6.24	23	3.97		
100-109	69	7.28	26	4.46		
90-99	112	11.80	39	6.69		
80-89	123	13.00	57	9.78	1	0.95
70-79	124	13.10	69	11.80	0	
60-69	116	12.20	91	15.60	5	4.72
50-59	78	8.23	102	17.50	12	11.30
40-49	56	5.91	82	14.10	27	25.30
30-39	20	2.12	42	7.21	29	27.40
20-29	4	0.42	7	1.20	21	19.80
10-19	2	0.21	4	0.69	8	7.54
0-9					3	2.83
N	947.0		583		106	
M	91.9		71.7		46.9	
σ	37.2		31.3		14.4	

TABLE IX

EFFECT OF ARTIFICIAL HYPERTHERMIA UPON VITAMIN A, CAROTENE AND XANTHOPHYLL OF PLASMA

DURATION HOURS	VITAMIN A UNITS PER 100 ML.							
	BEFORE TREATMENT	AFTER BEGINNING TREATMENT						
		IMMEDIATELY	1 DAY	2 DAYS	3 DAYS	4 DAYS	5 DAYS	7 DAYS
10	----	2.3	7.0	8.4	5.0	6.0		
14	7.1	5.0	17.6	13.8	12.0	11.4		
16	8.5	6.0						
15	8.6	5.8	15.6	18.2	22.8			13.6
16	10.8	3.5	4.5	4.7	13.5			
13	11.6	5.5	7.4	20.6	7.0			
19	12.4	3.4	7.4	7.4				
15	12.8	5.4	7.2	6.0	4.8			
16	13.6	19.8	29.3					
10	14.0	8.3	8.5	12.5	10.4	11.6		
14	16.0	9.2						
16	16.4	6.0			7.5		7.0	10.0
5	18.8	6.5	18.8					
16	25.0	14.0						
10	25.4	12.2	25.5					10.0
5	25.5	26.8	28.6	29.6				
16	26.2	7.8						
16	27.0	16.2						
14	41.5	13.5	9.4	20.5	33.5			
Mean decrement of carotene γ per 100 ml.		8.2	9.9	9.0	14.0	12.0		19.0
Mean decrement of xanthophyll γ per 100 ml.		15.0	8.7	13.0	13.0	11.0	6.0	-8.5

is considerable, as is shown by the large relative values of the standard deviations in all the distributions.

The fall in plasma carotinoids during infection is in part due to lowered intake, as already suggested by the effect of feeding diets low in carotinoid. But this effect does not account for the more rapid fall during infection. Another cause is fever. Through the kindness of Dr. Stafford Warren we have had the opportunity to observe the effect of artificial hyperthermia upon the carotene, xanthophyll, and vitamin A contents of the plasma. The results are shown in Table IX. The rapid fall in all three substances is apparent.

The concentrations of carotene and of xanthophyll fell in all cases for three days (on the average). At this time the patients resumed their normal diets. By the end of a week the xanthophyll content of the blood had risen above the initial value. The results of the analysis for vitamin A are given in detail. A marked fall occurred in 17 of the 19 persons examined; a rise occurred in 2, one of whom had had only a brief treatment. The fall is most evident as a rule immediately at the end of the treatment, and the lowest levels are found in the persons having the lowest initial levels of vitamin A. In 6 instances, the level of vitamin A increased above the initial level between the first and third day after beginning the treatment. A similar rise in the level of vitamin A of the plasma was observed after the fall of temperature in scarlet fever (Fig. 2) and in pneumonia. The rise after fever suggests either liberation from stores, increased ingestion due to improved appetite, or temporary inability to store the vitamin as rapidly as normally. It is obvious from the observations recorded here that the finding of a low level of vitamin A in the blood during infection docs not necessarily indicate low stores. It may, however, explain the occurrence of loss of visual acuity in dim light during prolonged fevers in persons with possibly normal stores of vitamin A. The decrease in plasma carotene, xanthophyll, and vitamin A during artificial hyperthermia is evidence that the low values found in infections result in part from fever.

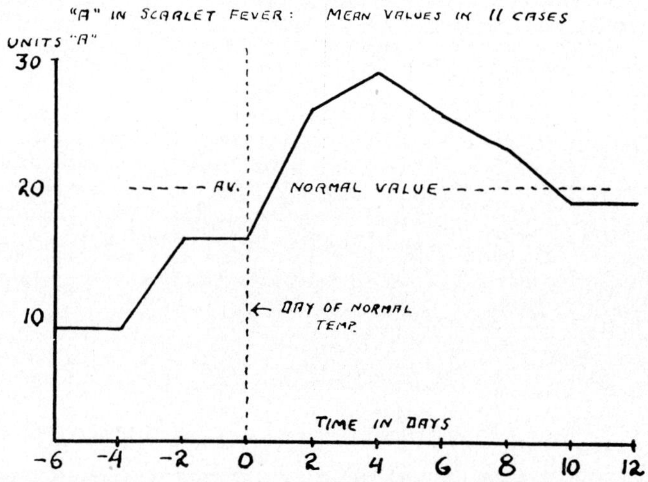

Fig. 2.—Rise in vitamin A of plasma after temperature became normal in scarlet fever reached a maximum in four days.

CAROTENE AND VITAMIN A IN DISORDERS OF METABOLISM

Xanthosis Cutis (Table X).—This name has been selected to describe those cases in which yellow discoloration of the skin is due to carotene or to xanthophyll. The term "carotinemia" is not appropriate, for two reasons: (1) The color may be due to xanthophyll; (2) the degree of pigmentation is not necessarily proportional to the concentration of carotene in the plasma. For example, no discoloration of the skin may occur in nephrosis or chronic nephritis even when the plasma contains a much higher concentration of carotinoid pigments than are found in xanthosis cutis. The condition is characterized by yellowness of the skin of the whole body, especially marked in the ears, the nasolabial folds, the palms, and the soles. The sclerae and the urine are normal. The condition has often been confused with jaundice. It need not be pathologic. It is frequently due to the ingestion of large quantities of vegetables containing carotinoids, or of eggs containing xanthophyll, and may be produced readily in many healthy persons by such diets. It is frequently observed in diabetics, often as a result of diet, sometimes as a result of the disease as well. Several of our patients had symptoms of hypothyroidism. Two of the subjects were suspected of having Addison's disease and may, in fact, have suffered from it, as they were asthenic and had hypotension. The plasma of one diabetic patient showed normal carotene but high xanthophyll. In another (a normal child) xanthosis cutis was produced by a diet rich in egg yolk. Our observations indicate that xanthosis cutis may be apparent, without Bright's disease, when the blood carotene or xanthophyll exceeds about

TABLE X

XANTHOSIS CUTIS

HOSPITAL NO. OR INITIALS	C	X	A	TOTAL C	REMARKS
62848			63	224	Recovering from xanthosis cutis
85103	640	112			Abnormal craving for carrots, raw or cooked
None	271	76			Took large amounts of carotene in oil; slight xanthosis
86814	183	35			Recovering; skin still yellow
28444	206	30			Addison's disease
I. McC.	346	231			Diabetic; diet mostly vegetables
I. McC.	364	340			Same patient, 15 months later; same condition
97552	170	328			Diabetes; arteriosclerosis
54371	416	232	80		Marked yellowness of skin
54371	258	124			Two months later; skin somewhat less yellow
44553				216	Moderately yellow skin; fever
Priv. pt.	316	135			Fond of vegetables; marked xanthosis
Priv. pt.	304	168	4.6		Fond of vegetables; marked xanthosis
143917	320	110	9.4		Fond of vegetables; marked xanthosis

250 micrograms per cent, or when the total carotinoids exceeds about 200 units per cent. Xanthosis may disappear within two weeks when the diet contains little carotinoid. The pigmentation of the skin, however, may persist for some time after the level of plasma carotinoids has become normal.

Diabetes (Table XI).—The carotene and xanthophyll content of the plasma was determined in 64 diabetics, mostly adults, whose disease was under good control. Those cases requiring more than 10 units of insulin per day were considered moderate or severe. Those patients receiving less than 10 units of insulin per day were considered as having mild cases. The cases with infection at the time of the determination

TABLE XI

CAROTENE AND XANTHOPHYLL OF PLASMA IN DIABETES

	CAROTENE γ PER 100 ML.			XANTHOPHYLL γ PER 100 ML.		
	INSULIN PER DAY			INSULIN PER DAY		
	OVER 10 UNITS		UNDER 10 UNITS	OVER 10 UNITS		UNDER 10 UNITS
	INFECTIONS		INFECTIONS	INFECTIONS		INFECTIONS
	NONE	PRESENT	NONE*	NONE	PRESENT	NONE*
N	29	7	28	29	7	28
M	128	104	112	103	74	87

*There were no infections at time of observation in persons receiving less than 10 units of insulin.

were tabulated separately. It will be observed that in each group both the carotene and the xanthophyll content of the plasma were higher than normal, and that the more severe group had the higher carotinoids. The elevation of carotinoids may be due in part to the high carotinoid content of the diet. But since the diet of the more severe diabetic cases did not contain more carotinoids than that of the milder group, it seems likely that in patients with diabetes the carotinoids are not so readily changed to colorless compounds as in normal persons. In 15 diabetic cases under good control the mean vitamin A content of the plasma was 19.7 units per 100 ml. In 2 diabetic cases not under good control, the vitamin A content of the plasma was below 10 units per 100 ml. More studies are needed before a low vitamin A content of plasma can be regarded as characteristic of diabetes.

Celiac Disease (Table XII).—As a rule, the serum and plasma in cases of celiac disease are practically colorless because of their low content of lipochromes. Analysis showed in only 2 of 12 of our cases a normal content of carotene or total carotinoid, and in only 3, normal vitamin A. The ingestion of halibut liver oil failed to cause a normal rise in the vitamin A of the plasma, probably as a result of poor absorption.[7, 10] The present observations indicate that when the plasma carotinoids are low in a person consuming a normal diet who, without fever or hepatic disease, is suffering from malnutrition, and in whom diarrhea may or may not be present, then the diagnosis of celiac disease must be considered. In such cases increased fat in the stool, "flat" blood sugar curves after standard doses of glucose, and "flat" vitamin A tolerance curves after ingestion of halibut liver oil will establish the diagnosis.

Jaundice (Table XIII).—During the acute stage of infectious hepatitis (catarrhal jaundice) the carotene, xanthophyll and vitamin A content of the plasma were found to be low. As the jaundice subsided and as the stools became colored with bile, the plasma returned to normal. The important cause for the abnormally low values is probably faulty absorption. During the acute period of the disease studied, the absorp-

TABLE XII

CELIAC DISEASE

HOSPITAL NO.	C	X	A	TOTAL C	REMARKS
50364			14.0		
50364			19.0	61	After 1 year
47229			8.0	7	
47229			14.0		After 2 years
47229			23.5	24	After 3 years
J. M.			9.0	0	
44698			13.0	30	
105685			12.0		
108537			6.0		
108537			30.0		After 1 month; improved
98940			12.0	0	
98940	54	24	13.2		After 10 months; not improved
69795			7.0		
102853			13.0	0	
99945	79	48	8.6		
122123	11	15	4.4		
Priv. pt.	42	32	3.5		
143163	58	75	8.3		

TABLE XIII

JAUNDICE

HOSPITAL NO. OR INITIALS	C	X	A	TOTAL C	REMARKS
					Acute infectious jaundice
39158				45	Third day
Priv. pt.				53	Fourth day
43007				25	Fifth day
41141				54	Eighth day
71671	79	62	15.0		Fourteenth day
65755	30	32			Second day
5050	50	57	5.0		Fourteenth day
5050			10.0		Twenty-fifth day
27681			1.6		During attack
27681	84	59	21.5		Eight days after
					Other types
17732			6.0	76	Icterus gravis
13436			0	29	Congenital obstruction, bile ducts

tion of vitamin A is almost entirely prevented. In the 2 cases studied during convalescence, we found that the ingestion of oils rich in vitamin A caused an abnormally high concentration in the plasma (5 to 8 times that expected in normal persons). It seems probable, therefore, that infectious hepatitis so affects the liver that the rate of storage for vitamin A is decreased for several weeks. In one case of congenital obstruction of the bile ducts, no vitamin A was found in the plasma. In one case of icterus gravis, the vitamin A content was low, but the carotinoids were abnormally high for the age. The stool contained xanthophyll in large amounts.

Disorders of the Thyroid.—Animals deprived of the thyroid gland are unable to convert carotene to vitamin A.[8] Such animals, after having received thyroxine, are again able to convert carotene to vitamin A. Large doses of thyroid substance or of thyroxine cause lowering of the vitamin A content of the liver. We might therefore expect to find low values of plasma vitamin A both in hypothyroidism and in hyperthyroidism, and high values of plasma carotene in hypothyroidism, and low values in hyperthyroidism. In the 2 cases of hyperthyroidism which we have observed, the carotinoids and vitamin A of the plasma were low.

Hypothyroidism (Table XIV).—In the majority of our cases high values for plasma carotene were found; in all cases low values for vita-

TABLE XIV

CAROTENE, XANTHOPHYLL AND VITAMIN A CONTENT OF PLASMA IN HYPOTHYROIDISM

HOSPITAL NO. OR INITIALS	C	X	A	REMARKS
62833	233	90		Myxedema
101922	344	66		Xanthosis
R. C.	238	100	10.4	Dry skin; lethargic
R. C.	203	64	18.1	Received thyroid 1 month
18441	88	66	2.1	Cholesterol 418
88501	87	40	12.6	Hypothyroidism; hypoglycemic convulsions; basal metabolic rate, -22%
107827	203	113	8.4	Plasma cholesterol 310; convulsions
105237	213	87		Hypothyroidism ?
126439	234	78	9.9	Hypothyroidism ? Plasma cholesterol 273
Priv. pt.	170	75	12.6	Basal metabolic rate, -37%
141713	126	58	7.0	Hypothyroidism ? Plasma cholesterol 216; basal metabolic rate, -27%
120514	121	44	13.7	Hypothyroidism ? Plasma cholesterol 184; basal metabolic rate, -32%
Priv. pt.	97	65	16.2	Hypothyroidism ? Plasma cholesterol 195; basal metabolic rate, -35%

min A were found. The peculiar yellowish discoloration of the skin in hypothyroidism may be due in part to xanthosis cutis. In several cases we have observed that when sufficient thyroid substance was administered to cause elevation of the basal metabolic rate and lowering of the blood cholesterol, the carotene and vitamin A content of the blood tended to become normal.

Nephrosis and Nephritis (Table XV).—The carotene, xanthophyll and vitamin A of the plasma may be considerably elevated in chronic

TABLE XV

CAROTENE, XANTHOPHYLL AND VITAMIN A CONTENT OF PLASMA IN NEPHROSIS AND NEPHRITIS

HOSPITAL NO. OR INITIALS	C	X	A	TOTAL C	REMARKS
62416			88		Chronic nephritis with edema
62416			71	226	Chronic nephritis with edema, 2 mo. later
110305	284	204			Chronic nephritis with edema
E. F.	117	60	99		Chronic nephritis with edema; terminal stage
E. B.	227	108	44		Chronic nephritis; no edema
E. B.	328	136	40		Chronic nephritis; no edema
98332	232	128			Nephrosis; inactive
74030			24	141	Nephrosis; recovered
88125			60	104	Nephrosis; active
88125	149	72			Nephrosis; recovered after 5 months
56752			23	206	Nephrosis; duration 4 months
56752			46	393	Nephrosis; duration 5 months
56752			151	283	Nephrosis; duration 5½ mo.; more edema and albuminuria
56752			184	300	Nephrosis; duration 5½ mo.; more edema and albuminuria
56752			87	268	Nephrosis; duration 6 mo.; improved
56752			55	285	Nephrosis; duration 7 mo.; greatly improved
56752			44	215	Nephrosis; duration 7½ mo., apparently cured (no recurrence in 6 years)
89870	238	185	15.6		Nephrosis; remission
89870	185	90	124		Nephrosis; relapse

glomerular nephritis—with or without edema—and in lipoid nephrosis. In our cases xanthosis cutis did not occur. We have no explanation for this observation. The concentration of vitamin A in the plasma may attain elevations which we have observed in no other disease—elevations which normally can be produced only temporarily by administering large doses of the vitamin. Two observations at autopsy, in cases of chronic glomerular nephritis, revealed high values of vitamin A in the plasma, in spite of very low values in the liver. This observation suggests that renal damage either may interfere with the capacity of the liver to store vitamin A or may cause liberation of the vitamin from the liver.

SUMMARY

The observations recorded in this paper clearly indicate the effect of the intake of carotene and xanthophyll upon the carotinoid content of the plasma. Relatively large amounts of those substances may pass through the placenta to the fetus. Vitamin A probably also passes through the placenta, but the fetus may also be able to form vitamin A from carotene. Normal infants and older persons readily absorb carotene from the diet or from solutions of carotene in oil, but the rate of absorption is slower than the rate of absorption of vitamin A. The low carotinoid content of the diet in early infancy and in the winter months explains the lower concentration of carotene and xanthophyll in the first six months of life and in the winter months. The mean vitamin A concentration of the plasma in normal persons reaches a constant level soon after birth and is not affected by season. The variations between single determinations are great. Infection causes a prompt and considerable fall in the concentration of carotene, xanthophyll and vitamin A in the plasma. This fall is due, in part, to low intake during infection, but is also due, in part, to fever. A few days after the temperature becomes normal, the vitamin A content of the plasma may rise considerably above normal.

Xanthosis cutis in normal persons, in diabetics, and in hypothyroidism is associated with an increase of carotene in the plasma, less often of xanthophyll. In severe untreated diabetes the tissues may not be able to metabolize carotene rapidly. In nephrosis and in severe chronic nephritis hypercarotinemia may occur without xanthosis cutis. In Bright's disease the level of plasma vitamin A may be greatly elevated, probably because the liver fails to store it. In hypothyroidism the carotinoids of the plasma may be elevated and the vitamin A may be low. Successful treatment with thyroid substance corrects the anomaly. In celiac disease the carotinoids and vitamin A are not readily absorbed.

REFERENCES

1. Moore, T.: Lancet **2**: 380, 1929.
2. Dániel, E. v., and Béres, T.: Ztschr. f. phys. Chem. **238**: 160, 1936.
3. Connor, C. L.: J. Biol. Chem. **77**: 619, 1928.
4. Clausen, S. W., and McCoord, A. B.: J. Biol. Chem. **113**: 89, 1936.
5. McCoord, A. B., and Luce-Clausen, E. M.: J. Nutrition **7**: 557, 1934.
6. Clausen, S. W., and McCoord, A. B.: J. A. M. A. **101**: 1383, 1933.
7. Chesney, J., and McCoord, A. B.: Proc. Soc. Exper. Biol. & Med. **31**: 887, 1934.
8. Fasold, H., and Heidemann, E. R.: Ztschr. f. d. ges. exper. Med. **92**: 53, 1933-34.
9. McCoord, A. B., and Clausen, S. W.: Paper read before the Section on Biological Chemistry, American Chemical Society Meeting, Kansas City, Missouri, April 14, 1936.
10. Breese, B. B., Jr., and McCoord, A. B.: To be published.

EXPERIMENTAL THERAPY OF ACUTE LEUCEMIA WITH EXTRACTS OF BONE MARROW

Jean V. Cooke, M.D.
St. Louis, Mo.

THE nature of leucemia and leucemic diseases has been the subject of much speculation, and the conceptions of its character have been based only on certain similarities between the symptoms or the pathologic lesions in the disease and those of other conditions the nature of which is somewhat better known. The two hypotheses which are most frequently mentioned have attributed the disease to a neoplastic change or to infection. Neither of these is supported by proof, and the analogies are not especially convincing.

The *neoplastic hypothesis* is founded on the presence of extensive active proliferation of cells in the marrow and blood, the secondary local tumorlike masses often containing mitoses in distant organs, and, in some cases, certain clinical symptoms such as anemia, asthenia, and loss in weight, which are common to malignant tumors. In addition, the proliferating cells in leucemia are usually radiosensitive as are certain neoplastic growths. On the other hand, leucemia differs considerably from malignant tumors in that the latter originate in a single group of cells which proliferate locally, while the stimulus to proliferation in leucemia is widespread and affects not a single group of marrow cells but most if not all of the marrow tissue of the body. The secondary organ and tissue metastases in leucemia, also, while composed of proliferating cells, do not tend to invade the surrounding tissue in the manner of malignant neoplasms. In those instances in which the leucemic cells spread from the edges into adjacent tissue, the morphologic appearance is not that of a malignant tumor but rather that seen in the slow infiltration of wandering inflammatory cells. The chief resemblance to a neoplastic type of disease is in those cases of leucemia with hyperleucocytosis while those without leucocytosis and with only slight or moderate infiltrations have little in common with newgrowths.

The *infective hypothesis* is suggested chiefly by those cases of acute leucemia in which such symptoms as toxemia and prostration, purpura, and fever often high and of a septic type have simulated the picture of an acute infection. This view has been apparently supported by the presence in certain instances of preceding or accompanying lesions of an infectious origin in the mouth or throat, although such recognizable infections are relatively inconstant. Chronic forms of leucemia show no

From the Department of Pediatrics, Washington University School of Medicine, and the St. Louis Children's Hospital.

striking clinical resemblance to infections. Against the infective hypothesis it has been urged that no bacteria have been isolated from the blood or tissues except in occasional instances in which obvious severe intercurrent or terminal secondary infection was present; that no organisms are visible in microscopic examination of leucemic tissues nor do the tissue lesions suggest infection; that although an invisible filtrable virus cannot be excluded as the causative agent, the symptoms and course of leucemia do not resemble those characteristic of virus disease; that there is no evidence of the transmissibility in human beings; and that in age and sex selectivity leucemia differs from those diseases resulting from infections.

The present paper concerns certain experimental observations made at the St. Louis Children's Hospital on patients with acute leucemia to test the validity of a new and different hypothesis as to the nature of the disease. This hypothesis assumes that acute leucemia is due to an acquired defect in normal marrow function characterized by the inactivation or destruction of one of the normal factors in hematopoiesis. Before stating the hypothesis in more detail, certain observations about acute leucemia will be reviewed.

The primary site of the disturbance in leucemia is the bone marrow. In the chronic myelogenous type this has never been questioned, since the cells involved are obviously myelogenic. In the acute forms of childhood, the hyperplastic abnormal nongranular leucocytes characteristic of the disease were earlier thought to be abnormal lymphocytes, and the disease was spoken of as "acute lymphatic leucemia." However, even in the acute forms the marrow is the principal seat of generalized and extensive cellular hyperplasia. In addition the abnormal cells in the circulating blood have been shown[1] to contain abundant proteolytic ferment and in this respect resemble closely myelogenous cells (granular leucocytes) and differ from lymphocytes which do not possess such proteolytic activity. This is additional evidence that the cells in acute leucemia are of myelogenous origin, probably myeloblasts, and that the bone marrow is the organ chiefly involved. The most constant characteristics of the blood in acute leucemia are associated with an aplasia of the normal formed elements, all of which have their origin in the bone marrow. Thrombopenia and anemia are constant as well as a marked decrease in the granular leucocytes. Of the few granular cells present, many are young and immature so that a disturbance in maturation of the granular leucocytes is one of the striking features of the disease.

In the mechanism of normal marrow hematopoiesis there must be certain chemical factors which regulate the development and maturation of the leucocytes. The delicate balance and lability of this mechanism are constantly demonstrated. It is possible that the production of these specific substances (maturation factors) controlling such development and maturation of marrow cells may be injured or inhibited by certain types of toxic injury. As examples of disturbances in such regulating mechanisms may be mentioned that involving the control of erythropoiesis by the liver fraction effective in the relief of pernicious anemia, the control of sugar metabolism by insulin, and the maintenance of calcium balance by parathormone. In poisoning by benzol, radium and roentgen irradiation, the resulting granulopenia is conceivably due to an injury of the enzymes or other factors which control the maturation of granular cells. The defective granulopoiesis constant in acute leucemia may therefore have its origin in the toxin-produced deficiency of a substance necessary to normal leucocytic development.

In attempting to explain the origin of such hypothetical toxic injury in acute leucemia, it is of interest that the disease has had a notable incidence among x-ray workers, and that acute bacterial infections have preceded the onset in a number of instances.

Regarding the proliferation of immature marrow elements and their appearance in the circulating blood in acute leucemia, it is possible that such a change is secondary to the disturbance in the mechanism of maturation mentioned, associated with failure of these young cells to mature, or to the eventual exhaustion of normal inhibiting factors. If one can assume that the physiology of normal blood formation depends on the continued presence of such specific actively secreted substances regulating cellular development and maturation, it is not difficult to conceive a later unrestrained proliferation of immature marrow cells such as are found in acute leucemia, when the normal control of the mechanism is lost and certain inhibiting factors are also lost or exhausted.

If one can attribute acute leucemia to toxic injury of a certain hypothetical factor concerned with maturation of the granular leucocytes, it follows that chronic myelogenous leucemia, in which there is an obvious overactivity in development and maturation of the granulocytes, might result from their excessive stimulation by a pathologic hyperfunction of the maturation process.

The conception of acute leucemia as a deficiency disease in which dysfunction of the marrow results from the absence of a secretion necessary for normal granulopoiesis suggested the possibility of testing such an hypothesis by attempting to supply the missing element through the parenteral injection of animal tissue extracts. After making a few observations with the use of extracts of liver, spleen, and thymus, without apparent effect, it was decided to study the effect of the injection of extracts of fresh red bone marrow on acute leucemia, and the results of these studies form the basis of this paper.

BONE MARROW EXTRACT IN ACUTE LEUCEMIA—EARLIER EXPERIMENTS

Preparation of Marrow Extract.—The earlier observations were made with several simple aqueous extracts prepared for me by Dr. G. H. A.

Clowes, of Eli Lilly and Company. These consisted of an aqueous extraction of finely ground beef ribs with a considerable volume of water, and later with 50 per cent alcohol. The extracts were combined, strained, evaporated to dryness *in vacuo* and defatted with gasoline. The residue was then taken up with water in proportion of about one part to ten and, after mixing twenty-four hours, was filtered through a Berkefeld candle. They were of a brown color and contained approximately 100 mg. of nitrogen per 100 c.c.

Injection into rabbits and guinea pigs showed no toxic effect and produced no constant change in the blood picture over several weeks. The action of two of the extracts on blood pressure was tested on dogs and one of them showed a definite pressor effect with increase in blood pressure of 12 to 15 mm. of mercury. The second extract had the usual depressor action of most tissue extracts. In children, subcutaneous or intramuscular injections were irritating and painful, the site often remaining tender and slightly swollen for a day or two, and at times a moderate febrile reaction lasting several hours followed the injections.

The effect of the marrow extracts on patients with acute leucemia in the St. Louis Children's Hospital was observed during a period of three years and brief summaries of several cases follow. In all summaries much irrelevant material and many details have been omitted although careful records were made over the many months of observation summarized.

CASE 1.—B. N., a 3-year-old boy, had been ill for three months when admitted on Sept. 9, 1931. He had had recurring fever, a poor appetite, and an increasing pallor. Within the previous month "bruised spots" had appeared on his legs from time to time, asthenia, some dyspnea, and enlargement of the cervical lymph nodes had developed, and four days before admission there had been a nasal hemorrhage lasting one hour. On examination, in addition to the skin hemorrhages, marked pallor and enlarged cervical nodes, the spleen and liver were both firm and easily felt below the costal margin, and the child was feverish and acutely ill. The blood showed 800,000 erythrocytes, 50,000 platelets, and 3,000 leucocytes of which 92 per cent were young nongranular mononuclear leucemic cells. The clotting time was 6 minutes and the bleeding time more than 10 minutes. One transfusion of 175 c.c. was given the day after admission following which the erythrocytes were slightly over one million.

On the fourth day after admission, marrow extract was given subcutaneously in doses of 2 c.c. and then increased to 5 c.c. daily. Little change was noted until the end of a week when the temperature, which had ranged from 38° to 40° C. (100.4° to 104° F.) and usually above 39° C. (102.2° F.), fell to normal (September 18), the enlargement of the cervical nodes disappeared, and the boy became alert, interested, and much improved clinically.

As clinical improvement continued, the spleen could no longer be felt (September 29), and he was able to be up in a wheel chair. During this time the red cells had gradually risen to 2,400,000 without further transfusion and the platelets were 150,000. The leucocytes, which had fallen to 1,500 a week after admission, had gradually risen to 6,200, and the granular cells were 45 per cent although abnormal leucemic cells were still present. Improvement continued during the next two weeks, and the child was able to walk around the ward. The temperature remained below 38° C. (100.4° F.), appetite was good, and the patient had gained 4½ pounds. There were no complaints except pain from the subcutaneous injections of marrow extract. The red count rose to 3,500,000, the platelets remained above 100,000, and the leucocytes varied from 9,500 to 12,700 with 34 to 41 per cent granular cells. Marrow extract injections which had been given daily for thirty days were discontinued on October 12.

A week later the patient had become cross and irritable, the spleen had increased in size to the level of the umbilicus, leucocytes had risen to 21,500 with only 3 per cent granular cells, and the erythrocytes had fallen to 2,300,000. Bone marrow extract injections were resumed in doses of 5 c.c. twice daily (Oct. 19), but the condition changed little except for the appearance of a number of skin hemorrhages, an epistaxis which required transfusion, and an increase in leucocytes to 35,000. By the end of two weeks (November 1), however, there was considerable clinical improvement, and the spleen had again receded in size and the leucocyte count had fallen to 3,000 with only 1 to 3 per cent granular cells. Clinical improvement continued, and by November 16 with increasing appetite the patient regained 3 pounds he had lost during his relapse, although blood during this time had remained leucopenic and granulopenic.

At this time the leucocytes began to rise and during the next month ranged from 6,000 to 12,000 with the granular cells varying from 16 to 24 per cent. The general clinical condition remained good, although the spleen became slightly larger. Shortly after the onset of this improvement in the blood, the marrow extract previously used became exhausted and a different preparation was employed. This second extract produced several somewhat severe and alarming reactions of an allergic type (edema of the face, hives, cyanosis and dyspnea) on several occasions and it was given only every second day in smaller doses. During the following month the leucocytes varied from 4,000 to 12,000 with the granular cells from 16 to 24 per cent, and the platelets from 50,000 to 80,000. There were no hemorrhages, and the patient was alert, active, and cheerful although the extract injections produced slight fever and occasionally allergic symptoms.

By December 14, the clinical condition was unchanged. There were no more allergic reactions, but, after each injection, the patient was feverish and listless and had just recovered from its effect by the time the next injection was given two days later. The extract produced very painful local reactions which persisted several days. The spleen had become considerably larger, but the blood continued essentially the same and erythrocytes had remained somewhat over 2,000,000 with no transfusions for more than two months. On December 28 he became much worse, with vomiting, fever which rose rapidly to over 40° C. (104° F.), and the granulocytes fell to 3 per cent of 7,000 leucocytes. Epistaxis and hematuria developed, high temperature continued, and death occurred Jan. 1, 1932. Necropsy showed leucemic infiltrations but no manifest evidence of infection.

Comment.—Distinct abatement of the leucemic toxic symptoms followed the continued use of bone marrow extract, and the blood also showed considerable improvement. There appeared to be a recession of the disease without true remission. The fact that the child recovered from a rather acute toxic phase of leucemia and lived four months with relatively mild symptoms from the disease was unusual and unexpected, and was attributed to the bone marrow therapy. The recurrence of acute leucemic symptoms shortly after injections were discontinued and their later recession, together with improvement in the blood after the extract was resumed, was also encouraging.

CASE 2.—B. B., a 5-year-old girl, had had scarlet fever 2 months before admission to the hospital on May 24, 1932. The cervical nodes had remained swollen, the child had lost weight and became progressively more pale; high fever together with large and small skin hemorrhages had been present for the week preceding. On examination, the patient was pale and acutely ill with fever of 40° C. (104° F.), cervical glands much enlarged, with axillary and inguinal glands and spleen slightly enlarged, many skin petechiae and ecchymoses. The blood showed anemia (2,700,000), thrombopenia, and 5,500 leucocytes of which 95 per cent were nongranular large leucemic mononuclear cells.

Bone marrow extract was started immediately in doses of 2 c.c. twice daily, and two transfusions were given. The temperature remained high for three days but thereafter fell to around 38° C. (100.4° F.), and the patient became clinically better. In the next two weeks this improvement continued, and the child was afebrile after a cervical abscess was incised and was able to be up in a wheel chair. The granulocytes rose to from 16 to 18 per cent without other change in the blood.

The child remained in the hospital six months with relatively slight change in her clinical state. She received marrow extract almost daily and several transfusions. During much of the time she was up in a wheel chair, cheerful, with good appetite and gaining slightly in weight. Once an abscess developed at the site of an injection and had to be drained. At times she was irritable and had some fever for periods of several days. There were no further hemorrhages, and the spleen remained only slightly enlarged. The leucocyte count varied from 5,000 to 12,000 except for one period of ten days during which it rose temporarily to 20,000 to 30,000 a few weeks after admission. The granular cells remained from 8 to 12 per cent, and the platelets continued to be less than 100,000. On Nov. 6, 1932, she developed a lobar pneumonia and died five days later. No necropsy was obtained.

CASE 3.—G. M., 5-year-old boy, had been pale and weak for three months when admitted to the hospital on Oct. 14, 1932. He had enlarged cervical lymph nodes, a palpable spleen, anemia (1,460,000 erythrocytes), decreased platelet count, and 9,000 leucocytes, of which 97 per cent were large nongranular mononuclear leucemic cells. Treatment consisted of several transfusions and, later, marrow extract injections. During the following six months there was only slight clinical improvement, but the patient remained cheerful and comfortable, although chronically ill. The blood continued typically leucemic, and once the leucocytes reached 46,000 although most of the time the count was less than 15,000. The granular cells remained low, and thrombopenia continued. Biopsy section of a cervical lymph node was typical of acute leucemia. In the seventeenth week he developed an acute otitis and temporary hemolytic streptococcus septicemia with the appearance a few weeks later of metastatic infectious foci near several joints which required incision, but which did not heal well. Death occurred in the twenty-seventh week after admission (April 19, 1933). No necropsy.

CASE 4.—B. B., a 2½-year-old girl, whose increasing pallor for three months had been the only symptom, was seen first on April 13, 1934, with a slightly enlarged spleen and a few small skin hemorrhages, leucocytes 5,500 with 96 per cent nongranular leucemic cells, platelets greatly reduced, and erythrocytes 1,700,000. Bone marrow extract injections were given daily, and the erythrocytes were brought to 3,000,000 by transfusion. She improved clinically and during the next three months was comfortable and without complaints, gained 3 pounds in weight; the erythrocytes remained about 3 million without transfusion. Occasionally transient fever was noted. Leucocytes showed little change, ranging from 3,000 to 6,000, although the granular cells at times increased slightly, at one time reaching 35 per cent but usually varying from 10 to 15 per cent

Marrow extract injections were discontinued after two months, and four weeks later fever appeared with subsequent skin petechiae and finally a severe intestinal hemorrhage followed by *B. coli* bacteremia, terminal bronchopneumonia, and death on July 14, 1934. No necropsy was obtained.

CASE 5.—C. M., 6-year-old boy, had had anemia for two months and slightly enlarged cervical lymph nodes for one month before admission on Feb. 25, 1934. He was asthenic and had a palpable spleen but no hemorrhages or fever. The blood was typical of acute leucemia without leucocytosis, and biopsy of an inguinal lymph node showed typical leucemic infiltration. During the following six months he received several transfusions and daily marrow extract injections for considerable periods, with no significant change in the blood picture at any time. Much of this time the patient was comfortable, happy, but moderately asthenic. At certain periods he was able to be up in a wheel chair. During the second month intercurrent hemolytic streptococcus infection of the ears and mastoid occurred and subsided, and in the third month a cervical abscess had to be incised. The spleen became moderately enlarged, but there were no hemorrhages.

Early in the sixth month the patient became rapidly much worse, the cervical nodes and spleen increased greatly in size, there developed obstructive orthopnea with inspiratory retraction of the interspaces, edema of the face, brassy cough, and slight cyanosis, and fluoroscopic examination showed an increased mediastinal shadow. Although he had been receiving injections of a marrow extract every second day during this time, the substitution of another extract in slightly larger daily doses was immediately followed by a somewhat dramatic clinical improvement. The orthopnea disappeared within a day or so, and there was very definite decrease in the size of the cervical and other nodes and the spleen. These changes seemed too prompt and striking to be merely coincidental. No alteration in the blood occurred although the enlargement of glands and spleen had receded. The patient remained listless and asthenic but without complaints. Appetite continued fairly good, and there were no hemorrhages. Three weeks later he died suddenly and somewhat unexpectedly (August 20) after an attack of vomiting and abdominal pain. There was no necropsy.

CASE 6.—C. M. L., a 6-month-old colored girl, with pallor of 2 months' duration was first seen June 12, 1934. All lymph nodes were visibly enlarged, spleen and liver greatly swollen, and the blood count showed 304,000 leucocytes all nongranular mononuclear leucemic cells. After three daily injections of marrow extract, the leucocytes were 5,000 with 13 per cent granular cells; the lymph nodes, liver, and spleen had decreased in size so strikingly that they were barely palpable. Fever, thrombopenia, and granulopenia persisted although the total leucocyte count remained low, and the infant died about four weeks after admission of bronchopneumonia and bullous impetigo. There was no necropsy.

Comment.—In Cases 2 to 6 the results of the marrow therapy were considerably less encouraging than in Case 1. In certain instances there was some increased maturation of granular cells, but the changes in the blood picture were relatively transient and not especially striking. Clinically, one patient (Case 2) recovered from a rather alarming acute, febrile, toxic state apparently caused by the leucemia in a short time after the injections were started, and in two other patients (Cases 5 and

6) there was rather prompt and striking shrinking of lymph nodes and spleen. Clinical improvement in the general condition was common, and four of the children lived somewhat longer periods (three for six months, and one for three months) in the hospital than is usual for patients with acute leucemia. They had relatively few acute symptoms and were comfortable and happy, although somewhat asthenic, for long periods. In one instance (Case 4) more acute symptoms recurred after the marrow extract was stopped, and two children (Cases 3 and 5) were able to resist severe acute streptococcus infections for a number of weeks. In these cases it seemed possible that the marrow extracts had been of some benefit in arresting the progress of the disease.

During this period several other children were admitted to the St. Louis Children's Hospital with acute leucemia but died in a few days or were removed when the diagnosis was made. The only patient under observation more than a week received marrow extract injections for 12 days with no apparent effect.

The results described were considered of sufficient interest to warrant further observation on the effect of marrow extracts but difficulty was encountered in devising a method by which red marrow could be secured sufficiently fresh and in adequate amount for preparing extracts. Eventually through the interest and cooperation of Mr. Charles Heim, Superintendent of the American Packing Company of St. Louis, such material became available. Mr. Heim devised and had made a machine for this work which would rapidly and cleanly break up fresh beef ribs into small bits; it was possible to start the preparation of an extract within 2 hours after the animal was killed.

BONE MARROW EXTRACTS IN ACUTE LEUCEMIA—LATER SERIES

Preparation of Later Extracts.—Ten pounds of fresh macerated beef ribs were extracted with 7,500 c.c. of water to which sufficient concentrated hydrochloric acid had been added to make 3 per cent by volume. After two hours the mixture was strained, and the residue again extracted for two hours with a like volume (7,500 c.c.) of 1.5 per cent hydrochloric acid. After straining off the coarse material, the residue was brought to pH 7.0 with sodium hydroxide. This appeared to be the isoelectric point for the protein present, and it was readily removed by filtration, leaving a water-clear filtrate. This filtrate was then concentrated rapidly in an evaporator, by which warmed air was fanned continuously over flat pans and drawn off by suction, the temperature of the extract being kept below 40° C. When the volume had been reduced to somewhat less than 10 per cent of the original, the extract was filtered and was sterilized by passing through a Mandler candle. Each 100 c.c. of the concentrated extract represented approximately one pound of the original ground ribs.

These extracts were clear, neutral, and of varying degrees of amber tint. They had a high content of sodium chloride and considerable calcium and phosphate. An analysis of five separate preparations showed a total nitrogen content varying from 128 to 265, nonprotein nitrogen from 93 to 151, and the coagulable protein nitrogen from 9 to 154 mg. per cent. They were not toxic when injected subcutaneously into laboratory animals in doses of 2 to 5 c.c.

Since subcutaneous injections in children were extremely painful and irritating, a very limited use of the extracts during the next year or so resulted because it did not appear justified to subject children regularly to so much pain and discomfort. During this time the irritating salts were dialyzed out of one extract, but a single patient treated with this preparation showed no apparent effect, and no further effort at purification was made. To avoid the local irritation, it was later decided to inject the extract intravenously, and in 1936 it was used in 10 c.c. doses diluted to 50 c.c. with sterile water in a patient with acute leucemia without any discomfort from the injection. He showed very slight clinical improvement following the injections but died from a severe pulmonary hemolytic streptococcus infection a few days later. In subsequent use of the extracts the intravenous route was employed routinely, usually in amounts of from 2 to 5 c.c. diluted several times with water and given slowly. The largest amount given has been 20 c.c.

Several case reports showing the results with these concentrated extracts follow:

CASE 7.—R. G., a 16-year-old boy, who had lost 25 pounds in a month and had several severe nosebleeds, was first seen Dec. 28, 1936, after having received several transfusions. There was no complaint except some weakness, and examination revealed a huge spleen which extended below the navel, enlarged inguinal lymph nodes and a slight erosion on the left nasal septum which had a tendency to bleed and require packing. There was no anemia but a definite thrombopenia, and the leucocytes numbered 105,000 with more than 90 per cent nongranular mononuclear leucemic cells. Daily injections of marrow extract were started and continued in doses of 2 to 3 c.c. intravenously.

During the following month the patient was quite comfortable, with fairly good appetite; he had no complaints but gradually lost weight. Severe epistaxis continued at intervals and necessitated several transfusions. There was no change in the size of the spleen. The erythrocytes remained around 2,000,000; the leucocytes fell gradually to 39,000, but the granulocytes increased to 25 per cent, although 8 per cent were immature forms; and the platelets remained low.

At one time during this period a transfusion of chronic myelogenous leucemia blood was given this patient. The donor was an adult in the same blood group (O) who had a total leucocyte count of 450,000 with typical clinical and blood picture of chronic myelogenous leucemia. No clinical change or detectable alteration in the blood picture of the recipient followed this transfusion.

In the second month there was little clinical change, and the patient remained cheerful, was without fever and spent much time sitting in bed reading. Because of severe nasal hemorrhage, transfusions had to be given several times to keep the red count above 2 million. The leucocytes continued to fall and reached 4,000 (February 28), but with 53 per cent granulocytes, while the platelets remained much decreased.

The third month in the hospital was complicated by several febrile infections, tonsillitis in the first week, from which he apparently recovered. The appetite became poor, weakness increased, hemorrhagic oozing continued from the nose, and after irregular fever for two weeks the patient died March 28 with hemolytic streptococcus sepsis. During the last month of life the leucocytes varied from 4,000 to 20,000 but the granular cells remained high (40 to 65 per cent) although pathologic leucemic cells were always present and thrombopenia persisted. Necropsy showed in addition to typical leucemic infiltrations of the viscera, bronchopneumonia with pulmonary abscess, serofibrinous pleurisy, and general peritonitis (hemolytic streptococcus).

Comment.—Although there was little clinical improvement in this patient and thrombopenia persisted, with recurring hemorrhage from an ulceration on the nasal septum, the hyperleucocytosis disappeared and there was a rather striking increase in granular cells in the blood, many of which were mature. Also, the disease did not progress as rapidly as was anticipated on admission, and three months elapsed before terminal intercurrent infection occurred. The transfusion of chronic myelogenous leucemic blood was tried only because of the possibility that the overactivity in maturation and development of the granular cells in chronic myelogenous leucemia might be associated with the presence in the blood of factors which could be transferred to a patient with acute leucemia. The experiment was apparently harmless and the result inconclusive.

CASE 8.—W. H., a 5½-year-old boy, first seen July 24, 1937, had a history of gradually increasing pallor and weakness for six weeks. There was a slight general glandular enlargement and the submandibular nodes were considerably swollen, firm and tender. Many petechiae and a few ecchymoses spotted the arms and legs. The liver extended two fingerbreadths below the costal margin, and the firm spleen reached below the umbilicus. The blood picture was typical of acute leucemia, with prolonged bleeding time (9 min.) and clotting time (4 min.); very few platelets; 2.5 million erythrocytes with 45 per cent hemoglobin; and 7,000 leucocytes of which 97 per cent were abnormal nongranular mononuclear cells of the leucemic type. On admission to the hospital he was acutely ill and moderately toxic, with fever of 39° C. (102.2° F.) On the face and scalp were a number of impetigo lesions of two days' duration, and the left knee was somewhat swollen and tender. During the following week hemolytic streptococci were grown from the blood on two occasions and additional localizations developed in the right shoulder and right leg. The picture then was that of streptococcus sepsis with severe toxicity and continued high fever (39° to 40° C.). An area of pneumonia had developed in the left lung by the end of the second week, and new skin lesions continued to appear; the arm and leg foci remained swollen and painful; and the fever and toxicity persisted unabated. There was little change in his condition during the third week except that the temperature was slightly lower and the pneumonic area cleared. The prognosis was considered hopeless and death imminent.

Two days after admission intravenous injections of marrow extract were started and continued daily in doses of 2 to 4 c.c. for four days. After the fourth injection the cervical nodes had regressed until they were no longer visible although they were still palpable. The spleen, which had been below the umbilicus, was barely palpable and three days later could not be felt. The extract injections were later continued every second or third day. The blood showed little change from the first examination except that a leucopenia varying from 600 to 3,000 developed, the thrombopenia continued, and the granulocytes were only 1 to 3 per cent. By the end of the first week when streptococcus sepsis was apparent, two transfusions were given, and sulfanilamide was started and continued in doses of 1.0 gm. (15 gr.) three times daily. Marrow extract injections were continued from two to three times weekly.

In the fourth week a series of remarkable changes occurred. The infectious focus in the right upper arm which had subsided somewhat, suddenly became more swollen and fluctuant, and those in the right and left legs simultaneously suppurated. The temperature fell to 38° C. (100.4° F.) within a few days, and the boy was definitely improved and more alert. On examination of the blood, it was found that the leucocytes had increased from 4,600 on August 18 to 14,000 on August 24 with abundant platelets (798,000), 73 per cent granulocytes, and no abnormal cells. The abscesses were incised and drained without excessive bleeding. Smears showed

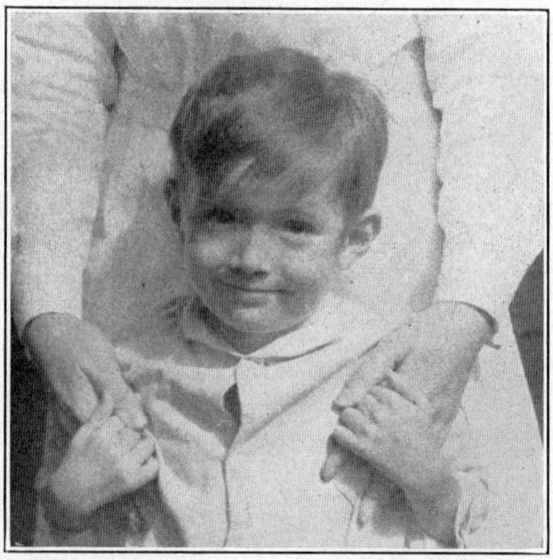

Fig. 1.—Five-year-old boy (Case 8) during remission of acute leucemia.

pus cells and many gram-positive cocci in chains and some in clumps, but on culture only *Staphylococcus aureus* was grown.

With the incision of the abscesses, improvement was continuous, the wounds healed, and the patient was happy and playful. The temperature remained below 38° C. (100.4° F.) After four weeks a mild pneumonitis with fever of 38° to 40° C. (100.4° to 104° F.) lasting a few days caused some concern, but the pulmonary signs and shadow disappeared within a week or so. For a period of two months the only other symptoms were moderate asthenia and slight fever. The boy gained several pounds, was cheerful and happy, and was able to walk around the ward (Fig. 1). The color remained good, and no transfusion was necessary for a period of six weeks. The blood examination continued to show abundant platelets; the total count varied from 8,000 to 19,000, the higher figure being obtained during the acute pulmonary infection. Granular cells varied from 40 to 80 per cent.

In the seventh week after the first sudden change in the blood picture the leucocytes began to increase in number and within a few days (Oct. 12) reached 50,000, with the granulocytes being reduced to about 10 per cent. A great reduction in platelets and the return of young nongranular mononuclear leucemic cells were noted. Following a increase in marrow extract injections, the leucocytes fell within a week to 9,000, but there was no change in the differential picture and the platelets remained low. During this time there was little change in the patient's clinical condition and he remained alert, playful and happy in spite of a fever of about 38.3° C. (101° F.) The spleen which had not been palpable for more than two months began to enlarge again and within ten days reached the umbilicus (Oct. 23). There was very slight enlargement of the axillary and cervical nodes, but a few ecchymoses were noted (October 25) on the legs. During the following week he became more irritable and feverish. The terminal picture was a *Staphylococcus aureus* septicemia with multiple skin and subcutaneous abscesses, and death occurred Nov. 13, 1937. No necropsy was allowed.

Comment.—The rather remarkable clinical and blood remission in this patient developed suddenly and the reappearance of granular leucocytes in the blood was accompanied by prompt suppuration of metastatic infectious foci which had previously been indolent. The recovery from a generalized streptococcus infection which appeared hopeless was also entirely unexpected and was attributed to sulfanilamide therapy. The recurrence of an acute leucemic blood picture almost two months later was soon followed by a return of clinical signs of the disease, and neither was affected by continued marrow therapy.

CASE 9.—I. M., a 3-year-old girl, was first seen Sept. 6, 1937, with high fever of several days' duration and anemia for two months. Physical examination was negative except for a fever of 40.7° C. (105.3° F.), and a mild tonsillitis of Vincent's type. There was no glandular or splenic enlargement. The blood revealed an anemia of 2,250,000 erythrocytes (40 per cent hemoglobin), thrombopenia (37,000), and 42,000 leucocytes, of which 98 per cent were nongranular mononuclear leucemic cells. Treatment with daily intravenous injections of marrow extract and transfusions was started immediately. The temperature remained above 40° C. (104° F.) for five days but fell to normal within the next four days; she remained afebrile thereafter, except for an occasional slight rise attributed to the intravenous injection. Within three days after admission the leucocytes had fallen to 3,200 without other change in the blood except an increase in erythrocytes to 3 million as a result of transfusions. Clinical improvement continued and two and one-half weeks after admission (September 22), the leucocytes were 8,200 with a normal-looking differential count in which there were 20 per cent relatively mature granular neutrophiles, and a very definite increase in platelets. At this time she was able to be up and was running about the ward (Fig. 2). The spleen was not enlarged but at times could be palpated at the costal margin. During the next four weeks, the patient continued active, afebrile, and without complaints except occasionally transient abdominal pain. The erythrocytes remained at 4.5 to 5 million without transfusion, and the leucocytes ranged from 6,800 to 13,000 with 22 to 30 per cent granular cells, most of which were segmented. Of the lymphocytes, only careful scrutiny prompted by a knowledge of the diagnosis of leucemia revealed that some still had characteristics suggestive of young nongranular leucemic cells. The platelets numbered 170,000, and many were of an abnormally large size. Marrow extract injection had been given about three times weekly. The weight increased 3 pounds while she was in the hospital.

Since the patient lived at a distance and had improved so much, it was decided to discharge her for a visit to her home; this was done on Oct. 15, 1937. A blood count made by her physician the following week showed 21,200 leucocytes with 92 per cent lymphocytes, and she was brought back to the hospital. During this week she had had no marrow therapy, but it was resumed on readmission (October 22) and continued in doses of 2 to 5 c.c. three or four times weekly for the next six weeks. During this time the child appeared well and was able to be up and about, had good appetite, no fever or other complaints, and gained 2½ pounds. The spleen remained just palpable, and one brief epistaxis occurred during this time. The blood, however, was definitely leucemic and apparently unaffected by the marrow injections. Leucocytes varied from 12,000 to 69,000 and were typical nongranular young leucemic cells, the granular cells being less than 5 per cent. The platelets continued to be of large size, and the count also remained very low (25,000).

The erythrocytes decreased gradually to 2 million, and two transfusions brought their number back to over 4 million but produced no change in the leucocytic picture. The leucocytes numbered 34,000 with 2 per cent granular cells at the time of discharge, on December 7, when the patient was again taken home and received no

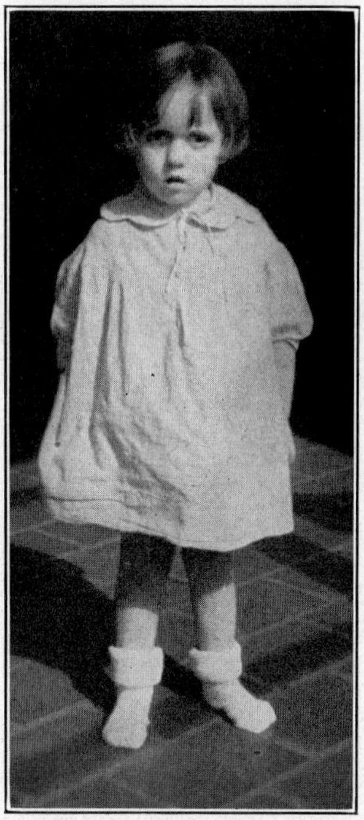

Fig. 2.—Three-year-old girl (Case 9) during remission of acute leucemia.

further treatment. She remained asymptomatic for a week and then became quite irritable, complained of abdominal and joint pains, and developed increasing asthenia and pallor. Three weeks after discharge (December 22) she had a profuse and continued epistaxis with fatal exsanguination.

Comment.—This patient recovered promptly from a toxic febrile attack, hyperleucocytosis disappeared, and the blood remission and clinical improvement which followed shortly were striking and persisted for several weeks. That the recurrence of a leucemic blood picture was related to the discontinuing of the marrow extract injections is doubtful although with their resumption the weight increased and there were no clinical signs of disease for a number of weeks.

CASE 10.—S. D., a previously healthy 18-month-old girl, was first seen Nov. 14, 1937, with multiple skin ecchymoses and fever of a week's duration. Very slight general glandular enlargement, a considerably swollen liver and spleen, and fever of 38.8° C. (101.7° F.) were the only physical signs. Leucocytes numbered 43,000 with 97 per cent nongranular mononuclear leucemic cells, platelets much reduced (58,000), and a slight anemia (4,000,000) with 8.5 gm. hemoglobin.

In the following two months, during which the patient was given two series of injections of marrow extract intravenously and several transfusions, there was continued anorexia with loss of weight, and a progressive anemia. A month after admission the leucocytosis had disappeared, and the total count was 1,500 to 3,000 with granulopenia and thrombopenia. Fever persisted and an acute bilateral otitis media developed followed by chronic ear discharge. At one time severe hematuria lasted several days.

In the tenth week (Jan. 19, 1938) after admission, the temperature fell to normal, and the blood, which on the previous day had shown thrombopenia, 5,200 leucocytes with 10 per cent granulocytes, was found to have 4,900 leucocytes with 68

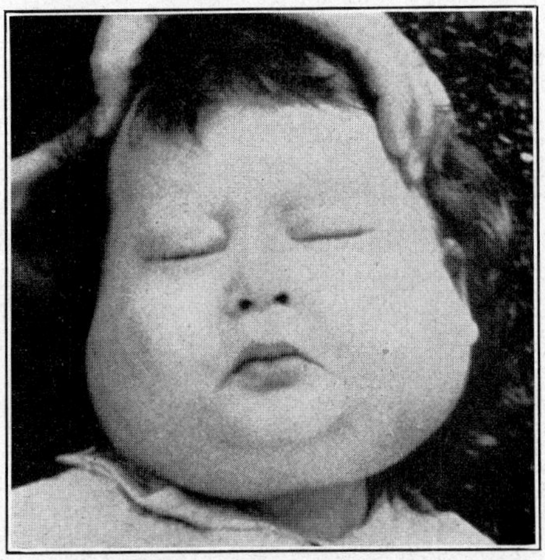

Fig. 3.—Extensive bilateral parotid swelling in 20-month-old girl (Case 10) during blood remission. (From 16 mm. film.)

per cent granulocytes and no abnormal cells. The platelets had become abundant (328,000). From this time the clinical improvement was rapid, and the patient was discharged two weeks later (Feb. 5, 1938) with a normal leucocyte count (7,900) and differential (6 stab, 48 segmented cells, 44 lymphocytes, and 2 monocytes), abundant platelets and no anemia.

The following eleven weeks the patient spent at home and was seen weekly at the hospital for observation, blood examination, and an injection of marrow extract. During the first month she gained 5½ pounds and was active, playful, and apparently in normal health although a slight chronic otorrhea persisted and both the liver and spleen remained considerably enlarged and firm. The erythrocytes rapidly rose to over 5,000,000 and leucocytes varied from 7 to 12,000 with a normal differential picture, the granulocytes ranging from 24 to 52 per cent. In the sixth week at home (March 16) a bilateral soft swelling of the parotid glands was first noted. These gradually increased in size and five weeks later they had become quite firm, as large as lemons, with much edema of the face and eyes, and with a similar swelling also of the submental tissues. The clinical appearance was that of Mikulicz's syndrome. She was readmitted to the St. Louis Children's Hospital (April 25), and for a period of two weeks large doses (5 to 20 c.c.) of the bone marrow extract were given intravenously each day with no apparent effect on the swellings which continued to enlarge until she could not open her eyes (Fig. 3). There was no fever, and the leucocytes still ranged from 6,800 to 8,000 with 44 to 60 per cent granulocytes and no detectable abnormalities in the smear.

Biopsy of a cervical lymph node in the region of the parotid was performed on May 5, and the pathologic report by Dr. H. B. McCordock follows:

"The original architecture of the lymph node is obliterated by a dense tumorlike growth of one type of cell which replaces the germinal centers and obscures the sinuses. Dense masses of new formed cells infiltrate the connective tissue framework of the node, but not the capsule. The infiltrating cells are slightly larger than small lymphocytes and contain coarsely reticular and deeply stained nuclei. The cytoplasm is so scant that it can be recognized with certainty only in isolated cells which infiltrate connective tissue spaces. Mitotic figures are numerous."

Although the danger of irradiation in acute leucemic states was appreciated, the continued growth of the parotid masses, the fact that the blood picture had been normal for more than three months, the microscopic appearance of the excised lymph node, together with parental insistence that something be done, combined to induce the trial of x-ray therapy over the tumor masses. During a period of ten days (May 9 to May 18) nine irradiations totaling 1,250 roentgen units were given. Ten days after the last irradiation the swellings had almost completely disappeared. No change occurred in the blood until the day of the last irradiation (May 18) when the leucocyte count dropped from 4,900 to 1,500, the granulocytes from 40 to 15 per cent, and the platelets became noticeably scarce. By the end of the following week (May 26) the leucocyte count was to 6,200 with only 3 per cent granulocytes, and another biopsy on a cervical lymph node showed (Dr. H. B. McCordock):

"Large masses of abnormal white cells replace the germinal centers and medulla. The trabeculae are thickened but not infiltrated. The peripheral lymph sinuses remain apparent and contain numerous leucocytes. The abnormal cells resemble immature lymphocytes or blast forms. The nucleus shows a fine chromatin structure, and there is a distinct nuclear membrane. A few eosinophilic myelocytes are found intermingled with the other cells. The changes resemble those seen in lymph nodes from cases of acute leucemia."

On June 1, leucocytes were 29,400 and on June 6, 34,200 all except one per cent being nongranular mononuclear leucemic cells. Death occurred on June 9, just one month after the first irradiation. During the last ten days of life, there developed fever, asthenia, irritability, and hemorrhages from the mouth and nose. No necropsy was permitted.

Comment.—Of special interest in this patient were the abrupt change in the blood picture with sudden loss of leucemic characteristics in a fashion similar to that observed in a patient cited previously (Case 8): the complete blood remission which lasted four months, the appearance of parotid and glandular swellings during the remission, which suggested a neoplastic growth, the rapid recession of these swellings after roentgen irradiation, and the recurrence of the clinical and blood picture of acute leucemia obviously produced by the irradiation.

The parotid tumors clinically were considered to be related to the leucemia-lymphosarcoma ("leucosarcoma") type but the biopsy section of an adjacent lymph node strongly suggested a metastatic neoplasm and appeared distinct from the usual picture of lymphosarcoma or leucemia.

Another node removed three weeks later, after irradiation, when the swellings had receded and the blood picture of leucemia had returned, showed only the characteristic appearance of an acute leucemic gland.

CASE 11.—L. M. G., a 13-year-old girl, was first seen Dec. 19, 1937, because of pallor and asthenia which had been increasing for three months. There had been pains in the extremities and within the week previous to admission, fever of 102° F. had been noted together with hemorrhagic areas in the skin of the legs and ankles and some bleeding from the gums. Examination showed, in addition to the hemorrhages, that the liver and spleen were greatly enlarged but there was no lymphatic glandular adenopathy. Bleeding time was 11 minutes; erythrocytes numbered 1,800,000; platelets, less than 50,000; leucocytes, 57,300 with only 1 per cent granulocytes and the remainder mononuclear leucemic cells.

She was immediately started on transfusions and daily intravenous injections of marrow extract. During the following two weeks uterine (menstrual) bleeding was so profuse that she had to be given 3,500 c.c. of blood. By this time the leucocytes had fallen to 3,500, and the granulocytes were 19 per cent without other change in the blood picture. Clinically she improved very little during the next month and required a total of 13,500 c.c. of blood in 40 transfusions because of continued profuse bleeding, chiefly from the nose, before her death on Feb. 2, 1938. The liver and spleen remained large. The marrow extract injections were continued daily except for two periods of several days each. The leucocytes varied from 2,000 to 14,000 but the granulocytes rose steadily so that during the last month they formed from 28 to 68 per cent of the total. Abnormal leucemic cells persisted, however; the platelets remained very low; and hemorrhages continued. Fever was present during most of the illness and about three weeks before death a severe streptococcus infection of the arm at the site of a venipuncture developed which showed little tendency to heal. Clinical signs of peritonitis were noted terminally, but permission for necropsy was not obtained.

Comment.—In this patient, as in Case 7, there was a marked decrease in the abnormal circulating leucemic cells, and the granular leucocytes showed an unusual rise. Both patients suffered from continued severe hemorrhages which persisted in spite of transfusions.

In addition to the patients whose cases have been summarized, several other children with typical acute leucemia were given marrow extract injections for periods of a week or less without apparent effect on the blood. In two children the injections were continued for from six weeks to two months. Neither showed any definite clinical improvement or change in the granulocytes. In one there was no significant alteration in the blood picture, while in the other, although well-marked reduction occurred in the number of leucocytes after a few weeks, this could not be fairly attributed to the bone marrow therapy. Both eventually died from intercurrent infection.

Besides the experimental observations on children with acute leucemia, five patients with typical chronic myelogenous leucemia were also given the marrow extracts. Three of these were children, and two were adults. In only one was any marked change in leucocytes observed. This patient, a child of 5 years, apparently early in the disease, showed on several occasions an increase in leucocytosis after the injections, followed by a decided drop in the count. A complete study of this patient with relation to the extract could not be made since irradiation therapy was later used, and he was not available for further observation. In view of the previously stated hypothesis, which assumes an increase in the leucocytic maturation factor for chronic myelogenous leucemia—the reverse of the condition in acute leucemia—no improvement in this type would be anticipated from the extract injections.

DISCUSSION

A review of the patients with acute leucemia treated with bone marrow extracts shows two (Cases 8 and 10) with complete remission of the disease of two and four months; two (Cases 1 and 9) with similar complete remissions for shorter periods; two (Cases 7 and 11) with marked increase in maturation of granular leucocytes; four (Cases 2, 3, 4, 5), in whom the disease remained clinically arrested or quiescent for from three to six months; two (Cases 5 and 6), in whom rather prompt decrease in size of leucemic enlargements of the lymph nodes and spleen was noted after the therapy was given; and other patients in whom neither the clinical course nor the leucemic blood picture was affected.

That the bone marrow extract therapy employed was responsible for any or all the favorable changes observed is without proof. All patients received transfusions at intervals, and other symptomatic treatment. It is true, however, that of 50 patients with acute leucemia reported[2] from the same clinic and under observation during the ten years preceding these experiments, who were also given frequent transfusions, none showed anything suggesting a remission or any increase in granular leucocytes to the degree observed in certain patients here reported. In these earlier patients, once the typical acute leucemic blood picture became evident, the blood remained leucemic, and the disease progressed, usually rapidly and without clinical arrest or remission, to a fatal termination.

The possibility that the favorable results in the patients reported might be related to fortuitous chance must be considered, and it is conceivable that certain of the instances of apparent general clinical improvement without blood change may have been merely coincidental. It is possible also that the instances in which toxic febrile states were alleviated and those in which leucemic swellings receded rapidly after the extract injections were chance observations. The increase in maturation of granulocytes, however, is more difficult to account for as accidental, and to include also the patients who had remissions in the leucemic blood picture would appear to stretch the already long arm of coincidence to an unusual degree. Remissions in acute leucemia have not been observed previously by the writer, and must be rare, since a single instance[3] was found in the literature. The general attitude of physicians regarding the improbability of remission in the disease is illustrated by the following experience: Two of the patients reported (Cases 8 and 9) were under observation in the hospital at the same time and were shown at a clinic attended by a number of physicians as examples of acute leucemia with complete clinical and blood remissions that had lasted a number of weeks. At this time both children appeared well (Figs. 1 and 2) and were able to walk into the room. The only comments elicited after their presentation indicated great skepticism as to the verity of the diagnosis of acute leucemia.

The abruptness with which the appearance of the blood may change is illustrated by the observations on two patients (Cases 8 and 10) who had complete restoration to a normal blood picture. In one (Case 8) the change was so unexpected that differential blood examinations had not been made for a week previous to the recognition of the blood remission, but in this period the granulocytes rose from 3 to 73 per cent, the platelets from less than 50,000 to 798,000 and the leucemic cells disappeared. In the second patient (Case 10) the blood had been leucemic on the day previous, and restoration to a normal blood picture occurred within twenty-four hours. Such abrupt changes in the circulating elements have been noted previously in the opposite direction with the development of leucemia in patients under observation in "preleucemic" states. In a previous report[4] such a patient was cited whose blood changed from 21,500 leucocytes with 72 per cent granulocytes to 140,000 with 11 per cent granulocytes a week later, while Borchardt[5] records a patient whose leucocytes rose within two days from 14,000 with 93 per cent polymorphonuclears to a leucemic picture of 91,800 leucocytes with 94 per cent "lymphocytes."

The evidence furnished by the experimental observations with bone marrow extract in acute leucemia in support of the hypothesis of dysfunction of the marrow related to maturation of the granular cells is, of course, inconclusive. It is of interest that in at least six instances (Cases 1, 7, 8, 9, 10, 11) there was an unmistakable and striking increase in granular leucocytes in the circulating blood during the treatment with the extracts.

It must be remembered that the extracts were prepared empirically and that, if they contained any specific substance, no test for potency was available. The only test was to determine whether patients with acute leucemia responded favorably to their administration; there was, therefore, always the possibility that certain patients showing no improvement may have received extracts with little activity or that age or other influences had altered their potency. A few observations of their effect on the blood of laboratory animals showed no constant changes in the leucocytes but this was not considered conclusive, since, for example, the liver fraction valuable in pernicious anemia produces no change in the erythrocytes of normal individuals.

If any specific potency is present in the marrow extracts used and if the changes observed were related to the replacement of some deficiency in a physiologic mechanism, it is obvious that the stimulation was inadequate and incomplete since even those patients with remissions relapsed and a later continuation of the injections was relatively impotent. Indeed the impression gained through many of the observations was that a definite effect on the disease was produced but that it was only partial and imperfect, as though only one of possibly several necessary substances was being supplied and that only sufficient to modify to a greater or less degree the progress of the disease.

Acute leucemia is universally considered a constantly fatal disease beyond the reach of therapy. It is hoped that the experiments here reported will appear sufficiently encouraging to warrant further investigation in the development of a potent biologic product which may be of value not only in treatment of the disease but in establishing its character.

SUMMARY

The hypothesis is suggested that acute leucemia may be related to a deficiency in physiologic factors which are necessary for the maturation of the granular leucocytes in the marrow.

A series of experiments is reported in which children with acute leucemia were treated by injection of extracts of bone marrow in an attempt to replace the missing maturation factors in hematopoiesis. Of the patients treated, four had more or less complete remissions of the leucemic state, and in several others there was evidence of considerably increased maturation of the granular leucocytes.

REFERENCES

1. Cooke, J. V.: Arch. Int. Med. **49**: 836, 1932.
2. Cooke, J. V.: J. A. M. A. **101**: 432, 1933.
3. Jackson, H., Jr., Parker, F., Jr., Robb, G. P., and Curtis, H.: Folia haemat. **44**: 30, 1931.
4. Cooke, J. V.: Am. J. Dis. Child. **44**: 1153, 1932.
5. Borchardt, H.: Verhand. d. deutsch. path. Gesellsch. **22**: 96, 1927.

500 South Kingshighway

THE IMPORTANCE OF DEFICIT OF SODIUM AND CHLORIDE IN DEHYDRATION

Daniel C. Darrow, M.D.
New Haven, Conn.

THE following two cases are reported to show that the central feature of the syndrome called dehydration is loss or deficiency of sodium and chloride. In the case of the burn, the mechanism of the loss of sodium chloride would not lead to loss of water; in the case of diarrhea the course during recovery indicated that there was a deficiency of salt but not of water. These cases will be used as a background for the discussion of certain newer concepts of dehydration, particularly as to the therapeutic implications.

CASE REPORTS

Case 1.—The patient, a boy slightly more than 3 years old, who had a severe burn with deficit of sodium and chloride, and acidosis, was admitted to the surgical service. An hour earlier he had overturned a pan of boiling water and scalded most of the skin of his right leg, about half of his left leg, and a large area on the lower part of his back. He was immediately placed in a continuous, warm tub of water to which salt was added. He was in the tub for about 60 of the first 64 hours. His temperature rose to 40° C. within 24 hours. About 12 hours after admission he

Table I

Concentration of Serum in Case 1

DAY	HCO_3 MEQ./1	CL. MEQ./1	PROT. %	N.P.N. MG. %
2.5	11	80	5.3	
3.5	22	96	4.9	16
12	20	69		
13	23	97	5.8	
17	22	100	6.8	23

had a convulsion lasting 15 minutes. A hypodermoclysis of 800 c.c. of physiologic saline solution was given at this time followed by a transfusion of 125 c.c. of blood 8 hours later. Again the next day (about 36 hours after admission) he had another convulsion and was again given a hypodermoclysis of salt solution. In the afternoon he was semicomatose and about 64 hours after admission in extremis. At this time the pediatric service was consulted. He was breathing rapidly and deeply, his eyes were sunken, his pulse rapid and feeble. A sample of blood showed marked decrease in concentration of chloride and bicarbonate (Table I). He was immediately given an infusion of hypertonic sodium chloride and bicarbonate (the sodium chloride and sodium bicarbonate contained in 1,000 c.c. of interstitial fluid added to 500 c.c. of normal saline) and 250 c.c. of compatible serum over a period of 5 hours. The drip was continued for a total of 42 hours with salt and glucose solutions. When the continuous infusion was started, the tubs were discontinued and the denuded areas

From the Department of Pediatrics, Yale University School of Medicine, New Haven.

sprayed with gentian violet (2 per cent). The temperature became lower and the boy looked much better within 12 hours. Chemical recovery was good the next morning (12 hours after starting the continuous drip). The treatment with gentian violet was continued for 6 days when the crusts were loosened by saline soaks and 15 minutes in a saline tub on the first day. The next day the tub was used for 4 hours and the following day for 9 of 12 hours during the day but not at night. During this day he lost his appetite and fever became higher (40° C.). The following day he was treated for only 4 hours in the tub when it again became obvious that he had developed severe salt deficit. The symptoms of circulatory collapse and dehydration were the same as before, but signs of acidosis were absent. (Breathing was Cheyne-Stokes.) The tubs were again discontinued and continuous infusion of hypertonic solution of sodium chloride and bicarbonate started. Recovery was again rapid. Thereafter his course was essentially satisfactory although he remained in the hospital for a total of ten weeks. The skin showed islets of epithelial tissues when the tubs were discontinued the second time. These were later supplemented by skin grafts.

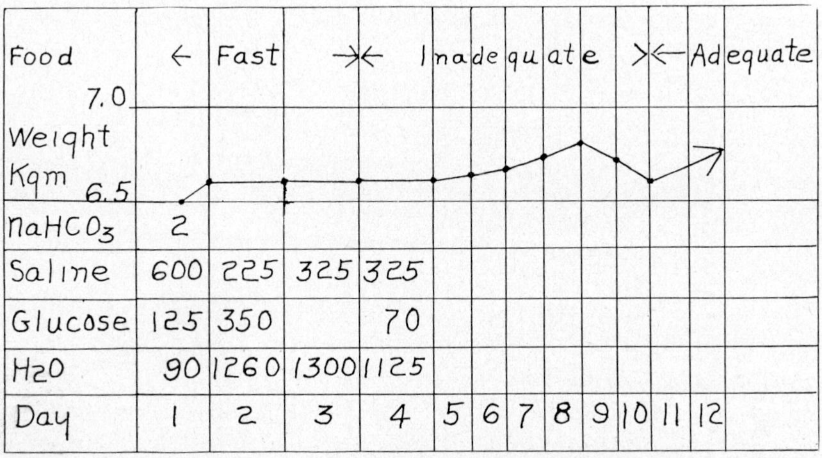

Chart 1.—The curve represents the course of the weight. The food intake is represented as "fast" when no food was given by mouth; by "inadequate" when the calories were less than 70 per kilogram, and "adequate" when over 70 calories per kilogram. One dose of 2 gm. of sodium bicarbonate was given by mouth. Saline is represented in cubic centimeters of 0.9 per cent sodium chloride by hypodermoclysis. Glucose is represented in cubic centimeters of a 10 per cent solution by intravenous infusion. Water is represented in cubic centimeters taken by mouth. Signs and symptoms of dehydration and acidosis were absent on the second day but diarrheal stools were still passed. On the third day the stools were practically normal.

During the first 10 days the white blood count was 25,000 to 30,000 per cubic millimeter. The urine was negative except that the specific gravity was always below 1.010 and on three occasions 1.005 during the first three days.

Summary.—A 3-year-old boy with an extensive burn developed symptoms of acidosis and salt deficit after spending about 60 of 64 hours in a tub containing salt. Improvement was rapid with continuous infusion of hypertonic sodium chloride and sodium bicarbonate. Symptoms of salt depletion again returned when the tub was again used for about 13 of 48 hours.

CASE 2.—The patient, 7½-month-old boy, had diarrhea with otitis media, acidosis, and deficit of sodium chloride. He had been artificially fed since birth and apparently was doing well until the present illness. Nine days before admission he developed a cold. Six days before admission he had many watery stools which did not contain blood. Two days before admission he started to vomit and probably vomited all his food and most of the water offered him during the two days before he was admitted to the hospital. On admission he was extremely sick, with greatly diminished skin turgor, sunken fontanels and eyes, Kussmaul breathing, and sunken abdomen. Both middle ears contained pus. The baby was treated with 2 gm. of sodium bicarbonate by mouth and was given subcutaneous injections of physiologic saline and blood transfusions. No food was given for three days, during which time urine and stools were collected for chemical analysis. Recovery was satisfactory. The course of the case is represented in Chart 1 and the metabolic results are given in Table II. Before treatment was started the serum showed the following concentrations: bicarbonate 14 mM. per liter; chloride, 108 mM. per liter; total base, 137 mM. per liter; total protein 6.8 per cent; and nonprotein nitrogen 65 mg. per cent.

TABLE II

OUTPUT IN CASE 2

	DAY	VOLUME C.C.	CL. MM.	P. MM.	FIXED BASE MEQ.	CA. MEQ.	N. GM.
Urine	1	380	12.0	10.1	7.1		3.4
Urine	2	214	4.2	2.4	0.1		0.6
Urine	3	214	4.8	1.1	1.6		1.0
Stool	1	350	28.1	3.0	47.9	3.1	1.8
Stool	2	250	13.2	2.8	18.7	2.3	0.6
Stool	3	76	1.8	0.4	2.3	0.0	0.1

The points to be noticed are: (1) marked decrease in concentration of serum total base on admission; (2) recovery from all symptoms and signs of dehydration within 24 hours; (3) excretion of negligible amounts of the administered sodium chloride and bicarbonate in the urine and stools; (4) retention of larger amounts of sodium and chloride not accompanied by a gain in weight. This last point is particularly important since no gain in weight indicates no increase in total body water. In other words retention of sodium chloride and sodium bicarbonate were responsible for re-establishing a normal distribution of body water.*

DISCUSSION

Underhill[1] first emphasized the significance in burns of the high concentration of hemoglobin and low concentration of blood chlorides. He later proved that the localization of chloride in the edematous reaction at the site of the burn was sufficient to explain the changes in the blood.

*The above argument neglects the water freed from the cells because no food was given except the intravenous glucose. While an exact calculation of the water freed from cells cannot be made, it is too small to affect the argument. Analyses were not made to demonstrate that recovery of normal concentration of serum sodium had taken place when clinical recovery was apparent. Furthermore the metabolic studies do not differentiate between sodium and potassium, and all conclusions assume that the excretions were largely sodium. We know that this was probably not the case but the assumption merely minimizes the amount of sodium retained. I have no real apologies for the plan of the metabolic work on this case since it was completed ten years ago shortly after I left Dr. Marriott's clinic. The work was never published because at the time I was unable to explain what recent experimental work has made obvious.

This work has been repeatedly confirmed[2, 3, 4] and Blalock has emphasized the importance of loss of plasma proteins as well as salt, in the production of shock in patients with burns. It was not surprising, therefore, to see obvious signs of acidosis, dehydration, and shock 60 hours after the burn. However, the marked reduction in concentration of chloride was not anticipated, since the patient had received 1,700 c.c. of physiologic saline in the previous 50 hours. Since this amount of saline is equivalent to one-half the sodium of the extracellular fluid of a boy of this size it is not likely that this quantity of salt was immobilized at the site of the burn. Before the second episode, no salt solution had been given, the inflammatory reaction about the burn was subsiding, and there was no vomiting, diarrhea, nor other of the usual means of salt loss. The mechanism of the loss of sodium chloride in the two episodes was not obvious until it was discovered that the tubs were only receiving enough sodium chloride to make a solution of about one-third physiologic strength. Obviously the surface denuded of skin permitted free diffusion of extracellular electrolyte from the tissue spaces and capillaries into the hypotonic water of the tub. By this process the body would lose sodium and chloride, but not water. Nevertheless, the patient showed symptoms and signs of loss of extracellular fluid, since the blood was concentrated with respect to hemoglobin and skin turgor was diminished. The low concentration of chloride was due to loss of sodium and chloride, but the evidences of loss of extracellular fluid and decrease in blood volumes were not due to loss of water from the body but rather due to shift of extracellular water into the cells.*

The state of the boy was analogous to that produced by Yannet and myself[5] in dogs. In these experiments, when loss of extracellular electrolyte was induced without change in total body water, the dogs developed all the symptoms and signs of clinical dehydration; the blood was concentrated with respect to red cells and serum proteins but the concentrations of serum sodium and chloride were reduced. Skin turgor was diminished. Analysis of red cells showed that water had gone into the red cells. It was shown that the changes in the volume of extracellular fluid indicated that water must have gone into other cells as well. This shift of water from extracellular spaces into the cells fits into prevailing concepts of the type of equilibrium that must exist between fluid on the two sides of cellular membranes. In other words basic and probably also acid ions do not cross cellular membranes in living cells in response to changes in osmotic pressure. Hence when loss of extracellular electrolyte (sodium and chloride) makes extracellular fluid hypotonic, osmotic equilibrium is attained by a shift of extracellular water into the cells.

*In view of the low concentration of serum chloride on the third day, it is likely it was equally low at the time of the two convulsions. If this be true, the convulsions were analogous to those seen in experimental water intoxication. The improvement after administration of physiologic saline solution fits in with this interpretation.

As has already been pointed out, the baby with "intestinal intoxication" was also not suffering from loss of total body water but rather from dehydration of extracellular fluids and increased hydration of intracellular fluids owing to loss of sodium and chloride. The observations upon which this concept rests are the low total base in serum on admission and the clinical recovery with retention of sodium and chloride but not of water.

It now seems clear that in most clinical types of so-called dehydration, the loss of sodium and chloride is greater than that of water. This is indicated by the fact that reduction in the concentration of sodium is more frequently encountered than normal or high concentrations. This is true in diabetic coma,[6, 7] diarrheal diseases,[8] nephritis,[9] miner's cramps,[10] Addison's disease,[11] etc. It follows, therefore, that physiologic saline or its equivalent is the most important therapeutic measure in dehydration. Experimental and clinical observations indicate that losses of sodium and chloride in cases showing marked dehydration may be equal to the amount contained in one-third of the extracellular fluid of the body, i.e., the amount contained in 70 c.c. of physiologic saline (or equivalent) per kilogram of body weight. In treatment this amount of salt may be necessary to restore body sodium and chloride and thereby re-establish normal distribution of body water.

Actually no rule can be given as to how much sodium chloride must be given to a dehydrated patient. Recovery from clinical evidences of dehydration and a diuresis containing chloride may be used as guides. However, in adrenal-cortical insufficiency and in certain cases of hyposthenuric nephritis, excretion of chloride occurs even when body chloride is deficient. For these reasons, in addition to the amount of saline necessary to produce a diuresis, estimations of the probable deficit of salt and of the probable amount which continues to be lost should be used in deciding on the dose of saline.

The above discussion brings out the reason why the administration of sodium and chloride as physiologic saline is the most important therapeutic procedure used for restoration of the normal distribution of body water in dehydration. The following paragraphs will point out briefly the treatment of renal insufficiency, disturbances in acid-base equilibrium, and shock, which frequently accompany deficiency of extracellular electrolyte.

Since the kidneys normally regulate the concentration of serum electrolyte as well as excrete nitrogenous waste products, the disturbances in acid-base equilibrium as well as elevation in nonprotein nitrogen may be regarded as brought about by renal insufficiency. If the abnormalities be considered as due to a deficit of body water, intravenous glucose and water by mouth should be the mode of treatment. Clinical experience and experimental studies[12, 13] show that the abnormalities of renal function continue to a greater or lesser degree as long as the deficiency of sodium and chloride persists, while administration of sodium chloride quickly restores renal function.

During deficiency of extracellular electrolyte, studies on dogs[12] and humans[13] indicate that the glomerular filtrate is reduced in volume, and urea is reabsorbed to a greater extent than normal by the renal tubules. This accounts for the high nonprotein nitrogen and perhaps also for the fact that water is excreted more slowly than normally. If small deficits of sodium exist, the kidneys may eventually restore electrolyte concentrations in serum by excreting water.[12, 14] However, if large deficits are allowed to persist the concentrations of serum electrolyte remain low because the kidneys do not diminish the volume of extracellular fluid in order to preserve concentrations. Nevertheless, large amounts of water may be excreted when the deficit of extracellular electrolyte remains marked, provided the intake is large. The disturbances in acid-base equilibrium are explained by the fact that, when large deficiencies of extracellular electrolyte are present, the kidneys fail to excrete the relative excess of chloride in acidosis and the relative excess of sodium in alkalosis. It is not clear what is the explanation of all these anomalies; in part they are dependent on the circulatory failure but in part they are also probably dependent on the fact that the function of renal tubules is best carried out when serum concentrations are approximately normal.

Experimental and clinical experience shows that sodium chloride quickly re-establishes normal renal function when this procedure brings about the correct volumes and concentration of extracellular electrolyte. Administration of large amounts of water for urine formation is of secondary importance and is probably taken care of by the water in physiologic saline. When kidney function is not disturbed by actual renal disease, physiologic saline alone will usually correct the disturbances in acid-base equilibrium, because the kidneys can excrete the relative excess of chloride in acidosis, and saline replaces the relative deficit of chloride in alkalosis. However, in cases with marked acidosis, or when losses of sodium and chloride are likely to continue, or when oliguria or disturbed renal function exists, the administration of physiologic saline without sodium bicarbonate may aggravate or produce acidosis.[15] This effect is brought about chiefly by diluting the bicarbonate already in the body at a time when the kidneys are not excreting the relative excess of chloride of physiologic saline. In acidosis this effect may be serious, even when renal function is fairly good, if loss of sodium in excess of chloride continues to occur as in diarrhea. Under these circumstances a solution resembling interstitial fluid more closely than physiologic saline has theoretic and practical advantages. Hartmann and I have both come to this conclusion and developed slightly different solutions resembling interstitial fluid.*† These solutions may be used in all types of dehydration.

The first patient illustrates the disadvantage of administration of physiologic saline while loss of extracellular electrolyte is taking place. Before the first episode, the boy received 1,700 c.c. of 0.9 per cent solution of sodium chloride. The salt solution undoubtedly postponed the development of alarming symptoms, but made it almost certain that deficit of sodium would be greater than deficit of chloride, and, hence, made acidosis a prominent feature. Before the second episode, no injections of salt solution were given and no acidosis developed. Confirming Hartmann,[15] we have observed analogous changes following administration of physiologic saline in diarrhea and renal insufficiency. For several years we have used a solution† resembling interstitial fluid in composition and have neither seen acidosis develop nor be aggravated during treatment. Administration of a balanced solution makes the use of special doses of bicarbonate (or its equivalent) seldom necessary.

Marriott[16] first pointed out the shocklike nature of dehydration, and Powers[17] brought out the importance of blood transfusions in therapy. This procedure is now recognized as the most important therapeutic measure for shock. Blalock[18, 19] and others have demonstrated that large amounts of extracellular electrolyte are immobilized at the site of traumatic injury and at the site of a burn. In this sense surgical shock is analogous to deficiency of extracellular electrolyte (dehydration) except that the sodium chloride is immobilized rather than lost from the body. Perhaps by shock one should refer particularly to the inability of the body to maintain blood circulation and blood pressure, not primarily because of cardiac failure, but rather on account of decreases in the volume of circulating fluids and loss of plasma proteins through capillary dysfunction. If plasma volume, blood pressure, and circulation remain insufficient for a few hours, secondary changes take place leading to dilatation of the capillaries and leakage of serum proteins into the tissue spaces. These features of shock may be prevented by blood (or plasma) transfusions and are sometimes corrected by the same means. However, if severe shock is allowed to persist several hours, no effective therapy is available. Since it is not possible to estimate which patients with dehydration will recover from shock with solutions of salt and glucose alone, it is necessary to give transfusions to many patients who would otherwise recover with only hypodermoclyses of saline and intravenous infusions of glucose.

Intravenous injections of glucose solutions produce such obvious improvements in many patients that their use is not always understood.

*Concentrated Lactate Ringers Solution, prepared by Eli Lilly and Company, Indianapolis, Ind.

†Concentrated Interstitial Salt Solution prepared by Sharp and Dohme, Philadelphia, Pa.

Glucose solutions supply the body with much needed food, and water without salt. Since excess of water over that in physiologic saline is not especially needed by a patient with low concentration of serum sodium, their use is chiefly as food and for treating shock by a temporary expedient while matching blood for transfusion, and perhaps as a general tonic through the effect of glucose on metabolism. Glucose solutions should not be given subcutaneously to patients with salt deficit since such injections immobilize the already depleted stores of sodium and chloride.[5] Glucose is specifically indicated in liver injury and perhaps in certain cardiac conditions.

SUMMARY

The case of a patient with severe burn is reported. Two episodes of symptoms of dehydration developed in which loss of sodium chloride without loss of water was produced by placing the boy in a continuous tub containing hypotonic salt solution. Symptoms of dehydration were due to loss of extracellular electrolyte without loss of body water.

Metabolic studies are reported on a patient with infantile diarrhea, which show that the symptoms of intestinal intoxication were brought about by loss of sodium and chloride without deficit of body water.

Therapeutic procedures for the treatment of dehydration are discussed in the light of recent concepts of the nature of dehydration.

REFERENCES

1. Underhill, F. R., Carrington, L., Capsinow, R.: Arch. Int. Med. **32**: 31, 1923.
2. Harkins, H. N.: Proc. Soc. Exper. Biol. & Med. **31**: 994, 1934.
3. Blalock, A.: Arch. Surg. **22**: 610, 1931.
4. Davidson, E. C.: Arch. Surg. **13**: 262, 1926.
5. Darrow, D. C., and Yannet, H.: J. Clin. Investigation **15**: 266, 1935.
6. Kidd, D. N.: J. Clin. Investigation **12**: 1169, 1933.
7. Atchley, D. W., Loeb, R. F., Richards, D. W., Jr., Benedict, E. M., and Driscoll, M. E.: J. Clin. Investigation **12**: 297, 1933.
8. Hamilton, B., Kajdi, L., and Meeker, D.: Am. J. Dis. Child. **38**: 314, 1929.
9. Peters, J. P.: Medicine **2**: 435, 1932.
10. Talbot, J. H.: Medicine **14**: 323, 1935.
11. Loeb, R. F., Atchley, D. W., and Stahl, J.: J. A. M. A. **104**: 2149, 1935.
12. Darrow, D. C., and Yannet, H.: J. Clin. Investigation **15**: 419, 1936.
13. McCance, R. A., and Widdowson, E. M.: J. Physiol. **91**: 222, 1937.
14. Kerpel-Fronius, E.: Ztschr. f. Kinderh. **57**: 489, 1935.
15. Hartmann, A. F.: Am. J. Dis. Child. **35**: 557, 1928.
16. Marriott, W.: Am. J. Dis. Child. **20**: 461, 1920.
17. Powers, G. F.: Am. J. Dis. Child. **32**: 232, 1926.
18. Blalock, A.: Surg., Gynec. and Obst. **58**: 551, 1934.
19. Mann, F. C., and Essex, H. E.: Am. J. Surg. **28**: 160, 1935.

ACCOMPLISHMENTS IN MATERNAL AND CHILD HEALTH AND CRIPPLED CHILDREN SERVICES UNDER THE SOCIAL SECURITY ACT

MARTHA M. ELIOT, M.D., JESSIE M. BIERMAN, M.D., AND A. L. VAN HORN, M.D.
WASHINGTON, D. C.

WITH the passage of the Social Security Act there again came into existence federal grants-in-aid to the states for maternal and child welfare. The program was broadened over that of the former Maternity and Infancy Act to include older children in the child health provisions, grants for medical and surgical care and hospitalization of crippled children, and grants for child welfare services for dependent and neglected children. The federal act makes it clear that the grants are intended to extend and improve conditions primarily for mothers and children living in rural areas or areas of economic distress. All states and territories are cooperating under the maternal and child health provisions, and all but one in services to crippled children.

MATERNAL AND CHILD HEALTH

Administration of Program.—Title V, Part 1, of the Social Security Act provides for the extension and improvement of maternal and child health services in the states through federal grants-in-aid administered for the Federal Government by the Children's Bureau of the Department of Labor and for the states by the state health agencies. Once the plan for services prepared by the state agency has been approved by the Chief of the Children's Bureau as in accordance with the Social Security Act, the program is directed and administered in its entirety by the state and local health agencies.

Of the $3,800,000 authorized for appropriation each year, $2,820,000 must be matched by the states; $980,000 is granted on the basis of the state's need for assistance in carrying out its plan and is not matched.[1]

In 1934 thirty-one state health agencies had bureaus or divisions of child health and of these only twenty-two were directed by full-time physicians.[2] Between 1929, when federal funds ceased to be available to the states under the Maternity and Infancy Act, and the passage of the Social Security Act in 1935, there had occurred a marked falling off in many states of both state and local appropriations for maternal and child health services and, because of the economic depression that was coincident, state health department budgets were cut, and general funds available previously for maternal and child health were reduced or entirely eliminated. On the other hand, it is encouraging to note that in a number

From the Children's Bureau, United States Department of Labor.

of states, maternal and child health activities established during operation of the Maternity and Infancy Act had been continued, indicating that the value of this work had been demonstrated to the people of these states.

In February, 1936, funds for maternal and child health services became available under the Social Security Act, and by June 30, 1936, 46 states, Alaska, Hawaii, and the District of Columbia had had plans approved and were receiving grants from the federal government. Plans for the two remaining states were approved before the end of the calendar year 1936.

Since, under the act, the responsibility for developing and submitting a plan is that of the state health agency, and since the needs of states vary widely because of special geographic, racial, agricultural, or industrial conditions, the plans that have been approved are very diverse in many respects. In certain respects, especially in regard to administrative features and types of basic services, the plans show similarities. The progress that has been made toward good administration, high standards of service, and a broader coverage for service may be briefly summarized.

All the forty-eight states, and Alaska, Hawaii, and the District of Columbia, have established divisions or bureaus of maternal and child health in the state health agency under the direction of a physician. In the spring of 1936, the Conference of State and Territorial Health Officers recommended to the Children's Bureau that the director of a division of maternal and child health in a state department of health should be a physician trained in pediatrics or obstetrics or both and preferably in public health as well. Today, of the 50 directors now in office, 30 have been trained in pediatrics, 5 in obstetrics, 6 have had previous experience in child health administrative positions, and 9 have had no specialized maternal or child health training or experience; all but 2 of these 9, however, have had general public health experience or training. Of the 50 directors, 22 have now had some training in a school of public health. Because of the many clinical features of a maternal or child health program, previous clinical training or experience has been considered by most state agencies to be a fundamental qualification for these positions. As the programs broaden and more and more local practicing physicians take part in rendering the service, this policy becomes increasingly important.

Additional physicians have been employed by forty-two states, either as administrative assistants or as clinical consultants. The plans for 1939 show that there will be twenty-eight pediatricians and thirteen obstetricians thus employed full time during the year.

Scope and Content of Program.—From the plans submitted by the several states, it becomes apparent that the functions of the state divisions of maternal and child health are as follows: (1) To seek the cooperation of the physicians of the state in extending statewide facilities for continuous health supervision throughout pregnancy, infancy, and childhood, and in providing care for sick children and for women at delivery; (2) to seek the cooperation of physicians and all other citizens of the state in informing the public as to what is good maternity care, infant care, and care of children at different stages of growth and development, and how facilities for such care may be made available in each locality of the state; (3) to develop maternity and child health services in all parts of the state through local health units; (4) to aid in the organization of local health units through the provision of child health or maternity services in areas not yet fully organized; (5) to be responsible for the establishing of high standards of service in the maternal and child health field; (6) to cooperate with all other bureaus of the state health agency in activities affecting the health and welfare of children and mothers, such as public health nursing, control of communicable diseases, including tuberculosis and syphilis, collection and study of vital statistics, control of the milk and water supply; (7) to cooperate with other state agencies concerned with problems of child health or welfare, as the bureaus of child welfare, departments of education and the agriculture extension service of the departments of agriculture; (8) to cooperate with medical and other professional groups in providing facilities for postgraduate education in maternity care and care of children and the related fields of nutrition and dental care, and (9) to promote health education through the schools and the general public.

The maternal and child health services that are carried out under state plans are basically those commonly described as health supervision:

(1) Prenatal clinics and child health conferences conducted by physicians with the aid of public health nurses; (2) home visiting by public health nurses for teaching maternal, infant, and child hygiene, and for instruction in bedside nursing care, and (3) nurses' classes or conferences with mothers for educational or follow-up purposes.

In addition, planning for care of the mother at delivery and of the infant in the neonatal period is becoming widely recognized as one of the important services to be rendered by the local staff. In an increasing number of local areas provision is being made for home nursing care at delivery of women attended by physicians and of their newborn infants, as well as the more usual prenatal and postnatal nursing care. In a number of states the problems of the medical and nursing care of prematurely born infants are being given special attention.

The services of consultant obstetricians and pediatricians to assist general practitioners with their individual cases are being made available in special regions or localities of certain states where such services are not available to women unable to procure them from their own resources. In at least one state such services are supplied on a state-wide basis. Though the number of such projects is still limited and the territory and population covered are relatively small, a variety of methods of meeting the need for case consultation service are being explored with a view to determining the most practical for use under different conditions. In eighteen states obstetricians or pediatricians are employed on a full-time salary basis for this purpose, usually to serve in a single district or county demonstration unit; in twenty-two states consultants are employed on a part-time salary or fee basis; and in four states specialists may be called for consultation from an approved list by general practitioners and payment is made on a case basis. Ultimately a study of the different methods in use should give information as to which conditions of employment and reimbursement permit a case consultant's services to be most fully and widely accepted, which conditions safeguard most surely the quality of the special consultation service, which plan of procedure defines most clearly the function of the case consultant as contrasted with the administrative consultant responsible for organization of the program, and most important of all, which plan results in raising most satisfactorily the general level of care rendered in the community.

During the current fiscal year, in 35 states, the District of Columbia, Hawaii, and Alaska, provisions are made for payments to practicing physicians for conducting prenatal and child health conferences and for school medical examinations. There is an increasing tendency on the part of the state agencies to enlist the aid of specialists in obstetrics and pediatrics in the state in setting up standards for the conduct of these conferences. A few states are establishing conference training centers for the general practitioners who will later take over the conduct of conferences in rural areas. If those conferences are to fulfill the purposes for which they are being established with regard to the individual served and to their influence on the character of medical practice in the community, they must measure up to the best practice in the community.

Last year under the provisions of the Social Security Act, prenatal clinics or conferences were conducted by physicians in 2,713 centers in thirty-six states. Child health conferences were conducted in 6,033 centers in forty-three states.

Interest in programs of postgraduate education for practicing physicians is increasing. In 1936 thirteen states conducted courses under the maternal and child health plan in cooperation with state medical societies; during the present fiscal year, 1939, thirty-nine states plan such courses. There is increasing evidence that the rural practitioners who care for such great numbers of mothers and children appreciate and are profiting by the courses which bring them not only factual information in obstetrics and pediatrics but stimulation to include health supervision and preventive procedures in their practices. The courses for local practitioners are creating a demand for short courses in obstetrics and pediatrics at medical centers where clinical observation and actual experience can supplement lectures.

Practically all state divisions of maternal and child health have conducted studies or surveys to better acquaint them with the health problems of mothers and children existing in their states. The majority of the studies have been concerned with infant and maternal mortality, a number of these in conjunction with the state medical societies; others have been special studies of the incidence of prematurity and stillbirths. Nutrition, immunization, and dental surveys have been conducted. These studies are all adding greatly to our knowledge of health conditions that actually exist in different parts of the country.

A steadily increasing number of states have added the services of one or more nutritionists to the staffs of the state health departments, usually in the divisions of maternal and child health, to serve as advisers to the medical, dental, and public health nursing staffs in matters related to nutrition of the family. On June 30, 1936, nine states had full-time nutritionists on their staffs. Today, twenty-four states employ forty-three full-time nutritionists, in most cases to serve in a statewide advisory capacity, in some to assist district or local staff in organizing local service or in rendering local service. The tendency is for the nutritionist engaged by the state to act as adviser to state and local staff and as a coordinator of service offered by different state or local agencies rather than to give individual case service. The value of a nutritionist in an urban health service has long since been proved, especially when there is coordination of service with the welfare agencies. In the rural areas the need is often greater than in the cities. Here the home economics specialist of the extension service may be working with many families, but her work may not be well coordinated with efforts of the health department staff. A nutritionist serving in a rural health unit can be of great assistance both in a general advisory and educational capacity and in giving case service when desirable. In a few rural areas service of this sort is being rendered.

The number of public health nurses probably constitutes a better index of actual services being rendered than any other one figure. To a great extent the effectiveness of the medical program depends upon the quality and the number of the public health nurses whose function it is to carry it into the home in understandable terms and techniques to the individual mother and child. This requires many skills and an understanding of human relationships which come only with proper training and experience under supervision. Most of the states have shown gratifying response to the recommendations of the state and territorial health authorities regarding the qualifications of the public health nurses employed by them. According to the 1939 maternal and child health budgets, the states have provided for the employment of 2,716 public health nurses or two-fifths of the total number of public health nurses working in the rural areas. In rural areas there is one public health nurse for every 11,000 persons in the population; in cities there is one for every 5,000 persons. The problem of adequate supervision and leadership for these public health nurses has been given serious consideration because of the need for special guidance and assistance in maternity nursing and in many of the problems of infant care and care of young children. For the year ended June 30, 1938, specialized public health nursing consultants in maternal and child health have been appointed to the staffs of twenty-one state health agencies and in twelve additional states the chief nurse or at least one of the generalized supervisors has had special work in maternity care or care of children.

Cooperation With Professional and Lay Groups.—One of the conditions specified in the Social Security Act that must be met before approval can be given to the state plan by the Chief of the Children's Bureau is that the plan must provide for cooperation with medical, nursing, and welfare groups and organizations. Up to the present time this condition has been met largely by the formation of state maternal and child health advisory committees made up of representatives from state medical associations, other medical organizations, the state nurses' associations, the state welfare departments, special organizations for child welfare or public health, lay organizations such as parent-teacher associations, state federations of women's clubs, and organizations of farm women. In some states technical subcommittees have been appointed to work with the divisions of maternal and child health in developing the medical phases of the program. In forty states members of the Academy of Pediatrics are represented on advisory committees. In thirty-three states the state medical societies have appointed committees to act in an advisory capacity to the state boards of health in their maternal and child health programs. There is need for improvement in the functioning of the technical committees in order to make sure that the members of the profession in each state who have a real interest in the program and have much of value to contribute may do so.

In addition to the function of giving technical advice through professional representation, the advisory committees in many states are proving invaluable in promoting the understanding of, and gaining the cooperation of, large groups of citizens through representation of lay groups on the committees.

Unmet Needs.—During the two years and eight months that federal funds have been available to the states for maternal and child welfare, steady progress has been made by the states and local communities in making services available to mothers and children. Many rural areas previously without such service have been reached; many groups in special need have been served; the quality of work in most places has been improved; standards of care have been established and extension of service into new fields has taken place; a basis for administrative procedure has been established on the federal-state level and in turn between the states and local communities; a basis for acquiring facts with regard to the need and the extent of service is being developed. However, as progress has been made in establishing services, recognition of the gaps in the total program and of specific needs has been inevitable. Facts regarding maternal mortality, mortality of infants on the first day and in the first month of life, and mortality and morbidity of older children are being widely studied. Ways to meet many of the needs are already well known, but resources are inadequate to provide the means to carry out the necessary steps in the program. That the amounts now available to the states are not adequate to fill their needs was made apparent by the state health agencies in submitting plans for maternal and child health services for the fiscal year 1939. In response to a question as to unfilled needs, twenty-eight states made statements of specific needs that in the aggregate amounted to $22,000,000 annually. These needs included funds for payment of physicians' fees for delivery and other medical care, hospitalization for maternity cases, additional public health nurses, additional prenatal and child health conferences, additional service of nutritionists, and additional public health units. Many other states made additional statements of need without specifying necessary personnel or costs.

The utter futility of providing means of assessing the health and welfare of children and of mothers and of not providing the means to maintain them in health or restore them to health if sick, or, in the case of maternity, to make available complete medical and nursing care of mother and infant has forced itself upon health and welfare workers and upon the people. The experience of two and a half years has made clear the great advances that could be made in maternity care, in the health supervision and medical care of children, and in the care of crippled children should facilities and resources for such care be made available to those unable to obtain good care.

Having come to the realization of the necessity for a courageous attack on the problem of maternity care and care of newborn infants that would meet the need with no half-way measures, national organizations and individual citizens have united in an effort to create public opinion favorable to action. The creation of the National Committee on Better Care for Mothers and Babies (now the National Council for Mothers and Babies)[3] early in 1938 was a timely development in view of the widespread public interest in the National Health Program presented by the Interdepartmental Committee to Coordinate Health and Welfare Activities at the National Health Conference[4, 5] in July, 1938. The need for an expanded program for maternity care and health supervision and medical care for children was included in the National Health Program as one of the major measures to be given precedence in the development of the proposed plan. Specific recommendations were made, following in general, as far as maternity care is concerned, the plan of action proposed at the Conference on Better Care for Mothers and Babies called by the Chief of the Children's Bureau in January, 1938.[3] Reference to the report of the Technical Committee on Medical Care to the National Health Conference shows that in the opinion of that committee a plan of gradual expansion over a ten-year period is desirable in order that administrative procedures may be sound and standards of care and qualifications of personnel be maintained at a high level.

CRIPPLED CHILDREN'S SERVICES

Administration of Program.—Under part 2 of title V of the Social Security Act, relating to services for crippled children, an appropriation of $2,850,000 annually is authorized "for the purpose of enabling each state to extend and improve (especially in rural areas and in areas suffering from severe economic distress), as far as practicable under the conditions in such state, services for locating crippled children and for providing medical, surgical, corrective, and other services and care, and facilities for diagnosis, hospitalization, and aftercare for children who are crippled or who are suffering from conditions which lead to crippling." The total amount of the sums made available by the federal government must be matched by the state.[1]

Prior to the passage of the Social Security Act in 1935, public provisions for the care of crippled children were sporadic and uneven and in many states totally inadequate, if not altogether lacking. In only 28 states was there an official state agency authorized by law to provide care and medical treatment for crippled children. In many of these states appropriations were small and services were greatly limited.

By June 30, 1936, state plans had been approved for the administration of services for crippled children for 38 states. At the close of the fiscal year 1937, every state had designated an official agency to administer services for crippled children, and state plans had been approved for forty-two states and Alaska, Hawaii, and the District of Columbia. At the present time, forty-seven of the forty-eight states, and Alaska, Hawaii, and the District of Columbia are conducting services for crippled children under the provisions of the Social Security Act. Louisiana is the only state which has not submitted a state plan, and it appears likely that as soon as certain financial and administrative problems have been clarified, a plan will be submitted, thus making state services for crippled children available throughout the country.

The programs for crippled children are being administered by several types of state agencies. At the present time the department of health is charged with the administration of crippled children's services in 24 states; in 15 states, the department of public welfare; in 4 states, the department of education; in 5 states, a crippled children's commission; in 1 state, a university hospital, and in 1 state, an interdepartmental committee administers the program through the crippled children's division of the department of education. It is interesting to observe that there has been an increasing trend toward establishment of new programs in state departments of health and, in a few cases, transfer of administrative responsibility to state departments of health from other state agencies. An appreciation of the inherent nature of the crippled children's program as one involving problems of medical care has undoubtedly influenced states in giving the administration of these services to the state health agencies. That the program for crippled children as set up under the Social Security Act is primarily one of medical care is also reflected in the types of personnel directing the state program of services. In 30 states a physician serves as director of the program; in 8 states, a nurse; in 3 states, a social worker; and in 9 states, a nonprofessional person.

Qualifications of Personnel.—Two years ago the Children's Bureau Advisory Committee on Services for Crippled Children appointed by the Secretary of Labor recommended that state agencies adopt standards for the selection of professional personnel which had been established by the various national boards for medical specialties such as the American Board of Orthopedic Surgery and the American Board of Pediatrics, or by recognized national professional organizations such as the National Organization of Public Health Nursing, the American Association of Medical Social Workers, and the American Physiotherapy Association. A review of state plans for the fiscal year 1938 showed that such standards were taken into consideration by state agencies in the selection of the various types of personnel as follows: surgeons, 24 states; nurses, 16 states; medical social workers, 19 states; and physical therapy technicians, 20 states. In many states, particularly those where difficulties have been encountered in obtaining local personnel who meet the qualification standards established by the national organizations, provisions have been made for further training of staff personnel.

A considerable number of public health nurses have received training in public health nursing, in orthopedic nursing, and in physical therapy. Several universities and schools of nursing have arranged their nursing curricula to serve to best advantage the trainee who is taking a supplementary course in public health nursing or in orthopedic nursing in order that she may return to the state equipped to serve as a consultant or to give direct service to crippled children. A number of social workers and physical therapy technicians have likewise been given additional training in their respective fields of work with crippled children. Educational centers have been interested in developing courses designed to equip workers in these special fields. The selection and training of personnel will require continuous attention if standards of service are to be maintained and steadily improved.

Standards for Hospitalization and Convalescent Care.—The recommendations which the Children's Bureau Advisory Committee on Services for Crippled Children made with respect to the selection of hospitals used for the care of crippled children have been of great assistance to the states in setting up standards for the selection of hospitals. With few exceptions the hospitals which are being used by the state agencies for the treatment and care of crippled children are those that have been registered by the Council on Medical Education and Hospitals of the American Medical Association and that have been approved for surgical service by the American College of Surgeons. Additional standards have been established by state agencies in line with those recommended by the advisory committee with regard to facilities and personnel to meet the special needs of crippled children. As a result of the increased interest in the care of crippled children and the additional funds made available under the Social Security Act, many hospitals have improved their equipment to give more adequate care to crippled children.

Standards for convalescent homes and for foster homes have not as yet been well defined. However, in the selection of convalescent and foster homes the majority of state agencies are cooperating closely with the bureaus of child welfare in the state department of public welfare that administer the program of child welfare services. The problem of convalescent care needs careful consideration with a view to developing satisfactory standards and increased facilities. The effective use of convalescent facilities meeting desirable standards provides a means of reducing hospital sojourn, and at the same time offers an opportunity for a more satisfactory transition from the period of active treatment in a hospital in readjusting a child to his return home.

Cooperation With Professional and Lay Groups.—Perhaps in no other type of service for children is there such a distinct need for a close correlation of all services affecting the program as in work for crippled children. The state agencies are utilizing extensively state and local services of both public and private agencies, and the outstanding work of private organizations and agencies has added much to the development of the program. In every state many valuable contributions are being made to the program by medical, health, nursing, education, welfare, and vocational rehabilitation agencies and organizations. This cooperation with various professional and lay groups is well exemplified in the representation of these groups on general and technical advisory committees which have been appointed by the majority of state agencies. In all states conducting services for crippled children a physician is serving on either the general advisory committee or the technical advisory committee. In 14 states a pediatrician is serving as a member of the technical advisory committee, and the remaining states are being urged to call upon pediatricians for service of this nature as well as for actual participation as consultants and clinic physicians in the program of care for crippled children.

Scope of Program.—No specific definition of "crippled child" was given in the wording of the Social Security Act, although several definitions had been proposed in the hearings before Congress. An investigation of the laws under which state agencies were operating showed variations extending from a very strict definition limiting the services to children with motor disabilities to a very broad definition and interpretation, which included all physically handicapped children who could be benefited by medical or surgical treatment. The various definitions of a crippled child incorporated in the laws of the several states have been accepted, for the present, with the idea that in actual practice definitions will be broadened gradually to include as wide a range of crippling conditions as is practicable within the limitations of the available funds. A few states have included such conditions as rheumatic heart disease and diabetes, but most of the cases accepted for care have been orthopedic and plastic conditions. As the peak load of children awaiting orthopedic care when the Social Security Act became effective is passed, it is possible that proportionately more care may be given to children crippled from cardiac conditions, especially in those states where rheumatic disease is common. Children whose chief disability is incurable blindness, deafness, or mental defect, and those having abnormalities requiring permanent custodial care are considered beyond the scope of this program.

When the Social Security Act was passed in August, 1935, there were marked differences in the extent and type of programs provided by state agencies. Only twelve states had developed services as broad in scope as those provided under the act. States that started with provision for little except diagnosis and hospitalization have recognized the shortcomings of such a program and have gradually broadened it to include a greater diversity of services. It was to be expected that some state plans in their initial stages would consist almost exclusively of services for physical restoration, but most of these plans are being expanded to provide for case-finding procedures, registration of crippled children, aftercare services and for coordination of health, welfare, nursing, and rehabilitation agencies. There has been observed a growing recognition of the fact that the crippled child needs these supporting services as well as skilled medical care.

Most of the states have taken steps to improve the quality of medical and surgical care and to provide the necessary auxiliary services to make care effective. There is, for instance, need of a continuing effort to bring children under care at an earlier stage, to keep them under continuous treatment and supervision as long as is necessary for their complete physical and social rehabilitation, and to make more readily available the essential aftercare services.

More effective methods for locating crippled children have been put into operation by state agencies during the past year through more systematic reporting by physicians, teachers, nurses, social workers, and others and through the use of epidemiologic reports and birth certificates. The use of epidemiologic reports in locating crippled children at present centers chiefly around the problem of providing prompt care to all needy cases of acute poliomyelitis, but they are also being utilized in a number of states in discovering cases of bone tuberculosis. The reporting of congenital defects, such as clubfoot, on the birth certificate is receiving consideration in a number of states. Such reporting is now required by law in six states.

Procedures with regard to acceptance of children for care and planning for care after discharge from the hospital have been reviewed in many states by social workers attached to the state staffs and a number of socially undesirable procedures have been corrected. The problems connected with court commitment are being given careful consideration. Requirements for economic eligibility are being more liberally interpreted so that any crippled child can be accepted for diagnostic service. Decision as to acceptance for treatment and other services following diagnosis is based on the social and economic condition of the family. The generally accepted principle is that no child whose parents are unable to provide adequate treatment from their own resources shall be denied service. Some progress is being made by several states in modifying or discarding certain undesirable requirements such as the signing of a pauper's oath or the signing of an agreement to repay, with interest, the cost of medical care.

A majority of the states have required residence in the state, but many of the official agencies are working out reciprocal relationships with other states for the care of children moving across state lines.

Diagnostic clinic services for crippled children have been greatly extended throughout the country, particularly in rural areas and in areas suffering from severe economic distress. State plans from twenty-seven states which gave information on the number of itinerant clinics scheduled for the fiscal year 1938 indicated that 456 such clinics were to be held during the year. These clinics are in addition to the large number of permanent clinics which are conducted at regular intervals at hospital centers in practically every state.

In 1938, 546 hospitals were approved by forty-eight state and territorial agencies for the care of crippled children. In the main, the special hospitals for crippled children, both public and private, and the general hospitals with orthopedic services located centrally in larger cities care for a majority of the children. There is, however, a trend toward decentralization of hospital services so that the crippled child can be hospitalized in an approved hospital near his own home. Furthermore, the procedures used by state agencies in the authorization of hospitalization and in the issuance of instructions to be carried out on the discharge of a patient have been further improved so that local health and welfare workers are better informed as to the aftercare necessary for good results.

Reports of Service Rendered.—Reports submitted by state agencies on the direct services actually rendered to crippled children have given additional valuable factual data on which to base plans for the future development of state services. The total number of children on the registers of 43 states, Alaska and Hawaii as of March 31, 1938, was 130,610. Table I presents a picture of certain activities for all the states from which reports were received during the calendar year 1937.

TABLE I

SUMMARY OF CRIPPLED CHILDREN'S SERVICES

REPORTS* FOR THE YEAR ENDED DECEMBER 31, 1937

TYPE OF SERVICE	NUMBER
Medical service in clinics (diagnostic or treatment):	
Individuals admitted	77,055
Visits	193,928
Care in hospitals:	
Children under care at beginning of year	3,796
Children admitted to care during year	38,277
Days' care	1,322,750
Care in convalescent homes:	
Children under care at beginning of year	1,337
Children admitted to care during year	3,831
Days' care	380,331
Care in foster homes:	
Children under care at beginning of year	350
Children admitted to care during year	757
Days' care	57,843
Field and office visits by:	
Public health nurses	212,248
Physical therapy technicians	187,250
Medical social workers (January-June)†	47,573
Other social workers (January-June)†	15,797
Individuals admitted by:	
Medical social workers (July-December)†	4,773
Other social workers (July-December)†	4,688
Children referred for vocational rehabilitation	3,654

*Figures are preliminary and incomplete. They represent primarily activities of the official state agencies but include some services provided by other public and private agencies in the various states. They include corrections received in the Children's Bureau through July 31, 1938.

†Owing to revision of report forms, effective July 1, counts of individuals admitted to case work service are available only for last six months of the year.

Unmet Needs.—In spite of the fact that considerable progress has been made in the extension and improvement of state services for crippled children, much remains to be done. If the program is to achieve the intent of the Social Security Act, some means must be found to bring to the attention of the state agency all crippled children. Methods previously employed have been unsuccessful in discovering the child of preschool age who is frequently missed in the school surveys upon which agencies have often depended. In addition to enlisting the interest and assistance of medical, health, nursing, welfare and educational agencies and organizations in reporting crippled children, it is important that some method be developed for informing the general public regarding the services for crippled children that are available and the method by which such services may be obtained. Restrictions imposed by state laws or administrative regulation with respect to residence requirements indicate that if services for crippled children are to be made available to the children of families moving across state lines, there is need for further development of reciprocal agreements between states with respect to responsibility for providing such services.

An outstanding need in many state programs appears to be the development of services for general diagnostic medical services and medical supervision of children suffering from orthopedic and plastic defects and from other physical handicapping conditions. In too few states have adequate provisions been made by the state agency for a general physical appraisal and medical supervision by qualified pediatricians of crippled children coming within the state plan of services.

Both convalescent and aftercare services in the child's home have been slower in development than services for physical restoration. The importance of adequate aftercare services following hospitalization cannot be emphasized too strongly. To be most effective, provisions should be made for adequate medical, nursing, physical therapy, and social services.

The facilities for psychometric examinations of crippled children do not appear to be adequate, and in some instances where such facilities are available, they are not being fully utilized. The whole field of mental hygiene with respect to the welfare of the crippled child has scarcely been touched.

Federal and state funds available for crippled children's services at the present time are wholly inadequate for providing diagnostic, treatment, and aftercare services for children suffering from such handicapping conditions as rheumatic fever, rheumatic heart disease, visual defects, and defects of hearing. Greater recognition should be given to the needs of this group as well as to those suffering from orthopedic and plastic defects.

Provisions for the care of the hopelessly crippled child are notably inadequate.

SUMMARY

There has been presented a review of accomplishments in maternal and child health and crippled children's services under the Social Security Act, including a description of administrative procedures, a brief presentation of the programs now being carried out by the states, the qualifications and training of personnel, and methods of cooperation with professional and lay groups.

REFERENCES

1. For detail with regard to terms of the Social Security Act, methods of allotment, amounts allotted and paid to states and description of services carried out, see Maternal and Child-Welfare Bulletins Nos. 1 and 2, U. S. Children's Bureau, Washington, 1935 and 1938.
2. Eliot, Martha M.: Child Health 1933-1934, J. PEDIAT. 4: 817, 1934.
3. Proceedings of Conference on Better Care for Mothers and Babies. U. S. Children's Bureau Publication No. 246, Washington, 1938.
4. Proceedings of the National Health Conference. In press (to be published by the Interdepartmental Committee to Coordinate Health and Welfare Activities).
5. Veeder, Borden S.: The National Health Conference, J. PEDIAT. 13: 400, 1938.

FURTHER OBSERVATIONS ON THE METABOLISM AND THE CLINICAL USES OF SODIUM LACTATE

ALEXIS F. HARTMANN, M.D., ANNE M. PERLEY, JACK BASMAN, M.D., MARTHA V. NELSON, AND CÉCILE ASHER, M.D., D.C.H.
WITH THE TECHNICAL ASSISTANCE OF MARIE MORTON
ST. LOUIS, MO.

IN A PREVIOUS communication, Hartmann and Elman[1] reported studies on the effects in dogs of loss of gastrointestinal secretions and demonstrated the therapeutic value of lactate-Ringer's solution* in various types of gastric and intestinal obstruction and fistula and in pancreatic duct fistula. At about the same time Hartmann and Senn[2] submitted data concerning the metabolism of sodium *r*-lactate in the human subject, both in health and in disease, and emphasized particularly the value of sodium *r*-lactate in the treatment of various types of acidosis, and recently Hartmann[3] compared the results in the treatment of diabetic acidosis (1) when no alkali was administered, (2) when *sodium bicarbonate* was used, and (3) when the alkali administration was *sodium lactate*, and emphasized the many ways in which the last mentioned treatment seemed superior to the others.

We now wish to report further observations concerning the metabolism of sodium lactate in the human subject, and its clinical uses in the relief and prevention of acidosis and in rendering the urine alkaline for therapeutic purposes.

I. METABOLISM OF SODIUM LACTATE IN THE NORMAL INDIVIDUAL

PLAN OF STUDY

In an investigation of the fate of intravenously injected sodium lactate in the normal human subject, the general plan of study was as follows: After a rest period of one hour, usually from 7:00 A.M. to 8:00 A.M., the subject's fasting oxygen consumption was determined by use of the Benedict-Roth metabolism apparatus. When two satisfactory tests had been completed, preliminary blood and urine specimens were obtained. On this and subsequent blood samples, serum carbon dioxide content, hydrogen ion concentration, lactic acid, dextrose, inorganic phosphate, and chloride were estimated. The urine samples were analyzed for carbon dioxide content, hydrogen ion concentration, and lactic acid. After the preliminary blood and urine specimens had been collected, the intravenous injection of sodium lactate was started. Five-

From the Department of Pediatrics, Washington University School of Medicine, and the St. Louis Children's Hospital.

*At times also designated as "combined solution," "Hartmann's solution," and "physiological buffer salts solution."

tenths molar solutions were used, the molar lactate being diluted with an equal volume of distilled water, Ringer's solution, or water containing 0.125 per cent calcium chloride. The calcium chloride was added in an attempt to lessen the discomfort due to tetany which sometimes accompanied the alkalosis developing in the normal subject following sodium lactate administration. The quantity of lactate injected varied from 3.2 to 8.1 c.c. of molar solution per kilogram of body weight, and the injection period ranged from 18 to 27 minutes with the exception of one experiment in which it was 37 minutes. In all of the experiments except the earliest ones, estimation of oxygen consumption was started shortly after the injection had begun and one or two tests of 6 to 7 minutes' duration were made during the injection, another shortly after it was over, then at half-hour intervals for 2 hours, and hourly for one to 3 hours more if the oxygen consumption had not already returned to the basal level. Blood and urine samples were collected immediately after the injection was over and blood again one-half, one, 2, and 3 or 4 hours later. Urine was collected at less frequent intervals until the excretion of lactic acid had become inappreciable.

Seven experiments were carried out with what we believed was racemic sodium lactate prepared from Mallinckrodt's "chemically pure" or "analytical reagent" lactic acid. Recently we were informed that the commercial lactic acid sometimes contains an excess of one isomer, so we may not always have been dealing with a true racemic mixture. Two experiments were carried out with *l*+ lactate, the sarcolactic acid used having been prepared by Peterson and Tatum, of the University of Wisconsin. In addition to the lactate studies, five experiments were carried out in which changes in the oxygen consumption associated with the intravenous injection of 0.5 molar sodium bicarbonate were observed.

RESULTS AND COMMENT

Chemical Changes in General.—The various chemical changes in blood and urine following the lactate injections will not be reported in detail, but Chart 1 gives these findings along with the oxygen consumption data in one representative experiment.

The intravenously injected lactate diffuses rapidly from the blood stream and, except for the portion which is excreted, is completely metabolized in from one to 2 hours. Plasma volume is increased temporarily by dilution, which is to be expected. Blood sugar increases slightly, then sinks to slightly hypoglycemic levels, the rise possibly being explained by a temporary decrease in the amount of dextrose being oxidized in the tissues because of partial substitution by the *d*-lactate as a substrate undergoing oxidation; the latter fall is possibly to be explained by a continuation of the glycogenic mechanism set in motion by the conversion of the *l*+ isomer into liver glycogen. The sodium ion liberated during the oxidation of lactate or its conversion into glycogen is transported to the kidneys for excretion largely as the bicarbonate salt, so that for several hours after the injection there exists a state of alkalosis of the base bicarbonate excess type with commensurate increase in the hydrogen ion concentration of the blood. Excretion into the urine of the excess base bicarbonate begins almost immediately and soon bicarbonate and the hydrogen ion concentration of the urine reach maximal values (500-600 volumes per cent, and 7.9-8.0, respectively). Within four hours more than one-half of the injected sodium is excreted in this way.

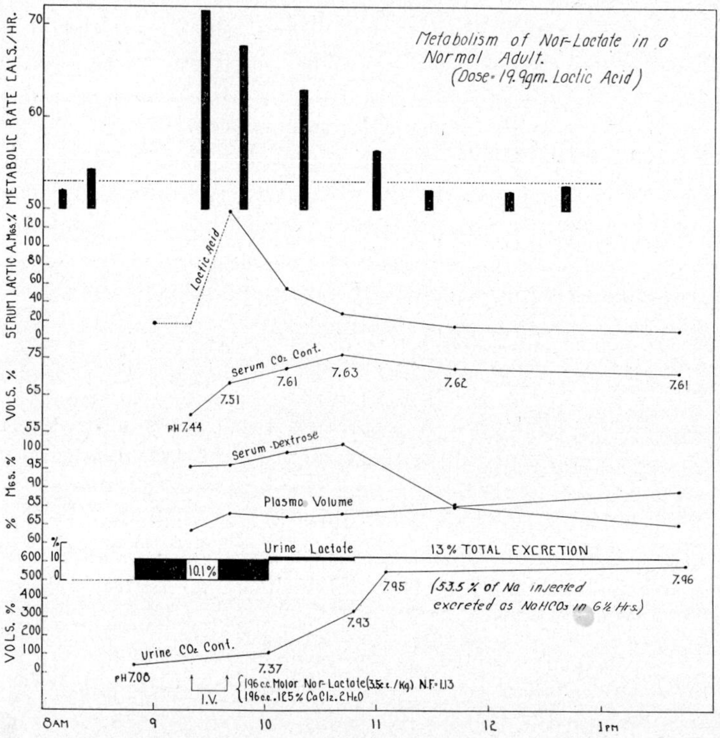

Chart 1.—Chemical changes in blood and urine and changes in oxygen consumption in response to the intravenous injection of sodium *r*-lactate.

Renal Excretion of Injected Lactate.—The quantities of lactic acid excreted in the urine are given in Table I. The small urinary losses of 1.5 per cent and 4.6 per cent of the amounts injected when sodium *l*+ lactate was given are in marked contrast to those of from 12.9 to 14.9 per cent when a corresponding amount of the "racemic mixture" was given. It is true that the injection periods were slightly longer when the *l*+ form was administered, but this difference in the rate of injection is not enough to explain the large differences in the quantities excreted.

Abramson and Eggleton[4] found that following the intravenous injection of sodium *r*-lactate the excreted lactate yielded a zinc salt which analyzed as racemic. Their observation suggests, of course, that the

TABLE I

LACTIC ACID EXCRETION AND CHANGES IN OXYGEN CONSUMPTION FOLLOWING INTRAVENOUS INJECTION OF SODIUM *r*-LACTATE AND SODIUM *l*+ LACTATE

DATE	SUBJECT	INJECTION PERIOD MIN.	M. NA LACTATE C.C. PER KG. BODY WT.	NA LACTATE INJECTED DECIMOLS	LACTIC ACID			PERIOD OF URINARY EXCRETION	BASAL O_2 CONSUMPTION CAL./HR.	EXTRA CAL. ABOVE BASAL	EXTRA CAL. PER DECIMOL NA LACTATE GIVEN
					GIVEN GM.	EXCRETED PER CENT	DISAPPEARED GM.				
1/ 8/32	C. A.	26	7.0(*r*)	4.20	37.8	30.0	26.5	4′21″			
1/20/32	C. A.	37	8.1(*r*)	4.87	43.8	15.6	37.0	2′47″			
1/13/32	A. P.	27	7.2(*r*)	3.30	29.7	29.6	20.9	5′7″			
2/17/32	C. A.	20	3.6(*r*)	2.11	19.0	14.9	16.2	2′33″	62.5	9.1	4.32
6/29/32	A. P.	18	3.5(*r*)	1.60	14.4				46.8	7.7	4.81
2/ 6/32	M. N.	19	3.9(*r*)	2.21	19.9	12.9	10.3	2′26″	53.1	18.2	8.24
6/27/32	M. N.	23	3.4(*r*)	1.90	17.1				53.5	4.4	2.32
2/10/32	C. A.	26	3.2(*l*+)	1.90	17.1	1.4	16.9	2′28″	53.7	16.6	8.74
2/12/32	M. N.	25	3.7(*l*+)	2.08	18.7	4.6	17.8	2′40″	57.8	10.3	4.86

two isomers were utilized equally well. Our finding that considerably less lactate was excreted in the urine after the sodium *l*+ lactate were injected than after a mixture of the two isomers was given, suggests on the other hand, that the *d*- form is utilized less readily than the *l*+ form. If this is the case, it is to be expected that the lactate excreted after the injection of a true racemic mixture would contain an excess of the less readily utilized *d*- isomer.

It will be noted that in two of the three experiments in which as much as 7 c.c. of molar sodium *r*-lactate per kilogram of body weight was given, the lactate excretion continued for a longer period than it did in those in which approximately 3 to 4 c.c. per kilogram were given, and the percentage of the injected lactate lost in the urine was considerably greater, being about 30 per cent of the amount given. This is to be expected because with the larger amounts of lactate a higher level of blood lactic acid was reached. In this connection, it should be remembered that in the normal subject diuresis promptly follows the intravenous injection, which is not always true in dehydrated individuals with acidosis who lose much less lactate in this way.

Changes in Oxygen Consumption During and After the Injection of Lactate and of Bicarbonate.—The data on changes in oxygen consumption are given in Table I and Chart 2. The extra calories burned from the beginning of the intravenous injection until the blood lactic acid had returned to the normal level were computed by plotting the calories per hour obtained in the oxygen consumption determinations against time and tracing with a planimeter, after connecting the points with straight lines, the area representing the calories above the basal level.

The blood lactic acid had usually returned to the normal level within one hour after the injection had started, always within two hours; therefore, in tracing the area of extra calories in the bicarbonate experiments a period of 1½ hours after the injection began was used.

TABLE II

CHANGES IN OXYGEN CONSUMPTION FOLLOWING INTRAVENOUS INJECTION OF SODIUM BICARBONATE

DATE	SUBJECT	MOLAR $NaHCO_3$ GIVEN C.C.	$NaHCO_3$ GIVEN DECIMOLS	$NaHCO_3$ GIVEN GM.	BASAL O_2 CONSUMPTION CAL. PER HR.	EXTRA CAL. ABOVE BASAL	EXTRA CAL. PER DECIMOL $NaHCO_3$ GIVEN
3/ 3/32	C. A.	3.5	2.02	17.0	55.1	11.0	5.45
3/25/32	A. P.	3.5	1.54	12.9	48.6	10.7	6.95
6/24/32	A. P.	3.5	1.54	12.9	45.1	6.4	4.16
3/23/32	M. N.	3.5	1.87	15.7	53.1	8.1	4.49
6/22/32	M. N.	3.5	1.83	15.5	54.1	6.1	3.34

It is apparent from the tables and charts that there was much variation in the extra oxygen consumption per decimol of lactic acid injected in the different experiments in which the sodium *r*-lactate was used. These values varied from 2.32 to 8.24 calories per decimol of sodium lactate given, and it will be noted that the extreme variations were obtained on the same subject. The two experiments with the sodium *l*+ lactate gave 4.86 and 8.74. With sodium bicarbonate the values ranged from 3.34 to 6.95 calories per decimol of alkali given. From the graphs it is obvious also that in several of the experiments with the "racemic" mixture and one with the *l*+ lactate, the oxygen consumption did not return to the basal level by the time the blood lactic acid had returned to normal. When sodium bicarbonate was given, in only one case had the oxygen consumption returned to the basal level within 1½ hours after the injection was started. In one experiment with the "racemic" mixture, subject C. A., February 17, the basal oxygen consumption was considerably higher than on other occasions, but the calories per hour had not fallen even to the basal level of the test day within 3½ hours after the beginning of the injection. In one case in which the *l*+ isomer was given, M. N., February 12, the basal oxygen consumption was also unusually high but fell approximately to the basal level of the preceding and subsequent experiments in slightly over 3 hours after the injection started. If this low level had been used as a base line, the extra calories per decimol of sodium lactate given would have amounted to 8.26 instead of 4.86. In one of the bicarbonate experiments, M. N., June 22, the two estimations of oxygen consumption made during the injection gave values actually slightly lower than the average of the basal oxygen consumption of that day. These low values are in marked contrast to the appreciable increases occurring during the injection in all of the other experiments with both bicarbonate and lactate.

Buchwald, Cori, and Fisher[5] in 1933 published their observations on the influence of intravenously injected *l*+ and *d*– sodium lactate on oxygen consumption in rabbits. When *l*+ lactate was injected the oxida-

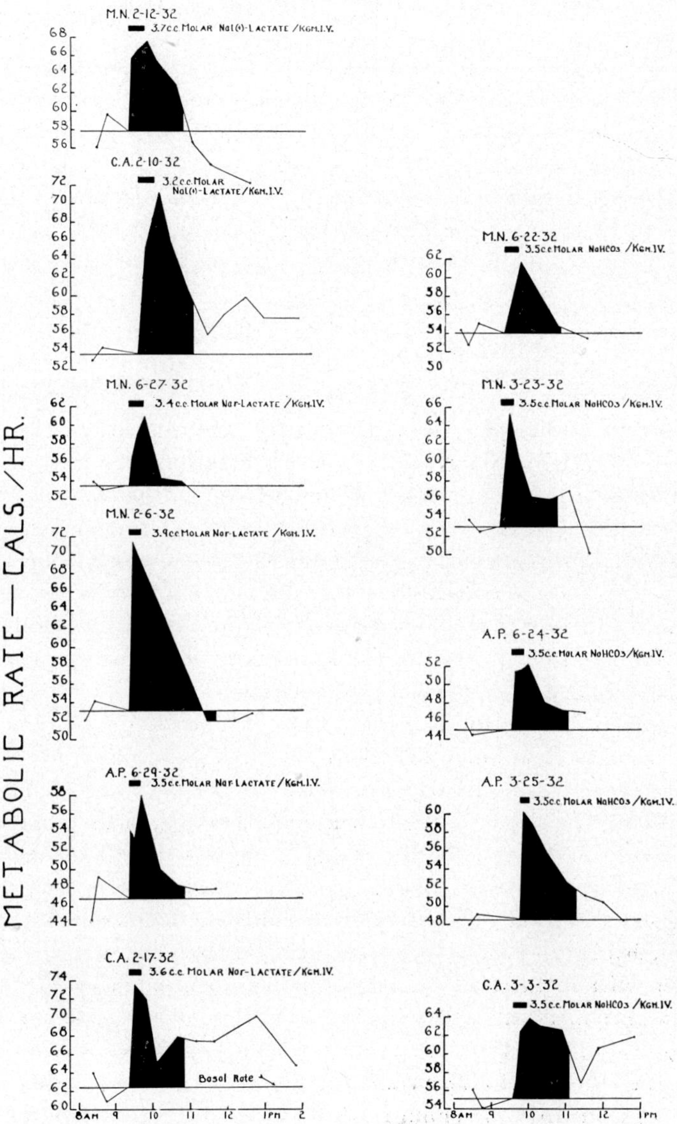

Chart 2.—Changes in oxygen consumption following intravenous injection of sodium *r*-lactate, sodium *l*+lactate, and sodium bicarbonate. The shaded areas include, in the case of the lactate experiments, the period elapsing from the beginning of the injection until the blood lactic acid had reached its normal level; in the case of the bicarbonate experiments, they include a period of one and one-half hours from the time the injection was started.

tion quotients obtained averaged 3.9, varying from 2.6 to 4.5, the extra oxygen consumption accounting for only one-fourth of the lactate which disappeared. They assume that the other three-fourths was converted to glycogen. Much smaller increases in oxygen consumption were obtained when sodium bicarbonate was injected in equivalent amounts than when sodium lactate was given. When correction was made for the slight bicarbonate effect which did occur, the oxidation quotient became 4.9. Injection of free *l*+ lactic acid which did not involve a bicarbonate error gave an average quotient of 4.4. They observed also that rabbits were able to utilize only one-fourth as much *d*– lactate as *l*+ lactate and the average oxidation quotient when *d*– lactate was given was 1.1. In an earlier investigation Cori and Cori[6] demonstrated glycogen deposition in the liver of rats following the injection of sodium *l*+ lactate but hardly any when *d*– lactate was given.

Abramson, Eggleton, and Eggleton[7] in 1927 reviewed the literature to date on the fate of injected lactate and reported their studies on anesthetized dogs. They did not find sufficient increase in oxygen consumption to account for the lactate which disappeared. The increases in oxygen consumption of 17 to 34 per cent which they obtained after the injection of sodium *r*-lactate they feel are due to the rise in plasma bicarbonate which follows lactate administration, for a similar rise in oxygen consumption occurred when corresponding amounts of bicarbonate were injected. They were unable to demonstrate glycogen synthesis in muscle or liver, and state that they doubt that this occurs in the intact animal, although it has been shown to take place in intact muscle. According to their viewpoint, as pointed out by Buchwald, Cori, and Fisher,[5] injected lactate acts like an easily oxidizable substrate which replaces other food stuffs in metabolism.

It is difficult to evaluate our oxygen consumption data in view of the variations and discrepancies which we have mentioned and in view of the fact that continuous oxygen consumption determinations were not made during the injections. In our experiments, as in those of Abramson and his co-workers, the increases in oxygen consumption when comparable amounts of sodium lactate and sodium bicarbonate were given on the whole did not differ greatly in contrast to the much smaller rises that Buchwald and co-workers obtained with bicarbonate as compared to those with lactate. If it is justifiable to assume that the effect of alkali administration on oxygen consumption is of the same magnitude whether the alkali is given in the form of sodium lactate or of sodium bicarbonate, it is quite apparent that the extra calories following lactate administration are not enough to account for the disappearance of the lactic acid on the assumption that the oxidation quotient of the *l*+ lactate is 4 or 5 and of the *d*– lactate is one. In the experiments in which the sodium *r*-lactate was given, assuming that it was a true racemic mixture and that the excreted lactate was largely the *d*– isomer, the extra oxygen consumption in some cases was not enough to justify the assumption of oxidation quotients of 4 and of one, even if we disregarded the alkali effect. In the two experiments with the *l*+ lactate which, as already pointed out, were rather unsatisfactory, if we assume an oxidation quotient of 4, the calories left to be considered as due to alkali effect are extremely small. It would seem probable, therefore, that at least part of both the *l*+ and *d*− lactate which disappeared replaced other food stuffs in metabolism.

II. ACIDOSIS OF RENAL ORIGIN

The acidosis of renal insufficiency, when the latter is extreme, seems always to be associated with a combination of phosphate and sulphate retention and loss of fixed base from the body fluids. In cases with less severe renal insufficiency, mild to moderate degrees of acidosis are sometimes encountered in the absence of such changes and seem to be the result of a new electrolyte pattern which is characterized by lower bicarbonate and higher chloride concentrations. It is quite possible that such an altered electrolyte pattern is merely the result of prolonged insufficient alkali intake, relative to its increased excretion with, however, adequate intakes of water and chloride and excessive retention of the latter.

To date (1937, inclusive) we have sixteen examples of this type of acidosis in eleven different infants or children treated with sodium *r*-lactate, in whom follow-up data were secured. The types of renal insufficiency included chronic active hemorrhagic nephritis, both with and without cardiac decompensation, acute and chronic suppurative nephritis, amyloid disease, nephrectomy, and an unusual case of tubular obstruction in an infant. In five instances, edema was present at the time that the acidosis was recognized and treated, and in three dehydration. As may be noted from Table III, in 15 of the 16 instances, the acidosis was relieved satisfactorily: i.e., the observed carbon dioxide content was raised within 12 hours (and usually much sooner) to a normal value, or to one that was in the zone of just mild acidosis (35-45 volumes per cent). In the single exception, a second administration of sodium lactate proved necessary. In comparing the observed rise in carbon dioxide content with that expected on the assumption that all of the sodium lactate is converted into sodium bicarbonate and distributed equally throughout the entire amount of body water (estimated as two-thirds of body weight), a calculation which has previously been described and made use of,[2] the following data are relevant:

Less than expected (−)			More than expected (+)
>20 vol. %	20-10 vol. %	10-0 vol. %	0-10 vol. %
(1) = 6.3%	(3) = 18.7%	(6) = 37.5%	(6) = 37.5%

Average = −5.7 vol. %

It should be mentioned that in the presence of edema, especially when cardiac decompensation is also present, the sodium lactate may be given in hypertonic strength: i.e., as one molar, one-half or one-third molar.

TABLE

RECOVERY FROM ACIDOSIS OF RENAL

No.	Case	Date	Age	Body			Serum†												
				Wt. Kg.	Water Liters	Edema	Vols. % CO_2 Content					NaCl Mg. %	Gm. % Protein			Lactic Acid Mg. %	Inorg. P. Mg. %	Ca. Mg. %	N.P.N. Mg. %
							Before	After	Hrs.	Ex-pected	Differ-ence		Total	Alb.	Glob.				
1	G- 198	10/24/30	7 yr.	16.9	11.3	0	20.8	51.3	4	43.0	+ 8.3	— —	8.50 —	— —	— —	12.0 —	5.0 —	12.0 —	87.0 —
2	G- 198	12/15/30	7 yr.	17.0	11.3	0	32.0	46.0	24	44.7	+ 1.3	—	— —	— —	— —	— —	— —	— —	75.0 —
3	I- 478	3/ 8/32	14 yr.	38.6	25.7	+++	26.0	40.0	6	43.4	− 3.4	— 585	6.95 —	1.99 —	4.96 —	28.5 —	8.8 —	8.8 —	186.0 —
4	I- 478	4/ 4/32	14 yr.	38.6	25.7	+++	44.9	49.9	22	66.7	−16.8	585	5.65 —	2.87 —	2.78 —	— 18.0	7.1 —	9.1 —	145.0 —
5	B- 707	5/ 2/32	8 yr.	42.2	27.7	+	28.0	67.5	20	67.7	− 0.2	608	7.60 5.00	— —	— —	— —	3.7 5.0	— —	133.0 110.0
6	J-2000	9/ 5/33	8 yr.	25.0	16.7	+	27.0	53.9	15	53.8	+ 0.1	608	7.15 —	3.90 —	3.25 —	— —	10.3 —	— —	180.0 —
7	L- 239	1/23/35	7 yr.	18.0	12.0	Dehyd.	22.3	57.1	12	55.9	+ 1.2	475	5.00 —	2.90 —	2.10 —	— —	17.5 —	7.8 —	197.0 215.0
8	E-1663	5/23/35	14 yr.	28.0	18.7	?	15.4	39.5	8	51.4	−11.9	590	6.10 5.32	— 1.66	— 3.66	— 28.0	20.0 19.7	8.1 7.5	135.0 125.0
9	L-2539	11/18/35	18 da.	2.5	1.7	Dehyd.	22.0	30.0	19	61.6	−31.6	708	— —	— —	— —	— —	— 8.6	— —	— 152.0
10	L-2539	11/19/35	19 da.	2.5	1.7	0	30.0	70.0	34	69.6	+ 0.8	725	— —	— —	— —	— —	— 8.0	— —	100.0 134.0
11	J- 201	10/26/36	7 yr.	20.0	13.3	Dehyd.	15.0	76.4	23	81.2	− 4.8	603	5.44 —	— —	— —	— —	9.7 —	— —	110.0 —
12	M- 830	2/25/37	3 yr.	12.2	8.1	++	21.0	55.9	14	62.9	− 6.6	634	— 3.93	— 1.00	— 2.93	— —	— 6.5	— 6.6	93.0 56.0
13	M- 830	3/ 2/37	3 yr.	13.2	8.8	++	31.0	58.2	6	64.5	− 6.3	595	— —	— —	— —	— —	— —	— —	49.0 60.0
14	N- 487	3/21/37	5 mo.	5.3	3.5	0	9.0	25.0	6	41.0	−16.0	351	— —	— —	— —	— —	— —	— —	— 247.0
15	N- 487	3/22/37	5 mo.	5.3	3.5	0	25.0	50.0	16	57.0	− 7.0	351	— —	— —	— —	— —	— 8.0	— 5.8	— 261.0
16	K- 508	7/12/37	7 yr.	16.0	10.7	++	11.2	46.4	9	44.6	+ 1.8	548	4.42 5.01	2.36 2.12	2.06 2.89	— —	4.5 4.5	5.1 5.2	140.0 112.0

*M. = Molar concentration. H. = Subcutaneously. D. = Died—No autopsy.
I.V. = Intravenously. R. = Ringer's solution. A. = Autopsy.
I.P. = Intraperitoneally. F.L.R. = Fortified Lactate-Ringer's solution. I. = Improved and still living.

†When double figures are given, the lower denote determinations after treatment.

In addition to these 15 instances in which follow-up data were secured, there have been many more occasions of apparently satisfactory relief, as judged by the amelioration of clinical symptoms of acidosis. Once, following the removal of most of the single remaining kidney in a child with chronic suppurative nephritis, the occurrence of acidosis was prevented for a period of almost a month by frequent administrations of sodium lactate solution. In the case with chronic amyloid disease (Case 8, Table III), as well as in Cases 1 and 2, recurrences of acidosis were frequent, and for a period of months were relieved by lactate administration.

It should also be mentioned that in three adults, the acidosis which followed prostatectomy and postoperative oliguria, vomiting, and dehy-

III

INSUFFICIENCY AFTER NA R-LACTATE THERAPY

Na r-Lactate*	Molar CC.	Molar CC./Kg.	Ringer's CC./Kg.	Dextrose CC.	Dextrose %	Diagnosis — Remarks	Outcome
112 cc. M.+225 cc. R. I.V.	112.0	6.6	13.3	—	—	Chronic suppurative nephritis (pyonephrosis).	
64 cc. M.+50 cc. R. I.V.	64.0	3.8	2.9	—	—		D. 6/ 5/31
200 cc. M. I.V.	200.0	5.1	—	—	—	Nephrotic stage of hemorrhagic nephritis and cardiac decompensation.	A. 4/ 7/32
250 cc. M.+50 cc. R. I.V.	250.0	6.4	1.3	—	—		
3000 cc. 1/6 M. I.V.+H.	500.0	11.8	—	300 I.V.	20	Anuria following removal of tuberculous kidney.	D. 6/27/32
400 cc. M. I.V.+600 cc. 1/6 M. H.	200.0	8.0	—	250 I.V.	20	Hem. neph. approaching terminal stage.	I.
1080 cc. F.L.R. I.V.+I.P.+H.	80.0	4.4	40.0	250 I.V.	10	Subacute hem. neph.	D. 1/25/35
1500 cc. F.L.R. I.V.+H.	300.0	10.7	42.9	—	—	Amyloidosis—chr. staph. suppuration.	A. 6/16/35
180 cc. 1/6 M. I.V.+H.	30.0	12.0	80.0	—	—	Multiple staph. abscesses of kidneys.	
180 cc. 1/6 M. I.V.+H.	30.0	12.0	—	—	—		A. 12/ 3/35
2400 cc. 1/6 M. I.V.+H.	400.0	20.0	80.0	—	—	Chr. suppurative neph.	A. 12/ 1/36
900 cc. F.L.R. I.V.+H.	150.0	12.3	92.0	150 I.V.	10	Nephrotic stage of chr. hem. neph.	
780 1/6 M. I.V.+H.	130.0	9.8	—	—	—		I.
300 cc. F.L.R. I.V.+H.	50.0	9.4	37.7	—	—	Oliguria—tubules filled and obstructed by precipitated material of undetermined composition.	A. 3/24/37
300 cc. F.L.R. I.V.+H.	50.0	9.4	37.7	—	—		
960 cc. 1/6 M. I.V.+H.	160.0	10.0	—	—	—	Hem. neph. approaching terminal stage.	I.

dration, was also relieved satisfactorily by this method. Satisfactory results were also secured in two adults who had developed acidosis following the development of anuria after transfusion reactions, and in one adult who had been given a fatal dose of diethylene glycol containing sulfanilamide ("Elixir of Sulfanilamide") and who had developed severe acidosis following almost complete suppression of urine.

In the chronic type of renal insufficiency when vomiting is absent or negligible, the continued oral administration of sodium lactate may be quite efficacious in relieving acidosis and preventing its recurrence. For this purpose, amounts of sodium lactate varying from 50 to 150 c.c. (1-5 c.c. of molar solution per kilogram) may have to be administered daily in three or four divided doses.

TABLE

RECOVERY OF ACIDOSIS OF DIARRHEAL ORIGIN

No.	Case	Date	Age	Body			Serum*												
							Vols. %		CO_2 Content			NaCl Mg. %	Gm. % Protein			Lactic Acid Mg. %	Inorg. P. Mg. %	Ca. Mg. %	N.P.N. Mg. %
				Wt. Kg.	Water Liters	Edema	Before	After	Hrs.	Expected	Difference		Total	Alb.	Glob.				
1	G-1608	8/10/30	6 mo.	6.6	4.4		37.7	45.0	2	47.6	−2.6	509 573							
2	G-2352	11/22/30	6 wk.	2.7	1.8		26.9	46.3	½	51.7	−5.4								
3	H- 479	2/28/31	8 mo.	6.3	4.2		23.6	46.5	3½	55.6	−9.1								
4	H- 669	3/14/31	5 wk.	2.7	1.8		23.9	48.3	3	61.2	−12.9								
5	H-1652	7/19/31	3 mo.	5.0	3.3		13.0	48.0	5½	40.1	+ 7.9								
6	H-2202	9/22/31	2 mo.	3.0	2.0		31.9	43.1	18	43.1	0	672 675	7.43				5.5		58.5
7	H-2641	11/27/31	8 mo.	7.6	5.0		27.4	69.5	14	67.7	+ 1.8	596 630 602	6.13				3.15		19.0
8	I-1728	9/15/32	16 da.	3.1	2.0		30.7	42.9	2½	69.8	−16.9								
9	I-1760	9/ 2/32	7 wk.	3.3	2.2		17.4	37.8	5	58.1	−20.4								
10	J- 219	1/23/33	6 mo.	6.5	4.3		23.7	41.6	3	58.3	−16.7	872 655	7.60 4.47			63.5 98.6 26.8			127.0 34.0
11	J-1574	7/22/33	9 mo.	5.2	3.5		28.0	72.0	15	70.2	+ 1.8	661 596						10.0	
12	J-2009	9/ 5/33	7 mo.	5.0	3.3		36.8	52.5	14	77.5	−25.0								
13	J-2168	9/26/33	6 wk.	3.1	2.1		16.5	61.8	10	59.2	− 2.6	665 667	9.05 5.61						120.0 47.0
14	J-2350	10/18/33	5 mo.	4.3	2.9		37.0	53.3	11½	44.9	+ 3.4	608 567	8.74 5.67			49.8			47.0 20.8
15	J-2292	11/ 7/33	5 wk.	2.8	1.9		23.1	48.5	13	43.1	+ 5.4	678	6.95						33.0 28.0
16	J-2713	12/10/33	2 mo.	3.5	2.3		30.2	53.4	15	49.6	+ 3.8	745	7.95			40.9			60.0
17	L- 377	2/15/34	10 mo.	8.8	5.9		33.6	58.7	4½	55.6	+ 3.1	748 655	7.95 6.83						45.0 48.0
18	K-2378	10/29/34	11 da.	3.3	2.2		17.2	36.8	24	47.7	−10.9	725					4.7	11.9	32.0
19	K-2264	10/24/34	16 da.	2.6	1.7		16.2	43.2	22	55.7	−12.5	700	9.18			40.6	7.2		103.0
20	K-2432	11/ 5/34	7 mo.	6.5	4.1		37.5	74.1	24	73.0	+ 1.1		5.35						40.0
21	K-2730	1/15/35	4 wk.	2.9	1.9		20.0	26.0	2½	55.3	−29.3	785							53.5
22	K-2730	1/15/35	4 wk.	2.9	1.9		26.0	32.0	2¼	61.3	−29.3	765							53.5
23	L- 116	1/18/35	1 mo.	2.8	1.9		12.9	46.3	20	43.5	+ 2.8	675	6.03						30.0
24	L- 203	1/23/35	7 mo.	5.8	3.9		19.1	24.6	7	78.3	−53.7	715							
25	L- 327	2/ 8/35	5 mo.	5.9	3.9		18.0	56.3	9	55.3	+ 1.0	503 643	4.96						22.0
26	L- 687	4/ 3/35	6 wk.	3.8	2.5		19.0	40.7	16	37.0	+ 3.7		5.60			28.7	5.0	9.0	52.0
27	L- 995	5/21/35	5 mo.	5.4	3.6		17.0	71.0	29	79.2	− 8.2	705	8.70 7.30			21.5 72.4			217.0 204.0

*When double figures are given, the lower denote determinations after treatment.

†M. = Molar concentration.
I.V. = Intravenously.
I.P. = Intraperitoneally.

H. = Subcutaneously.
C.I.V. = Continuous intravenous.
R. = Ringer's solution.

F.L.R. = Fortified Lactate-Ringer's solution.
D. = Died—No autopsy.
A. = Autopsy.
I. = Improved and still living.

IV

AFTER NA R-LACTATE—NONSPECIFIC DIARRHEA

Na r-LACTATE†	Molar CC.	Molar CC./Kg.	RINGER'S CC./Kg.	DEXTROSE CC.	DEXTROSE %	DIAGNOSIS — REMARKS	OUTCOME
20 cc. M.+130 cc. R.+100 cc. 10% dextrose I.V.	20.0	3.0	20.0	150	10	Convulsions, circulatory failure—moribund at time of treatment.	A. 8/10/30
20 cc. M.+400 cc. R. I.V.	20.0	7.4	148.0	40 80	5 10	B. coli septicemia, otitis media, broncho-pneumonia.	D. 12/ 4/30
60 cc. M.+100 cc. 5% dextrose I.V.	60.0	9.5		100	5	Mastoiditis, broncho-pneumonia, necrosis of colon.	A. 3/ 1/31
30 cc. M.+50 cc. 20% dextrose I.V.	30.0	11.1	129.0	50	20	Athrepsia, thrombosis of longitudinal sinus, circulatory collapse.	A. 3/16/31
40 cc. M.+205 cc. 5% dextrose I.V.	40.0	8.0	50.0	205	5	Broncho-pneumonia, moribund at time of treatment.	A. 7/21/31
10 cc. M.+300 cc. R. I.P.	10.0	3.3	100.0			Otitis media, broncho-pneumonia, circulatory collapse.	D. 10/ 6/31
30 cc. M.+60 cc. dextrose I.V. 60 cc. M.+R.+D. C. I.V.	90.0	11.8	110.0	860	10	Otitis media, mastoiditis—continuous I.V. drip for 31 hrs.; equal parts 10% dextrose and lactate Ringer's.	I.
210 cc. ⅙ M. I.V.+I.P.	35.0	11.2	241.0			Spina bifida, hydrocephalus, otitis media, broncho-pneumonia.	A. 9/17/32
20 cc. M.+100 cc. R. I.V. 20 cc. M.+100 cc. R. H.	40.0	12.1	61.0			Spina bifida, hydrocephalus, otitis media, sclerema.	A. 9/ 8/32
180 cc. ⅙ M. I.V. 220 cc. ⅙ M. H.+I. P.	66.0	10.1	62.0			Nutritional edema, convulsions.	I.
400 cc. ⅙ M. I.P.	66.0	12.6	77.0			Carpopedal spasm, cardiac dilatation.	A. 7/24/33
360 cc. ⅙ M. I.P.	60.0	12.0	80.0	200	10	Pertussis, meningismus, circulatory collapse.	A. 9/ 6/33
240 cc. ⅙ M. I.V.	40.0	12.9	258.0	238 C. I. V.	10	Otitis media, 10% Dextrose for 58 hrs. by continuous intravenous drip.	I.
10 cc. M.+283 cc. R.+282 cc. 10% Dextrose	10.0	2.1	66.0	282	10	Otitis media.	I.
100 cc. ⅙ M. I.V.	16.0	6.0	30.0			Otitis media, mastoiditis, ulcerative enteritis.	A. 11/17/33
120 cc. ⅙ M. I.V.	20.0	5.7	228.0			Otitis media.	I.
120 cc. ⅙ M. I.V. 150 cc. ⅙ M. I.P. 80 cc. ⅙ M. H.	58.0	6.5	47.0			Otitis media.	I.
180 cc. ⅙ M. H.	30.0	9.0	38.0	125	5		I.
90 cc. ⅙ M. I.V. 90 cc. ⅙ M. H.	30.0	11.5	46.0	60	10	Broncho-pneumonia, thrombosis renal vein.	A. 10/15/34
195 cc. ⅙ M. I.V. 195 cc. ⅙ M. H.	65.0	10.0	101.0	140	20	Pharyngitis, pyelitis, mental deficiency.	I.
180 cc. ⅙ M. H.+I.P.	30.0	10.3				Birth injury, cyanosis, convulsions, otitis media.	I.
60 cc. ⅙ M. I.V. 120 cc. ⅙ M. H.	30.0	10.3					I.
35 cc. ⅙ M. I.V. 120 cc. ⅙ M. I.V.+H.	26.0	9.2	153.0	80	20	Cyanosis, circulatory collapse.	I.
450 cc. 1/5 M. H.+I.P.	103.0	17.7		100	10	Congenital heart disease, broncho-pneumonia, mental deficiency.	D. 1/23/35
5 cc. M.+120 cc. R.+120 cc. 10% Dextrose I.V. 360cc.⅙M.H.+I.P.	65.0	11.0	20.0	120	10	Broncho-pneumonia, staphylococcus septicemia, moribund at time of treatment.	A. 2/19/35
20 cc. M.+100 cc. 10% Dextrose I.V.	20.0	5.2	26.0	100	10	Degeneration of cerebral cortex, convulsions, broncho-pneumonia.	A. 4/ 8/35
100 cc. M.+750 cc. R. I.V.+H.+ I.P.	100.0	18.5	138.0	300	10	Thrombosis transverse sinus, meningitis, broncho-pneumonia.	A. 5/23/35

TABLE IV—

RECOVERY OF ACIDOSIS OF DIARRHEAL ORIGIN

No.	Case	Date	Age	Body: Wt. Kg.	Body: Water Liters	Body: Edema	Serum*: Vols. %: Before	Vols. %: After	CO_2 Content: Hrs.	CO_2 Content: Expected	CO_2 Content: Difference	NaCl Mg. %	Gm. % Protein: Total	Gm. % Protein: Alb.	Gm. % Protein: Glob.	Lactic Acid Mg. %	Inorg. P. Mg. %	Ca. Mg. %	N.P.N. Mg. %
28	L-1394	7/11/35	11 da.	3.1	2.1		27.9	56.6	19	59.9	− 4.3								
29	L-1406	7/12/35	3 wk.	2.7	1.8		14.8	58.0	12	114.3	−56.3								
30	L-1511	7/26/35	4 wk.	2.5	1.7		24.1	56.0	24	50.4	+ 5.6								113.0 60.0
31	L-1522	7/28/35	2 wk.	3.1	2.1		12.0	55.0	21½	54.6	+ 0.4					44.1 60.5			
32	L-1554	8/ 1/35	2 wk.	2.2	1.5		12.9	30.1	13	42.7	−12.6								
33	L-1564	8/ 2/35	2 wk.	2.1	1.4		22.9	39.8	20	86.9	−47.1								
34	L-2600	12/ /35	6 wk.	3.1	2.1		17.0	46.2	5	59.6	−13.4								
35	M- 137	1/ 7/36	8 mo.	5.4	3.6		22.0	42.4	14	50.6	− 8.2	650	6.19						29.0
36	L-2448	1/ 9/36	3 mo.	3.7	2.5		18.0	49.8	30	63.6	−13.8	579	7.30				9.3	7.5	26.5 31.5
37	M- 155	1/10/36	14 mo.	8.3	5.5		20.5	43.5	5	53.0	− 9.5						4.0	10.2	
38	M- 188	1/15/36	20 mo.	13.0	8.6		28.9	52.1	17	46.7	+ 5.4								
39	M- 663	4/30/36	3 wk.	2.6	1.7		21.2	48.1	5½	60.7	−12.6								47.0 35.5
40	M-1789	9/21/36	2 mo.	4.2	2.8		20.0	50.6	12	52.0	− 1.4								
41	M-2061	11/15/36	9 mo.	4.9	3.3		32.0	39.5		65.9	−26.4						3.1	9.2	20.0
42	L-2210	11/15/36	3 mo.	3.0	2.0		13.1	33.7	12	50.0	−16.3	854 790	7.63						66.0 74.0
43	N- 525	3/29/37	8 da.	2.0	1.3		17.4	44.0	20	101.8	−57.8								
44	N- 595	4/11/37	3 wk.	1.9	1.2		9.5	22.5	2½	65.5	−43.0								

TABLE

CASES OF

No.	Case	Date	Age	Body: Wt. Kg.	Body: Water Liters	Body: Edema	Serum: Vols. %: Before	Vols. %: After	CO_2 Content: Hrs.	CO_2 Content: Expected	CO_2 Content: Difference	NaCl Mg. %	Gm. % Protein: Total	Gm. % Protein: Alb.	Gm. % Protein: Glob.	Lactic Acid Mg. %	Inorg. P. Mg. %	Ca. Mg. %	N.P.N. Mg. %
1	G-1683	8/20/30	3 yr.				25.0	66.4											
2	G-2058	10/28/30	16 mo.	7.2	4.8		27.5	44.6	3	69.5	−24.9								
3	L-1431	7/16/35	2 yr.	11.4	7.6		31.5	54.5	13	50.6	+ 3.9								
4	L-1859	9/ 8/35	5 yr.	17.0	11.3		30.0	61.0	12	63.6	− 2.6								
5	L-2455	10/30/35	10 mo.	8.8	5.9		15.0	63.4	21	66.2	− 2.8								
6	M-1253	7/11/36	2 yr.	11.0	7.3		10.0	78.0	14	56.0	+22.0								
7	M-1411	8/ 1/36	5 mo.	4.7	3.1		12.0	16.0	13	55.3	−39.3								
8	N-1126	7/ 1/37	18 mo.	7.9	5.2		38.0	44.6	7	72.4	−27.8								

*When double figures are given, the lower denote determinations after treatment.

†M.=Molar concentration.
I.V.=Intravenously.
I.P.=Intraperitoneally.

H.=Subcutaneously.
C.I.V.—Continuous Intravenous
R.=Ringer's solution.

F.L.R.=Fortified Lactate-Ringer's solution
D.=Died—No Autopsy.
A.=Autopsy.
I.=Improved and still living.

CONT'D

AFTER NA R-LACTATE—NONSPECIFIC DIARRHEA

Na r-Lactate†	Molar CC.	Molar CC./Kg.	Ringer's CC./Kg.	Dextrose CC.	Dextrose %	Diagnosis — Remarks	Outcome
60 cc. 1/6 M. I.V. 20 cc. M.+400 cc. R. H.	30.0	9.6	129.0	75	10	Streptococcus and B. coli septicemia.	A. 8/ 4/35
70 cc. M.+550 cc. R. I.V.+H.	80.0	29.6	333.0	75	10	Cellulitis, septicemia, moribund at time of treatment.	A. 7/14/35
20 cc. M.+200 cc. R. H.	20.0	8.0	80.0	65	10	Impetigo, moribund at time of treatment.	A. 8/ 1/35
40 cc. M.+380 cc. R. I.V.+H.	40.0	12.9	122.0			Comatose at time of treatment.	I.
120 cc. 1/6 M. I.V.+I.P.	20.0	9.0	45.0	50	10	Prematurity.	D. 8/ 2/35
240 cc. 1/6 M. I.V.+H.	40.0	19.0	87.0	60	10	Otitis media—moribund at time of treatment.	A. 8/16/35
280 cc. 1/6 M. I.V.+H.	40.0	12.8	80.0	50	10	Otitis media.	I.
275 cc. 1/6 M. I.V.+H.	46.0	8.5	37.0			Otitis media, rickets.	I.
300 cc. 1/6 M. I.V.+H.	51.0	13.8	54.0			Impetigo, broncho-pneumonia, otitis media, convulsions.	A. 1/19/36
480 cc. 1/6 M. I.V.+H.	80.0	9.6	39.0	100	10	Spastic paralysis, otitis media, rickets.	I.
420 cc. 1/6 M. H.	70.0	5.4	31.0	150	10	Otitis media, ketosis.	I.
180 cc. 1/6 M. I.V.+H.	30.0	11.5	153.0	70	10	Otitis media, thrush.	I.
40 cc. M.+400 cc. R. I.V.+H.	40.0	9.5	95.0	80	10	Otitis media.	I.
50 cc. M.+250 cc. R. I.V.+I.P.	50.0	10.2	81.0			Athrepsia, otitis media, broncho-pneumonia.	I.
200 cc. 1/6 M. I.P.	33.0	11.0	133.0	70	10	Impetigo, otitis media, broncho-pneumonia.	A. 11/17/36
30 cc. M.+360 cc. R. I.V.+H. 19 cc. M.+75 cc. 5% Dextrose H.	49.0	24.5	180.0	75	5	Prematurity, peritonitis, broncho-pneumonia, circulatory collapse.	A. 3/ 3/37
180 1/6 M. I.V.+P.	30.0	15.7	210.0			Moribund at time of treatment.	D. 4/14/38

IV-A

BACILLARY DYSENTERY

Na r-Lactate	Molar CC.	Molar CC./Kg.	Ringer's CC./Kg.	Dextrose CC.	Dextrose %	Diagnosis — Remarks	Outcome
40 cc. M.+1700 cc. R. H. 20 cc. M.+200 cc. Dextrose I.V.	60.0			400	10	Cellulitis, hemolytic streptococcus septicemia.	A. 8/28/30
360 cc. 1/4 M. H.	90.0	12.5				Hiss-Russell, hemolytic streptococcus septicemia, otitis media, mastoiditis, pyuria.	D. 10/28/30
65 cc. M.+800 cc. R. I.V.+H.	65.0	5.7	70.0	250	10	Hiss-Russell, parotitis.	I.
1020 cc. 1/6 M. I.V.+H.	170.0	10.0	40.0	250	10	Hiss-Russell.	I.
810 cc. 1/6 M. I.V.+H.+I.P.	135.0	15.3	51.0	115	10	Hiss-Russell, scarlet fever, septicemia, meningitis, peritonitis.	D. 12/13/35
660 1/6 M. I.V.+H.	150.0	13.6	73.0	100	10	Hiss-Russell, acute parotitis.	I.
360 cc. 1/6 M. I.V.+H.	60.0	12.8	85.0	100	10	Shiga, sclerema, moribund at time of treatment.	D. 8/ 2/36
480 cc. 1/6 M. I.V.+H.	80.0	10.0	40.0	100	10	Hiss-Russell, otitis media, encephalitis.	A. 7/ 4/37

III. ACIDOSIS OF DIARRHEAL ORIGIN

This form of acidosis, compared with that of renal origin, is somewhat more complex in that contributory factors are: (1) loss of base bicarbonate from the body as the result of failure to reabsorb alkaline digestive juices; (2) renal insufficiency due partly merely to oliguria, the result of anhydremia, and partly also to acute degenerative renal changes; (3) circulatory failure, particularly the result of anhydremia which leads to tissue anoxia and permits such acids as lactic acid to accumulate, and (4) ketosis, the result of starvation or infection, seen especially when the diarrhea is the result of acute ileocolitis due to the dysentery bacillus.

As in a previous communication,[8] we prefer to classify the acute diarrheas under two main types: (1) the so-called nonspecific diarrhea, and (2) acute bacillary dysentery. As may be noted from Tables IV and IV-A, we now (inclusive of 1937) have 60 cases of acidosis associated with nonspecific diarrhea treated with sodium lactate solution, and 8 due to acute bacillary dysentery, in whom follow-up data have been secured. It may also be noted that all but 3 were satisfactorily relieved. In addition, we have treated apparently successfully, but without confirmatory follow-up laboratory data, 100 more cases of acidosis associated with nonspecific diarrhea and 41 with acute bacillary dysentery. The initial carbon dioxide contents in these cases without follow-up data varied from 10 to 39 volumes per cent, and 44 were under 28 volumes per cent. In comparing the observed effects in 64 cases with the calculated, the following data are of interest:

Less than expected (−)				More than expected (+)	
>30 vol. %	30-20 vol. %	20-10 vol. %	10-0 vol. %	0-10 vol. %	10 vol. %
(7) = 10.9%	(8) = 12.5%	(16) = 25.0%	(17) = 26.5%	(15) = 23.5%	(1) = 1.6%

Average = −11.8 vol. %

It should be mentioned that the success in the relief of acidosis in such cases was much better than the success of treatment as a whole. The eventual mortality in this group of patients was 51 per cent. In many instances the patients were moribund at the time of admission to the hospital, but despite their moribund state they metabolized sodium lactate fairly normally and were completely relieved of acidosis before death. It should also be mentioned that in this type of case there is a strong tendency for recurrence of acidosis, and lactate-Ringer's solution has to be given after the initial relief of acidosis in amounts sufficient to prevent recurrence of dehydration if recurrence of acidosis is to be avoided. Such fluid administration may be given with interrupted injections subcutaneously, intraperitoneally or intravenously in the usual amounts, or as a continuous intravenous drip.

IV. DIABETIC ACIDOSIS

Inclusive of 1937 we have treated 55 cases of diabetic acidosis with sodium lactate, and in Chart 3 and Table V the results of treatment are

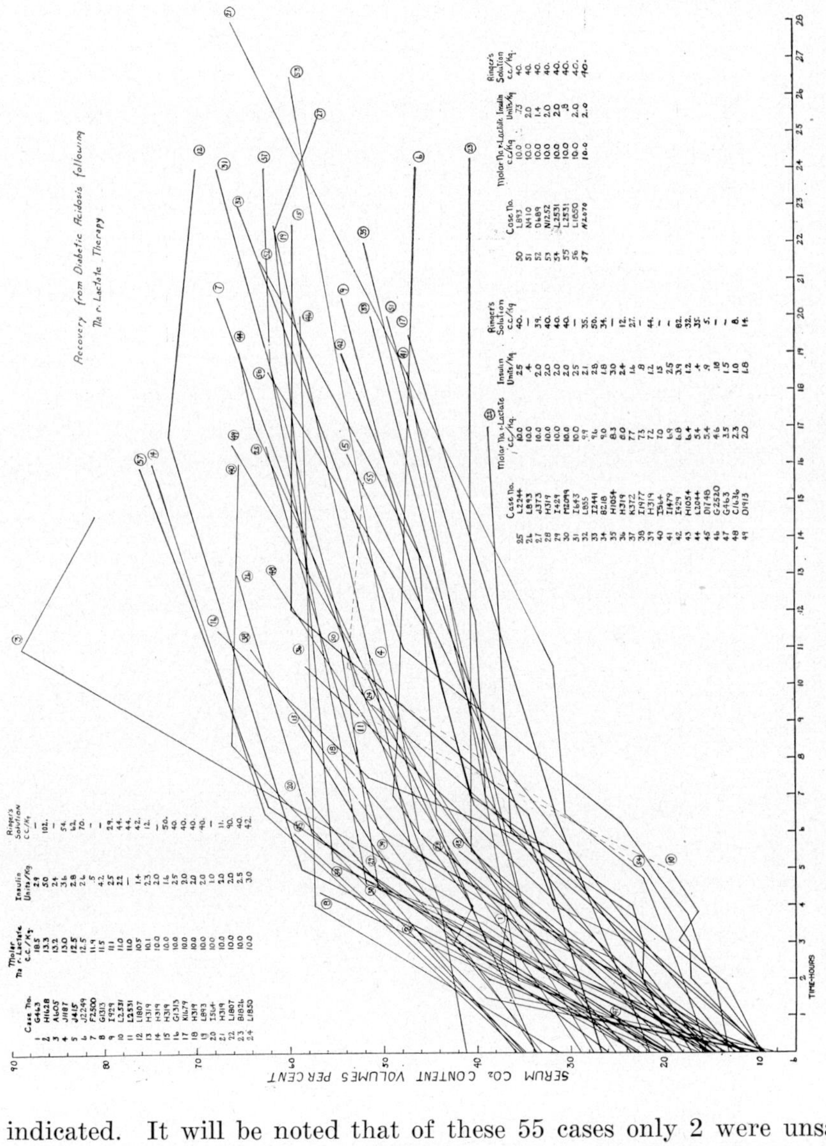

Chart 3.—Rise in serum carbon dioxide content in cases of diabetic acidosis following sodium r-lactate therapy.

indicated. It will be noted that of these 55 cases only 2 were unsatisfactory by definition, and in only one case did the carbon dioxide content rise to more than 80 volumes per cent after the successful relief of acidosis. Furthermore, only two deaths occurred in the group, a mortality of 3.6 per cent.

TABLE V

Data Incident to Recovery from Acidosis of Diabetic Origin After Na r-Lactate Therapy

No.	Case	Date	Age	Body: Wt. Kg.	Body: H_2O Liter (Estimated)	Serum: CO_2 Content—Vols. %: Before	After	Hrs.	Expected	Difference	Nacl. Mg. %	Protein G.%	Alb. G.%	Glob. G.%	Lactic Acid Mg. %	Inorg. P. Mg. %	N.P.N. Mg. %	Dextrose Mg. %	Therapy: Na r-Lactate*	Molar: CC.	Molar: CC./Kg.	Ringer's Solution CC./Kg.	Insulin 1st 8 Hrs. U./Kg.
1	G- 463	12/28/30	11 yr.	35.0	23.3	8.5	36.0 37.6 36.8	2 3 4	71.0	−35.0 −33.4 −34.2	660 655 669	10.5 6.68 5.95 5.29			100.8 75.6 55.0	5.7 1.4 1.0	47.0 55.0 45.0 53.0	432 407 498 131		650	18.5	—	2.9
2	H-1628	7/14/31	6 yr.	15.0	10.0	10.8	39.0 47.0	1¾ 3½	55.6	−16.6 − 8.6								560 360 296	200 cc. M.+ 200 cc. R. I.V.	200	13.3	102	5.0
3	A- 605	5/30/33	21 yr.	44.0	29.3	14.4	88.7 80.9 70.4	11 14½ 36	58.9	+29.8 +22.0 +11.5	562 468 456 520	10.7 7.05					49.0 38.8	588 29 250 397	1350 ⅙ M. I.V. 2150 ⅙ M. (H.)	583	13.2	—	2.4
4	J-1187	6/12/33	11 mo.	5.7	3.8	15.0	39.0 52.0	3 11	59.2	−20.2 − 7.2								300 172 58	75 cc. M.+375 cc. H_2O-½ I.V. ½ H.	75	13.0	54	3.6
5	J- 415	2/23/33	8 mo.	4.6	3.1	12.8	24.5 38.3 53.9	4 8 16	55.0	−30.5 −16.7 − 1.1	696	9.02			32.2 49.7 33.8	4.7	37.5	628 645 312 75	130 cc. ⅙ M. I.V. 220 cc. ⅙ M. (H.)	58.3	12.5	62	2.8
6	J-2249	10/ 6/33	2¼ yr.	11.3	7.5	10.4	29.2 38.6 42.5 40.4 49.0 46.4	1½ 2½ 3½ 4½ 7½ 24	52.6	−23.4 −14.0 −10.1 −12.2 − 3.6 − 6.2	596	8.72 7.48 7.02 7.65 7.56			32.8 58.0 35.2 26.5 20.2		25.0 25.0 25.0 25.0 25.0	525 237 115 56 48 56		141	12.5	70	2.6
7	F-2500	4/ 4/33	7 yr.	21.0	14.0	41.2	44.0 67.3	6 20½	81.2	−37.2 −13.9							69.7	176 109 162	1500 cc. ⅙ M. I.V.—H.	250	11.9	—	0.5
8	G-1313	7/ 7/30	13 yr.	9.6	6.4	20.3	29.0 56.9	1½ 4½	58.7	−29.7 − 1.8	521				26.4 34.0		22.0	410 508 335		110	11.5	—	4.2

9	I- 929	5/12/32	14 yr.	27.0	18.0	11.4	20.3 22.2 22.1 23.5 40.7 54.0	2½ 3½ 4½ 6 8½ 20½	48.7	−28.4 −26.5 −26.6 −25.2 − 8.0 + 5.3	595 544	6.70 6.35 5.42					32.0	360 263 195 168 150 133	200 cc. ⅙ M. I.V. 800 cc. ⅙ M. I.P. 800 cc. ⅙ M. (H.)	300	11.1	29	2.5
10	L-2531	3/30/36	6½ yr.	18.1	12.0	9.7	13.5	2	47.0	−33.5	658 615	10.4			27.7 83.4		27.0	405 266	200 M.+1000 cc. H_2O −I.V.+H.	200	11.0	44	2.2
11	L-2531	3/30/36	6½ yr.	18.1	12.0	19.1	18.2 16.3 52.8 52.8	3 3¾ 5 9¼ 22	56.4	−28.8 −30.7 − 3.6 − 3.6	623 603 612 527 533	8.75 7.65			41.6 33.0 32.2		20.0 17.0	199 166 113 284	200 M.+1000 cc. H_2O I.V.+H.	200	11.0	44	—
12	L-1807	8/ 5/36	5 yr.	19.0	12.6	19.8 pH. 700	58.5 72.8 69.9	5 17 24	55.4	+ 3.1 +17.4 +14.5								290 250 55 80	200 cc. M.+1000 cc. H_2O I.V.+H.	200	10.5	42	1.4
13	H- 319	2/ 2/34	12 yr.	32.6	21.7	19.0	49.8 59.0	5 9	53.0	− 3.2 + 6.0					54.8 40.2 18.9			775 292 181	1980 cc. ⅙ M. Continuous Drip	330	10.1	12	2.3
14	H- 319	12/26/33	12 yr.	32.0	21.3	35.5	62.5 74.7	6½ 16	69.2	− 6.7 + 5.5	515 486	10.2			38.9 30.8 21.4		48.0 52.0	492 197 60	960−⅙ M. I.V. 960−⅙ M. H.	320	10.0	—	2.0
15	H- 319	3/19/34	12 yr.	31.0	20.6	26.7	34.1 59.8 59.6	6½ 12 22½	60.4	−26.3 − 0.6 − 0.8					27.7 64.3 23.9 29.9			525 347 184 98	310 cc. M.+1550 cc. R. I.V.−H.	310	10.0	50	1.6
16	G-1313	6/ 5/34	7 yr.	20.0	13.3	15.8	31.6 51.7 67.8 71.5	5½ 7½ 11½ 30½	49.5	−17.9 + 2.2 +18.3 +22.0	567 575	7.93 6.27			51.7 64.2 49.1 41.6 28.9		56.3 32.4	857 614 536 399 234	480 cc. ⅙ M. I.V. 720 cc. ⅙ M. H.	200	10.0	40	2.5
17	K-1679	7/31/34	2 yr.	11.5	7.6	21.7	31.6 47.6	6½ 19½	55.7	−24.1 − 8.1	585 585				37.6			376 222 126	690 cc. ⅙ M. I.V.+H.	115	10.0	40	2.0
18	H- 319	10/25/34	13 yr.	40.0	26.7	12.2	24.4 33.5 45.4 54.9	2 3 5 8	45.8	−21.4 −12.3 − 0.4 + 9.1	479 521 550 560	9.96 8.40 8.05 7.85			45.4 71.8 63.0 42.8 25.2		49.0 44.0	1160 659 578 398 325 114	2400 cc. ⅙ M. I.V.+H.	400	10.0	40	2.0

*M.=Molar concentration.
I.V.=Intravenously.
I.P.=Intraperitoneally.

H.=Subcutaneously.
R.=Ringer's solution.
F.L.R.=Fortified Lactate-Ringer's solution.

D.=Died—No autopsy.
A.=Autopsy.
I.=Improved.

TABLE V — Continued

DATA INCIDENT TO RECOVERY FROM ACIDOSIS OF DIABETIC ORIGIN AFTER Na r-LACTATE THERAPY

				SERUM															THERAPY				
				Body		CO_2 Content—Vols. %					Nacl.	Protein	Alb.	Glob.	Lactic Acid	Inorg. P.	N.P.N.	Dextrose		Molar			
No.	Case	Date	Age	Wt. Kg.	H_2O Liter (Estimated)	Before	After	Hrs.	Expected	Difference	Mg. %	G.%	G.%	G.%	Mg. %	Mg. %	Mg. %	Mg. %	Na r-Lactate*	CC.	CC./Kg.	Ringer's Solution CC./Kg.	Insulin 1st 8 Hrs. U./Kg.
19	L- 893	5/ 6/35	17 mo.	10.0	67.0	11.5	25.0 34.0 40.5 47.0 61.0	2½ 3½ 4½ 5½ 22½	45.0	−20.0 −11.0 − 4.5 + 2.0 +16.0					29.0 40.0 34.6 29.8 21.0 22.1			375 252 174 135 91 185	600 cc. ⅙ M. H.+I.P. +I.V.	100	10.0	40	2.0
20	I- 564	1/31/34	13 yr.	30.0	20.0	34.9	59.0	7	68.5	− 9.5								242 580 410	1800 cc. ⅙ M. I.V.+H.	300	10.0	—	1.0
21	H- 319	8/14/35	14 yr.	35.0	23.3	15.4	18.9 22.2 30.7 31.9 66.0	2½ 5 6½ 10½ 28	49.1	−30.2 −26.9 −18.4 −17.2 +16.9								727 520 228 133	2100 cc. ⅙ M. I.V.+H_2O	350	10.0	11	2.0
22	L-1807	9/ 1/35	4 yr.	15.0	10.0	13.1	14.6 24.9 36.1 38.6	2 4 6 17	46.7	−32.1 −21.8 −10.6 − 8.1								455 381 273 216 162	70 cc. M.+800 R. I.V. 80 cc. M.+550 R. I.P.	150	10.0	90	2.0
23	B-1826	9/27/35	14 yr.	40.0	26.7	14.5	40.8 40.5	5½ 24	48.1	− 7.3 − 7.6					47.8 57.9 44.1			502 155 375	400 cc.M.+2000 cc. H_2O I.V.+H	400	10.0	40	2.5
24	L-1850	9/6/35	8 yr.	18.8	12.5	9.1	51.0	9½	43.2	+ 7.8								478 55	190 cc. M.+950 cc. H_2O I.V.+H.	190	10.0	42	3.0
25	L-2244	10/31/35	5 yr.	15.0	10.0	11.1	50.6 62.1	6 16½	44.7	+ 5.9 +17.4		5.30 5.21 5.25	2.77		23.0 30.0 27.7		22.2 17.0 13.5	503 87 41	450 cc. ⅙ M. I.V. 450 cc. ⅙ M. H.	150	10.0	40	2.5
26	L- 893	7/20/36	3 yr.	12.0	8.0	26.0	57.6 65.5	5½ 13	59.7	− 2.1 − 2.1 + 5.8								215 72 75	720 cc. ⅙ M. I.V.−H.	120	10.0	—	0.4

27	J- 373	8/ 6/36	10 yr.	22.5	15.0	20.2 pH. 7.01	55.5 61.3 57.0	5¼ 22 25½	53.8	+ 1.7 + 7.5 + 3.2		5.35					18.0	372 90 375 77	220 cc.M.+ 1125 cc. H_2O I.V.+H.	220	10.0	39	2.0
28	H- 319	8/12/36	15 yr.	40.0	26.7	23.5	44.3	5½	57.1	−12.8								554 220	400 cc. M.+ 2000 cc. H_2O I.V.−H.	400	10.0	40	2.0
29	I- 429	8/20/36	13 yr.	40.4	26.9	19.5	50.3	5	53.6	− 3.3								562 74	410 cc. M.+2025 H_2O I.V.+H.	410	10.0	40	2.0
30	M-2099	11/ 6/36	10 yr.	23.0	15.3	15.0	50.2	4½	48.7	+ 1.5		7.97 7.43					30.0 26.0	330 167 336	230 cc. M.+1150 cc.H_2O I.V.−H.	230	10.0	40	2.0
31	I- 643	4/ 4/32	13 yr.	45.0	30.0	17.0	18.1 24.9 33.3 39.5 51.7 62.0 67.5	1½ 2 3 4 5 18½ 24	50.6	−32.5 −25.7 −17.3 −11.1 + 1.1 +11.4 +16.9	573	8.85			22.1 — 39.5 30.2 27.8 25.0 22.7 20.5	4.5	30.0	470 — 308 301 270 252 218 214 185	450 cc. M.+ 2400 cc. H_2O I.V.+H.	450	10.0	—	2.5
32	L- 855	4/29/35	11 mo.	8.0	5.3	9.6	14.5 16.0 17.5 20.5 24.5 47.9 65.0	2 3 4 5 6½ 11 23	39.3	−24.8 −23.3 −21.8 −18.8 −14.8 + 8.6 +25.7					22.0 12.6 6.0 12.6 6.0 10.0 13.0			553 378 275 215 163 105 180 149	70 cc. M.+ 350 cc. H_2O I.V.−H.	70	9.9	35	2.1
33	I-2441	12/20/32	6 yr.	17.7	11.8	15.1	25.7 35.2 51.2	2 4 20	47.3	−21.6 −12.1 + 3.9	579	8.99			30.2 39.4 23.4		31	500 287 89 60 56 50.5	170 cc. M.+ 900 cc. R. I.V.+H.	170	9.6	50	2.8
34	B- 218	8/21/36	13 yr.	46.3	30.9	13.5	54.2	5	43.9	+10.3								540 288	420 cc. M.+ 2100 cc. H_2O I.V.−H.	420	9.0	34	1.8
35	H-1054	5/ 1/31	12 yr.	30.0	20.0	16.1	35.2 52.0	4 22	44.1	− 8.9 + 7.9	603 556 538	8.58 7.33 8.76			64.3 51.5 42.3	3.9 2.0 3.0	27.0	508 278 40	250 cc. M.+ 600 cc. 5% glucose	250	8.3	—	3.0
36	H- 319	1/28/31	10 yr.	25.0	16.6	14.4	59.0	10½	41.4	+17.6	503 504	8.41 7.30				2.0	53.5 30.0	655 70	200 cc. M.+ 300 cc. R. I.V.	200	8.0	12	2.4
37	K- 372	2/11/34	10 yr.	18.6	12.4	25.2	52.8 62.5	10 24	51.9	+ 0.9 +10.6					18.9 28.9			240 154 87	500 cc. ⅙ M. I.V. 364 cc. ⅙ M. (H.)	148	7.7	27	1.6

*M. = Molar concentration.
I.V. = Intravenously.
I.P. = Intraperitoneally.

H. = Subcutaneously.
R. = Ringer's solution.
F.L.R. = Fortified Lactate-Ringer's solution.

D. = Died—No autopsy.
A. = Autopsy.
I. = Improved.

TABLE V — Continued

Data Incident to Recovery from Acidosis of Diabetic Origin After Na r-Lactate Therapy

				Serum															Therapy				
				Body		CO_2 Content—Vols. %					Nacl.	Protein	Alb.	Glob.	Lactic Acid	Inorg. P.	N.P.N.	Dextrose		Molar		Ringer's Solution	Insulin 1st 8 Hrs
No.	Case	Date	Age	Wt. Kg.	H_2O Liter (Estimated)	Before	After	Hrs.	Expected	Difference	Mg. %	G.%	G.%	G.%	Mg. %	Mg. %	Mg. %	Mg. %	Na r-Lactate*	CC.	CC./Kg.	CC./Kg.	U./Kg.
																		293	635 cc. ⅙ M. I.V.				
38	I-1977	10/ 6/32	10 yr.	25.0	16.6	33.8	64.0	11	68.8	− 4.8								144	460 cc. ⅙ M. (H.)	182	7.3	—	0.8
																		489	260 cc. M.+				
39	H- 319	6/14/34	13 yr.	36.0	24.0	32.0	50.7	5½	56.3	− 5.6								166	1300 cc. R. I.V.+H.	260	7.2	44	1.2
												7.50	3.33	4.12			40.0	475	140 cc. M.+				
40	I- 564	3/21/32	11 yr.	20.0	13.3	35.0			58.6									63	800 cc. H_2O	140	7.0	—	1.5
							66.0	8		+ 7.4									H.				
							65.4	16		+ 6.8								365					
																		60					
											608	6.96			23.9		37.0	437	200 cc. ⅙ M., I.V.				
41	I-1479	7/26/32	4½ yr.	14.4	9.6	16.2	35.8	2	39.6	− 3.8					32.8			150		100	6.9	—	2.5
							47.2	18½		+ 7.6								243	400 cc. ⅙ M. (H.)				
																		543					
42	I-429	2/29/32	9 yr.	21.9	14.6	13.6			36.6		544	7.60			32.0	4.2	33.0		150 cc. M.+	150	6.8	82	3.9
							18.8	2		−17.8					63.0			427	900 cc. R., I.V. H.				
							22.4	3		−14.2					35.0			357					
							23.5	4		−13.1					33.2			300					
							31.8	5		− 4.8								300					
							54.2	19		+17.6					29.6			172					
																		316	210 cc. M.+440 cc.				
43	H-1054	8/21/31	12 yr.	33.0	22.0	15.0	42.0	5½	36.4	+ 5.6								135	R., I.V. H.	210	6 4	32	1.2
																		359	125 cc. M.+				
44	L-2044	10/ 3/35	7 yr.	22.9	15.3	33.8			52.1									41	625 cc. H_2O, I.V. H.	125	5.4	35	0.4
																		42					
							63.8	16		+11.7								151					
							65.7	19		+13.6								424					
45	D-1748	12/25/30	6 yr.	23.0	15.3	34.0	59.6	6	52.5	+ 7.1									120 cc. M.+125 cc.	120	5.4	5	0.9
																			R. I.V.				
																		40	250 cc. M.+				
46	G-2520	5/22/33	14 yr.	54.0	36.0	31.3	57.2	4	46.8	+10.4								56	800 cc. H_2O I.V.+H.	250	4.6	—	0.18
							58.9	20		+12.1								383					

48	C-1636	2/ 7/32	17 yr.	56.8	37.9	29.0	61.5	13	36.7	+24.8								135 70	130 cc. M.+ 400 cc. H_2O I.V.+H.	130	2.3	8	1.0
49	D-1913	3/ 9/31	15 yr.	50.0	33.3	27.5	56.0	16½	34.2	+21.8								678 66	100 cc. M.+300 cc. R. I.V.	100	2.0	14	1.8
50	L- 893	1/25/37	3½ yr.	15.2	10.1	23.0	51.0 54.4	4 11	56.0	− 5.0 − 1.6								223 201 189	152 cc. M.+ 760 cc. H_2O I.V.−H.	152	10.0	40	0.73
51	N- 410	3/ 5/37	2 yr.	9.1	6.0	18.0	39.0 40.0 49.5	7 11 20	51.7	−12.7 −11.7 − 2.2								456 860 40 52	182 ⅙ M. I.V. 364 ⅙ M. H.	91	10.0	40	2.0
52	D- 689	3/ 7/37	12 yr.	31.1	20.7	19.0	44.0 46.0 63.0	6½ 13½ 21½	52.6	− 8.6 − 6.6 +10.4								452 199 50 186	310 cc. M.+ 1550 cc. H_2O I.V.+H.		10.0	40	1.4
53	N-1252	7/19/37	23 mo.	9.0	6.0	9.0	29.2 36.6 46.1 59.8	2 4 6 26½	42.6	−13.4 − 6.0 + 3.5 +17.2								532 234 187 163 126	90 cc. M.+ 450 cc. H_2O, I.V.+H.	90	10.0	40	2.0
54	L-2531	9/ 5/37	8 yr.	25.0	16.6	9.9 pH. 7.24	17.1 17.3 22.4	2 3 5	43.6	−26.5 −26.3 −21.2		6.34			26.8 52.7 26.2		26.0	334 308 180	250 cc. M.+ 1250 cc. H_2O I.V.+H.	250	10.0	40	2.0
55	L-2531	9/ 5/37	8 yr.	25.0	16.6	22.4 pH. 7.33	53.7 52.0	5½ 10½	56.1	− 2.4 − 4.1					20.6			122 20.4	250 cc. M.+ 1250 cc. H_2O I.V.+H.	250	10.0	40	0.8
56	L-1850	10/ 5/37	10 yr.	23.2	15.5	9.5 pH. 7.08	40.2 45.3 62.0	6¾ 11½ 18½	43.3	− 3.1 + 2.0 +18.7		6.74 5.50			29.1 42.0 36.8		27.0 20.0	345 64.4 58 62	232 cc. M.+ 1150 cc. H_2O ½ I.V. ½ H.	232	10.0	40	2.0
57	N-2070	11/11/37	12 yr.	40.0	26.2	29.3 pH. 7.30	62.5 76.0	6½ 16	62.9	− 0.4 +13.1		7.41 6.57			24.0 29.0 16.4		27.0 17.5	355 120 108	400 cc. M.+ 2000 cc. H_2O I.V. H.	400	10.0	40	2.0

*M. = Molar concentration.
I.V. = Intravenously.
I.P. = Intraperitoneally.

H. = Subcutaneously.
R. = Ringer's solution.
F.L.R. = Fortified Lactate-Ringer's solution.

D. = Died—No autopsy.
A. = Autopsy.
I. = Improved.

It is of interest to compare the observed rises in carbon dioxide content with those calculated at different times after the commencement of treatment:

3 Hours After Beginning Treatment (53 Cases)

Less than expected (−)				More than expected (+)
>30 vol. %	30-20 vol. %	20-10 vol. %	10-0 vol. %	0-10 vol. %
(2) = 3.8%	(19) = 35.8%	(21) = 39.6%	(10) = 18.9%	(1) = 1.9%

Average = 17.4 vol. %

6 Hours After Beginning Treatment (48 Cases)

Less than expected (−)				More than expected (+)	
>30 vol. %	30-20 vol. %	20-10 vol. %	10-0 vol. %	0-10 vol. %	10 vol. %
(1) = 2.3%	(5) = 11.3%	(11) = 25.0%	(19) = 43.2%	(7) = 15.8%	(1) = 2.3%

Average = 8.1 vol. %

12 Hours After Beginning Treatment (34 Cases)

Less than expected (−)			More than expected (+)		
30-20 vol. %	20-10 vol. %	10-0 vol. %	0-10 vol. %	10-20 vol. %	20-30 vol. %
(1) = 2.9%	(3) = 8.8%	(10) = 29.4%	(12) = 35.2%	(7) = 20.6%	(1) = 2.9%

Average = +1.2 vol. %

18 Hours After Beginning Treatment (23 Cases)

Less than expected (−)		More than expected (+)		
20-10 vol. %	10-0 vol. %	0-10 vol. %	10-20 vol. %	20-30 vol. %
(2) = 8.7%	(5) = 21.7%	(8) = 34.8%	(7) = 30.4%	(1) = 4.3%

Average = +4.0 vol. %

24 Hours After Beginning Treatment (8 Cases)

Less than expected (−)	More than expected (+)	
10-0 vol. %	0-10 vol. %	10-20 vol. %
(2) = 25.0%	(3) = 37.5%	(3) = 37.5%

Average = +5.9 vol. %

V. ACIDOSIS OF SEVERE INFECTIONS AND MISCELLANEOUS CAUSES

Here also pathogenesis may be complex, and contributory factors frequently are ketosis, circulatory or renal failure, either of which may be organic or functional, and loss of gastrointestinal secretions by vomiting, diarrhea or fistula, and acid administration. We have 26 examples of acidosis of this type, 20 being relieved satisfactorily (Table VI). Of the 6 exceptions, one (Case 7) is to be explained by the inadequate dose of sodium lactate, 5.8 c.c. molar per kilogram body weight; in cases 12, 19, and 22, second therapeutic injections of lactate proved effectual. The following data compare the observed values following institution of treatment with those expected:

Less than expected (−)				More than expected (+)
30 vol. %	30-20 vol. %	20-10 vol. %	10-0 vol. %	0-10 vol. %
(3) = 12.0%	(7) = 28.0%	(7) = 28.0%	(4) = 16.0%	(4) = 16.0%

Average = −15.4%

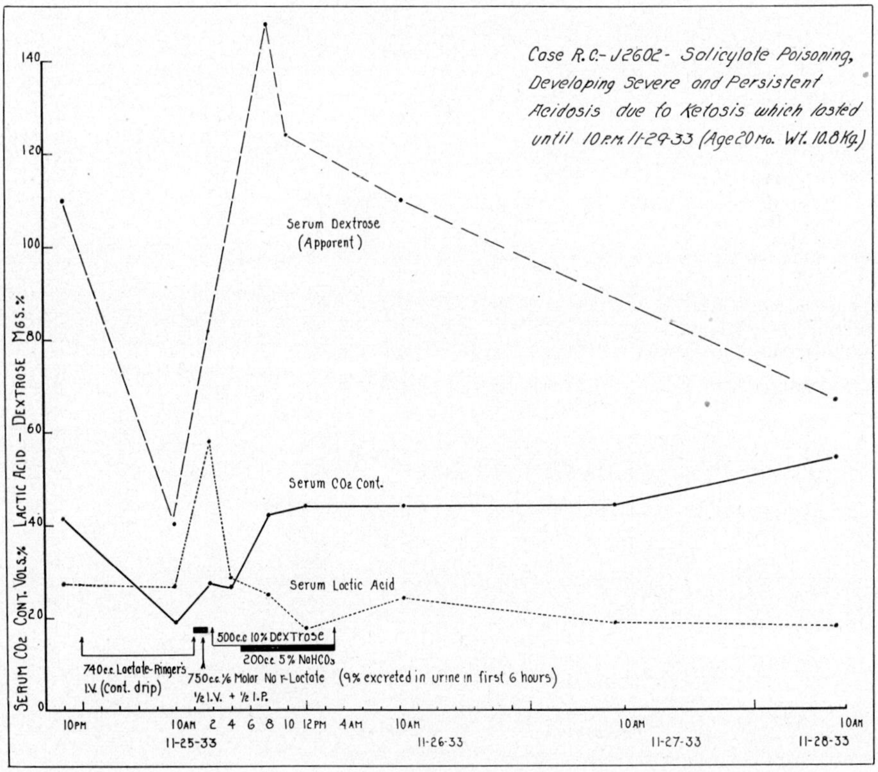

Chart 4.—Case of salicylate poisoning with severe ketosis and acidosis treated successfully with sodium *r*-lactate, dextrose, and sodium bicarbonate.

The underlying infections in this group included various types of severe upper respiratory tract infections with blood stream involvement, meningitis, septic thrombophlebitis, and suppurative nephritis. It should also be mentioned that many of these patients were moribund at the time of treatment of the acidosis.

The case of salicylate poisoning (Cases 12 and 13, Table VI, and Chart 4) is of special interest:

This infant aged 20 months was brought to the hospital one night with the history that following the ingestion of 14-16 tablets, later found to be

TABLE

RECOVERY FROM ACIDOSIS OF SEVERE INFECTIONS AND

No.	Case	Date	Age	Body			Serum*												
				Wt. Kg.	Water Liters	Edema	Vols. %		CO₂ Content			NaCl Mg. %	Gm. % Protein			Lactic Acid Mg. %	Inorg. P. Mg. %	Ca. Mg. %	N.P.N. Mg. %
							Before	After	Hrs.	Expected	Difference		Total	Alb.	Glob.				
1	G-2127	12/14/30	5 wk.	4.7	3.1		23.5	42.5	4	54.2	−11.7								
2	G- 814	8/ 5/30	2 yr.	9.4	6.2		29.5	49.8	5	58.4	− 8.6	632							
3	H- 778	4/ 3/31	3 wk.	2.8	1.8		12.4	28.8	20	49.7	−20.9	747				40.1			
4	H- 992	4/24/31	2 wk.	3.6	2.4		19.8	36.2	2	75.8	−39.6	684 585							
5	H-1047	5/22/31	6 wk.	3.2	2.1		16.4	45.0	13½	88.4	−43.4	747				40.0			
6	H- 978	5/ 9/31	4 da.	2.6	1.7		25.0	56.9	3	75.5	−18.6								
7	H-2457	10/28/31	3 mo.	3.6	2.4		28.0	32.0	18	47.6	−15.6	813 784				56.7 26.5			105.0 77.0
8	H-2457	10/28/31	3 mo.	3.6	2.4		28.3	54.0	12	60.9	− 6.9	796 702	7.45 7.20			21.0 15.0			56.0 67.0
9	I-1193	6/19/32	1 yr.	8.0	5.3		16.7	46.0	15	41.0	+ 5.0								
10	I-2159	10/31/32	21 mo.	7.8	5.2		26.7	40.6	12	45.2	+ 4.6	632	5.20				4.5		90.0 79.0
11	I-2017	10/12/32	5 yr.	12.0	8.0		18.7	44.2	16	52.3	− 8.1								
12	J-2602	11/24/33	20 mo.	10.8	7.2		18.8	26.2	4	57.8	−31.6								
13	J-2602	11/25/33	20 mo.	10.8	7.2		26.2	42.2	3	62.5	−20.6								
14	J-2499	12/ 6/33	5 mo.	4.7	3.1		23.9	51.9	6	59.9	− 0.8	668	4.95				9.0		198.0
15	K-2038	9/12/34	4 mo.	5.0	3.3		14.3	35.9	8	51.4	−11.7		7.28			32.0	5.8		34.0
16	K-2038	9/30/34	4 mo.	4.4	2.9		18.3	41.9	23	41.4	+ 0.5	608							21.0
17	K-2789	12/31/34	19 mo.	6.7	4.5		18.7	31.0	5	51.0	−20.0								
18	L-2633	1/ 1/36	19 mo.	12.0	8.0		20.1	43.5	17	53.6	−10.1								
19	M -246	1/26/36	15 da.	2.4	1.6		16.5	30.5	25	54.3	−23.9								50.0
20	M- 246	1/27/36	16 da.	2.6	1.7		30.5	52.0	26	62.1	−10.1	661 683	 5.30			66.5 65.4			32.0
21	—	10/ 8/37	24 yr.	50.0	33.3		15.5	38.4	16½	49.2	−10.8								
22	N-1993	10/31/37	2 wk.	2.2	1.4		14.3	19.5	5	49.4	−29.9						9.2		91.3
23	N-1993	10/31/37	2 wk.	2.2	1.4		19.5	22.1	12	51.5	−29.4	655							80.5
24	N-1993	10/31/37	2 wk.	2.2	1.4		22.1	55.3	17½	77.5	−22.2								80.5
25	N-2072	11/11/37	11 mo.	6.5	4.3		10.7	17.8	6	44.2	−26.4					35.5			51.8
26	N-2072	11/12/37	11 mo.	6.5	4.3		17.8	35.0	15	52.2	−17.2								

*When double figures are given, the lower denote determinations after treatment.
†M.=Molar concentration.
I.V.=Intravenously.
I.P.=Intraperitoneally.
H.=Subcutaneously.
R.=Ringer's solution.
L.R.=Lactate-Ringer's solution.
F.L.R.=Fortified Lactate-Ringer's solution.
D.=Died—No autopsy.
A.=Autopsy.
I.=Improved.

sodium salicylate, he developed a convulsion and began to vomit. Because of the presence of mild acidosis and persistent vomiting even after gastric lavage, it was decided to give him lactate-Ringer's solution throughout

VI

MISCELLANEOUS CAUSES AFTER SODIUM R-LACTATE THERAPY

Na r-LACTATE†	Molar CC.	Molar CC./Kg.	RINGER'S CC./Kg.	DEXTROSE CC.	DEXTROSE %	DIAGNOSIS — REMARKS	OUTCOME
45 cc. M. I.V.	45.0	9.5		170	10	Acute mastoiditis—streptococcus hemolyticus; diarrhea.	D. 2/15/30
80 cc. M.+120 H_2O	80.0	8.5				Mastoiditis.	I.
30 cc. M.+60 cc. H_2O I.V.	30.0	10.7	14.0			Extensive thrombophlebitis, gangrene, septicemia, circulatory failure.	A. 4/ 7/31
60 cc. M.+400 cc. H_2O H.	60.0	16.6				Otitis media, pneumonia, diarrhea, incomplete fluid absorption.	D. 4/26/31
67.5 cc. M.+H_2O I.V.+H.	67.5	21.0		200	5	Mastoiditis, hemolytic streptococcus, circulatory failure.	D. 5/23/31
240 cc. $\frac{1}{6}$ M. I.V.	40.0	15.4				Spina bifida, neurogenic bladder, cystotomy, anuria.	D. 5/ 9/31
21 cc. M.+50cc.—5% Dext. I.V.	21.0	5.8	19.0	50	10	Thrombophlebitis of lateral sinus, athrepsia, vomiting, diarrhea.	A. 11/ 1/31
20 cc. M.+100 cc. Dextrose 15 cc. M.+75 cc. Dextrose I.V.	35.0	9.7		975	10		
H.	60.0	2.5	37.5	240	5	Starvation ketosis following attempt at weaning.	I.
43 cc. M.+165 cc. Dextrose I.V.	43.0	5.5	51.0			Otitis media, laryngitis, pneumonia, athrepsia, anemia.	A. 11/ 5/32
120 cc. M.+800 cc. H_2O I.V.+H.	120.0	10.0				Scarlet fever, mastoiditis, thrombophlebitis of lateral sinus.	A. 12/17/32
	135.0	11.6				Salicylate poisoning, ketosis, see Chart 4.	I.
50 cc. M. I.V.	50.0	10.6				Otitis media, erysipelas, thrombophlebitis, pyonephritis with infarcts, septicemia—strep. hemo.	A. 12/ 6/33
150 cc. $\frac{1}{6}$ M. I.V. 150 cc. $\frac{1}{6}$ M. I.P.	50.0	10.0	40.0			Acute suppurative nephritis—B. coli.	D. 10/11/34
185 cc. $\frac{1}{6}$ M. I.V.+H.	31.0	7.0					
$\frac{1}{6}$ M. I.V.+H.	65.0	9.7	39.0			Pneumonia, jaundice, circulatory failure. Fluids incompletely absorbed.	D. 12/31/34
$\frac{1}{6}$ M. I.V.+H.	120.0	10.0	33.0			Acute laryngotracheal bronchitis—strep. hemo.	I.
$\frac{1}{6}$ M. I.V.+H.	27.0	11.2	52.0			Prematurity, diarrhea, jaundice, fatty infiltration of liver, cardiac dilatation, circulatory collapse.	A. 3/24/36
$\frac{1}{6}$ M. I.V.+H.	24.0	9.2	38.0				
$\frac{1}{6}$ M. I.V.+H.	500.0	10.0	40.0			Diethylene glycol poisoning, adult.	D. 10/12/37
200 cc. $\frac{1}{6}$ M. I.V.+H. 200 cc. R. H.	22.0	10.0	40.0			Thrombi in veins of kidney, adrenal, brain and spleen with early infarcts of brain and kidney, broncho-pneumonia, septicemia—B. coli.	A. 10/ 8/37
200 cc. F.L.R. H.	20.0	10.0	80.0				
220 cc. F.L.R. I.V.+H. 200 cc. L.R. H.	40.0	15.3	11.0				
390 cc. $\frac{1}{6}$ M. I.V.+H.	65.0	10.0	40.0			High fever of undetermined origin, vomiting, starvation, dehydration.	I.
390 cc. $\frac{1}{6}$ M. I.V.+H.	65.0	10.0	40.0				

the night by the continuous intravenous drip method. Much to our surprise the next morning we noted signs of severe acidosis and stupor. Despite the administration of 740 c.c. of lactate-Ringer's solution during the night, the serum carbon dioxide content had dropped from 42.0 to

18.8 volumes per cent. During the same interval the "apparent" blood sugar had dropped from 110 to 40 (26 "true") mg. per cent, and acetone could be detected on the breath and in the urine. Strongly positive tests for both aceto-acetic acid and salicylate in the urine were also obtained. Seven hundred and fifty cubic centimeters of one-sixth molar sodium *r*-lactate were then given, half intravenously and half intraperitoneally, and much to our uneasiness, the serum carbon dioxide content rose only to 26.2 volumes per cent (expected 57.8). At this time we wondered whether with the enlarging liver and the severe ketosis the metabolism of lactate might have been interfered with, and consequently decided to add sodium bicarbonate to the 10 per cent dextrose which was being given by the continuous drip method, because of the hypoglycemia and ketosis. When 200 c.c. of 5 per cent sodium bicarbonate had been given, the serum carbon dioxide content had risen only to 42.2 volumes per cent (expected 62.5). Later when lactic acid was determined in the blood and urine, and the duration and extent of ketosis followed, the explanation of the apparent partial failure of both sodium *r*-lactate and sodium bicarbonate to relieve completely the acidosis became clear (Chart 4): Lactate was metabolized normally but the amount of sodium released as well as the amount of sodium administered as the bicarbonate salt was quantitatively insufficient to balance completely the base binding effect of the ketone acids, which continued to be formed in large amounts for about five days. Undoubtedly larger amounts of sodium *r*-lactate were indicated both for its anti-acidotic and glycogenic effects.

COMMENT

In considering the efficiency of sodium lactate therapy for different types of acidosis from the quantitative viewpoint, we note that in the group of diabetics, after twelve hours values expected from our method of calculation were almost exactly realized, but "undershooting" tended to occur in the other groups. Such "undershooting" was minimal and generally negligible for the group with renal insufficiency, but was considerable and frequently of some consequence in the groups with diarrhea and severe infections. Before attempting to explain such discrepancies as did occur, we should first point out that our method of calculating expected values of bicarbonate concentration is at the best only a very rough one. In the first place, the amount of sodium lactate excreted into the urine is not considered. Such a loss is appreciable in normal individuals in whom diuresis with the excretion of highly alkaline urine follows promptly the intravenous injection. The situation is quite different, however, in subjects with severe acidosis, particularly when dehydration is also present. In such individuals diuresis, if it occurs to any extent at all, is usually not attended by the excretion of significant amounts of lactate because the delay in its appearance is usually long enough to permit the level of blood lactate to fall to ap-

TABLE VII

DATA ON URINARY EXCRETION OF LACTATE IN CASES OF DIABETIC ACIDOSIS

SUBJECT	MOLAR SODIUM r-LACTATE GIVEN				EXCRETED	
	C.C. TOTAL	C.C./KG.	ROUTE	TIME (MIN.)	PER CENT	(HR.)
P. K.	150	7.0	I.V.	(60)	6.5	(6)
D. B.	310	10.0	I.V.-I.P.-H.		9.3	(11)
W. T.	150	10.0	I.V.-I.P.-H.		8.8	(13)
D. B.	400	11.5	I.V.-H.		15.2	(9)

proximately normal values (Table VII). Furthermore, in subjects with severe acidosis, the urine is not immediately rendered alkaline by the injection of the usual therapeutic dose of sodium lactate, and it is probable that for that reason there is even relatively less loss of sodium than lactate. It would seem, therefore, that no serious discrepancy in the calculation of the theoretical rise of bicarbonate should result from failure to consider the amount of injected lactate escaping into the urine. Failure to consider, however, the base-claiming effect of buffer substances other than bicarbonate would seem to be a much more important omission. During the development of acidosis, should the pH of the blood and body fluids fall from 7.4 to 7.0 (which frequently happens), we should expect from the work of Van Slyke, Hastings, and Neill[9] that about 10 milliequivalents of alkali per liter of blood would be yielded by buffers other than bicarbonate, when the latter would be yielding approximately 18 milliequivalents, and similarly would be claimed by such buffers during the recovery process. Tissue buffers would be expected to behave similarly, and the net result should be a dissipating effect by such buffers on the conversion of sodium lactate into sodium bicarbonate when severe acidosis is completely relieved. By such a mechanism itself it is conceivable that as much as 35 per cent of a "therapeutic" dose of lactate may fail to be converted into bicarbonate. In the extremely dehydrated individuals, furthermore, the injection of fluid is usually followed by permanent water retention which goes to re-establish a normal body water content. Such a gain in the volume of body water, if the dosage of lactate were based on the original weight, would further widen the difference between expected and actual rises of bicarbonate. These two last mentioned factors seem to account for the poor agreement between actual and calculated bicarbonate concentrations noted in the subjects with severe acidosis associated with diarrhea, dehydration, and severe infections (Tables IV and VI). Furthermore, such discrepancies should be magnified if the dosage of sodium lactate were enough to have resulted in alkalosis of the base bicarbonate excess type, for in such a case a restraining effect on the rise of base bicarbonate would result from its rapid compensatory excretion into the urine.

While such factors as the above mentioned would tend to lead to a lower bicarbonate concentration than that expected by our method of calculation, at times there might be at least two operating in the opposite direction. In subjects in whom ketosis contributed to the acidosis, antiketogenic measures operating simultaneously with the liberation of sodium from combination with lactate would certainly tend to favor bicarbonate restoration, and so also would any renal activity concerned with the excretion of acid in an unneutralized state, or bound to ammonia.

With such modifying factors in mind, we may now consider and compare results actually obtained with those calculated. In the group of cases with renal insufficiency (Table III), ketosis is either nonexistent or is negligible; dehydration, while occasionally present and severe, is usually absent—in fact, edema is not uncommonly present; there can be little excretion of ammonia bound to acid, and there is also a reduced ability to excrete urine of high acidity. We would, therefore, expect good agreement between calculated and realized increases of bicarbonate except in the cases with very low blood hydrogen ion concentration and except in those with significant dehydration. Such seems to be the case (Table I). In the group with diarrhea, except when the latter was due to infection with the dysentery bacillus, modifying factors would tend to restrict bicarbonate increase and in this group we frequently see substantial discrepancies between expected and realized values. On the other hand, in the group with diabetes, ketosis is usually of a degree sufficient to balance or even slightly overbalance dissipating factors, and good agreement usually existed after twelve hours between calculated and realized bicarbonate concentrations (Table V). The poorest agreement is to be found in the group with severe infections (Table VI). Many of these patients were moribund at the time of treatment, and in addition to the possibility of operation of some or all of the "dissipating" factors mentioned above would also be circulatory failure leading to retarded absorption of fluid injected subcutaneously, tissue anoxia, and liver damage, all conceivably leading to some delay in the metabolism of lactate.

Actual failure to restore within twelve hours even very low bicarbonate values to 35-70 volumes per cent occurred in only 8 cases out of a total of 273 treated. These apparent failures are shown in Table VIII. In 4 instances, it should be noted, however, that after a second dose of sodium lactate had been given, satisfactory relief occurred. The explanation almost certainly is that with the development of very severe acidosis which permits the pH of the blood and body fluids to fall to the neighborhood of 7.0, buffer substances yield base to support the falling bicarbonate, claiming base again as it is released from metabolism of sodium lactate during the recovery process, and in that way dissipate the effect of the conversion of sodium lactate into sodium bicarbonate. Taking this into consideration, together with the fact that in general the most severe degrees of acidosis are to be found associated with dehydration of diarrheal origin in young infants, especially in the presence of

TABLE VIII

CASES OF ACIDOSIS FAILING TO RECOVER PROMPTLY AFTER SODIUM *r*-LACTATE THERAPY

CAUSE OF ACIDOSIS	HIST. #	AGE	SERUM CO_2 CONTENT VOLS. PER CENT				MOLAR NA LACTATE C.C. KG.	PROBABLE EXPLANATION
			BEFORE	AFTER (HRS.)	EXPECTED	DIFFERENCE		
Starvation and dehydration (premature)	M-246	15 da.	16.5 30.5	30.5(25) 52.0(26)	54.3 62.1	−23.9 −10.1	10.0	
Diabetes	L-2531	6 yr.	9.7 19.1	19.1(5) 52.8(4½)	55.0 64.4	−35.9 −11.6	11.0 11.0	Fixed base depletion?
Infection and renal insufficiency	L-2359	18 da.	22.0 30.0	30.0(19) 70.0(34)	61.6 69.6	−31.6 + 0.8	12.0 12.0	Second dose of lactate in each instance gave better response than first.
Renal insufficiency	N-487	5 mo.	9.0 25.0	25.0(6) 50.0(16)	41.0 57.0	−16.0 − 7.0	9.5 9.5	
Salicylate poisoning (ketosis)	J-2602	20 mo.	18.8 26.2	26.2(4) 42.2(3)	57.8 62.5	−31.6 −20.3	11.6 11.0 ($NaHCO_3$)	Continued acid formation.
Diarrhea (premature)	L-1554	14 da.	12.9	30.1(13)	42.7	−12.6	9.0	Moribund; died 15 hours later.
Ac. Bacillary dysentery	M-1411	5 mo.	12.0	16.0(11)	55.0	−39.0	12.8	Died 17 hours later.
Diarrhea and infection	H-778	21 da.	12.4	28.8(20)	49.7	−20.9	10.7	Base depletion (?) plus circulatory failure.

serious infection, and because in comparing expected rises of blood bicarbonate with those actually occurring in such cases of acidosis, an appreciable "undershooting" was noted in approximately half of the cases and no appreciable "overshooting" occurred, it has been our policy for some time to make 15 c.c. of molar sodium *r*-lactate per kilogram our routine dose in such cases (i.e., 90 c.c. of isotonic or ⅙ molar per kilogram) instead of 10 c.c. which we had first recommended and which still seems best for cases of acidosis of renal or diabetic origin. With the 50 per cent increase in dosage, initially very low carbon dioxide contents are much more consistently being brought to normal with the single initial administration of sodium lactate. In one instance, the case of salicylate poisoning, it should be noted that an unusual form of acidosis was present in that acid was being generated at an unusually rapid rate, and that repeated administration of alkali was necessary. In 2 cases (L-1554 and M-1411), however, the failure cannot be explained on any such ground and seems due to the fact that the infants were moribund at the time, and perhaps for that reason lactate metabolism was ineffectual. In such infants failure to respond properly to sodium lactate therapy might be due, as suggested by Minot, Dodd, and Saunders,[10] to liver damage and derangement of lactic acid metabolism secondary to guanidine intoxication. If such were the case, however, one would expect initially high blood lactic acid levels to increase and remain even higher after injections of sodium lactate, which we have not observed. Perhaps such cases could be better treated with at least an initial dose of sodium bicarbonate.

SUMMARY AND CONCLUSIONS

1. Following the intravenous injection of sodium lactate the urinary excretion of lactic acid was considerably greater when the "racemic" mixture was given than when a corresponding amount of the *l*+ isomer was administered. This observation suggests that the *l*+ isomer is utilized more readily than the *d*– form.

2. The increases in oxygen consumption during and after intravenous injection of both "racemic" and sodium *l*+ lactate were quite variable but were not enough larger on the whole than the increases with the injection of an equivalent amount of sodium bicarbonate to account for the disappearance of the lactic acid on the basis of an oxidation quotient of 4 for *l*+lactate and of one for the *d*– isomer. It seems quite probable, therefore, that part of both the *l*+ and *d*– isomers which disappeared replaced other food stuffs in metabolism.

3. By means of the intravenous injection of sodium *r*-lactate the acidosis of renal origin was satisfactorily relieved; that is, the observed carbon dioxide content was raised within twelve hours to a normal value or to one in the zone of just mild acidosis (35-45 volumes per cent) in 11 patients on whom follow-up data were obtained in 15 out of 16 instances. In the single exception a second injection was necessary. In many more cases, without follow-up data, apparently satisfactory relief was obtained. In the chronic type of renal insufficiency when vomiting is absent or negligible, the continued oral administration of sodium lactate may be effective in relieving acidosis and in preventing its recurrence.

4. Sixty cases of acidosis associated with nonspecific diarrhea and 8 associated with acute bacillary dysentery were treated with sodium lactate, and follow-up data indicated that all but three of these were satisfactorily relieved. One hundred more cases with acidosis associated with nonspecific diarrhea and 41 with acute bacillary dysentery were treated with apparent success, but without follow-up data.

5. Fifty-five cases of diabetic acidosis were treated with sodium lactate, only 2 being unsatisfactory by definition, and in only one case did the carbon dioxide content rise to more than 80 volumes per cent. Two deaths occurred in the group, a mortality of 3.6 per cent.

6. In a group of 26 patients with acidosis of severe infections and miscellaneous causes, 20 were relieved satisfactorily of their acidosis. In one of the unsatisfactory cases, less than the usual dose of lactate was given, and in 3 others, a second injection proved effectual.

7. Actual failure to restore within twelve hours even very low bicarbonate values to 35 to 70 volumes per cent occurred in only 8 out of a total of 273 cases. The reasons for these apparent failures are discussed. It is suggested that in cases of very severe acidosis with the serum pH value probably approaching 7.0, 15 c.c. of molar sodium lactate per kilogram be given (i.e., 90 c.c. of isotonic or one-sixth molar per kilogram) instead of 10 c.c. which was first recommended and which still seems best for acidosis of renal or diabetic origin.

REFERENCES

1. Hartmann, A. F., and Elman, R.: J. Exper. Med. **50**: 387, 1929.
2. Hartmann, A. F., and Senn, M. J. E.: J. Clin. Invest. **11**: 327, 1932; ibid. **11**: 337, 1932; ibid. **11**: 345, 1932.
3. Hartmann, A. F.: Arch. Int. Med. **56**: 413, 1935.
4. Abramson, H. A., and Eggleton, P.: J. Biol. Chem. **75**: 753, 1927.
5. Buchwald, K. W., Cori, C. F., and Fisher, R. E.: J. Biol. Chem. **103**: 763, 1933.
6. Cori, C. F., and Cori, G. T.: J. Biol. Chem. **81**: 389, 1929.
7. Abramson, H. A., Eggleton, M. G., and Eggleton, P.: J. Biol. Chem. **75**: 763, 1927.
8. Marriott, W. McK., Hartmann, A. F., and Senn, M. J. E.: J. Pediat. **3**: 181, 1933.
9. Van Slyke, D. D., Hastings, A. B., and Neill, J. M.: Quoted by Peters and Van Slyke in ''Quantitative Clinical Chemistry,'' p. 894, Baltimore, 1931, Williams & Wilkins Company.
10. Minot, A. S., Dodd, K., and Saunders, J. M.: J. Clin. Investigation **13**: 917, 1934.

500 South Kingshighway

ACUTE EPIDEMIC ENCEPHALITIS IN ST. LOUIS

THEODORE C. HEMPELMANN, M.D.
ST. LOUIS, MO.

FOREWORD

THE epidemic of acute encephalitis which occurred in St. Louis in 1933 called attention to a serious infectious disease the presence of which had not been previously recognized in the western hemisphere. In a volume such as this, dedicated to the late Dr. W. McKim Marriott, it is interesting to note that Marriott himself was one of the first sufferers from the disease, the diagnosis being further complicated by the fact that he had left the city when the initial symptoms arose. Fortunately, after a stormy illness, his recovery was complete.

* * *

In the last five years St. Louis and its suburbs has been visited by two severe epidemics of encephalitis. The first of these occurred in the summer of 1933 and the next in the summer of 1937. In the earlier epidemic over 1,100 cases of the disease were reported, with a mortality rate of about 20 per cent (22.5 per cent in the city proper), whereas in 1937 only 431 cases were reported with 107 deaths (24.8 per cent mortality). The two epidemics ran a parallel course so far as seasonal incidence and symptomatology were concerned, but the 1937 cases showed a slightly higher mortality rate, and children were somewhat oftener affected than was the case in 1933. In contrast to most infectious diseases, both incidence and mortality rate increased with advancing age, the latter being markedly affected by the presence of other pathologic processes such as cardiorenal disease, which might be present. It is interesting to note that Japan has had at least thirteen epidemics of a clinically similar disease, in one of which, in 1924, the number of cases reached almost 7,000 with a mortality rate of nearly 60 per cent.

ETIOLOGY

Early in the 1933 epidemic Muckenfuss, Armstrong, and McCordock, and later Webster and Fite succeeded in isolating a filtrable virus which, when injected intracerebrally into monkeys and mice, or instilled into the nostrils of the latter, produced the disease. Serum from patients recovering from the disease shows neutralizing properties for the virus, whereas that obtained from individuals who have had the so-called lethargic (von Economo) encephalitis fails to neutralize. Up to the present time, nine strains of the virus have been isolated in the laboratories of Washington University School of Medicine and the viruses

From the Department of Pediatrics, Washington University School of Medicine, and the St. Louis Children's Hospital.

recovered in 1933 and 1937 have been shown to be immunologically identical. The mode of transmission appears to be through contact infection rather than by way of food, water, or insects. Multiple cases in one family occurred but were very unusual.

INCUBATION PERIOD

By direct intracerebral inoculation this was usually eight to fourteen days in monkeys and five days in mice. Although not definitely established in human beings, the incubation period is probably between eight and fourteen days.

PATHOLOGY

The characteristic lesions are in the central nervous system and consist of intense congestion with petechial hemorrhages, cellular infiltration, and degenerative changes in the nerve cells. There occurs a cufflike infiltration of round cells about the blood vessels and small focal collections of cells elsewhere in the cortex, midbrain, medulla, pons, and upper levels of the cord. In contrast to the picture in lethargic encephalitis, except in the severest cases, the basal nuclei often escaped involvement.

SYMPTOMS

The symptoms commonly observed are in part those frequently found in many infectious diseases, plus another group indicative of involvement of the central nervous system. Briefly, the onset is usually abrupt with high fever and pronounced meningeal symptoms, but the latter were often masked by muscular aches, vomiting and abdominal pains, or other signs of a general infection. Despite the serious and often alarming picture presented by the patient in the early stages of the illness, recovery was ordinarily rapid and sequelae of an objective nature rare. For purposes of description it is convenient to discuss the clinical course of the disease by dividing the cases into three different groups although frequently one type of the disease merged indistinguishably into another.

Type I.—The most frequent clinical course of the disease was that in which the encephalitic symptoms dominated the picture from the very beginning. The onset was usually sudden, ushered in by malaise and perhaps chilly sensations, or occasionally convulsions, to be followed in rapid succession by headache, vomiting, and high fever (103° to 105° F.—39.4° to 40.6° C.). Such patients as were sufficiently rational frequently complained of muscular pains, abdominal cramps, and, in some instances, of sore throat and photophobia. Stiffness of the neck and even of the lower spine was frequent but may be absent even in cases of considerable severity. At the same time, in all but the mildest cases, some degree of mental confusion, sluggishness, or increasing drowsiness was present, although rarely was the coma so deep that the patient could not be aroused momentarily at least. At times mild delirium and insomnia or hyperexcitation replaced apathy and somnolence. Moreover, many patients were disoriented as to time and place and had no recollection of events during the early stages of the illness. Tremors, involving especially the hands, tongue, and lips, were common, and speech was thick, slurred, and often unintelligible. Less frequently, however, complete aphasia occurred. In a few cases, too, there was a marked cerebellar type of ataxia present, which had usually disappeared by the end of the second week.

The neurologic examination further revealed that the Kernig sign was frequently positive but not always in proportion to the amount of neck rigidity present. Absence of the abdominal reflexes was the rule in adults, but in children these were often normally present throughout the entire illness. The knee jerks were irregular, being normal at some times and perhaps absent or exaggerated at others, even in the same cases. Similarly, plantar reflexes might be normal at one examination and abnormal a few hours later.

It is interesting to note that in contrast to the lethargic encephalitis of von Economo, marked ocular disturbances, such as ptosis and double vision, were quite rare, although slight blurring of vision and even diplopia were occasional transient manifestations at the onset of the disease. Nystagmus and changes in the pupillary reflexes or in accommodation were uncommon. Fundus examination was usually negative.

Among other but less frequent manifestations was paralysis, consisting oftenest of mild or occasionally persistent facial weakness. In other instances spasticity of one or more of the extremities was observed, but such paralytic symptoms as developed usually disappeared within one or two weeks of the onset. Mild exophthalmos was observed in some patients, especially in adults, and in one case was so extreme as to cause complete forward dislocation of the globes. Changes in the pulse rate also occurred, producing such variations as a bradycardia or in other instances a tachycardia. Fever, usually highest in the first few days of the disease, as a rule fell by rapid lysis or even by crisis within eight to ten days of the onset. In exceptional instances, fortunately rare, it persisted of an irregular type, for several months. Improvement usually coincided with the fall in temperature, but occasionally mental confusion or tremor persisted long after the fever had reached normal. Headache and nausea were present only in the early stages of the disease, and vomiting was rarely of a projectile type. Considering the serious nature and situation of the pathologic lesions with their concomitant symptoms, it was amazing to find that most patients had apparently recovered entirely by the end of the arbitrarily determined isolation period of three weeks.

Spinal Fluid: In all types of the disease the spinal fluid as revealed by lumbar puncture was moderately increased in amount and pressure during the acute stages of the illness. The cell count was increased, numbering as a rule from 50 to 300, or occasionally as high as 500 to 1000 cells, but always predominantly mononuclears. The globulin showed a moderate increase, and the sugar content remained normal or slightly above this level.

Leucocyte Count: The blood count in all types of the disease showed such variations as to make it of little value in diagnosis. As a rule, there was a slight leucocytosis present, but occasionally a well-marked leucopenia was observed. The Schilling hemogram usually showed a slight shift to the left.

Type II.—In this group, the symptoms of encephalitis were preceded by a definite *period of invasion.* During this time, usually one to four days, but lasting occasionally a week or longer, the patient complained of headache, malaise, chilliness or even definite rigors, nausea, abdominal pain, and almost invariably muscular aches in the back and extremities. When it is added that occasionally there was photophobia, and sore throat or other signs of a mild upper respiratory infection, it is not surprising to find that the initial diagnosis in such instances was more likely to be influenza than encephalitis. Moreover, such individuals usually had moderate to high fever, as well as the above mentioned evidences of a generalized infection. During the next few days, however, the temperature fell toward normal and all the symptoms were markedly ameliorated, so that convalescence seemed established. Suddenly, however, the fever again rose abruptly, headache became much worse, and drowsiness, mental confusion, tremors, and nuchal rigidity developed. Thereafter, the course was similar to the Type I infection, the presence of invasive symptoms apparently not affecting the prognosis.

Type III.—In this group are placed the mild or abortive forms of the disease in which the diagnosis would probably never have been suspected but for the fact that there was an epidemic of encephalitis in the community at the time. At best, it seems probable that more such cases were overlooked than recognized. Some degree of fever and headache was ordinarily present, and perhaps transient nausea, chilliness, and abdominal or muscular pains were present. Frequently a slight tremor of hands and tongue, with perhaps absence of the abdominal reflexes, suggested the possibility of encephalitis, although the sensorium was usually clear. Rigidity of the neck or a positive Kernig sign was, of course, of great significance if present. Again, a few patients complained of mild transient vertigo or blurred vision, but drowsiness and mental confusion were slight or entirely absent. Despite these mild symptoms, lumbar puncture revealed typical changes in the spinal fluid. As was to be expected, recovery was very rapid, the symptoms rarely lasting more than a week or ten days. That these were really cases of encephalitis seems amply attested not only by the clinical course and spinal fluid findings, but also by the presence in the blood of such patients of neutralizing substances for the virus isolated and recognized as the specific cause of the disease.

COMPLICATIONS

These were much more common in adults than in children and increased in frequency and seriousness as the older age levels were reached. Pathologic conditions antedating the onset of the encephalitis (e.g., cardiorenal disease, arteriosclerosis, hypertension), greatly increased the gravity of the disease. The most frequent immediate cause of death, however, aside from the toxemia of the infection, was bronchopneumonia or lobar pneumonia.

PROGNOSIS AND SEQUELAE

As mentioned above, the mortality rate in 1933 was 20 per cent, but in 1937 with a smaller total of cases the rate reached almost 25 per cent. It was lowest in children (slightly over 5 per cent) and rose with advancing age, being markedly influenced by the presence of other pathologic processes which were present at the time of onset of the encephalitis. In nonfatal cases, however, recovery was usually surprisingly rapid and ordinarily complete. Sequelae, such as commonly follow the so-called lethargic type encephalitis, were conspicuous by their absence. In a recent follow-up study of 331 patients of the 1933 epidemic there was found no single instance of definite parkinsonism although 11 per cent had some type of muscular tremor. When it is realized that about 40 per cent of the patients re-examined were over fifty years of age, when tremors from other causes become increasingly common as the age advances, it is evident that this type of sequel is less frequent than was to have been expected from previous experiences with other varieties of encephalitis. It is noteworthy that other organic residual effects actually observed on physical examination were present in but 5.7 per cent of the cases. Forty-two per cent of patients reported no complaints of any nature, but about a similar number reported subjective nervous complaints such as nervous excitability, irritability, headaches, and slight loss of memory. Only rarely were such complaints of a serious nature, and it is significant that they were much less frequent in children than in adults. Indeed, it seems quite probable that in many instances the changes found on physical examination or mentioned as subjective complaints were the result of age rather than the attack of encephalitis. It cannot be gainsaid, however, that in certain instances the central nervous system suffered irreparable damage during the acute phase of the illness, and in consequence permanent sequelae have remained.

TREATMENT

There is at present no specific treatment for acute epidemic encephalitis. Although patients who have recovered from this disease usually have neutralizing substances for the virus in their blood streams, it seems doubtful whether knowledge of this fact will ever prove useful as a therapeutic measure, for once a virus disease becomes established and produces clinical symptoms, specific sera are usually ineffective. Prophylactic injections of such a specific serum would seem scarcely warranted as long as the disease affects only one in a thousand population, as was the case in the St. Louis area.

Lumbar puncture often affords lasting relief from the headache, but further treatment must be entirely symptomatic in the present stage of our knowledge. Especial attention should be given to the prevention of dehydration of the tissues through the use of Hartmann's or Ringer's solution administered subcutaneously and dextrose or sucrose solutions intravenously. Stuporous patients may have to be fed by gavage, although blood transfusions may act as general supportive measures and supply food as well.

REFERENCES

Hempelmann, T. C.: J. A. M. A. **103**: 733, 1934.
Hempelmann, T. C.: M. Clin. North America **20**: 415, 1936.
Hempelmann, T. C.: Encephalitis, Brennemann's Practice of Pediatrics, Vol. IV, Chap. 7.
McCordock, H. A., Collier, W., Gray, S. H.: The Pathological Changes of the St. Louis Type of Acute Encephalitis, J. A. M. A. **103**: 822, 1934.
Muckenfuss, R. S., Armstrong, C., McCordock, H. A.: Pub. Health Rep. **48**: 1341, 1933.
Muckenfuss, R. S., Armstrong, C., Webster, L. T.: Etiology of the 1933 Epidemic of Encephalitis, J. A. M. A. **103**: 731, 1934.
Report on the St. Louis Outbreak of Encephalitis, Pub. Health Bull., No. 214, January, 1935.
Webster, L. T., Fite, G. L.: Science **78**: 463, 1933.
Webster, L. T., and Fite, G. L.: Proc. Soc. Exper. Biol. & Med. **31**: 344, 1933.
Kaneko, R., and Aoki, Y.: Ergebn. d. inn. Med. u. Kinderh. **34**: 342, 1928.
McCordock, H. A., Smith, M. G., and Moore, E.: Proc. Soc. Exper. Biol. & Med. **37**: 288, 1937.
Bredeck, J. F., Broun, G. O., Hempelmann, T. C., McFadden, J. F., and Spector, H. I.: J. A. M. A. **115**: 17, 1938.

THE EFFECT OF VITAMIN D ON LINEAR GROWTH IN INFANCY

II. The Effect of Intakes Above 1,800 U.S.P. Units Daily

P. C. Jeans, M.D., and Genevieve Stearns, Ph.D.
Iowa City, Iowa

ALTHOUGH a large quantity of data concerning growth of infants must be analyzed in order to determine standard rates of growth, much can be learned by following carefully the growth rates of small groups of infants, living under carefully controlled conditions of housing and diet. During the past ten years the growth of more than 100 infants has been so watched, many of the infants being studied during the greater part of the first year of life. For a large number of these infants the major differences in the dietary regimen have been in respect to the source and quantity of the vitamin D supplement, changes which necessarily involved also alterations in the vitamin A intake.

The first publication of this series[1] demonstrated that infants given a good diet containing approximately 340 units of vitamin D daily from cod-liver oil,* grew at rates faster than the averages reported in the recent literature.[2, 3] It was shown also that infants given the same dietary regimen but obtaining all their vitamin D from milk containing 135 units to the quart, grew at rates average by the above mentioned standards. These standards, in turn showed rates of growth more rapid than the averages reported in 1920 or earlier.[4] The evidence indicated that vitamin A was not the important factor, and it was concluded that the increased rate of skeletal growth was due to the effect of vitamin D. These findings were subsequently confirmed by Slyker and coworkers[5] in a well-controlled outpatient study of a large number of infants.

The present report discusses factors affecting the interpretation of growth rates of individual infants and extends the study to include a group of infants given from 1,800 to 4,600 units of vitamin D daily.

In a study of a large group, individual variants may be disregarded as being relatively unimportant. In studies of small groups, these variants may lead to erroneous conclusions. For example, it is well known that tall babies tend to grow faster than short ones. A baby 55 cm. long at birth will grow 27 cm. during the first year if his growth is average,[2, 3] but the average increase in length of a baby 45 cm. long at

From the Department of Pediatrics, State University of Iowa.
This study was aided by grants from Mead Johnson & Company, Evansville, Ind., and National Oil Products Company, Harrison, N. J.
*The term units throughout this article refers to U.S.P. units.

birth is only 22 cm. If the infants of a small group are predominantly either large or small, the growth results must be interpreted accordingly.

Illness also influences the rate of growth in length. In our experience, illness seems always to cause a slowing of growth, but the retardation may be of short or long duration, may occur during the illness, or after the infant has recovered. This period of slower growth is usually followed by a period of more rapid growth, which usually compensates entirely for the earlier slowing. Curves illustrative of these differing effects of illness on growth rate are shown in Fig. 1. The solid lines indicate periods of health, the dotted lines show acute illness, and broken lines a mild middle ear infection. The fine lines represent average growth for infants of the given age. It will be observed that following

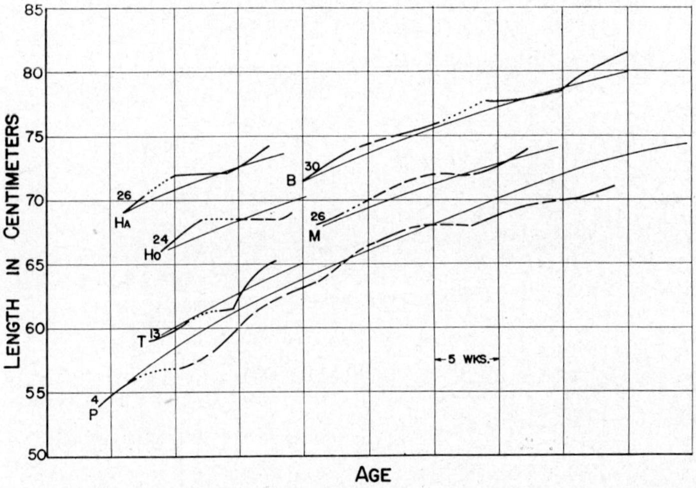

Fig. 1.—The effect of illness upon rate of growth in infancy. The solid lines indicate periods of health; dotted lines, acute illness; broken lines, mild chronic illness, usually otitis media. The age of each infant in weeks is given in numerals at the beginning of the curve, and fine lines represent average growth rate of infants of the given age.

an attack of acute bronchitis of two weeks' duration, the growth of infant Ha completely ceased for a period of four weeks; a similar cessation of linear growth was observed in infant B after acute laryngitis requiring tracheotomy. Both infants subsequently compensated entirely for the temporary slowing of growth. Bronchitis followed by mild middle ear infection caused cessation of growth for six weeks in infant Ho. On the other hand, acute bronchitis in infant T and pneumonia in infant P, both young infants, caused a slowing of growth for only about two weeks, while bronchitis followed by middle ear infection caused little or no slowing of growth until after seven weeks of illness for infant M. The last named infant resumed growth as soon as he recovered from the middle ear infection. The entire growth curve of infant P illustrates the fact that a chronic low-grade middle ear infection may have a far more marked and lasting effect on the growth rate than a single acute illness of much greater severity. In order to judge the effect of nutrition on the growth of a baby who has been ill, the growth rate should be followed for a sufficient period after illness to include both the compensatory period of more rapid later growth and also a period wherein growth occurs at the baby's normal rate.

Detailed and careful observation of infants under controlled conditions often indicates an apparent lack of relationship between the rate of growth during the first six to eight weeks of infancy and the dietary regimen given the infant. Fig. 2 shows the growth rates of three infants given as the sole source of vitamin D milk containing 135 units to the quart. Curves A and B indicate a steady rate of growth; curve C shows a much more rapid growth rate until the eighth week of life, after which this growth curve parallels the other two. All three infants were given the same dietary regimen throughout. The growth

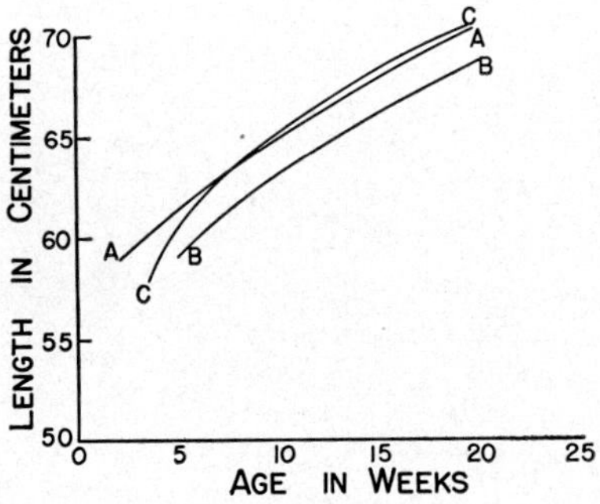

Fig. 2.

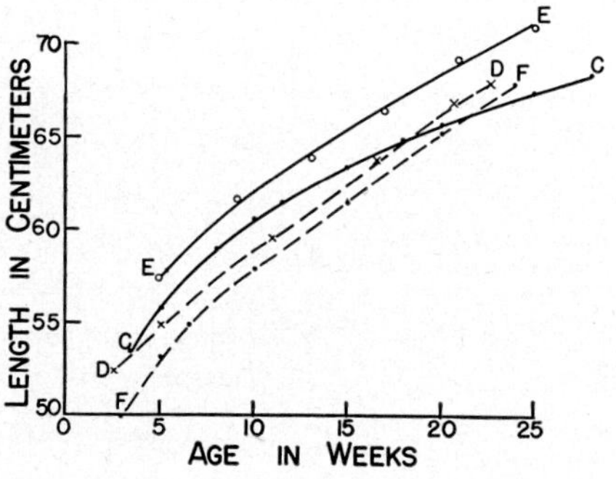

Fig. 3.

Fig. 2.—Growth rates of three infants given milk containing 135 units of vitamin D to the quart as the sole source of the vitamin. The growth rates of all three infants were similar after 8 weeks of age; the rapid earlier growth of infant C indicates the influence of factors other than diet.

Fig. 3.—Growth rate of infant C (Fig. 2) compared with those of three infants given 340 units of vitamin D daily as cod-liver oil. Curves D, E, and F show parallel growth rates after eight weeks, at a rate more rapid than the growth of infant C who received the lower unitage of vitamin D. Curves C, E, and F show rapid early growth, apparently not related to dietary regimen. Curves C and D illustrate the erroneous conclusions which may be drawn when only two measurements of growth are considered; actual rates of growth of the two infants are equal at 18 weeks of age; the growth of infant C is influenced by two factors, that of infant D apparently by only one.

of infant C after eight weeks shows that, throughout the entire period of infancy, his growth rate would probably approximate that of the other two infants. A short term study of this infant, particularly if measurements were taken only at the beginning and end of the study, might lead to very erroneous conclusions concerning the efficacy of the diet.

Fig. 3 shows the growth curve C in contrast to growth curves of three infants given 340 units of vitamin D daily as cod-liver oil. It will be noted that curves E and F show rates of growth previous to eight weeks which are more rapid than during the later period, whereas the growth rate illustrated in curve D is consistent throughout. After the eighth week, the rates of growth of the three infants given 340 units of vitamin D daily (curves D, E, and F) are very similar and noteworthily greater than the rate of growth of infant C, who was given milk containing 135 units of vitamin D to the quart. A comparison of curves C and D illustrates the error which might easily arise if growth rates of curves C and D were compared only at first measurement and at or near the eighteenth week of life. Such comparison would show equal growth which might be wrongly ascribed to diet. While growth of the two infants is actually equal up to the eighteenth week the growth rate of infant C is the resultant of two factors; that of infant D is apparently affected by only one. Both infants C and F, on the other hand, show rapid early growth. The two curves are approximately parallel to the eighth week, but thereafter the rate of growth depends directly upon the dietary regimen. It seems, therefore, safer when studying growth of individual infants in relation to dietary regimen to consider only the rate of growth after the eighth week of life although the regimen should be instituted as soon after birth as possible.

We are as yet unable to state exactly the cause of these differing rates of growth during the first two months. In the few cases wherein accurate dietary and medical histories of the mother could be obtained, the rate of growth of the infant during the first two months correlated well with the nutritional and physical status of the mother at the time of the child's birth.

In studying the rate of growth of infants given large amounts of vitamin D, the entire growth curve of each infant is presented, but only the part of the curve after the eighth week of life is considered indicative of the effect of diet.

In this study vitamin D was given from three sources, two of which contained also vitamin A. A high unitage cod-liver oil* was given two infants in the amount of three standard teaspoonfuls daily, which allowed an intake of about 1,800 units of vitamin D and 6,300 units of vitamin A. A cod-liver oil concentrate emulsified in cream† was used as the second source; 3 c.c. were added to the daily feedings of each of three infants, permitting a daily intake of 2,200 units of vitamin D and 1,400 units of vitamin A dispersed in the milk. During the last three weeks of the study the vitamin A content of the concentrate was increased tenfold, allowing 14,000 units daily, the vitamin D content remaining constant. Viosterol in oil was given to four babies in amounts allowing about 4,500 units of vitamin D daily; this group of infants received no vitamin A in addition to that of the food. The studies were carried out without regard to season, and during the summer months

*Obtained through the courtesy of Mead Johnson & Company, Evansville, Ind.

†Obtained through the courtesy of the National Oil Products Company, Harrison, N. J.

the infants were outdoors when weather permitted. While the group studied is small in number, the degree of dietary control was excellent, and the growth rates observed differed consistently from those of infants fed 300 to 400 units of vitamin D daily.

The growth rates of the infants are shown in Figs. 4, 5, and 6 in comparison with the Kornfeld standard curves as background. Fig. 4 shows the linear growth of two girls, one given cod-liver oil (1,800 units of vitamin D daily), and the other viosterol (4,600 units of vitamin D daily). Neither child showed extremely rapid growth during the first two months; both grew consistently faster than the average rate until 20 to 25 weeks of age. At that age a short period occurred wherein growth ceased entirely, after which linear growth was resumed at a rate

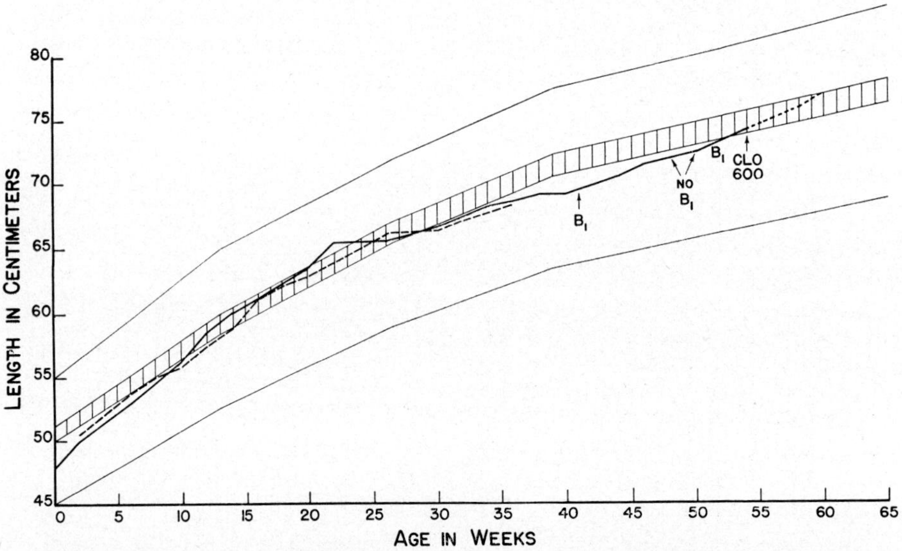

Fig. 4.—Linear growth of two girl infants given very high vitamin D dosage. The fine lines represent the average rates of growth by the Kornfeld standard. Baby B received 1800 units daily as cod-liver oil; Baby S was given 4600 units a day as viosterol. The period B_1 marks the term of thiamin therapy. The dotted line shows the growth rate when the vitamin D dosage was decreased to 600 units as cod-liver oil; rate of growth increased. (Broken line, Baby B; solid line, Baby S.)

below the average normal. Infant S who received viosterol was studied under this regimen until 40 weeks of age. As some decrease in appetite had been observed, thiamin (vitamin B_1) was added to the daily diet in the form first of an extract of rice polishings, later in a form combined with the carbohydrate (a dextrin-maltose mixture) of the milk feeding. Some increase in growth rate followed, but as both forms of the vitamin addition proved laxative, necessitating rest periods, the use of the thiamin addition was discontinued and the vitamin D dosage was changed to one teaspoonful of cod-liver oil, containing about 600 units of vitamin D. Growth was maintained at greater than average rate for a period of six weeks, when the study of the infant was concluded.

The second infant (B) whose growth rate is shown in Fig. 4, was given three teaspoonfuls of cod-liver oil daily, permitting an intake of 1,800 units of vitamin D and 6,300 units of vitamin A. This infant also showed evidence of decreased growth after about 6 months of age. The study of baby B could be continued only until the thirty-sixth week of age; the feeding instructions at discharge allowed only one teaspoonful of cod-liver oil daily. The baby visited the ward on her first birthday. At this age she was considerably taller than baby S., who was the same age. As will be seen from the chart, the two were of almost identical height at 36 weeks of age. The rate of growth of baby B, therefore, must have been above normal after the vitamin D dosage was decreased.

Four other girl infants have been studied (Fig. 5), but only one could be studied throughout the major part of infancy. This infant (Sa) had been used as a subject for a study of the effect on growth and

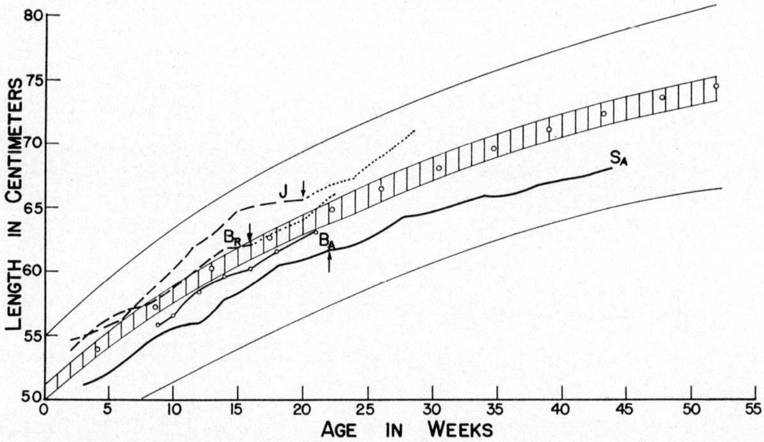

Fig. 5.—Linear growth of four girl infants given very high vitamin D dosage compared to standard Kornfeld rate. Dotted portions of curves represent growth rates observed when the vitamin D dosage was decreased to 400 units daily as cod-liver oil. Babies Br and J were given 2200 units of vitamin D daily as the cod-liver oil concentrate dispersed in the feeding; growth increased when the dosage was decreased to 400 units daily. Baby Ba was given 4600 units daily as viosterol. Baby Sa was given 270 units daily as viosterol until 21 weeks of age, at which time the dosage was increased to 4600 units. The slowing of growth with high dosage contrasts with the increase of growth rate of baby J when the vitamin D intake was lowered. The circles represent average lengths observed by Peatman and Higgons[6] for girl infants given 1600 to 9000 units of vitamin D daily.

mineral retention of a vitamin D intake of 270 units daily as viosterol. That study had been discontinued in the spring and the baby, then 21 weeks old, was thereafter given 4,600 units of vitamin D as viosterol. The rate of growth to 21 weeks had been average; after this period, the rate was considerably below average, remaining so throughout the study. The failure of the high vitamin D dosage to increase growth rate is in contrast to the increase in growth rate noted in baby S when 600 units of vitamin D were substituted for 4,600 units.

Baby Ba was given 4,600 units of viosterol daily from the date of her admission at the age of 9 weeks. At 21 weeks, the baby left the hospital.

Growth was about 1 cm. greater than the average rate and had not yet showed evidence of slowing, a result similar to those observed with infants S and B at the same age.

Two girl infants were given the "high vitamin D milk" made in the laboratory by adding to each day's feeding enough cod-liver oil concentrate dispersed in cream to give a total day's intake of 2,200 units. These infants could be studied for less than six months. No decrease in appetite was observed. One infant, Br, grew at a little less than average rate at the beginning of the study, and at average rate after the age of eight weeks. The growth of the other baby, J, was faster than average from the eighth to the fifteenth week, then showed a definite slowing for the succeeding five weeks. The vitamin D intakes of both infants

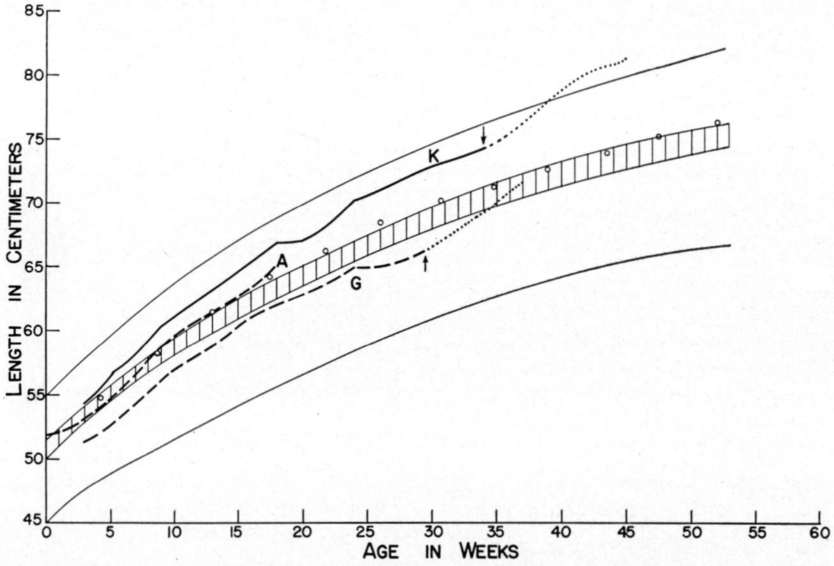

Fig. 6.—Linear growth of three boy infants given very high vitamin D dosage compared to standard Kornfeld rate. Dotted portions of curves represent growth rates observed when the vitamin D dosage was decreased to 400 units daily as cod-liver oil. Baby G received 2200 units daily as the cod-liver oil concentrate dispersed in the feeding; Baby A, 1800 units daily as cod-liver oil; and baby K, 4600 units a day as viosterol. The rates of growth of babies G and K were increased when the vitamin D intake was decreased to 400 units a day. The circles represent average lengths observed by Peatman and Higgons[6] for boy infants given 1600 to 9000 units of vitamin D daily.

were then changed to 400 units daily as cod-liver oil. Subsequent growth is shown as dotted lines. Baby J showed average growth for four weeks, then sharply accelerated growth for the succeeding four weeks. Baby Br's growth was maintained at average for four weeks, and then the rate increased somewhat.

The growth rates of the three boy infants are shown in Fig. 6. The lowest curve, G, indicates the growth of the baby given 2,200 units of vitamin D in the milk, as the cod-liver oil concentrate dispersed in cream. Growth proceeded at better than normal rate until 16 weeks of age and from then to 24 weeks at barely normal rate. After the twenty-fourth week growth was definitely slowed. At 29 weeks of age the high vitamin D feeding was discontinued, and 400 units of vitamin D as cod-liver oil were given daily. The growth rate showed an almost immediate increase, which was maintained for a period of six weeks, until the study was concluded.

A second boy, A, was given 1,800 units of D daily as cod-liver oil. This baby left the hospital at 18 weeks of age, before any slowing of growth was observed. The child's appetite was excellent throughout the study.

The third boy, K, was remarkable for his excellent appetite throughout the entire study. His food intake was always above average. His rate of growth was excellent up to 24 weeks of age, except for one temporary slowing due to an upper respiratory infection. From the twenty-fourth to the thirty-fourth week growth continued at average rate. Slowing of growth in this child could not be considered as due to decreased ingestion of food caused by lack of appetite. The child's hands and feet were very large compared to his body size, so that, even though the baby's length was above average, it was felt that stunting might have occurred. The vitamin D dosage was therefore decreased to 400 units daily, given in the form of cod-liver oil. After two weeks the growth rate increased, and in ten weeks the body length had increased 6.6 cm. or 3.2 cm. above the expected increase of 3.4 cm. in this period.

Summarizing, each infant given the high D dosage and studied up to 25 weeks of age or longer showed a slowing of growth to or below average rate by the standard used. Each of these infants who was then given a lower dosage of vitamin D, 400 to 600 units daily, showed an increased rate of growth, four of the five growing at markedly greater than average rates for periods of four to ten weeks.

In some of the infants the decrease in rate of growth observed when the very high dosage of vitamin D was given could be ascribed to decreased appetite with consequent food refusals; other infants, however, showed excellent appetites throughout the study, but the growth rate could still be increased by decreasing the daily vitamin D ingestion. The depression of appetite occurred as often when the vitamin was given in concentrated form, as when it was ingested as three teaspoonfuls of oil.

Four infants were given no vitamin A in addition to that of the food; of these, two grew at less than average rate and one at average rate during later infancy, while the study of the fourth was concluded at twenty-one weeks, at which time she was growing at average rate. Two of these babies were later given cod-liver oil containing 400 and 600 units of vitamin D, 2,800 and 4,200 units of vitamin A, respectively. Both babies showed a definite increase in rate of growth.

Two babies were given three teaspoonfuls of cod-liver oil, containing 12,000 to 13,000 units of vitamin A in addition to that of the food. One baby grew at less than average rate after 25 weeks of age; at 34 weeks of age the cod-liver oil dosage was decreased to one-third of its former level, thus decreasing the intake of both vitamins A and D; growth proceeded more rapidly. The second infant was studied only to 18 weeks of age; the rate of growth was above average at that age.

Three babies were given 1,400 units of vitamin A daily in addition to that of the food. During the last few weeks of the vitamin D study the vitamin A content of the diet was increased tenfold, the vitamin D ingestion remaining constant. The growth rate of two of the three infants continued to decrease, that of the third remained approximately the same. When the vitamin D intake was decreased to 400 units daily and the vitamin A intake to 2,800 units, the rate of growth increased for all infants.

Of the five infants studied to thirty weeks or later, four presented a very definite slowing of growth, one grew at average rate. The infant who grew at average rate and two of those whose growth rate was below average received no vitamin A in addition to that of the food. One infant whose later growth was below average, received 6,300 units of vitamin A in addition to the vitamin D; her rate of growth was practically identical with that of one of the infants given no added vitamin A. The fifth infant was given a tenfold increase in amount of vitamin A for three weeks of the study without any observable increase in growth rate occurring, in contrast to the prompt increase in growth rate when the vitamin D intake was lowered. Thus, the slowing of growth, when observed, was noted in infants given additional vitamin A or only that of the diet. The increased rate of growth which followed the lowering of the vitamin D intake occurred whether the vitamin A intake was lowered markedly or increased. Vitamin A, in amounts above those supplied by the food, apparently does not affect linear growth in infancy.

The study of these nine infants indicates that when vitamin D is fed to infants in amounts over and above 1,500 units daily, growth proceeds at average or greater rate up to about 6 months of age, and that after 6 months of age, increase in length occurs at average or less than average rate. The rate of growth with very high vitamin D dosage is thus about the same as had been observed for sixteen infants given vitamin D milk containing only 135 units to the quart, and is definitely slower than the growth rate observed in thirty-six infants given 340 units of D daily.

Very similar results in growth rate with high vitamin D intake are reported in a large outpatient study by Peatman and Higgons.[6] These authors report growth rates of 1,112 subjects (577 boys and 535 girls) of whom 60 per cent came from the middle or wealthy classes. The infants were of American parentage, with northern European stock predominating. The dietary regimen was very carefully supervised and included vitamin D as follows: "Cod-liver oil or one of its substitutes is started at four weeks. By two months each child receives daily 9,000 or more units of vitamin A (U.S.P. XI) and 1,600 or more units of vitamin D (U.S.P. XI). At 4 months this dose is increased to a minimum of 20,000 units of vitamin A and 3,200 of vitamin D. After 8 months the amount varies from this minimum to a maximum of three times this quantity, depending on the condition of the child."

The average lengths observed by these investigators are shown in charts 5 and 6 as circles. It will be noted that the average growth rate for the boys is almost identical with the "upper average" line of the Kornfeld standard, and for the girls, exactly average according to the standard. That average growth was achieved by the outpatient group and less than average growth was observed for many of the infants of the present study may be attributed to the better degree of control always possible in inpatient studies. The data presented by Peatman and Higgons thus support admirably the data presented in this paper.

The effect of vitamin D on linear growth apparently reaches a maximum and further increases in intake result in decreased, rather than increased rates of growth. The rate of growth of infants given 135 unit vitamin D milk is greater than that of infants given no vitamin D;[1, 5] infants given 340 units[1] or 600 units[5] of vitamin D daily grew at noteworthily greater rates than those receiving only 135 units. No definite difference in growth rate appeared between the groups given 340 and those given 600 units of D daily. Infants given very high dosage of vitamin D (1,800 to 5,000 units daily), however, grew at rates definitely less rapid than those given 340 to 600 units, and approximately equal to those of the group fed milk containing 135 units to the quart. A few infants given these high dosages grew no faster than infants receiving no additional vitamin D.[4, 5]

This study of growth of infants with a high intake of D brings out an additional factor which must be considered in studying the growth of individuals, namely, that some factors of diet definitely affecting growth may not show a noticeable effect until the infant is more than 6 months of age. In order to determine the effect of a given dietary regimen upon the rate of growth and development of the infant, it appears necessary to study the infants throughout the greater part of the first year of life.

SUMMARY

The rate of linear growth of nine infants given from 1,800 to 4,600 units of vitamin D daily has been compared with standard rates of growth, and with the growth of infants given the same dietary regimen but amounts of vitamin D varying from 135 to 340 units daily. The rates of growth with the very high vitamin D intake were similar to or less than those of infants given 135 units daily, and definitely lower than the growth rates of infants given 340 units of vitamin D daily.

It is concluded that the effect of vitamin D on increasing linear growth reaches a maximum when the vitamin D intake is greater than 135 and less than 1,800 units, probably in the neighborhood of 340 to 600 units daily.

Vitamin A in amounts exceeding those of the food (milk, vegetable, and fruit purées) apparently does not affect linear growth of infants.

Factors affecting growth rates of individual infants are discussed. It is concluded that in order to determine the effect of the dietary regimen, growth should be studied well past 6 months of age, preferably during the greater part of infancy. Growth during the first 8 weeks of life may be affected by factors other than the dietary regimen of the infant.

REFERENCES

1. Stearns, G., Jeans, P. C., and Vandecar, V.: J. Pediat. **9**: 1, 1934.
2. Kornfeld, W.: Ztschr. f. Kinderh. **48**: 188, 1929-30.
3. Stuart, H. C.: J. Pediat. **5**: 194, 1934.
4. Baldwin, B. T.: Physical Growth of Children, Birth to Maturity, University of Iowa Studies, Iowa City, 1921.
5. Slyker, F., Hamil, B. M., Poole, M. W., Cooley, T. B., and Macy, I. G.: Proc. Soc. Exper. Biol. & Med. **37**: 499, 1937-38.
6. Peatman, J. G., and Higgons, R. A.: Am. J. Dis. Child. **55**: 1233, 1938.

ENCEPHALITIS RHEUMATICA
(CHOREA MINOR OF SYDENHAM)

Its Diagnosis and Course

Hugh McCulloch, M.D.
St. Louis, Mo.

INTRODUCTION.—Chorea continues to be a disease of great pediatric interest and discussion because of its frequency of occurrence and its uncertain etiology and relation to rheumatic fever. Because of the nature of the condition there is great difficulty in securing direct evidence of its cause, course, and relationship. It is the purpose of this paper to discuss, first, the concept of the disease formed from an experience during the past twenty years at the St. Louis Children's Hospital, in the Children's Cardiac Clinic, and, second, to describe the common conditions occurring in pediatric practice which simulate the disease and may be confused with it.

Dr. Marriott was always interested in each case of chorea on the wards and stimulated others about him in the subject. Probably the elusive, unknown, uncertain features challenged his scientific mind to search for something new.

History.—Since Sydenham's original description of chorea[1] in 1686, very little important information has been added. Cheadle[2] pointed out clearly and definitely the close relationship between chorea and rheumatism in children and probably was the first to emphasize the peculiar manifestations of rheumatism in children as compared with adults. His description of chorea supplements Sydenham's with accurate clinical observations based on principles of modern medicine. Since Cheadle's work nothing has been added to our knowledge.

Pathologic reports are extremely meager, there being no mention of the disease in most text books of pathology. Clinical studies and reports of importance during the past twenty years come from either neurologists and psychiatrists,[3-6] with emphasis on the symptoms and relation to other types of incoordinate movements of children, or from pediatricians,[7, 8, 9] and cardiologists,[10-13] with more emphasis on the relation of the disease to the rheumatic state and its manifestations elsewhere in the body. These reports describe less the symptoms and more the underlying cause of the disease, the widespread lesions of rheumatism in children, and the high incidence of heart disease in the general group. Many of these reports are concerned with the direct relationship

From the Department of Pediatrics, Washington University, and the Cardiac Clinic of the St. Louis Children's Hospital.

Presented in part at the joint Meeting of Regions II and III, American Academy of Pediatrics, in St. Louis, Nov. 18, 1935.

between chorea and rheumatic heart disease in children. Most of the general literature is concerned with the treatment of the disease, and in this connection reference may be made to Sydenham's original statement that "purging and *alternating medicine* are to be used until he [the patient] is quite well." And from the current literature, it is apparent that there seem to be many alternative remedies.

Clinical Picture.—The clinical appearance of children with chorea is well known generally. There is a history of gradual onset of several days or weeks of "nervousness," or "twitching," or "irritability" and "peevishness," or "being tired," and irregular movements occurring during the waking hours, of all parts of the body under voluntary control. The severity of jerking and incoordinate movement progresses in degree together with appearance of a more or less marked emotional instability and imbalance characterized by irritability, more often crying, less often laughing about irrelevant details. All the semivoluntary functions, such as speech and respiration, may be involved to some degree. There may be such incoordination as to simulate paresis of a limb or part. Not only does the child make purposeless, aimless, involuntary movements, but there is a great degree of incoordination and confusion of purposeful movements. These movements show no intention intensification. They are never present during sleep, which is usually undisturbed though restless. Due to difficulty in feeding and walking, there is loss of weight and malnutrition after the first few weeks. There is usually a history of acute rheumatism, either a previous attack of chorea or some other rheumatic manifestation, such as arthritis, heart disease, or tonsillitis. Often an upper respiratory infection has preceded the onset of the chorea, though this may be so insignificant as to escape notice. A history of fright or some other emotional strain can be obtained usually, though logically a mental shock may be only the first consciousness of the family that the child is "nervous." In all probability the emotional strain is the result rather than the cause of the attack of chorea.

The attacks are more frequent in girls than boys; more frequent in the spring of the year than at other times; commoner in older children than younger children; commoner in blonds than in brunets; and commoner in children with frequent "colds" and "sore throats." All races seem equally affected when living under the same conditions. The Negro race[14] in the northern cities, is particularly subject to chorea as a manifestation of rheumatism. The patient's mental and emotional development varies, and it may be said that chorea develops only in those children who have some weak point where the manifestation starts. The familial socio-economic background is generally faulty and furnishes a fertile soil for emotional disturbances to appear. The intelligence quotient determined in choreic children may be low or high but is usually an irregular curve, independent of performance tests based on muscular coordination. It has been shown by many workers, that rheumatism is increasingly frequent in the lower social strata, particularly when the family is impoverished in ability to make the best of poor circumstances or to provide proper health and environmental facilities for their children. This implies an intellectual poverty as well as an economic poverty. Chorea may be an exception to this feature of rheumatism, for one is likely to encounter chorea rather frequently in private practice.

Few positive, objective findings can be observed in a child with active chorea. There is no fever; the blood picture is usually normal, though eosinophilia of 5 to 10 per cent has been found in a surprising number of children. There is no leucocytosis, but the sedimentation rate of red blood cells may be prolonged.[15] Findings in the heart as well as changes in other parts are a concurrent result of rheumatism. The neurologic examination is normal except for the movement. The reflexes are inconstant, but in no way suggest an anatomic lesion of the brain or spinal cord. No satisfactory explanation has been offered for the movement of the body which could be caused by the known changes in the brain. The pattern of the movement at no time is constant as in paralysis agitans, nor does the movement suggest a chorea major (Huntington's chorea). X-rays, spinal fluid examinations, and chemical studies of the blood and body tissues have shown no consistent changes. The basal metabolic rate when determined before or after the period of chorea is normal, and there is no other evidence of internal gland disturbance.

Brain specimens examined postmortem are rare since the patients usually recover. Specimens which have been described show increased vascularity, a few plasma cells scattered irregularly, and slight edema of the glial structures. These changes may be found generally but are located chiefly about the basal nuclei. No structures resembling rheumatic nodules have been described, and no changes suggesting scar tissue formation have been seen. These findings, even in the few cases, seem important in that they are characteristic features of rheumatic fever found elsewhere in the body, especially in the joints. It is also well known that rheumatic nodules are not often found in children about the joints or elsewhere during an attack of acute arthritis with periarticular swelling. These observations should serve to classify the disease as one of the exudative manifestations of rheumatic fever, rather than as a proliferative one. When the proliferative changes occur, there are invariably scars resulting in the tissue in which the nodules occur, such as the heart. This is probably the explanation of why chorea is not followed by permanent paralysis, weakness, or other neurologic changes in the body or brain.

In this respect too, there are essential differences from other types of encephalitis where permanent damage to brain tissue is the rule in many cases. But the same findings occur in the joint when one contrasts attacks with acute rheumatic fever, with either chronic rheumatoid arthritis in children (Still's disease) or in adults. In both of these conditions there are progressive structural changes in the joints, involving periarticular tissue as well as cartilage, bone, and joint capsule. The changes in the brain in chorea, therefore, represent a type of inflammatory process or a response of that tissue to the agent of rheumatic fever and should be classed as a true encephalitis.

Chorea patients usually recover completely without residual injury of any kind. After several weeks a slow improvement is noted, and the symptoms disappear. The recovery may be spontaneous, occasionally may occur rapidly, or may result from the many available forms of therapy. If the rheumatic process progresses in other parts of the body, especially the heart, the picture changes. Reoccurrence is frequent, especially during the spring season, or the next manifestation of the rheumatic process may be in some other region.

Differential Diagnosis.—Among the conditions occurring in children, chorea must be distinguished from poliomyelitis, encephalitis lethargica in its several forms, psychogenic motor disorders, hysteria and habit spasms, occasionally brain injuries and tumors, and from physiological myxedema of adolescence.

Children with hemichorea often suggest poliomyelitis when the incoordination is so pronounced as to interfere with walking, or the use of the arms and legs. The differential diagnosis is easy to make as there are neurologic findings of importance in poliomylitis, such as nerve trunk pain, changes in reflexes, and objective weakness of the affected part. In all doubtful cases spinal fluid examinations should be made to establish the diagnosis.

Encephalitis lethargica, in its early stages, may resemble chorea because of the delirium, confusion, incoordination, and weakness. The rapidly progressive course of encephalitis lethargica tells the story in a day or so. Fever, slight leucocytosis and lymphocytosis, the absence of eosinophilia, and the organic neurologic findings are observed in the acute cases of encephalitis lethargica, and the examination of spinal fluid makes the diagnosis.

It has been suggested that choreiform movements may occur in children as a late result of an attack of encephalitis lethargica so mild as to be missed at the time; or an attack of encephalitis of a milder form, such as the St. Louis type, or a postinfectious encephalitis following measles, whooping cough, chicken pox, or mumps. In the latter group there are many children who may have a mild encephalitic change at the time of the initial disease, who later develop encephalitis recognizable at the time, or the changes may be delayed for months or years. It has been the observation in this clinic that numerous children, with so-called idiopathic chorea in the absence of history or findings of rheumatic fever, give a history of a severe attack of one of the children's contagious diseases or a combination of several in rapid succession. Such children are usually in the younger age group, from 6 to 10 years.

Psychogenic motor disorders offer the most frequent, difficult differential diagnosis. Among adolescents, especially girls, hysteria may simulate chorea closely, and considerable examination may be required to distinguish the two conditions. Habit spasms in the younger age group must be distinguished, but there is rarely any difficulty. The pattern of the habit spasm is constant, though the pattern may change from one to another. Habit spasm is usually limited to an affected part, and there is no emotional disturbance and no other signs of rheumatic fever. Habit spasms last for a longer period of time, are often imitative, are contagious, and have a purposeful, even though misdirected character.

We have also observed choreiform movements frequently in children with crossed cerebral dominance, as described by Orton and other workers. The history of reading and spelling difficulties, especially disturbances of speech, crossed handedness and eyedness, most apparent in the early school age, together with emotional disturbance at home and behavior difficulties should suggest the psychic nature of the choreiform movement and serve to distinguish these children from those with rheumatic chorea.

Careful neurologic examination will reveal sooner or later the presence of tumors and of brain injuries at birth and subsequently, though these findings should be suspected in all cases of chorea even of known rheumatic origin.

We have observed, in increasing numbers in the older age group of 10 to 15 years, children with choreiform movements who have body pains especially in the legs at night; school difficulties, especially a slight but definite deterioration in the quality of school work, usually in the spring of the year; lack of appetite; an increasing laziness both mental and physical; a definite tendency to obesity; a retardation of linear growth with increasing gain in weight; a slightly lowered basal metabolic rate, and a progressive myopia. Such children have what has been termed ''physiologic myxedema of adolescence,'' and on administration of thyroid gland substance these signs and symptoms quickly respond and disappear. The choreiform movement which these children manifest is indistinguishable from true rheumatic chorea. The story of body pains also makes the differential diagnosis somewhat difficult. However, the absence of objective joint signs, the occurrence of pain at night and only in the legs, and the ill defined nature of the pain serve to classify them. Careful consideration of the clinical picture of this type of adolescence disturbance and the absence of psychogenic factors and rheumatic history or findings should point the way. The similarity of the two groups of cases is striking, and repeated examinations are necessary.

It is probably true that every child with chorea has some lowered resistance of a structural somatic defect in the portion of the brain which gives rise to choreiform movements and that the associated occurrence of an etiological factor only serves to bring to light the encephalitic injury. This injury or change in the brain must determine the incidence of chorea in rheumatic children since only a portion of such children develop chorea. There has been no evidence that the agent of rheumatic fever, toxin, virus, or bacterial product of any nature, has a neurotropic quality other than a general affinity for all endothelial tissue of highly specialized function.

Relation to Rheumatic Fever.—It has been implied throughout this discussion the chorea minor of Sydenham is a rheumatic manifestation, and it is believed in this clinic that such is the case. For this reason the term *encephalitis rheumatica* is suggested as proper and more descriptive. It should serve to distinguish such cases from all others with a more obvious etiology or from those with idiopathic chorea of unknown etiology. Since the attack of chorea may be the first manifestation of the rheumatic state in a child, all cases must be watched for further or the later development of the usual picture of rheumatic fever. Also the usual number of rheumatic children may have the factors described above to cause the development of chorea and likewise children with chorea due to those same factors mentioned above may develop rheumatic fever. Therefore, there will always be a certain overlapping in the diagnosis of all children.

It would be difficult to estimate in any statistical way, the relationship of chorea to rheumatic fever. Clinical observations of large groups of children with either rheumatic fever or chorea show strikingly a close relationship. The lack of anatomic observations on brain tissues results from the nature of the situation, the lack of opportunity to secure brains for examination at autopsy, and from the inaccessibility of the brain for any examination other than an indirect one. The unknown nature of the etiologic agent of rheumatic fever makes it impossible to carry out tests or experimental studies for the classification of chorea. It is suggested that the encephalitis of rheumatic fever is similar in its anatomic process to the arthritis, the acute pericarditis, and myocardial changes of an exudative attack of rheumatic fever. The erythemas and urticarias of rheumatic fever are of this same order. The occurrence of an attack of chorea following an acute upper respiratory infection, or tonsillitis, in the same way attacks of other manifestations of rheumatism occur, also should serve to emphasize the causal relationship.

CONCLUSION

The term *encephalitis rheumatica* is suggested for chorea minor of Sydenham in order to emphasize the relationship of chorea to rheumatic fever and to describe the nature of the process in the brain. It is suggested that encephalitis rheumatica (chorea) is an exudative manifestation of the rheumatic state. The nature of the lesions in the brain in this type of encephalitis is similar to those occurring in the joints, heart, and other parts of the body.

Careful study of all cases of encephalitis rheumatica should be made to distinguish them from brain injuries and tumors, from encephalitis due to other causes, especially postinfectious encephalitis of childhood, from psychogenic motor disorders of children and adolescents, and from physiologic myxedema of childhood.

REFERENCES

1. Quoted by Still, Sir Frederick: History of Pediatrics, p. 276, 1931, Oxford University Press.
2. Cheadle, W. B.: Harveian Lectures of 1888, London, 1889.
   Idem: System of Medicine by Albott and Rolleston, Vol. II, part 1, p. 645, New York, 1908, The Macmillan Company.
3. Gerstley, J. B.: J. PEDIAT. **6**: 42, 1935.
4. Guttmann, E.: J. Neurol. & Psychopath. **17**: 16, 1936.
5. Martin, J. P.: Brain **57**: 504, 1934.
6. Bradshaw, D. A.: J. Exper. Psychol. **20**: 84, 1937.
7. Irish, I. A.: J. PEDIAT. **5**: 654, 1934.
8. Glover, J. A.: Proc. Roy. Soc. Med. **27**: 953, 1934.
9. Lucas, W. P.: Am. Heart J. (in press).
10. Parrish, P. L.: J. PEDIAT. **11**: 617, 1937.
11. Schwarz, H.: Am. J. Dis. Child. **49**: 952, 1935.
12. Coburn, A. F.: Am. J. M. Sc. **193**: 1, 1937.
13. Jones, T. D.: J. A. M. A. **105**: 571, 1935.
14. Lueth, H. C.: J. PEDIAT. **3**: 775, 1933.
15. Struthers, R. R., and Bacal, H. L.: Canad. M. A. J. **35**: 258, 1936.

THE IRREGULAR EXTENSIONS OF THE END OF THE SHAFT IN THE X-RAY PHOTOGRAPH IN CONGENITAL SYPHILIS, WITH PERTINENT OBSERVATIONS

Edwards A. Park, M.D., and Deborah A. Jackson, B.S.
Baltimore, Md.

THE x-ray changes at the ends of the long bones in congenital syphilis are subject to great variation. Actual changes in the bone may be too slight to show in the x-ray picture. On the other hand, they may be so developed as to disfigure and deform the x-ray image to an extent not equaled in any other disease. Moreover, they vary greatly in kind. Either the *Spirochaeta pallida* must be subject to variation in its growth requirements, or bones in different infants must vary much in their different parts with respect to growth favorableness, or circulatory conditions must vary. At any rate, in some infants it is the cartilage cells which seem to bear the brunt of the invasion, and in others it is the osteoblasts which are especially affected; in some destructive processes appear as the predominant feature, in others an irregular new bone formation in the periosteum. In this article, which is presented as a very small token of respect for the memory of Dr. McKim Marriott, who exerted so powerful an influence in pediatrics in this country and abroad, we call attention to an x-ray phenomenon of congenital syphilis which in some cases is very striking. We refer to the irregular projections of the dense shadows of the end of the shaft into the cartilage which give to the end such a jagged appearance in the x-ray film. What is their cause? This is the question which we shall answer. Before we do that, however, it will be necessary to describe in some detail the vascular supply of the epiphyseal cartilage, the cartilage canals, and the changes produced in them by syphilis, and also to make clear the changes in the cartilage itself produced by the disease, since the formation of the projections is dependent on them. Inasmuch, also, as the projections seem to vary with the rate of growth, not only in different bones but in the skeleton as a whole at different age periods, it seems advisable to say something on that subject.

The irregular projections of the end of the shaft into the cartilage are not always present in congenital syphilis. They are usually absent if the syphilitic involvement is slight, and they may be absent, even though the involvement is extremely severe. When the condition is well developed in a long bone of an extremity, the end appears jagged, irregularly serrated, or marked by wedgeshaped, thornlike, or completely irregular projections; in some instances it looks irregularly scalloped

From the Harriet Lane Home of the Johns Hopkins Hospital, the Department of Pediatrics of the Johns Hopkins University School of Medicine and the Children's Bureau of the United States Department of Labor.

(Figs. 1 and 2). In the ribs the picture is somewhat different. The extensions into the cartilage are longer and sharper (Fig. 3). The

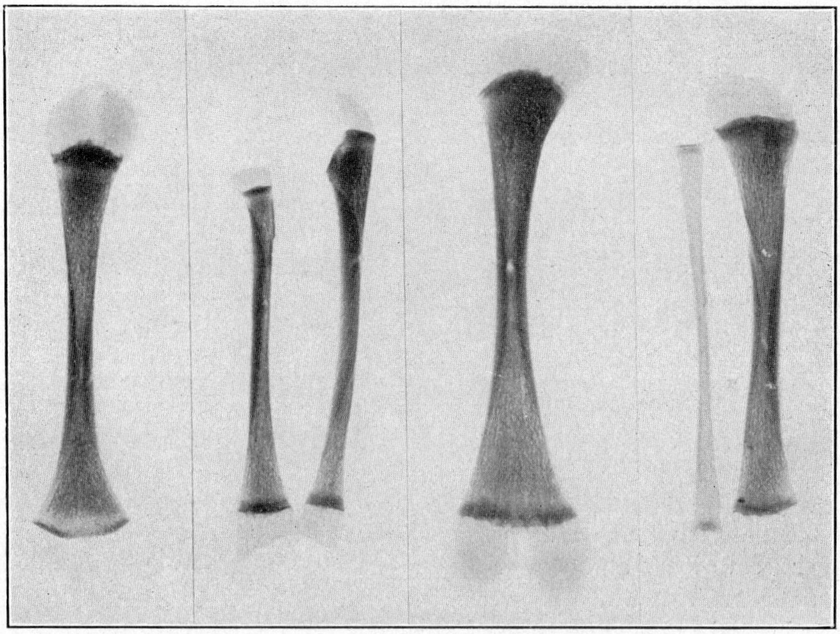

A. B. C. D.

Fig. 1.—X-ray photographs of the humerus, radius, ulna, femur, tibia and fibula taken from Baby T., No. 599, stillborn. The ends of the bones show the characteristic projections with which this paper deals. Notice that they are absent at the slow growing ends of the upper ulna, upper radius and lower humerus.

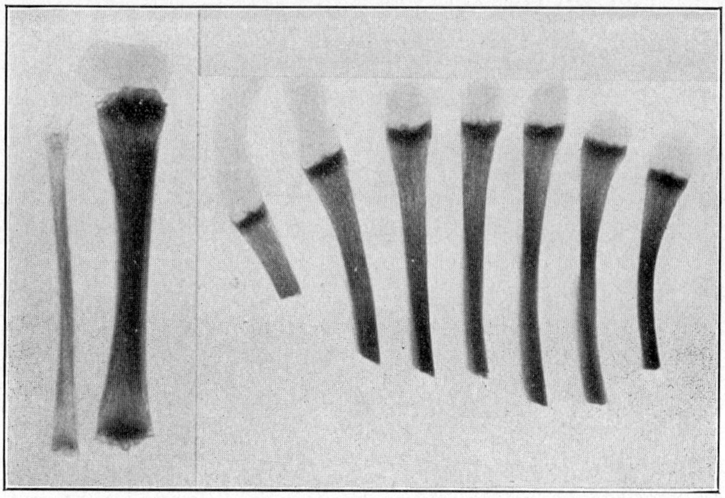

Fig. 2. Fig. 3.

Fig. 2.—X-ray photograph of the tibia and fibula of a syphilitic infant, Baby B., No. 300, aged 6 hours. The ends show a scalloped type of irregularity.

Fig. 3.—X-ray photograph of the middle tier of ribs taken after death from I. N., No. 517, aged one day, showing a sample of the kind of changes at end of ribs which occur in congenital syphilis.

appearance is often as if the rib were barbed or pronged. Whether rib or long bone of the extremity, the end appears to be abnormally dense and the prolongations under discussion seem to have the same density as the end. The impression is obtained that some abnormal formation occupies the end of the bone and that it is this which juts out irregularly into the cartilage.

An analysis of the x-ray films in our series of cases of congenital syphilis, exhibiting the phenomenon, shows that the bone ends most commonly affected are the rapidly growing ones. The slow growing ends do not show it at all or do so indistinctly. The almost stagnant upper end of the ulna does not develop it; the upper end of the radius may show it occasionally. The lower end of the humerus shows it rarely, though at the same time it may be extremely developed at the fast growing end. In general the development is in proportion to the rate of growth. For this reason in our series it was greatest at the anterior ends of the middle ribs, next at the lower end of the femur, next at the upper end of the femur, both ends of the tibia and the upper end of the humerus, and next at the lower ends of the radius and ulna.

But the relationship to growth rate is not a constant one, as in certain other conditions, and ceases to be clearly evident soon after birth. Rickets, which is a disturbance in metabolism, involves the ends of the long bones in exact proportion to their rate of growth. As might be expected, the heavy metals which form insoluble compounds with phosphates and at the same time happen to cast shadows in the x-ray film, for example, lead, are deposited at the ends of the bones exactly according to the rate of growth. Elementary phosphorus, which stimulates bone production and causes shadows to appear in the x-ray film solely by increasing the density of structure of the bone, also affects the ends of the long bones exactly in proportion to their rates of growth. One can actually measure the abnormal bone produced under the influence of rickets or during the administration of the metals and in that way determine the growth rate. One would scarcely expect that congenital syphilis, a disease produced by living things which move about and multiply according to various conditions of vascularization and tissue favorableness, would manifest itself in the skeleton symmetrically or according to any growth scheme. Nevertheless, it is true that in fetal syphilis the affection of the ends of the bones is in general proportional to the rate of growth. Indeed, by actual measurement of the depth of the syphilitic formations in stillborn children it can be demonstrated that the upper end of the ulna grows relatively faster during intrauterine life than after birth. After birth has occurred, the bones are no longer affected by congenital syphilis according to the rate of growth. Why this is so, we do not know, but we surmise that factors coming into being with extrauterine existence, such as trauma, muscle strain and strain resulting from gravity, all become operative, alter the vascularity or other conditions and predispose toward the lodgement, multiplication and activity of the spirochetes in them. The closer, then, to birth, the greater the approximation of involvement of the ends of the bones to the rate of growth. The older the infant, the less the correspondence, until there is none at all. In our analysis of 77 cases of congenital syphilis, in which the bones were studied both by means of x-ray and histologic methods, the phenomenon was noted 48 times. In 20 instances the infant was stillborn and in 18 was 2 weeks of age or under. When the syphilis makes its appearance at the ends of the long bones for the first time at the end of the first or second month, the phenomenon does not usually develop. The oldest infant showing it, however, was 6 months of age, so there are exceptions.

Growth in length occurs faster in fetal life than ever again. Inasmuch as growth in length depends on proliferation of the epiphyseal cartilage, it would seem probable that the phenomenon under discussion was connected with the rapid growth of the cartilage and that its occurrence chiefly in connection with intrauterine syphilis is explicable on that ground. Indeed, it is in the infections already well developed at the time of birth that one finds the widespread affections of the cartilage presently to be briefly described.

When one studies the bones of congenital syphilitics after death in order to ascertain the cause underlying the x-ray phenomenon, one finds that the projections are about the nutrient vessels of the cartilage, known as the cartilage canals, and that in many instances the proliferative cartilage itself shows extreme degenerative changes. It seems likely that the two phenomena are related. First, then, what are the cartilage canals and what is the effect of the disease upon them and, second, what are the degenerative changes in the cartilage produced by the disease?

The cartilage canals (Fig. 4) are the nutrient vessels of the cartilage *plus their connective tissue sheaths.* The connective tissue sheaths are very thick and make the canals appear as large structures. The sheath probably acts as an insulation, protecting the cartilage from the direct contact with the blood. In the specimen cleared with oil of wintergreen, so that both cartilage and connective tissue become transparent but the outline of the vessels still remains visible often by virtue of their contained blood, the canals appear as tunnels in the middle of which lie the artery and entwined about it one or two veins. The blood vessels are branches of the perichondrial network of arteries and veins. The arteries enter from all sides. It is as the result of this penetration that the interior of the epiphyseal cartilage becomes vascularized and the nucleus of ossification of the epiphysis forms. The canals persist only for a time which varies with the particular bone. But we are interested only in the cartilage canals which supply the generating zone of the proliferative cartilage and shall limit our descriptions to them.

In the ribs and certain other long bones (but not in the femur) the vessels which form the nutrient supply of the proliferative cartilage penetrate the perichondrium and enter the resting cartilage just on the distal side of the generating zone of the proliferative cartilage. They run perpendicularly into the cartilage along the distal surface of the generating zone and converge toward the center. Before arriving at the center, however, they end and, before ending, give off branches which descend a short distance toward the shaft. They are end vessels, not anastomosing with each other or with the vessels of the shaft. Occasionally it happens in the normal bone that a branch of a cartilage canal

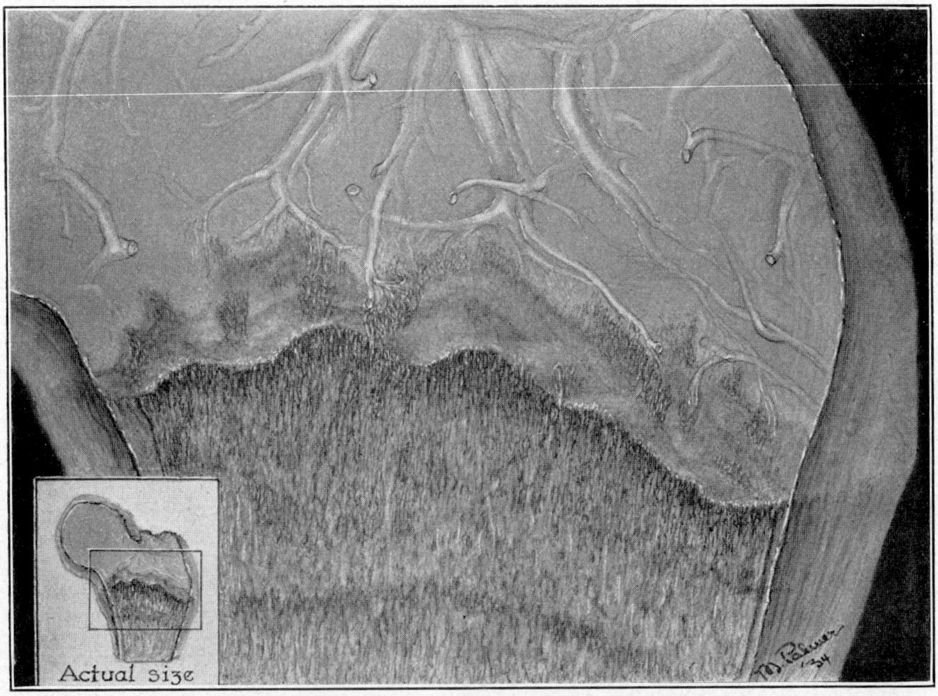

Fig. 4.—Drawing from the upper end of the femur, cleared in oil of wintergreen, to show the relationship of the cartilage canals to the projections from the end of the shaft. When a canal approaches the end of the shaft, the shaft seems to mound up or ridge in order to meet it.

directed toward the shaft may be very large and may even reach the shaft. However, this is a rare exception. Undoubtedly the function of the cartilage canals lying along the generating zone of the proliferative cartilage is to supply nutrient material to it. As long as growth in length lasts, the cells in the generating zone keep multiplying, just as the epithelial cells in the basal layers of the skin keep multiplying throughout the life of the individual. It is as a result of the multiplication of the cells in the generating zone of the proliferative cartilage that the bone grows in length. It is natural, therefore, that it should have a special nutrient supply. The vessels in the cartilage canals seem to end in bulbous terminations. The bulbous endings perhaps represent filtration mechanisms, comparable to the glomeruli of the kidney.

In congenital syphilis the cartilage canals are not always affected. They are very frequently affected, however, in particular when the disease becomes well developed during intrauterine life. When affected, they become extremely large, several times their normal size. When one examines with the microscope, one finds that the tissue of the cartilage canal is composed of fibroblasts with rather large nuclei which are oval shaped and that all through the interstices are capillaries distended with red blood cells. We think it probable that the insulation of the blood vessels breaks down in congenital syphilis when the cartilage canals become so vascular and the cartilage cells forming the walls of the

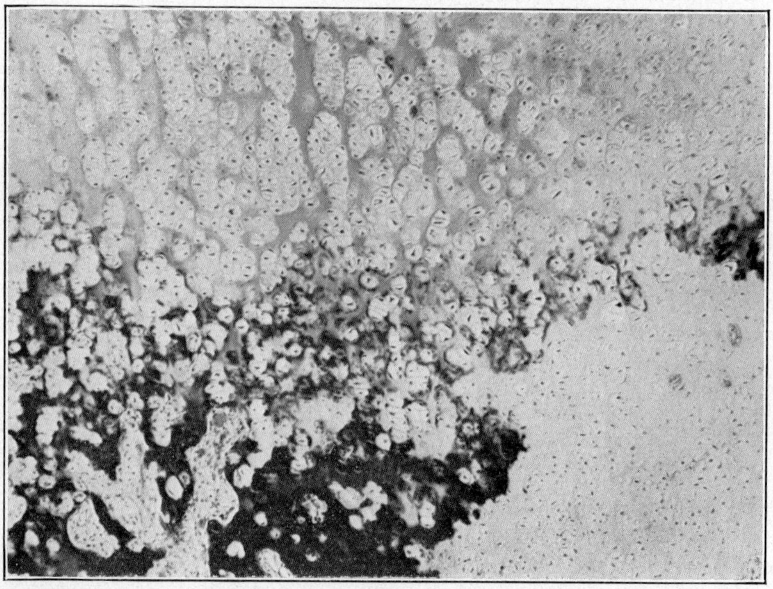

Fig. 5.—Photomicrograph (high power view) from a microscopic section, taken from rib of R. P., No. 1018, aged 4 months. The section shows the extreme degeneration of the cartilage which so often occurs when the disease becomes advanced in fetal life. The cartilage at the right lower corner is badly affected. The cells are small, orderly alignment does not exist, the matrix substance is much increased and there has been failure to take up calcium. At the left, calcification (black) has occurred. But the disorderly pattern of the lattice is enough to show the extreme state of disorder and degeneration, which existed in the cartilage at the time when the lime salts deposited.

tunnels are attacked and destroyed and the tunnels themselves in that way become enlarged. The hypertrophy of the cartilage canal in congenital syphilis is made possible only as the result of destruction of the cartilaginous walls. The descending branches of the cartilage canals which often become enormous, pass through the proliferative cartilage to the shaft as broad channels and meet the vessels of the latter.

Just as the cartilage canals may or may not be attacked by the syphilis, so the proliferative cartilage may or may not be affected. In some cases of severe syphilitic infection the cartilage appears to escape;

in other instances it is attacked and undergoes degenerative change to a degree not seen in rickets, scurvy, or any other disease (Fig. 5). When the cartilage is severely affected, the cells do not develop normally and rapidly undergo degenerative changes. In the severest involvements many of the older cells, those nearest the shaft, seem to be dead. Production of matrix substance seems to be much increased so that in general it seems much more abundant than normal. Large masses of matrix substance appear in the histologic preparations without cells or containing degenerated remains. Column formation of the cells becomes very irregular or stops altogether. The greatest variation in the state of individual cells exists. Some appear swollen and large, while adjacent cells remain as small as osteoblasts. As already indicated, dead and living cells seem to occur close together. The architectural arrangement has gone.

It is thought that the change in the cartilage cells is not a late development, that is, it does not begin in the old cartilage near the cartilage-shaft junction, but has its origin where proliferation begins to take place. In other words, we think that the cells in the generating zone itself must be affected by the disease so that the newly formed cells which are produced are abnormal at the time of their formation. The reason for thinking this is that in typical cases the young cartilage seems abnormal. The family groups appear irregular and distorted and the matrix substance abnormally developed.

When the cartilage is very seriously affected in congenital syphilis, it may not calcify at all or not in the normal way. Either the lymph carrying the inorganic material cannot penetrate or else the cartilaginous material has lost the power to produce the "local factor," phosphatase or some other enzyme, or the pH necessary to give it the property of taking lime salts selectively out of the blood. Large masses of degenerated cartilage remain calcium-free, though lying close to the shaft. One often finds under the microscope that the lime salts deposit only at the margin of the degenerated cartilage, commonly as a continuous layer, or they deposit in the immediate periphery of the cell but not in the matrix substance a short distance away from the cell. In some cases lime salts deposit in the cells themselves, a condition which never happens normally. When the calcification occurs in the cells, the inference seems justified that the cells are dead. Indeed, the very abnormal cartilage in congenital syphilis often calcifies not after the manner of living but of dead tissue.

A proof that the changes which we have described in the cartilage in congenital syphilis are true ones which existed during life and are not artifacts from poor fixation or post-mortem change is furnished by the pattern of the lime salt deposits. If the structure of the cartilage has been abnormal either in rickets, scurvy, or congenital syphilis, the pattern of the lime salt deposits will show it. The depositing lime salts

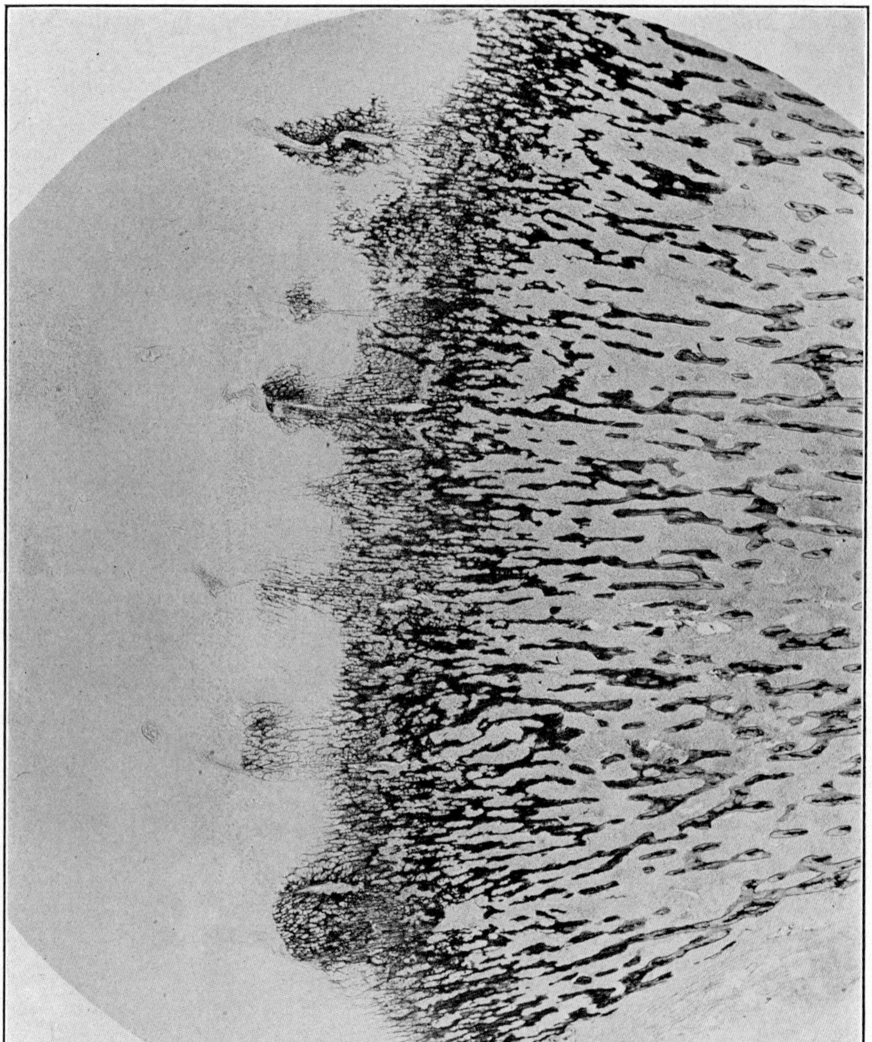

Fig. 6.—Photomicrograph (low power view) of a microscopic section of the lower end of the femur, seen in Fig. 1. It shows plainly the cause of the irregular projections of the end of the shaft into the cartilage. They are due obviously to building up of calcification about the vertical branches of the cartilage canals in advance of elsewhere. The canals are much hypertrophied, as is evidenced by the fact that they show so well at all places in a section in a single plane. The calcified matrix stains black. The network formed by it *in toto* is the syphilitic lattice. The preparation makes clear that the projections are merely extensions of the lattice.

petrify and perpetuate the pattern of the cartilage. If the formation of matrix substance is irregular or if the matrix substance develops in excess, the pattern of the calcification, i.e., the calcified lattice can be relied upon to tell the tale.

The involvement of the cartilage in any given bone is most irregular, just as the involvement of the cartilage canals is irregular. One may find the proliferative cartilage fairly normal in one place and extremely abnormal in an adjacent one.

We are now prepared to return to our original task and undertake to explain the reason for the irregular extension of the shadows of the end of the shaft into the cartilage, as seen in the x-ray film. Examina-

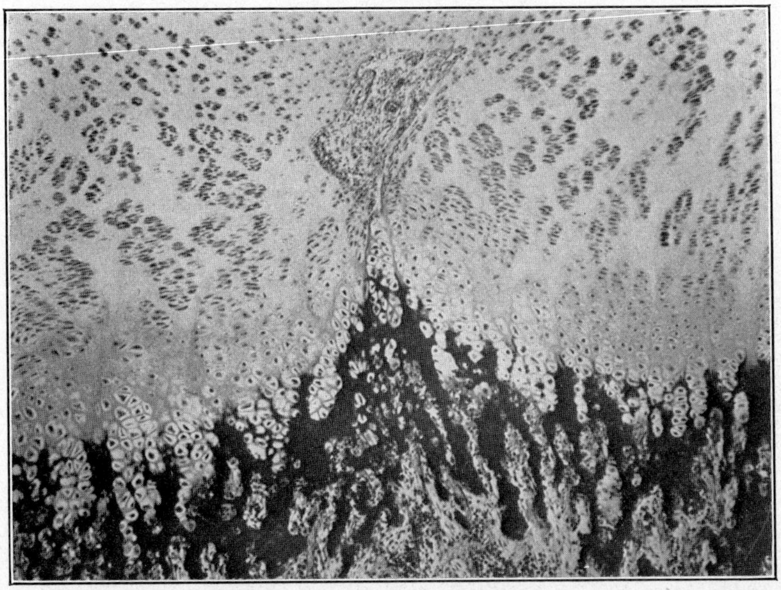

Fig. 7.—Photomicrograph (high power view) of a microscopic section taken from upper end of tibia of Baby C., No. 1110, aged 5 days. This shows that the proliferative cartilage has matured more rapidly around the cartilage canal than at a distance from it. Notice that the clear cells, the cells occupying the regions where calcification is impending, extend high along it. We have explained the extensions of the calcification around the cartilage canals on the ground that the cartilage in proximity to them undergoes the cycle of maturation necessary for calcification at a more rapid rate.

tion under the microscope shows that calcification of the cartilage adjacent to the cartilage canals occurs in advance of calcification of the cartilage between the cartilage canals. The projections from the end of the shaft are nothing more than the extensions of the calcification around the cartilage canals (Fig. 6).

The phenomenon is explained in this way. The cartilage in immediate proximity to the cartilage canals matures much more rapidly than normal and remains more nearly normal in appearance, whereas the cartilage at a distance from the cartilage canals does not or undergoes the degenerative changes described (Fig. 7). The result is that in the cartilage around the canals calcification occurs faster than normal, whereas between it occurs much more slowly or not at all. The result

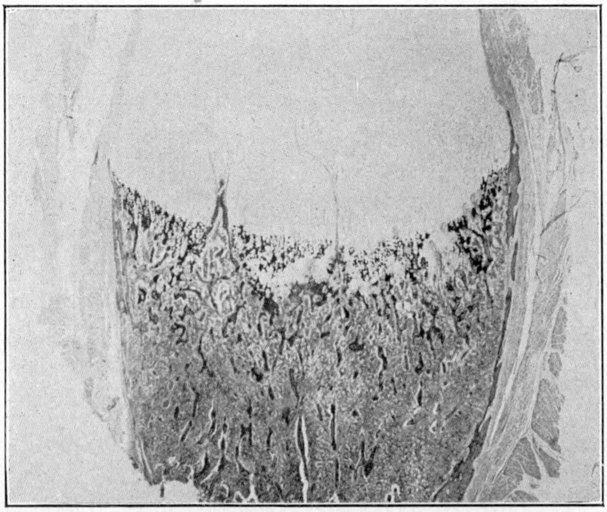

Fig. 8.—Photomicrograph (low power view) of a microscopic section taken from a rib of W. M., No. 1055, aged 9 weeks. It shows metaplastic bone formation in a cartilage canal (the inverted V). Since the formation contains calcium, it casts a shadow and will appear in the x-ray photograph as a projection from the end of the shaft. Metaplastic bone formation in a hypertrophied cartilage canal is a rare sole cause of a projection shadow. Extensions of the syphilitic lattice around the vertical branches of the canals are the common cause. But both conditions may be present in combination.

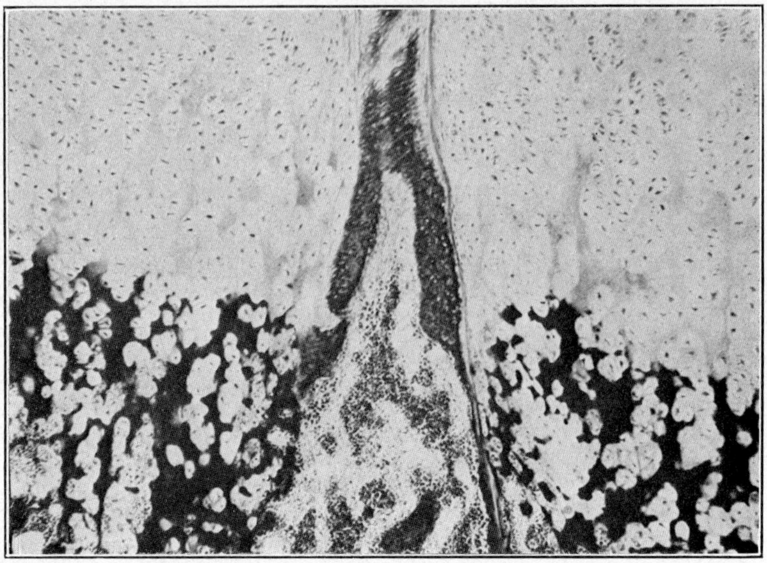

Fig. 9.—Higher power of preceding, showing the metaplastic nature of the inverted V formation in the canal.

is that lattice formation (calcification of the matrix frame) occurs around the cartilage canals in advance of lattice formation between.

The projections are the result, then, of the extensions of the lattice around the cartilage canals and they are rendered even more prominent by the lagging or failure of calcification in the regions between. When one examines the proliferative cartilage through the microscope, one can see that the cartilage around the cartilage canals has not only matured earlier but that the cells have a much more normal appearance than the cells at a distance. The microscope reveals, then, that the generating zone of the proliferative cartilage is not higher placed around the cartilage canals but rather that the cartilage matures in those regions at a greatly increased rate and develops and remains more nearly normal. Under the binocular in the cleared specimen the extensions of the calcification around the cartilage canals appear as mounds or ridges (Fig. 4). These mounds or ridges of calcified material give rise to the characteristic appearance of extensions from the end of the shaft in the x-ray film.

However, another factor may enter into the formation of these projections. It is this. When the branches of the cartilage canals directed toward the shaft become very large in congenital syphilis and the connective tissue contained in them very abundant, it often happens that the connective tissue calcifies and forms metaplastic bone (Figs. 8 and 9). These bands or columns of metaplastic bone, occupying the interior of the canal, are parallel to the long axis of the shaft. They cast shadows and are oftentimes partly, sometimes entirely, responsible for a projecting shadow seen in the x-ray photograph.

In some instances the lattice is built up around all the cartilage canals; in others only around some. The reason for this is not entirely clear.

The description which has just been given explains why the projecting shadows from the end of the shaft have the same consistency in the x-ray film as the end of the shaft itself. The shadow at the end of the shaft is produced by the syphilitic lattice. The projections are nothing more than extensions of the lattice.

The final question is why the cartilage matures more rapidly and calcification occurs higher up around the cartilage canals than elsewhere. We do not have any exact information and are forced to reply in conjecture. It seems altogether probable, however, that the more rapid maturation of the cartilage in the neighborhood of the canals is due to the increased vascularity of the cartilage canals and the breakdown of the normal insulation. In congenital syphilis it is plausible to think that the diffusion mechanism by which the generating zone is supplied with nutrient material becomes disabled. We should suppose that the supply of lymph to the cells immediately adjacent to the canals was increased, so that they matured with an increased rapidity, whereas the cells of the generating zone between received an insufficient or inferior supply and developed more slowly or even underwent degenerative changes. One reason for thinking that this may be the case is the analogous phenomenon observed in rickets and concerned with the phenomenon of cupping. The cells of the proliferative cartilage lying immediately under the perichondrium develop more rapidly than the cells in the interior. The result of the more rapid development of the cartilage cells in the subperiosteal layer is that their destruction and the calcification of the matrix and conversion into shaft occur earlier. Consequently, the shaft forms more rapidly at the extreme periphery than centrally, and cupping develops. The reason which we have assigned for the increased and more rapid maturation of the cartilage cells lying immediately under the perichondrium is that because of their situation they receive under the strain of rickets additional nutrient material from the perichondrial blood vessels.

The question arises whether the condition more responsible for the development of the projections from the end of the shaft in congenital syphilis is the accelerated development of the cartilage around the cartilage canals or the lagging of calcification as the result of the degeneration of the cartilage in the regions between. The reply is that the phenomenon is due primarily to the more rapid maturation of the cartilage around the canals, but that it may be intensified by the failure of calcification of the cartilage between. The reason for this answer is that the phenomenon may occur in congenital syphilis even when the cartilage between the canals does not show much or any degeneration. But under those circumstances the projections are not so well developed.

REMARKS ON A CASE OF CONGENITAL IDIOPATHIC HYPERTROPHY OF THE HEART

GROVER F. POWERS, M.D., AND PHILIP M. LECOMPTE, M.D.
NEW HAVEN, CONN.

THESE remarks will deal with one of the many subjects upon which the pediatric clinic of the Johns Hopkins Medical School focused study, so-called congenital idiopathic hypertrophy of the heart. Professor John Howland[1] wrote one of the early papers on this condition, his contribution being published in the memorial volumes of 1919, commemorating the seventieth birthday of Sir William Osler. The case report and studies which we shall give demonstrate the important place which, in the past quarter century, chemical techniques have taken in clinical studies, a development fostered by Dr. Howland when he early established a chemical laboratory as an integral part of his department and placed it under the supervision of the late Williams McKim Marriott. Dr. Marriott was ever a dynamic member of the group in the Harriet Lane Home, and his leadership continued to inspire the pediatric department in Baltimore long after he went to St. Louis as Professor of Pediatrics in Washington University.

CASE REPORT

A male baby, aged 8 months, was admitted to the pediatric service of the New Haven Hospital on Dec. 26, 1937, and died the following day, having been in the hospital thirty-two hours (N. H. H. No. A-77231).

The family history was noncontributory: there were two pregnancies, the first resulting in a male child now living and well at the age of 19 months; the patient was the product of the second pregnancy.

The patient was born after a normal delivery and weighed 6 pounds 14 ounces. The outstanding feature of the past history was that the child never had thriven; vomiting, coughing, and irritability were the outstanding characterizations given by the parents regarding the patient's ill health. There was never adequate explanation for the vomiting, which varied in occurrence and amount but was often severe. The birth weight was doubled at 7½ months of age and had not increased since. Cough was sometimes present and sometimes absent; it was hacking and nonproductive in nature when present. The symptoms grew worse during the two weeks prior to admission; vomiting and coughing along with alternating drowsiness and irritability became alarming on the day preceding admission. No solid food and only little milk or water were taken. The referring physician diagnosed pneumonia of the left lower lobe.

On admission the patient was observed to be a well-formed child but undernourished (weight, 14.6 pounds and length, 71 cm.). The head was not remark-

From the Departments of Pediatrics and Pathology, Yale University School of Medicine, and the Pediatric and Pathological Services of the New Haven Hospital and Dispensary.

Presented at a joint session of the Johns Hopkins Medical and Surgical Associations, Baltimore, Feb. 26, 1938. The program consisted of contributions by members of the Medical School, Class of 1913.

able. The temperature was normal (37.3° C.), and the child was quiet, slightly cyanotic, but not dyspneic. There was no clubbing of fingers or toes. The significant findings were those relating to the lungs and heart. There was dullness of the percussion note and suppression of breath sounds over the left chest, most marked posteriorly; there were no râles and no bronchial breathing. The heart was enlarged to the right and left of the sternum. The rate was not rapid nor sounds remarkable in intensity; both systolic and diastolic murmurs were heard by a junior observer only. The liver was palpable just below the costal margin, but the spleen was not palpable. The blood pressure was 100/70. The red blood cells were 5,400,000, hemoglobin 13 gm., and white blood cells 6,100, with 42 per cent polymorphonuclears.

A fluoroscopic examination at this time showed a very large heart with variations in density described as a ''heart within a heart,'' findings which suggest pericardial effusion. On the film these differences in density were not easily made out, but the striking enlargement of the heart in all diameters was obvious (Fig. 1). There was some infiltration of the right upper lobe of the lung.

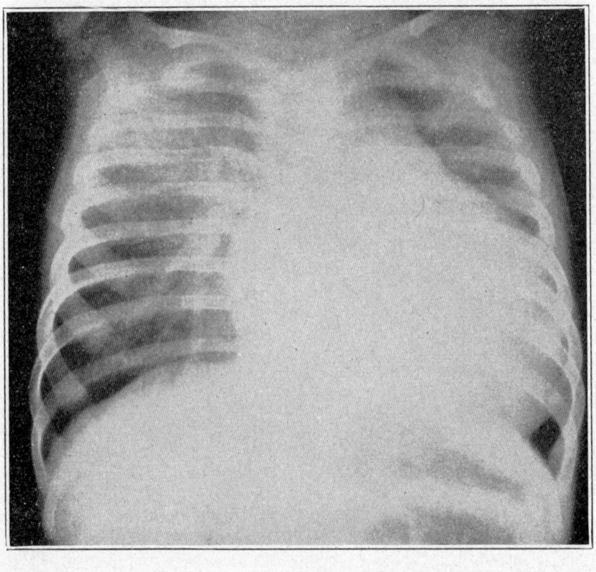

Fig. 1.—Roentgenogram of thorax. Transverse diameter of thorax, 14.7 cm. and of heart, 9.6 cm.; in lateral projection, anteroposterior diameter of heart, 8 cm.

The patient became rapidly and progressively worse. The temperature rose steadily to 40.6° C., and the child became increasingly restless and dyspneic; he seemed to be in very great distress, the cause of which was not obvious. A second white blood count showed 7,100 cells, 48 per cent being polymorphonuclears. Examinations a few hours before death showed signs suggestive of consolidation in the left lower lung posteriorly and right upper lung anteriorly and a heart enlarged in all diameters, extending on the left to the lateral chest wall. The rate was 180 per minute; there were no murmurs, and the sounds were not remarkable. The liver was felt one fingerbreadth below the costal margin in the mid-clavicular line.

An electrocardiogram (Fig. 2) was taken a few hours before death. The rate was 200 and the time interval 0.2 seconds. Dr. Arthur J. Geiger's interpretation was as follows: ''The rapid and regular ventricular rate of supraventricular origin is noted. Since no auricular waves are discernible, the tachycardia probably originates in the A-V node. Two aberrant beats, probably of ventricular origin, were seen in Lead III. The QRS complexes and T-waves are normal. Impression: paroxysmal tachycardia probably of A-V nodal origin.''

The urine showed a slight reduction for sugar, no acetone; the quantity was not sufficient for further study. Blood culture (post-mortem) showed no growth in either blood broth or on blood agar plate. The spinal fluid (post-mortem) contained a few red blood cells; no organisms were seen. The Kahn test was negative.

The clinical diagnosis was congenital idiopathic hypertrophy of the heart; the possibility of glycogen storage disease of the heart, so-called cardiomegalia glycogenica, was suggested.

The autopsy was performed eight hours after death by Dr. Philip LeCompte; the body had been kept in a refrigerator at 32° to 35° F. Only relevant data are presented concerning post-mortem findings.

There was no excess of free fluid in the peritoneal cavity. The anterior edge of the liver extended 2 cm. below the costal margin in the right mid-clavicular line

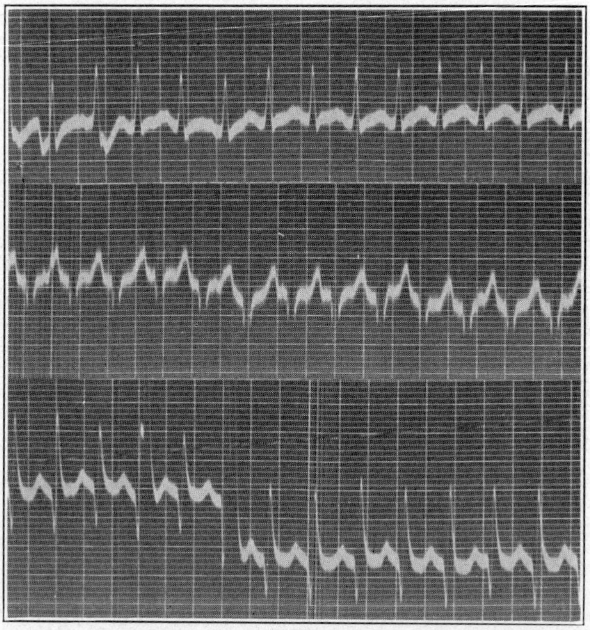

Fig. 2.—Electrocardiogram taken a few hours before death.

and not at all in the left mid-clavicular line. When the chest plate was removed there were found about 20 c.c. of clear straw colored fluid in the right pleural cavity and 2 or 3 c.c. in the left. The striking feature of the appearance of the thoracic cavity was the enormous size of the heart, which occupied most of the left hemithorax and extended well over to the right. The transverse diameter of the heart in situ was 9 cm., while that of the chest was 13 cm. The left lung was markedly compressed and its atelectatic lower lobe lay like a flap over the left side of the heart. Only 3 or 4 c.c. of pale, clear fluid were found in the pericardial sac.

The heart weighed 93 gm., in contrast to 37 gm.,[2] the average for an 8-months-old child. The organ was globoid in shape and appeared to be made up largely of firm, rounded left ventricle. The epicardium was smooth and glistening. No anomalies of the great vessels or valves were present, although special search was made for malformations. The entire aorta and the main branches of the pulmonary artery were carefully examined and did not appear unusual. The coronary vessels were normal in origin, distribution, and appearance. The right auricle was moderately large, but the walls were not greatly thickened. The cavity of the right ventricle was moderately large, and the walls were 2 to 3 mm. in thickness. The endocardium of the right heart was smooth, thin, and glistening. The left auricle was very large and lined by smooth, glistening endocardium, through which could be seen gray-white opaque material suggesting diffuse fibrous tissue (Fig. 3). The cavity of the left ventricle was very large with flattened trabeculae carneae and

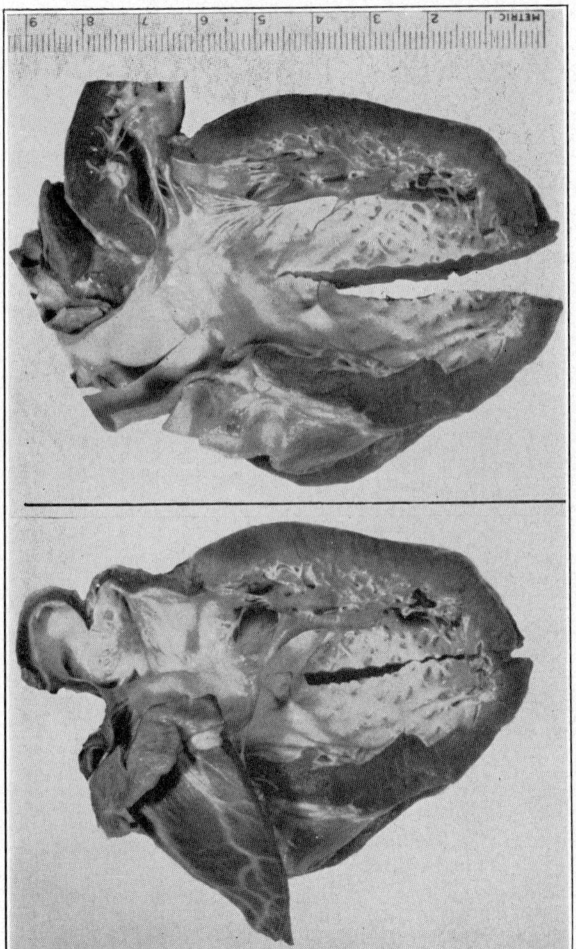

Fig. 3. Fig. 4.

Fig. 3.—Left auricle and ventricle showing large chambers, thickened walls, and gray-white, opaque, diffusely thickened endocardium.

Fig. 4.—Left ventricle and aorta showing large chamber, thickened walls. Note absence of narrowing of vessel and gray-white, opaque, diffusely thickened endocardium.

diffuse gray-white, opaque tissue beneath the endocardium like that seen in the left auricle (Fig. 4). The wall of the left ventricle was 8 to 9 mm. thick. On section the muscle was very firm and pale reddish brown with definite yellow-pink areas near the endocardium. The foramen ovale was open to a probe in an oblique manner; the ductus arteriosus was closed.

The upper lobe of the right lung was deeper red than the remainder. On section this portion was mottled with small ill-defined pale yellow-gray areas. The left lung was not remarkable except for complete atelectasis of the lower lobe.

The liver weighed 125 gm. as compared with 254 gm.,[2] the average for an 8-months-old child; the organ was not remarkable except for its relatively small size.

The adrenals (combined weight 2 gm.), the kidneys (combined weight 44 gm.), and the thymus were not noteworthy.

Examination of the brain was not permitted.

Histologic examination of the heart showed a uniform and orderly fibrous thickening without cellular infiltration of the endocardium of the left auricle and

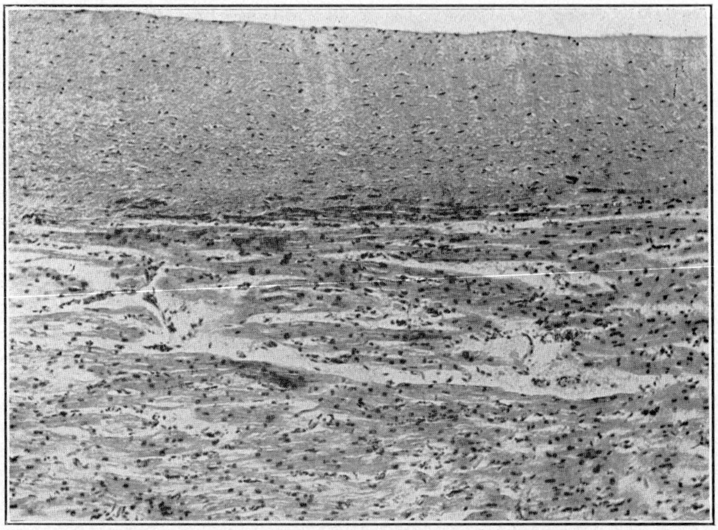

Fig. 5.—Photomicrograph of section of left ventricle showing uniform thickening of subendocardial connective tissue. Elastic as well as collagenous fibers were demonstrated. Note absence of cellular infiltration in both endocardium and myocardium. Hematoxylin-eosin stain was used. (×125.)

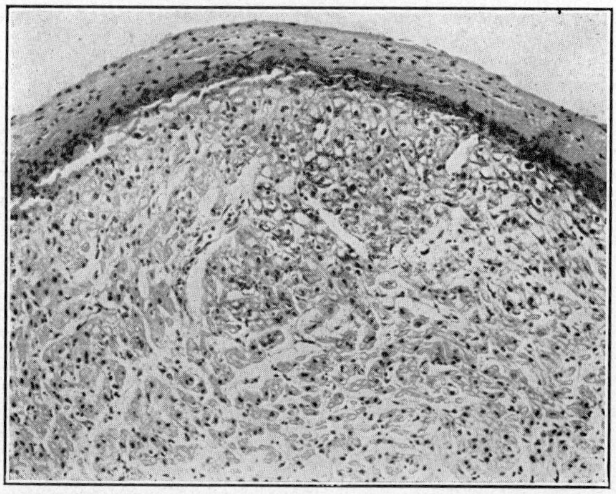

Fig. 6.—Photomicrograph of portion of left ventricle, fixed in absolute alcohol and stained by Best carmine method. Just beneath the thickened endocardium there is a bundle of vacuolated fibers containing black granules (red in original stain). Only in such fibers as these, which are presumably Purkinje fibers, was glycogen demonstrable. Note the absence of granules in surrounding muscle. (×90.)

ventricle (Fig. 5). Elastic fibers were demonstrable in these tissues. There was a questionable slight increase in interstitial fibrous tissue of the myocardium of the right ventricle; there was no cellular infiltration and no scarring of the myocardium. There was no abnormal vacuolization and no fragmentation of the muscle fibers; no mitotic figures[34] were seen. The diameter of the individual heart fibers did not seem unusual; the average of fifty micrometer measurements of individual fibers gave a value of 9.2 microns as compared with a similar average of 8 microns for the fibers of the heart of average weight of a child of comparable age. The fibers of a heart of average weight of an adult measured 12 microns in diameter.

After fixing the tissues in absolute alcohol, sections of the heart made from both paraffin and celloidin blocks were stained by the Best carmine method for glycogen, and none showed red granules except in a few fibers just beneath the endocardium of the left ventricle, presumably the normal[3] Purkinje fibers (Fig. 6). The stain was checked with saliva-digested controls and tissue known to contain glycogen, as well as by chemical analyses (see Table I).

Sections of the lungs showed congestion and edema. Sections of the right upper lobe showed in the alveoli many large mononuclear cells with vacuolated cytoplasm. Best carmine stains of tissue from this area showed no glycogen.

Sections of other organs, including adrenals, showed nothing remarkable. Best carmine stains of the liver, skeletal muscle, and kidneys showed no evidence of glycogen, and there was no vacuolization in any organs suggestive of glycogen storage.

Sudan III stains showed no fat in the myocardium or kidneys and only a small amount in the liver cells. In some of the alveoli of the lungs, especially in the right upper lobe, large vacuolated mononuclear phagocytes were seen. The sudan III stain showed that these vacuoles contained fat.

Fresh tissue from the heart, liver, and kidneys was taken at the time of autopsy for chemical analyses for glycogen. Four hours later a piece of the right upper lung was taken from modified Kaiserling solution for similar investigation. The determinations were made according to a modification of the method of Pflüger by Dr. Herman Yannet and showed less than 0.1 per cent of glycogen in heart, liver, kidneys and lung.

COMMENT

The post-mortem study of this case thus demonstrated the presence of an enlarged heart with fibrotic thickening of the endocardium of the left auricle and ventricle. The chemical as well as histologic studies gave no support to a diagnosis of glycogen storage disease of the heart or other organs. The clinical and pathologic findings agreed in supporting the diagnosis of idiopathic hypertrophy of the heart. Presumably, since no hypertrophy of the muscle fibers could be demonstrated, there must have been cardiac hyperplasia to account for the enlargement. Three obvious clinical questions were left unanswered: why was there a sudden unfavorable change in the child's condition a few hours before death? Why did the infant have high fever without leucocytosis? What was the actual immediate cause of death? It might be pointed out here that dramatic exitus is the characteristic termination of patients with congenital idiopathic hypertrophy of the heart.

DISCUSSION

In general it may be said that there are five main cardiac abnormalities with which so-called congenital hypertrophy in infants has been associated when that hypertrophy is not due to malformation or disease of the heart or to extracardiac disorders such as anemia, increased metabolism, renal disease, or hypertension. The associated conditions referred to are: (1) abnormalities of the great vessels;[4, 5, 32, 45] (2) abnormalities in origin or distribution of the coronary vessels;[6, 47] (3) glycogen storage disease, i.e., von Gierke's disease;[8, 20, 39] (4) rhabdomyoma;[21-23, 42] and (5) myocardial and endocardial "degeneration," atrophy, cellular infiltration, and fibrosis.[4, 5, 24, 45] Fewer cases than formerly are now finally diagnosed as congenital idiopathic hypertrophy because the hearts of many patients so diagnosed clinically fall into one of these five groups and are perhaps not strictly idiopathic. The case we have described showed none of these conditions; there was only cardiac enlargement and endocardial fibrosis which is described in many of the cases diagnosed as congenital idiopathic hypertrophy of the heart and may be an integral part of that disorder rather than a cause of it. Writing in 1936, Mahon[24] states: "Of the sixty-three autopsied cases of so-called 'idiopathic hypertrophy' reported to date, twenty-two have shown, in addition to the cardiac enlargement, endocardial and myocardial changes occurring either singly or in combination, and being the 'simple cardiac defects' most frequently associated with the hypertrophy."

In regard to glycogen disease of the heart there are several cases of cardiac hypertrophy in infants in which this etiology for the hypertrophy has been given.[7-19] It has long been known that in normal animals glycogen promptly disappears from body cells after death. In glycogen storage disease as described by von Gierke and others there are abnormal deposits of glycogen in various organs, notably liver, skeletal muscle, and kidneys, and this glycogen does not disappear promptly after death. Were this not true, probably no description of glycogen disease would have been made, since the first and most of the subsequent studies are based on autopsy examinations made a variable number of hours post mortem; the disorder has been diagnosed also from biopsy material from the liver. No one knows the cause of this failure of normal glycogenolysis; the glycogen itself does not seem to differ from that ordinarily found, and it has seemed obvious to various workers to suggest absence, or failure in some way, of the glycogenase of the organ or blood to function.

Hypertrophy does not always accompany glycogen deposition in the heart. In the 19-month-old patient reported by Unshelm[9] and by Kimmelstiel[18] glycogen was said to be abundant in the heart, yet clinically the organ was not enlarged and post mortem it weighed 50 gm. in comparison with the average for that age of 56 gm.

The emphasis which recent reports in the literature have placed on glycogen disease as an explanation for certain cases of congenital idiopathic cardiac hypertrophy and indeed of focal and diffuse rhabdomyomata has prompted us to report this case. Our purpose in presenting the material is not so much to point out that our patient did not have glycogen disease chemically or pathologically, but to emphasize the necessity for more comprehensive investigations in the future; all cases of von Gierke's disease should be studied from the cardiologic standpoint, and all cases of idiopathic cardiac hypertrophy should have, if possible, the benefit of the most searching metabolic inquiry. It is not enough, as has been done several times, to restudy the hearts of previously reported cases of idiopathic hypertrophy and state that because of vacuolization of heart muscle fibers or of carmine staining granules in the cells, the essential disorder was glycogen disease of the heart.[6, 8, 13, 14, 25] The tissues for adequate glycogen study must be fixed promptly in absolute alcohol, since glycogen is dissolved, in part, at least, from material which has stood in formalin, leaving empty vacuoles. In our opinion, all of the cases of glycogen disease of the heart which have been comprehensively studied have shown that involvement of the heart was but a part of a general metabolic disorder in which other organs shared, although in some instances possibly to a lesser degree than the heart. Just as the striking clinical symptoms may have pointed to the heart, so the most extensive but not sole pathologic involvement may have been in that organ. The glycogen deposit in von Gierke's disease may be a by-product, so to speak, of disturbances in function of some organ not now identified with the pathology of the disease.[36] For example, in their studies of experimental pituitary basophilism, Thompson and Cushing[37] found that at post mortem dogs which had been injected with gonadotropic extract showed liver cells "highly distended with glycogen. Professor Wolbach states that he has encountered a similar change only in von Gierke's disease. A remarkable change was also apparent in the test animals' *striated muscle,* both cardiac and peripheral. Whereas in the muscle of the control animal the striations are sharply shown, in the test animal they are scarcely distinguishable. Unfortunately no pieces of muscle were fixed in alcohol so that staining for glycogen was precluded."

In contrast to the findings of Dr. Yannet in this case the following data on the glycogen content of organs in other reports are presented for comparison (Table I).

Cardiac rhabdomyoma has been suggested as etiologically responsible for some cases of congenital hypertrophy of the organ. These tumors may be nodular or diffuse and they contain glycogen. They are associated sometimes with tachycardia and arrhythmia and with tuberous sclerosis of the brain. It was natural, therefore, that it should be suggested that diffuse rhabdomyomata of the heart might really be von Gierke's disease of that organ and that glycogen deposits in the brain might account for the associated cerebral disorders. We have a little material bearing on this point. In a patient 9 months of age (N.H.H. No. A-54477), who had multiple nodular cardiac rhabdomyoma and tuberous sclerosis of the brain, a belated, and, therefore, inconclusive examination of formalin preserved tissue showed in the heart a positive Best carmine stain of the tumor tissue only. There was some carmine staining of the liver cells, but the kidneys and skeletal muscles were negative. Chemical analyses of brain and heart disclosed glycogen content of less than 0.1 per cent. Also, in a recent case of tachycardia in the newborn infant (N.H.H. No. A-76460), in which a small nodule,

TABLE I

GLYCOGEN STUDIES ON PATIENT AND DATA FROM CASES IN THE LITERATURE

	CONGENITAL IDIOPATHIC HYPERTROPHY	HYPERTROPHY OF HEART WITH PATENT INTERVENTRICULAR SEPTUM	GLYCOGEN DISEASE			
	PRESENT CASE	VAN CREVELD[11]	VAN CREVELD[11] (POMPE)	SCHÖNHEIMER[10]	UNSHELM[9]	ANTOPOL[15] ET AL.
Heart	<0.1%	0.55% L.V. 0.05% R.V.	7.96%	–	–	3.57%
Liver	<0.1%	0.103%	9.13%	10.43%	14.2%	3.25%
Muscle	–	0.011%	9.39%	–	–	–
Spleen	–	0.01 %	1.46%	–	–	–
Kidney	<0.1%	0.062%	–	6.53%	–	4.34%
Brain	–	–	–	–	–	–

possibly a rhabdomyoma, was found at the top of the interventricular septum, only small amounts of glycogen and fat were found in focal areas of the myocardium (Best carmine and sudan III stains). Chemical analysis of the heart showed less than 0.1 per cent glycogen.* We believe the subject of cardiac rhabdomyoma is not understood to the satisfaction of all pathologists, but it seems probable, despite the suggestion of Virchow,[21] that while this tumor, whether or not it be a true neoplasm, is associated with certain cases of cardiac disorder, it is not to be very seriously regarded in etiological relationship to the special condition under discussion in this paper.

In respect to the reported lesions in the myocardium of some cases of congenital hypertrophy of the heart, we find ourselves quite perplexed as to their significance. These lesions are usually described by such terms as fibrosis, cellular infiltration, hydropic degeneration.†[13, 25] In our case these changes were looked for in many sections taken from various parts of the heart, including those recommended by Gross.[38] No definite changes, other than the endocardial fibrosis which has been described, were found. Failure to do well, vomiting, coughing, en-

*Analysis by Dr. Yannet in 1938 of the formalin preserved brain of the patient with rhabdomyoma reported by Wegman and Egbert[42] (N.H.H. No. A-32505) showed glycogen content of less than 0.1 per cent.

†Hydropic degeneration is usually described in cases where no attempt was made to demonstrate glycogen at the time of autopsy. It may be that tissue from which glycogen has been dissolved by a formalin solution appears in sections in such manner as to warrant description as hydropic degeneration.

largement of the heart without signs of malformation, dramatic exitus with unexplained fever, and little or no leucocytosis, constitute the usual and characteristic clinical pattern of these cases irrespective of the presence or absence of myocardial lesions post mortem. This causes one to wonder whether the myocardial changes when present are really significant in an immediate etiological sense. In the case reports one sees photomicrographs of myocardial lesions, but from the text it is not always clear whether the pictured lesion is from a small localized area or is representative of widespread damage to the heart. In a limited degree the changes described are common post-mortem findings when carefully searched for in many and various cases in which the question of serious cardiac disease does not arise. It would not seem that these changes, whatever their etiology, could be the cause of the cardiac enlargement or of death in cases of congenital idiopathic hypertrophy.

It is evident that this subject of congenital hypertrophy of the heart in children has been advanced somewhat since the early papers by Howland and others, but many cases classified under this designation are certainly idiopathic. Levy[26] and associates have described similar cases in young adults, and here also the cardiac hypertrophy is unexplained for the most part. Hypertrophy is usually ascribed to increased work[17, 40] which the heart for one reason or another is forced to do. In congenital idiopathic hypertrophy the cause of the increased work is not apparent. One possible cause of "work" hypertrophy in this disorder not yet adequately investigated, however, is arteriovenous fistula or arteriovenous anastomosis.[27, 28, 44] Arteriovenous aneurysms could probably be determined usually by careful physical examination, but anastomoses might be discovered only by means of special methods of vascular visualization. Constriction of the capillary bed is mentioned[46] in some articles without proof of such constriction.

In contrast to the work theory of hypertrophy we should like to call attention to Eyster's extension of the conception of heart injury with dilatation as the etiology of hypertrophy. This theory has recently received favorable clinical appraisal by Davis and Blumgart,[29] particularly in regard to coronary atherosclerosis and congestive heart failure. Eyster produced cardiac dilatation in dogs, in some by means of a constricting band placed for a few days on the aorta, in others by injury of the aortic valves,* and in still others by massive and repeated transfusions. The hearts dilated but soon returned to normal size. However, in about three months they were found to be greatly hypertrophied, a result believed due to the original injury caused by dilatation and stretching. We suggest that something of this nature might have hap-

*It should be pointed out that the operative procedures involved a wider disturbance of structure than just that implied by descriptive statements about obstructive bands and valvular injury. One cannot perform such operations without serious trauma to nerve, cardiac, and other tissue with consequent disturbances of function in addition to those attributed to the principal operative procedure.

pened in some of the patients under consideration.[41] In newborn infants, Dunham and D'Amico[31] showed that the heart is relatively but temporarily enlarged. This enlargement seems adequately explained by postnatal cardiac-respiratory readjustments, but it may be that in some infants the myocardium is damaged in uterine life or in the process of birth and shows subsequent hypertrophy. It is germane to point out that idiopathic hypertrophy of the heart has been described in newborn infants[35] and that most of the cases are described in children less than 1 year of age (forty-one of Kugel and Stoloff's[5] fifty-nine cases were less than 1 year old; the mean age of Abbott's[32] fifteen cases is ten months, the youngest being a newborn infant and the oldest, 4 years of age).

To many physiologists, clinicians, and pathologists the explanation of cardiac hypertrophy is not yet wholly understood.[43] On this subject Sir Thomas Lewis[33] remarked in 1933: "There is still much that remains to be explained; it is clear that there must be hidden sources of increased work or the conclusion that increased work is the cause of hypertrophy needs revision."

Finally, in view of the explanation of some cases of cardiac hypertrophy on the basis of glycogen disease, it is wise to consider that other types of metabolic disturbance might be etiologically operative in certain other cases. The metabolic disorder might be in the cardiac tissue itself, perhaps something to do with chemical changes in contraction; less is known about the physiology of the contraction of heart muscle than of skeletal muscle. Or the stimulus to hypertrophy might arise in other organs or tissues whose functional derangement reacted upon the heart. These are speculations, but in any case it behooves us to go further afield in our search for a solution of congenital idiopathic cardiac hypertrophy than post-mortem studies of the organ itself, valuable as are such investigations.

CONCLUSIONS

A case of idiopathic hypertrophy of the heart in a male child 8 months of age is reported together with pathologic and chemical studies.

Best carmine stains and chemical analyses of tissue from the heart, liver, kidneys, lungs, and striated muscle (no chemical study of the latter) showed no evidences of glycogen storage disease.

The bearing of this case study on the subject of congenital idiopathic hypertrophy of the heart is discussed.

REFERENCES

1. Howland, John: Contributions to Medical and Biological Research, Vol. 1, p. 582, New York, 1919, Paul B. Hoeber, Inc.
2. Coppoletta, J. M., and Wolbach, S. B.: Am. J. Path. **9**: 55, 1933.
3. Todd, T. W.: Special Cytology. II. Edited by Cowdry, p. 861, New York, 1928, Paul B. Hoeber, Inc.
4. Stoloff, E. G.: Am. J. Dis. Child. **36**: 1204, 1928.
5. Kugel, M. A., and Stoloff, E. G.: Am. J. Dis. Child. **45**: 828, 1933.

6. Carrington, G. L., and Krumbhaar, E. B.: Am. J. Dis. Child. **27**: 449, 1924.
7. Pompe, J. C.: Ann. d'anat. path. **10**: 23, 1933.
8. Humphreys, E. M., and Kato, K.: Am. J. Path. **10**: 589, 1934.
9. Unshelm, E.: Jahrb. f. Kinderh. **137**: 257, 1932.
10. Schönheimer, R.: Ztschr. f. physiol. Chem. **182**: 148, 1929.
11. Van Creveld, S.: Acta Brevia Neerlandica **3**: 77, 1933.
12. Van Creveld, S.: Arch. Dis. Childhood **9**: 9, 1934.
13. Kato, K.: Practice of Pediatrics. Edited by Brennemann, Vol. 3, Hagerstown, Md., 1937, W. F. Prior Company, Inc.
14. Finkelstein, L. E.: Am. J. M. Sc. **191**: 415, 1936.
15. Antopol, W., Heilbrunn, A., and Tuchman, L.: Am. J. M. Sc. **188**: 354, 1934.
16. Putschar, W.: Beitr. z. path. Anat. u. z. allg. Path. **90**: 222, 1932.
17. White, P. D.: Heart Disease, ed. 2, New York, 1937, The Macmillan Company.
18. Kimmelstiel, P.: Beitr. z. path. Anat. u. z. allg. Path. **91**: 1, 1933.
19. Bishoff, G.: Ztschr. f. Kinderh. **52**: 722, 1932.
20. Von Gierke, E.: Beitr. z. path. Anat. u. z. allg. Path. **82**: 497, 1929.
21. Virchow, R.: Berl. klin. Wchnschr. **33**: 679, 1896.
22. Schmincke, A.: Beitr. z. path. Anat. u. z. allg. Path. **70**: 513, 1922.
23. Farber, S.: Am. J. Path. **7**: 105, 1931.
24. Mahon, G. S.: Am. Heart J. **12**: 608, 1936.
25. Sprague, H. B., Bland, E. F., and White, P. D.: Am. J. Dis. Child. **41**: 877, 1931.
26. Levy, R., and Rousselot, L. M.: Am. Heart J. **9**: 178, 1933; Levy and von Glahn, W. C.: Tr. A. Am. Physicians **52**: 259, 1937.
27. Holman, E.: Arteriovenous Aneurysm, New York, 1937, The Macmillan Company.
28. Seegar, S. J.: Surgery **3**: 264, 1938.
29. Davis, D., and Blumgart, H.: Ann. Int. Med. **11**: 1024, 1937.
30. Eyster, J. A. E.: Tr. A. Am. Physicians **42**: 15, 1927; Eyster, J. A. E., Meek, W. H., and Hodges, F. J.: Arch. Int. Med. **39**: 536, 1927; Eyster: J. A. M. A. **91**: 1881, 1928.
31. Dunham, E. C., and D'Amico, M.: Yale J. Biol. & Med. **6**: 385, 1934.
32. Abbott, M. E.: Loose Leaf Living Medicine, Vol. 4, p. 207, New York, 1931, Thomas Nelson & Sons.
Idem: Internat. Clin. **3**: 15, 1934.
33. Lewis, Sir Thomas: Diseases of the Heart, London, 1933, The Macmillan Company.
34. MacMahon, H. E.: Am. J. Dis. Child. **55**: 93, 1938.
35. Simmonds: München. med. Wchnschr. **46**: 108, 1899.
36. Wilder, R. L.: J. Pediat. **7**: 214, 1935.
37. Thompson, K., and Cushing, H.: Proc. Roy. Soc. London, s. B. **115**: 88, 1934.
38. Gross, L., Antopol, W., and Sacks, B.: Arch. Path. **10**: 840, 1930.
39. Ellis, R. W. B., and Payne, W. W.: Quart. J. Med. **29**: 31, 1936.
40. Leaman, W. G.: Internat. Clin. **3**: 1, 1934.
41. Farber, S., and Hubbard, J.: Am. J. M. Sc. **186**: 705, 1933.
42. Wegman, M. E., and Egbert, D. S.: J. Pediat. **6**: 818, 1935.
43. Golden, J. S., and Brams, W. A.: Am. Heart J. **13**: 207, 1937.
44. Porter, W. B.: Tr. A. Am. Physicians **52**: 41, 1937.
45. Levine, H. D.: Am. J. Dis. Child. **48**: 1072, 1934.
46. Emerson, P. W., and Green, H.: Am. Heart J. **4**: 116, 1928.
47. Bland, E. F., White, P. D., and Garland, J.: Am. Heart J. **8**: 787, 1933.

DIABETES AND PREGNANCY

Observations on the Offspring With a Pathologic Report

Francis Scott Smyth, M.D., and Mary B. Olney
San Francisco, Calif.

OBSTETRICIANS are not in agreement regarding pregnancy in diabetic women. In the preinsulin era most diabetic women were sterile; now there are numerous reports on diabetes and pregnancy. The apparent frequency with which the pregnancy is complicated by toxemia has led some investigators to a pessimistic outlook (Wiener).[1] Other reports (Peckham)[2] emphasize the successful gestation where a careful diabetic regime is followed. Isolated case studies, such as that of Lawrence,[3] have called attention to improvement in the maternal carbohydrate tolerance after the twenty-eighth week. Lambie,[4] reviewing the whole subject, points out that either aggravation or improvement of the maternal diabetes may take place at any stage of pregnancy. Lambie discusses the possible significance of renal and alimentary glycosurias in relation to temporary diabetes of pregnancy, which has a relatively good prognosis. He advocates induction of premature labor if hyperglycemia has not been controlled, as macrosomia is to be expected. More recently Sherrill[5] has discussed the role of diabetes and pregnancy. Citing the experiments of Carlson and Drennan[6] as well as his clinical experience with diabetes, Sherrill doubts the likelihood of fetal insulin affecting the maternal diabetes.

Since 1922 nineteen infants have been born of women whose pregnancy was considered complicated by diabetes. In fourteen of the mothers glycosuria appeared only with gestation and was controlled by diet or by diet and temporary use of insulin, which suggests glycosuria from causes other than diabetes mellitus. Of the entire group, eleven gave birth to excessively large infants. One mother gave a history of having had nine children: one, by her first marriage, was of normal weight; the other eight, by two subsequent marriages, all weighed 10 pounds or more at birth. Another macrosomic infant was stillborn in the home. The post-mortem changes were so marked that pathologic studies could not be interpreted.

The condition of the newly born infants of diabetic mothers demands special care, not only because of insulin given just before delivery, but also because of the possibility of essential hyperinsulinism as reported by Gray and Feemster.[7] Hence, we have made special studies on those infants born of diabetic mothers in the last few years. Sugar determinations have been made on the blood of the

---

From the Department of Pediatrics, University of California Medical School.

CHART I

Mother S.

Aged 21 years
Diabetes for 2½ years
Insulin for 2½ years
Diet: C 110 P 80 F 80
(During most of pregnancy)
Insulin:

Before gestation	– 40 u./24 hr.
6 months gestation	– 30 u./24 hr.
7 months gestation	– 70 u./24 hr.
At term	– 30 u./24 hr.
Post partum	– 30 u./24 hr.

Breast milk:

5/21/1931	– 3.5	per cent sugar
5/25/1931	– 3.1	per cent sugar
6/ 1/1931	– 5.38	per cent sugar

Infant S. (Boy)

Weight at birth 3650 gm.
5/20/1931—Maternal blood sugar: 482 mg. per cent
Infant blood sugar: 244 mg. per cent
5/21/1931—Infant blood sugar: 79 mg. per cent
CO_2 36 vol.
Vomiting repeatedly, clyses of 5 per cent glucose daily for 6 days
5/23/1931—Infant blood sugar: 64 mg. per cent
5/27/1931—Infant blood sugar: 75 mg. per cent
6/11/1931—Infant blood sugar: 89 mg. per cent
Discharged on breast feeding in good condition

11/3/1934

	Blood:	Urine:
Fasting	79.2 mg. per cent	blue
½ hour	108.0 mg. per cent	blue
1 hour	84.6 mg. per cent	blue
2 hour	70.2 mg. per cent	blue
3 hour	75.6 mg. per cent	blue

CHART II

Mother R.

Aged 41 years
Diabetes for 12 years
Insulin for 8 years
Diet: C 170 P 70 F 100
Insulin:

Before gestation	– 30 u./24 hr.
6 months	– 40 u./24 hr.
8 months	– 80 u./24 hr.
Post partum	– 35 u./24 hr.

Infant E. R. (Girl)

Weight at birth 3030 gm.
6/ 8/31—Maternal blood sugar: 155 mg. per cent
Cord blood sugar: 133 mg. per cent
Infant blood sugar: 95 mg. per cent
6/ 9/31—Infant blood sugar: 57 mg. per cent
6/11/31—Infant blood sugar: 82 mg. per cent
Clyses of glucose 3 per cent in Ringer's solution daily for 16 days
6/ 9/31—Cyanotic; vomiting; required Drinker respirator
6/11/31—Vomiting, suggestive of obstruction; fed thickened lactic acid formula
6/25/31—Discharged in good condition

11/19/34

	Blood:	Urine:
Fasting	86.4 mg. per cent	blue
½ hour	140.4 mg. per cent	blue
1 hour	100.4 mg. per cent	blue
2 hour	93.6 mg. per cent	blue
3 hour	82.8 mg. per cent	blue

Reaction
10/17/35

	Blood:	Urine:
Fasting	55 mg. per cent	blue green
½ hour	140.4 mg. per cent	blue
1 hour	178 mg. per cent	
2 hour	142 mg. per cent	blue green
3 hour	135 mg. per cent	blue

mother, the cord, and the infant. The use of 3 per cent glucose in Ringer's solution has been routine when the infant arrived in the nursery. It should be mentioned that the normal newly born infant has an expected blood sugar level lower than that of older infants and children, usually 85 to 100 mg. per cent. Premature infants have even a lower level. The Hagedorn-Jensen capillary sugar determination usually gives values 15 to 20 mg. per cent higher than the macrodetermination (venous blood).

Charts I, II, and III summarize the important features of the three cases studied under the above regime.

CHART III

Mother R.

Aged 42 years
Diabetes for 13 years
Insulin for 9 years
Diet: C 170 P 70 F 100
Insulin:

Before gestation	– 30 u./24 hr.
7 months gestation	– 40 u./24 hr.
7½ months gestation	– 70 u./24 hr.
8 months gestation	– 105 u./24 hr.
Post partum	– 40 u./24 hr.

Infant W. R. (Boy)

Weight at birth (one month premature) 2640 gm.
3/ 8/32—Maternal blood sugar: 87 mg. per cent
Cord blood sugar (micro): 67 mg. per cent
Infant blood sugar (micro): 53 mg. per cent
3/29/32—Infant blood sugar (micro): 72 mg. per cent
3/31/32—Infant blood sugar (micro): 111 mg. per cent
Clyses of glucose 3 per cent given first four days
Blood sugar on 3/31/32 taken after clysis
For shallow breathing on 3/31/32 given CO_2 and O_2

11/19/34

	Blood	Urine:
Fasting	81.0 mg. per cent	blue
½ hour	140.4 mg. per cent	blue
1 hour	75.6 mg. per cent	blue
2 hour	79.2 mg. per cent	blue
3 hour	72.0 mg. per cent	blue

10/ 5/35

	Blood	Urine:
Fasting	73.8 mg. per cent	blue
½ hour	163.8 mg. per cent	blue
1 hour	144.0 mg. per cent	blue
2 hour	84.6 mg. per cent	blue
3 hour	82.8 mg. per cent	blue

The infant's blood sugar, even allowing for the effect of predelivery insulin, may be very low. The cord blood sugar may anticipate this finding by showing a much lower level than that of the maternal blood taken simultaneously. In two of the infants projectile vomiting and cyanosis were striking features, quite possibly related to persistent hypoglycemia. This interpretation circumvented pyloroplasty which was suggested for one of the infants. The use of subcutaneous glucose appeared extremely valuable in carrying the infants through a critical period, after which an apparent adjustment was made.

The following report* concerns the autopsy findings of an infant born of a diabetic mother. During a gestation period of eight months the maternal diabetes was poorly controlled. The report is made because there are complete studies, not only of pancreatic tissue, but also of the other endocrine glands.

CASE REPORT

Family History.—The father, aged 28 years, living and well, and mother, aged 26 years, diabetic, were parents of Baby G., a girl (mother's first pregnancy). There was no family history of diabetes; the mother had eight siblings, living and well.

Present Illness.—Mother had nocturia and polyuria two or three years before discovering she had diabetes. Two and a half years before her pregnancy she was started on a diabetic regime with 40 units of insulin. Reactions caused the dosage to be reduced to 30 units daily. The dosage was 20 units daily for the first seven months of pregnancy, then it was reduced to 10 units a day because of a low fasting blood sugar. Glycosuria necessitated increasing the insulin to 40 units a day at seven and one-half months of pregnancy. One week later vomiting and epigastric pain developed, and at eight months of pregnancy she was hospitalized for treatment of marked acidosis and dehydration.

She continued to vomit in the hospital and it was six days before the acidosis was cleared. Because of cardiac dilatation she was digitalized in preparation for termination of the pregnancy by cesarean section. The infant was delivered without difficulty and after carbon dioxide and oxygen inhalation, had good color for about an hour.

Physical Examination.—Weight 2840 grams; length 48.5 cm. There was marked cyanosis. Respiration was difficult and crying feeble. Heart sounds were normal; lungs atelectatic. Muscles were limp; there was no excessive perspiration and no bulging of fontanels.

Course: Carbon dioxide and oxygen inhalations did not clear the cyanosis. Three hours after delivery the infant was placed in the Drinker respirator and caffeine and continuous inhalations were given. Two and one-half hours later one ounce of breast milk was given by lavage. It was regurgitated with mucus. A change was made to oxygen inhalation despite which the feet and legs became mottled nine hours after delivery. Caffeine and epinephrine were given four times in the next three hours. The infant expired thirteen hours after delivery. A cardiac puncture was done for blood sugar determination immediately after death (value 38 mg. per cent).

Autopsy.—Autopsy was begun six hours and twenty minutes after death. The usual ventral and scalp incisions were made. The organs were normally situated. The umbilical structures were not unusual. Bilateral ovarian cysts protruded above the pelvis into the abdominal cavity. The thymus showed a few punctate asphyxial type subscapular hemorrhages. The heart showed a few petechial subepicardial hemorrhages. The foramen ovale was anatomically open. The ductus arteriosus was widely open. The lungs were unexpanded and showed multiple subpleural petechial extravasations of blood. The thyroid gland was well developed. It was sliced until it revealed a normal appearing parathyroid body. Opening of the gastrointestinal tract revealed meconium from the duodenum downward. The liver revealed recent congestion. The biliary system was patent. Bile was expressed through the cystic and common ducts into the duodenum. The pancreas was situated between the curve of the duodenum and the hilus of the spleen; it was a pink-

*These findings were discussed briefly at the 1934 meeting of the Society for Pediatric Research.

ish-gray color and had the usual cellular consistency. The adrenal glands appeared normal in size, shape, and situation and were heavily coated with white granular fetal-type fat. The inner cortical and central medullary tissue showed a fresh hemorrhagic zone 2 mm. in thickness. The kidneys showed fetal lobulation and were red and congested. The bladder had the usual fetal pointed dome with the urachal top well closed.

The uterus was of the usual newborn infant shape and size. The endometrium appeared blood stained and quite soft. The tubes were draped over large bilateral fluid-filled ovarian cysts resembling Graafian follicle cysts of the adult. In the cyst walls was a plainly visible anastomosing vascular network. The ovary was a polar spongy condensation of tissue which on section was seen to be made up of multiple cysts with rather thick walls.

The meninges were clean and the tentorium cerebelli and supracortical vessels intact. The brain was symmetrical and well formed. The ventricular system appeared normal. The venous sinuses of the skull and the middle ear structures were normal. The pituitary gland was normally situated and was one-fourth or one-fifth the normal size of the adult gland.

The breasts were flat and the nipples barely discernible.

Representative sections were taken for preparation for microscopic examination.

Organ:	*Actual Measurements From Baby G.*	*Standards According to Abt and Grulee**
Thymus	12 gm.	8 to 15 gm., usually 12 gm.
Heart	27 gm. (with aorta)	20 to 25 gm.
Lungs (together)	57 gm.	50 gm.
Liver	135 gm.	120 to 150 gm.
Spleen	9.5 gm.	5 to 20 gm., average 13.5 gm.
Kidneys	28 gm. (together with ureters and bladder)	13 gm. (left), 12 gm. (right)
Brain	440 gm.	220 to 400 gm., average 350 gm.
Adrenals (together)	8 gm.	2 to 16 gm., usually 8 gm.
Pancreas:	4.5 gm.	2.5 gm.
Head	1.5 cm. diameter	1.2 cm. breadth
Tail	0.5 cm. diameter	0.6 cm. thickness
Length	4.0 cm.	5 to 8 cm.
Pituitary	7 by 6 by 4 mm. (one-fourth to one-fifth adult size)	0.1 gm. (one-sixth adult size)
Uterus with tubes and cystic ovaries	30 gm. Left ovary 4.5 by 4 by 3 cm. Right ovary 3.5 by 3 by 2.5 cm.	

*Abt: Pediatrics, W. B. Saunders Co.; Grulee: Clinical Pediatrics, New York, 1926, D. Appleton-Century Co.

Microscopic Description.—The lungs contained congested and unexpanded lung tissue in which fetal plicated bronchioles were empty and clean. There were subpleural petechial, asphyxial type hemorrhages. Interstitia showed no evidence of inflammation.

Heart.—The usual infantile myocardium showed marked interstitial congestion, vacuolated muscle cells; there were scarcely perceptible cross striations.

Liver.—The lobules and cylinders of hepatic cells were well formed and vascular congestion was intense. Immature blood cells were diffusely scattered through the interstitia of the portal channels and along the sinusoids of the lobules. Immature erythrocytic tissue was prominent. Erythroblasts and nucleated erythrocytes were abundant. Giant cells and small groups of myeloblasts and myelocytes were found. Comparison was made with sections of liver from fetuses 11.5 cm. (3.5 months), 15.5 cm. (4 months), 27 cm. (5 months), and five normal term infants. The hemopoietic function was nearest that of the 3.5-month fetus although the lobules were better developed. The scattered groups of myeloblastic tissue and the eosinophilic granular cells were much more prominent than in any of the sections examined. Except for the number of myeloblastic elements present the picture seemed to be that described in the liver of the third to fifth month.* A search of the literature brings no more recent or different account from this and no reference to its pathologic persistence except in congenital syphilis. MacCallum† describes in the liver in congenital syphilis general retardation of development with the

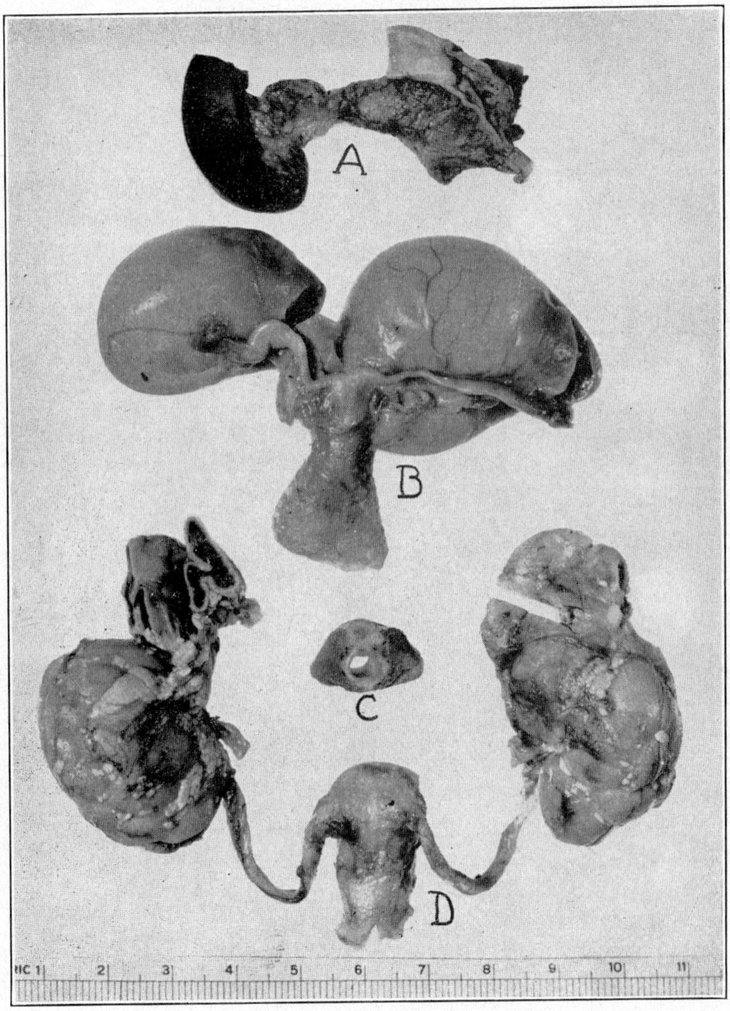

Fig. 1.—Gross appearance of spleen and pancreas. Uterus enlarged; cystic ovaries. *A*, Spleen and pancreas; *B*, uterus and cystic ovaries; *C*, thyroid with tracheal cartilage; *D*, adrenals, kidney, ureters, and bladder.

whole organ engaged in blood formation. This liver was like the ones he describes except there was no fibrosis in the liver or in the bone marrow for which the bone marrow might be compensating, nor was there evidence elsewhere of infection. No spirochetes were found in Levaditi silver-stained sections of the liver. It might

*Kiebel and Mall: Human Embryology, Vol. 2, Philadelphia, 1912, J. B. Lippincott Company.

†Textbook of Pathology, Ed. 3, p. 745, Philadelphia, 1924, W. B. Saunders Company.

be speculated that there was long continued hyperinsulinism in this baby with excess glycogenetic activity and a stimulation for retained hemopoiesis.

Spleen.—The tissue was well formed with normal capsule, trabeculae, vessels, sinusoids, and white and red pulp. There was a normal number of cells of the myeloblastic series in the Malpighian bodies. There was intense recent vascular congestion.

Kidneys.—There was well-formed infantile parenchyma with the usual fetal lobular grouping of glomeruli. No hemopoietic collections of cells were in the interstitia.

Femur.—There was normal fetal bone marrow and well-formed cortical and cancellous bone.

Brain.—Tissue was well formed and without discoverable alteration.

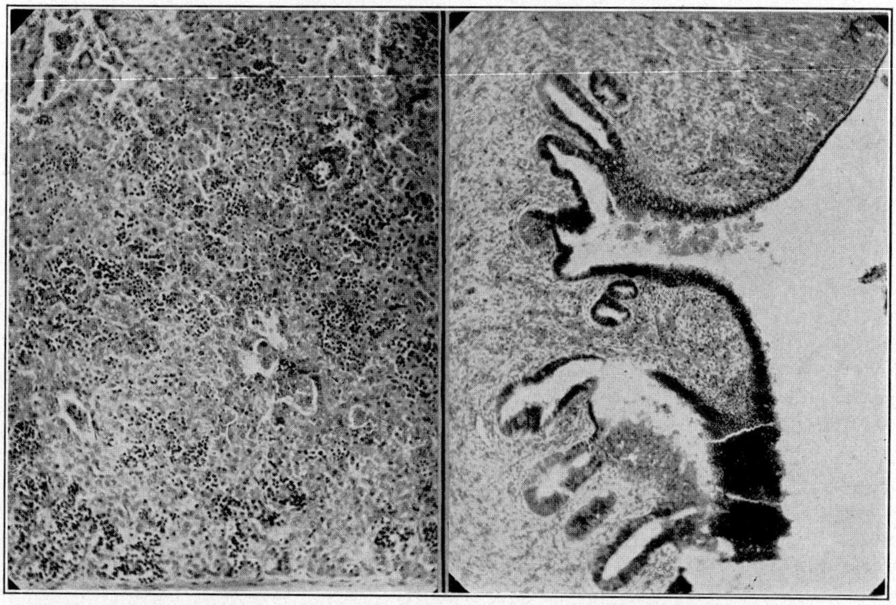

Fig. 2. Fig. 3.

Fig. 2.—Microscopic view of liver showing abundant islands of extramedullary hemopoiesis.

Fig. 3.—Endometrium which is thicker than usual for this age as is the deeper and more complicated endometrial gland formation.

Uterus.—Fetal cervix and infantile myometrium were normal. The endometrium was thicker than in the usual term infant and endometrial glands were deeper and more complicated. The stroma contained many extravasated erythrocytes and a few lymphocytes. A little of the surface epithelium was separating. The picture was that of advanced development. The congestion suggested that of early menstruation.

Placenta and Cord.—The cord showed only the usual physiologic endarteritis. The placenta was free from any inflammatory change except that of endarteritic narrowing of the vessels in the large villous branches. The smaller villi for the most part were quite delicate and well vascularized.

Circulating Blood.—The blood cells studied in the larger vascular spaces in the various organs appeared well formed. In the liver there seemed to be an excessive number of nucleated red blood cells but the average of counts in various organs placed the relative number at about 1 per cent. There was no disproportion of white to red cells. Polymorphonuclear leucocytes made up about 50 per cent of the white cells.

Pancreas.—Sections from the head, body, and tail of the pancreas all showed a remarkable hyperplasia of the island tissue. In the head region particularly the bulk of the tissue was insular and the islands were not confined but diffuse, often growing about well-formed ducts. Slides stained for reticulum by the silver method used by Otani showed the island cells in places apparently budding from the ducts and having a common basement reticulum. In the head region a capsular membrane seldom was demonstrable about the overgrown island. In the body and tail more discrete islands were present; by comparison with islands in the pancreas of ten normal term infants they were much more numerous and considerably larger. A section from the head region and surrounding tissue showed many normal nerves and lymph nodes and a normal appearing duodenum near the site of the ampulla. The acinous tissue appeared normal.

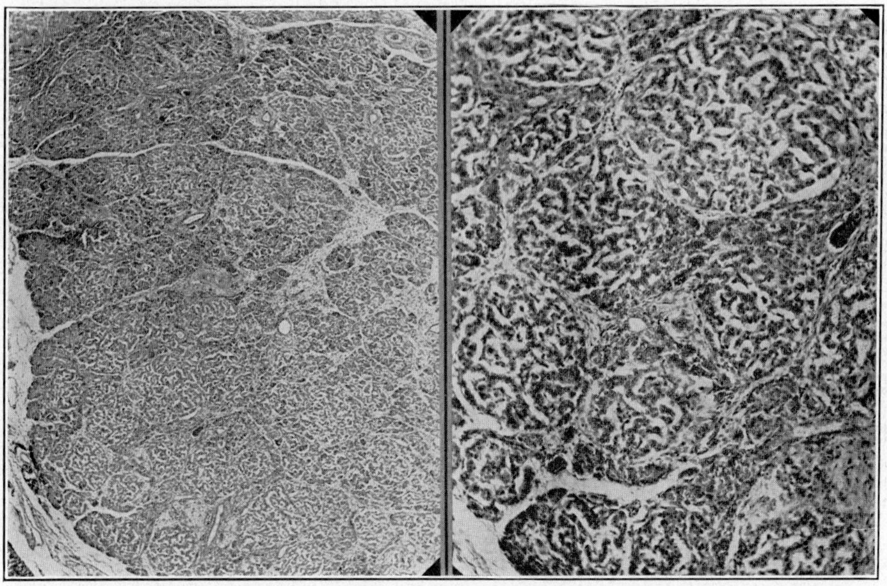

Fig. 4.—Low- and high-power field views of pancreas showing increased number and size of islets of Langerhans.

Gray and Feemster[7] counted and measured the islands in the normal pancreas and in that of an infant of a diabetic mother. They found an average of 184 islands per 50 sq. mm. in sections from all parts of the pancreas in their case and an average of sixty-four islands in six normal cases. In Baby G. the islands of a large part of the head region were not sufficiently delimited to allow counting. Entire lobules appeared as adenomatous formations of island tissue. In many counts from other regions of the head and from the body and tail the average was 196 islands per 50 sq. mm. The count of islands in sections of the pancreas of ten normal term infants (those dying from asphyxia in long labors or from intracranial hemorrhage) agrees remarkably well with that of Gray and Feemster. The average was sixty-two islands per 50 sq. mm. Counts by regions in three of the ten cases were fifty-six for the head, fifty-nine for the body, and seventy-nine for the tail. Gray and Feemster found the average diameter of the islands in their case to be 213 by 182 microns. The largest island measured 726 by 324 and the smallest 104 by 104. This is in marked contrast to their normal figures of average 115 by 102, largest 206 by 198, and smallest 55 by 50. Islands in the head region of the Baby G. pancreas made up without delimiting reticular membranes practically all of whole lobules measuring up to 3.36 by 4.48 mm. in cross section. The average diameter of the delimited islands was 242 by 190, the largest 880 by 560 microns. As the islands were not followed through serial section the true diameters of the smallest delimited islands could not be determined. In the ten normal sections the average diameter was 114 by 112 and the largest 225 by 192. Gray and Feemster calculated the quantity of island tissue in their case as twenty-four times normal. Disregarding the adenomatous islands in the head of the Baby G. pancreas, by comparison of counted and measured islands the increase in volume was thirty or more times normal.

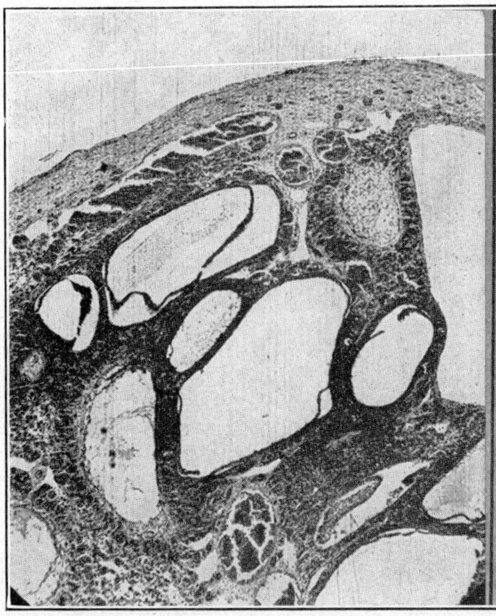

Fig. 5.

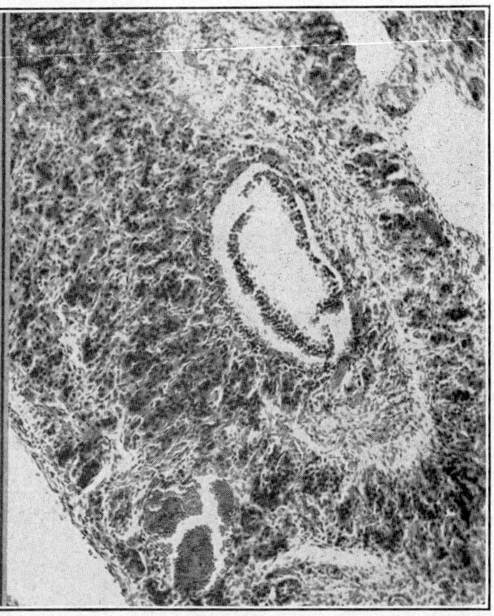

Fig. 6.

Fig. 5.—Section of ovary showing walls of cysts and interstitial cells.

Fig. 6.—Section of adrenal gland showing wide fascicular zone and scattered medullary cells near central blood vessel.

Otani* describes three types of islands. With silver staining of reticulum to check reticular island capsules, he describes: Type A, islands connected with acini; Type B, with ducts; Type C, entirely separate from exocrine tissue. In reticulum stains by the Otani method 90 per cent of the islands were of Types A and B. More than half were of Type A which perhaps indicates the very embryonal, rapidly growing nature of the islands.

Bloom† advises a Mallory Azan stain to differentiate the island cells. Differentiation in this case has not yet succeeded but studies indicate these islands are mostly A cells.

Ovaries.—The ovarian parenchymal zone was made up largely of large atretic follicles with an intervening stroma filled with large interstitial cells. As compared with sections from ovaries of newborn infants the resting primordial follicles

*Studies on Islands of Langerhans, Am. J. Path. 3: 1, 1927.

†Anat. Rec. 49: 363, 1931.

of the cortex were reduced greatly in number and appeared to be used up in an unusual abortive development which has proceeded en masse. Each atretic follicle has a thin thecal coat, a granulosa layer two or three cells deep, and a degenerate ovum with a pyknotic or fragmented nucleus. These atretic follicles described by Maximov* are found in sparse numbers in the ovary of the newborn infant but are more numerous in the first year of extrauterine life. The thecal cells appear to undergo an abortive lutein change and after the follicular outlines are lost they are found as large polyhedral cells with eosinophilic cytoplasm filling the interstitia. Maximov (p. 655†) states that it is an established fact that the interstitial cells of the ovary in postembryonic life originate from the theca interna of the atretic follicles. The ovaries in this case seem to be an exaggerated illustration of this fact. The larger cystic processes as judged by their wall tissue were abortive follicular cysts.

Breasts.—There was no evidence of undue development or activity in the rudiments of the mammary gland.

In the histologic description of the adrenal, thyroid, parathyroid, thymus, and pituitary glands comparison was made with tissue from term infants. The work of E. R. A. Cooper is used as a reference.†

Adrenal Glands.—The sections showed the usual newly born adrenal gland with a wide fascicular zone. The cortical cell columns became blunt and doubled on the periphery to form a thin, imperfect, glomerular zone. The inner ends of the fascicular columns merged into the boundary zone where they often reached the large vascular channels. The reticular zone was not well separated, though the outer fascicular cells were somewhat more vacuolated. The separate medulla was not present, but scattered medullary cells were seen near the central blood vessels. There were a few large ganglion cells in the same central regions. The inner cortex was extremely vascular.

Cooper points out that the initial sympathochromaffin cells may differentiate into either medullary or ganglion cells and that small numbers of each of the latter cells may be found at birth though no true medulla has separated. Study of sections of natal and postnatal adrenal glands shows the hemorrhagic boundary zone very commonly, the medulla differentiating at about four months, and widely varying numbers of large ganglion cells. The large cells described by Gray and Feemster in the adrenals of the infant born of a diabetic mother probably are ganglion cells. The photomicrograph in their report shows cortical cells of the boundary zone with scattered larger ganglion cells.

Thyroid Gland.—Well-formed tissue made up the well-vascularized interstitia which supported closely packed colloid-containing acini. These acini were small for the most part and lined by cuboidal epithelium. There were many rather dilated acini which approached in size those of the adult gland. The gland in no way differs from Cooper's description of the gland at term except for the dilated, colloid-filled acini. The Baby G. thyroid, compared with term thyroid glands, seemed to have more stored colloid. This may be considered an index of overdevelopment if the gland is considered to have been producing so much colloid it had a surplus to store within acini.

Parathyroid.—The oval body attached to the thyroid capsule at the posteromedian pole of the thyroid was 1 mm. long and 0.4 mm. wide in section. The parenchymal cells were supported by a delicate capsule, trabeculae, and a finer reticulum meshwork. Thin walled capillaries followed the trabeculae. The parenchymal cells formed loosely winding and anastomosing cords. The small round nuclei were the most important feature as the cytoplasm was vacuolated and indefinite in outline.

*Textbook of Histology, p. 650, Philadelphia, 1930, W. B. Saunders Company.

†The Histology of the More Important Human Endocrine Organs at Various Ages, London, 1925, Oxford University Press.

There were scattered chief cells having a finely granular eosinophilic cytoplasm. Judged by Cooper's description the gland was normal.

Thymus.—The cortical and medullary portions were well defined. The Hassall corpuscles were small, separate, and did not reach the periphery. The fibrous septa were not unduly wide. The gland was normal judged by Cooper's description and his quotation of Hammar (Endocrinology, September, 1921).

Pituitary Gland.—The most numerous cells of the anterior lobe were the oxyphils. The cells were grouped about the congested vascular sinuses as in the adult gland. There were a few chromophobe cells on the periphery of the larger cell group. Basophilic cells were very infrequent and showed no tendency toward concentration in any one zone. By comparison with available descriptions the anterior lobe approached the development of a puberty gland. The little posterior and intermediate lobe tissue present appeared quite normal. There was a little less intermediate lobe tissue than would be expected at birth.

Cooper states that undifferentiated nongranular cells are in the majority until the end of fetal life. The oxyphil cells are described at birth as being found gathered in the dorsal and posterior portions of the anterior lobe. The few basophil cells present at birth are at the anterior pole and the anterior part of the ventral margin of the lobe. The neutrophil or chromophobe cells vary greatly in number; they are more numerous than the basophils but tend to be grouped with them. During early postnatal life the epithelial cells of the anterior lobe are well separated from each other and later become closely packed in dense solid masses.

Anatomic and Pathologic Diagnosis.—1. A premature female infant, weight 2835 gm., height 48.5 cm., was estimated to be 9.5 lunar months of age by Haase rule. Lower epiphyseal centers of ossification in the femur were well developed, which places fetal age at over 9 months. There was asphyxia with multiple subpleural, subepicardial and thymus subscapular petechial hemorrhages. Passive congestion of viscera and fetal pulmonary atelectasis were present.

2. There were hypertrophy and hyperplasia of islands of Langerhans.

3. Cystic degeneration of ovaries had occurred and there were large and small abortive Graafian follicle cysts. There was wholesale atresia of follicles with widespread interstitial cell development in the ovaries.

4. Pituitary gland, thyroid gland, and endometrium had relatively advanced development.

5. There was unduly persistent and widespread early fetal type hematopoiesis in the liver. The liver was of normal weight and size for a term infant. The hematopoietic stage was that of a 3.5-month fetus.

DISCUSSION

Some confusion is found in the literature regarding the pathology occasionally seen in infants born of diabetic mothers. Ambard, for example, reported as "congenital diabetes" the case of an infant born of a diabetic mother. His diagnosis was based on finding 1.2 per cent sugar in the infant's urine. Feldman reported the postmortem study of a diabetic woman in the ninth month of pregnancy. The maternal pancreas was definitely atrophic and the bladder urine contained excess sugar and acetone. Microscopic section of the maternal pancreas showed a decrease in island tissue and increased connective tissue. The fetus weighed 3100 gm.; the spleen, liver, adrenals, and kidneys seemed not unusual, and the bladder urine showed excess sugar but not acetone. The fetal pancreas was of normal size but on microscopic section showed many islets two or four times the normal size, which Feldman interpreted as edematous and associated with an interstitial pancreatitis. In the absence of evidence of syphilis, Feldman concluded that the toxic factor which produced degenerative changes in the maternal pancreas was active in producing changes in the fetal pancreas. The findings then represented an earlier stage of the same process.

The presence of sugar in the bladder of the unborn fetus is admittedly not diagnostic, yet he submits obviously hyperplastic tissue as evidence of diabetes. It is our contention that had the child been delivered hyperinsulinism might have ensued.

Schretter and Nevinny's reports[10] likewise are open to a different interpretation than the one they present. The infant born of a diabetic mother was oversized and had blood sugar of 52 mg. to 62 mg. in the first five days but reached as high as 172 mg. per cent on the sixteenth day. Urinary sugar and acetone determinations were not reported for the infant. The baby died on the thirty-second day with incomplete heart block, which post-mortem examination revealed was probably related to a septal defect of the heart. A later report by the same authors offers more detailed pathology and a valuable comparison with "normal" tissue. "The number of islands were increased over and above the well-recognized increase in the first quarter year of postnatal life. While hypertrophic 'giant islands' occurred only occasionally in the normal control, they dominate the picture in this case." In addition to the pathologic findings in the pancreas there was found an enlarged anterior hypophyseal lobe with an increase in eosinophilic cells. The ovaries were laden with large follicle cysts. The adrenals, although small, showed wide cortices in three cell layers. The thyroid showed poorly developed spaces with but little light staining colloid. Although it is conceivable that during gestation in a diabetic woman there might be initial stimulation of the fetal pancreas and a later "exhaustion phenomenon," the pathological picture must be recognized as distinctly different from that more commonly found in diabetes. In other words, enlargement and hyperplasia usually are evidence of increased function; they may represent depressed function only after an attempted compensation.

The isolation of insulin removed some of the mysteries with regard to the endocrine factors in the maintenance of blood sugar, but the interrelation of pituitary, thyroid, adrenal and liver cannot be denied. (Wauchope[11] and Harris.[12])

The report of Dubreuil and Anderodias[13] recognized hypertrophy and hyperplasia of the insular tissue and postulated a compensatory mechanism. In our own country the study of Gray and Feemster[14] is more convincing. The infant that lived four days had a blood sugar of 67 mg. per cent on the third day. The persistent vomiting which may be considered characteristic of this condition was present.

In addition to hypertrophy and hyperplasia of the insular tissue, there were hypertrophy and hemorrhage of the adrenal glands. Unfortunately no mention is made of other endocrine glands.

Since this last report, Heiberg[15] has published his study of the tissues of an infant born of a diabetic mother. At birth the blood sugar was 88 mg. per cent (method?) but fell to 60 to 70 mg. per cent save for a slight rise after a single clysis of dextrose. The child died on the second day. Island counts showed no increase compared with normal controls, and Heiberg interprets the case as functional hyperinsulinism despite an increase in the size of the pancreas approximately three times that of the control. This latter fact would suggest to us increased function and hypertrophy. The condition of the infant also suggests that perhaps heroic administration of dextrose might have carried the infant over the period of adjustment, such as apparently took place in three of our cases.

With a recent review of the literature, Nothmann and Hermstein[16] discuss the relation of diabetes and pregnancy. In their own case study there was no apparent effect on the maternal diabetes, but in the fetus there were found hypertrophy and hyperplasia of the pancreatic islets.

Correlation of function and pathology is not always easily demonstrable. In diabetes hyalinization, fibrosis and lymphocytic infiltration in the young are found not uncommonly. Hydropic degeneration emphasized by Allen[17] is not frequent in Warren's[18] experience. A few instances of island hypertrophy were found by Warren. Heiberg[19] some years ago reported adenoma of the pancreas in diabetes. Yet we believe such instances are exceptional and that they may relate to extrapancreatic pathology and should not be cited as illustrative pathology.

With regard to the significance of island counts, which Lawrence and McCance[20] chose to disregard, the careful studies of Nakamura[21] are valuable. The latter has shown that in the newborn infant they are normally increased and that definite decrease takes place with age. From a functional point of view we have already mentioned the characteristic low blood sugar of newborn infants, which facts may be related. In the pathology of our fourth case, however, even recognizing the expected increase in number of the islands in infants, the overgrowth of insular tissue, together with the hypoglycemia, leaves little doubt as to correlated hyperplasia and hyperfunction.

Macrosomia of infants born of diabetic mothers mentioned by Dubreuil and Anderodias,[22] and Lambie,[23] suggests that where the maternal hyperglycemia is not controlled an excessively large infant may be expected. (The family cited earlier in our report is striking.)

It will be noted in our report that the cesarean section was performed before term but that by measurements the baby was not premature. This is further corroborated by the skeletal roentgenogram which showed bone growth compatible with 9.5 months' gestation. We may then assume the infant to be relatively macrosomic. The role of glycogen deposition and hypertrophy of tissue has recently attracted attention. In his description of "hepatonephromegali glycogenica," von Gierke[24] postulates a duration of the fetal condition in which the glycolytic ferment is at fault. It is known that glycogen can be accumulated in large amounts in fetal tissue. Van Creveld[25] has suggested this as a basis for hypertrophy of tissues and possibly such conditions as idiopathic hypertrophy of the heart. However, in addition to the overgrowth possibly due to excess glycogen, mention should also be made of the possible endocrine factors. Kraus[26] has emphasized the pluriglandular pathology which he considers secondary to pancreatic insufficiency in diabetes. He found small atrophic adrenals, a small pituitary body, and changes in the thyroid gland. Some change in these endocrine glands might reasonably be expected in essential (pancreatic) hyperinsulinism of the young.

Hydramnios has been reported of frequent occurrence in pregnant diabetic women. Wiener[27] mentions it as an indication for premature induction of labor. It was apparently not an important factor in Peckham's[28] series and there is evidence cited by Lambie[29] that it is related to faulty control of the diabetes. We mention it here, not because of its occurrence in our small series, but because it has been associated with infantile developmental defects.

Sagal[30] has called attention to the frequency of congenital anomalies in children born of diabetic mothers. We were unable to obtain Sagal's article so we do not know whether hydramnios or endocrine factors were blamed for the developmental aberrations.

SUMMARY

There is considerable evidence that under rigid control during pregnancy, the diabetic woman may have a satisfactory course and gestatory product. Although reports vary it is difficult to prove that the infantile insulin production has any effect on the maternal blood sugar. Where the maternal diabetes has not been adequately controlled, the newborn infants may present temporary symptoms referable to hypoglycemia. In some cases these symptoms of cyanosis, vomiting, and feeding difficulty may persist for as long as three weeks and necessitate parenteral glucose administration for that time. A follow-up of one patient showed a hyperinsulin-like sugar curve at 4 years of age.

Reports of postmortem studies of infants born of diabetic mothers vary. In some no hyperplasia of islet tissue has been found, and the hypoglycemia must be considered functional in type. In others the finding of hypertrophy and hyperplasia of the islets of Langerhans makes the correlation obvious.

One study is made in which the relative macrosomia, advanced bone age, and more mature genital tract suggest a pituitary effect. Complete endocrine pathology is reported but with our present limited knowledge the interrelationship is best described as dysfunction. Perhaps some interrelationship will be found to account for the mild as well as the fatal hypoglycemia of the newborn infant. Fetal glycogen storage hypertrophy also is postulated as a possible etiology for some of the pathology.

The authors wish to acknowledge the assistance of the late Dr. Alfred H. Heald, who compiled the pathologic report.

REFERENCES

1. Wiener, H. J.: Am. J. Obst. & Gynec. **7**: 710, 1924.
2. Peckham, C. H.: Bull. Johns Hopkins Hosp. **49**: 184, 1931.
3. Lawrence, R. D.: Quart. J. Med. **22**: 191, 1929.
4. Lambie, C. G.: J. Obst. & Gynaec. Brit. Emp. **33**: 563, 1926.
5. Sherrill, J. W.: California & West. Med. **40**: 321, 1934.
6. Carlson, A. J., and Drennan, F. M.: Am. J. Physiol. **90**: 466, 1929.
7. Gray, S. H., and Feemster, L. C.: Arch. Path. & Lab. Med. **1**: 348, 1926.
8. Ambard, L., and others: Bull. et mém. Soc. méd. d. hôp. de Paris **49**: 547, 1925.
9. Feldman, I.: Centralb. f. allg. Path. u. path. Anat. **42**: 435, 1938.
10. Schretter, G., and Nevinny, H.: Arch. f. Gynäk. **140**: 397, 1930; ibid. **143**: 465, 1930.
11. Wauchope, G. M.: Quart. J. Med. **2**: 117, 1933.
12. Harris, S.: J. A. M. A. **101**: 1958, 1933.
13. Dubreuil, G., and Anderodias: Compt. rend. Soc. de biol. **2**: 1490, 1920.
14. Gray, S. H., and Feemster, L. C.: See reference 7.
15. Heiberg, K. A.: Virchows Arch. f. path. Anat. **287**: 629, 1933.
16. Nothmann, M., and Hermstein, A.: Arch. f. Gynäk. **150**: 287, 1932.
17. Allen, F. M.: J. Metabolic Research **1**: 193, 1922.
18. Warren, S.: The Pathology of Diabetes Mellitus, Philadelphia, 1930, Lea & Febiger.
19. Heiberg, K. A.: See reference 15.
20. Lawrence, R. D., and McCance, R. A.: Arch. Dis. Childhood **6**: 343, 1931.
21. Nakamura, N.: Virchows Arch. f. path. Anat. **253**: 286, 1924.
22. Dubreuil, G., and Anderodias: See reference 13.
23. Lambie, C. G.: See reference 4.
24. von Gierke, E.: Ziegler's Beitr. **82**: 497, 1929.
25. Van Creveld, S.: Maandschr. v. kindergeneesk. **2**: 123, 1932.
26. Kraus, E. J.: Virchows Arch. f. path. Anat. **247**: 1, 1923.
27. Wiener, H. J.: See reference 1.
28. Peckham, C. H.: See reference 2.
29. Lambie, C. G.: See reference 4.
30. Sagal, S.: Concerning the Influence of Pregnancy on the Development of Diabetes. Ginek (russ.) **7**: 697, 1928; with summary in German. Ber. ü. d. ges. Gynäk. u. Geburtsh **16**: 187, 1929. Quoted by Schretter and Nevinny: See reference 10.

CONGENITAL HYPERTROPHIC PYLORIC STENOSIS

With Special Reference to Surgical Treatment

Kenneth H. Tallerman, *M.C.*, M.D., F.R.C.P.
London, England

THE question of the treatment of pyloric stenosis is one on which a great deal of discussion still takes place. In England there is, generally speaking, a preference for surgical treatment, but this is by no means universal. A paper published by Svensgaard[1] in 1935, in which treatment with eumydrin is discussed, focused attention once more on the value of medical as opposed to surgical treatment for this condition.

In view of the interest and importance of this subject, it was felt that it would be of value to analyze from a clinical standpoint a series of cases dealt with during the last ten years, keeping in mind especially considerations of treatment and prognosis. The material on which this study is based consists of all patients with pyloric stenosis admitted to the Children's Department of the London Hospital during the period of ten years from Jan. 1, 1928, to Dec. 31, 1937, together with all such patients admitted to the Infants' Hospital, London, under the care of the writer during the time of his association with that hospital, a period of three years. The former group numbers 70, the latter, 32 patients. One other case occurred, with recovery, the diagnosis being confirmed at operation, but, since the case notes have been mislaid and details are not available, it has had to be excluded from the series. During this period there were in addition 2 cases which might be regarded as examples of pylorospasm.

In the matter of diagnosis, rigid criteria were adopted throughout, these being the universally accepted clinical features of the disease, together with the palpation of a pyloric tumor. In 96 patients the tumor was definitely felt, i.e., in 94 per cent of the series; in 2 its detection was doubtful, and in only 4 was it not felt. In each of these six cases where no tumor was definitely felt, the diagnosis was made because of the symptoms being typical and gastric peristalsis being observed, and in each it was confirmed at operation.

Of these 102 patients, 80 of whom were males and 22 females, 4 were treated medically and 98 surgically; 15 died, giving a total mortality rate of 14.7 per cent. In each of the 4 patients treated medically, gastric peristalsis was seen and a pyloric tumor palpated. Three of these recovered, and one died as a result of gastroenteritis; the diagnosis of pyloric stenosis was confirmed at autopsy. As their

From the Children's Department of the London Hospital, and from the Infants' Hospital, Vincent Square, London, England.

number is so small, further detailed comment will not be made on these patients who were treated medically.

The following analysis deals particularly with the 98 patients who were treated surgically. In each of these the diagnosis was confirmed at operation. Treatment was in general conducted on similar lines throughout the series at both hospitals. Many of the infants were given some form of adjuvant preoperative medical treatment, such as a sedative mixture of chloral hydrate and tincture of belladonna before feeding, and, usually for those who were definitely dehydrated, subcutaneous injections of physiologic saline solution; gastric lavage with saline solution was carried out as a routine. Artificially fed infants were usually given a partially skimmed dried milk mixture with added sugar, acidified with lactic acid. In all cases Rammstedt's operation was performed. Many of these infants were given a rectal injection of physiologic saline solution immediately after operation, before receiving any food by mouth, and this was repeated later if necessary. In every case feeding commenced 3 to 4 hours after operation. Small feeds of a glucose solution were given at first, and these were followed by gradually increasing quantities of breast milk or of an artificial feeding mixture similar to that given before operation, the acid being omitted in most cases after a short period. Breast-fed infants were actually sucking from the breast within 27 hours, and those fed artificially were taking an adequate feed within 36 hours of operation.

Of the 98 patients operated upon, 68 were treated at the London Hospital, with 9 deaths, and 30 at the Infants' Hospital, with 5 deaths. When the 98 cases are considered together, there were thus 14 deaths, giving a mortality rate of 14.3 per cent for the patients treated surgically. Four deaths can be regarded as surgical fatalities, and of the remaining ten children who died, seven succumbed to gastroenteritis subsequent to operation. Fifty-three of the operations were performed under general anesthesia, 2 under a combination of general and local anesthesia, and 43 entirely under local anesthesia; 7 deaths occurred subsequently in each of the first and third groups. At the time of admission 17 of the 98 infants were recorded as being less than 4 weeks of age, 69 from 4 to 8 weeks inclusive, and 12 over 8 weeks of age. All those who died were aged 4 weeks or more at the time of admission; 4 of them were 8 weeks or more, one, the oldest of them, being 12 weeks of age.

It is often difficult to be certain, from the history, of the exact duration of symptoms, but, so far as any definite statement seems justifiable, 56 of the patients who recovered may be regarded as having had symptoms for less than 3 weeks prior to admission, and in 7 cases symptoms had been present for 5 weeks or longer. Of those that died six had exhibited symptoms for less than 3 weeks, and 3 for more than 5 weeks. The longest apparently definite duration of symptoms was 8 weeks, in the case of a child who recovered.

Some idea of the general condition of the infants may be conveyed by stating that 57 of the 98 who were operated upon weighed less than at birth when admitted to the hospital; in a few of the remaining 41 infants the birth weight was not recorded. Ten of the 14 who died subsequent to operation are known to have weighed less than their birth weight when admitted to hospital.

Of the 98 infants treated surgically, 34 were breast-fed, 48 were artificially fed, and 16 were fed partly on breast milk and partly on artificial food. It is interesting to note that 12 of the 14 deaths occurred in artificially fed infants, and these included all the cases of gastroenteritis; the 2 breast-fed infants who died fall into the group classed as surgical fatalities. This emphasizes the importance of breast feeding as regards prognosis.

Average figures for length of stay in hospital are purposely not given, as they are likely to convey a totally false impression. The majority were in the hospital for 1 to 3 days before operation; in only 26 cases was operation delayed for more than 3 days after admission. For the 84 surgically treated patients in this series who recovered, the minimum total length of time in the hospital was 6 days, 9 having been in the ward for this short period only. The longest time spent in the ward by any child who recovered was 35 days, this case being complicated by the presence of pyelitis and a rectal abscess. The longest period of hospitalization for any infant in the whole series was 59 days; this particular infant, who died of pneumonia which developed 3 weeks after operation, was actually in the ward for 28 days before operation, owing to the fact that the diagnosis was not established for some time. Thirty infants were in the hospital for less than 10 days, 59 for less than 14 days, and only 25 for a period of 2 weeks or longer. No infant was ever discharged until progress from every standpoint was regarded as satisfactory. As regards the 14 fatalities, 7 infants died within 14 days of admission, and 7 after a longer period in the hospital.

The short time spent in hospital by the majority of these infants treated surgically is in marked contrast to the long periods usually required for medical treatment. Svensgaard,[1] for example, reports having kept her 61 patients treated with eumydrin in hospital for an average period of 77 days, although she admits that they were purposely kept not only until the symptoms had disappeared, but until they had been gaining weight satisfactorily for a long time. In her reported series of patients treated prior to the introduction of eumydrin, the periods of inpatient treatment were even longer. Monrad[2] also gives as average periods of time spent in the hospital 65 and 122 days for breast-fed and artificially fed infants, respectively. In Eckstein's paper,[3] in which he contrasts the medical and surgical treatment of patients with pyloric stenosis within the same clinic, he shows that on an average the former required that infants should remain nearly three times as long in hospital as the latter, and his recorded period of time in hospital even after surgical treatment was considerably longer (an average of 34 days, with 13 days as a minimum) than in the series here reported. The question of possibly treating some cases of pyloric stenosis medically as outpatients, must not, however, be overlooked.

Although the advantage of a short period of treatment and early discharge from a hospital ward is unquestioned, the time required for medical treatment would be relatively unimportant if this offered a much better chance of recovery than operative treatment. It is not, however, certain that the case for medical treatment is as yet definitely proved. The evaluation of the comparative advantages of these two main types of treatment is not by any means a simple matter, and critical consideration is necessary in assessing the reports found in the literature.

The differences in the details of treatment adopted by the many physicians working in different clinics naturally introduce variable physical factors. In addition, there is some difficulty in assessing and comparing the results of treatment in the various series of cases that are reported. For example, there is the question of the physical condition of the patients when they are first seen. It will be found that some observers do not record in any detail such data as age and weight of the infants, the duration of their symptoms, and the degree of emaciation at the time of the commencement of treatment. In reporting large series of cases it is admittedly impracticable as a rule to give complete protocols, and average figures are likely to be very misleading, but these comments are made in order to draw attention to a factor which makes for difficulty. The better the condition of a child when he comes under treatment, the better are his chances of recovery, hence the importance, when trying to compare different results, of knowing the duration of the illness and exact details of physical condition. In the absence of complete data it is hardly possible to make a truly critical comparison between the results of different methods of treatment adopted in different reported series. Taking the reports published during the last eleven years by some representative observers, most of whom record a series of not less than 100 patients treated either medically or surgically (the consideration of really small series from this point of view being of little value), it is found that most striking differences occur in mortality rate.

Monrad[2] feels that 24 of his cases should be excluded from the series, as 17 of the patients were moribund and 7 others were suffering from severe complicating conditions such as pyelitis, which made their case

TABLE I

	YEAR OF PUBLICATION	NUMBER OF CASES	MORTALITY
Medical Treatment			
Monrad[2]	1928	223	14.8%
Wolff[4]	1930	92	2.2%
Faxén[5]	1933	126	5.5%
Svensgaard[1]	1935	179	5.5%
Surgical Treatment			
Tisdall, Poole, and Brown[6]	1927	120	13.2%
Haberer[7]	1934	102*	6.9%
Wallace and Wevill[8]	1934	145	24.8%
Thompson and Gaisford[9]	1935	209	14.4%
Jewesbury and Page[10]	1937	303	12.5%
Medical and Surgical Treatment at the Same Clinic			
Eckstein[3]			
Medical cases	1934	92	18.4%
Surgical cases		110	3.4%

*Fifty-eight of these cases are apparently also included in Eckstein's series of 110 surgically-treated patients.

hopeless. If this is done his series is reduced to 199 cases, with a mortality rate of 4.5 per cent. Faxén[5] also thinks that 3 of his patients might well be excluded, as they died of conditions other than pyloric stenosis; he therefore regards his mortality rate as being 3.3 per cent. Such exclusion of cases from these series is not, however, really justifiable, as it would mean that in drawing conclusions from these reports prognosis would be based on the results obtained from the treatment of selected cases.

Eckstein's figures[3] are especially interesting, as they pertain to infants treated in the same clinic, one group by medical and the other by surgical methods; of his reported patients, those submitted to surgical treatment show an outstandingly superior rate of recovery.

Although at first sight it appears from reference to the figures in Table I that the death rate in those treated surgically is on the whole much higher than in those treated medically, certain points should be considered in further detail. Svensgaard,[1] in the paper already mentioned, records a total of 179 patients treated medically. They fall into three groups: 71 cases, with 5 deaths (1911 to 1922); 47 cases, with 3 deaths (1922 to 1927); and 61 cases, with 2 deaths (1927 to 1934). The total mortality, as is shown in Table I, was 5.5 per cent. In the group from 1927 to 1934, however, the mortality was only 3.3 per cent, and if one of the recorded deaths in this group, due to pyelonephritis, is excluded, it is then found that only one child out of 60 died, giving a mortality rate of 1.6 per cent. During each of these three periods referred to, a different method of medical treatment was employed. In the last period, to which Svensgaard[1] draws special attention, eumydrin was prescribed, and in her opinion this was responsible for the lowering of the mortality rate. Excellent though these results appear to be, it should be borne in mind that consideration of a large series of cases is necessary in order that the treatment of this condition may be viewed in true perspective. Any experienced pediatrician knows that he may have thirty or forty cases without a death occurring, and yet three or four may be lost from the next score or so, although the treatment is similar. On this account it will be necessary to review in the future the results of treatment with eumydrin on a much larger series of patients, before drawing a final conclusion. It may be mentioned here that Braithwaite[11] has just recorded a series of 21 patients treated with eumydrin, 3 of whom died. This might be said to show a mortality rate of no less than 14.3 per cent, but it is of course hardly justifiable to speak of percentages in so small a series.

Furthermore, the question of diagnosis arises, for without a record of very strict criteria it is difficult to be certain that all cases included in any series are actually true examples of congenital hypertrophic pyloric stenosis. In most of the surgically-treated patients in the series quoted, either the diagnostic criteria adopted or the findings at operation appear to put the diagnosis beyond question. Regarding those treated medically, however, it should be noted that Monrad[2] does not consider the palpation of a pyloric tumor to be essential for diagnosis, and Svensgaard[1] does not insist upon it. Faxén[5] does not state his diagnostic criteria at all. It is possible, therefore, that some infants who would be regarded by other observers as suffering from habit vomiting or pylorospasm may be included in such series as these. This would naturally be partly responsible for some of the low mortality rates reported, since these conditions yield readily to medical treatment, which for them is the correct procedure. Wolff's diagnostic criteria[4] appear to be quite rigid and definite. From the fact that only 18 of his patients were treated as inpatients, it might be inferred that the majority of his cases were relatively mild; he states, however, that 56 were severe or very severe. In all probability a factor contributing to the low mortality rate was freedom from the cross-infections which are liable to occur in a hospital ward. From his results it would appear that outpatient treatment by medical methods of, at any rate, the milder cases of pyloric stenosis is worthy of serious consideration, with a view to its more general adoption.

Whether or not pylorospasm, which has already been alluded to, is a clinical entity distinct from pyloric stenosis, is a debatable point. Holt and McIntosh[12] state that a temporary pylorospasm undoubtedly occurs in some young infants, but that the existence of persistent spasm of the pylorus without hypertrophy has still to be proved. They consider that pylorospasm is quite different from hypertrophic pyloric stenosis. Parsons[13] holds that a good case can be made out for the existence of pylorospasm, and Tisdall, Poole, and Brown[6] believe that the two diseases are clinically distinct and able to be recognized. The writer holds the same view and agrees with these observers that the really important point in differential diagnosis is the palpation of a pyloric tumor. This can be accomplished, as is shown by the series reported in this paper, in about 95 per cent of all cases if careful examination is made, but it is necessary to pay attention to certain points in technique. The observer should sit to the left of the infant, place the whole of his left hand, previously well warmed, on the abdomen, and palpate with the fingers *while the infant is being fed.* If, after examining for about ten minutes, he fails to detect the hard pylorus, which can often be felt to contract and relax under the fingers, it is advisable to try again in the same way during one or more subsequent feeds. In cases of pyloric stenosis, patient repeated examination will almost invariably reveal this physical sign, which should be considered of the greatest importance in making a correct diagnosis. If the tumor cannot be palpated after repeated efforts, the writer feels that a diagnosis of pyloric stenosis can only be justified if the infant, while under careful expert observation, is found to show every other typical symptom and sign. Sometimes the tumor may elude palpation owing to the fact that it is tucked up under the liver. In doubtful cases radiography is often helpful, but it cannot replace physical examination in making a diagnosis. The comments made by Higgins[14] in regard to the pyloric tumor in this condition are of interest and importance to the clinician. He not only lays great stress on the palpation of the tumor, which he regards as decisive in the diagnosis of pyloric stenosis and as the distinguishing feature between this condition and pylorospasm, but he also discusses the development of the hypertrophic process through an evolutionary cycle, resolving in the direction of natural cure. This offers an explanation of the spontaneous recovery which may occur after the age of about three months.

Further factors of importance in assessing the comparative advantages of different methods of treatment are the type of feeding and the length of stay in hospital. Breast-fed infants are known to show a higher recovery rate from pyloric stenosis than those who are artificially fed, and the longer an infant is kept in hospital the greater is the risk of intercurrent infection and resulting death. Early diagnosis and the initiation of treatment while the child is still in good condition has a significant influence upon the prognosis. This is well illustrated by the figures of Tisdall and his co-workers,[6] who point out that, if they excluded from their series those patients admitted to hospital in poor condition, their mortality rate would be reduced to 8 per cent, instead of their stated figure of 13.2 per cent quoted in Table I.

It is not out of place to remark that the surgical treatment discussed in connection with pyloric stenosis usually consists of a combination of surgical and medical treatment, since such medical procedures as gastric lavage, administration of physiologic saline if the infant is dehydrated, and careful adjustment of the diet, form a most important adjuvant to surgical treatment.

In the light of his experience the present writer considers that pyloric stenosis should not be regarded as a true surgical emergency and that a short period of preliminary medical treatment is desirable in order to counteract, not only dehydration, but also the alkalosis and gastritis which accompany this condition if symptoms have persisted for any length of time. Unless, however, symptoms cease within a day or two, and the infant begins to gain weight satisfactorily, there is a good case for operating at once rather than waiting until the infant, owing to further loss of weight, becomes a bad operative risk. It is important to realize that operation should never be withheld on the grounds of the serious condition of an infant; the worse the condition, the more urgent is the need for early operative intervention. It is in older infants, who are first seen at about 3 months of age and are in relatively good condition, that medical rather than surgical treatment seems especially indicated, since it is generally recognized that after this age the condition is likely to improve spontaneously and eventually to subside of its own accord. Two of the 4 medically treated patients mentioned above were of this age and responded well. Only 2 of those operated upon had reached the age of 3 months on admission, all the others being younger.

The importance of breast feeding in relation to prognosis is generally accepted and is borne out in this series. A further important factor, as already stated, is of course the general condition of the child at the time treatment is commenced; therefore, the earlier the diagnosis is made the better. It must also be emphasized that an infant already suffering from the results of partial starvation should be fed normally as soon as this can be safely accomplished, and the older methods of giving a low diet for a considerable period after operation are unnecessary and not without risk.

The longer an infant remains in hospital the greater is the chance of his acquiring an infection which may prove fatal, and this is particularly the case regarding those fed artificially. In this connection it should be noted that infants suffering from pyloric stenosis who are treated in private practice are found to show a higher recovery rate than those treated in hospital, the lesser risk of cross-infections being an important factor in influencing their course favorably, in addition, naturally, to the advantage of individual nursing. Rapid discharge from a hospital ward is therefore advantageous, and our tendency recently has been to discharge these infants earlier than was usually the case some years ago. From time to time a relatively long stay in hospital is required, as, for example, when there has been delay in arriving at a definite diagnosis, or when the mother's secretion of breast milk is insufficient and it is thought advisable to keep her and the infant in the hospital until an adequate secretion has been established. Our present aim, however, is to discharge the child 5 or 6 days after operation, arranging for the mother to bring him back for the removal of stitches on the ninth day, and subsequently for supervision in the outpatient department as long as this is deemed necessary.

Early diagnosis, a short period of preoperative medical preparation, close cooperation between physician and surgeon (the primary responsibility for the conduct of the case resting with the former) and early discharge from hospital after operation are considered essential if good results are to be obtained. Finally, it should be emphasized that breast feeding has a most favorable influence upon prognosis.

SUMMARY

One hundred and two cases of congenital hypertrophic pyloric stenosis are reported. Ninety-eight of these patients were operated upon, of whom fourteen died, giving a mortality rate of 14.3 per cent.

An analysis of these cases is given, and certain points are commented upon with special reference to treatment and prognosis.

The question of the comparative advantages of surgical and medical treatment of this disease is critically discussed.

It is a pleasure to acknowledge my indebtedness to those of my colleagues who were responsible for the surgical treatment, especially Sir James Walton, who operated on nearly all the London Hospital patients, and Mr. D. Levi, who carried out all the operations on those patients treated by myself at the Infants' Hospital. I wish also to thank Dr. A. G. Maitland-Jones for permission to report such cases as came under his care at the London Hospital.

REFERENCES

1. Svensgaard, E.: Arch. Dis. Childhood **10**: 443, 1935.
2. Monrad, S.: Proc. Scand. Ped. Cong., Acta Paediat. **7**: Supplement 2, 16, 1928.
3. Eckstein, A.: Klin. Wchnschr. **12**: 295, 1934.
4. Wolff, S.: Jahrb. f. Kinderh. **128**: 287, 1930.
5. Faxén, N.: Acta Paediat. **14**: 388, 1932-3.
6. Tisdall, F. F., Poole, M. W., and Brown, A.: Am. J. Dis. Child. **34**: 180, 1927.
7. Haberer, H. v.: München. med. Wchnschr. **81**: 903, 1934.
8. Wallace, H. L., and Wevill, L. B.: Brit. M. J. **1**: 1153, 1934.
9. Thompson, W. A., and Gaisford, W. F.: Brit. M. J. **2**: 1037, 1935.
10. Jewesbury, R. C., and Page, C. M.: St. Thomas's Hosp. Rep., Second Series **2**: 141, 1937.
11. Braithwaite, J. V.: Brit. M. J. **1**: 334, 1938.
12. Holt, L. E., and McIntosh, R.: Holt's Diseases of Infancy and Childhood, p. 275, New York, 1933, D. Appleton-Century Company, Inc.
13. Parsons, L. G.: Diseases of Infancy and Childhood, Parsons and Barling, Vol. I, p. 739, London, 1933, Oxford University Press.
14. Higgins, T. T.: Brit. M. J. **1**: 502, 1935.

SYSTEMATIC HEALTH WORK FOR MOTHER AND CHILD

Kirsten Utheim-Toverud, M.D.
Oslo, Norway

HEALTH WORK in early childhood has been developed in Norway, as in nearly all other countries, as isolated infant welfare work, with supervision of the infant throughout the first year. This supervision, performed chiefly by private health organizations in the larger cities, has been an important factor in reducing the infant mortality to the low figures of 39 per 1,000 live births for Norway in the year of 1934 and 44.2 per 1,000 live births in 1935.

Nevertheless, we have various deficiency diseases in this country: in infancy mostly in the form of rickets in the rural districts, up to 43 per cent in the north part of our country, and in later years as dental caries, which affects 99 per cent of our school children.

Furthermore, it is evident from our statistics that our neonatal mortality is relatively high. For Norway as a whole it comprises 50 per cent of the total infant mortality, and for the city of Oslo, with a total infant mortality of 30 per 1,000 in 1935, it accounted for 71 per cent.

From previous work[1] we know that most of the stillborn infants are prematurely born and that the premature infant deaths consititute the greatest percentage of the neonatal deaths.

It has been shown[2] that prematurity may be prevented to a certain extent by a systematic supervision of the mother throughout pregnancy. This is particularly true for unmarried mothers. Supervision in a home for unmarried mothers reduced premature births from 25 per cent in mothers admitted to the home after delivery to 3 per cent in mothers admitted in good time before delivery.

By experimental and clinical work we have found that pregnancy, considered as the essential growth period it is, quite often gives a negative balance as far as certain important nutritional factors are concerned.[3] Out of 27 metabolism experiments performed on 17 women, pregnant from six to nine months, 21 experiments showed a negative calcium balance and 12 a negative phosphorus balance. Furthermore, we found an iron retention below the fetal need in 13 experiments out of 20 performed on 15 women from 25 to 39 weeks pregnant.[4] This negative calcium and phosphorus balance may result, as it is shown by histologic work, in a deficient structure of bones[5] and teeth.[6] It is also found from clinical analysis[7] that the low iron retention may result in a low iron content in the fetal organism, a condition of importance for the development of the infant.

From the Children's Department, Norway Dental School.

By regulating the diet of the mothers so that it contains at least 1.6 gm. calcium, 2.2 gm. phosphorus, and 20 mg. iron daily, the balance of these nutritional factors were made positive when the diet was otherwise sufficient. It was also found that the newborn infant's store of vitamins A,[8] C,[9] and D[8] was low in many cases and that this store varied according to the diet and regime of the mother throughout pregnancy.

In the lactating period a negative calcium balance was also found quite frequently, and the vitamin content of the breast milk was found to vary considerably, particularly as to vitamin C. From Gaehtgens' experiments[10] we know the vitamin A content varies also.

Experimentally, as well as clinically, it has been shown that these diet deficiencies during fetal life and early infancy may influence the infants and render them more susceptible to the development of manifest deficiency diseases in postnatal life, as rickets, anemia, tetany, and scurvy, if the postnatal diet as well is insufficient. This is particularly true for premature infants.

These diet deficiencies throughout fetal life and early infancy may be prevented, but only if prophylactic work is started early enough, that is to say, not at the birth of the infant but at the time of conception. This means that a complete prophylactic work in childhood must consist of supervision of the mother throughout the entire period of pregnancy, the following of the infant throughout the first year, and continued supervision throughout the preschool age.

Such a prophylactic health work was planned for the country of Norway two years ago as the only sound basis for the health work in schools, which was started years ago and has spread extensively throughout the country. The whole growth period of the individual will in this way be supervised, and, when the work is well organized, most of the determining factors in general hygiene are thus under control.

Nearly two years ago, September, 1936, this plan was put to work in a rural community just outside Oslo, and it is the preliminary result of this health work since that time which is recorded in the following pages.

The plan worked out by the local physician, Dr. A. Henriksen, in cooperation with Professor Toverud and the author consisted of supervision at a health station throughout pregnancy, once a month in the first seven months, twice during the eighth month and once a week during the ninth month. The infant is likewise examined by the physician once a month during the first half of the first year and every other month during the second half. After the first year the examination is performed three times a year. In addition to this, the teeth are examined and treated from the third year on, in children whose parents have followed the directions of the health station. At the same time intensive propaganda has been carried on in the district for the purpose of making the mothers understand the importance of a proper diet.

When the work was started in September, 1936, we wanted to get an impression of the nutritional state of the population, particularly the state of the pregnant women. For this reason determinations of blood calcium, hemoglobin, ascorbic acid in the blood, and the "distinction power" were performed in all pregnant and in some lactating women.

The methods used in these determinations are the following: for serum calcium, the micromethod described by Nordbö[11] and for hemoglobin, the Zeiss-Ikon colorimeter previously standardized. The mark 100 on this colorimeter corresponds to 100 per cent hemoglobin, or 13.8 gm. per 100 c.c. of blood. For vitamin C in the blood serum we used the methylene blue method of Lund and Lieck[12] based on the principle first described by Martini and Bonsignore, that ascorbic acid can decolorize a methylene blue solution in light. A modification of this method worked out as a micromethod by Elmby and With[13] was used in this work. The "distinction power" was determined according to Edmund,[14] using Tscherning photometric glasses and letters of various gray intensity previously standardized. The so-called long test, blindfolding the eye one-half hour before the performance of the test, was used in this service. The normal dark vision was, according to Edmund and other investigators, considered to be the power of reading at least the first three letters corresponding to the figure of 1.25.

The community in which this work was started has a population of 8,000 inhabitants. From 100 to 120 births a year has been the average figure during recent years in this district. During the twenty months this work has been going on, 117 pregnant women have visited the health center. When examined, the mothers have been given directions as to diet and general hygiene. They have all been told to take 1 tablespoonful of cod liver oil, 1 quart of milk, vegetables, and fruit corresponding to about 75 to 100 mg. of ascorbic acid each day, meat and fish both twice a week, liver and blood at least once a week, besides egg, and whole wheat bread daily. When the hemoglobin was low, iron as ferrichloride was given, and, if milk was not well tolerated, calcium phosphate was added to the diet in an amount calculated to correspond to the calcium content of 1 quart of milk (1.2 gm. calcium).

The nutritional status of these women may be seen from Table I, where the hemoglobin values, calcium content and ascorbic acid content of serum, and the dark vision of these women are recorded. In such determinations the question arises where to put the border line between normal and subnormal values.

As to hemoglobin, the women 15 per cent below the normal figure of 100 per cent, that is, women with a hemoglobin of 85 per cent, and the women 20 per cent below the normal value, that is, women below 80 per cent, have been recorded as subnormal. According to the first calculation, 37, or 31.6 per cent, are subnormal; according to the second calculation, 20, or 17.1 per cent. Repeated determinations were performed in 24 out of these 37 women, and 16 (or 67 per cent) of them returned to the normal value before delivery (Table II).

As far as the "distinction power" is concerned, all previous investigators seem to agree on the figure of 1.25 as the first normal value. From Table I it is seen that 36, or 30.8 per cent, of the women examined showed subnormal values. Thirty-two of these 36 women were followed

TABLE I

THE HEALTH CONDITION OF PREGNANT WOMEN IN THE RURAL COMMUNITY OF SKEDSMO

NO. OF WOMEN EXAMINED	NO. OF WOMEN WITH HEMOGLOBIN BELOW		NO. OF WOMEN WITH DISTINCTION POWER BELOW 1.25	NO. OF WOMEN WITH SERUM CA BELOW		NO. OF WOMEN WITH SERUM ASC. ACID BELOW 0.5 MG. %
	85%	80%		9.5 MG. %	9 MG. %	
117	37 31.6%	20 17.1%	36 30.8%	46 39.3%	18 15.4%	
49						24 49 % 0.3 – 1.2 mg. % lowest and highest figures

TABLE II

PREGNANT WOMEN WITH SUBNORMAL VALUES OF HEMOGLOBIN, DISTINCTION POWER, CALCIUM AND ASCORBIC ACID IN BLOOD SERUM EXAMINED REPEATEDLY DURING PREGNANCY

	NO. OF WOMEN WITH SUBNORMAL VALUE	NO. OF WOMEN REACHING NORMAL VALUE BEFORE DELIVERY
Hemoglobin %	24 (below 85%) 16 (below 80%)	16 (above 85%) 13 (above 80%)
Calcium in serum	36 (below 9.5 mg. %) 16 (below 9.0 mg. %)	31 (above 9.5 mg. %) 25 (10 mg. % or above) 11 (above 9.5 mg. %) 15 (above 9.0 mg. %)
Distinction power	32 (below 1.25)	29 (1.25 or above)
Ascorbic acid in serum	16 (below 0.5 mg. %)	15 (above 0.5 mg. %)

regularly throughout pregnancy, and 29 of them developed a normal "distinction power" during the time of supervision; in only 3 cases did the "distinction power" fail to reach normal before delivery (Table II).

When serum calcium is considered, it is more difficult to fix the limits of normal values. If 9.5 mg. per 100 c.c. of serum is stated as such, 46, or 40 per cent, of the pregnant women were found to have a serum calcium below normal. If only values below 9.0 mg. are noted, 18, or 15.4 per cent, of the women may be considered as having subnormal values. Thirty-six of the 46 women examined were followed with repeated analyses throughout pregnancy; 31 reached values above 9.5 mg. per cent, and in the majority of cases (25) values of 10 mg. per cent and above were found (Table II).

Ascorbic acid in the blood serum was also determined in 49 pregnant women, and values below 0.5 mg. per cent were found in 24, or 49 per cent. Of these 24 women 16 were followed with repeated analyses throughout pregnancy, and all except one reached values above 0.5 mg. per cent. It is not clear where to fix the limit of normal values. Lund has mentioned the value of 0.3 mg. per cent as normal in Denmark. It was found in this series that only women on diets with low vitamin C contents showed similar values, and an increase of the content of the diet to about 75 mg. per day readily raised the content to above 0.5 mg. per cent. All determinations were made three to four hours after breakfast.

Thus we see that evidence of deficiencies in various nutritional factors has been present in 30 to 40 per cent of the pregnant women in this district—deficiencies which in the majority were corrected by diet regulation.

In 147 lactating women "distinction power" was determined, and low values were found in 53 (36 per cent). Thirty-seven of these 53 women were followed with repeated examinations during the lactation period, and 31 of them reached normal values under supervision. Only 6 women remained at the low distinction value of 1.00 (Table III).

Table III

"Distinction Power" in Lactating Women

NO. OF WOMEN EXAMINED	NO. OF WOMEN WITH DISTINCTION POWER BELOW 1.25
147	53 (36%) Of these 37 were followed with repeated tests during lactation 31 reached normal values during control

Table IV

Health Condition of Mother and Child in the Community of Skedsmo

	NO. OF BIRTHS	ECLAMPSIA IN MOTHER	NO. OF STILLBIRTHS	NO. OF PREMATURE BIRTHS
Records from Sept. 1, 1934, to Sept. 1, 1936	219	3 (all died) 1.4%	5 2.3%	11 5%
Records from Sept. 1, 1936 to June 1, 1938 Mothers not visiting the health station	93	2 (alive) 2.2.%	2 2.2%	8 8.6%
Records from Sept. 22, 1936, to June 1, 1938 Mothers visiting the health station regularly	105	0	0	2 1.9%

In order to see what effect this systematic health work has had on the mother and child in this community, we have tried to compare the results achieved at the health station with material from previous years in the same community.

From Table IV it is seen that in the two preceding years, 1934-1936, 3 women out of 219 delivered died of eclampsia. During the last two years 2 out of 93 women who have not visited the health station developed eclampsia. Of the 105 mothers who have been delivered and have visited the health station regularly during pregnancy, not one developed eclampsia, and no stillbirths have occurred. As to the number of premature births 11 infants, or 5 per cent, were born prematurely in the period 1934-1936, and in the period 1936-1938 8 of 93 infants were born prematurely of mothers who had not visited the health center. All had birth weights below 2500 gm. Of 105 mothers attending the center, only 2 were delivered prematurely. One case was a twin birth, and in the other case the infant had a birth weight of 2150 gm. All infants were followed closely and they developed very well.

At this point we may note that the decrease in the number of premature infants as a result of a systematic prenatal control is considered to be of great importance. This fact is illustrated by material from a home for unmarried mothers where the diet and general hygienic control for the last seven years have been raised to meet the actual need during pregnancy as far as we know it today (Table V). Premature birth is a somewhat vague term. The premature infants from this home are therefore classified in three ways. As we see from Table V, a distinct decrease in the number of premature births has taken place in this material, whether it is classified according to the obstetrician's diagnosis, or according to the birth weight (below 2750 gm. or below 2500 gm.). The high incidence of prematurity in these women without prenatal supervision is explained by the fact that we in this home are dealing with unmarried young mothers.

Table V

Premature Births at Sebbelow Stiftelse From August, 1931, to June, 1938

	Total No. of Infants Born	No. of Infants Born Prematurely According to the Diagnosis of the Obstetrician	No. of Infants With Birthweight Below 2750 gm.	No. of Infants With Birthweight Below 2500 gm.
Infants born of mothers admitted previous to delivery	224	7 (3.1%)	9 (4%)	5 (2.2%)
Infants born of mothers admitted after delivery or just before	124	33 (26.6%)	30 (24.2%)	19 (15.3%)

From Table VI it will be seen that the incidence of rickets, judged from the examination of infants visiting the center sometime during the first year, was 20 per cent in this district. The diagnosis was made by clinical examinations, and the diagnostic symptoms were craniotabes,

TABLE VI

THE HEALTH CONDITION OF INFANTS IN THE COMMUNITY OF SKEDSMO, SEPTEMBER, 1936, TO JUNE, 1938

	NO. OF INFANTS EXAMINED	NO. OF INFANTS WITH RICKETS
Infants whose mothers were not controlled during pregnancy	152	30 (19.9%)
Infants whose mothers were controlled during pregnancy	105	4 (3.8%) (3 had only an early osteoporotic craniotabes, 1 bowing of the legs)

rachitic rosary, and bowlegs. If roentgenologic studies could be made on these infants, this figure would certainly have been considerably higher. It has also to be mentioned that about one-third of the infants examined were overweight.

Of the group of infants who had been under systematic prenatal as well as postnatal control at the center, 4 showed disturbance in calcification. Temporary and strictly localized craniotabes was observed around the third month in 3 infants. One of these infants was a twin, and another was born in a very poor home where vegetables and fruit could not be provided in sufficient amount. The second and third infants were born of a mother whose prenatal control had only lasted the three last weeks of pregnancy. The fourth infant showed bowlegs at 10 months of age and was suffering from a hereditary adipositas which was so marked that the infant weighed 13.5 kg. at 10 months of age. (Father and grandfather were both very fat.) If we consider the symptoms of the latter group as due to rickets, a lowering in the incidence of rickets had taken place from 19.9 per cent to 3.8 per cent in this district.

We have also been interested in the lactating function of the mothers in this district. We know that inability of many mothers to nurse their infants is a general feature in modern life. The frequency of this inability varies from place to place. It is often said to be unwillingness on the part of the mothers, but this is true certainly in only the minority of cases. All facts today indicate that this inability is a symptom of a deficiency of some unknown nutritional factor or hormone which is the determining one in this process.

The figures in Table VII seem to show that the inability to nurse becomes less frequent when the general hygiene of the mothers is raised. This is even more the case when a closed prophylactic system is in effect. The various health factors, particularly the nutrition of the mother, are then more controlled, with the result that 90 per cent of the unmarried mothers in the last group under the best general hygienic control are able to nurse their infants, as compared with the first group of married mothers in the rural district showing a nursing ability in only 55 per cent.

TABLE VII

		TOTAL NO. OF MOTHERS	NO. OF MOTHERS NURSING THEIR INFANTS EXCLUSIVELY AT LEAST 4 MOS.	PER CENT NURSING ABILITY
Women from Skedsmo without supervision during pregnancy	Open prophylactic system	128	70	54.7
Women from Skedsmo supervised during pregnancy	Open prophylactic system	105	70	66.7
Women admitted to Sebbelow St. after delivery June 1, 1936, to June 1, 1938	Closed prophylactic system	37	27	73.0
Women adm. to Sebbelow St. in good time before delivery June 1, 1936, to June 1, 1938	Closed prophylactic system	78	70	89.7

As far as the teeth are concerned, only the children from 2 to 3 years old are recorded; this is the oldest group of children controlled, as the center has been functioning only 21 months. The examinations were performed by Professor Toverud and his assistants at the Children's Department of the Norway Dental School. It is seen from Table VIII

TABLE VIII

THE DENTAL CONDITION IN THE FIRST GROUP OF CHILDREN IN THE COMMUNITY OF SKEDSMO

	NO. OF CHILDREN EXAMINED	NO. OF CHILDREN WITH CARIES	NO. OF CARIOUS TEETH PER CHILD
2 to 3 year old children not belonging to the health station	33	27 (82%)	5
2 to 3 year old children visiting the health station	40	12 (30%)	1.2

that the number of children with carious teeth has decreased from 82 per cent in the group outside the health center to 30 per cent in the children who have visited the center regularly. In this connection it must be mentioned that in regulating the diet, factors influencing the teeth both generally and locally have been heeded, that is, an optimal diet for the mother and infant has been provided. Cod liver oil and orange juice have been given to the infants beginning at 1 month of age, and fruits and vegetables were added at 4 months of age whether breast milk or a cow's milk mixture has been given. After 8 months of age sugar was not given to the infant.

The work described in this paper has been an attempt to see what a systematic health work plan starting at the very first beginning of the individual with attention to all known nutritional factors is able to secure for the mother and child in a poor rural district. The newer knowledge of nutrition makes us understand that many of the morbid conditions in mother and child are deficiencies, some of them are understood but many of them are not. We certainly do not know yet what is the "normal" nutrition of a pregnant and lactating woman, her optimal need of the various food factors, nor do we know that so far as the child is concerned. Pathologic conditions in teeth, particularly the widespread dental caries, a striking feature in our modern life, proves this. Any attempt, even small, to put out in practical life a systematic prophylaxis may be of interest.

REFERENCES

1. Utheim-Toverud, K.: Acta paediat. **18:** 249, 1936.
2. Utheim-Toverud, K.: Am. J. Dis. Child. **46:** 954, 1933.
3. Utheim-Toverud, K., and Toverud, G.: Acta paediat. **12:** Suppl. II, 1931.
4. Utheim-Toverud, K.: Norsk. mag. f. lægevidensk., 177, 259, 381, 1935.
5. Utheim-Toverud, K.: Ztschr. f. Kinderh. **56:** 66, 1934.
6. Utheim-Toverud, K., Häupl, Toverud, G.: Den Norske Tannl. for. Tid. 1934.
7. Utheim-Toverud, K.: Norsk. mag. f. lægevidensk. **96:** 468, 1935.
8. Utheim-Toverud, K.: Acta paediat. **18:** 174, 1935.
9. Utheim-Toverud, K.: Arch. Dis. Child. **10:** 313, 1935.
10. Gaehtgens, G.: Med. Prax., Bd. 24, 1937.
11. Nordbö: Biochem. Ztschr. **246:** 460, 1932.
12. Lund and Lieck H.: Hospitals-tidende, 798, 1936.
13. Elmby and With: Bibliot. f. læger, 85, 1937.
14. Edmund, C., and Clemmensen: On Deficiency of Vitamin A and Visual Dysaptation.

The Journal of Pediatrics

Vol. 13 | December, 1938 | No. 6

Original Communications

THE TREATMENT OF NEUROGENIC MEGACOLON WITH SELECTIVE DRUGS

Walter O. Klingman, M.D.
New York, N. Y.

A REVIEW of the literature on the subject of megacolon or dilatation of the colon leaves one without a clear understanding of both the pathology and etiology.[1] Since Hirschsprung's[2] original description of hypertrophy and dilatation of the colon in children, in 1888, many possible causes have been advanced, and a variety of therapeutic regimes have been tried.[3, 4] The more recent successful procedures in the treatment of megacolon have been those in which a better functioning of the bowel has resulted when part of the innervation of the colon has been surgically interrupted.

Originally the cause of megacolon was obscure, and it was known as congenital idiopathic dilatation of the colon. Congenital hypertrophy was thought to be the primary condition and spasm secondary, but both factors were present in all cases. Later neuromuscular unbalance was proposed as a primary cause, produced by a disturbed equilibrium between the two autonomic nervous systems supplying the gut and resulting in a paralysis of a segment of the colon. Fraser and Hunt[5] and others had felt that congenital idiopathic megacolon had a neuropathic cause resulting in a disturbance in the coordinating mechanism of the rectosigmoid and the anal sphincter. A theory originally expressed by Gaskell[6] and Sherrington[7] was later revived by Wade and Royle,[8] who felt that congenital dilatation of the colon was due to a postural tone being superimposed on the rectal mechanism which disturbed the coordination function of the sphincter. Fraser and Hunt were under the impression that the disturbed mechanism of the rectosigmoidal region was caused by a failure of the sphincter to relax.

From the Babies Hospital, New York City.

Bartle[9] in his excellent review of the literature which followed Hunter and Royle's work on the effects of sympathectomy for reduction of spasticity in the muscles of limbs paralyzed through a central or cortical lesion, proposed a new theory. He had studied the theories of the function of the sympathetic nerve supply of the bowel as propounded by Bayliss,[10] MacLeod,[11] Gaskell,[6] Langley,[12] and others.[13, 14, 15, 16] Bartle concluded that the neurogenic mechanism causing megacolon resembled the neurogenic mechanism responsible for the spastic extremities seen after central paralyses. He called attention to a case of Royle's where relief from an obstinate constipation of long standing had resulted, after the white ramus of the second lumbar had been cut.

Stimulated by the results obtained by Wade and Royle and the satisfactory results in two of Wade's patients, Judd and Adson proposed a new etiology for megacolon from their own investigations and operative experience. They stated that congenital megacolon and megacolon acquired in early life without obvious mechanical obstruction are due to hyperactivity of the sympathetic innervation of the rectum. This theory was based upon the dual innervation of the rectum and anus with parasympathetic and sympathetic fibers. The motor impulses to the longitudinal muscle fibers of the rectum were known to be transmitted by the parasympathetics and the motor impulses to the circular muscles of the rectum by the sympathetics, partially arising from the lumbar rami communicantes passing down through the sympathetic trunks, the hypogastric and pelvic plexuses. Conversely, the inhibitory impulses to the longitudinal muscle fibers were supplied by the sympathetics, the inhibitory impulses to the circular fibers being supplied by the parasympathetics. It was not possible for them to deduce whether the hyperactivity of the sympathetics postulated in cases of megacolon was due to an irritating lesion of the ganglia of the postganglionic or the preganglionic fibers or was of central origin; but they favored the latter view. Therefore, they proposed and performed lumbar sympathetic ganglionectomy and ramisectomy for congenital idiopathic dilatation of the colon. They felt that the resulting improved colon emptying was not necessarily due to division of the white ramus or to removal of the lumbar ganglia but to a thorough interruption of the sympathetic chain below the last white ramus, preganglionic fiber to the ganglia. The division of the lumbar sympathetic chain diminished the sympathetic stimuli to the circular muscles of the rectum and, when symptoms of obstruction and toxicosis developed, division of the lumbar sympathetic trunks should be considered.[17] Their results were very encouraging.

Learmonth, in reviewing operations on the sympathetic nerves of the terminal portion of the bowel and of the bladder, stated later that a surgical procedure confined to the lumbar sympathetic trunks and their branches does not interrupt all the sympathetic fibers passing to the terminal part of the bowel.[18] Judd and Adson had felt, however, that interruption of the sympathetic influence, as achieved by their operation, resulted in a better functional balance between sympathetic and parasympathetic systems. Learmonth preferred to interpret the operative outcome as a better integration of the different functions of the nervous system.

From Judd and Adson's report it was assumed that there was a type of megacolon which was due to autonomic nervous system unbalance in the nature of hyperactivity of the sympathetic system resulting in tonic spasm of the sphincter or rectosigmoidal apparatus. Fraser and Hunt had already suggested that a similar condition might be due to lack of inhibition of the sphincter. Prompted by these studies, we considered attacking the problem on the premise that some types of megacolon might be due to an inability of the sphincter or rectosigmoidal apparatus to be properly inhibited or that the unbalance resulted from faulty inhibition.

In the light of the newer knowledge of the physiology of nerve control of the rectosigmoid, a rational therapeutic approach with properly selected drugs has been attempted. Atropine has been used for years, but the rather undesirable toxic atropine effects have discouraged its use. Furthermore, lack of classification of the types of neurogenic disturbance has hindered a solution of the problem from the pharmacodynamic standpoint, and until these types of megacolon could be distinguished clinically, selective drug therapy was not possible.[19-21]

Clinically, idiopathic or acquired megacolon, we believe, falls into one of two groups, excluding mechanical obstruction of the colon. First, there is a group called rectosigmoidal achalasia, in which one finds a failure of the rectosigmoidal apparatus to relax. Secondly, there is a group in which one finds a failure of the motor function of the parasympathetic system to act effectively above the rectosigmoidal region. Rectosigmoidal achalasia may arise from two causes: one due to overactivity of the sympathetic system resulting in spasm of the rectosigmoidal apparatus, and the other due to failure of the parasympathetic system to properly inhibit the rectosigmoidal apparatus.

A series of seven cases was studied. All of these cases were being considered for surgical treatment. At first no definite plan of medication was carried out, but we tried one drug and if that did not work we tried another. Benzedrine sulfate, ephedrine sulfate, and atropine sulfate were all tried. Atropine had been effective for intervals in the first cases studied but the by-effects were so annoying that it had to be discontinued. In view of the satisfactory response to atropine sulfate, despite the unpleasant toxic effects, we felt that the parasympathetic system undoubtedly played a considerable part in the production of disturbed neuromuscular function. Therefore, in searching for a selective drug, it seemed advisable to choose one which would act exclusively on the parasympathetics. Just how atropine or one of its derivatives or a drug acting exclusively as a paralysant of the parasympathetics becomes effective in establishing better bowel function in megacolon is difficult to explain. One working hypothesis is that with overaction of the parasympathetics retention in the colon occurs from inability of the longitudinal muscle fibers to expel the feces without help of the circular fibers, which in neurogenic megacolon are too completely relaxed. A parasympathetic paralysant would lessen this inhibiting effect and one then might get some circular muscle fiber action. Gaskell and Sherrington suggested that megacolon was a disturbance of postural tone of the gut. With a disturbance of this kind one might expect some interferences in the coordinating function of the rectal sphincter mechanism. A parasympathetic paralysant in that event would help the motility of the colon even if the posture of the gut were not helped.

Still another thought in explanation of the action of a parasympathetic paralysant is given by Loewi,[22] who says that a drug like atropine inhibits the action of the parasympathetic nervous system not by paralyzing, as has been supposed, but by stopping or preventing the action of acetylcholine in or near the reacting cell. He also states that when a balance obtains between cholinergic and adrenergic substances, atropine, by removing the cholinergic factor, acts as a synergist to the adrenergic factor. Myerson's experiments would also lead one to accept this view.[23] In particular reference to the gastrointestinal tract, the tonus of the rectosigmoidal apparatus may be diminished by adrenergic action, following administration of a parasympathetic paralysant.

Yet another explanation may come from the effect that a parasympathetic paralysant may have when it acts by inhibiting the liberation of acetylcholine. Aside from being liberated in very small quantities ordinarily at the terminations of the parasympathetics, acetylcholine is also present in small quantities at the terminations of the sympathetic fibers at the junction of the preganglionic and postganglionic fibers. A drug reducing the liberation of acetylcholine at this junction might sufficiently reduce the overactivity of the sympathetic innervation and lead to a better balance (Fig. 1).

In some respects the use of a parasympathetic paralysant is almost paradoxical, and one is forced to accept it on the grounds that it is effective, the means by which it acts being as yet unexplained. Rather contradictory findings from atropine are being observed elsewhere by investigators, especially where an unbalance exists or is artificially produced by other drugs.

Whatever the explanation may be, drugs acting exclusively on the parasympathetics as paralysers are beneficial in establishing better emptying of the bowel in certain cases of megacolon.

The drug of choice to inhibit liberation of acetylcholine should be atropine but, as already mentioned, its highly toxic effects contraindicate its administration. In a search, therefore, for a less toxic atropine-like compound, syntropan was selected because of its inhibiting effect, similar to atropine on the reacting cells, at the parasympathetic nerve endings.

Syntropan is the ester of 3- diethylamino-2, 2- dimethyl-1 propanol and tropic acid and is marketed under the name of syntropan (Roche). It was selected because it controls tonus without interfering with the peristaltic reflex. It also has a much greater safety ratio than atropine sulfate, the toxic dose being more than twice that of atropine. Likewise, its administration is not accompanied by the disagreeable effects on circulation, the pupil, and the glandular secretions. Its effect on the colon is also much greater than that of atropine and it has no atropine-like action on the small intestine. The effective dose of syntropan is also much more easily reached without appearance of any toxic symptoms, which is not true of atropine. In all cases it was given by mouth.

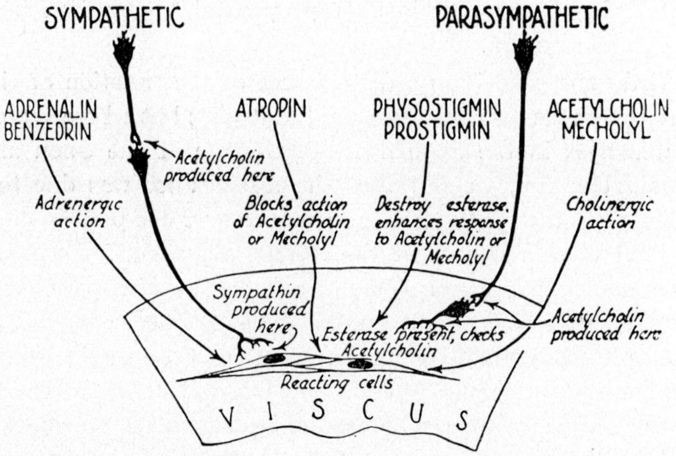

Fig. 1.—Myerson's schematic illustration of the points of action of various adrenergic and cholinergic drugs. (J. A. M. A. **110**: 102, 1938.)

All of the cases treated were first tried with syntropan. Of the seven cases treated, five of them responded to such treatment. The exceptions are mentioned in detail later. The patients ranged in age from 8 months to 14 years. All of them had preliminary barium studies to demonstrate the existence of megacolon (see x-ray plates).

The result of treatment has been excellent. The case reports below show a satisfactory bowel function which has continued throughout the follow-up period in all suitable cases, with no indications of loss of effectiveness of the drug. On the contrary, some of the patients are doing very well on reduced dosages, and two patients are no longer taking syntropan and have normal bowel function.

In the group of rectosigmoidal achalasia, a single case is presented, Case 1, in which we felt that the condition was due to motor hyperactivity of the sympathetics. There was in this instance a similar failure of the rectosigmoidal apparatus to relax, but the condition did not respond to syntropan therapy. The dosage was increased as high as we felt it was safe to do so, being uncertain when toxic central symptoms might appear. Because of lack of a safe and practical drug for reducing sympathetic function, we thought it right to advise a presacral nerve resection and ganglionectomy on this patient. Perhaps we were too hasty in abandoning ephedrine or benzedrine sulfate drug therapy in the treatment. Ergotamine tartrate was not tried because of the impractical feature of giving it subcutaneously, as its effectiveness by mouth is rather dubious. It is quite possible that this is the type of case (hyperactivity of the sympathetics) that ultimately one would select for surgical treatment, whereas the other types may be treated medically. The other cases in the group of rectosigmoidal achalasia were all in patients who showed a failure of the rectosigmoidal apparatus to relax because of lack of proper inhibitory function of the parasympathetic system.

In a third type, showing no disturbance of the function of the rectosigmoidal apparatus by roentgenographic studies but where there was an obvious weakness in the expulsive musculature of the colon above the rectosigmoidal region, we felt that the disturbance was due to failure of the parasympathetics to initiate or maintain the expulsive mechanism (longitudinal muscle fibers) of the colon. The drug of selection here should be one which again acts exclusively on the parasympathetic system. Physostigmine would be the drug of choice, were it not too toxic. A physostigmine-like preparation was selected, prostigmine, which supposedly intensifies the action of acetylcholine at the terminations of the parasympathetic fibers. Acetylcholine is normally rapidly destroyed in the tissues by an esterase. Because physostigmine and prostigmine utilize in their own hydrolytic destruction much of the esterase that would otherwise be left free to destroy the minute amounts of acetylcholine constantly being liberated by the parasympathetics, there is a diversion of the esterase from the acetylcholine which allows it to accumulate in larger quantities and thus produce greater pharmacologic effects.[22] The single patient treated has made a very satisfactory response and has continued good bowel function on a gradually diminishing dosage of medication. The medication was given by mouth.

So far, we have encountered no cases where there has been overactivity of the sympathetic innervation of the colon above the rectosigmoidal apparatus. It is our impression, however, that this condition does exist and that there is a group of disturbances due to faulty balance of the autonomic innervation of the colon above the rectosigmoidal apparatus in which either parasympathetic or sympathetic elements are the offenders. It is possible that the classical types of atonic and spastic constipation belong to this group. Studies on these latter conditions are now being pursued with hope of determining their etiology from the standpoint of the neuromuscular mechanism.

We propose the following classification of the neurogenic disturbance resulting in megacolon with constipation, based on the reported experiences in the literature and on our own clinical studies:

1. Cases of rectosigmoidal achalasia: (a) Those caused by motor hyperactivity of the sympathetic innervation to the rectosigmoidal apparatus (cases which are not influenced by any known or tried medications); (b) those caused by ineffective inhibitory function of the parasympathetic innervation to the rectosigmoidal apparatus (cases which respond to parasympathetic paralysants).

2. Cases of deficient motor function of the innervation of the colon above the rectosigmoidal apparatus: (a) Those caused by deficient parasympathetic motor function (cases which respond to parasympathetic stimulants); (b) those caused by deficient sympathetic motor function.

Clinically, the two types of rectosigmoidal achalasia cannot be distinguished except after trial of appropriate drug therapy, as outlined above, but by barium enema study it is frequently possible to demonstrate whether or not there is rectosigmoidal spasm with or without delayed emptying of the colon. In cases of rectosigmoidal achalasia there is marked delay in emptying, whereas in the cases where there is deficient motor function on the part of the parasympathetics of the colon above the rectosigmoidal apparatus there is good emptying of the lower colon but retention of the barium in the upper colon.

Based on the above classification, we propose a selective form of treatment for each of the conditions classified. When x-ray interpretation makes it possible to establish that the rectosigmoidal apparatus is functioning, one should try prostigmine. If the rectosigmoidal apparatus is not functioning one tries first benzedrine sulfate and then syntropan. If there is no response to either of the latter drugs, we propose continuing the present surgical treatment of lumbar ganglionectomy and presacral resection, until more satisfactory selective drug action can be found.

COMMENT

In a review of the literature on megacolon with constipation, whether congenital or acquired, it is evident that the theories postulating a neurogenic origin of the condition have gained strong support from accumulated clinical and experimental evidence. This support was largely given by the development of a form of treatment consisting of lumbar sympathectomy and ganglionectomy. The recent advances in pharmacology and also in the studies of the autonomic nervous system have opened new avenues for attacking the problem of megacolon with drugs of the cholinergic and anticholinergic type. One cannot at this time be too dogmatic as to the anatomic or pharmacologic theories supporting the explanations given for the results obtained in the cases mentioned in this paper. However, the clinical results of effective bowel functioning must be considered as a strong argument in favor of the theories expressed. Many factors must be taken into consideration in the treatment of constipation with megacolon. Change of environment by placing patients under hospital routine and type of diet might be stressed by some as a deciding factor in establishing good bowel functioning. However, objection may be raised against this as being a factor in that most of the cases were observed in the hospital for a sufficiently long period without acquisition of good bowel function before treatment was started. One patient had been in the hospital for two observation periods of several weeks with no beneficial results.

Several points of interest should be mentioned. All of the cases studied showed the same symptoms, namely, severe constipation, usually bowel movement by enema only, abdominal distention, visible peristalsis, muscle atrophy of the abdominal wall, toxic symptoms, spastic or hypertonic anal sphincter, and x-ray findings of megacolon after barium enema.

After treatment, the majority of the cases did well on reduced dosage of medication, two patients no longer requiring any medication. It is quite possible that the drugs used have been beneficial in setting up acquired reflexes which are constantly at work regulating the bowel actions.

Neither surgical nor medical treatment sheds any light on the etiology of megacolon other than to demonstrate that it probably arises from an autonomic nervous system unbalance. Most probably the dilatation and hypertrophy of the colon, which constitute the characteristic morphology, are compensatory changes that arise in an attempt to remove the fecal content of the sigmoid.

SUMMARY

1. An attempt has been made to attack the problem of megacolon on the basis of neurogenic unbalance.

2. A classification of neurogenic disturbances resulting in megacolon with constipation has been proposed on the basis of barium enema study and a trial of appropriate drug therapy.

3. Surgical treatment of neurogenic megacolon is advisable for those cases where there is extreme overactivity of the sympathetic innervation to the rectosigmoidal apparatus.

4. Selective drug therapy has proved effective where neurogenic unbalance exists because of faulty inhibitory or motor function of the parasympathetic system.

ABSTRACTS OF CASES STUDIED

1. Cases of rectosigmoidal achalasia.

a. Those caused by motor hyperactivity of the sympathetic innervation to the rectosigmoidal apparatus.

CASE 1.—M. D., Babies Hospital, No. 525528, male, aged 10 years, was admitted Aug. 21, 1937, and discharged Dec. 5, 1937.

At the age of 2 or 3 weeks the mother noted that the child had become very constipated and rarely, if ever, had a normal bowel movement. He had been given an enema almost daily since then and for two months before admission, received along with various dietary measures directed at control of constipation, one tablespoonful of mineral oil each day and an oil enema every other night. His appetite was never good. His abdomen had always been prominent and changed its shape

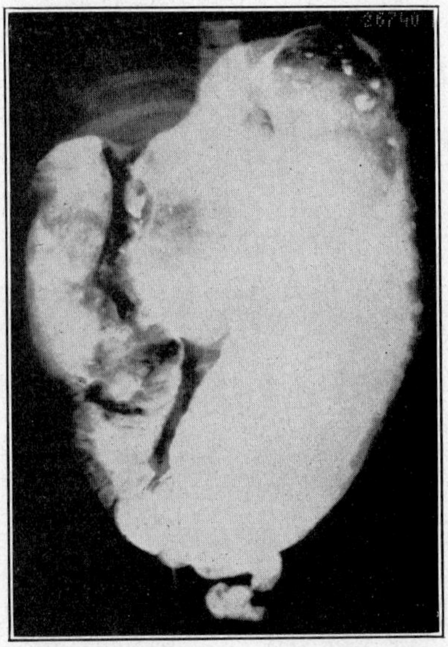

Fig. 2.—Case 1. Barium enema study made before operation. A case of hyperactivity of sympathetic innervation to rectosigmoidal junction resulting in tonic spasm of that region.

frequently. Five months before admission, at the age of 10, he had an attack of extreme constipation, with vomiting and abdominal distention, which required an operation for acute intestinal obstruction at the Hackensack Hospital. The type of operation performed was not determined.

The patient was started on syntropan by mouth and was given gradually increasing doses, receiving up to 165 mg. per day, but without any effect (Fig. 2).

He was operated on Nov. 13, 1937, having a presacral neurectomy done. He had his first bowel movement spontaneously on the sixth day after the operation. Six months later he was having daily bowel movements without help of any kind.

b. Those caused by lack of proper inhibitory function of the parasympathetic innervation of the rectosigmoidal apparatus.

CASE 2.—A. A., Babies Hospital, No. 403707, male, aged 27 months, was first admitted Dec. 29, 1933, at the age of 2 years and 3 months. He was discharged Jan.

19, 1934. He was admitted the second time on Jan. 28, 1937, at the age of 5 years and 4 months; he was discharged March 21, 1937.

The child had been constipated since birth; the bowels had never moved without either an enema or a cathartic and often even with these measures the patient would go a week without a satisfactory spontaneous movement. The stools then were unusually small and ribbonlike. The abdomen was always large. Vomiting would occur about every two weeks. His appetite had always been good. Examination showed a distended, protuberant abdomen and the transverse, descending, and sigmoidal colon were palpated. The internal sphincter was quite spastic.

Barium enema at the time the patient was 27 months old (Fig. 3) showed a greatly elongated and dilated sigmoid and colon; the rectum remained undilated. After twenty-two hours, a large amount of retention was present in the dilated and elongated sigmoid. The patient was then discharged as being too young to be operated upon. He was readmitted to the hospital on Jan. 28, 1937. He had been receiving a milk and molasses enema each evening for eighteen months after the time of his first discharge, and then a simple enema almost every night, but he never had a stool unaided by enema.

The patient was tried on benzedrine sulfate with no effect, receiving up to 10 mg. a day. Then he was placed on syntropan starting with 5 mg. by mouth, three times a day and gradually increasing up to 150 mg. a day, when satisfactory bowel movements were established. After his discharge from the hospital the dosage was gradually reduced to 50 mg. in the morning and 25 mg. in the afternoon, and at the present time he is maintained on 25 mg. once daily.

Barium enema after syntropan administration disclosed that the colon still was markedly dilated; it showed marked improvement in the emptying time, and the colon was free from barium after five hours.

CASE 3.—J. F., Babies Hospital, No. 517616, male, aged 8 months, was admitted June 4, 1937, and was discharged June 18, 1937.

There was a history of no spontaneous bowel movements since birth. After birth the abdomen was very distended and there was a very tight anal sphincter. A daily enema was given since birth, laxatives being ineffectual. If enemas were not given daily at first, distention would always result. Vomiting had occasionally been present. Rectal examination showed a constricted ring at the upper rectum. The abdomen was moderately distended and the sigmoid was easily outlined.

Barium enema showed megacolon of moderate degree (Fig. 4). Retention of the barium was still present after forty-eight hours.

The patient was started on syntropan, 5 mg. three times a day and the dosage was increased gradually to 18 mg. three times a day, when regular bowel function of three or four stools was established. Then the bowel movements became so frequent that the medication was reduced and then discontinued. Normal bowel function has continued up to this time.

CASE 4.—P. K., Babies Hospital, No. 510468, female, aged 8 years, was admitted Feb. 15, 1937, and discharged March 6, 1937.

There was a history of constipation since infancy. Vomiting had frequently occurred in the neonatal period and a pylorospasm was suspected. Constipation was so severe that enemas and mineral oil were used very frequently. She was subject to attacks of abdominal pain. The stools were ribbonlike. Barium enema showed an enormous increase in caliber and length of colon, the rectum being of normal size (Fig. 5). There was a constriction above the rectosigmoidal junction at the approximate level of the fourth lumbar vertebra.

She was started on benzedrine sulfate, receiving up to 17 mg. per day with no effect. Then she was placed on syntropan, and bowel function was established on a dosage of 25 mg. in the morning, 12.5 mg. at noon, and 25 mg. in the afternoon. Bowel function was maintained on an average dose of 50 mg. per day. Follow-up barium enema showed a dilated colon as before, but there was a markedly improved emptying time.

Fig. 3.

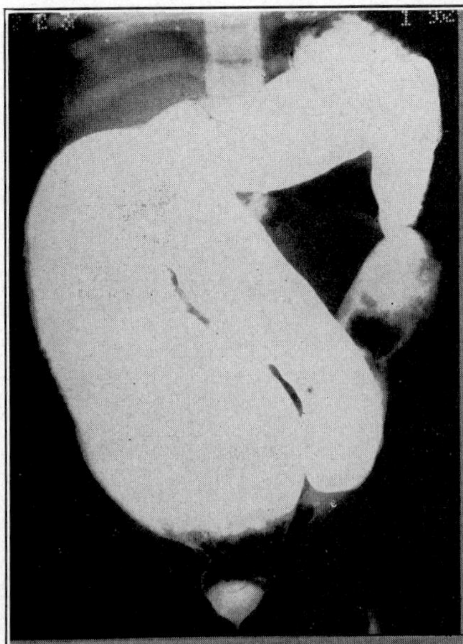

Fig. 4.

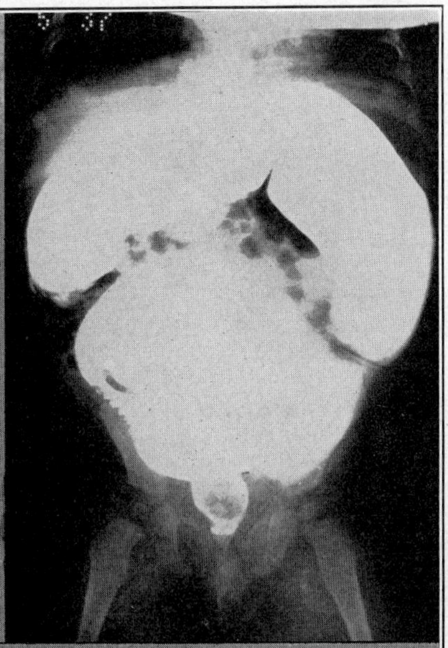

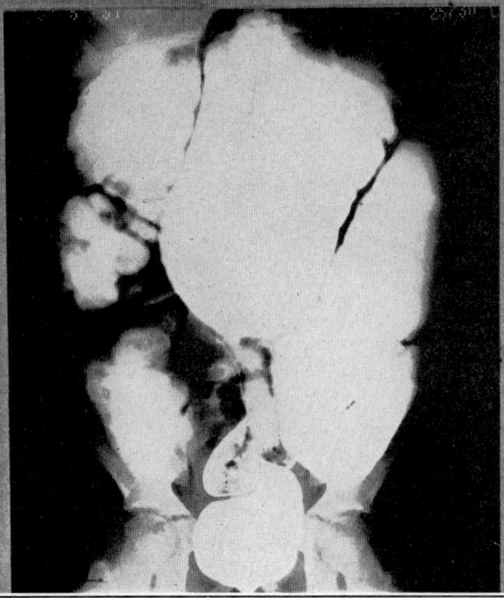

Fig. 5.

Fig. 3.—Case 2. Barium enema study made before treatment. A case of faulty inhibitory function of parasympathetic innervation to the rectosigmoidal region.

Fig. 4.—Case 3. Barium enema study made before treatment. A case of faulty inhibitory function of parasympathetic innervation to the rectosigmoidal region.

Fig. 5.—Case 4. Barium enema study made before treatment. A case of faulty inhibitory function of parasympathetic innervation to the rectosigmoidal region.

CASE 5.—M. W., Babies Hospital, No. 517596, male, aged 5 years, was admitted May 27, 1937, and discharged June 18, 1937.

The patient had been very constipated since birth and had never had a spontaneous bowel movement. Diets and medications had been tried and enemas were eventually relied upon. The stool had always been of small caliber. On one occasion he had been admitted to a hospital because of obstruction but was not operated upon. He had been receiving five tablets three times a day of 1/1000 grain of atropine and 5 ounces of olive oil per rectum each night, before coming to the hospital. Examination revealed a protuberant abdomen and easily palpated sigmoid and colon. It proved impossible to pass a proctoscope more than 5 cm. beyond the anal ring.

Barium enema revealed a marked elongation and dilatation of the colon above the rectosigmoidal region, extending for a short distance in the terminal portion of the sigmoid and giving the appearance of a rectal stenosis (Fig. 6).

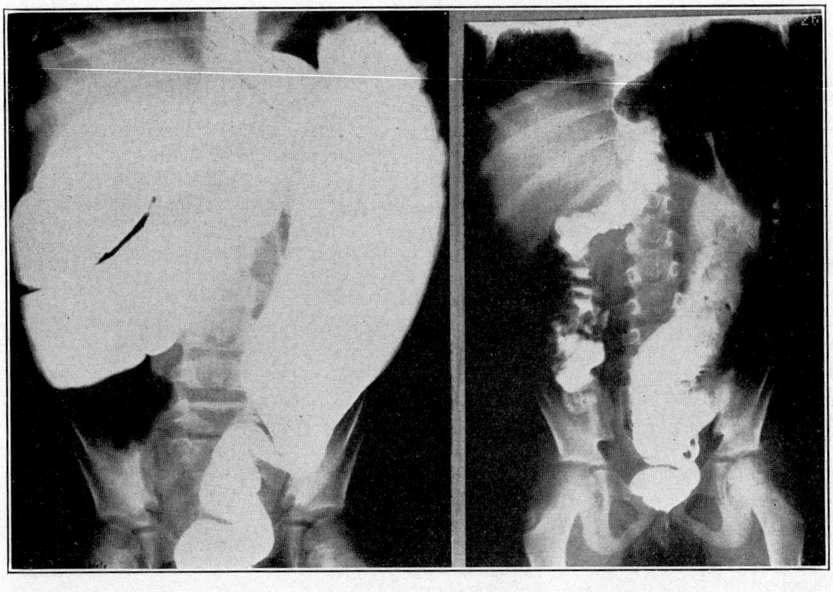

Fig. 6. Fig. 7.

Fig. 6.—Case 5. Barium enema study made before treatment was started. A case of faulty inhibitory function of the parasympathetic innervation to the rectosigmoidal region. The region of constriction here has the appearance of a stenosis.

Fig. 7.—Case 5. Barium enema study made after successful treatments with syntropan, showing improved emptying after the first defecation within an hour after barium enema was given.

He was started on syntropan by mouth, and at a dosage of 25 mg. three times a day regular bowel function was established and has persisted. A follow-up barium enema showed no significant changes in the outline of the bowel but good emptying of the colon (Fig. 7).

CASE 6.—F. D., outpatient, female, aged 14 years.

There was a history of severe constipation since birth, with no spontaneous bowel movements. Enema had been relied upon entirely at first with a trial of most of the cathartics and oils from time to time. Eventually a routine was established for an enema every other day. On some rare occasions, by taking cathartics, she had successful daily emptying for as long as four or five days.

Barium enema showed an enormously dilated sigmoid and descending colon with normal rectum (Fig. 8). The rectosigmoidal junction was stricturelike, and there was marked delay in emptying.

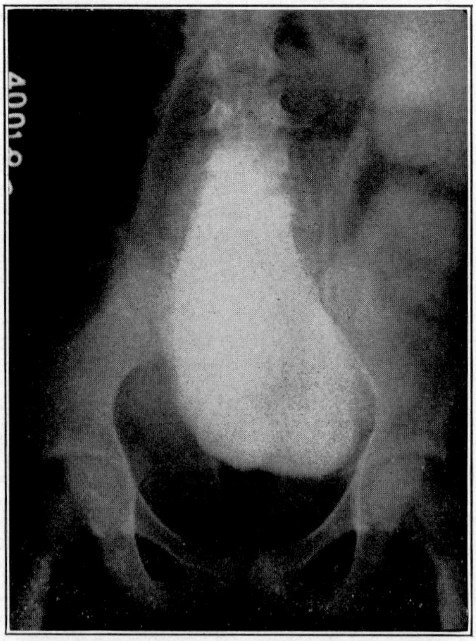

Fig. 8.—Case 6. Barium enema study made before treatment was started. A case of faulty inhibitory function of the parasympathetic innervation to the rectosigmoidal region.

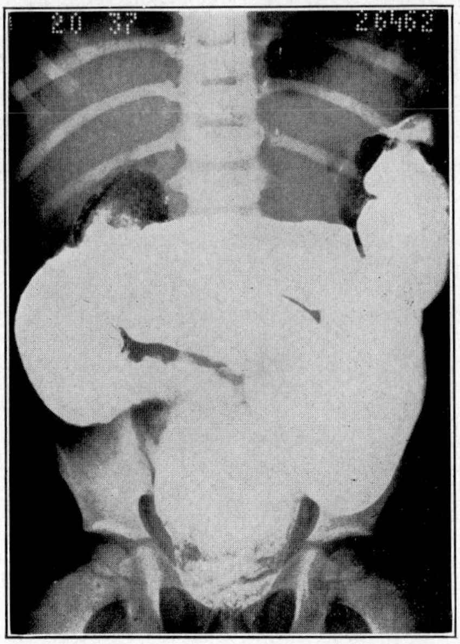

Fig. 9.—Case 7. Barium enema study made after treatment with prostigmine. A case of deficient parasympathetic motor function of the colon above the rectosigmoidal region.

The patient was placed on syntropan and became regulated as to bowel movements after reaching a dosage of 50 mg., three times a day. Barium enema taken three months after normal bowel function was established still showed the colon to be markedly enlarged but there was a distinct improvement in the emptying.

2. Case of deficient motor function of the parasympathetic innervation of the colon above the rectosigmoidal apparatus.

CASE 7.—C. Q., Babies Hospital, No. 517662, male, aged 3 years, was admitted June 21, 1937, and discharged July 20, 1937.

The patient had always been severely constipated and had seen many doctors from the age of 1 month on. Many laxatives and cathartics had been tried; finally soapsuds enemas and olive oil enemas were used. Spontaneous movements sometimes occurred on a day after enema and when Ex-lax had been given. The stool was always of large caliber and never of pencil form. Barium enema showed an elongated sigmoid, with good evacuation of the barium. The patient was started on prostigmine 5 mg. three times a day and increased by 2 mg. every two days. He became regular in his bowel movements after a dosage of 12 mg. three times a day was reached.

Follow-up barium enema one month later showed no appreciable change in the size of the transverse diameter of the large bowel and no evidence of delay or obstruction. The redundant sigmoid was present as before. A second follow-up barium enema four months after treatment was started (Fig. 9) showed elongated sigmoid as before and a satisfactory emptying of the colon, but no evidence of dilatation of the colon. The patient has been having two or three evacuations a day since leaving the hospital. The mother gradually reduced the dosage of prostigmine and when last seen she had discontinued it entirely and was giving small amounts of mineral oil only.

REFERENCES

1. Finnery, J. M. I.: Surg., Gynec. & Obst. **6**: 6, 1908.
2. Hirschsprung, H.: Jahrb. f. Kinderh. **27**: 1, 1888.
3. Hughes, W. E.: Tr. Philadelphia Path. Soc. **13**: 40, 1887.
4. Formad, H. F.: Tr. Philadelphia Path. Soc. **16**: 23, 1893.
5. Fraser, J.: Brit. M. J. **1**: 359, 1926.
6. Gaskell, W. H.: The Involuntary Nervous System, London, 1916, Longmans, Green & Co.
7. Sherrington, C. S.: Proc. Roy. Soc. London **40**: 411, 1896; Quart. J. Exper. Physiol. **2**: 109, 1909; Brain **39**: 191, 1915.
8. Royle, N. D.: M. J. Australia **1**: 77, 1924.
9. Bartle, H. J.: Am. J. M. Sc. **171**: 67, 1926.
10. Bayliss, W. M.: Principles of General Physiology, London, 1924, Longmans, Green & Co.
11. MacLeod, J. J. R.: Physiology and Biochemistry in Modern Medicine, St. Louis, 1922, The C. V. Mosby Company.
12. Langley, J. N.: Textbook of Physiology, Edited by E. A. Schaefer, **2**: 616, 1900.
13. Osler, W.: Arch. Pediat. **10**: 111, 1893.
14. Neugebauer, F.: Ergebn. d. Chir. u. Orthop. **17**: 598, 1913.
15. Duval, M.: Rev. de chir. **40**: 506, 1905.
16. Barrington-Ward, L.: Brit. J. Surg. **1**: 345, 1913-14.
17. Judd, E. S., and Adson, A. W.: Collected Papers of the Mayo Clinic **20**: 1928.
18. Rankin, F. W., and Learmonth, J. R.: Collected Papers of the Mayo Clinic **20**: 1928.
19. Berger, H. C.: M. Clinics N. America **7**: 1175, 1924.
20. Meyer, A. E.: Am. J. Dis. Child. **19**: 167, 1920.
21. Kuntz, A.: J. A. M. A. **106**: 345, 1936.
22. Loewi, O.: Arch. f. d. ges. Physiol. **237**: 504, 1936.
23. Myerson, A.: J. A. M. A. **110**: 101, 1938.

OBSERVATIONS ON CONGENITAL MEGACOLON

Geza de Takats, M.D., and Alfred D. Biggs, M.D.
Chicago, Ill.

Congenital megacolon, frequently referred to as Hirschsprung's disease, had been described by more than twenty authors before Hirschsprung's communication in 1886.[1] Nevertheless, he has popularized this clinical entity and has given a description of the disease to which little can be added today. Because of the rarity of the condition, reports of single or a few cases have appeared from time to time and have been ably summarized in collective reviews by Finney[2] in 1908, by Neugebauer[3] in 1913, by Fowler, Davidson, and Mellon[4] in 1922, and by Ask-Upmark[5] in 1930. A recent monograph of Pässler[34] brought the bibliography up to date.

In 30,000 autopsies in the London Hospital for Sick Children, Fenwick could find only three cases, an incidence of 1:10,000.[1] At a later date, R. C. Lightwood found that one in every 2,620 patients at the same institution suffered from megacolon.[6] In a general hospital, Walton found an incidence of four to 131,000. We found nine cases at St. Luke's Hospital in the years between 1931 and 1937, during which time 79,035 admissions occurred; this would give an incidence of 1:9000. Uniformly, the prevalence of males over females has been stressed, in a ratio of 3:1 to 5:1. Megacolon may be present at delivery; in fact it has been reported in a 7-month-old fetus (Von Ammon, 1842); but of 223 cases, reported by Patel, seventy-three were in adults. Corbin reports 200 cases from the Argentine among adults who have come under his personal supervision.[7] Whether these cases may be truly regarded as megacolon or simply are due to long sigmoid loops with atonic constipation is debatable. Our fifth, eighth, and ninth cases were in adults lacking a history of constipation in childhood.

Many theories have been advanced as to the causes of this disease, and we have summarized the most important ones in Table I. It is quite likely that several factors may contribute to this intractable hypertrophy and dilatation of the colon and that the etiology may vary. It is obviously important to study the etiology of the disease if we are to evolve logical and satisfactory methods of management. For this reason some clinical and experimental data which have a bearing on etiology must be discussed.

THE MECHANICAL FACTOR IN CONGENITAL MEGACOLON

While the original definition given by Hirschsprung really excludes all patients with a demonstrable rectal obstruction, nevertheless, cases

From the Department of Surgery, University of Illinois, College of Medicine and St. Luke's Hospital. Presented before the Chicago Pediatric Society, March 15, 1938.

TABLE I

POSSIBLE CAUSES OF MEGACOLON

TABULATION OF THE THEORIES ADVANCED	
A. Congenital Anomalies	*C. Other Causes*
Dilatation and hypertrophy (Hirschsprung)	Lymphangiectasis resulting in gigantism (Finney)
Dilatation and hypertrophy (Mya)	Chronic colitis (Walker and Griffith)
Hypertrophy, secondary dilatation (Fenwick)	Diastasis of rectus muscles (Levi)
Congenital defect (Bailey)	Atony associated with wasting disease (Griffith)
B. Mechanical Obstruction	*D. Neuromuscular Dysfunction*
Too long mesosigmoid (Barth)	Neuromuscular segmental defect (Formad, Hawkins)
Too long sigmoid loop (Marfan)	Segmental paralysis (Pennato)
Obstruction in terminal bowel (Treves, V. David)	Defective muscular tone (Murray)
Obstruction at Houston's valves (Perthes)	Lesion of sympathetic nerves (Bing)
Distention of colon by meconium (Wilkie)	Reflex spasm of sphincters (Fenwick)
	Failure of coordination (W. J. Mayo)
	Achalasia of terminal bowel (Hurst)
	Delay of inhibition (Fraser)
	Increased plastic tone (Royle)

presented by Treves,[8] Vernon David,[9] and Brenneman[10] amply demonstrate the importance of bearing an anorectal stricture in mind. One of our own patients (Case 2) had a diaphragmatic type of stricture one inch above the anocutaneous zone. In spite of daily dilatations, which finally resulted in a complete disappearance of the stricture, the megacolon progressed. Case 6 had an imperforate anus, which ultimately resulted in fecal incontinence.* In Brenneman's two cases, which came to autopsy after two weeks of dilatation, no trace of any diaphragm could be found at post mortem, nor could Dr. C. J. de Bere find any stricture by proctoscopic examinations in our patient a few weeks after birth. One wonders whether or not a tight sphincter might occasionally give the impression of a partial atresia and also whether in the presence of a true atresia the megacolon might not be due to a loss of reflexes from the anal canal.

A long sigmoid loop or a long mesentery of the sigmoid have been accused of being the causes of megacolon. True enough, some patients suffering from megacolon have abnormally long sigmoid loops; this was found also in six of our patients. But it must be stated that: (1) the elongation of the loop may be the result and not the cause of colonic stasis; (2) not all cases of megacolon have long sigmoid loops—Case 3 had a very short, spastic sigmoid loop; (3) there are many cases of dolichocolon (long sigmoid loop) seen in the x-ray department which have never given rise to colonic dilatation and hypertrophy or constipation.

The possibility of kinks and valvular mechanisms, especially at the sigmoid flexure, has been emphasized ever since the careful study of a colostomized patient by Perthes[11] in 1905. He found that while an

*This was true of a recently observed, tenth case, which is not reported here.

enema could easily pass the Houston valves from the rectum through the colostomy, nothing would pass in the opposite direction. Following division of the folds in the mucosa, marked improvement resulted. It is probable that these valvular mechanisms do play a role, but only after the colonic stasis and distention have become established. Hurst,[6] whose views on megacolon will be quoted repeatedly, believes that the pelvirectal sphincter of O'Beirne is a myth; but he does state that the three Houston valves, which are normally easily overcome by the gastrocolic reflex, may produce mechanical obstruction in the previously distended and kinked bowel.

The occurrence of a volvulus of the long and distended sigmoid loop has been reported; Case 2 showed such a partial volvulus on one admission, but high colonic enemas relieved it. Case 1 had a huge fecal impaction in a long sigmoid loop, which was resected.

Thus, it may be said that while mechanical factors may play an important role in the production of symptoms, and especially as secondary complications, there exists a group of cases in which the underlying, primary mechanism must be elsewhere.

CONGENITAL ANOMALIES

That megacolon is present at birth and sometimes in the fetus has been repeatedly reported. Most case histories, if carefully analyzed, reveal the fact that distention and intractable constipation were obvious in the first weeks after birth. Six of our cases give such a history. Other congenital anomalies, such as imperforate anus, pyloric stenosis, rectovaginal fistula, or bicornuate uterus, may be present. Case 6 had a transposition of the heart, lungs, and liver to the opposite side. The anomaly producing the disease was said by Hirschsprung, Mya, Fenwick, and Bailey to be a congenital dilatation and hypertrophy, but this, of course, does not explain the mechanism of its production. Other causes, such as lymphangiectasis resulting in gigantism, chronic colitis, diastasis or absence of the rectus muscles, and atony of the bowel, have been suggested but have not been generally accepted.

NEUROMUSCULAR DEFECT

That a segment of the colon, mostly the sigmoid, might be paralyzed or have a defective muscular tone has been advanced early among the theories of megacolon. Fenwick spoke of a spasm of the anal sphincter and hypertrophy of the colon proximal to the obstruction. Lately much interest has been focused on the role of the visceral motor mechanism in the production of megacolon. Hurst,[6] one of the most experienced clinicians in this field, who has seen thirty-two cases and studied them with great care, feels that megacolon is due to an absence of relaxation of the sphincter ani, when the normal colonic peristalsis reaches the rectum. This achalasia, which is analogous to the so-called cardiospasm, is not a rectal spasm, nor is there an overactivity of the sympathetic nervous system, but rather a diminished tonus of the sacral, parasympathetic outflow. Inflammatory reactions around the anus may produce such achalasia by degeneration of the Auerbach plexus. Thus the stimulus for the act of defecation is poorly transmitted (Brown[12]).

The theory of Hurst, which has been expressed by others as failure of coordination, delay of inhibition or neuromuscular dysfunction, has much experimental and clinical support. In the first place, it is obvious to anyone who has had the opportunity to study any of these children that the colon of the patient, in spite of its dilatation, is not paralyzed. In fact, vigorous and painful peristaltic movements are always seen, especially when the colon is hypertrophic. The intestinal obstruction of these patients has all the earmarks of a mechanical obstruction, and yet at autopsy no such obstruction can be found. The bowel then must be contracting, either against the closed sphincter, which fails to relax, or against a valvular obstruction or kink. When the sphincter is dilated manually or by systematic use of conic bougies, which are passed every morning and kept in for half an hour, improvement frequently results.[6]

The last theory, which was proposed by Wade and Royle,[13] postulates an increased postural or plastic tone of the bowel which is mediated by the sympathetic nervous system, just as in striated muscle. This principle, which was equally adapted to the treatment of spastic paralysis, has since been definitely shown to be incorrect; nevertheless, it opened a vast field for the surgery of the sympathetic nervous system. While the theory of the operation is not tenable, the results were surprising.

THE PERVERTED PHYSIOLOGY OF MEGACOLON

If, as emphasized in the above analysis of hypotheses, the lack of coordination between proximal and distal parts of the colon seems to be the most likely cause of the congenital primary megacolon, it seems profitable to summarize briefly the knowledge concerning the innervation of the distal colon. Peristalsis is a neuromuscular phenomenon dependent on a nervous reflex and subserved by the intrinsic plexuses of the gut. The upper set of lumbar nerves carries the sympathetic impulses, and the lower set of sacral nerves carries the parasympathetic fibers.[14] A diagram illustrates this extrinsic innervation (Fig. 1). Stimulation of the sympathetic outflow inhibits peristalsis; it also tightens the internal sphincter as observed in man by Learmonth,[15] who stimulated the presacral nerve by a faradic current. One of us has repeatedly observed that grasping the hypogastric plexus with a forceps will constrict the anus around the inserted finger. Parasympathetic stimulation, on the other hand, will increase peristalsis and relax the sphincter. Acetylcholine, prostigmine, or physostigmine act through these nerves. The third set of nerves is somatic; they are paralyzed in lesions of the cord or cauda equina.

Aside from animal experiments, in which Adamson and Aird were able to produce megacolon in cats by dividing the parasympathetic sup-

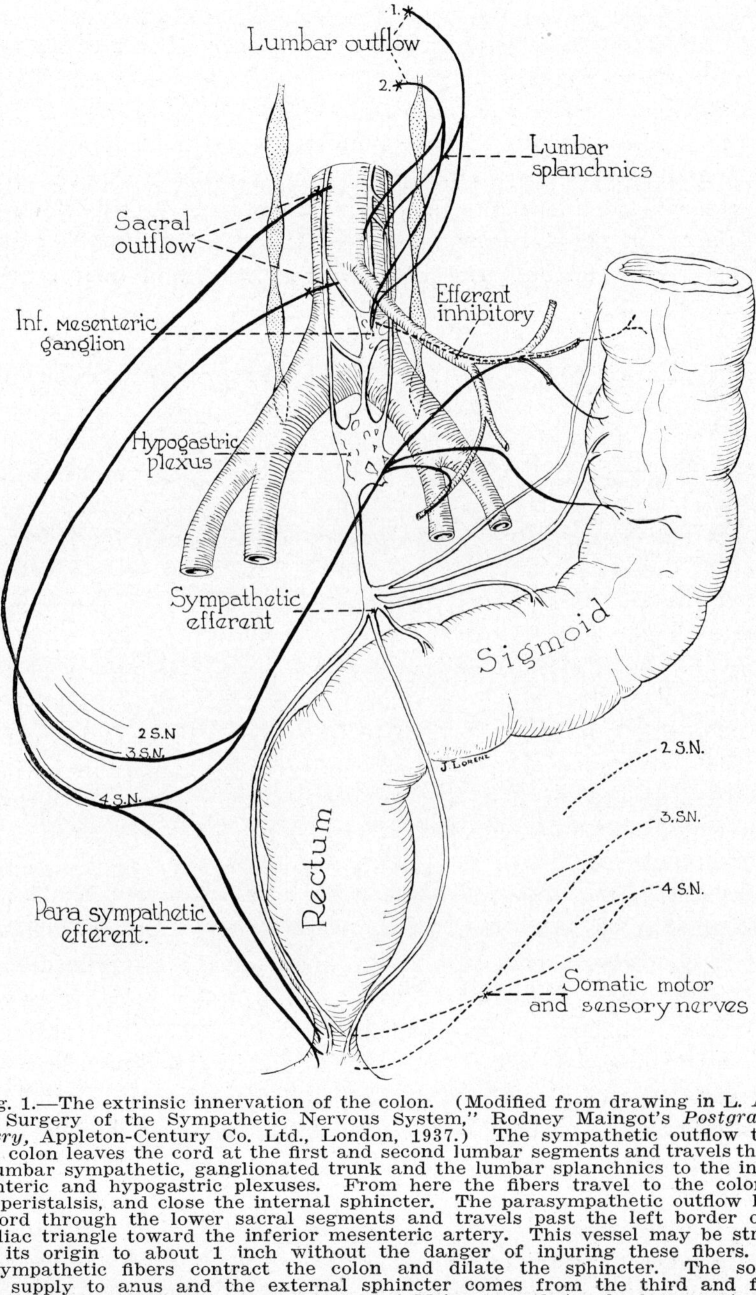

Fig. 1.—The extrinsic innervation of the colon. (Modified from drawing in L. Abel's "The Surgery of the Sympathetic Nervous System," Rodney Maingot's *Postgraduate Surgery*, Appleton-Century Co. Ltd., London, 1937.) The sympathetic outflow to the distal colon leaves the cord at the first and second lumbar segments and travels through the lumbar sympathetic, ganglionated trunk and the lumbar splanchnics to the inferior mesenteric and hypogastric plexuses. From here the fibers travel to the colon, inhibit peristalsis, and close the internal sphincter. The parasympathetic outflow leaves the cord through the lower sacral segments and travels past the left border of the interiliac triangle toward the inferior mesenteric artery. This vessel may be stripped from its origin to about 1 inch without the danger of injuring these fibers. The parasympathetic fibers contract the colon and dilate the sphincter. The somatic nerve supply to anus and the external sphincter comes from the third and fourth sacral segment. The intramural plexuses of Meissner and Auerbach are not shown in the diagram. This failure to convey a normal impulse for defecation has been one of the theories of megacolon.

ply to the colon,[16] and Burrows, by irritating the lumbar sympathetic ganglia with silica,[17] there are a number of observations on man to illustrate the effect of the two antagonistic sets of nerves. Thus, patients suffering from peripheral vascular disease, in whom lumbar sympathectomies are done frequently, show increased peristalsis as a result of a release from sympathetic inhibition. In patients with cauda equina lesions, in whom the lumbar sympathetic outflow is intact but the sacral parasympathetic outflow is destroyed, the rectal sphincter is usually patulous, the sensation of the lower rectum is lost, and the capacity for storage and thus for massive bowel movements is absent. Such a patient passes small fecal masses at frequent intervals. When all extrinsic nerves are lost, peristalsis in the gut continues satisfactorily, and even continence may be slowly restored. Obviously none of these conditions exist in megacolon.

The unquestionably favorable effects of sympathectomy in cases of megacolon have been explained by (1) diminution of plastic tone of the colon,[13] (2) allowing the weakened pelvic parasympathetic nerves to exert their action unopposed by the antagonistic sympathetic innervation, and (3) the release of a reflex sympathetic inhibition.[14] From a physiologic standpoint, this latter explanation seems the most probable. Be that as it may, it is easy to show that in man as well as in the animal, the section of the sympathetic nerve supply to the distal colon results in a release of inhibition and often in a massive defecation with a relaxation of the sphincter ani.

One final point should be made, which has a bearing on prognosis and emphasizes the urgency of combating persistent colonic distention with all available measures, and that is the unfavorable effect of maximal distention on the bowel. These effects have been summarized with the addition of many original contributions in the recent monograph of Wangensteen on intestinal obstruction.[18] The gaseous content of the bowel after obstruction of the sigmoid colon contains small amounts of O_2 and CO_2 but an overwhelming amount of nitrogen (80 per cent). We shall return to this point in our therapeutic suggestions. The other effect is the diminution of blood flow when intracolonic pressure rises. This pressure may rise from 12 to 52 cm. of water, which may exert, as Wangensteen has calculated, around 735 cm. of water pressure per centimeter surface in the cecum to 340 cm. in the descending colon. The frequency with which perforation occurs in the cecum in late or neglected cases of obstruction is immediately apparent because of the different amount of stress exerted on different segments of the bowel.

Increased intracolonic pressure influences absorption from the bowel. Absorption through the veins, through the lymphatics, and transperitoneally is greatly modified following distention. Lymphatic absorption of dyes or bacteria is greatly enhanced by obstruction. One of us has encountered large lymph channels and lymph nodes in explorations for megacolon, and this finding may explain Finney's theory of lymphangiectasis in cases of megacolon. That these patients are toxic, dehydrated, and anemic is sufficiently known and should be remembered in outlining treatment.

DIAGNOSIS

The diagnosis of megacolon, except in early infancy, is easy and depends on the three cardinal symptoms of obstinate constipation, marked enlargement of the abdomen, and visible peristalsis. Spontaneous bowel movement is rare, and sometimes weeks may go by without evacuation. Periods of constipation may be followed by diarrhea, which may persist in spite of massive fecal impaction.

The abdomen may assume tremendous proportions especially in the upper part above the navel. The skin is thin and shiny. Tympanitic sounds are obtained, but occasionally large fecal masses may be palpated and percussed. No free fluid is present. Deep peristaltic waves are often visible, and gurgling sounds may be heard with or often without the stethoscope. The sigmoid colon is often redundant, and the loop may be visible even under the right lobe of the liver. The abdominal distention compresses the contents of the chest. The costal arches are widely separated, the diaphragm is high, the heart and lungs are pushed up, interfering with respiration and circulation. Because of the poor intake and utilization of food and liquids, the child is emaciated and dehydrated. A marked secondary anemia is often present. Sudden complications may occur in the form of ulcerations, perforation of the bowel, or volvulus of the sigmoid loop, which may cause death of the child unless promptly recognized.

In the neonatal period the diagnosis may be difficult. However, the abdomen is large and close observation will usually reveal peristaltic waves. Diarrhea may alternate with constipation, or diarrhea may predominate for the first few weeks of life, as in Case 2. Persistent vomiting during the first weeks of life is likely to occur.

This condition should not be confused with any other. However, at times congenital duodenal obstruction, early cases of celiac disease, tuberculous peritonitis, or rickets must be considered. Mechanical obstruction of the bowel should be ruled out by digital or proctoscopic exploration of the rectum. A thin barium mixture, slowly instilled under fluoroscopic control, gives an idea of the size and location of the distended loops and helps to rule out congenital strictures or bands. For a satisfactory barium enema the colon should be as thoroughly evacuated as possible. In older children a barium meal gives a better idea of the amount of stasis than the enema. The barium, however, should be diluted with equal amounts of petrolagar and may have to be evacuated with some of the parasympathetic drugs or with spinal anesthesia.

From the study of some of our cases appearing in adult life, the conclusion must be drawn that congenital megacolon may exist in a latent, symptomatic stage for many years, during which time the neuromuscular dysfunction is compensated and spontaneous bowel movements are possible. In spite of this the anatomic changes may be quite extensive (Case 9).

MEDICAL MANAGEMENT

In undertaking the medical management of congenital megacolon one has to assume that congenital strictures of the rectum are absent or, should they be demonstrable, have been dilated by daily digital dilatations which can be carried out after proper instructions to the child's mother or nurse. These strictures, as reported by Vernon David[9] and by Brennemann,[10] are situated from 1 to 2 cm. above the anus. Occasionally they must be divided surgically. It must be emphasized, however, that megacolon may persist or even progress after the removal of these obstructions, and this occurred in Case 1 of our series. Five such cases were reported by Judd and Thompson.[19]

Rectal dilatations have been systematically employed by Hurst,[6] who uses increasing sizes of conic bougies in order to induce better relaxation of the internal sphincter. That this is of great value is best demonstrated by our experience with Cases 2 and 3, both of whom have always experienced weeks of relief following manual disimpaction of the rectum. This procedure carried out under a general anesthetic naturally dilates and stretches the sphincter and may even lead to a short period of incontinence.

A number of various diametrically opposed measures have been advocated to facilitate the emptying of the colon. Some authors advocate a rough, high residue diet to promote peristalsis, others order a bland diet so that fecal accumulation may be reduced. Some urge the elimination of animal protein to decrease putrefaction, while others prescribe a buttermilk diet. Some advise abdominal massage, and others disapprove for fear of perforating a thin colon. Some push carbohydrates to restore liver glycogen, and others are afraid of increasing fermentation. Some give cathartics; others feel that they are useless, may bring an impaction, and favor ulceration in the colon.

Equal, if not more numerous, are the suggestions for drug therapy. Atropine has been given in large doses with the idea of relaxing the spasm of the sphincter; so have opium and papaverine. Saturated solutions of magnesium sulfate have been used for rectal instillations which, according to Bonar,[20] irritate the local neuromuscular mechanism. Hot tap water enemas have been found useful by Fridell.[18] Pancreatic, insulin-free tissue extract[21] and parathormone[22] have been found to empty the distended colon under roentgenologic control. The parasympathetic drugs, such as pilocarpine, eserine, prostigmine, and acetylcholine, have been employed. The latter drug is highly advocated by Abel[23] for improving atonic constipation or postoperative ileus.

Of all these suggestions the use of high, warm colonic irrigations, the administration of mineral oil, systematic rectal dilatations, and a well-balanced diet, avoiding extremes of high or low residue, seem logical. Obviously in case of acute obstruction or as a preoperative measure, the low residue diet is preferable. When, however, with the aid of enemas and mineral oil, fairly regular evacuations have been obtained, a certain amount of roughage may be of advantage. We have seen help from small doses (1/150 gr.) of eserine administered with mineral oil, especially following sympathectomy, when such a parasympathetic drug can act without the opposition of sympathetic influence on the bowel.

In studying the possible effect of sympathetic denervation on the emptying of the bowel, spinal anesthesia has been advocated as a preoperative test.[24] It has also been noted that sometimes spinal anesthesia alone will restore functional activity for many weeks and months. Such a case has been reported by Stebins, Morton, and Scott.[25]

The indications for medical management may be briefly summarized as follows: (1) in an effort to minimize distention of the bowel and prevent nutritional changes in all infants and children up to the age of 3 years; (2) in all mild and latent cases, even after that age, if response to treatment is satisfactory and the child is growing normally; (3) as a preoperative measure, once it is recognized that the case is not medically tractable. Obviously this is the point on which most pediatricians and surgeons have disagreed in the past, all the more as the mortality of bowel resections and the frequent recurrences did not encourage pediatricians to refer their cases to surgery. With the introduction of sympathectomies in the treatment of megacolon, many of the objections against surgery will have to be revised.

We also feel that most cases of atonic constipation with long, redundant sigmoid loops, seen in adults, do not really belong to the category of congenital megacolon. Spinal anesthesia does not evacuate this colon well, and it is held by Learmonth[26] that sympathectomy is not indicated. Skillful medical management may relieve constipation. Adson,[31] however, has recently reported an excellent result in one case of adult atonic constipation by the use of splanchnic nerve section and upper lumbar sympathectomy.

SURGICAL TREATMENT

As Rankin[27] has pointed out, in deciding between medical and surgical measures, three important factors must be considered, namely, the extent of the lesion, the age of the patient, and the presence or absence of obstruction. Obviously there are many constipated children, in some of whom the x-ray may reveal anatomic anomalies such as undescended cecum, mobile cecum, and redundant sigmoid loop, who are readily treated with simple training and medical measures. Learmonth[26] has recently studied material from the Royal Hospital for Sick Children in Aberdeen and feels that in constipated children, in whom there is an elongated and distended colon, in whom medical measures do not result in satisfactory evacuation, and in whom a barium meal reveals an intractable colonic stasis, a neurologic operation is indicated. We shall refer to the various types of sympathectomy later.

The age of the patient often contraindicates anything but emergency surgery. In our series the youngest child operated on was 5 years old, but surgical procedures have been reported at an earlier age. Obviously, in infants colonic distention must be combated with conservative measures, in spite of which they may succumb (Case 4). Whether in the future a combination of oxygen inhalations,[28] parasympathetic drugs, and continuous colonic suction will be effective in the refractory cases in infants remains to be seen. We would hardly advise surgery of any sort before 4 years of age.

TABLE II

MORTALITY STATISTICS FOLLOWING CONSERVATIVE AND SURGICAL TREATMENT EXCLUSIVE OF SYMPATHECTOMY

AUTHOR	NUMBER OF CASES	MORTALITY FOLLOWING	
		CONSERVATIVE TREATMENT PERCENTAGE	SURGICAL TREATMENT PERCENTAGE
Danziger	94	75	34
Lowenstein	2	88	22
Schmidt	119	60	40
Neugebauer	254	68	5
Schneiderlöhn	268	79	52
Judd and Thompson	42	19	23
Ask-Upmark	102	37	52

The presence of acute intestinal obstruction produced usually by volvulus of the elongated sigmoid loop may call for an immediate operation. Untwisting of the volvulus with or without ileostomy, appendicostomy, or cecostomy is imperative and may be lifesaving. Most of the acute intestinal obstructions, however, are relieved by high colonic irrigations.

Before the advent of sympathectomies for megacolon, difference in mortality following medical and surgical management was very slight. We have summarized some of the older statistics not containing sympathectomies in Table II. The last review of Ask-Upmark was based on 102 cases collected from Swedish hospitals between 1895 and 1928. Some of the patients have been followed for as long as twenty-five years. Because of these and other statistics both pediatricians and surgeons have been reluctant to advocate surgical procedures removing parts of or the entire colon. Many years ago Von Eiselsberg stated that one should either resect the colon or close up the abdomen, as sidetracking operations seemed of no avail. In a recent report on colonic resections for Hirschsprung's disease, Laqua[29] stated that the immediate mortality of one-stage resections was 25 per cent; that of several stage resections was 6 per cent.

The disconcerting phase of colonic resections, however, should not be the immediate mortality. With adequate preparation, multiple-stage operations and extensive resections are well tolerated, especially in children. However, a progressive dilatation of the segment, proximal to the resection, has been reported too often to be ignored. Even when the entire colon was removed, the dilatation extended to the ileum.[6] Our Case 1 showed this kind of secondary dilatation following resection of the sigmoid loop.

We do not wish to imply that colonic resections have no place in the treatment of megacolon for the reason that even when medical therapy or sympathectomy have been successful, the elongated, redundant sigmoid loop with its occasional kinking and twisting may produce attacks of acute intestinal obstruction. Case 2 illustrates this point because after a successful sympathectomy, which resulted in daily spontaneous bowel movements, two attacks of partial volvulus have so far occurred. Under such circumstances the resection of the redundant sigmoid loop may prevent a great deal of future trouble. In Case 1 the resection was well tolerated, but the megacolon still persists.

We now come to the indications and results of sympathectomy in congenital megacolon. The operation was first done for this condition in 1927 by Wade and Royle,[13] who did a lumbar ramisection. During the last ten years several modifications of the original operation have been described. While Learmonth and Rankin have attacked the presacral nerve and inferior mesenteric plexus,[15] Judd and Adson[30] used a lumbar sympathectomy, and lately Adson[31] suggested for severe cases the resection of the splanchnic nerves and two upper lumbar sympathetic ganglia. While both procedures interrupt the sympathetic fibers to the colon, both have effects on other organs. The Learmonth operation abolishes the contraction of the seminal vesicles and thus produces sterility in the male, although orgasm is present. The lumbar sympathectomy, if done high enough, will not affect ejaculation, but denervates both lower extremities so that they become hot and dry. In our experience this produces no discomfort or disadvantage. Finally, Telford and Stopford[32] devised the section of the medial branches of the lumbar sympathetic nerves, which avoids sterility in the male and vasoparalysis in the lower extremities. This is undoubtedly the optimal type of operation, although for a thorough denervation the lumbar sympathectomy seems preferable.

Morton and Scott[24] have made a very important contribution to the selection of the suitable cases for sympathectomy. They proposed the use of spinal anesthesia to inhibit the sympathetic outflow to the colon and demonstrated the evacuation of the colon under the anesthetic. We have made use of this test in Case 2. However, in Case 3, a nervous, anxious child, it was impossible to get a satisfactory spinal tap, and hence, instead of inhibiting the sympathetics, we resorted to stimulating the pelvic parasympathetic outflow. This was done with an ampule of prostigmine given subcutaneously, but acetylcholine could be used equally well.[31*] In this case the response was only slight owing to the loss of contractile power of the colon, demonstrated later at operation.

In studying the musculature of the colon in Hirschsprung's disease, it becomes evident that while some cases show marked muscular hypertrophy (Cases 1, 2, and 4), some patients come to the autopsy table or are seen on the operating table (Case 3) with extreme thinning-out of the colonic wall and a complete loss of the musculature.

Whether this is a congenital defect or a result of exhaustion, muscular decompensation, and nutritional effect of constant distention, is difficult to say. But the fact remains that when the muscle power of the colon is lost, no type of sympathectomy can help, nor can rectal dilatations be of any avail. The urgency of decompressing the colon from early infancy is obvious. Our second patient, with hypertrophy of the musculature and prompt response to a spinal anesthetic, made a far more spectacular recovery after sympathectomy than the third patient, who responded poorly to prostigmine and showed a thin transparent membrane instead of a hypertrophied colon.

The results of sympathectomy for megacolon have been very promising. Provided suitable cases are selected and aftertreatment is scrupulously carried out, it offers today the best method of regulating defecation and avoiding future complications.

The preoperative evacuation of the colon is important. The patient is placed on a low residue diet with daily high enemas, mineral oil, and acetylcholine. It may take two weeks to get the colon comparatively empty. In case of fecal impaction, the rectum is dilated under general or spinal anesthesia. In a maximally distended colon, the inhalation of 95 per cent oxygen may be helpful.[28] As the children are often dehydrated, toxic, and anemic, dextrose given intravenously and blood transfusion diminish the surgical risk. While both of our sympathectomies have been done in one stage, it might be advantageous occasionally to operate in two stages by an extraperitoneal route.[31] The mortality of sympathectomies is small. Adson[31] reported two deaths following the operation. Compared with colonic resection it is a harmless procedure.

Following operation, we have placed these children on a general diet, mineral oil, and physostigmine (gr. 1/150, three times a day). They were urged to move their bowels right after breakfast. The training

*In a recent case the response to acetylcholine was used for a preoperative test.

of this habit is usually absent in these patients. Hot enemas must be kept up daily until the contractile power of the colon is regained. In Case 2 this occurred a few weeks after operation; in Case 3, only six months later. Even so, sudden impactions or incomplete volvulus may occur (Case 2).

Because the operation has only been practiced for the last ten years, it is difficult to obtain late results. Up to date over 100 sympathectomies have been performed for megacolon, but late results are not available.[34] In our own work forty-eight lumbar sympathectomies performed for other reasons resulted in one death, a mortality of 2 per cent. The best follow-up studies were presented by Ross,[33] who reviewed the end re-

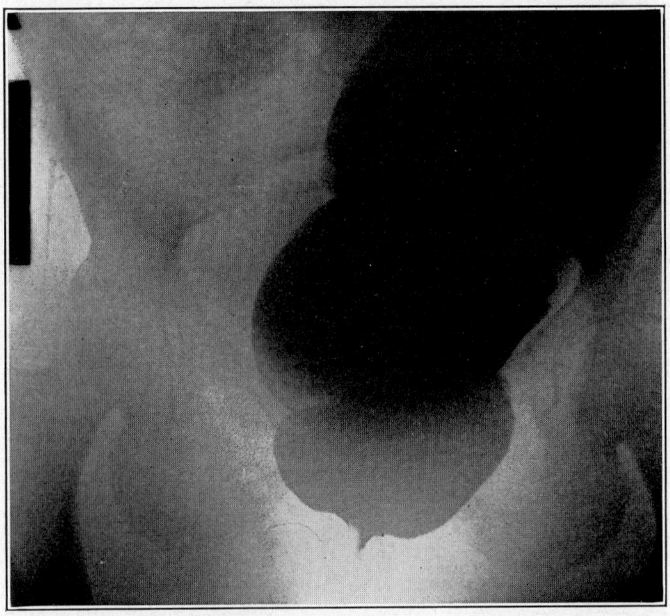

Fig. 2.—Case 1. Barium enema six years following resection of the sigmoid loop. Note the huge rectal ampulla and rectosigmoid loop.

sults in seventeen cases done by the Fellows of the Association of Surgeons of Great Britain. Fifteen of these operations were completely successful, and in the other two, the condition of the patients was much improved. Generally speaking, when early results were good the benefit seemed to be lasting.

CASE HISTORIES

CASE 1.—C. S., 17-year-old girl, entered St. Luke's Hospital on April 6, 1931, complaining of belching, distention, and inability to move bowels spontaneously.

Past History.—At age of 6 years the patient was operated on for intestinal obstruction, and again at 11 years of age. Following that she had to have cathartics and enemas daily.

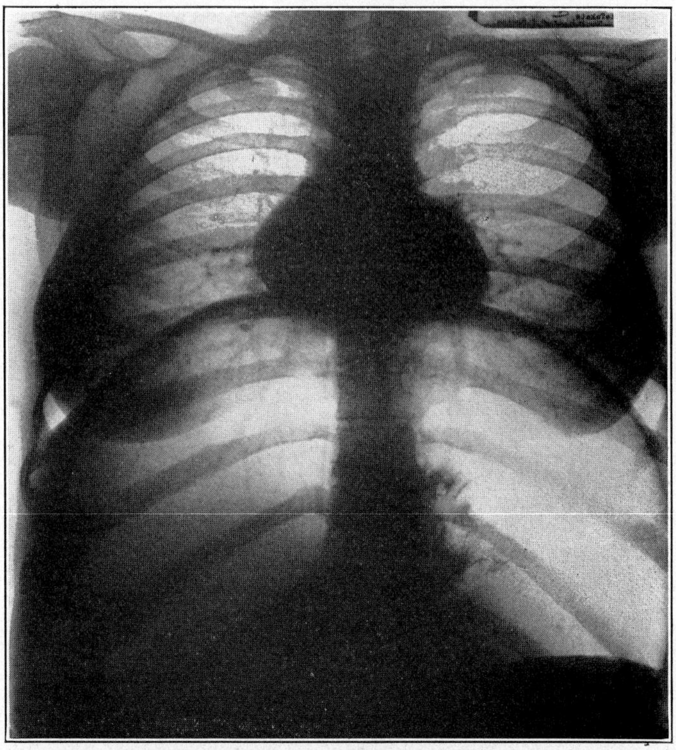

Fig. 3.—Case 1. Flat plate six years following partial colectomy. Note the high diaphragm, the compression of the chest and the pressure on the heart, increasing its transverse diameter.

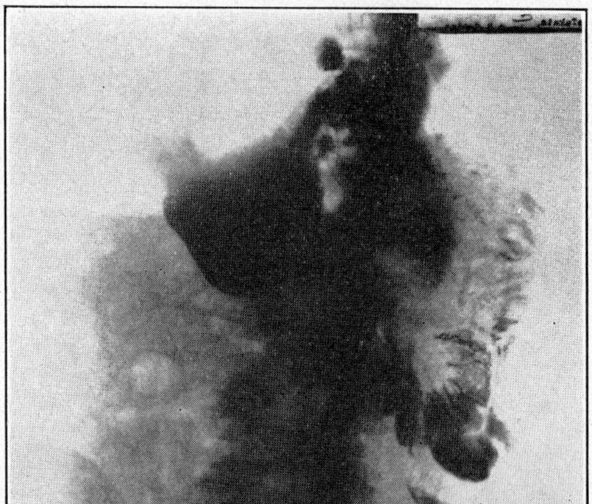

Fig. 4.—Case 1. Five-hour gastric residue. This patient had frequent attacks of nausea and upper abdominal distress without a demonstrable organic obstruction.

Examination revealed an emphysematous chest, a right rectus scar, and a symmetrical, right-sided distention which would partially disappear after belching and passing flatus. There were no abnormal points of tenderness. A neurologic examination was negative. X-ray examination revealed an enormous dilatation of undetermined portions of the bowel.

Operation on April 24, 1931, by Dr. L. L. McArthur revealed an enormously dilated sigmoid loop, which was resected. The small bowel and the rest of the colon were not distended. An end-to-end anastomosis restored the continuity of the bowel. The resected bowel weighed 12 lbs. 14 oz. It had the shape of a huge U-shaped

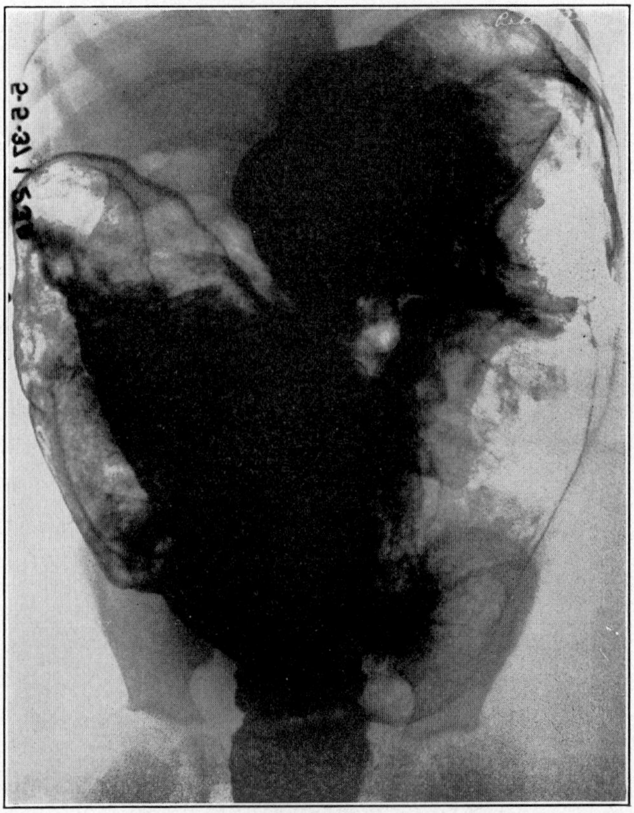

Fig. 5.—Case 2. Barium enema before spinal anesthesia. Note the elongated sigmoid loop extending to the right hypochondrium. There is an acute angle at the sigmoid flexure, below which the sigmoid is narrow, and above which the bowel is dilated.

sausage. The individual arms were 40 and 30 cm. long. The longer arm had a diameter of 15 cm. the smaller, 9.5 to 9.8 cm.

The postoperative course was uneventful. She left the hospital on the eighteenth day. Six years later, on Aug. 19, 1937, she was readmitted, 8 months pregnant, and was greatly troubled with distention and emesis since onset of pregnancy. Enemas and knee-chest position slightly relieved the distention. A month later a normal spontaneous delivery followed. X-ray pictures taken on Oct. 9, 1937, five weeks after delivery, revealed a sigmoid and descending colon of normal caliber; at the splenic flexure the colon suddenly lost its tone and dilated to four to five times its normal size. At no point was there an obstruction (Figs. 2, 3 and 4).

Summary.—Patient with congenital megacolon was operated on twice for intestinal obstruction; sigmoid loop was resected in 1931, there was a normal delivery in 1937. Colon shows progressive dilatation above site of anastomosis. A sympathectomy is being considered.

CASE 2.—R. P., boy, was born at St. Luke's Hospital on Jan. 27, 1932, somewhat cyanotic and with a distended abdomen. He vomited since birth; atropine and a special milk formula were of little avail. The greater portions of the feeding were returned. On Feb. 14, 1932, Dr. L. L. McArthur made the diagnosis of a megacolon and felt that sympathectomy was indicated. At first, digital dilatation of the rectum was practiced several times a day, later less frequently. Three weeks after birth,

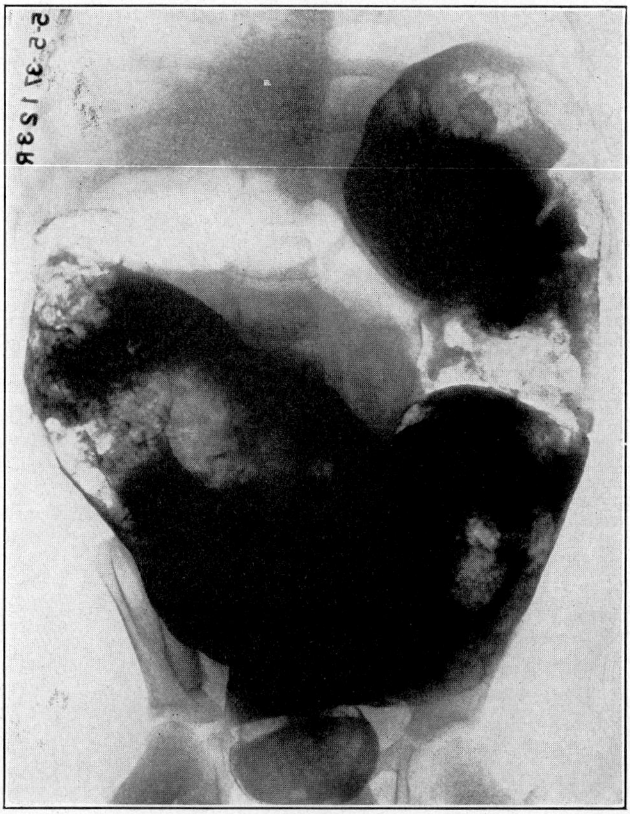

Fig. 6.—Case 2. Barium enema one-half hour after spinal anesthesia had been induced. Note the contraction of the right half of the transverse colon, the smaller diameter of the descending colon, and the proximal loop of the sigmoid. The distal loop is spastic. The child evacuated much of the barium on the fluoroscopic table.

the infant's weight dropped from 8 pounds and 3 ounces to 7 pounds and 11 ounces. At this time a fibrous ring was discovered about an inch above the anus, which constricted the tip of the fifth finger. However, rectal examination by Dr. de Bere showed a normal anus and rectum on March 15, 1932. The patient was discharged in an improved condition on March 19, 1933, and was on a Carnation milk diet. There was still diarrhea, but no vomiting. Attempts to obtain a visualization of the rectum and colon were unsuccessful.

Second admission occurred on Dec. 6, 1932, at the age of 10 months. In the interval rectal dilatations were done daily and later were reduced to once every two weeks. Three days before admission the child refused to eat, and vomited; the abdomen had become distended and marked peristaltic waves were visible. The child was pale and emaciated. Tap water, peroxide enemas, and suppositories being of no avail, the fecal impaction was removed through a proctoscope followed by enemas. A barium enema showed a great deal of distention in the colon, especially on the right side. He was discharged and placed on a low residue diet.

Third admission was on May 14, 1934, at the age of 2 years and 4 months, for persistent constipation. A barium enema at this time revealed a colonic dilatation, especially of the transverse colon. Repeated enemas gave temporary relief.

Fourth admission, Oct. 5, 1934, revealed the same status. Bowel movement occurred only after enemas. The patient had had an acute respiratory infection.

Fifth admission was on April 3, 1935, at the age of 3 years and 1 month. He had been getting a tap water enema every second day; his bowels had never moved

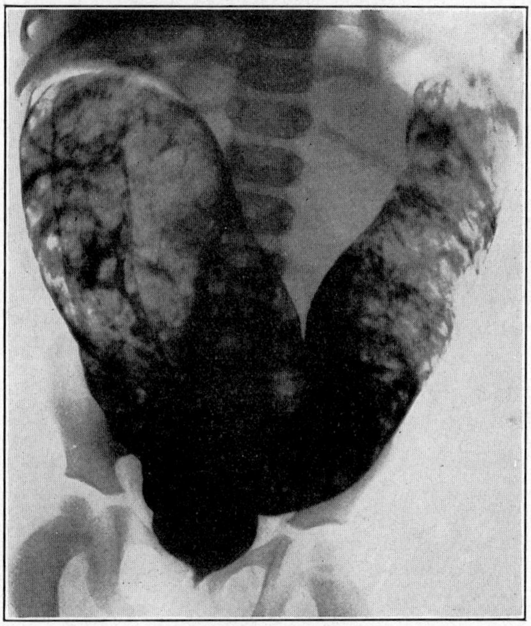

Fig. 7.—Case 2. Barium enema one month after bilateral lumbar sympathectomy and resection of the inferior mesenteric and superior hypogastric plexuses. The colon has much better tonus, the diameter has markedly decreased. The elongated sigmoid loop is in evidence. Again the sharp angulation of the sigmoid loop causing a secondary mechanical obstruction is obvious.

spontaneously. Three days prior to admission he began to vomit. Oil and hot water enemas relieved the impaction.

Sixth admission occurred on April 23, 1937, at the age of 5 years. He had in the meantime been to the County Hospital for another episode, and there developed scarlet fever. He re-entered County Hospital in January, 1937, where he stayed for more than two months. At this entrance the rectum was again disimpacted, but manually. Fluoroscopic observation indicated a definite angulation of the sigmoid in the right upper quadrant, a markedly redundant sigmoid loop, and a dilatation of the large bowel extending throughout the colon. Following a spinal injection of 35 mg. of novocain, there resulted a massive evacuation of the bowel with a diminution of the size of the colon (Figs. 5 and 6). Sympathectomy was suggested, but because of the redundant and angulated sigmoid loop, it was thought that an anastomosis between the cecum and sigmoid might become necessary.

On May 20, 1937, a bilateral lumbar sympathectomy and presacral nerve section were performed by one of us (G. de T.). The small intestine was collapsed. The entire large intestine was tremendously hypertrophic and dilated. The sigmoid loop was abnormally long with a long mesentery, and it angulated in the right upper quadrant. The abdominal wall was closed with silk. There was remarkably little postoperative reaction. A month later a barium enema showed a much smaller diameter of the colon (Fig. 7). The child still needed enemas twice a week. Three months later the patient's abdomen was flat, but he still had spells of retention. The sphincter was quite relaxed.

On Nov. 18, 1937, the patient was readmitted to the hospital because of vomiting, diarrhea, and sore throat. The abdomen was greatly distended, and visible peristalsis

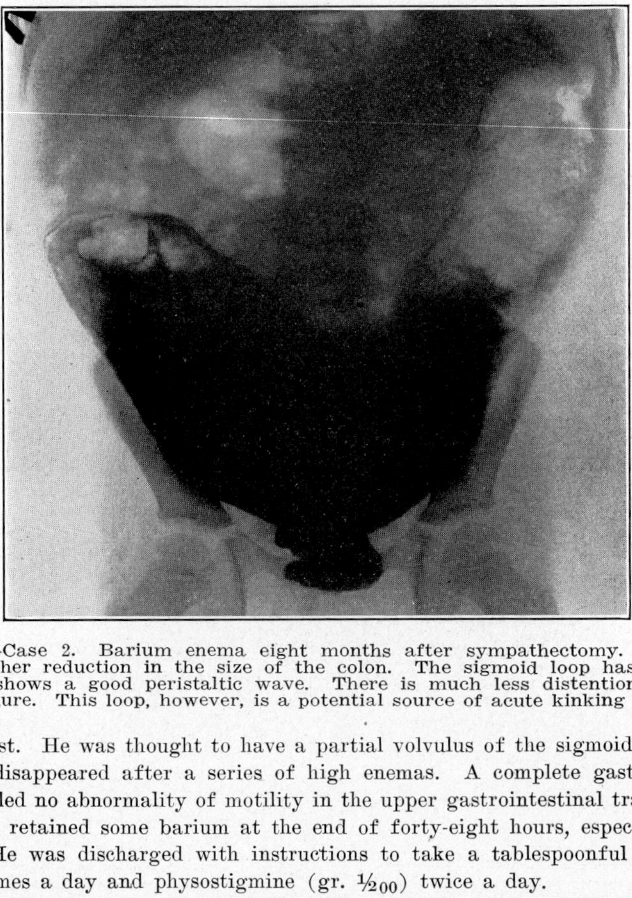

Fig. 8.—Case 2. Barium enema eight months after sympathectomy. There has been a further reduction in the size of the colon. The sigmoid loop has contracted down and shows a good peristaltic wave. There is much less distention above the sigmoid flexure. This loop, however, is a potential source of acute kinking or volvulus.

was manifest. He was thought to have a partial volvulus of the sigmoid loop. The distention disappeared after a series of high enemas. A complete gastrointestinal series revealed no abnormality of motility in the upper gastrointestinal tract, but the large bowel retained some barium at the end of forty-eight hours, especially in the sigmoid. He was discharged with instructions to take a tablespoonful of mineral oil three times a day and physostigmine (gr. $\frac{1}{200}$) twice a day.

On Dec. 23, 1937, the patient still had much distention, but had had five spontaneous bowel movements in one week. Eserine was increased to $\frac{1}{150}$ gr. three times daily.

On examination on Jan. 13, 1938, eight months after operation, the patient was having two spontaneous bowel movements daily with the aid of eserine (Fig. 8). He weighed 43 pounds, a gain of 5 pounds, looked strong, and was not dehydrated.

He was last examined on March 4, 1938. Continued improvement was noted. During the previous month he had had spontaneous daily movement without the use of eserine or other medication except mineral oil. The mother had not been able to detect visible peristalsis for two months previously.

CASE 3.—W. Q., 8-year-old boy, was admitted to St. Luke's Hospital on Aug. 4, 1937, referred by Dr. E. McEnery. Since the child's birth, the mother had difficulty with his persistent distention and constipation. During the first week he began to have fecal vomiting. Repeated enemas overcame the obstruction, and he was discharged from St. Elizabeth Hospital. He failed to gain regularly. Dr. I. Abt placed the child on a buttermilk diet, which was not well tolerated. On protein powdered milk he did better. At the age of 5 years the child was at the Children's Memorial Hospital because of a convulsion. Dr. McEnery referred the patient, as distention and constipation continued to persist. Deformity of the thorax was marked.

After emptying the colon as well as possible, a thin barium-petrolagar mixture was given by rectum. The rectum and sigmoid were not dilated, in fact, looked

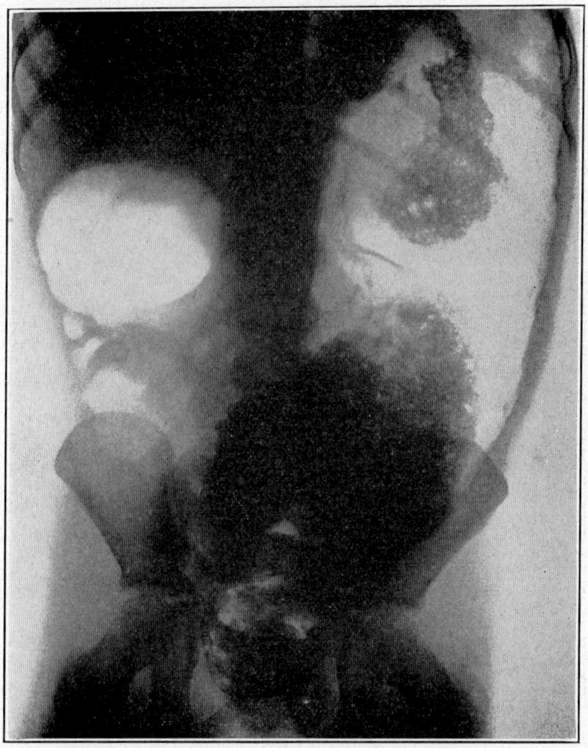

Fig. 9.—Case 3. Barium enema before operation. Note the short spastic sigmoid loop and the sudden dilatation at the angle between the sigmoid and descending colon. There is a huge gas bubble in the left half of the colon, elevating the diaphragm. There is a large air pocket in the ascending colon.

rather spastic. The dilatation began at the junction of the sigmoid with the descending colon and extended over to the cecum. The caliber of this dilated bowel was approximately five times the normal size. Spinal anesthesia was contemplated but was impossible because of the child's extreme anxiety and restlessness. Instead, prostigmine (1 c.c.) was given subcutaneously, which made very little difference in the caliber of the bowel (Figs. 9 and 10).

It was felt that the muscle power of the colon was seriously impaired, but a sympathectomy was still preferable and less dangerous than a total colectomy. Accordingly, on Aug. 9, 1937, through a midline laparotomy, both lumbar sympathetic chains and the presacral nerve were resected (G. de T.). The colon was enormously dilated; the dilatation started at the pelvirectal junction and ended abruptly at the ileocecal valve. Below the pelvirectal junction the bowel seemed spastic. However, there was no mechanical obstruction at this point. The muscular coat of the colon seemed to have disappeared; the bowel was transparent and had the appearance of a fish bladder. On the left side a number of lymph glands were encountered, making a complete dissection above the second lumbar ganglion impossible.

The patient had a stormy convalescence; only repeated injections of pitressin and continuous colonic suction could relieve the distention. However, the wound healed firmly, and he was discharged two weeks after the operation and instructed for a general diet, mineral oil, eserine, and daily enemas.

There was little change in the motility of the bowel during the first two months. On Nov. 11, 1937, he had a bowel impaction, which had developed along with an anal fissure as a result of daily rectal catheterizations. The sphincter was dilated under a general anesthetic, and large quantities of inspissated feces were removed manually.

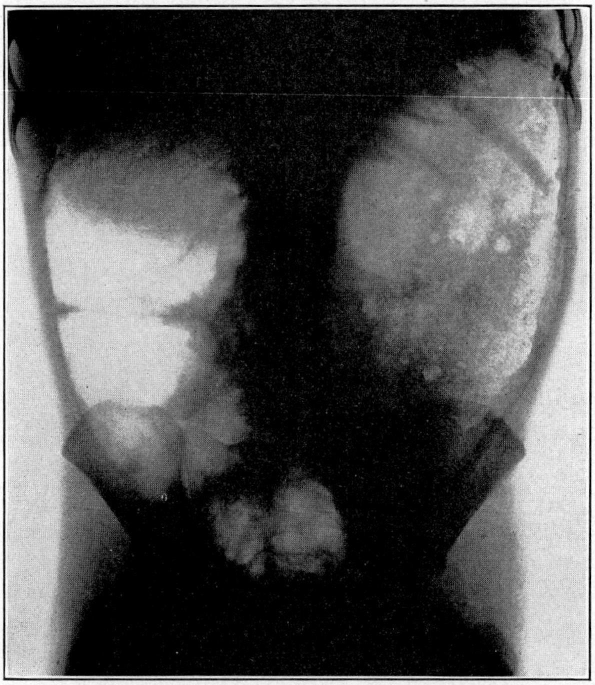

Fig. 10.—Case 3. Barium enema one-half hour after the administration of one-half an ampule of prostigmine. The air bubble in the descending colon is somewhat smaller, and there is a slight haustration visible on the medial side over the lower half of the left colon. Some of the barium in the sigmoid has been pushed into the rectal ampulla. There is, however, a very slight response to parasympathetic stimulation.

Following this, bowel movements became regular and spontaneous. On March 9, 1938, the child's abdomen was flat, and he had daily bowel movements. The rectum did not feel spastic, the fissure had healed. Enemas by catheter did not seem necessary. The child lost his toxic appearance and gained 4 pounds in three months. Barium enema seven months after operation revealed less distention and more contractility (Fig. 11).

CASE 4.—J. W., 5-week-old male infant, was admitted to St. Luke's Hospital on Sept. 22, 1935, on the service of Dr. S. C. Henn. The patient's abdomen had been distended since birth, accompanied by severe constipation; two days before admission diarrhea and vomiting set in.

Present Status.—The patient was a poorly developed male infant with a markedly distended abdomen and visible peristalsis just above and to the left of the umbilicus. He seemed in great agony. After enema and rectal tube, he had an explosive evacuation of flatus. There was no mass or stricture on rectal palpation. There was marked secondary anemia with 50 per cent hemoglobin. X-ray examination revealed no slowing of the passage of barium and a marked dilatation of the distal half of the colon (Fig. 12).

Course.—Following daily enemas, a formula of condensed milk, and rectal tube, distention and vomiting subsided for a week. On Sept. 30, 1935, he began to vomit again, and his temperature rose to 100.2° F. His diet was changed to include ten daily feedings of 2 ounces each of Eagle Brand condensed milk, diluted

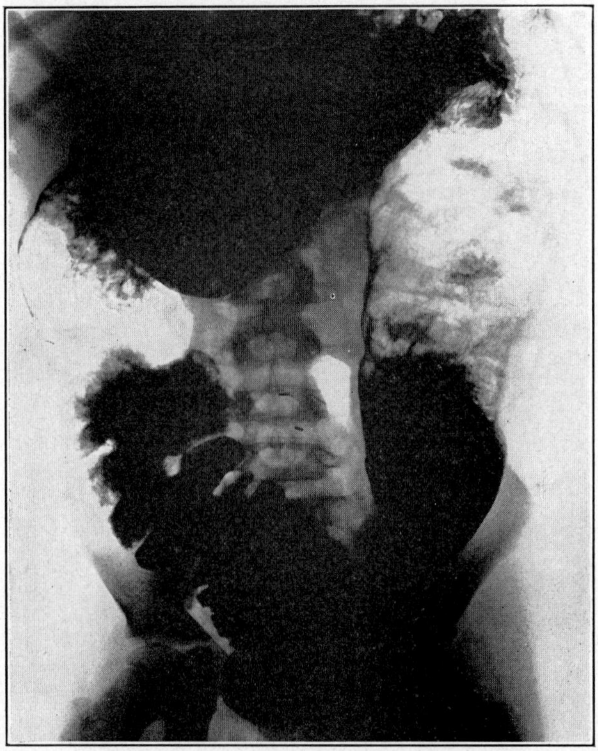

Fig. 11.—Case 3. Barium enema seven months after sympathectomy. The ascending colon shows marked activity. Both ascending and descending colons have a smaller diameter. The transverse colon is still markedly dilated.

1:8. On Oct. 6, 1935, 15 c.c. of the father's blood was given intramuscularly. On Oct. 9, 1935, his red blood count was 2,080,000, white blood count 17,500, and Hb. 6.4 gm. per 100 c.c. There was anisocytosis of the red cells, normoblastic, polychromatophilic, and basophilic stippling. On Oct. 15, 1935, 60 c.c. of citrated blood was given into the left saphenous vein, and 35 c.c. was injected into the buttocks. The patient gradually went downhill, and death occurred on Nov. 23, 1935, at the age of 13 weeks (Fig. 13). Autopsy revealed a congenital dilatation and hypertrophy of the wall of the large bowel, marked anemia, marked emaciation, fatty changes in the liver, and petechial hemorrhages of the lining of the large bowel. There were no other anomalies and no mechanical obstruction of the bowel.

Case 5.—Miss B. C., 28 years old, entered St. Luke's Hospital on the service of Dr. H. I. Meyer on Feb. 26, 1937, complaining of intermittent abdominal distention and cramping for the past year. She had always been constipated and used cathartics habitually.

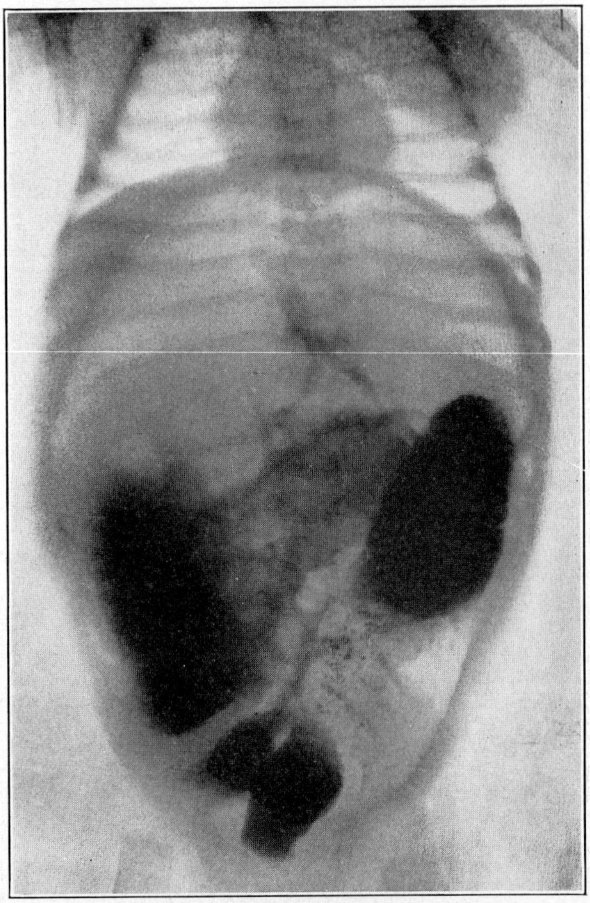

Fig. 12.—Case 4, following barium enema. Note the areas of spasm between the dilated colonic segments. Fluoroscopy in such a case is far more informative. The diaphragm is high, and the organs of the chest are compressed.

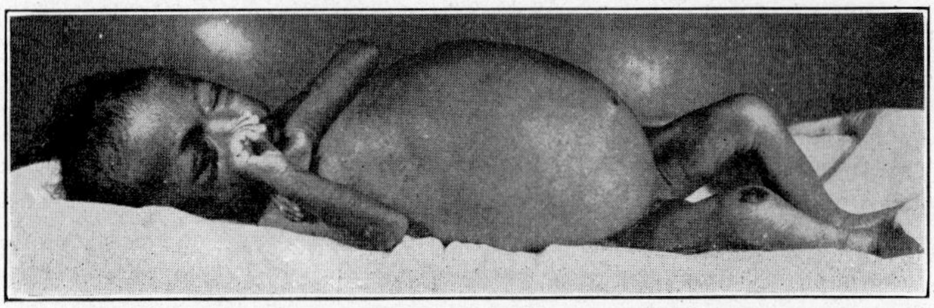

Fig. 13.—Case 4. J. W. shortly after death. Note the extreme emaciation and that the maximum of distention is above the navel.

Past History.—Following a tonsillectomy, catharrhal jaundice of 12 weeks' duration occurred. The appendix was removed in 1912.

Examination.—There was tenderness in right lower quadrant. No mass palpated and no peristaltic waves were visible.

Operation was performed on Feb. 27, 1937, by Dr. H. I. Meyer. An exploratory laparotomy revealed a dilatation and abnormal mobility of the entire colon. There was a small band of adhesions at the site of the previous appendectomy but this was causing no obstruction. The colon was dilated to about three times its normal size but was not indurated, inflamed, or obstructed. The small bowel was also distended with fluid and gas. The abdomen was closed in layers.

Postoperative Course.—Patient made a smooth convalescence and left the hospital on the fourteenth day. She remained constipated but can be regulated by enemas and cathartics.

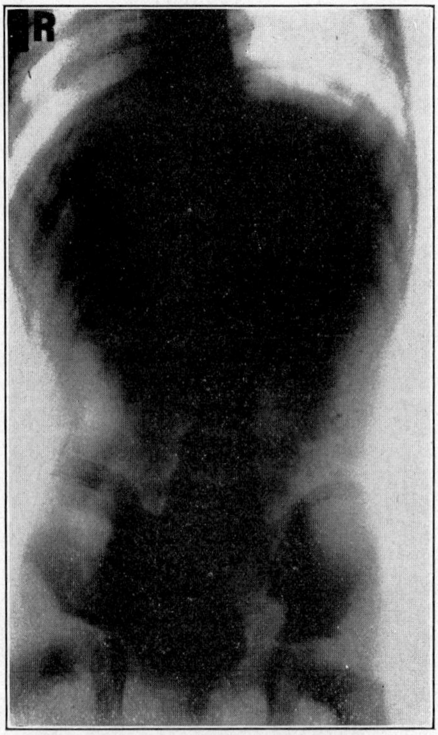

Fig. 14.—Case 6. Cystogram reveals the bladder pushed over to the right by a fecal mass in the sigmoid. The bladder seemed to fill easily without producing a desire for micturition. Megacystis?[34]*

CASE 6.—R. B., 5 years old, entered St. Luke's Hospital on April 17, 1937, on the urologic service of Dr. Harry Culver, because of fecal incontinence and intermittent abdominal distention.

Past History.—Seven days after birth an imperforate anus was operated upon at another hospital. Following this the patient developed fair control of his bowels until November, 1936, when he had no bowel movements for ten days. After several cathartics were given, the patient developed a fecal incontinence and had five to eight bowel movements daily, which persisted ever since. At the age of 1 year the patient feli out of his buggy and was unconscious for ten days, with a resulting total blindness.

*In a tenth case, not reported, the bladder could be filled to 500 c.c., without producing a desire for micturition.

Examination revealed an alert but totally blind child with a dextrocardia, eccentric right pupil, bilateral cataracts, absence of normal anus, an artificial anus anterior to normal location, a penoscrotal fistula, and a large accumulation of fecal masses in the left lower quadrant. Cystoscopy revealed a normal urinary bladder and vesical neck. The penoscrotal fistula admitted a probe which reappeared at the anus. Cystogram showed a normal bladder pushed to the right by a mass in the sigmoid (Fig. 14). X-ray examination of the chest, abdomen, and pelvis revealed a transposition of the lung, heart, and liver to the opposite side and a typical megacolon (Fig. 15). The large bowel seemed to be in normal position.

Course.—The patient was discharged from pediatric service.

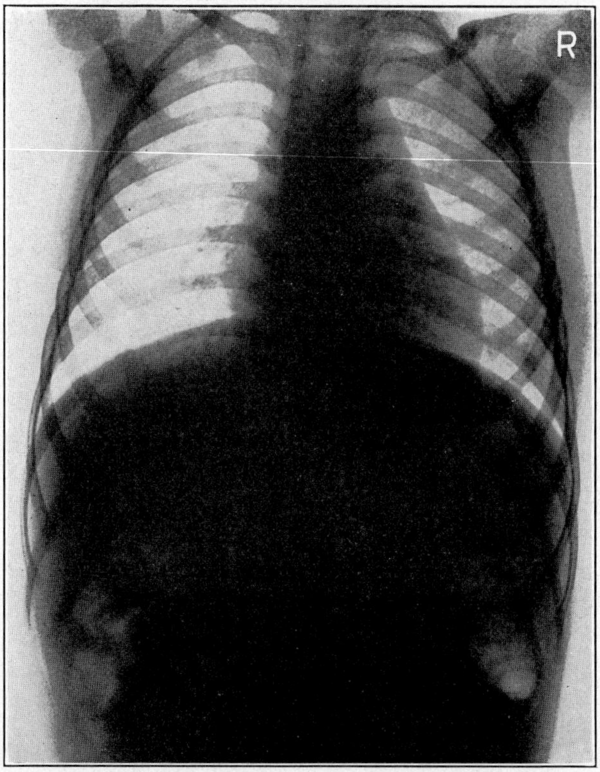

Fig. 15.—Case 6. Flat plate showing the heart on the right, the liver predominantly on the left side. The large bowel seemed to be in the right position.

CASE 7.—M. J. R., 4-year-old girl, entered St. Luke's Hospital on the service of Dr. H. E. Jones, because of distention and constipation of two weeks' duration.

Past History.—At the age of 3 years, with a high intestinal obstruction, the patient was under the care of Dr. H. E. Jones, who found a duodenal compression at the superior mesenteric vessels and performed a gastroenterostomy. She had intermittent attacks of constipation since the last admission.

Examination revealed a well-nourished child with palpable, soft masses in the right and left colon and audible peristaltic sounds. Rectal examination was negative. A barium enema showed no filling defect or obstruction in the colon. The rectum was normal. The sigmoid was located high in the midline; the left half of the colon and the sigmoid were redundant, freely movable, and enlarged. The transverse colon was high and dilated. The cecum was located in the right upper quadrant (failure of migration).

Course.—Child was discharged after the temporary obstruction subsided. Later course is unknown.

CASE 8.—A. L., 47 years old, entered St. Luke's Hospital on July 30, 1936, on the service of Dr. H. E. Mock, complaining of severe constipation for the past ten years and spells of fainting.

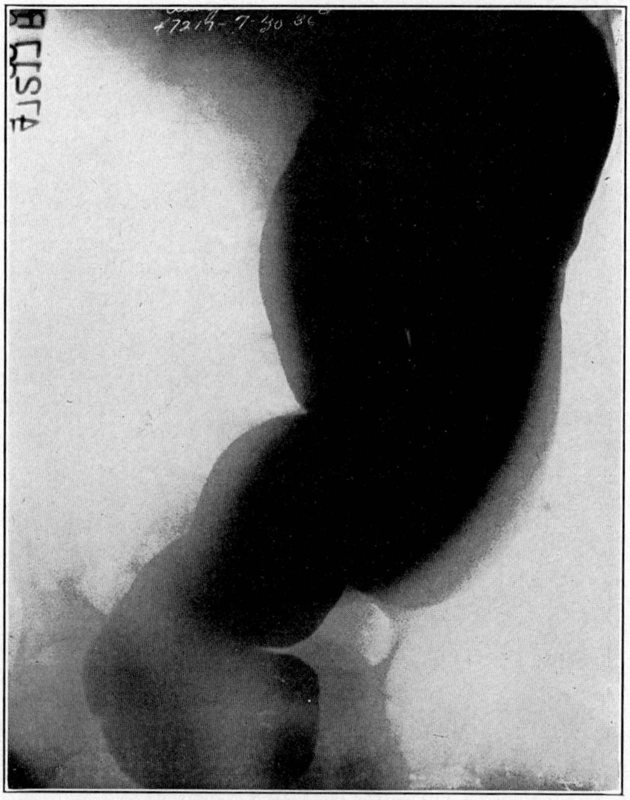

Fig. 16.—Case 8, following barium enema. The distal colon is approximately five times its normal size. The sigmoid loop is very short. The barium stopped abruptly at the distal third of the transverse colon. Subsequent examinations revealed no mechanical obstruction at this point.

Past History.—Prior to 1917, patient had two daily bowel movements. From then on he had to use laxatives. The interval between bowel movements increased to four to five days, together with decrease in appetite and difficulty in breathing. Diet, cathartics, and large amount of water were of no avail.

Examination revealed a distended abdomen with a tight rectal sphincter. Examination by Dr. T. L. Fentress elicited a good history for genuine epilepsy. Barium enema showed that the color filled very slowly; one gallon was used to fill the distal half of the colon. The bowel was dilated five times its normal size; no barium could be forced beyond the distal half of the colon because the patient could not retain any more barium (Fig. 16). Diagnosis of megacolon was made. Dr. C. G. Brown advised bland, bulky diet, oil retention enemas, phenobarbital, and possible sympathectomy.

CASE 9.—R. C., aged 43 years, came to St. Luke's dispensary on May 2, 1937, complaining of having lost 50 pounds in the last year and a dull pain in left chest. A physical examination revealed no significant findings. Under the care of Dr. C. G. Brown he was placed on a bland diet and sedatives. X-ray examination by barium enema revealed a huge dilatation of the distal half of the colon. The barium would not pass the splenic flexure, and at first it was thought to be caused by an organic obstruction at this level. Re-examination on June 21, 1937, showed some narrowing in the descending colon, which was thought to be the result of spasm (Fig. 17). On a bland diet and mild sedatives, the patient was symptom-free. He had never been constipated.

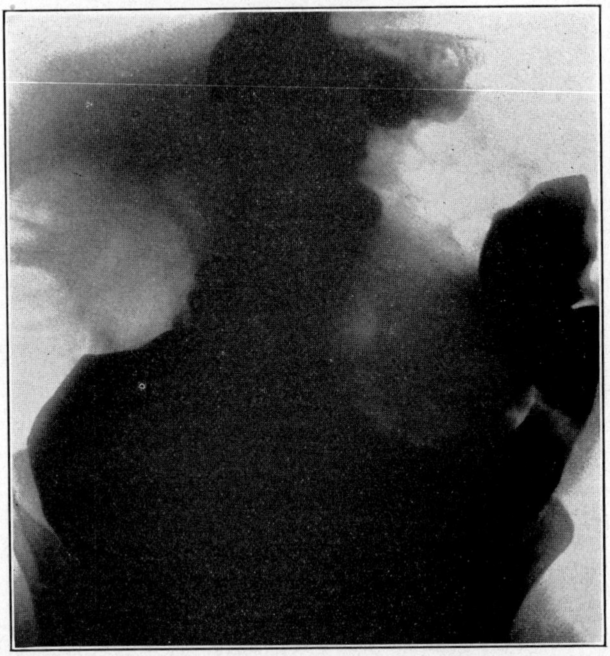

Fig. 17.—Case 9, following barium enema. There is a huge sigmoid loop and a marked narrowing of the descending colon, which, however, is not constant. Patient had segments of narrowing and dilatation, possibly indicative of a faulty neuromuscular mechanism.

COMMENT

It was not our purpose to give a detailed review of the present status of the knowledge on congenital megacolon; rather we wished to record certain observations which may contribute to the better understanding and more rational therapy of the disease. Obviously these patients are seen by the pediatrician in early infancy. At least 70 per cent of the cases appear within the first few weeks of life.[2] If intensive, conservative therapy is instituted, including daily irrigations, rectal dilatations and parasympathetic drugs, many children respond well. For the intractable cases, after the age of 3 years, sympathectomy offers real help. However, it also has its limitations and may have to be followed by removal of parts of the colon, usually the sigmoid loop. Table III tabulates our cases.

TABLE III

CASES OF MEGACOLON

St. Luke's Hospital, Chicago, 1931 to 1937.

CASE NO.	NAME	AGE	SEX	DURATION OF SYMPTOMS	TREATMENT	RESULT
1	C.S.	17 yr.	F	Since birth	Partial colectomy	Recurrence after 2 years
2	R.P.	5 yr.	M	Since birth	Sympathectomy	Successful 18 months postoperative
3	W.Q.	8 yr.	M	Since birth	Sympathectomy	Successful 14 months postoperative
4	J.W.	5 wk.	M	Since birth	Conservative	Died at 13 weeks
5	B.C.	28 yr.	F	One year	Exploratory laparotomy	No change
6	R.B.	5 yr.	M	Since birth	Imperforate anus incised 7 days after birth	Megacolon persists
7	M.J.R.	4	F	2 years	Conservative	Intermittent fecal impactions
8	A.L.	47	M	20 years	Conservative	Not traced
9	R.C.	43	M	Sternal pain Fullness No constipation	Dietary	No change in symptoms

SUMMARY

The incidence, theories concerning its causation, and the perverted physiologic mechanisms responsible for the production of congenital megacolon have been discussed. The medical and surgical treatment, with indications and results, have been described. Nine case histories have been briefly presented. An early intensive treatment by the pediatrician in conjunction with surgical methods for the resistant cases has been emphasized.

Our thanks are due to the pediatric, surgical, and urologic staffs of St. Luke's Hospital for the permission to study the above reported cases.

REFERENCES

1. Bartle, H. J.: Am. J. M. Sc. **171**: 67, 1926.
2. Finney, J. M. T.: Surg., Gynec. & Obst. **6**: 624, 1908.
3. Neugebauer, F.: Ergebn. d. Chir. u. Orthop. **7**: 598, 1913.
4. Fowler, W. F., Davidson, S. C., and Mellon, R. D.: Surg., Gynec. & Obst. **34**: 601, 1922.
5. Ask-Upmark, E.: Beitr. z. klin. Chir. **151**: 73, 267, 1930.
6. Hurst, A. F.: Guy's Hosp. Rep. **84**: 317, 1934.
7. Corbin, F. G.: Surg., Gynec. & Obst. **35**: 23, 1922.
8. Treves, F.: Intestinal Obstruction. Its Varieties With Their Pathology, Diagnosis and Treatment. New York, 1899, William Wood & Company.
9. David, V. C.: Surg., Gynec. & Obst. **37**: 197, 1923.
10. Brennemann, J.: J. A. M. A. **89**: 662, 1927.
11. Perthes, G.: Arch. f. klin. Chir. **77**: 1, 1905.

12. Brown, D., and Robertson, E. G.: Brain **58**: 256, 1935.
13. Wade, R. B., and Royle, N. D.: M. J. Australia **1**: 137, 1927.
14. Trumble, H. C.: Brit. J. Surg. **23**: 214, 1935.
15. Rankin, F. W., and Learmonth, J. R.: Ann. Surg. **92**: 710, 1930.
16. Adamson, W. A. D., and Aird, J.: Brit. J. Surg. **20**: 220, 1932.
17. Burrows, H.: Brit. J. Surg. **31**: 577, 1934.
18. Wangensteen, O. M.: The Therapeutic Problem in Bowel Obstructions. A Physiological and Clinical Consideration. Springfield and Baltimore, 1937, Charles C. Thomas.
19. Judd, E. S., and Thompson, H. L.: Minnesota Med. **11**: 439, 1928.
20. Bonar, B. F.: Am. J. Dis. Child. **48**: 123, 1934.
21. Reeves, R. J., and Harrison, E. K.: Radiology **28**: 731, 1937.
22. Sheldon, L., Kern, R. A., and Hakonsson, E. G.: Am. J. M. Sc. **184**: 94, 1932.
23. Abel, L.: Lancet **2**: 1247, 1933.
24. Morton, J. J., and Scott, W. J. M.: Ann. Surg. **92**: 919, 1930.
25. Stebins, S. J., Morton, J. J., and Scott, W. J. M.: Am. J. Surg. **27**: 107, 1935.
26. Learmonth, J. R.: Brit. M. J. **2**: 154, 1937.
27. Rankin, F. W., Bargen, J. A., and Buie, L. A.: The Colon, Rectum and Anus. Philadelphia and London, 1932, W. B. Saunders Company.
28. Fine, J., Hermanson, L., and Frehling, S.: Ann. Surg. **107**: 1, 1938.
29. Laqua, K.: Beitr. z. klin. Chir. **151**: 471, 1931.
30. Judd, E. S., and Adson, A. W.: Ann. Surg. **88**: 479, 1928.
31. Adson, A. W.: Surgery **1**: 859, 1937.
32. Telford, E. D., and Stopford, J. S. B.: Brit. M. J. **1**: 572, 1934.
33. Ross, J. P.: Brit. J. Surg. **23**: 433, 1935.
34. Pässler, H. W.: Megacolon und Megacystis. Entstehung, Erkennung und Behandlung. Leipzig, 1938, J. A. Barth.

THE TREATMENT OF HYPOGONADISM IN THE ADOLESCENT MALE

Bruce Webster, M.D.
New York, N. Y.

WHEREAS the majority of cases of suspected hypogonadism in the adolescent boy are in reality only instances of delayed puberty which will eventually result in spontaneous recovery,[1] it must be recognized that a few cases have true hypogonadism which will, if untreated, persist into adulthood. The difficulties of the early separation of this group from that which will make a spontaneous recovery have led to much of the confusion in evaluating endocrine therapy in adolescent hypogonadism. The former group will recover if untreated. Yet the medical literature for the past thirty years contains innumerable reports of the cure of this condition by substances which later have been proved to be biologically inactive. A lack of knowledge of the exact mechanism of normal puberty has further complicated this differentiation. Longitudinal studies of normal adolescent boys have recently shown that the anatomic changes which constitute puberty occur in a definite sequence. Deviations from this sequence usually mean abnormality. With the development of our knowledge along these lines, it is to be expected that the recognition of the group which may persist into adulthood will be made much easier. At present these cases are rarely detected before the age of twelve or thirteen.

Although clinical endocrinologists in the past have devised many classifications of hypogonadism, most of them are without much meaning since our knowledge of the underlying pathologic processes is very slight. Clinically, these cases seem to fall into a few simple groups. The majority of cases appear to be of the so-called Fröhlich's or adiposogenital dystrophy type.[2] These cases are characterized by obesity, hypogonadism with lack of development of secondary sexual characteristics, and in many instances hypothyroidism. There exists considerable discussion in the medical literature as to whether the so-called Fröhlich's syndrome is a purely functional disturbance of the anterior lobe of the pituitary, whether a chromophobic adenoma is present, or whether there is an involvement of the adjoining hypothalamic region of the brain. From the standpoint of physiologic disturbances, it would seem that the obesity, the hypofunction of the thyroid, and the absence of gonadal development all indicate a state of hypofunction of the carbohydrate or fat metabolizing factors, the thyreotropic hormone, and the gonadotropic fractions of the anterior lobe of the pituitary. Whatever the

From the Barbara Henry Endocrine Research Laboratory of the Department of Medicine of the New York Hospital and Cornell University Medical College.

underlying etiological factor, it would appear to have produced an anterior lobe insufficiency which manifested itself by lack of development of its various functions.

The second type encountered is the so-called primary hypogonadism. These cases are characterized by overgrowth of the long bones, undernutrition, and lack of development of primary and secondary sexual characteristics. Some of these cases give a definite history of injury to, or infection of, the testes during childhood. Trauma, interference with the blood supply during operations for bilateral hernia or undescended testes, and bilateral orchitis due to mumps are the commonest causes. There are, however, other cases which appear to be due to an absence or deficiency of the secretion of the gonadotropic fraction of the anterior pituitary, with consequent testis atrophy. Why this one fraction should be deficient while the remaining ones are normal is difficult to explain.

A third type of gonadal insufficiency in the adolescent is encountered in children who have had, during adolescence, some severe constitutional disease. Severe bronchial asthma, colitis, and tuberculosis may bring about nutritional disturbances which result in lack of development of primary and secondary sexual characteristics. These cases are characterized, not by testis atrophy, but by a general arrest of genital development. Recent work would suggest that this may be due to a vitamin insufficiency.

Attempts at therapy of delayed puberty in the adolescent male have been largely along two lines. Gonadotropic substances in the form of pregnancy urine extracts and anterior pituitary extracts have been given in an attempt to stimulate the testes to secrete androgenic hormones. Thompson and his collaborators[6] reported increase in size of the genitals in adolescent boys following the administration of pregnancy urine extracts. Such therapy must be carried out over long time periods and has met with varying degrees of success. If sufficient amounts were given, and if adequate normal testis tissue was present, development of primary and secondary sexual characteristics occurred. Since many of these boys have little or no normal testis tissue, such therapy was successful in only a limited number of cases. Further, it must be remembered that many of the individuals in whom this form of therapy is successful are the ones with some functioning testis tissue which may eventually bring about spontaneous puberty.

The second form of treatment of gonadal insufficiency consisted of attempts at replacement of the androgenic or testis hormone. Koch[3] and more recently Vest and Howard[4] have reviewed the development of the androgenic hormones from the crude transplantation experiments of the early workers to the synthesis of androsterone in 1934 by Ruzicka and his co-workers.[5] Until these synthetic androgenic hormones became available, attempts at replacement therapy met with but feeble success, due largely to the difficulty of obtaining adequate amounts of the hormone. McCullagh,[7, 8] Hamilton,[9] Vest and Howard,[4] Kenyon and his co-workers,[10] and others have reported genital growth and manifestations of secondary sexual characteristics following the administration of testosterone propionate to adult eunuchoids. Hamilton[9] gave testosterone propionate to five cryptorchid children. An increase in the number of erections noted was reported, but anatomic changes were not recorded. Vest and Howard[4] induced increases in size of the external genitals and the development of secondary sexual characteristics in two normal boys, aged 3½ and 9 years. Moricard and Bize[11] reported an increase in size of the penis in three children during the administration of testosterone propionate.

In the light of our rapidly increasing knowledge of the role of the androgenic hormones in the development of puberty, it seemed advisable to begin replacement therapy* in hypogonadism in the adolescent male as soon as the condition could be definitely detected. By so doing, the psychic trauma which these individuals usually undergo could be prevented, and, it was hoped, normal anatomic conditions could be brought about. Because of the known wide variation in the development of sexual maturation in the normal adolescent boy and the tendency of minor degrees of hypogonadism to undergo spontaneous recovery,[1] an attempt was made to select for this study only cases of true hypogonadism which in our opinion were likely to result in adult hypogonadism. Six cases were chosen. The majority of these individuals had been under our observation for periods varying from one to three years before the beginning of the experiment. In three cases therapy with pregnancy urine extracts had been carried out for several months without success. In each case this had been stopped for six months or longer before the present period of observation began. Of the six cases, two were typical of the so-called Fröhlich's syndrome; one was considered an instance of primary hypogonadism without history of previous disease or trauma of the testes and without evidence of other endocrine disorder; two were bilateral cryptorchids, both of whom had had previous operative procedures; and one was an example of a severe constitutional disease causing retardation of sexual development.

CASE 1.—N. Y. H. No. 154-333. J. W., of Czechoslovakian parentage, was referred to the clinic in January, 1937, at the age of 14 years because a school physician had made a diagnosis of obesity and ''genital infantilism.'' The boy had always been healthy. He was active and moderately athletic. The father and three sisters were tall and thin. The mother was obese. Physical examination of the patient at that time showed an obese boy—weight, 69.2 kg., height, 161 cm. The breasts were prominent. The abdomen and hips were very obese. The penis was infantile, measuring 3 cm. The testes were small and soft. The prostate could not be felt. There was no axillary or pubic hair. The voice was juvenile. The basal metabolism was −18 per cent by the Aub-DuBois standard, with a pulse rate of 60. Measurements and photographs were taken and the patient was placed

*We are grateful to the Ciba Pharmaceutical Products, Inc., for the testosterone propionate (perandren) used in these studies.

on a 1000 calorie diet. There was a gradual weight loss until, in October, 1937, he weighed 64.9 kg. and was 163 cm. tall. The breasts had increased somewhat in size but there had been no other change in the physical condition. The boy was then nearly 15 years old and showed very little evidence of the increase in size of the testes which usually occurs as the first external indication of beginning puberty. Assay of the urine for androgenic hormones showed 136 color units per 24 hours. Estrogenic hormones could not be detected in his urine by our methods of assay. These hormone levels were far below the normal for boys of that age period. At this time it was felt that the boy had definite hypogonadism and would probably not undergo spontaneous recovery. He was started, therefore, on intramuscular injections of testosterone propionate in 5 mg. doses three times a week. This was continued until Dec. 16, 1937. No change in physical appearance could be detected.

On Dec. 16 the dosage was increased to 25 mg. three times a week. His weight at this time was 69.3 kg. and his height was 163 cm. By Jan. 4, 1938, a striking change in physical appearance had occurred. The weight was 73 kg. Pubic hair was beginning to grow. The penis measured 6 cm. in length. The breasts had decreased in size. Treatment was continued at the same dosage. On March 15 it was noted that the voice was deeper. Axillary hair was beginning to grow. The dosage was reduced to 25 mg. weekly. This was continued until June 20, 1938. At that time he weighed 72.5 kg. and was 169 cm. tall. The obesity of the abdomen and hips had disappeared. Pubic hair was abundant as was the axillary hair. Coarse hair had appeared on the face. The voice was deep and of adult type. The penis was 9 cm. in length. The scrotum and testes had enlarged. There was considerable increase in the degree of firmness of the testes. The prostate was palpable. In general, he exhibited a typical picture of a normal boy of 15½ years. Treatment was discontinued on June 20. One month later no evidence of regression had occurred.

CASE 2.—N. Y. H. No. 197-416. E. N. was admitted to the clinic in April, 1938, at the age of 14 years. The mother, who was of Irish extraction, was obese. The father was of normal size. The child was healthy until the age of 12 years, when he began to gain weight. At the time of admission, he weighed 52.3 kg. and was 153 cm. tall. The hips and abdomen were obese. The breasts were prominent. The penis was 3 cm. in length. The testes were small and soft. The prostate could not be detected. A few pubic hairs were present. A diagnosis of Fröhlich's syndrome was made. Because of the soft consistency and small size of the testes, it was felt that this case offered a poor prognosis for spontaneous recovery. Accordingly, beginning April 25, testosterone propionate in 25 mg. amounts was given intramuscularly three times a week. One month later, on May 24, the penis had increased markedly in size and was 6 cm. long. Pubic and axillary hair was present. The scrotum had darkened in color and was corrugated. On July 5 the penis was 8 cm. long. The testes were firm and had increased slightly in size. The voice was deep and coarse hair was present on the legs and face. The prostate was barely palpable.

CASE 3.—N. Y. H. No. 80-190. D. R., of Scotch parentage, was first admitted to the clinic in November, 1934, at the age of 10 years. The mother stated that the child was born with bilateral undescended testes and bilateral congenital hernias. At the age of 9 years, a left-sided herniotomy was performed. The hernia recurred, and he was again operated upon six months later. On admission to the clinic, a recurrent inguinal hernia was present on the left. There was a right-sided inguinal hernia. The scrotum was undeveloped. Neither testis could be felt. Pregnancy urine extracts were given daily in 100 unit doses, for six months. No change occurred.

In June, 1935, an operation was performed in which the left inguinal hernia was repaired. An atrophic testis was found in the canal and was placed in the scrotum. On the right side, no evidence of testis tissue could be found. The patient was seen at intervals until January, 1938. During the entire interval

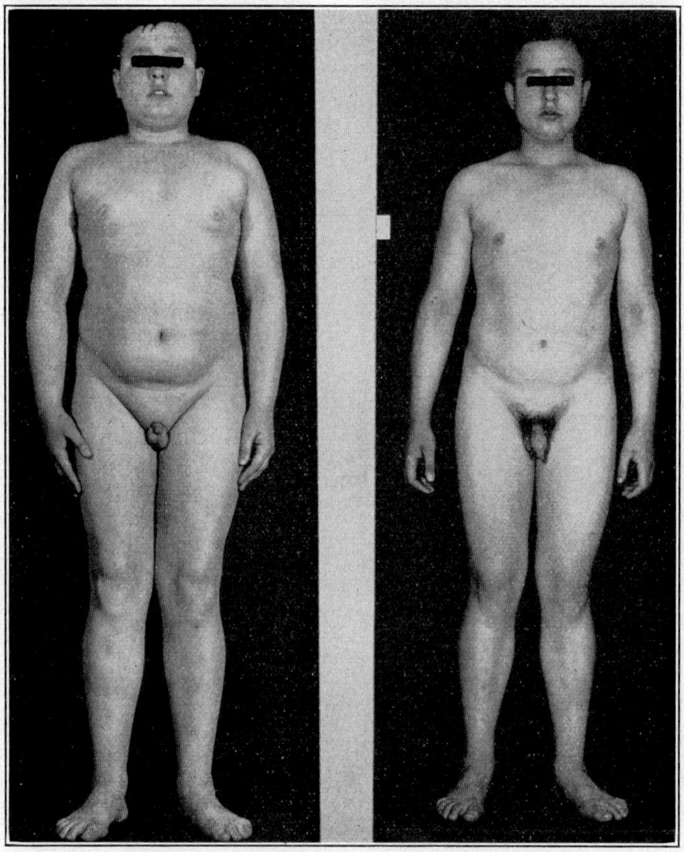

A. *B.*

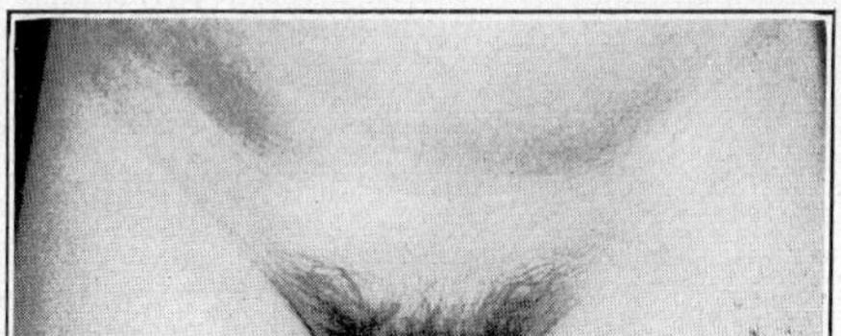

C.

Fig. 1.—Case 1. Photograph showing the appearance of the patient before beginning treatment on Oct. 20, 1937, aged 14 years and 10 months. The second photograph shows the appearance on June 20, 1938, eight months later. The third picture shows the normal genitals at the cessation of treatment on June 20, 1938.

he remained very much underweight, in spite of high calorie feeding. He was then 13 years and 6 months of age. His weight was 39.2 kg. His height was 154 cm. An atrophic left testis could be felt. The prostate could not be detected.

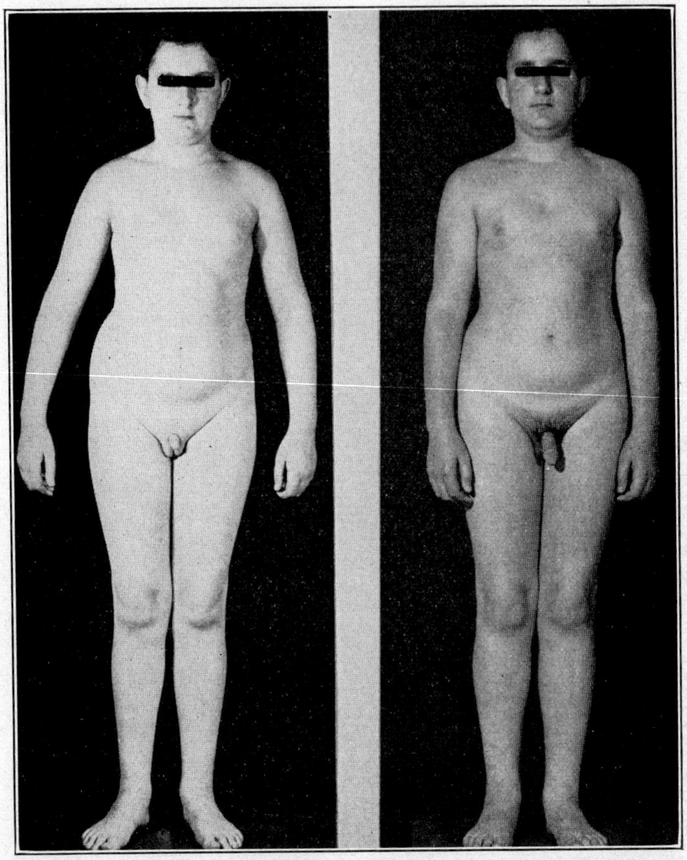

A. *B.*

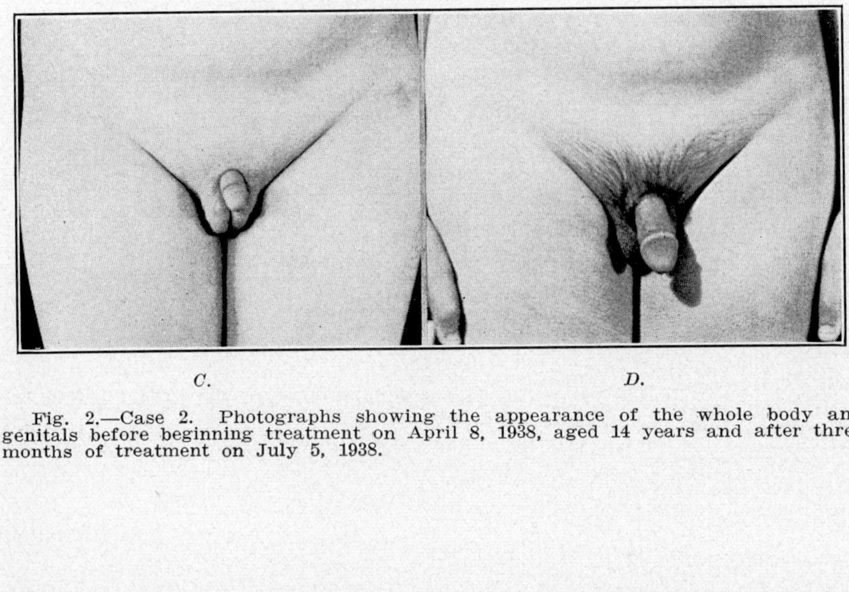

C. *D.*

Fig. 2.—Case 2. Photographs showing the appearance of the whole body and genitals before beginning treatment on April 8, 1938, aged 14 years and after three months of treatment on July 5, 1938.

The penis was 4.5 cm. long. No pubic or axillary hair was present. At this time 25 mg. testosterone propionate was given intramuscularly three times a week. Four weeks later, on February 24, a striking change was noted. The body weight

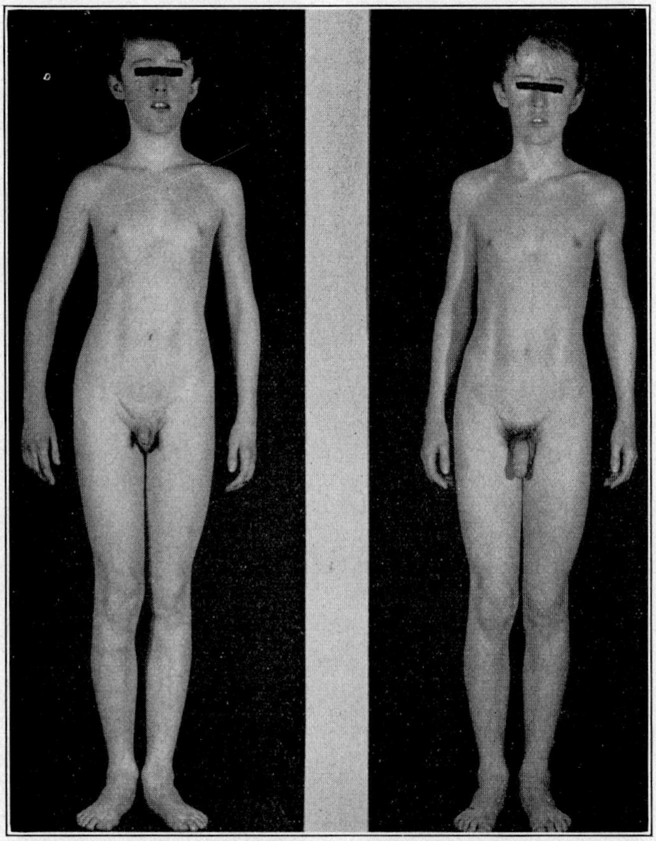

A. *B.*

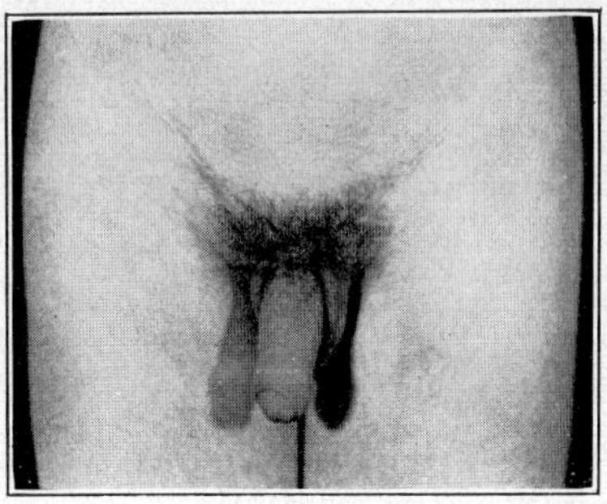

C.

Fig. 3.—Case 3. Photographs showing the appearance of the patient before treatment on Feb. 1, 1938, aged 13 years and 6 months, and on May 19, 1938, after three and a half months of treatment. The third photograph shows the appearance of the genitals on May 19, 1938.

was 45 kg. There had been a marked increase in the size of the penis, and the voice had deepened. Pubic hair was present. The mother remarked that the boy exhibited much more energy than ever before in his life. On March 17 the voice was of the adult type. The penis was 8 cm. long and pubic and axillary hair was abundant. Very little change could be noted in the atrophic left testis. The dosage was reduced to 25 mg. once a week. On June 30 the weight was still 45 kg. He had grown to 162 cm. The general feeling of well-being continued. The penis was 10 cm. in length. The prostate was readily felt. There was a heavy growth of hair on the legs and face.

CASE 4.—N. Y. H. No. 42-262. F. F., of English parentage, was first seen in 1934 at the age of 9 years. He weighed 10 pounds at birth and had always been a fat child. The father and mother were both normal. There were no brothers or sisters.

At the age of 8 years and 6 months, it was noted that the patient was a bilateral cryptorchid and that the penis was infantile. An exploratory operation was done at this time. No testis tissue could be found in either inguinal canal.

When first seen in the clinic the patient weighed 37.7 kg. and was 130 cm. tall. He was obese. There were bilateral inguinal scars. The penis was infantile. The scrotum was undeveloped. No testes could be felt. Basal metabolism was -1 per cent. Assay of the urine for androgenic hormones gave a negative result. Pregnancy urine extract was injected daily in 1 c.c. doses for an entire year beginning in June, 1935. No gonadotropic effect occurred. On Oct. 19, 1937, the patient was 13 years and 6 months old. His weight was 49.0 kg. He was 146.7 cm. tall and was still obese. The penis was infantile, being 3.5 cm. long, and the scrotum was undeveloped. At that time testosterone propionate in 5 mg. doses was given intramuscularly three times per week. By December 17, no appreciable change had occurred. The dosage was then increased to 25 mg. three times per week. Within three weeks pubic hair had appeared. On February 3, 1938, the penis was 5.5 cm. in length. Pubic and axillary hair was present. There had been considerable development of the scrotum. The prostate was palpable. The voice was deeper. On June 9 the patient was 153 cm. tall. The penis was 7.5 cm. long, and pubic hair was abundant. No testis tissue could be palpated. The voice was masculine in type, and there was hair growth on the face, arms, and legs. The dosage was reduced at that time to 10 mg. twice a week. The patient is still under observation.

CASE 5.—N. Y. H. No. 179-480. H. W. was admitted to clinic in September, 1937, at the age of 14 years and 8 months. The patient was of Austrian-Jewish parentage. The mother was obese and had a tendency to hypertrichosis. The father was tall and thin. The child appeared normal until the age of 13 years, when he began to gain weight. At that time a diagnosis of bilateral undescended testes was made, and he received injections of pregnancy urine extract for two months.

On admission to clinic he weighed 63 kg. and was 158 cm. tall. He was slightly obese. The breasts were prominent. There was some pubic hair. An infantile penis, 1.5 cm. long, was present. The scrotum was small. Two atrophic testes, approximately 1 cm. in length, could be palpated. The prostate could not be felt. A diagnosis of hypogonadism was made. There was no evidence of an intracranial tumor. Testosterone propionate in 5 mg. doses was given intramuscularly three times a week from October 21 until December 16 with no appreciable change in his condition. At that time the dosage was increased to 25 mg. three times a week. Three weeks later, on January 4, 1938, marked development of the scrotum was noted. The testes were firmer and larger. The penis had enlarged slightly. On March 3 the breasts were normal. The scrotum and testes had continued to enlarge, and the penis was 4 cm. in length. On May 1, the voice was deep and coarse hair was present on the face, legs, and arms. On June 30, the boy weighed 71 kg. and was 166 cm. tall. There was a heavy growth of axillary and pubic hair. The penis was 6 cm. in length and the testes were approximately 3 cm. long. The prostate was palpable. The boy's features had "coarsened" and were definitely masculine. The patient is still under treatment.

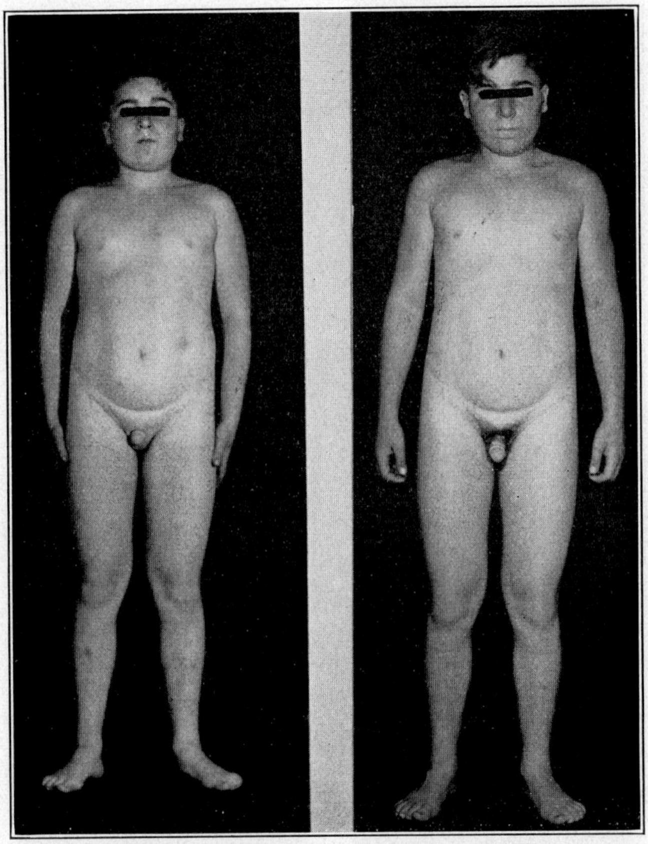

A. *B.*

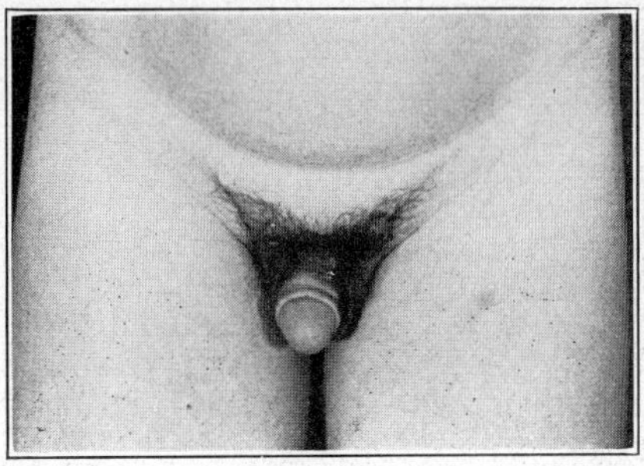

C.

Fig. 4.—Case 4. Photograph showing the appearance of the patient on Oct. 20, 1937, aged 13 years and 6 months. The second photograph shows his appearance on June 30, 1938, after eight months of treatment. The third picture shows the appearance of the genitals on the latter date.

CASE 6.—T. G. was referred for opinion by his physician in September, 1937, when he was 17 years of age. The boy was of English parentage. Both the father and mother were normal. The patient was a normal infant and was healthy until the age of 11 years. At that time, he developed a severe ulcerative colitis. From the age of 11 until 17 years, the patient was constantly undernourished

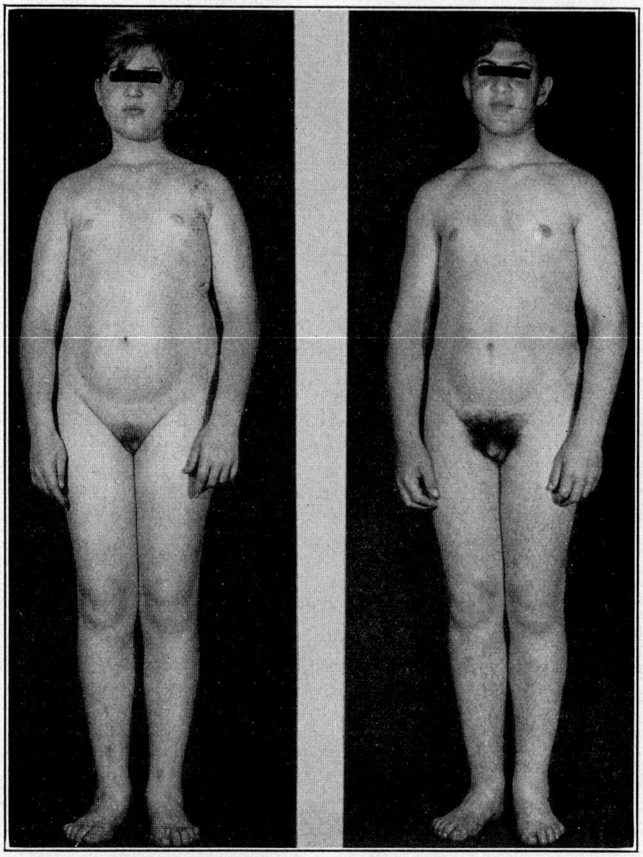

A. *B.*

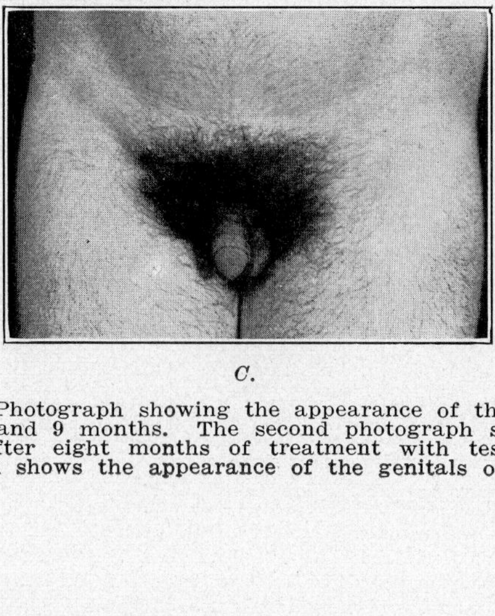

C.

Fig. 5.—Case 5. Photograph showing the appearance of the patient on Oct. 20, 1937, aged 14 years and 9 months. The second photograph shows his appearance on June 30, 1938, after eight months of treatment with testosterone propionate. The third photograph shows the appearance of the genitals on June 30, 1938.

and almost continually had a severe secondary anemia. His growth and physical development became arrested. When seen in September, 1937, he had the appearance of a child of 12 or 13. He was 158 cm. tall and weighed 50 kg. The face was juvenile. There was no evidence of beard growth. No axillary hair and but scanty pubic hair was present. The breasts were slightly enlarged. The penis was 4.5 cm. long. The testes were moderately firm but were approximately only 1.5-2 cm. long. The prostate was barely palpable. The pelvis was of the broad juvenile type. This case was considered an instance of delayed growth and puberty due to the nutritional disturbances resulting from a prolonged illness. Assay of the urine for androgenic hormones showed only 120 color units for twenty-four hours. During the autumn of 1937, the colitis subsided slightly but no change in growth or development occurred.

On Jan. 6, 1938, intramuscular injections of testosterone propionate, 25 mg. three times a week were started. This treatment was carried out by the referring physician. By May 16, 1938, four months later, a striking change had occurred. He had gained 8 kg. in weight and 4 cm. in height. Hair was present on the face requiring him to shave twice a week. Axillary hair was present. Pubic hair had increased in amount and was spreading over the legs and abdomen. The penis was 10 cm. long. The scrotum had developed, and the testes had increased in size. The prostate was readily palpable. The patient reported marked increase in sexual drive as well as an increase in general well-being. During this time period the colitis was only moderately active, being in much the same state as it had been in the autumn of 1937. On May 16 the dose was reduced to 10 mg. twice a week.

DISCUSSION

A consideration of the above protocols would seem to show that treatment of adolescent hypogonadism with testosterone propionate will bring about increased genital growth and the secondary sexual characteristics usually associated with normal puberty. Whether or not this form of treatment must be continued for the remainder of the individual's life, remains to be seen. Although regression of genital growth probably will not take place after the cessation of treatment, it is to be expected that small maintenance doses must be given in order to maintain libido, hair growth, and the various other functions apparently dependent upon a normal level of androgenic hormones in the blood. Although it is difficult to determine the optimum dosage of testosterone propionate necessary to bring about or maintain puberty, it was apparent from our study that 5 mg. three times a week exerted very little effect. Twenty-five milligrams three times a week seemed to be an adequate dosage. In no instance was excessive libido apparent. Smaller doses of 10 mg. two or three times a week appear to be adequate to maintain beard growth, libido, etc., after they have been established. A careful study of more cases is necessary in order to obtain additional data on the subject of clinical dosage.

Assay of the urine and blood* for androgenic and estrogenic hormones was carried out before and during treatment of these cases. These studies are as yet incomplete and will be reported elsewhere. In

*These studies were made with the collaboration of Dr. Ralph Oesting and Miss L. M. Wright.

general all six cases showed low levels of urinary androgens before treatment. After therapy there was a tendency for blood androgens and urinary estrogens to increase.

The first change which occurred in these cases following the injection of testosterone propionate was the appearance of pubic and axillary hair. An increase in size of the penis, development of the scrotum, and deepening of the voice soon followed. Growth of beard and increase in size of the prostate occurred only after several weeks' treatment. It was thought, in three cases, that an increase in size of the testes occurred. The gain in weight in Cases 3, 5, and 6 was striking and warrants further study. Although an increase in total weight occurred, these patients looked less obese at the end of the period of treatment than at the beginning. There was a decrease in size of the mammary region and abdomen. Growth spurts were noted in each case during the period of the administration of testosterone propionate. In the short time during which these patients were under treatment, no x-ray evidence of epiphyseal closure could be detected.

Because of the age of these patients, data were not elicited as to the frequency of erections and emissions. Case 6, the oldest boy of the group, reported a marked increase in the number of erections. Emissions occurred for the first time in his life. The parents of cases 3, 4, and 5 reported a marked increase in energy of these children during the period of treatment.

CONCLUSIONS

The use of testosterone propionate in six cases of adolescent hypogonadism is reported. It appears to bring about striking anatomical changes resulting in the growth of the penis, scrotum, and prostate. Secondary sexual characteristics such as hair growth and voice change occur as in the normal process of puberty. It would seem that this substance offers a means of inducing, in hypogonadal adolescent males, the anatomical changes which normally occur at puberty.

REFERENCES

1. Webster, Bruce: In press.
2. Fröhlich, A.: Wein. klin. Rundschau **15**: 883, 1901.
3. Koch, F. C.: J. Urol. **35**: 382, 1936.
4. Vest, S. A., and Howard, J. E.: J. Urol. **40**: 154, 1938.
5. Ruzicka, L., et al: Helvet. chim. acta. **17**: 1395, 1934.
6. Thompson, W. O., Heckel, N. J., Thompson, P. K., and Dickie, L. F. N.: Endocrinology **22**: 59, 1938.
7. McCullagh, E. P.: Med. clin. North America **17**: 769, 1933.
8. McCullagh, E. P., McCullagh, D. R., and Hicken, N. F.: Endocrinology **17**: 49, 1933.
9. Hamilton, J. B.: Endocrinology, **21**: 744, 1937.
10. Kenyon, A. T., Sandiford, I., Bryan, A. H., Knowlton, K., and Koch, F. C.: Proc. Soc. Exper. Biol. & Med. **37**: 683, 1938.
11. Moricard, R., and Bize, R.: Compt. rend. Acad. d. Sc. **204**: 1044, 1937.

THE HISTOPATHOLOGY OF CONVULSIVE DISORDERS IN CHILDREN

H. M. Zimmerman, M.D.
New Haven, Conn.

CONVULSIVE attacks accompany many different diseases in infancy and childhood. In such conditions as tetany, hyperinsulinism, and asphyxia, to mention but a few, the exact mechanism of the convulsions is poorly understood, but can hardly be attributed to a preexisting organic cerebral lesion. When they occur in the course of such an infectious disease as pertussis, they are frequently attributed to cerebral inflammation. In other infectious illnesses, such as pneumonia and dysentery, their mechanism is again obscure. Under such circumstances inflammatory changes in the nervous system can undoubtedly at times be demonstrated, but in a far greater number of instances no lesions are found which would produce convulsions. The changes which are seen with great regularity in the brain following such attacks are noninflammatory and are the result rather than cause of the convulsions. The presentation of evidence for this conclusion is the prime reason for the present communication.

In part, this study deals with the histopathologic findings in a group of seven children, each of whom died during or after severe convulsions or respiratory failure which occurred in the course of a serious infectious illness. An inflammatory lesion of the nervous system was considered as a possible explanation for the convulsive attacks in these patients. The post-mortem findings, however, did not substantiate this conclusion in a single instance. They did reveal a type of noninflammatory change in the brain which Spielmeyer and his co-workers have associated with epileptiform attacks, a change which they believed resulted from but did not cause the attacks.

Another part of this paper is concerned with the presentation of the anatomic findings in the nervous systems of nine other children who died as the result of either severe convulsions or asphyxia but did not have an associated infectious illness. In these cases a diagnosis of encephalitis was not ventured clinically, yet the lesions encountered during the post-mortem examinations were entirely similar to those observed in the first group. Being uncomplicated by infectious illnesses, the second group of cases more readily permitted an analysis of the pathogenetic factors underlying the cerebral lesions. When these fac-

From the Department of Pathology, Yale University School of Medicine, New Haven, Conn.

This study was aided by a grant from the Research Funds of the Yale University School of Medicine.

tors were determined with some certainty, it became apparent that they were equally applicable to the first group of cases. They will be discussed in some detail in the body of this paper.

On several occasions Spielmeyer[1-3] emphasized the role which functional vascular disturbances plays in the production of lesions in the nervous systems of epileptics. The lesions consist of necrobiotic foci in the cerebral and cerebellar cortices and especially in the cornu ammonis formations of the temporal lobes. In the cerebral cortex the ischemic necrosis of the ganglion cells has a pseudolaminary distribution and is followed by gliosis in cases of long standing. The glial scarring is

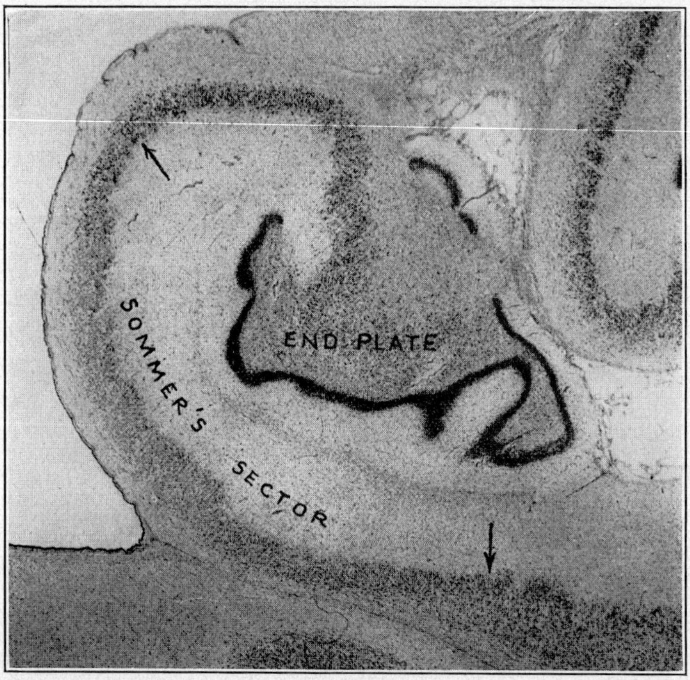

Fig. 1.—Normal cornu ammonis formation of a child 2½ months old. Between the arrows lies the vulnerable Sommer's sector. A resistant band of cells connects the latter with the end plate. Nissl stain. (×14.)

especially prominent in the subpial layer. The structures which suffer most in the cerebellum are the Purkinje cells and the small cells of the granular layer. Arborizations of microglia occur early in the molecular layer of the cerebellum, and ultimately a condition of lobular atrophy results if the cellular destruction which preceded it was extensive. The changes which occur in the cornu ammonis formations are perhaps the most important, because they are most constant and appear earliest. They also consist of ischemic necrosis of the ganglion cells, particularly of those in the vulnerable band known as Sommer's sector (Fig. 1). The vulnerability of the cornu ammonis formation was shown by Uchimura[4] to be a factor of its relatively inadequate blood supply. To these zones of predilection Scholz[5] added the thalamus and, on the basis of his findings in idiopathic as well as symptomatic epilepsy, he concluded that the child's brain in the first year of life was especially susceptible to these lesions.

By "functional vascular disturbances" Spielmeyer meant any interference with circulation capable of producing cerebral anoxemia, exclusive of organic vascular occlusion as produced by thrombosis or embolism. He considered angiospastic phenomena to be the functional factors of prime significance, but he included also capillary and venous stasis. He was of the opinion that organically diseased blood vessels, including those that are altered by atheromatous changes, are particularly prone to vasomotor disturbances.[6] The histopathologic residua of these functional vascular disturbances are vascular stasis, capillary and "ring" hemorrhages, and the necrobiotic lesions previously mentioned.

CONVULSIONS IN THE COURSE OF INFECTIOUS ILLNESSES

Pneumonia

CASE 1.—A white male child, 4½ years of age, whose illness began with coughing and drowsiness, had generalized convulsion lasting one-half hour, followed by two similar ones and a fourth which lasted over one hour. Coma, fever, cyanosis, large, fixed right pupil, and retinal hemorrhages were present. The reflexes were sluggish. Death occurred two and one-half days after onset of illness. The case was diagnosed as bilateral diffuse pneumonia and pleurisy. Macroscopic examination showed cerebral edema and petechiae; also widespread destruction of nerve cells of cerebral cortex.

Clinical History.—The patient was born in the New Haven Hospital at full term by cesarean section. His development was normal until the onset of the last illness, which began with poor appetite and drowsiness two days before his readmission to the hospital. A slight cough appeared, but he was not particularly ill until ten o'clock the next morning when he had a generalized convulsion which lasted about one-half hour. The same afternoon two more severe generalized convulsions occurred which were treated with sodium bromide and chloral hydrate. At eleven o'clock that evening he had his fourth convulsion which lasted for more than one hour. The pupils were markedly dilated, but there was no nystagmus and no retraction of the head.

On admission to the hospital the child was comatose and cyanotic. Respirations were rapid and the temperature was 40.6° C. The right pupil was larger than the left and did not react to light. The fundi showed tremendous engorgement of the veins and several large hemorrhages. Signs of pneumonia were found in the lower lobe of the left lung. The deep reflexes were sluggish; the Babinski and Kernig signs were negative.

The child was placed in an oxygen tent, but he continued in coma and had repeated convulsions. The pneumonia spread to the right lung. In spite of intravenous glucose infusions and digitalis, he expired two and one-half days after the onset of illness.

The blood Kahn and Wassermann tests were negative. A blood count revealed 4,400,000 red blood cells and 14,200 white blood cells and a differential count of 90 per cent polymorphonuclear leucocytes. Blood culture revealed pneumococcus Type I in both the blood agar plates and the broth. The cerebrospinal fluid was under increased pressure and contained forty-five cells per cubic millimeter, of which twenty-five were of the mononuclear variety. Pandy reaction was negative.

Necropsy.—Post-mortem examination was performed by Dr. David M. Grayzel three hours after exitus.

The bronchi and bronchioles were the seat of an acute inflammatory process. Most of the left lung, with the exception of the anterior margin, was consolidated and gray in color. The upper and lower lobes of the right lung were firm and deep red. Both pleural cavities contained a fibrinopurulent exudate. On microscopic examination the pulmonary alveoli were filled with fibrin and leucocytes.

A large amount of freshly clotted blood was present in the stomach and filled the entire intestinal tract. The only possible source of this hemorrhage was an ulcerative process in the first part of the duodenum. The ulceration was superficial, involving only the mucosa and a portion of the submucosa, and no large ruptured blood vessels were found. There was, however, a considerable amount of blood throughout the submucosa in the region of the ulceration. The latter appeared to be of recent origin since there were but few leucocytes and no fibrosis at the base.

Brain.—On macroscopic examination the only abnormalities noted in the nervous system were the presence of widespread edema and small clusters of petechial hemorrhages in the occipital lobe cortex. Histologically extensive lesions were seen throughout the cortical gray matter and even in the central gray. These consisted of destruction and disappearance of ganglion cells without any apparent changes in the glia. Entire convolutions were seen to be totally depopulated of their nerve cells (Fig. 2). Sommer's sector in the cornu ammonis formation had completely disappeared (Fig. 3). Some convolutions revealed the destructive process in zones limited to one or two laminae. The frontal, temporal, and parietal lobes were more seriously involved than the occipital. In those regions where the cellular destruction was not complete, there was, nevertheless, extensive cellular injury characterized by swelling and nuclear and cytoplasmic disintegration. This type of change was seen in nearly all the basal ganglions and was particularly striking in the hypothalamic nuclei.

CASE 2.—A white male infant, 28 months of age, whose illness began with profuse nasal discharge, fever, cough, and vomiting, had generalized convulsion lasting five minutes, followed by repeated convulsions and stupor. There was bilateral positive Babinski sign. Status epilepticus, dysphagia, papilledema and irregular respirations were followed by death on the seventh day of illness. Pneumococcus pneumonia was present. There was widespread destruction of nerve cells of the cerebral cortex.

Clinical History.—The patient, a 28-month-old white male infant, was the product of a normal pregnancy which was terminated by cesarean section because of a contracted pelvis. Subsequent development was that of a normal child.

Two days before his admission to the New Haven Hospital he developed a moderately profuse nasal discharge. Food was poorly taken that day, and by evening an elevated temperature was first noted. That night the child coughed frequently. The cough and fever persisted throughout the following day, and almost all food given was vomited. On the morning of the day of admission to the hospital he had a generalized convulsion lasting about five minutes. During the afternoon he had three or four convulsions of a similar nature.

The temperature on admission was 39.8° C. Respirations were rapid and labored. There was frequent nonproductive coughing. Stupor was so marked that it was impossible to rouse the child even with painful stimuli such as pinpricks. An occasional twitching of the right side of the face was noted. The right arm and leg were spastic, the left, flaccid. The tendon reflexes were in general sluggish, less active on the left than on the right. There was a bilateral extensor Babinski phenomenon. Abdominal reflexes were absent. There was moderate dullness to percussion over the entire right side of the chest, and over this area the breath sounds were diminished. Roentgenographic evidence of consolidation in the lung was demonstrated for the first time on the third day after admission.

The subsequent course in the hospital was exceedingly stormy. The child had frequent convulsions which were difficult to control with the usual sedative drugs. During the nonconvulsive periods there was a persistent twitching of the facial muscles and a definite tendency for the eyes to deviate to the right. During the

Fig. 2.

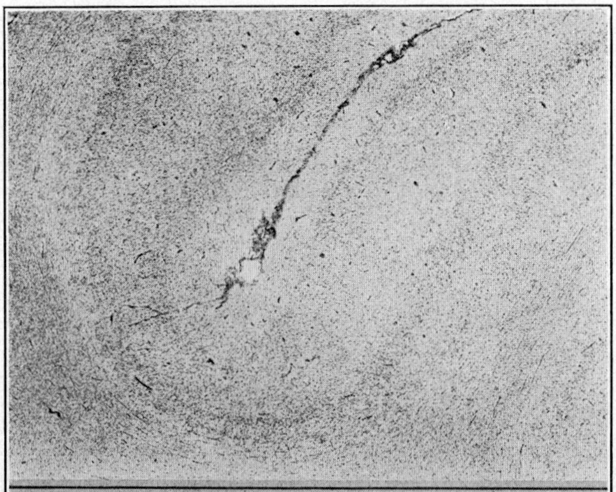

Fig. 3.

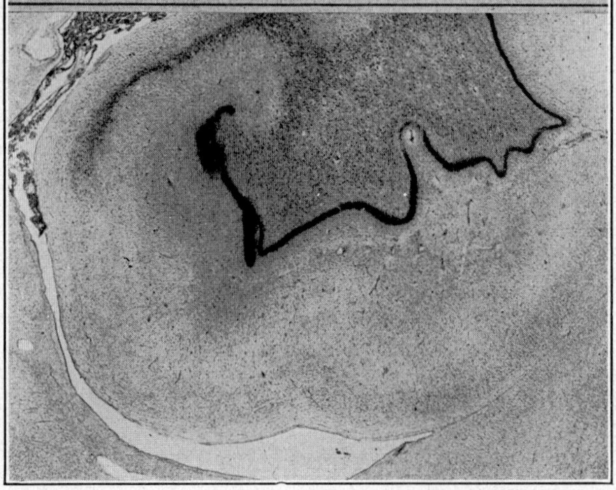

Fig. 2.—Case 1. Photomicrograph of the cerebral cortex at the depth of a sulcus. The usual lamination is obliterated because of the disappearance of nearly all the ganglion cells. The glia alone remains uninjured. Nissl stain. (×16.)

Fig. 3.—Case 1. The entire Sommer's sector is devoid of ganglion cells, but the resistant band persists. Nissl stain. (×11.)

succeeding days the spastic condition of both right extremities became more marked. Dysphagia developed on the fifth day. Papilledema gradually appeared. The day before the death of the child, which occurred seven days after the onset of the illness, respirations became very shallow and irregular.

The important laboratory data were as follows: Red blood count 5,800,000; hemoglobin 100 per cent (Sahli); white blood count 22,000; leucocytes 75 per cent;

lymphocytes 25 per cent. The spinal fluid was normal except for moderately increased pressure. The blood cultures were repeatedly positive for pneumococcus Type IV. The Kahn test on the blood was negative.

Necropsy.—A complete examination was performed seventeen hours post mortem. The tracheal mucosa was congested; the peritracheal lymph nodes were large and succulent. Both lungs contained extensive zones of consolidation in which fibrin and leucocytes were present in abundance microscopically. The pleural cavities contained a fibrinopurulent exudate.

Brain.—The cerebral parenchyma was of the usual consistency and revealed neither congestion nor hemorrhages. Microscopically, the cortical cytoarchitecture was destroyed by degenerative lesions which varied in extent from place to place but were everywhere essentially of the same type (Fig. 4). They consisted of necrosis of the ganglion cells, involving sometimes one and sometimes another of the cortical laminae. Frequently all the ganglion cells of several contiguous convolutions were wiped out. The cells which had not disappeared completely were swollen and showed chromatolytic changes. In hematoxylin-eosin preparations these cells showed

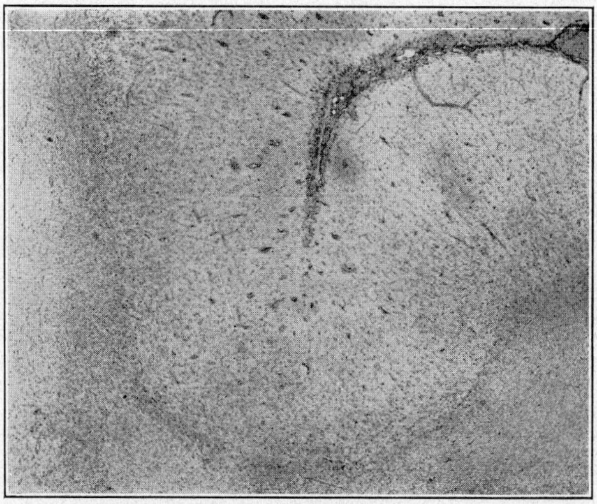

Fig. 4.—Case 2. The ganglion cells in all six cortical layers are destroyed. There is some proliferation of the subpial protoplasmic glia. Nissl stain. (×25.)

marked eosinophilia as well as pericellular edema. The capillaries in the cortex had a thickened, hyaline appearance. Associated with the ganglion cell damage was a proliferative response on the part of the glia. The protoplasmic astrocytes were particularly numerous beneath the pia and the microglia, in the deeper layers. Destroyed myelin fibers were found in the cerebral cortex and subcortex.

Comment.—Convulsive episodes are not infrequently encountered in the course of pneumonia in children. When they assume the nature of status epilepticus, and especially when coma and changes in the reflexes supervene, the suspicion of an inflammatory encephalitic process is aroused. This diagnosis was not confirmed in either of these two cases, for the cerebral lesions found at necropsy were not of an exudative nature. They corresponded in every important detail rather to the lesions which have been described in cases of epilepsy where they have been attributed, as already briefly outlined, to vascular disturbances of a functional nature. In the first case, that of the child who survived the onset of convulsions for two and one-half days, the presence of cerebral edema and petechiae tended to support this view. In the second case, which has been reported previously in more detail,[7] there was already considerable evidence of glial proliferation in addition to the widespread cortical necrobiosis. This could easily be accounted for by the fact that the child did not die until seven days after the onset of convulsions.

Pertussis

CASE 3.—A poorly developed white female child, aged 18 months, had pertussis which lasted five weeks and culminated in generalized convulsions and loss of certain reflexes, resulting in death after eighteen hours. Microscopic examination revealed organizing bronchiolitis and pulmonary emphysema. There was destruction of nerve cells in the cerebral cortex, vascular congestion, and "ring" hemorrhages.

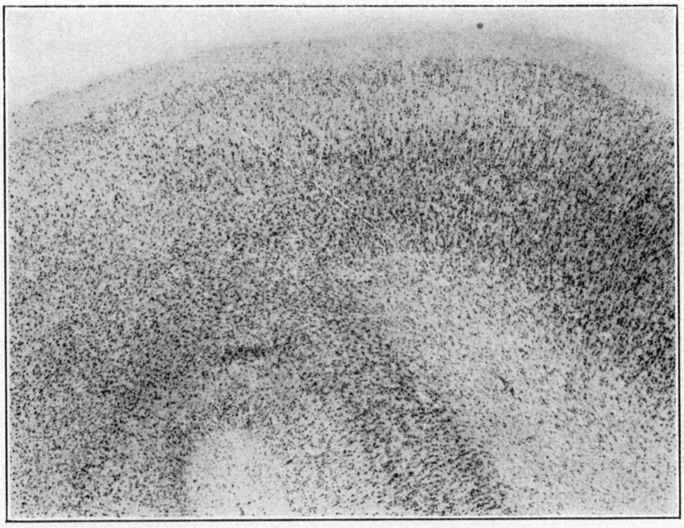

Fig. 5.—Case 3. The third layer of the temporal lobe cortex has a bleached appearance due to the loss of ganglion cells. Nissl stain. (×25.)

Clinical History.—The patient was an 18-month-old white female who presented a feeding problem almost from birth. She was breast-fed only for the first three weeks of life and was then given a formula. She remained rather weak and poorly nourished and was backward in her development. The first tooth appeared at thirteen months; she did not sit up until 14 months of age and never learned to creep or walk.

The present illness began with an attack of whooping cough from which three other children in the family were suffering. The illness was moderately severe but progressed without untoward symptoms for five weeks. At three o'clock one morning, however, she had a generalized convulsion and shortly after that began to convulse almost constantly. In this condition of status epilepticus she was brought to the New Haven Hospital where her temperature was found to be 40.8° C. She was semicomatose. The pupils were large and fixed; there were no hemorrhages in the fundi. Bronchial breathing and coarse râles were heard in the chest. All the extremities were flaccid and the reflexes were sluggish.

Clyses and infusions of saline and glucose were given soon after admission. A slight internal strabismus developed. Ocular movements were conjugate, and there was no nystagmus. Corneal reflexes were absent. A response to noise could not be elicited, but responses were made to painful stimuli. The deep reflexes in the arms as well as in the abdominal region disappeared. Generalized convulsions continued in spite of avertin, and the patient suddenly expired after a particularly severe convulsive attack. This occurred eighteen hours after the initial convulsion.

Laboratory examinations revealed a negative blood Kahn test and a negative blood culture. Red blood cells numbered 4,100,000; white blood cells were 43,000 per cubic millimeter; the differential count showed 49 per cent leucocytes and 43 per cent lymphocytes.

Necropsy.—The necropsy was performed by Dr. David M. Grayzel one and one-half hours post mortem.

The anterior margins of both lungs contained subpleural emphysematous bullae. There were no zones of frank consolidation in either lung. Microscopic examination revealed ruptures of many alveolar walls permitting interalveolar communication. A few bronchioles were seen to contain an exudate of leucocytes in their lumina, and in some bronchioles the exudate was being organized.

Brain.—Both cerebral hemispheres were well developed. The meninges were thin and translucent. Macroscopic examination of the brain revealed no abnormalities, and histologically the meninges and cerebral parenchyma contained no exudate of any sort. The vessels in the occipital cortex were engorged with blood, and there were even a few "ring" hemorrhages present in this part of the brain. In the insular cortex the vessels were surrounded by greatly dilated Virchow-Robin spaces. Large zones of injured ganglion cells were seen in the vulnerable bands of both cornu ammonis formations. The third and fifth layers of the hippocampal cortex lacked many of the ganglion cells, producing a bleached or faded appearance in Nissl preparations (Fig. 5). Some of the remaining nerve cells in these parts of the brain were shrunken and hyperchromatic, and a few showed pericellular incrustations.

CASE 4.—A white female infant, 11 months old, contracted pertussis along with three other siblings. There were rapid and difficult respirations, fever, cyanosis, and disorientation. The head was retracted, the back arched, and the extremities spastic. There was coma, breathing was gasping and irregular. The eyes deviated to the left. Death occurred twenty-four hours after onset of respiratory difficulty. The case was diagnosed as pulmonary emphysema and focal pneumonia. There was destruction of ganglion cells of the cerebral cortex.

Clinical History.—The child contracted a cold and pertussis two weeks before admission to the New Haven Hospital. Two older sisters and a brother had whooping cough at the same time. One week after the onset of illness the patient began to whoop and vomited about once a day with her paroxysms of coughing. She developed a high fever associated with labored and rapid respiration. On the day of admission to the hospital the mother found the infant motionless and staring off into space. The physician who sent the child in to the hospital diagnosed the condition as pneumonia and meningitis.

The temperature was 39.5° C., and the pulse rate 180 per minute. The child appeared seriously ill, disoriented, and out of touch with the environment. Breathing was laborious, and cyanosis was present. The head was retracted, and the back arched; the extremities were slightly spastic. A few scattered petechiae were present on the sclerae and trunk. The anterior fontanel was large and sunken. Both eardrums were red and bulging. For the most part, the lungs were hyperresonant, but dullness was found over the right base.

Gram-positive diplococci were present in the purulent exudate obtained by myringotomy. Dyspnea and cyanosis persisted, requiring adrenalin and carbon-dioxide therapy. The child lapsed into coma and failed to respond even to painful stimuli. Breathing became gasping and irregular, and the eyes deviated to the left. At no time during the course of the illness were any actual convulsions noted, but the body was held in tonic contraction for several hours before exitus, which occurred twenty-four hours after admission to the hospital.

The spinal fluid was clear and contained no leucocytes and only one lymphocyte per cubic millimeter. Blood culture revealed pneumococcus Type IV.

Fig. 6.

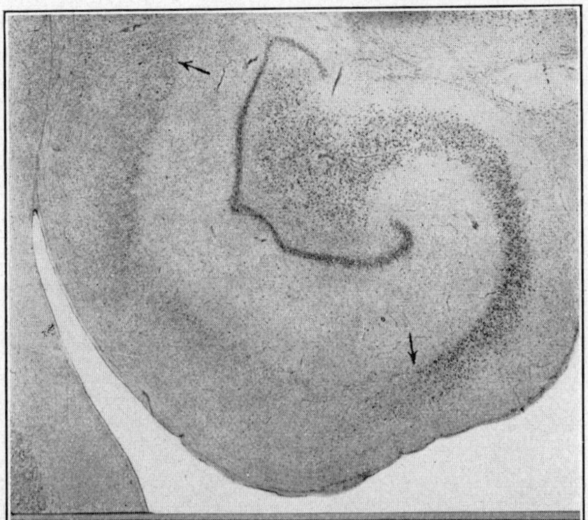

Fig. 7.

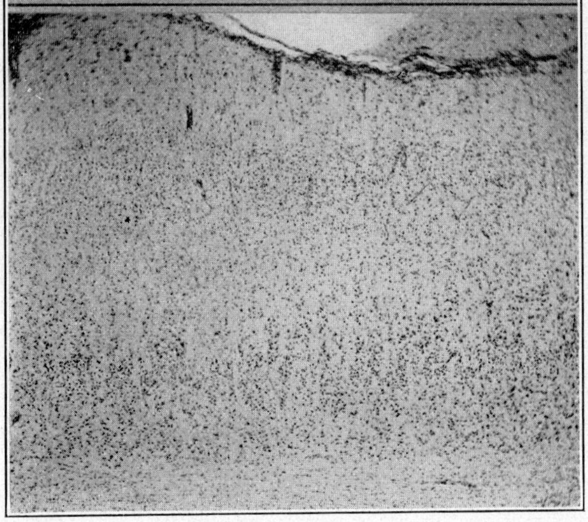

Fig. 6.—Case 4. Many of the ganglion cells in Sommer's sector (between arrows) of the cornu ammonis formation have disappeared, but those in the resistant band are well preserved. Nissl stain. (×13.)

Fig. 7.—Case 4. The cytoarchitecture of the cerebral cortex is altered by an almost complete loss of ganglion cells in the third layer. There is a moderate increase in the glia of the subpial layer. Nissl stain. (×40.)

Necropsy.—Post-mortem examination was performed by Dr. Lincoln Opper twelve hours after exitus.

Both lungs were extremely emphysematous except for the lower lobe of the right lung which was consolidated, deep red in color, and friable. Small fresh hemorrhages were scattered through the parenchyma of both lungs. The bronchi and bronchioles were filled with tenacious purulent exudate and their mucosa was deeply congested. Microscopic examination of the pneumonic lobe of the right lung revealed leucocytes and fibrin in the alveoli.

Brain.—There were no lesions found on macroscopic examination of the brain. The leptomeninges over the left postcentral gyrus were discolored with a small amount of blood, but there was no evidence of exudate anywhere in the subarachnoid space.

On histologic examination some ganglion cells in almost every cerebral gyrus were altered by an ischemic type of change. This cellular injury reached its maximum in the cornu ammonis formations, the calcarine regions of the occipital lobes, and the postcentral gyri. In the cornu ammonis formations the ischemic change progressed to a point where many nerve cells disappeared completely (Fig. 6). Even the end plate had many ischemic ganglion cells. In other cerebral gyri it was usually the cells of the third cortical layer which were most severely injured (Fig. 7). An occasional Purkinje cell in the cerebellar cortex was similarly affected, but the granular cells were well preserved.

Comment.—Changes such as these two cases presented were described by both Husler and Spatz[8] and Neubürger[9] in the nervous systems of children who succumbed to pertussis with convulsions. Whereas Husler and Spatz considered the etiology of these changes to be some form cf toxin and the whole process a toxic encephalitis, Neubürger felt that the lesions could be explained on the basis of air emboli. He believed that the increased pulmonary pressure in whooping cough led to rupture of the delicate lung capillaries through which large amounts of air were introduced in the cerebral circulation. Spielmeyer,[1] however, felt that the lesions were best explained on the basis of functional vascular changes.

In our third case the presence of vascular congestion and "ring" hemorrhages supports this view of Spielmeyer. It is not difficult to see how the severe convulsions would affect the intrathoracic pressure in a manner conducive to venous and capillary stasis and hence cerebral ischemia. All the circumstances in this case were similar to those in the first two. But the fourth case is not as readily explained inasmuch as the child did not convulse. Nevertheless, respiratory difficulty and cyanosis were prominent features in this child's clinical history and apparently were as effective in inducing cerebral ischemia as are convulsions. That this is actually so will be demonstrated in some of the subsequent cases.

Peritonsillar Abscess

CASE 5.—A white male infant, 6½ years old, suddenly developed status epilepticus which ended fatally in about six and one-half hours. He lost consciousness and became cyanotic. There was fever. Necropsy revealed peritonsillar abscess, capillary stasis and hemorrhages in the brain, ischemic cell changes, and destruction of ganglion cells in the cerebral cortex.

Clinical History.—On arising from bed about ten hours prior to admission to the hospital, this 6½-year-old child said that he did not feel well and wanted no breakfast. Shortly afterwards he complained of being chilly and toward evening, rather suddenly, had a generalized convulsion which lasted one and one-half hours.

He was sent to the Meriden Hospital, Meriden, Conn., where the ordinary sedatives and a spinal puncture were of no avail in stopping the convulsions.

The child was fairly well nourished and well developed. He was unconscious and cyanotic; breathing was stertorous. The temperature on admission was 107.6° F.; the pulse rate was 156 per minute and irregular. The heart was pounding, but there were no murmurs and no enlargement. The throat could not be examined because the jaws were tightly closed.

The spinal fluid was under normal pressure and fell rapidly when 10 c.c. were withdrawn. It was clear and contained only two lymphocytes and one leucocyte per cubic millimeter. At the end of about five hours of constant convulsions, the child died.

Necropsy.—The examination was made by Dr. J. A. Ferguson about twelve hours after death.

The only lesions encountered outside the nervous system were in the posterior pharynx, which was swollen and intensely congested. Both tonsils were deep red,

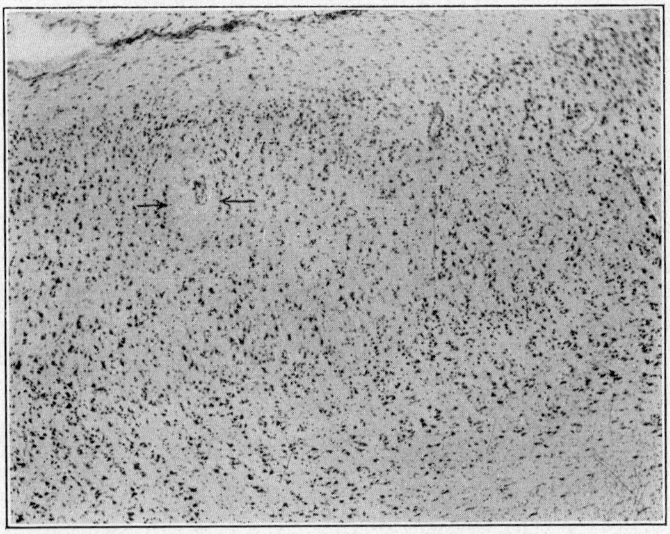

Fig. 8.—Case 5. The arrows point to a "ring" hemorrhage in the cerebral cortex. The cellular architecture is somewhat altered by the disappearance of ganglion cells. Nissl stain. (×65.)

and the left one contained a small quantity of pus which was easily expressed from it and the peritonsillar tissues.

Brain.—The cerebrum was covered by intensely congested leptomeninges. There was no cerebral swelling or edema. The subcortical vessels were engorged and many petechial hemorrhages were found in the white matter of the brain. Abnormalities were not discovered macroscopically in either the basal ganglions, cornu ammonis formations, or occipital cortex.

Many pial and parenchymal arterioles and capillaries were found congested on histologic examination. Small hemorrhages were found widely distributed in the cerebral cortex and subcortex as well as in the medulla (Fig. 8). Some of these were of the ''ring'' type. The ganglion cells of the cortex in general had a shrunken appearance, but only in the temporal and occipital lobes had they disappeared in sufficiently large numbers to alter the cytoarchitectural appearance. Ischemic cell change was present in the cornu ammonis formations and occipital lobes. Capillary stasis only was present in the cerebellum.

Comment.—In this instance the necrobiotic changes in the cerebral cortex were less conspicuous, and the capillary congestion and hemorrhages were more striking than in the previous cases. The survival of the child for only six and one-half hours after the onset of the convulsive attacks undoubtedly influenced the limitation of the necrobiotic lesions.

Bacillary Dysentery

CASE 6.—The patient was a white male child whose illness began with a chill lasting five minutes. Three hours later stupor, delirium, fever, and rapid pulse rate developed, along with bacillary dysentery, with mucus and blood in the stools. Generalized tonic convulsion, lasting twenty minutes, was followed by a similar convulsion two hours later. There was a succession of tonic and clonic convulsions, each lasting about two minutes and more marked on right side. Respirations were labored and rapid; there was cyanosis. Death occurred four hours after the initial convulsion. Cerebral edema and destruction of nerve cells in cerebral cortex, especially cornu ammonis formations, were noted.

Clinical History.—Two weeks before admission to the New Haven Hospital the patient had a cold, rhinitis, and an elevation of temperature. He was in bed for four days and then apparently recovered. At 8:30 P.M. of the day of admission to the hospital the child had a chill which lasted five minutes, following which he slept restlessly. At 9:00 P.M. he vomited and appeared flushed. At 11:00 P.M. the father noted that the child failed to recognize him. He became stuporous, irrational, and delirious, and was brought to the hospital in this condition.

It was learned that the patient's brother was hospitalized three days previously with bacillary dysentery. The parents had both had diarrhea, and the father was still suffering from this ailment. In the summer of the preceding year the patient and his oldest sister, aged 11 years, had diarrhea for three or four days. A cousin, 1½ years old, visited the family that summer and developed a diarrhea the following day. The family's drinking water is obtained from a well.

On admission the patient's temperature was 40.4° C., the pulse rate 180, and the respirations 36 per minute. He appeared acutely ill and was stuporous but could be aroused. Reflexes were normal.

He remained semicomatose until noon of the following day, when he appeared brighter and took fluid by mouth. Frequent loose stools containing mucus, pus, and streaks of blood were passed. He did well until 4:00 P.M. of that day, when he vomited and again lapsed into coma. At 7:00 P.M. he had a generalized tonic convulsion lasting twenty minutes, which was relieved with intravenous magnesium sulfate. Two hours later a similar seizure occurred, followed by a period of quiet until 11:30 P.M., when he began to have tonic and clonic convulsions in succession, each lasting about two minutes. These seizures continued with more marked involvement of the right side of the body. Respirations became more rapid and labored, and cyanosis appeared. Following a vomiting spell at 1:00 A.M., respirations ceased, death occurring four hours after the initial convulsion and approximately thirty hours after the onset of the present illness.

Urinalysis revealed three-plus sugar but no acetone and no cells in the sediment. A blood count showed 5,170,000 red blood cells and 39,800 white blood cells. The differential count was 89 per cent leucocytes and 9 per cent lymphocytes. Blood Kahn test was negative. Stool culture yielded dysentery bacilli, but blood culture was negative. The spinal fluid was not examined.

Necropsy.—Post-mortem examination was performed by Dr. Robert Tennant, Jr., eight hours after exitus.

There was a generalized lymphoid hyperplasia, with especial involvement of Peyer's patches and solitary lymph follicles of the intestines. The mesenteric lymph nodes were enlarged, measuring 1 to 1½ cm. in diameter. In the collapsed intestinal tract there was found a small quantity of milky white, tenacious mucoid material. The mucosa of the intestines was injected, and on microscopic examination was seen to contain numerous small ''punched out'' ulcers which were localized to the regions of the Peyer's patches and lymph follicles. The whole wall was edematous and infiltrated with mononuclear cells and eosinophilic leucocytes.

Brain.—The brain was edematous and its convolutions were flattened. A well-marked cerebellar pressure cone was present. The cerebral meninges were free of exudate and hemorrhage. The vessels in the centrum ovale were quite congested. In several gyri the normal cortical cytoarchitecture was blurred. This was caused by the fact that many of the ganglion cells were shrunken and stained poorly, whereas others had completely disappeared. Some appeared waterlogged and showed extensive chromatolytic changes. In the cornu ammonis formations many of the ganglion cells of Sommer's sector were absent (Fig. 9).

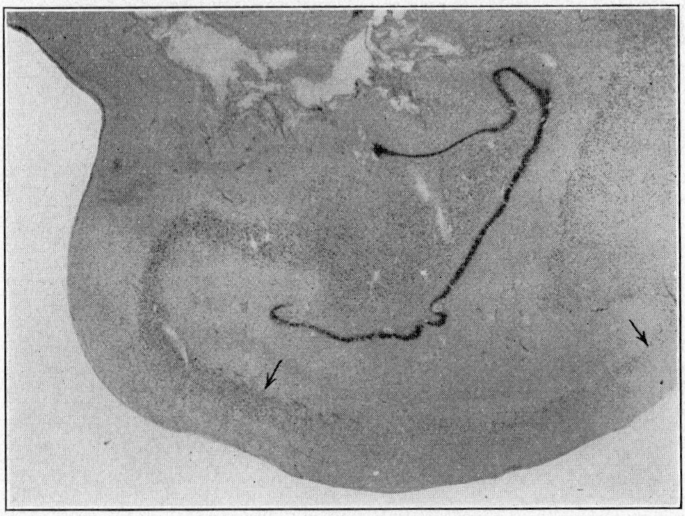

Fig. 9.—Case 6. The bleaching of Sommer's sector (between arrows) is due to destruction of its cellular components. Some of the injured cells, however, still persist (death of child only four hours after initial convulsion). Nissl stain. (×11.)

Comment.—As in Case 5, the full extent of the cortical cellular destruction was not reached because the survival of the child was a matter of only four hours from the initial convulsive attack. The cerebral edema and subcortical vascular congestion, as well as the necrobiotic changes which were present, were referable to the convulsive attacks and their concomitant intracranial vascular disturbances.

Upper Respiratory Tract Infection

CASE 7.—A 5-year-old white girl became anorexic, feverish, and drowsy; she vomited once, had generalized convulsions, and lost consciousness. The pupils were unequal. Repeated generalized convulsions were followed by status epilepticus. Death came on the thirteenth day of illness, with fever of 107° F. There was destruction of nerve cells of the cerebral cortex.

Clinical History.—This 5-year-old white girl was well until about five days before admission to the Children's Hospital, Boston, when she became anorexic and feverish and vomited once. She then recovered and felt better until the day before admission, when she became drowsy and slept a considerable part of the time. Two hours before admission she had a generalized convulsion and lost consciousness.

The child was well developed and well nourished. The eyes were pulled over to the left and occasionally rolled back. There was no acetone on her breath. Her color was good and respirations were normal. Nevertheless, she was semicomatose and did not respond to stimuli. The left pupil was slightly larger than the right; both fundi showed slight haziness of the disks. A moderate amount of postnasal discharge was noted, and the pharynx was slightly injected. She had had no exposure to contagious diseases.

Soon after her admission to the hospital she began having generalized convulsions which could be controlled only with sodium luminal, avertin, or paraldehyde. When not under the influence of these sedatives, the child convulsed almost constantly. She

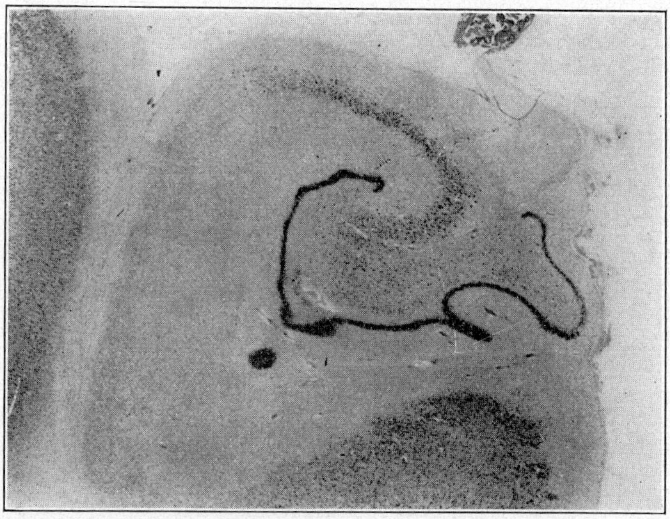

Fig. 10.—Case 7. Extensive destruction of ganglion cells is present in Sommer's sector. The end plate is similarly involved, but to a lesser degree. Nissl stain. (×11.)

never regained consciousness after the onset of the illness and died on the thirteenth day. Her temperature rose on that day to 107° F., but it had been between 101° and 102° F. throughout most of the illness.

Laboratory examinations revealed four-plus acetone in the urine. Red blood cells numbered 4,360,000 per cubic millimeter; white blood cells were 5,800 per cubic millimeter, with a normal differential count except for a high lymphocytic-monocytic ratio. The spinal fluid on repeated examination, which included culture, was entirely normal. The blood Wassermann reaction and the tuberculin test were negative. Repeated blood cultures were negative; blood calcium was 9.7 mg. per cent; blood sugar was 129 mg. per cent.

Necropsy.—Post-mortem examination was limited to the intracranial contents and was performed at the Children's Hospital, Boston, under the direction of Dr. Sidney Farber. Fresh tissue from the cerebellum and occipital lobes was injected into monkeys, with negative results.

There was no macroscopic evidence of meningitis or a parenchymal inflammatory lesion. On microscopic examination, also, the meninges were found to be free from exudate. The cortex of all the cerebral lobes, except the temporal, presented a normal cytoarchitectural appearance. In the cornu ammonis formations there was extensive necrosis of the ganglion cells in Sommer's sector (Fig. 10). The blood vessels in this part of the brain were not altered, and there was no proliferation of the glia. Many of the Purkinje cells in the cerebellum had disappeared, leaving behind focal glial proliferations in the molecular layer. The putamina also showed destruction of their ganglion cells, and here the lesion was associated with vascular thickening and hyalinization and with the proliferation of microglia.

Comment.—A limited post-mortem examination precluded the determination of the exact nature of the underlying infectious disease. The symptoms pointed so overwhelmingly to the nervous system that they overshadowed the clinical picture. There is thus left the meager evidence of a postnasal discharge and an injected pharynx to indicate an upper respiratory tract infection as the illness which initiated the repeated generalized convulsive attacks. The changes in the nervous system, contrary to indicating an inflammatory condition, which could cause these attacks, were of a type which has been shown in all six previous cases to have resulted from cerebral ischemia and, except in one instance (Case 4), from the convulsions themselves.

CONVULSIONS WITH MALNUTRITION

CASE 8.—A black male child, 3 months old, had marasmus from improper nutrition. Stimulants were required after the sudden cessation of respiration. There was a generalized convulsion, and respiratory difficulty for twenty-two hours resulted in death. There was widespread destruction of nerve cells of the cerebral cortex.

Clinical History.—The patient was a black male infant, 3 months of age, who was born in the ambulance on the way to the hospital after a normal pregnancy and with a breech presentation. The birth weight was 3,700 gm.

The mother, aged 18 years, was a known syphilitic who had received treatment in the New Haven Hospital. Her serology was negative at the time this child was born. She had one other child, a boy 2 years old, who was well; she had no other children or pregnancies.

The patient was breast-fed for the first 3 weeks of life and was then placed by the mother on a formula of 1 tablespoon of condensed milk in 32 ounces of water. Of this, he received 8 ounces every four hours for a period of five weeks. He then began to vomit and took but four ounces of the formula at a feeding. One teaspoonful of cod-liver oil and one-half glass of orange juice were given twice daily. He is said to have done well on this regime except that he gained no weight. At the age of 8 weeks, when he began refusing half his formula and to vomit, the loss of weight became continuous.

On admission to the hospital the infant was poorly developed, poorly nourished, and extremely dehydrated. The temperature was 95.4° F., and his weight was 3,000 gm. The skin was loose and flabby, and the eyelids were puffy.

Immediately after admission he was started on parenteral fluids, saline and glucose, and was given a transfusion of 75 c.c. of blood. On the morning after admission the infant suddenly stopped breathing for several moments and then breathed shallowly and slowly. Caffeine sodiobenzoate, adrenalin, carbon dioxide, and artificial respiration were employed, with little success. Four hours later he had a short period of tonic contractions of the entire body, the hands being held in carpal spasm. Five c.c. of calcium gluconate were given intramuscularly. The following morning, some twenty hours after the onset of respiratory difficulty, he once more developed weak, shallow respirations which became Cheyne-Stokes in type; he died two hours later.

The blood Kahn and Wassermann reactions were both negative. The red blood cells numbered 4,290,000 and the hemoglobin 76 per cent on admission. There was no albumin, sugar, acetone, or diacetic acid in the urine.

Necropsy.—Post-mortem examination was performed by Dr. David Gaiser within three hours after exitus.

The body weighed 2,910 gm. and measured 55½ cm. in length. Practically no subcutaneous adipose tissue was present. Examination of the accessible bones, including the skull, ribs, and left femur, revealed no abnormalities in the periosteum, costochondral junctions, and diaphysis. Congestion was found in the lower lobes of both lungs but there was no pneumonic exudate or hemorrhage. The duodenum was filled with a large fresh blood clot which originated from an ulcer on the posterior surface of the duodenum 2 cm. from the pylorus. The base of the ulcer lay in the head of the pancreas, was granular, and contained a small thrombus which was attached to an eroded blood vessel. Numerous leucocytes infiltrated the walls and base of the ulcer. The entire intestinal tract was filled with dark, gelatinous blood clots.

Brain.—Macroscopic examination of the brain revealed no abnormalities, but on histologic examination there appeared widespread changes in the cerebral cortex. Most extensively involved were the insular, occipital, and hippocampal gyri, which showed ischemic necrosis of the ganglion cells, sometimes involving one and sometimes all of the laminae. The third cortical layer, however, was most frequently destroyed. The same ischemic involvement of nerve cells was seen in the claustrum and pallidal nuclei. The cornu ammonis formations had lost all but a few cells of the Sommer's sector (Fig. 11). None of the nuclei in the medulla were injured.

CASE 9.—A white male infant, 6 months old, with history of intractable diarrhea from birth. There was respiratory difficulty, followed by cessation, requiring stimulants and artificial respiration. Death occurred after twelve hours. There was cerebral edema and destruction of nerve cells of the cerebral cortex associated with glial proliferation.

Clinical History.—The patient was a white 6-month-old male infant who began having five to seven loose green stools daily from the age of three days until his admission to the hospital, twenty-five days before death. The intractable diarrhea was seemingly uninfluenced by any methods of feeding, although these were repeatedly changed. The child was breast-fed during the first three months of life, then received breast and supplementary feedings for the next two months. At this time a series of experiments in feeding was begun by the mother, who changed the diet whenever she heard of some new food or when she suspected that the old was injuring the baby. The child was finally brought to the New Haven Hospital because of the diarrhea, extreme pallor, emaciation, and unexplained fever.

The birth of the child was said to have been normal and spontaneous. There were no convulsions or cyanosis. This was the first child of a 26-year-old mother who had no other pregnancies.

The diarrhea could not be controlled in the hospital, even when all food by mouth was stopped for a while and the child was given parenteral fluid, intravenous glucose, and transfusion. As soon as the food by mouth was increased above 30 calories per kilo, the diarrhea recurred. The temperature was elevated throughout the course, sometimes reaching 39° C.

At 8:30 one evening, the child developed Cheyne-Stokes respiration and became anotic. One hour later he suddenly ceased breathing entirely, and the heart sounds ame very faint. Stimulants revived him somewhat, but the Cheyne-Stokes breath-

ing continued. Again one-half hour later the respirations ceased, necessitating artificial respiration. The child seemed then to have revived, although he remained cyanotic, but at nine o'clock the following morning he died.

Repeated blood cultures yielded no growth of organisms. The white blood cells were always above 14,000, and the differential count showed 73 per cent leucocytes and 23 per cent lymphocytes. The blood Kahn reaction was negative, as was also the tuberculin reaction.

Fig. 11.

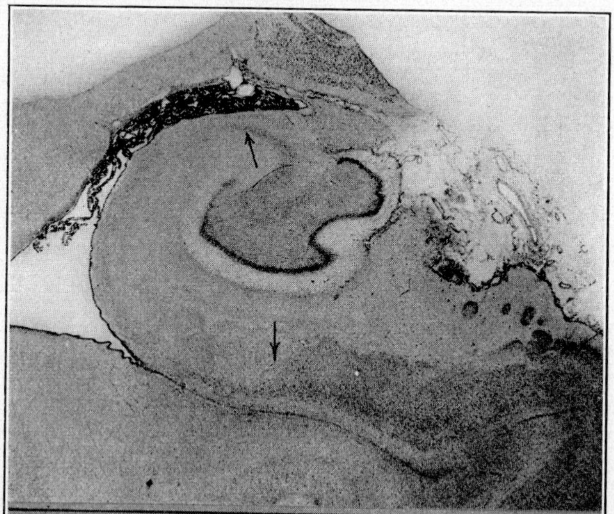

Fig. 12.

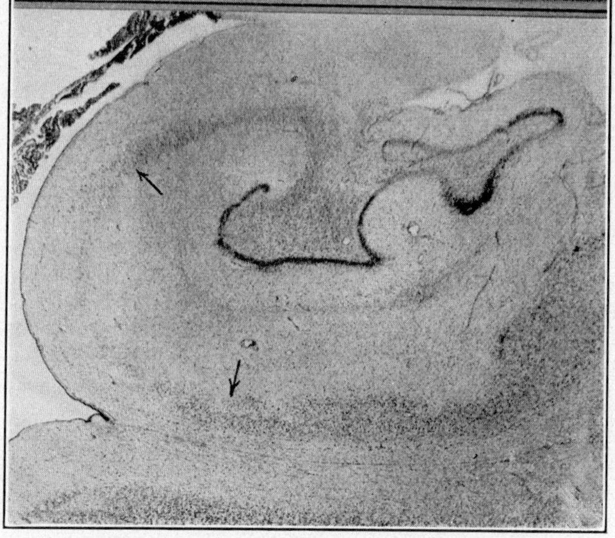

Fig. 11.—Case 8. There is a disappearance of all but a few nerve cells in Sommer's sector of the cornu ammonis formation. Nissl stain. (×11.)

Fig. 12.—Case 9. Part of Sommer's sector (between arrows) is devoid of ganglion cells. Nissl stain. (×18.)

Necropsy.—Necropsy was performed by Dr. Dan Egbert five hours post mortem.

Aside from the lesions in the nervous system, the only positive findings were the emaciation and a fibrosis of the pancreas. The fibrous tissue in this organ was infiltrated with large numbers of lymphocytes.

Brain.—Macroscopic examination of the nervous system revealed no abnormalities. Histologically there was seen widespread cortical damage characterized by a diminution in the number of ganglion cells in the superficial laminae. This was associated with a proliferative response on the part of the glia, chiefly of the astrocytic variety. The chief damage had occurred in the cornu ammonis formations (Fig. 12), but the cortex of the frontal, parietal, and occipital lobes was also involved. The basal ganglions were spared.

Many of the nerve cells which still persisted were shrunken and hyperchromatic; others showed ischemic necrosis; some were surrounded by pericellular incrustations. There was evidence of edema throughout the brain, as manifested by greatly dilated perivascular spaces which imparted a spongy appearance to some portions.

CASE 10.—A 5-month-old white male infant was presumably well until sudden onset of illness with vomiting, drowsiness, and generalized convulsions. Respiratory difficulty and retinal hemorrhages culminated in death, in twenty-four hours. The infant had rickets and cerebral and subdural hemorrhages; there was destruction of nerve cells of the cerebral cortex.

Clinical History.—The patient, a white male infant, 5 months of age, was born to healthy parents following the first pregnancy, the course and termination of which were entirely normal. The child had been well until the onset of the present illness which started with forceful vomiting. He became increasingly drowsy, and there was generalized stiffening with twitchings of the right eye and the right hand. Breathing became stertorous, and the pupils were dilated.

On admission to the New Haven Hospital respirations were noted to be of the Cheyne-Stokes type. The skin was extremely pale, except for one small hemorrhagic nodule over the lower ribs in the right axillary line. Both fontanels were open and very tense. The pupils were dilated and fixed. The fundi, especially the right, showed a number of small fresh hemorrhages, and the right disk was obscured by a massive hemorrhage. The heart sounds were rapid and high-pitched. The blood pressure was 105 mm. of mercury systolic and 70 mm. diastolic. There was a positive Babinski sign on the left, but the deep reflexes were normal. Death occurred eighteen hours after admission to the hospital and about twenty-four hours after the first generalized convulsion.

Lumbar puncture revealed xanthochromic fluid with an initial pressure of 350 mm. of water. The rapidly fatal termination precluded any laboratory examinations.

Necropsy.—Post-mortem examination was performed by Dr. Lincoln Opper four and one-half hours after exitus.

The body was well nourished and well developed. The occipital and parietal bones of the calvarium were extremely soft to palpation. Small, sharply circumscribed fenestrations were found everywhere in the calvaria, which was peculiarly square-shaped due to the prominences of the frontal and parietal bosses. The lower ribs were flared in bell fashion. A microscopic preparation of an osteochondral junction of a rib showed a typically rachitic zone containing strands and clusters of large vesicular cartilage cells in place of osteoid tissue. This junction also showed an increased vascularity. There were no subperiosteal hemorrhages, but petechiae were found in the splenic capsule, thymus, and pleurae.

The liver was normal in size, weighing 205 gm., but it was mottled externally and on section with irregular green-yellow patches. Microscopically there was noted a diffuse hepatic fibrosis which was most marked in the periportal zones. Small round cells and plasma cells were seen in the proliferating connective tissue which replaced cords of liver cells. There was marked stasis in the bile capillaries.

Brain.—A large subdural hematoma of recent origin was present over the right parietal lobe. This appeared to arise from a massive hemorrhage in the right temporal lobe which ruptured through the superior temporal gyrus (Fig. 13). There

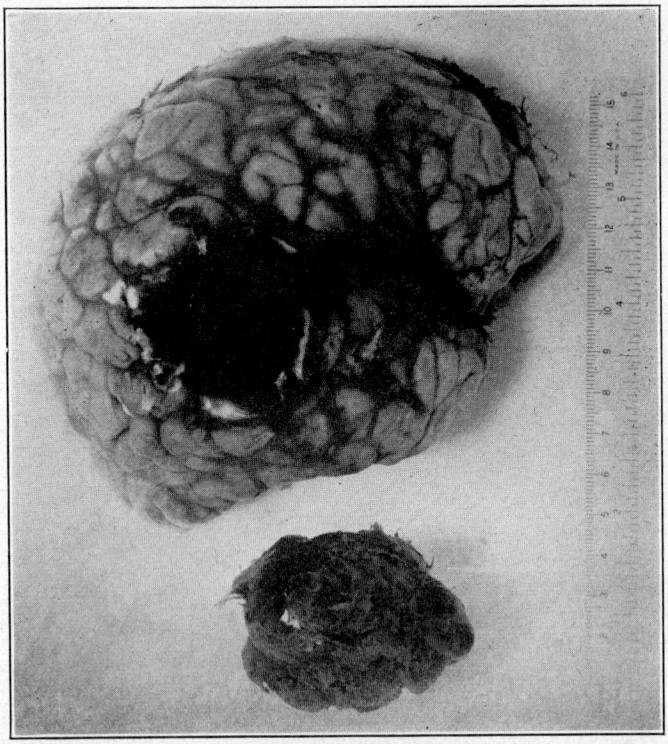

Fig. 13.—Case 10. Photograph of the brain showing the site of hemorrhage in the right temporoparietal region. The blood clot, which has been removed, lies below.

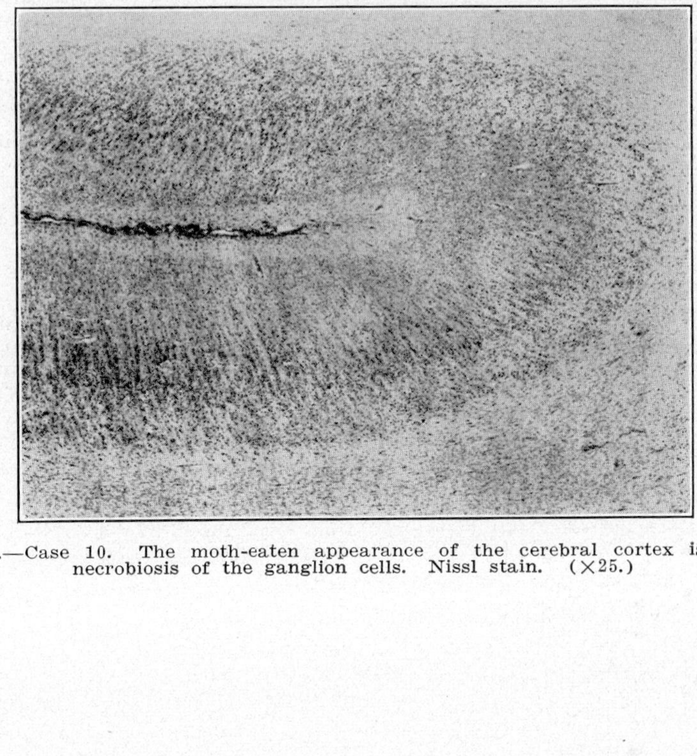

Fig. 14.—Case 10. The moth-eaten appearance of the cerebral cortex is due to necrobiosis of the ganglion cells. Nissl stain. (×25.)

was nothing to indicate the source of the hemorrhage either in the gross or on microscopic examination. It was of recent origin, as indicated by the well-preserved red blood cells of which it was composed. The remainder of the parenchyma of the temporal lobe contained numerous small petechiae.

Throughout the cortex of the cerebrum and particularly in the occipital lobes there were found foci of necrosis involving the ganglion cells. These foci had no predilection for any particular cortical layer, being so widely disseminated in all the layers as to impart a moth-eaten appearance to the cortical cytoarchitecture (Fig. 14). In most instances the cells had completely disappeared without leaving any trace. The glia cells did not participate in the reaction.

Comment.—Each of the three infants in this group had a severe grade of malnutrition to which the final illness, which was characterized by Cheyne-Stokes respiration or convulsive seizures, was attributable. In Case 9 only was there any fever, and this was due to dehydration. Acute infection was not a part of the clinical course in these children, yet the cerebral lesions demonstrated at necropsy were similar in kind and distribution to those found in the children who succumbed during acute infections. The cerebral edema in Case 9 and the hemorrhages in Case 10 were evidences of disturbed cerebral circulation resulting from respiratory difficulty or convulsions, having the same pathogenesis, therefore, as the necrobiotic lesions themselves.

CONVULSIONS FOLLOWING ICTERUS GRAVIS

CASE 11.—A white male child, 11 months old, who had icterus gravis neonatorum accompanied by generalized convulsions and followed by repeated spasmodic attacks and mental retardation, had a sudden onset of respiratory difficulty, resulting in death nine hours later. There was widespread destruction of nerve cells in the cerebral cortex, basal ganglions, and nuclei of the medulla and cerebellum.

Clinical History.—The patient, a white male child aged 11 months, was born by low forceps delivery following a normal pregnancy. There was no history of birth injury. At the age of 5 days he developed jaundice, which became very severe during the course of the next few days and was accompanied by convulsions. He remained in the hospital for six weeks, at the end of which time the jaundice had completely disappeared, and he was discharged.

At home he continued to have daily spasmodic attacks and appeared to be definitely retarded mentally. For this reason he was admitted to the New Haven Hospital where physical examination revealed a well-developed and well-nourished child who was spastic, apathetic, and out of touch with the environment. The head was held slightly retracted, though it could readily be flexed on the neck. The reflexes were hyperactive, and there was a questionable bilateral Babinski sign. Encephalography revealed a moderate increase in the size of both lateral ventricles and, to a lesser degree, of the third and fourth ventricles. There appeared to be some cortical atrophy.

Once more the child was discharged from the hospital to his home where his course remained uneventful until the day of death. On the morning of that day, at 11:30, he was apparently doing well, but at 12:10 he was found limp and cyanotic. He was not breathing, and his heart was not beating. At 12:20 adrenalin was injected intracardially, and artificial respiration was started. The heart began to beat a few minutes later, and at 12:40 he gradually began to breathe. He remained limp and motionless until 2:30 P.M., when the muscle tonus gradually increased. The child became spastic and had a well-sustained ankle clonus. There were occasional twitchings of the jaw. At 9:20 P.M., he became cyanotic and died of respiratory failure without having regained consciousness since noon.

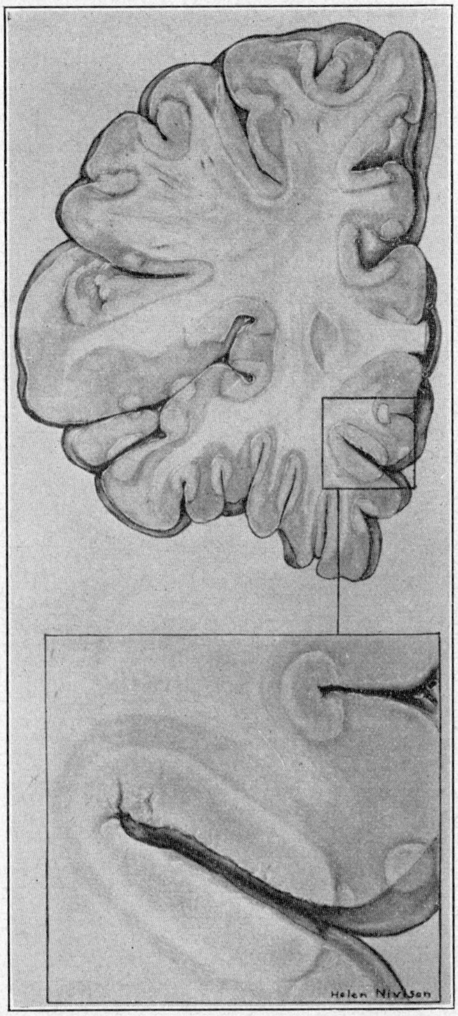

Fig. 15.—Case 11. Patches of discoloration due to necrobiosis are seen in the cortical gray matter in the troughs and at the sides of the sulci. Drawing of frontal lobe.

Necropsy.—Post-mortem examination, which was limited to the intracranial contents, was performed by Dr. David M. Grayzel one hour and twenty minutes after exitus.

Brain.—The brain was well developed, and there was no apparent atrophy of the cerebral convolutions. There was likewise no evidence of internal hydrocephalus. An amazing picture of yellow, patchy discoloration was seen in the cortical gray matter, occurring in the majority of instances in the troughs of the cerebral sulci and extending occasionally along the sides of the sulci (Fig. 15). The lesions were sharply limited to the cortical gray matter and did not appear to extend to the subcortex. Similar discolorations were seen in the central gray matter, particularly in the thalami and putamina. The cortex of the occipital lobes showed the most extensive involvement.

On microscopic examination the cortex presented a moth-eaten appearance due to the disappearance in patches of many of the ganglion cells (Fig. 16). Sometimes this lesion involved one and sometimes another of the cortical laminae, but more often all six layers were involved. When one layer alone was destroyed, it was usually the third. The involvement was predominant in the depths of the cerebral sulci, but in rare instances the crests of the convolutions were also implicated. The lesions were more extensive in some of the gyri than in others. Thus the entire cornu ammonis formations were destroyed, and the cortex of the occipital lobes was much more extensively involved than the cortex of any other lobe. Similar

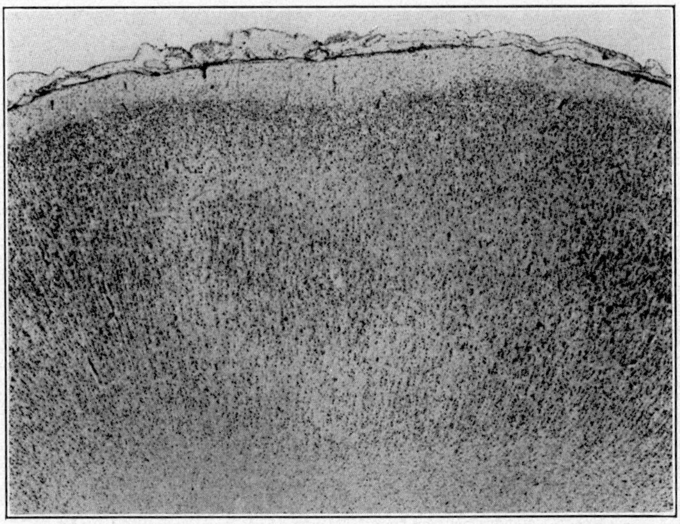

Fig. 16.—Case 11. The photomicrograph shows a peculiar ringlike, bleached zone in which there is necrobiosis of ganglion cells. Motor cortex. Nissl stain. (×25.)

lesions were present in the caudate nuclei, the putamina, the inferior olives of the medulla, and the dentate nuclei of the cerebellum.

The surviving nerve cells in the foci of injury were altered in a variety of ways. Often they were ischemic. Occasionally they showed hydropic degeneration and contained one or more vacuoles in their cytoplasm. Many of the cells were surrounded by pericellular spaces of edema. Chronic cell damage was found in almost every focal lesion. Some cells were shrunken and hyperchromatic, and there was a loss of distinct demarcation between nucleus and cytoplasm. Pericellular incrustations were found outside some of the cell bodies and their processes. The glia was not involved in either degenerative or proliferative responses. There was no evidence of bile pigments or bile salts in any part of the brain.

Comment.—This child undoubtedly had jaundiced basal ganglions during the course of the icterus gravis, for the lesions in the caudate nuclei, putamina, inferior olives, and dentate nuclei are the well-recognized residua of this condition. The mental retardation and the spasticity likewise fit in with this assumption. The hyperchromic cell change and the more recent necrobiosis, however, are to be accounted for on the basis of the convulsive attacks during the neonatal period and the respiratory collapse during the final nine hours of life.

BIRTH INJURY AND ASPHYXIA

CASE 12.—A white female infant, 3 days old, born to 19-year-old primipara after moderately severe labor lasting 19 hours, was covered with meconium. Alternating periods of pallor and cyanosis were associated with irregular respiration. There were right facial paralysis, spasticity of the left arm, bilateral ankle clonus, and dissociation of ocular movements. There was destruction of nerve cells of cerebral cortex, associated with glial proliferation.

Clinical History.—The patient was a white female infant born to a 19-year-old primipara. Birth followed a nineteen-hour labor of moderate severity, and delivery was spontaneous. At birth the infant was covered with meconium and breathed poorly. Stimulants were administered and the baby was placed in a respirator when breathing became more regular. About six hours after birth a right facial paralysis was noted. Three times during the following morning the baby vomited tarry material, which gave a positive guaiac reaction. Periods of pallor alternating with periods of cyanosis were present.

The patient was pale and drowsy and had irregular, rapid, and deep respirations which alternated with periods of apnea and cyanosis. At times the eyes deviated to the left. The fundic veins were full, but there were no retinal hemorrhages. The mouth was pulled to the left, and there was right facial weakness. The left arm was held in flexion and was slightly spastic; the right was almost flaccid. Reflexes of the lower extremities were not abnormal, but there was a slight increase in the right knee jerk.

On the day following birth, a bilateral ankle clonus was noted. The anterior fontanel felt boardlike, but was not full. The next day complete dissociation of ocular movements appeared. An odor of acetone was detected on the breath, and a urine specimen at that time showed four-plus acetone, two-plus albumin, and one-plus sugar. In spite of clyses and gastric lavage, the child did not improve. The respirations became shallow, grunting, and irregular, and the fontanel bulged slightly. A few râles at the right base were noted, and the child vomited bloody material. Death occurred on the third day.

Bleeding time was three minutes, and clotting time was three minutes. Blood culture was positive for *Streptococcus hemolyticus*. Spinal, cisternal, and ventricular punctures were attempted without success.

Necropsy.—Post-mortem examination was performed by Dr. David Dial one hour after exitus, and the following is an abbreviated transcript of his protocol.

The body was well developed and appeared well nourished, measuring 51 cm. in length and weighing 3,450 gm. About 10 c.c. of clotted blood were present in the left thoracic cavity, and a smaller quantity was found in the pericardial sac. The lungs were mottled alternately with light and dark red patches of consolidation. These were most numerous in the lower lobes and showed, on microscopic examination, a pneumonic exudate of leucocytes, fibrin, and red blood cells. Amniotic material was not to be seen in either the bronchioles or the alveoli.

Brain and Spinal Cord.—The cerebral convolutions were distinctly flattened; otherwise there were no changes noted on macroscopic examination. Microscopically, the usual cortical cytoarchitecture was obliterated in large numbers of cerebral gyri (Figs. 17 and 18). Marked astrocytic proliferation was seen in the first cortical lamina; occasionally such cells were in mitotic division. In the deeper laminae, the rod-shaped Hortega cells were most numerous. The nerve cells of these layers, however, had completely disappeared. In a few isolated zones groups of nerve cells persisted uninjured in the midst of wide fields of cellular destruction.

Fig. 17.

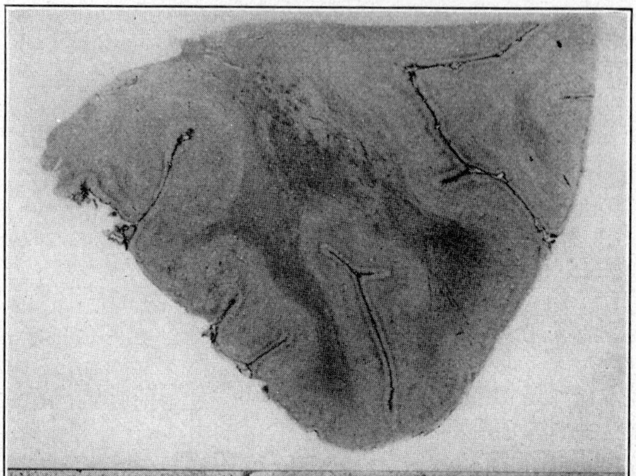

Fig. 18.

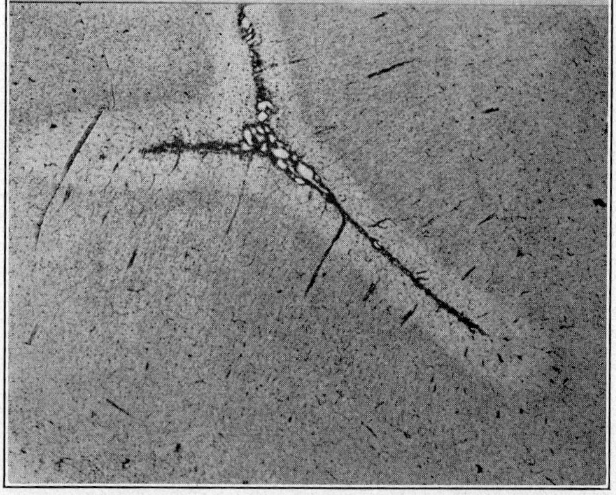

Fig. 17.—Case 12. Photomicrograph of part of the occipital lobe. The entire cortical cytoarchitecture is obliterated and there is a reversal of the staining properties, the subcortical white matter being stained darker than the cortical gray. Nissl stain. (×2.)

Fig. 18.—Case 12. The ganglion cells of the cortex of three adjacent gyri in the occipital lobe have completely disappeared. The glia has proliferated to a mild degree. Nissl stain. (×25.)

In the subcortical white matter the glial reaction was more widespread, more active, and more varied. Glia in mitotic division were more frequently encountered here than in the cortex. Phagocytic cells filled with fat were present in abundance, and there was evidence to indicate that some of the myelinated fibers were undergoing destruction.

In several places in the centrum ovale as well as in the reticular formation of the pons, several small hemorrhages were found, in which the red blood cells had become laked and had liberated their pigment.

CASE 13.—A black male infant, 3 days old, was born to 16-year-old primipara after induced labor in the eighth month of gestation. He was apparently normal

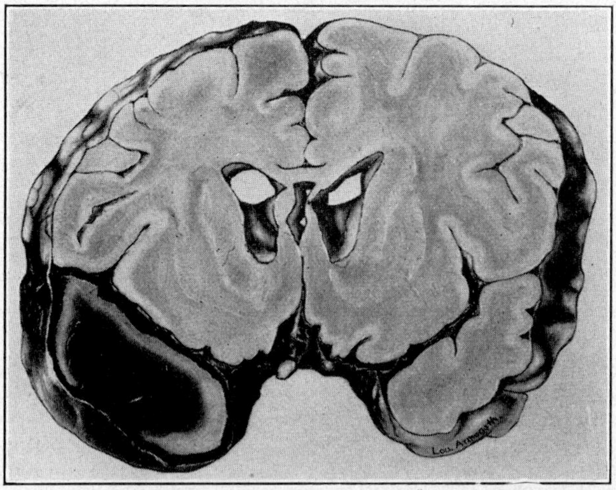

Fig. 19.—Case 13. Drawing of a section of the brain to show the hemorrhage in the right temporal lobe.

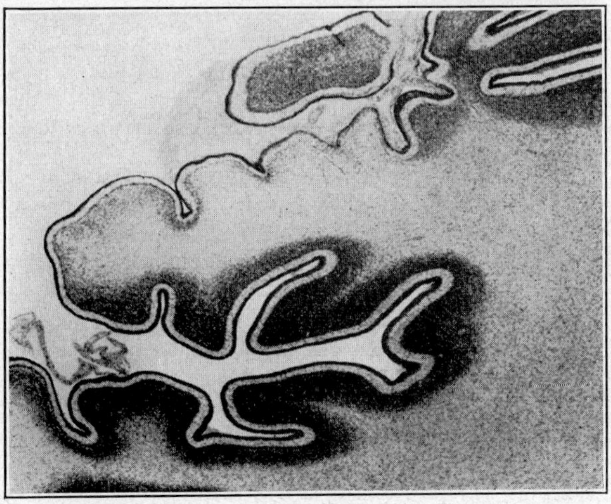

Fig. 20.—Case 13. The Purkinje and granular cells of several lobules of the cerebellum have disappeared. Nissl stain. (×25.)

until five hours preceding death, when feebleness, respiratory difficulty, facial weakness, and retraction of the head were noted. There were massive intracerebral and subarachnoid hemorrhages; nerve cells of the cerebral and cerebellar cortex were destroyed.

Clinical History.—The patient was a 3-day-old black male infant born to a primipara who was 16 years of age. Roentgen-ray pelvimetry revealed a small pelvis in the mother and a large fetus, consequently it was considered advisable to induce labor in the eighth month of gestation. Quinine and castor oil were used without effect. Finally, pitocin was employed intranasally, and pains began. The delivery was normal and spontaneous and the child cried well following delivery. First stage of labor lasted seventeen hours and second stage, forty-five minutes.

For the next three days the child seemed to be doing well. His birth weight was 3,360 gm., and he lost only 235 gm. He was nursing poorly, but the mother had not begun to lactate well. Temperature and respiration were normal. There were no restlessness, irritability, or convulsions.

At midnight of the third day he appeared feeble and seemed unable to grasp the nipple when put to breast. Four hours later the respirations became very irregular, and the color was poor. A questionable facial weakness was noted, but there were no convulsions. The head was retracted and the fontanel was full. Supportive treatment was without avail, and the child died one hour later.

The Wassermann reaction on the mother's blood was negative.

Necropsy.—Post-mortem examination was performed by Dr. John Mendillo six hours after exitus. The findings other than those in the nervous system were not contributory.

Brain.—A massive subarachnoid hemorrhage, which had its origin in the underlying parenchyma, covered the entire right temporal lobe (Fig. 19). Hemorrhage was also found in both sylvian fissures and over the orbital surfaces of the frontal lobes. A large blood clot was found in the right cerebellar lobe, which compressed the pons and in part destroyed the vermis cerebelli. The lateral ventricles were dilated as the result of the compression of both the aqueduct of Sylvius and the fourth ventricle. Clotted blood was found in the right lateral and in the third ventricles.

In several places near the sites of the parenchymal hemorrhages, greatly dilated blood vessels with thin walls were encountered, which were markedly congested. It appeared that some of these, by rupturing, had produced the extensive hemorrhages. The cerebral cortex was the seat of widespread destruction of ganglion cells. These cells alone had been injured and had disappeared; the glia remained intact. The cerebellar cortex also contained small zones of necrosis which destroyed Purkinje cells and the small granular cells (Fig. 20).

CASE 14.—A white male infant, 2 days old, was born after induced labor when fetal movements nearly ceased. He was pale, cyanotic, anemic, and had respiratory difficulty. There was a true knot in umbilical cord and destruction of nerve cells of the cerebral cortex.

Clinical History.—The patient was a white male infant, 2 days of age, who was born at full term to a 35-year-old para ii. Three days before delivery, the fetal movements became less marked, but the heart beat was audible in the left lower quadrant and was strong and regular. Labor was induced with castor oil and quinine, and pains started after several hours. The descent of the head was slow so that low forceps were employed.

At birth the infant was pale and cyanotic, and although the lungs were well expanded, there was a low respiratory grunt. A true knot was found in the cord when the placenta was delivered, but the placenta itself appeared to be normal. The infant had a blood count of 2,700,000 red blood cells and 50 per cent hemoglobin. Because of this, he was transfused with 80 c.c. of the mother's blood, to which he reacted well. Without showing any untoward signs, he expired on the second day of life.

Necropsy.—Post-mortem examination was performed by Dr. Knox H. Finley eight hours after exitus. The necropsy revealed no unusual findings except in the nervous system.

Brain.—On macroscopic examination there could be seen no abnormalities in the meninges and cerebral parenchyma. Microscopically, both the parietal and occipital cortex contained large zones in which there was an almost complete absence of the ganglion cells in the third, fourth, fifth, and sixth layers (Fig. 21). The second layer was nearly normally preserved. Those ganglion cells which still persisted in the involved zones showed a loss of the Nissl bodies and indistinctness of the nuclei. The glia was altered by a degenerative change somewhat similar to that in the nerve cells; the nuclei were shrunken, irregular, and granular.

CASE 15.—An 18-month-old white male child, born after instrumental delivery, had a convulsion lasting ten minutes on third day of life. Well until the onset of irritability, there were repeated convulsions, vomiting, and loss of consciousness, which resulted in death at the end of twenty-four hours. There was destruction of nerve cells of the cerebral cortex.

Clinical History.—The patient was a white male infant, 18 months of age, who was born following a labor of four hours which was terminated with the aid of

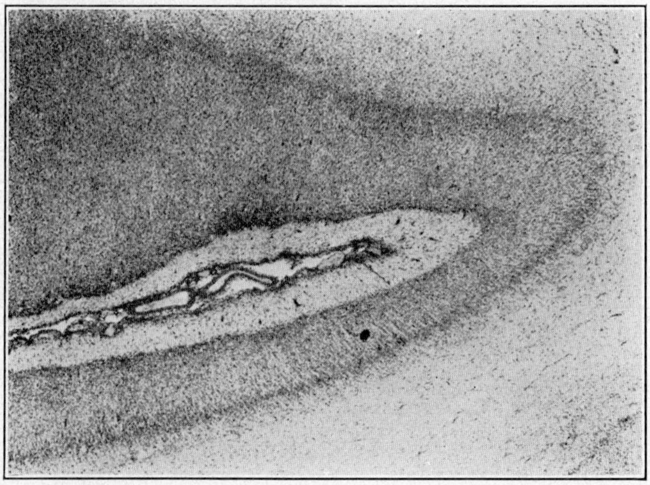

Fig. 21.—Case 14. The cortical cytoarchitecture of the occipital lobe is blurred as the result of extensive necrobiosis of the ganglion cells. Nissl stain. (×25.)

forceps. The birth weight was 9 pounds, 4 ounces. The infant cried well following delivery and appeared to be perfectly well until the third day, when he had a generalized convulsion lasting ten minutes. From this he recovered without apparent ill effects and developed normally, sitting up at 4 months and walking at 12 months. Teething started when the child was 5 months old and just beginning to talk.

The illness had its beginning one evening when the child accidentally struck his head several times on a carpeted floor. He picked himself up on each occasion but appeared slightly dizzy. At bed time, two hours later, he appeared somewhat irritable but fell asleep fairly promptly. Early the following morning the child became very irritable and cried considerably. His eyes rolled upward, and the mother thought he was having a convulsion. Following this he had a peculiar "stare," and it was noted that he was unconscious. Before his admission to the New Haven Hospital he had a series of twenty convulsions spaced about twenty minutes apart, each convulsion lasting about five seconds. The legs and arms were in flexion. The child vomited frequently. The temperature was normal throughout.

On admission to the hospital, the child was still unconscious. He had a convulsion which was characterized by a turning of the head to the left and extension of the feet and legs, with the toes assuming a fanlike position; the arms were flexed and the eyes turned upward. The Babinski sign was positive bilaterally.

A bilateral subtemporal decompression was made soon after admission in view of the history of repeated head trauma. Nothing was found. Following the operations the convulsions ceased, but the child still did not regain consciousness. Three hours later the respirations became labored and finally stopped, twenty-four hours after the onset of the illness.

Lumbar puncture revealed an initial spinal fluid pressure of 250 mm. of water, which rose to 300 mm. when the child was crying. The fluid was clear and contained but two cells and no albumin. Blood culture yielded negative results. The blood Kahn test was negative.

Necropsy.—Post-mortem examination, which was limited to the intracranial contents, was performed by Dr. Knox H. Finley five hours after exitus.

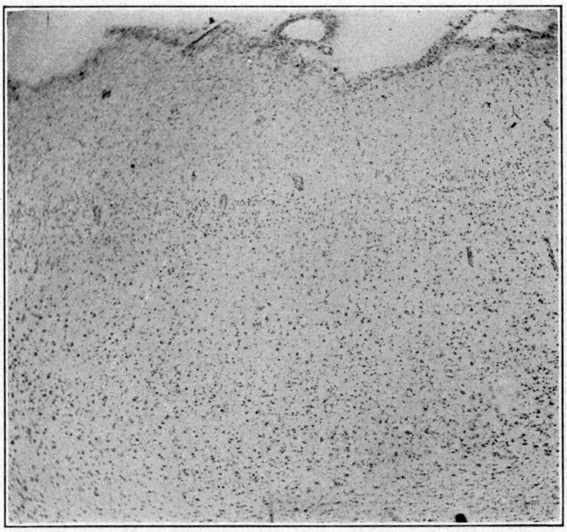

Fig. 22.—Case 15. The bleached appearance of the cerebral cortex is due to necrobiosis of the ganglion cells. Nissl stain. (×40.)

The defects in the parietal bones, which were made during the craniotomy procedures, each measured 2 cm. in diameter. There was no evidence of subdural hemorrhage. The leptomeninges were pale and translucent everywhere. Macroscopic examination of the brain revealed normal structures.

On histologic examination nearly all the ganglion cells of the cerebral cortex appeared swollen and lacked Nissl granules. Their nuclei were shrunken and hyperchromic and failed to show nucleoli. In some gyri the nerve cells had completely disappeared, altering to a marked degree the laminar appearance of the cortex (Fig. 22). To a less degree these same cellular changes were present in the basal ganglions, pons, and cerebellum.

Comment.—The histories of birth injury or asphyxia cannot be disputed in Cases 12, 13 and 14, and the pathogenesis of the cerebral lesions is, therefore, a matter of simple deduction. These cases are of the utmost importance in illucidating the pathogenesis of the lesions in all the other cases. There is only presumptive evidence that the child described as Case 15 suffered a birth injury, this evidence consisting of the facts that the child was large at birth, was delivered by forceps, and had a severe generalized convulsion on the third day of life. There can be no doubt, however, that the cerebral lesions found on postmortem examination had resulted from the repeated convulsions which occurred during the final twenty-four hours of life. Unfortunately, a partial examination precluded the discovery of the cause of these convulsions and the widespread distribution of the recent cerebral changes could have obscured any older lesions.

PNEUMOTHORAX WITH PARTIAL ASPHYXIA

CASE 16.—A 6-month-old white female child developed neurogenic fibrosarcoma in left kidney region. There was surgical shock and left pneumothorax following operative removal of tumor. The pulse rate was rapid and feeble, and respirations, slow

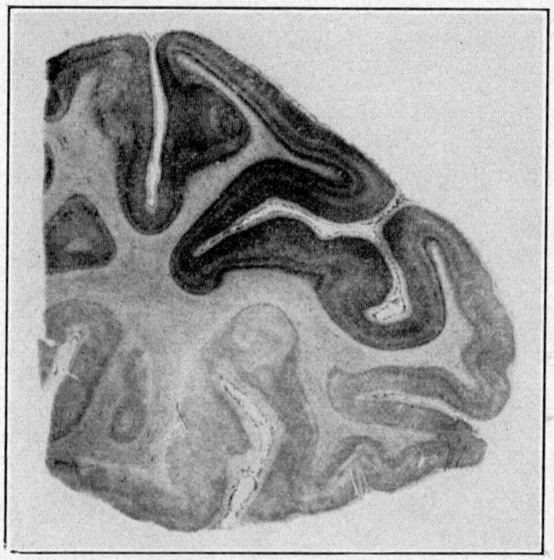

Fig. 23.—Case 16. Photomicrograph of occipital cortex showing faded appearance of several gyri due to necrobiosis. Nissl stain. (×2.)

and shallow. There were twitches of the right arm and lips. Large and petechial hemorrhages were scattered in the brain; there was destruction of nerve cells in the cerebral cortex.

Clinical History.—The patient was a white female child, 6 months of age, who was born following high forceps delivery after about one-half hour of labor. The membranes had ruptured three hours previously. The child appeared normal at birth and had a normal feeding and developmental history.

In the course of a routine physical examination at 3 months of age, the child was found to have a firm mass in the left upper quadrant of the abdomen. This was found to be a renal tumor, and after a course of deep roentgen-ray therapy it was decided to perform a nephrectomy. Accordingly, under ethylene and ether anesthesia the left kidney and adrenal were removed together with the adherent spleen and a portion of the pancreas. During the course of the dissection the left costophrenic sinus was cut, and although the rent in the pleura was immediately sutured, the patient went into "surgical shock." The heart shifted to the right. A needle was inserted into the left pleural cavity at the seventh interspace and 75 c.c. of air were removed. The child grew worse; the pulse rate rose to 200 per minute; the respirations became slow and shallow. Slight twitches of the right arm and lips occurred, and the child expired approximately thirty hours after the operation.

Examination of the tumor revealed a fibrosarcoma of neurogenic origin.

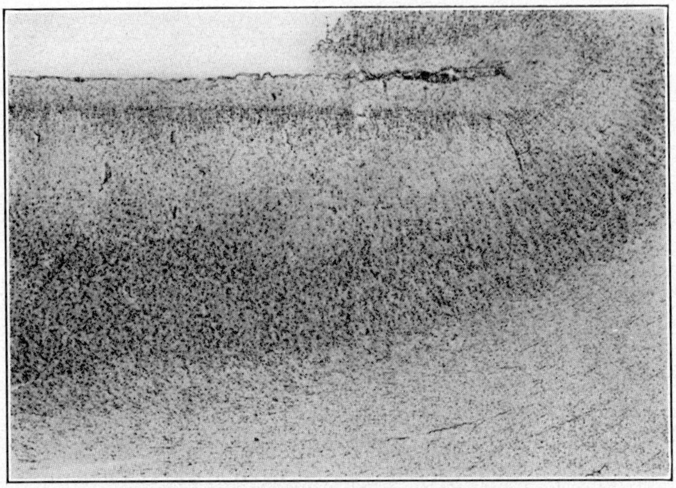

Fig. 24.—Case 16. The ganglion cells of the cortical layers, especially the third, have completely disappeared. Nissl stain. (×25.)

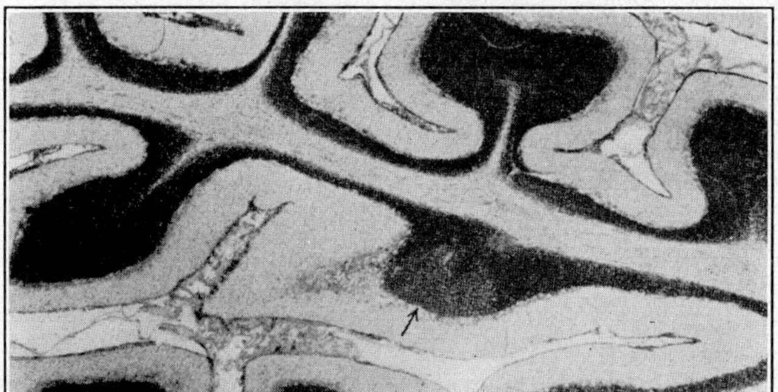

Fig. 25.—Case 16. Photomicrograph of cerebellar cortex. Note faded appearance of the granular cell layer due to necrobiosis. Nissl stain. (×25.)

Necropsy.—The necropsy was performed by Dr. David M. Grayzel one and one-half hours post mortem. Aside from the evidence of the recent surgical procedure, the important findings were confined to the nervous system.

Brain.—A small fresh blood clot was seen in the subdural space between the two cerebral hemispheres. A focus of hemorrhagic discoloration measuring 8 mm. in diameter was present in the cortex of the left occipital lobe at the base of one of the sulci. This had the appearance of an hemorrhagic infarct and represented the only macroscopic abnormality noted in the entire brain.

In addition to the hemorrhage in the left occipital lobe, microscopic examination revealed numerous petechiae and congested vessels in other parts of the brain. In many places the cerebral cortex had lost its nerve cell elements, this lesion being confined to the third layer in some gyri and involving all the layers in other gyri (Fig. 23). The necrobiosis had a pseudolaminary distribution, especially in the occipital lobe cortex (Fig. 24). A moth-eaten appearance was presented by the cerebellar cortex where the granular cells had a faded appearance in the Nissl preparations (Fig. 25). The Purkinje cells were either entirely absent in circumscribed zones or were swollen, round, and vesicular.

Comment.—In no case of this whole series is the pathogenesis of the cerebral injury more certain than in this one. The pulmonary collapse designated as ''surgical shock,'' with its attendant respiratory failure and cerebral ischemia, accounts for the histologic lesions, which are clear-cut and in every way comparable to those in the other cases.

GENERAL COMMENT

Analysis of the clinical histories and histopathologic changes in the nervous systems of this group of children, which succumbed to severe convulsive disorders, respiratory failure, or asphyxia, leads to the conclusion that the lesions resulted from cerebral anoxemia. This point of view is in agreement with that expressed by Spielmeyer and his school. Little need be added in explanation of the method by which cerebral anoxemia is produced as the result of respiratory collapse or asphyxia. Nor is it particularly difficult to understand how the ganglion cells, which are peculiarly susceptible to anoxemia, are injured, especially in young children. It is not as readily understood how convulsive attacks produce the anoxemia.

As already mentioned, Spielmeyer felt that cerebral angiospasm in many instances preceded or accompanied the convulsion. This could readily produce anoxemia, but the proof for such a mechanism is difficult to deduce from necropsies. In our cases it appears rather that the convulsive attacks, which were associated with great respiratory distress, produced venous stasis in the brain as the result of increased intrathoracic pressure, and this led to cerebral anoxemia.

This paper does not deal with the pathogenesis of convulsions, but rather with the histopathologic changes which these produce in the nervous system. The changes are to be regarded solely as the result of the convulsive attacks; it is not conceivable that they were preexisting and initiated the attacks. It must be emphasized that in no instance in this series was an encephalitis responsible for them.

SUMMARY

Extensive necrobiotic changes of the ganglion cells were found in the cerebral cortex, especially the cornu ammonis formations of the temporal lobes, the basal ganglions, and the cerebellar cortex of a group of sixteen children ranging in age from early infancy to 6½ years. The lesions were similar to those described by Spielmeyer and others in cases of epilepsy. Severe convulsions and prolonged periods of respiratory difficulty or asphyxia dominated the clinical pictures in these cases. Although seven of the children had an underlying infectious illness which suggested the possibility of encephalitis as the cause of the symptoms, the other nine were free from infection. None of the children had inflammatory cerebral lesions which could have accounted for the symptoms. It was concluded that cerebral anoxemia, resulting either from the convulsions, the respiratory difficulty, or the asphyxia, was responsible for the lesions in the nervous systems.

REFERENCES

1. Spielmeyer, W.: Ztschr. f. d. ges. Neurol. u. Psychiat. **109**: 501, 1927.
2. Spielmeyer, W.: Arch. Neurol. & Psychiat. **23**: 869, 1930.
3. Spielmeyer, W.: Ztschr. f. d. ges. Neurol. u. Psychiat. **148**: 285, 1933.
4. Uchimura, J.: Ztschr. f. d. ges. Neurol. u. Psychiat. **112**: 1, 1928.
5. Scholz, W.: Ztschr. f. d. ges. Neurol. u. Psychiat. **145**: 471, 1933.
6. Spielmeyer, W.: Monatschr. f. Psychiat. u. Neurol. **68**: 605, 1928.
7. Zimmerman, H. M., and Yannet, H.: J. Nerv. & Ment. Dis. **75**: 386, 1932.
8. Husler, J., and Spatz, H.: Ztschr. f. Kinderh. **38**: 428, 1924.
9. Neubürger, K.: Klin. Wchnschr. **4**: 113, 1925.

NICOTINIC ACID IN THE TREATMENT OF ACRODYNIA

Frederick F. Tisdall, M.D., F.R.C.P.(C.), T. G. H. Drake, M.B., F.R.C.P.(C.), and Alan Brown, M.D., F.R.C.P.(C.)
Toronto, Ont.

In September, 1937, Elvehjem et al.[1] reported the cure of black tongue in dogs by the administration of nicotinic acid. For many years it has been known that black tongue in the dog and pellagra in the human being respond favorably to the same dietary procedures. Following this lead, Spies et al.[2] and Fouts et al.[3] in November, 1937, and later others, reported spectacular results in the treatment of pellagra with nicotinic acid. Thus a chemical compound known for some seventy-five years has now been shown to be essential for human nutrition.

Although acrodynia and pellagra are distinct clinical entities, there is a superficial resemblance between the two diseases. They both have skin lesions and they both may have involvement of the mucous membranes of the mouth. Until the discovery of the role of nicotinic acid in pellagra, they both responded very slowly to dietary or other therapeutic procedures.

The etiological factors in the development of acrodynia are unknown. In view of the similarity of the symptoms of acrodynia and those which can be produced in animals by dietary deficiencies, one view is held that acrodynia is due to a defect in the utilization by infants and children of some essential food element, probably belonging to the vitamin B complex. Another widely held view is that acrodynia is a particular and unusual response to a toxemia, as practically all these children have evidence of throat infection with involvement of the tonsils. These two views, however, can be reconciled. On one hand it is recognized that almost any dietary deficiency results in a lowered resistance to infection; therefore, these children would be more susceptible to infection than the average child. On the other hand, the presence of an infection interferes with the utilization by the body of many of the nutritional factors, including members of the vitamin B complex.

In view of these facts, an attempt was made to determine whether nicotinic acid, now known to be a member of the vitamin B complex, is of value in the treatment of acrodynia. Accordingly, the acid was administered to six infants suffering from this disease. Their ages were 8, 11, 12, 12, 17, and 24 months. They all had typical symptoms of acrodynia, namely, marked irritability, loss of appetite, rash and redness of the skin, the redness involving particularly the hands and feet,

From the Hospital for Sick Children, Toronto, and the Department of Paediatrics, University of Toronto.

later desquamation of the skin of the hands and feet, increased perspiration, so that the skin had the typical damp clammy feel, redness of the end of the nose, photophobia, and in the more severe cases redness of the gums and mucous membranes, with exfoliation of some of the teeth. In every instance there was redness of the pharnyx and involvement of the tonsils.

The nicotinic acid used was kindly furnished by Dr. Nielsen of the Abbott Laboratories. Two forms were used, pure nicotinic acid and the monoethanolamine salt of nicotinic acid. No difference was found in the action of these two substances. In regard to dosage, the only information we had to go on was Spies' experience that he was able to administer 500 mg. daily to adults, in five divided doses. In order to obviate any possibility of defective absorption from the intestinal tract, we gave the nicotinic acid intravenously by means of a continuous intravenous injection of a solution of one part normal saline and two parts 5 per cent glucose. The initial dosage was 20 mg., given over a period of about twelve hours. The method of administration was then changed to intramuscular injections, which were given twice daily the first day, 20 mg. each time, then the dose increased to 40 mg. twice a day. No local reaction occurred. In one or two instances the babies developed a definite skin reaction a short time after the injection. The skin became red and blotchy, but this passed off in the course of half an hour. In other instances, the infants were given the nicotinic acid by mouth, a total of 100 mg. a day being given to the younger infants, and 125 mg. a day to the older ones. The daily amount was given in three divided doses. Only occasionally was nicotinic acid found in the urine.

In view of the severity of the symptoms in most of the cases and the seriousness of the disease, we did not feel justified in eliminating the ordinary therapeutic procedures which in the past had been found to give the best results. Accordingly, all these infants, in addition to the nicotinic acid, received a diet which included milk, egg yolk, a mixture of equal parts of Pablum, wheat germ, and a finely ground green oat grass very rich in the vitamin B complex, oleum percomorphum, orange juice, and, in the older infants, liver. After the infants had been observed for a time, the tonsils and adenoids were removed.

With the first infant to receive the nicotinic acid, the photophobia largely disappeared in twenty-four hours. In the other cases, we could detect no evidence of any effect on photophobia. With the second infant, the rash dried up comparatively rapidly and at the end of four or five days had largely disappeared from the body; and the hands and feet instead of being a cyanotic, reddish color, became a light brick red, with the skin dry and starting to desquamate. At the end of two weeks the redness was barely perceptible. We gained the impression in practically every instance that the skin lesions tended to dry up and the skin to desquamate somewhat more quickly than we had observed without the use of nicotinic acid. However, in one case the redness of the hands and feet returned during an exacerbation of the throat infection, although the infant was receiving 100 mg. of nicotinic acid daily. The mouth lesions did not heal any quicker than ordinarily. The rate of improvement of the infants was very slow, being interrupted at intervals by exacerbations of the nasopharyngitis, which evidenced itself not only by the redness of the nasopharynx but by irritability of the infant and almost complete loss of appetite, so that all feedings had to be forced.

It was evident that the nicotinic acid had no demonstrable effect on the clinical course of the disease as a whole.

CONCLUSIONS

Although nicotinic acid when combined with the therapeutic procedures usually employed in this clinic in the treatment of acrodynia seemed to hasten the healing of the skin lesions, no evidence was found that it shortened the period of recovery from the disease.

REFERENCES

1. Elvehjem, C. A., Madden, R. J., Strong, F. M., and Wooley, D. W.: J. Am. Chem. Soc. **59**: 1767, 1937.
2. Spies, T. D., Cooper, Clark, and Blankenhorn, M. A.: J. A. M. A. **110**: 622, 1937.
3. Fouts, P. J., Helmer, O. M., Lepkovsky, S., and Jukes, T. H.: Proc. Soc. Exper. Biol. & Med. **37**: 405, 1937.

INJURY OF THE CHILD BY ROENTGEN RAY DURING PREGNANCY

Report of a Case

F. Elmer Johnson, M.D.
New York, N. Y.

In the neurological and gynecologic literature many requests have been made for additional reports of infants born with abnormalities following irradiation of the fetus in utero. I shall report a case complete with details of dosage of roentgen ray and necropsy to add to the growing list. I am further motivated because the pediatric literature, including textbooks, pays so little attention to radiogenic anomalies.

Driessen[1] demonstrated in 1924 with experiments on rabbits that with exposure of one-half of the uterus to roentgen ray, the pregnancy on that side was terminated while the ovum on the other side continued to develop unmolested. This suggested to him that the effect of the radiation is a direct action on the ovum and cannot be ascribed to injury of the ovary. The earlier in pregnancy the radiation is given and the greater the intensity of the exposure the more the fetus is injured. Driessen concluded that exposures to radium or roentgen ray in the first half of pregnancy cause retrogression while those in the later half do not terminate pregnancy, but the newborn infants are subnormal in some way. The malformations are most liable to occur in the central nervous system, eyes, and blood vessels.

Murphy[2] in 1929 reported fifty-three women who received postconception radiation. Twenty-three of these aborted, but the others who went to term gave birth to children who were unhealthy according to the definition arbitrarily determined upon for the purposes of his study. Most of the pregnancies were unsuspected at the time of treatment. These defects were: underweight at birth, microcephalus, blindness, hydrocephalus, Mongolian idiocy, and other gross defects of structure and function, the majority of them involving the central nervous system.

Goldstein and Murphy,[3] in 1929, reported the results of a questionnaire sent to 1700 gynecologists and radiologists throughout the United States. With those found in the literature, they collected 106 case reports of women who had received radiation therapy during pregnancy. Seventy-four of these women were delivered of full-term children, but thirty-eight of the children presented disturbances of health or development of more or less serious nature. There was a high incidence of grave mental and gross anatomic defects. Sixteen were microcephalic idiots. The authors reported one patient of their own with microcephalic idiocy born to a mother irradiated for carcinoma of the cervix late in pregnancy. They mention a similar case of Petenyi's born after roentgen ray therapy for carcinoma in the fifth and sixth months of pregnancy. Goldstein and Murphy conclude that no pregnancy should be allowed to continue to term when radium or roentgen ray therapy has been employed on the pregnant uterus.

Goldstein,[4] in 1930, published a paper which is more germane to our discussion in which he coined the term "radiogenic microcephaly." In this paper he dealt with nineteen microcephalic out of seventy-six infants born to mothers who were irradiated during pregnancy (25 per cent). He stressed particularly the ocular defects associated with microcephalus which occurred in a large number of these children. In many he observed disturbances of the eye ranging from abnormalities to inflammatory conditions. He suggested that some of these malformations, notably the microphthalmia, might be pathognomonic of radiogenic microcephalus. Heredity, syphilis, the previous general health of the mother prior to and during pregnancy, and the circumstances incident to labor were among the conditions studied. The cause of microcephalus in sixteen cases in this series could not in any way be ascribed to these factors.

Goldstein also found that the mothers had received relatively large doses, thirteen receiving more than one dose. Seven of the latter were given three or more treatments with a maximum in one case of seventeen. Sixteen were treated with roentgen ray, two with radium, and one with mesothorium. In general, pregnancy was unsuspected when the treatment was given. Ten were irradiated for myomas, three for carcinomas, two for sterilization, and four for miscellaneous reasons.

Of the fourteen children whose weight at birth was known, all but one were decidedly small, and four were premature. The head varied in shape and was small where measurements were recorded. The typical small round head of microcephalous infants occurred in nine. Three were oxycephalic, the type of head also known as "tower head" or "turmschaedel" and four children had flattened occiputs.

In fifteen children in whom the condition of the eyes was recorded, twelve had pathologic lesions. Although microphthalmia is found only once in 300,000 births in the general population, it was present in seven of these infants. In fifteen exposed to radiation in the first four months of gestation, eleven (73.3 per cent) manifested disturbances of the eyes. Only one of the other four irradiated after the fourth month showed an ocular defect. Defects other than neurological and ocular were not encountered consistently enough to classify. All of the children who lived were later classed as imbeciles or idiots.

Goldstein in his article compiled a table entitled, "Recorded Experiments Showing Irradiation Effects on Nervous System and Eyes." In four of the ten articles abstracted, by Bagg,[5] Hanson,[6] Hippel and Pagenstecker,[7] and Tribondeau and Belley,[8] microphthalmia was produced quite regularly in the offspring when their mothers were irradiated. Goldstein summarized the experiments as follows: "The intimate etiologic relationship between embryonal irradiation and developmental anomalies in the visual organs is further exemplified by observations made on the eyes of animals irradiated in utero and of young animals irradiated after birth. It is my belief that the method of irradiation employed experimentally in the pregnant animal or in the newborn offspring is comparable with the therapeutic method employed in the pregnant woman, especially as the types of defects observed clinically are similar to those observed experimentally. The table shows that optic atrophy and microphthalmia were produced in the young animal receiving irradiation of the eyes, and that, in experimental studies, cataracts were observed in the offspring of animals irradiated during pregnancy.

"The experimental studies recorded in the table demonstrate conclusively the facility with which serious diseases of the eye may be produced in young animals, either by maternal irradiation during gestation or by direct treatment of the head or eyes after birth. The eyes of the young animals and the embryonal optic anlage, therefore, appear to be very sensitive to irradiation. If fetal irradiation and irradiation of the eyes of the animal shortly after birth may be assumed to correspond with the irradiation received by the human embryo, it is obvious that the developing optic apparatus is especially sensitive to the injurious influence of radiant energy. This would account for the frequent occurrence of congenital microphthalmia, optic atrophy, and amaurosis in children with radiogenic microcephaly, particularly since nonradiogenic microcephaly is not associated with these types of defects of the eyes."

Goldstein and Wexler[9] have noted the constancy with which rosettes occurred in the retinas of the eyes of human embryos when large doses of roentgen rays were applied to the uterus during the first two months of pregnancy. The ciliary body and iris were also found to be rudimentary. They summarize by stating that the effect is stimulation or proliferation of the posterior segment, and inhibition or retardation of the growth in the anterior segment of the globe. The time of exposure in relation to the development determines the defect.

Ernest Farber,[10] in 1933, brought up to date the general conclusion of gynecologists on the effects of roentgen ray to the germ cells and fetus as follows:

"Roentgen irradiation of the ovaries does not seem to prevent the birth of a healthy child. However, irradiation of the pregnant uterus causes severe injury of the fetus, at least if it is done in the first months of pregnancy. In 50 per cent of the cases the injury consists in what Zappert calls 'roentgenogenic fetal microcephalia' associated with severe malformations of the eyes, the same as observed in the animal experiments. The effect of irradiation on the fetus when other organs of the pregnant woman are exposed may or may not affect the fetus." Farber, however, mentions seven cases reported from the literature by Scholl in which microcephalus and eye defects occurred in children born of mothers irradiated for cancer of the breast, sarcoma of the thigh, etc. Farber also reports a case of his own which deserves reporting here. A woman was irradiated for cervical adenitis. She was amenorrheic during the entire treatment. She had often missed her menses before and being 30 years old and married eight years without children had not suspected that she was pregnant. She received ten treatments in three months, allegedly with the body shielded up to the breast. Increasing indisposition following the treatments was believed to be roentgen toxemia. The diagnosis of pregnancy was made soon afterwards. The baby was born six months later and weighed 2,600 gm. There was microphthalmia, complete coloboma, and at 21 months of age the baby was very backward mentally and physically. He concluded that "in any case the greatest precaution is indicated in irradiating sexually mature women who may possibly be pregnant not only when an irradiation of the uterus is intended but also for general and remote local irradiations."

Miller et al.,[11] in the latest article available, give the following summary quoted in part:

"It seems reasonable to advise that the use of radium and x-ray during pregnancy for treatment purposes be restricted to very clear and urgent indications and that the use of diagnostic x-ray examinations be not too frequently repeated during pregnancy.

"It seems advisable to interrupt any pregnancy which has been subjected to therapeutic radiation, for it is generally admitted that serious radiation effects on the offspring will result in a high percentage of cases. These effects are proportioned to the amount of radiation and are more serious in early pregnancies, though the fetus may be seriously injured at any stage of development."

CASE REPORT

A male infant, 6½ months old, was admitted to St. Luke's Hospital, New York City, on July 23, 1934. He weighed 2700 gm. at birth and had gained only 420 gm. He had always been weak, and the mother had noticed that his head was peculiarly shaped. For three days previous to admission he had vomited everything eaten. He had been fed since birth on the breast and supplementary cow's milk formulas. There was nothing abnormal about his birth history or in the examination of the alimentary tract.

The mother had had nine pregnancies. The first and eighth were miscarriages. The fourth pregnancy resulted in twins, one of whom died at 6 months of age with convulsions. The other children are well. Both parents had been treated for syphilis since 1927, and Wassermann tests on parents and baby on admission were negative. The parents were symptom-free at time of infant's admission.

In January, 1933, the mother visited a gynecologic clinic and was advised to have radiotherapy for fibroids of the uterus but was not treated until the following September. She was treated three times in fifteen days, receiving 1150 roentgen units in air. In utero it was estimated that the mother received 400 roentgen units. Later in November an Aschheim-Zondek test was positive for pregnancy. The baby was born June 8, 1934, at full term. It was estimated that the treatments were given approximately seventeen, twenty-four, and thirty-two days after conception.

Upon examination the baby was found to be feeble although he had a fairly good cry. He preferred to lie on his side with his head retracted, arms flexed on chest and legs crossed. The head was relatively large, measuring 38.2 cm., while the chest was 33 cm. in circumference. The anterior fontanel measured 4 cm. longitudinally, and the tension was increased. The posterior fontanel was open, and the sutures were slightly separated. The eyes were small showing the sclera above the cornea. The pupils were dilated and eccentric with very little iris showing on the nasal side. The corneas measured only 6 mm. There was continual slow lateral nystagmus. The fundi were negative. The extremities were stiff, and the deep reflexes were increased. The infant's head was easily transilluminated.

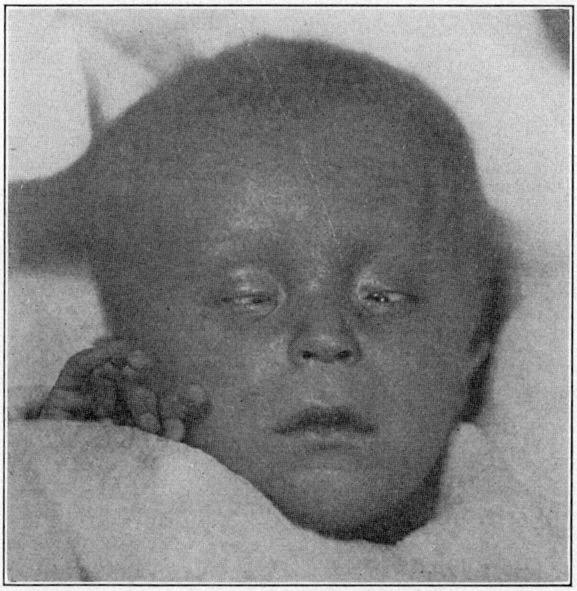

Fig. 1.—Picture of child, showing microphthalmia and shape of head.

Repeated spinal punctures were done and, when the baby was not crying, showed a maximum pressure of 24 mm. of mercury. Examination of the fluid was negative.

Because of the translucency and shape of the head, a needle was inserted through the external horn of the anterior fontanel and 350 c.c. of fluid withdrawn and replaced with 350 c.c. of air. Roentgenograms were taken showing an external hydrocephalus and a small brain (Fig. 2). The needle wound continued to drain, and an infection of the meninges with *Staphylococcus aureus* resulted.

The salient features of the necropsy are in the examination of the head. Necropsy was done by Dr. Leila C. Knox. On opening the skull about 50 c.c. of yellowish flocculent fluid was found free about the brain surface beneath the dura. The brain was small and only filled the lower half of the entire cranial vault. It measured 28 cm. in its occipitofrontal circumference and weighed 225 gm. The pia and arachnoid, covering the entire surface of both hemispheres, were covered by a thick purulent, yellowish-white, foul-smelling exudate. This extended beneath the tentorium and to a lesser extent across the pons and medulla. Both cerebral cortices were flattened over their superior surfaces; their convolutions were small and poorly demarcated. The frontal lobes showed marked agenesis, their anterior tips extending only 1 cm. beyond the anterior end of the temporal lobes. The sylvian fissures were poorly demarcated. The corpus callosum was rudimentary; the fornix and mammillary bodies were absent. On section the anterior and temporal horns of the lateral ventricles were narrowed and flattened; the occipital horns were somewhat dilated. Their ependymal lining was covered with soft, reddish, granular exudate. The choroid plexus of the lateral, third, and fourth ventricles was friable and showed severe inflammatory changes. The third ventricle

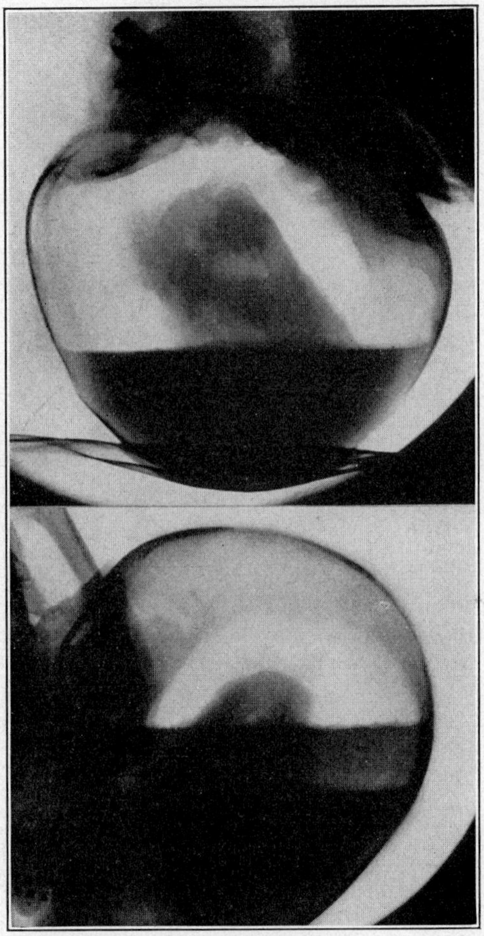

Fig. 2.—Roentgenograms of the head after displacement of spinal fluid with air, showing external hydrocephalus and small brain.

was very indistinctly defined, being a mere slit between the poorly developed optic thalami, posterior portion of which could not be defined. There was no aqueduct of Sylvius or any direct communication between the third and fourth ventricles. The fourth ventricle was wide, and its floor was covered by thick exudate. The olfactory bulbs were present and small. Considerable thick exudate was present over the optic chiasm. The optic tracts posterior to their decussation became flattened and merged into the pes pedunculi. The geniculate bodies cannot be defined.

The *anatomic diagnosis* was: agenesis of frontal cerebral hemispheres, maldevelopment of the third ventricle, geniculate bodies, optic thalamus, optic tracts, corpus callosum, and fornix, absence of aqueduct of Sylvius, microphthalmus, external hydrocephalus, purulent meningitis, and bronchopneumonia.

Microscopic examinations.—In the brain, sections through the cortex of the frontal lobes showed some proliferation of the glial cells in the superficial layers and invasion with small round cells. There was a marked deficiency and defective growth of the ganglion cells, while in the deeper portion of the entire cerebral tissue there were many vacuolated areas, apparently due to degenerative changes in the neurones. The blood vessels throughout the brain showed no pathologic changes, except a slight hyaline degeneration of their walls. Levaditi's stains did not reveal the presence of spirochetes. The leptomeninges throughout the cortex, midbrain, and pons were invaded by an acute suppurative process. The ependymal lining of the lateral ventricles was destroyed and the subependymal tissue invaded with round cells and polynuclears, which in areas formed cuffs about the blood vessels. The third ventricle was small and patent, its lumen partially filled with albuminous material; the lining ependymal cells were intact. The quadrigeminal bodies appeared to have an increase in the glial tissue.

The venous sinusoids of the spleen were dilated with red cells, the pulp reticulum containing an increased number of monocytes. The remaining organs showed no remarkable changes.

The microscopic diagnosis was: agenesis of cerebral hemispheres, malformation of brain, acute suppurative meningoencephalitis, and septic spleen.

COMMENT

In the literature there is an accumulation of evidence over the past seventeen years, since Aschenheim[12] reported the first case, that irradiation of a pregnant woman is fraught with danger to the fetus. Either abortion results, or in over 50 per cent of the live births there will be gross defects of the central nervous system and eyes.

The fact that many normal children are born after irradiation of the mother may be explained at least in part by physical factors. The fetus may be protected by the thickness of the mother's abdominal wall, the amount of amniotic fluid, or the position of the fetus in relation to the placenta and source of radiation. The high percentage of lesions of the central nervous system and eyes and the astonishing relative absence of other anatomic defects makes one think that the sensitivity of fetal nervous tissue to roentgen ray and radium is most important. The eyeballs of the early fetus are relatively larger and less protected than later. The chance of injury is proportional to the size of the dose and nearness of treatment to conception and probably to other factors, as intercurrent infections and individual variations in radiosensitivity. On the other hand, some infants are not harmed if the dose of radiation is small and if they are exposed later in pregnancy. It is a generally recognized fact that early fetal nervous and optic tissues are very susceptible to radiation. There is also evidence that irradiation of the mother in places remote from the uterus may also be harmful to the fetus.

The case reported bears out the generally accepted opinion at the present on the harmful effects of irradiation on the fetus. The very rudimentary brain in a skull of normal dimensions suggests that the fetal nervous tissue was injured but the bones were unaffected. The microphthalmia and small brain in this case are in accord with the association so well shown by Goldstein in human offspring and by many experimenters in animals.

It seems reasonable to believe that after more cases have been reported, certain lesions, particularly in the eyes, will be found pathognomonic of irradiation of the fetus. Microphthalmia is so rare in the general population and in ordinary cases of microcephalus, that its common occurrence in radiogenic microcephaly suggests that it represents a specific lesion of radiation.

REFERENCES

1. Driessen, L. F.: Nederl. maandschr. v. geneesk. **12**: 239, 1924.
2. Murphy, Douglas P.: Surg., Gynec. & Obst. **48**: 766, 1929.
3. Goldstein, Leopold, and Murphy, Douglas P.: Am. J. Obst. & Gynec. **18**: 189, 1929.
4. Goldstein, Leopold: Arch. Neurol. & Psychiat. **24**: 102, 1930.
5. Bagg, H. J.: Am. J. Anat. **30**: 133, 1922.
6. Hanson: Proc. Ann. Philos. Soc. **62**: 301, 1923.
7. Hippel and Pagenstecker: München. med. Wchnschr. **54**: 452, 1907.
8. Tribondeau and Belley: Arch. d'électric. méd. **15**: 907, 1907.
9. Goldstein, Isadore, and Wexler, David: Arch. Ophth. **7**: 434, 1932.
10. Farber, Ernest: Jahrb. f. Kinderh. **89**: 33, 1933.
11. Miller, James R., Corscaden, James A., and Harrar, James A.: Am. J. Obst. & Gynec. **31**: 518, 1936.
12. Aschenheim, E.: Arch. f. Kinderh. **68**: 131, 1920.

1160 Park Avenue

OXYGEN THERAPY BY THE OPEN BOX METHOD

Daniel J. Pachman, M.D.
Chicago, Ill.

THE open box method of administering oxygen was first described a few years ago by Burgess.[1] When oxygen was allowed to flow at a steady rate into the bottom of an open top box whose sides and floor were impermeable to air, it was found that oxygen concentrations as high as 60 per cent could be obtained within the box. Since the publication of the first description of this method, various changes in the original apparatus have been made.[2, 3]

At the present time, the type of apparatus described below is being used at this hospital to administer oxygen to young children and infants (Figs. 1, 2, 3).

The sides and back are made of a light nonporous wood. Cleaned, noninflammable x-ray films are used as transparent windows in the sides. Rubberized cloth forms the bottom of the box, but in front is replaced by a transparent rubber material, Pliofilm.* The removable bottom and front is made in one piece and is fastened in place by strips of wood and thumb screws. In this manner the entire bottom is made airtight. In the lower front is placed the aperture for admitting the head of an older child, or the head, thorax, and arms of a small infant. A nine-inch zipper allows this opening to be made larger.

In the rear of the apparatus is the ice compartment which aids in maintaining a comfortable temperature and humidity within the box. Rubberized cloth acts as a baffle plate, separating the ice compartment from the front portion. A metal ice container which has a tube in its base is suspended from a cross bar and is filled with ice about the size of refrigerator cubes. Melted ice is drained from the tube of the container through the sides of the box by means of rubber tubing into a collecting pail on the floor. The container also has a false bottom, and within it is a sponge to absorb condensed moisture. A hinged board acts as a cover to the ice cooler compartment. The oxygen inflow from a tank and regulator enters the side of the box directly on one side and the outlet for the drain is on the other.

The oxygen content within the box can be determined fairly accurately by means of a simple oxygen analyzer. This apparatus is a modification of the method described by Henderson and Greenberg and measures the sum of oxygen and carbon dioxide.[4] However, the carbon

---

*Pliofilm is manufactured by the Goodyear Rubber Company, Akron, Ohio. Double thickness No. 250 is used.

From the Department of Pediatrics, University of Chicago.

Presented in part at the meeting of Region III of the American Academy of Pediatrics, Chicago, Oct. 15, 1937.

dioxide content of the bottom of the box has been found to be below 2 per cent and is therefore of little practical significance.

Three inches of the lower end of a six-inch tube are blown so that the end will contain approximately 20 c.c. of air.* Steel wool is then lightly

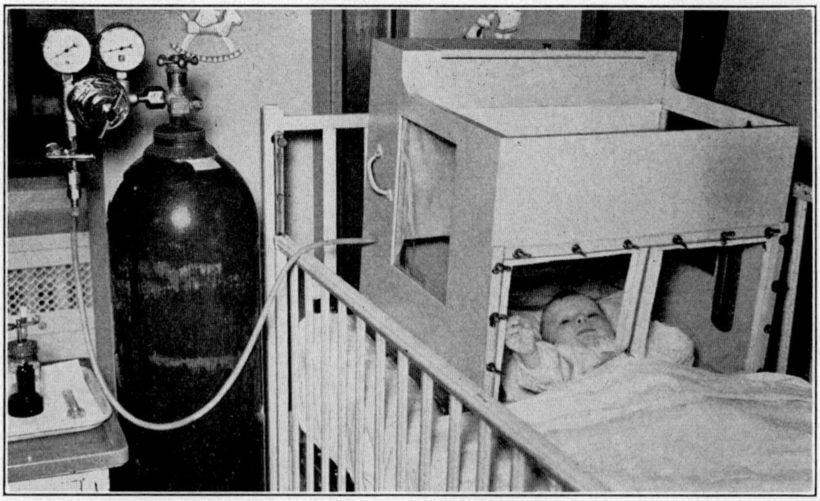

Fig. 1.—View of box in use showing a 4-month-old infant within it. The oxygen analyzer is seen at the left.

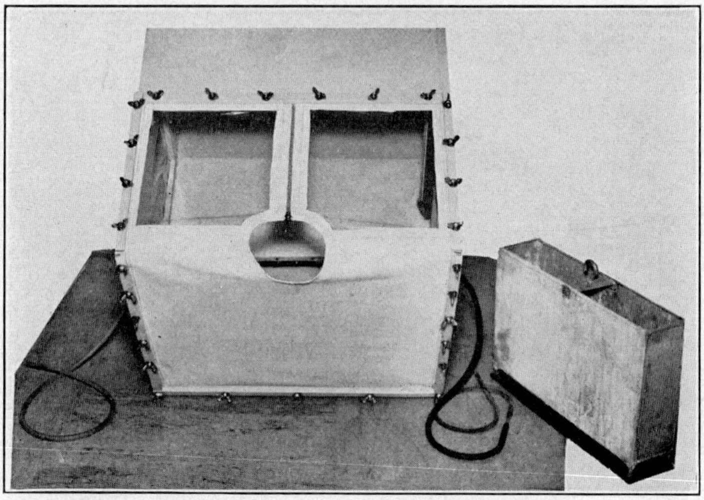

Fig. 2.—View of box showing the floor and the front piece. The ice cooler is pictured at the right.

packed into the wide end of the tube. The narrow end of the tube is pushed through a two-hole rubber stopper. The apparatus is inserted into a wide mouthed glass bottle (180 c.c.). The bottom of the wide

*Gooch crucible holders (25 mm. width), obtainable from E. H. Sargent Co., Chicago, Ill., may be used instead.

end of the tube rests about one-fourth inch from the bottom of the bottle. A rubber tube (one and one-half inches) is then attached to the glass tube protruding through the rubber stopper, and a pinch clamp is

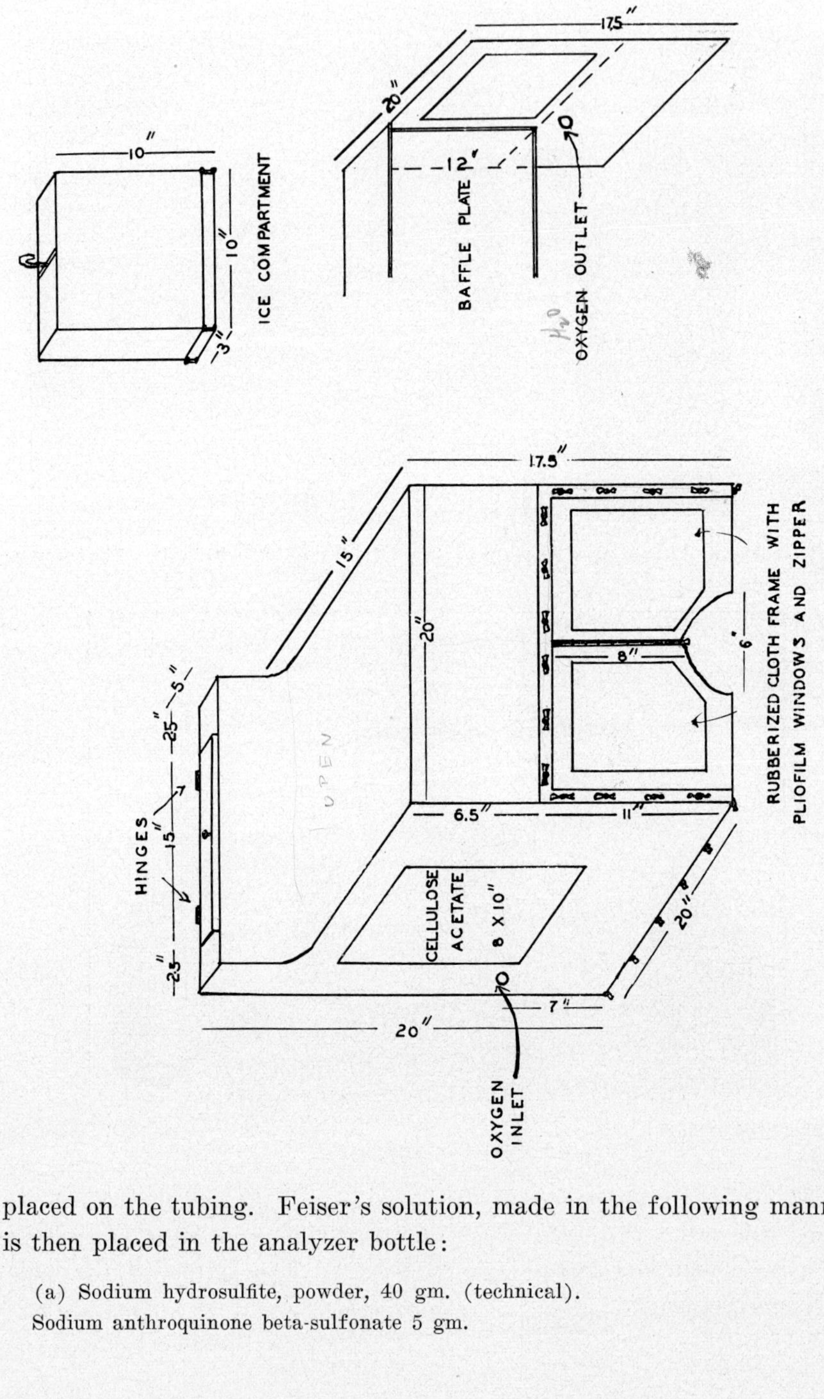

Fig. 3.—Dimensions of the various parts of the apparatus.

placed on the tubing. Feiser's solution, made in the following manner, is then placed in the analyzer bottle:

(a) Sodium hydrosulfite, powder, 40 gm. (technical).
Sodium anthroquinone beta-sulfonate 5 gm.

These are mixed together and 11 gm. are placed in each of four well-stoppered bottles.

(b) Sodium hydroxide (6 per cent solution) 60 c.c.

When ready for use, contents of one small bottle containing mixture described in (a) is mixed with this sodium hydroxide solution (b).

A 10 c.c. syringe is then attached to the open end of the rubber tubing, the clamp released, and fluid drawn up to a marker on the glass tube. The clamp is then replaced, and the analyzer is ready for use.

Procedure.—After releasing the clamp, 10 c.c. of atmospheric air (oxygen concentration 18 to 20 per cent) is placed by syringe into the analyzing solution through the rubber tube. The clamp is then replaced. The level of the fluid in the glass tubing will be changed and after three to four minutes, the syringe is attached, the clamp released, and suction applied until the initial level is reached. The oxygen content is then read from the syringe. For example, if the plunger is at 8 c.c., then 2 c.c. has been absorbed (oxygen) and there is an oxygen concentration of 2/10 or 20 per cent in the air. The air within the box is then tested. A 10 c.c. sample is obtained at the level of the patient's nose, and the procedure outlined previously is carried out.

CHART I

Name: R. H. Unit No.: 183421
Division: BR-3 Clinic or Service: Pediatric

DATE	TIME	OXYGEN CONCENTRATION IN AIR	OXYGEN CONCENTRATION IN TENT	LITERS PER MINUTE ON GAUGE	TEMP. WITHIN BOX	ROOM TEMP.	REMARKS
6-13-38	Oxygen Started 2:15 P.M.			6			
6-13-38	2:30 P.M.	20%	48%	6	76	78	Reduced to 5 liters.
6-13-38	3:30 P.M.	20%	60%	5	76	78	Rm. humidity 36; box humidity 42. Oxygen reduced to 4½ liters.
6-13-38	7:30 P.M.	20%	48%	4½	78	78	Oxygen reduced to 3½ liters.
6-13-38	11:30 P.M.	22%	62%	3½	76	76	Rm. humidity 40; box humidity 40.
6-14-38	3:30 A.M.	22%	64%	3½	78	76	Rm. humidity 42; box humidity 41.
6-14-38	7:30 A.M.	20%	43%	4	76	76	Left at 4 liters.
6-14-38	11:30 A.M.	20%	43%	4	74	74	Left at 4 liters.
6-14-38	3:30 A.M.	20%	50%	4	74	74	Patient coughing a good deal.
6-14-38	7:30 P.M.	20%	50%	4	74	74	Oxygen reduced to 3½ liters. Patient comfortable.
6-14-38	11:30 P.M.	20%	48%	3½	74	74	Rm. humidity 48; box humidity 48. Oxygen increased to 4 liters.
6-15-38	3:30 A.M.	20%	60%	4	74	74	Oxygen reduced to 3½ liters. Child comfortable.
6-15-38	7:30 A.M.	20%	58%	3½	74	74	Left at 3½ liters.
6-15-38	11:30 A.M.	20%	50%	3½	76	76	Oxygen increased to 4 liters.
6-15-38	3:30 P.M.	20%	50%	4	76	76	Left at 4 liters.
6-15-38	7:30 P.M.	20%	48%	4	80	80	Child comfortable.
6-15-38	11:30 P.M.	20%	40%	4	78	78	Oxygen increased to 4½ liters.
6-16-38	3:30 A.M.	20%	48%	4½	76	76	

Humidity recorded as relative humidity.

The air within the box is analyzed every four hours and is recorded on a special oxygen therapy chart (Chart 1). The oxygen content of atmospheric air is constant (18 to 20 per cent) and can be used as a check on the accuracy of the analyzer.* The liters of oxygen used per minute are read off from the gauge. The remarks column is used for any notes such as, oxygen inflow increased, child cyanotic, humidity within the box, etc.

Using the open top method, with an inflow of 4 to 5 liters of oxygen per minute, oxygen concentrations as high as 64 per cent have been obtained at the level of the patient's nose.

A cover is necessary for the ice water compartment as it is believed that convection currents, attracted by the cold, would otherwise force oxygen-rich air upwards from the bottom. The presence of leaks in the floor of the box, or in the lower portion, have a decided effect upon the concentration of oxygen. Oxygen-rich air may escape from around the collar and lower the oxygen concentration. Cotton gauze or batting around the child's neck or chest may be used to prevent leakage. Drafts of air in the room may interfere with the proper operation of the apparatus, and can be prevented by placing a metal screen between the box and the open window.

The explanation of the mechanism of this method of oxygen therapy has been given as follows: (1) There is a balance between inflow of oxygen and its diffusion upward; (2) oxygen is slightly heavier than air; and (3) when cooled tends to sink to the bottom. Removal of the ice cooler, however, has little effect on the oxygen concentration. The end result may be due to a combination of (1) and (2).

The advantages of this type of apparatus are many:

1. It is very inexpensive to make and to operate.
2. It is very simple to operate as no motors are needed.
3. The apparatus is portable and can be used in the home.
4. Children can be fed without removal from the box.
5. The pliofilm windows allow for clear vision from within as well as from without. The children are not apprehensive.
6. Examinations and treatments can be carried out without removal of the patient from the box.

REFERENCES

1. Burgess, A. M., Briggs, Asa S., and Burgess, A. M., Jr.: New England J. Med. **210**: 254, 1934.
2. Burgess, A. M., and Chaffee, F. H.: New England J. Med. **216**: 203, 1937.
3. Burgess, A. M.: New England J. Med. **216**: 467, 1937.
4. Henderson, Y., and Greenberg, L. A.: J. A. M. A. **96**: 1474, 1931.

*New solutions are necessary about every three to four days or when a white film appears.

Critical Review

IMMUNITY AND SUSCEPTIBILITY TO DISEASE IN EARLY INFANCY

Charles F. McKhann, M.D., and Israel Kapnick, M.D.
Boston, Mass.

THE distribution and severity of disease in early infancy would appear to be affected by climate, local environment, race, and family as well as by the nutrition and the individual physical characteristics of the infant, all acting more or less through the immune responses of the patient to the frequency and closeness of contact with the disease. Infrequency of exposure may affect the incidence of disease in the newborn infant, yet it fails to account for the remarkable resistance to certain diseases and fails to prevent a sizable incidence of other diseases within a few weeks of birth. Thus not the least important factor is the immunologic make-up of the infant.

Clinical observations have established that the newborn infant is immune to certain disease processes and susceptible to others. Furthermore, it is evident that infants develop resistance to disease poorly and that the characteristic manifestations of some disorders are greatly influenced by this lack of immunologic response. Also we may derive from the immunologic response indications as to the optimal time to begin active immunizations.

The newborn infant is immune up to several months of age to measles, scarlet fever, poliomyelitis, and diphtheria, but is susceptible to pyogenic infections, colon bacillus infections, and to pertussis; a transient immunity of a few weeks may be observed to chicken pox, vaccinia, and to pneumococcus and influenza bacillus infections. Allergic manifestations appear rarely before the fourth month; hemorrhagic nephritis is observed uncommonly under 18 months of age; and rheumatic fever is seldom encountered in children under 2 years of age. It is further well known that arthritis of rheumatic type or atrophic character or even proliferative type is almost never encountered in infancy whereas suppurative involvements of the joint are seen comparatively frequently.

Certain diseases such as typhus and undulant fever occur in infants less commonly and in less severe form than in adults. Although the incidence of yellow fever has been noted to be greater in children than in adults, the course is usually mild.

Infants under a few months seem definitely resistant to the common cold. Pneumonia is uncommon in the early weeks of life but thereafter rises rapidly in incidence. Pneumonia in infants is often not of lobar distribution but is of diffuse infiltrating type. The interstitial pneumonitis so frequently observed may well be due to the inability of the patient to localize the pneumonic process. Staphylococcal infections are virulent in early infancy and frequently cannot be dis-

From the Department of Pediatrics, Harvard Medical School, and the Infants' and Children's Hospitals, Boston.

tinguished from streptococcal infections. Thus cellulitis in the newborn infant may be due to the staphylococcus, and dermatitis exfoliativa and pemphigus neonatorum may represent unopposed staphylococcic skin infections.

The incidence and character of meningitis in infants have been studied by Fothergill and Sweet.[1] Apparently the transient resistance present at birth to the pneumococcus and influenza bacillus is lost within a few weeks and the patient then becomes extremely susceptible to meningeal involvement with these organisms. Colon bacillus meningitis is observed infrequently but because of its age distribution may be considered a disease of the neonatal period. Newborn infants are susceptible to pertussis, which is particularly dangerous at this age. Only infrequency of exposure prevents a sizable death rate of infants from pertussis.

The immunity of the newborn infant is derived from the mother and is mostly passive in character. However, unlike passive immunity following an injection of serum, which immunity lasts only three or four weeks, that observed in the newborn infant lasts in the case of measles for five months, for scarlet fever, six to eight months, and for diphtheria and poliomyelitis equivalent times. Antibacterial immunity is of shorter duration and more nearly simulates artificial passive immunity. After the passive immunity is lost a period of susceptibility ensues greater usually than that shown by older children.

Thus a consideration of resistance to disease in early infancy may be broken down into two phases: (1) the immunity of the newborn infant, transient and passive in character; and (2) the immunologic responses, active in character, which occur in the newborn and young infant.

IMMUNITY IN THE NEWBORN

The basis of the selective immunity to disease that is observed in newborn infants might be due to:

1. Transplacental transmission of (a) antigen from the mother, resulting in active intrauterine immunization of the fetus, and (b) antibodies from the mother, producing passive intrauterine immunization.
2. Transmission of antibodies from the mother to the infant through colostrum and milk.
3. Tissue immunity of the rapidly growing infant.

PERMEABILITY OF THE PLACENTA TO BACTERIA AND VIRUSES

Many observations have been made on the permeability of the placenta to bacteria and to viruses. A secondary question has been whether the placenta is normally permeable to bacteria, or whether lesions must occur locally for transmission to take place. It seems probable that organisms cannot pass through the healthy placenta, but that they can pass after pathologic processes have damaged the organ.

The transmission of syphilis is well established and is unfortunately common. It is possible that the morphology of the *Treponema pallidum* allows it to penetrate the placenta more easily than can other organisms. Congenital malaria must also be considered as proved, judging from reports in the literature.[2]

The leprosy organism reaches the fetus in a considerable number of cases, and intrauterine infection in leprosy must be considered, particularly when the disease develops in early infancy.[3]

Congenital pneumonia has been observed repeatedly and may be a cause of stillbirth.[4] Placental transmission of gonococcic infection apparently can occur, as indicated by the appearance of gonococcic polyarthritis in the newborn infant.[5] One of us has observed two such cases.

Congenital tuberculosis probably occurs in rare instances; however, infection is usually by postnatal contact and if the infant of a tuberculous mother is removed from the infective surroundings immediately after birth, tuberculosis usually does not develop.

The filterable viruses readily penetrate the placenta. Infants have been born showing definite signs of measles, chicken pox, and smallpox, evidences of intrauterine infection with these diseases. The authors have observed instances of chicken pox and smallpox in the newborn infant. There are several reports in the literature of intrauterine poliomyelitis. However, a case observed by the authors as well as consideration of the distribution of the poliomyelitis virus in the body indicates that such transmission probably does not occur. In our case a mother who had had poliomyelitis when five months pregnant was delivered of an infant who showed no evidence of the disease and who was only passively immune to it. The failure of the virus to enter the blood stream would account for this lack of similarity to other virus diseases. The transmissibility of rabies virus has been demonstrated in dogs and rabbits,[6] and Herrmann[7] has confirmed the passage in man by inoculating animals with brain emulsion of fetuses from pregnant women that had died of rabies infection. However, the virus in the brain of the fetus was decreased in virulence.

Experimental studies have been made on changes in placental permeability due to damage by various agents. Ueda[8] found that the toxins produced by the typhoid and dysentery bacilli, streptococcus, pneumococcus, and staphylococcus contracted the blood vessels of fresh mature human placentas. Ueda suggested that the interruption of pregnancy frequently seen in acute infectious diseases may be due to the action of bacterial toxins on the placenta.

PLACENTAL TRANSMISSION OF ANTIBODIES

An extensive literature exists on the transmission of antibodies through the placenta. The human placenta is permeable in variable degree to antitoxins, precipitins, bacteriolysins, complement-fixing antibodies, and to some of the natural antibodies. All of these yield a purely passive immunity which disappears within periods of time varying somewhat with the specific antibody.

The placental transmission of diphtheria antitoxin in the human has been studied repeatedly.[9] The passage of tetanus antitoxin has also been established.[10] In most cases the blood of the infant at birth contains the same concentration of diphtheria antitoxin as the mother's blood, but gross divergences have been noted. Kuttner and Ratner[11] made accurate quantitative determinations of diphtheria antitoxin in infant's, mother's, and cord blood by the Kellogg method, and found no loss of antitoxin by passage through the placenta. The concentration of antitoxin in the cord blood corresponded to that in the blood of the mothers.

The antitoxic substance to scarlet fever is also present in the umbilical cord blood. The blanching of scarlet fever rashes with placental serum was found by Toomey[12] with 79 per cent of 227 serums.

Some serums blanched the scarlet fever rashes as well as did convalescent scarlet fever serum. The ability to neutralize Dick toxin in vitro was demonstrated in these same bloods. The conclusion that the immunity of the newborn infant to scarlet fever represents in large part a passive transfer of antitoxin from the mother seemed justified.

The serum of infants contains little opsonin for virulent hemolytic streptococci, and even this small amount is lost in a few weeks.[13] The age distribution of antistreptolysin is similar to that of naturally acquired diphtherial and scarlatinal antitoxin.[14] The infants' titer, equal at birth to that of the mothers', diminished rapidly during the first few weeks of life. Lippard and Wheeler[15] made the interesting observation that antifibrinolytic substance was usually present in the newborn infant in much higher concentration than in the mother. Lippard and Johnson[16] found that children under 3 years of age lacked the capacity to develop resistance to fibrinolysis.

The neutralization of poliomyelitis virus by umbilical cord blood has been adequately demonstrated.[17]

The newborn infant is immune to measles if the mother has experienced the disease. The passive character of the immunity was shown by Herrmann[18] and by Debré and Joannon.[19] Finkelstein,[20] Jorge,[21] and de Souza[22] have reported the use of placental blood serum in dosage of 10 to 60 c.c. in prevention of measles.

Bryce and Burnet[23] also note that apparently the placenta becomes less permeable for maternal antibodies during the later months of pregnancy.

Umbilical cord blood and the blood of newborn infants contains staphylococcus antitoxin in practically the same amounts as the maternal blood.[23] This is lost during early infancy and is followed by a gradual rise in antitoxin during later years to what is assumed to be a normal level. Agglutinins against typhoid were found to pass the placenta by Scholtz,[24] Schumacher,[25] Staubli,[26] Mosse and Daunie,[27] and more recently by Peduzzi.[28] Timmermann[29] found that the H and O agglutinins pass unequally through the placenta. The H form passes in most cases and the O passes seldom if at all. The authors have witnessed two cases of typhoid in pregnant mothers whose infants had negative agglutination reactions in cord blood. A similar case was reported by Neff and Schwartz.[30] An infant was born three weeks prematurely of a mother in the third week of typhoid fever. The mother's Widal reaction was positive in 1:2560. The infant's cord blood was negative; culture of cord blood was also negative. One month after birth the infant's Widal was positive in 1:20,480, the highest dilution ever observed in that laboratory. The infant was formula-fed and had had no contact with the mother after delivery. This case suggests that the antigen rather than the antibody passed the placenta and that the infant within a few weeks developed antibodies of his own. Cooke[31] has shown the complement-fixing antibody of tuberculosis to be transferred from mother to offspring. Halban and Landsteiner[32] found maternal bacteriolysins in the infant's serum but in a lesser concentration than in the mother's. The isoagglutinins in the newborn infant are not developed by the fetus but are derived from the mother and transmitted through the placenta, and agree closely with the level found in the mother's serum.[33] The isoagglutinins present at birth disappear within ten days to two or three weeks and are gradually replaced by the child's own, which then remain throughout life. Occasionally isoagglutinins may be present in the newborn which were lacking in the maternal blood so that they must be derived from the infant's organism.[34] Probably there is a transmission of this natural antibody through the placenta, and the fetus can also elaborate isoagglutinins of its own, providing they are compatible with the mother's blood. Nattan-Larrier[35] found that fetal blood does not contain natural antisheep hemolysin, although it can be demonstrated simultaneously in mother's blood. Artificially produced hemolysin, on the other hand, passes through the placenta. He found also[36] that pseudoglobulin was the principal if not the only carrier of the antitrypanosomic substance of the human serum, while euglobin was the carrier of the antisheep hemolysins of human blood. Both the antitrypanosomic and hemolytic substances were incapable of traversing the placenta. Nattan-Larrier took this as evidence of the nonidentity of natural and artificial hemolysin. Nattan-Larrier and Richard[37] found that maternal alexin did not pass the placenta. Von Oettingen and Witebsky[38] have presented evidence to show that the tissues of the placenta show no group characteristics. The placenta acts apparently as a neutral organ between mother and fetus and hence in heterospecific pregnancies the fetus cannot be injured by the mother tissues.

The possibility of both active and passive sensitization in utero brings up the question of the transmission of proteins through the placenta.

Infants may be born of nonsensitive mothers and yet manifest profound anaphylactic symptoms when they ingest some protein food for the first time.

Ratner[39] presents clinical evidence for the possibility of active sensitization in utero in cases where the mother had overindulged in certain protein foods, such as nuts, eggs, and wheat, during her antepartum period. After birth the infant, with a predisposition for allergy, manifested some form of allergic phenomenon when coming in contact with this food for the first time. The antigenic proteins enter the maternal circulation in an unchanged state from the intestinal tract and thereby gain entrance to the fetal circulation.[40]

Cooke and Vander Veer,[41] Spain and Cooke,[42] and Clarke, Donnally, and Coca[43] have shown that there is a tendency for the children of asthmatic parents to develop asthma and for those of parents suffering from hay fever to develop hay fever. This led Bell and Eriksson[44] to study the transfer of skin-sensitizing antibodies from mother to offspring in cases of asthma and of hay fever. Direct testing and the Prausnitz-Küstner method of passive transfer were used. Mother's sera reacted positively in all cases, and cord and infant's blood, negatively. Presumably skin-sensitizing antibodies were not transferred through the placenta.

From the available evidence it may be concluded that active and passive sensitization in utero can occur.[45]

TRANSMISSION THROUGH COLOSTRUM AND MILK

The role of colostrum in the transmission of antibodies in animals was noted by Famulener[46] and was emphasized by the work of Smith and his collaborators[47] who found that colostrum was essential to the newborn calf in the prevention of colon bacillus septicemia. Howe[48] demonstrated that the serum of the calf was deficient at birth in both pseudoglobulin and euglobulin and that after the ingestion of colostrum these globulins, the antibody carrying proteins of the blood, rose rapidly to normal levels. Lewis and Wells[49] and Boyd[50] showed that the human placenta allows the passage of pseudoglobulin in undiminished quantity, and only euglobulin is held back. Kuttner and Ratner[11] found that transitional milk and later milk did not contain antitoxin. Human colostrum occasionally contained small amounts of antitoxin, but the antitoxin content of infant's blood showed no increase attributable to colostrum feeding. Ratner, Jackson, and Gruehl[51] reviewed the evidence and concluded that colostrum was essential for the transmission of immunity in goats and cattle, but that it played a negligible role in man. There is also inadequate evidence for the passage of sensitizing proteins through the human colostrum or milk.[52] The transmission of antibodies through the later milk was also studied without evidence for this mode of transmission in humans.[52] However, Toomey[53] has recently studied the agglutinins against the enteric group of organisms in mother's blood, baby's blood, mother's milk, and placental blood. The agglutinins were transmitted through the placenta, but the amount was small and much less than the titer shown by the mother's serum which usually contained massive agglutinins against the enteric group. The blood serum of the infant, 10 days after birth, showed a marked increase in agglutinin titer over the placental serum. Since the titer of the infant's serum approximately paralleled that of the mother's milk, it seemed probable that the milk was the source of the agglutinins.

TISSUE IMMUNITY

Instances are recorded of infants who were immune to scarlet fever and to diphtheria whose mothers were demonstrated to be susceptible to these diseases. Placental or mammary transmission of immunity does not explain these phenomena; so a third possibility has been suggested, designated "tissue immunity" of the young.[54] The ability of embryonic tissue to neutralize diphtheria toxin as well as the resistance of embryonic tissue to tumorous growths is pointed to as evidence of this.[55]

PRACTICAL APPLICATION

Two practical applications have been made of the transplacental transmission of antibodies.

Nattan-Larrier, Ramon, and Grasset[56] have shown that it is possible to protect the newborn infant against tetanus by injecting the mother with tetanus toxoid before the birth of the infant; the protection derived from his procedure lasts for about two months, suggesting that the antibody developed by the mother rather than the injected toxoid traverses the placenta. This method of rendering infants temporarily immune has been used in Africa and in China, where childbirth tetanus is very common.

Placental extracts have been made and used effectively in the prevention and modification of measles.[57] In addition to measles antibody these extracts contain diphtheria antitoxin, scarlet fever antitoxin, antistreptolysin, and antibodies neutralizing poliomyelitis virus. Variable amounts of antibacterial substances are also demonstrable. An effect of placental extract on the inhibition of vaccinia in chick embryo cultures has recently been demonstrated. An interesting observation resulting from the studies of placental extract has been that the antibodies occur not only in the blood serum of the placenta but throughout the tissues of the organ. This storage of antibodies in the tissue may reflect a similar condition in the infant and might account for the long passive immunity in infants to certain diseases.

DEVELOPMENT OF IMMUNITY IN INFANTS

The respiratory and gastrointestinal tracts of newborn infants are sterile[58] but soon become the habitat of a variety of organisms. Kneeland[59] followed the bacteriology of the nose and throat in infants throughout the first year of life and found that the respiratory tract, sterile at birth, soon reflected the flora of normal adults. Pathogens were usually absent till the infant was 2 or 3 months of age, suggesting that type of contact may play a role in the bacterial seeding process. The first colds of infants were mild and were accompanied by no alterations in normal bacteriology. Barenberg, Greene, and Abramson[60] reported that institutional children were more susceptible to pneumonia between the ages of 6 months and 2 years, and that the case rate below 6 months was very low. Kneeland and Dawes[61] followed a similar group of infants and also found that infants in the first few months were comparatively immune. After 18 months children had many colds but were moderately resistant to pneumonia. Infants from 8 to 14 months had fewer colds but were highly susceptible to serious respiratory disease, especially pneumonia. Sutliff and Finland,[62] working along the same lines, found that bactericidal power against the pneumococcus was present in many infants in the first ten days of life but from two months was absent or very rare. From two to eleven years pneumococcidal power again returned. The bactericidal power of infants' blood was less in degree but reflected qualitatively the mothers' bactericidins. Negative skin tests to protein and to autolysate in the newborn infant indicated that reactivity to specific antigens was not passively transferred from the mother.

Fothergill and Wright,[63] studying influenza meningitis, pointed out the relation of the age incidence to the bactericidal power of the blood against the causative organism. These authors found that *influenza* meningitis is rarely seen under 2 months of age or beyond 6 years. Eighty per cent of reported cases have occurred between ages of 2 months and 3 years. Cord blood and blood of infants under 2 months had considerable bactericidal power while that of infants between 2 months and 3 years had practically none. After 5 years the bactericidal power gradually rose to adult levels. Davies[64] tested the response of infants to inoculation with Type I pneumococcus carbohydrate and found the reaction much less than that observed in older children and adults.

These results are in agreement with a considerable amount of evidence which indicates that the development of immunity in infants differs from that in older children and in adults.[65] The development of natural antibodies such as isoagglutinins may be taken as indicative of the ability of the infant to develop immune bodies. The patient's own isoagglutinins are seldom apparent under one month and do not usually reach their adult titer until 2 years.[66] Natural hemolysins to heterologous red cells are absent from the blood of newborn infants, even though present in the mother. They develop gradually in the infant, reaching about 20 per cent of the adult level by the end of the first year of life.[67]

The same general tendency for the development of antibodies with advance of age is seen in the case of diphtheria antitoxin.[68] Very young children not only develop diphtheria antitoxin slowly from spontaneous contact with the organism, but they respond in less degree to the injection of toxoid or of toxin-antitoxin mixtures than do older children.[69] At the end of the second year of life, when the great majority of children have developed their particular blood group, the proportion whose serum contains protective amounts of diphtheria antitoxin is almost at its minimum. That lack of contact with the antigen is probably of influence in the slow development of immunity to diphtheria is indicated by observation of persons isolated from large groups who develop immunity only in adult life. The results of large numbers of Dick tests indicate a definite relation of age to the development of immunity to scarlet fever even slower in its appearance than that to diphtheria.[70] The situation with respect to poliomyelitis would seem also analogous to that of diphtheria, although the data on immunity to this disease are not extensive.[71]

Freund[72] has been interested in the problem of age and immunity, and has studied the subject experimentally finding that the formation of agglutinins against typhoid bacilli, of hemolysins against sheep cells, and of precipitins against horse serum and egg white was less intense in young animals than in adult animals immunized in the same way. Frankenstein[73] found in infants that only an occasional subject produced agglutinins after inoculation with typhoid vaccine. Other workers have found that the response to typhoid vaccine occurs but is definitely less marked than in older children.[74]

Age is also of significance in the development of skin reactivity as has been noted in the slow development of a positive tuberculin reaction in young infants[75] and in a tendency to be nonreactive to Dick and Schick tests even in the absence of the specific antibody from the blood stream.[76] Reactions to skin tests with pneumococcic antigens were also minimal in infants[77] as were those to intradermal injections of colon, typhoid, streptococcus, and other bacterial extracts.[78]

The factors which influence the rapidity and extent of development of natural and artificially stimulated antibody response in infants are little known, and considering the importance of this subject in the field of pediatrics the attention devoted to it has been inadequate. Nutritional habits, types of food, character of environment, the endocrine make-up of the patient, family or racial differences may be among the forces operative.[79]

Racial resistance, examples of which are numerous, will be reflected in the individual, yet the infant often shows least of the evidences of the racial immunity. The importance of diet is exemplified in the infected corneal or pulmonary lesions in Vitamin A deficiency and has been further defined in experimental studies of the relation of diet to infection.[80] An endocrine maturation phenomenon may be indicated by the experiments of Jungeblut who rendered normal young monkeys insusceptible to poliomyelitis through repeated injections of pituitary extracts.[81] The influence of one disease in predisposing to another by increasing the individual susceptibility is too well known in pediatrics to require more than mention. Certain types of infants seem to be even more susceptible than the group as a whole. Thus in an epidemiologic survey[82] of infections arising in a group of hospitalized infants only 5.5 per cent of previously well infants became infected, whereas 19 per cent of premature infants, 35 per cent of chronically malnourished and 17 per cent of luetic, eczematous, and congenitally defective infants were involved. Scorbutic infants were highly susceptible to infection while rachitic infants were no more so than normal infants. Little is known of the immune responses of premature infants and whether debilitated patients and those suffering from deficiency diseases develop the ability to produce antibodies at times chronologically comparable to normal infants. Here is a large field awaiting exploration. It is hardly more than necessary to indicate the general influences of overcrowding, poverty, and other social and environmental factors.

Hirszfeld[83] has introduced the concept of serologic maturity which does not deny the influence of antigenic stimulation but assumes that the age or constitutional nature of the individual must be of the state to permit the immunologic response. Grasset[84] with a similar concept speaks of a curve of aptitude to acquire immunity. It is interesting to note that a disability to produce immune bodies similar to that in infants occurs in aged persons

We may tentatively conclude that immunity in the young differs from immunity of later ages (except possibly advanced age) through the interaction of two factors: (1) the specific antigen; (2) a state of immunizability, reflecting the capacity of the infant to respond to contact with the antigen. The failure of a response to contact with the antigen may result from its neutralization by the passively acquired antibody derived from the mother or may be traceable to the absence in the infant of the development permitting antibody production. Until immunologic maturation has taken place natural antibodies do not appear, and attempts at artificial immunization may have little result. If the antigenic stimulus is great, antibodies may be formed even during this early period, but they seldom reach any magnitude and tend to sink rapidly to low levels. The time of appearance and the strength of the reaction vary somewhat with the individual. Most infants respond slowly to antigenic stimulation yet a rare patient will have a rapid or efficient response, even in earliest infancy.

The necessity of contact with the antigen is shown by the tendency of antibody titers to fall unless antigenic stimulus is repeated at intervals. In infants, however, the factor of immunizability deserves more careful study. One should not be satisfied with the term serologic immaturity but must attempt to establish by chemical and physiologic studies the basis of such immaturity. Is the genesis of plasma proteins the important factor? Do dietary deficiencies or endocrine development play roles? As yet these are questions that cannot be fully answered but which should be objectives of persistent research.

Although the basis of the immunologic response of infants is poorly defined, a survey of the situation may serve to guide certain parts of daily practice.

The newborn infant is immune to many diseases by reason of passive transfer of antibodies from the mother. After the passive immunity is lost the infant becomes susceptible—more susceptible than the older child. This susceptibility appears to depend on a deficiency in the ability to produce antibodies. The deficiency is associated with a similar low level of natural antibodies such as isoagglutinins and heterophile antibodies.

From this we may derive that a lessened response to active immunization must be expected in infants and that a further diminution in response occurs if immunization is attempted before the natural immunity is lost. Thus a toxoid immunization against diphtheria will secure a larger percentage of solid immunizations if it is done after the passive immunity derived from the mother is gone and further if it is done late in infancy, when immunizability is rising. The young child responds even better than the infant, but undue delay must be weighed against the possible dangers of exposure in the older patient. Thus immunization against diphtheria, scarlet fever, and smallpox may all be delayed until late in the first year of life without material increase in danger to the infant and with a much greater immune response than would be obtained from earlier inoculation.

In view of the susceptibility of the infant to certain diseases and the character and severity of the disease process at early ages, therapeutic measures available for adults should be extended to infancy. We are now in such a transition in the treatment of pneumococcus pneumonia. A few years ago serum was employed in the treatment only of lobar pneumonia. Now serum treatment has extended to treatment of all pneumococcus pneumonias, and as serum becomes available for the types found in infants, serum therapy has been extended with very gratifying results into this age group.

SUMMARY

The immunity of the newborn infant to certain diseases is passive in character and is soon replaced by susceptibility more marked than that of older individuals. This great susceptibility may account for many of the unusual characteristics of disease in infancy and is dependent apparently on a deficiency in the capacity of the infant to produce antibodies.

This deficiency requires that more intensive therapy be applied toward infectious disease in infancy wherever such therapy is available, e.g., as in serum treatment of pneumonia.

Also the inadequate antibody response in early infancy should lead to delay in the active immunizations at least until the second half year of life when passive immunity derived from the mother has been lost and immunizability of the infant is rising.

REFERENCES

1. Fothergill, L. D., and Sweet, L. K.: J. Pediat. **2:** 696, 1933.
2. Forbes, R. P.: Am. J. Dis. Child. **25:** 130, 1923.
   Wislocki, G. B.: Bull. Johns Hopkins Hosp. **47:** 157, 1930.
3. Pineda, E. V.: J. Phillipine Islands M. A. **8:** 67, 1928.
4. Müller, C.: Arch. f. Gynäk. **150:** 482, 1932.
5. Slobozianu, H., and Herscovici, P.: Gynéc. et obst. **28:** 601, 1933.
6. Lanfrenchi, S., and Lenzi, S.: Ann. d'ig. **28:** 233, 1918.
7. Herrmann, O.: Ztschr. Immunitätsforsch. u. exp. Therap. **58:** 371, 1928.
8. Ueda, K.: Jap. J. Obst. & Gynec. **14:** 502, 1931.
9. Fischl, R., and Wunscheim: Ztschr. f. Heilk. **16:** 249, 1895.
   Kayser, H.: Ztschr. f. klin. Med. **56:** 17, 1905.
   Polano, O.: Ztschr. f. Geburtsh. u. Gynäk. **53:** 456, 1904.
   Ruh, H. O., and McClelland: Am. J. Dis. Child. **25:** 59, 1923.
   Neill, J. Y., Gaspari, E. L., Richardson, L. V., and Sugg, J. V.: J. Immunol. **22:** 117, 1932.
10. Tenbroeck, C., and Bauer, J. H.: Proc. Soc. Exper. Biol. & Med. **20:** 399, 1923.
11. Kuttner, A., and Ratner, B.: Am. J. Dis. Child. **25:** 413, 1923.

12. Toomey, J. A., and August, M. H.: Am. J. Dis. Child. **38**: 953, 1929.
13. Ward, H. K., and Lyons, C.: J. Exper. Med. **61**: 515, 1935.
14. Wilson, M. G., Wheeler, G. W., and Leask, M. M.: Proc. Soc. Exper. Biol. & Med. **31**: 1001, 1934.
15. Lippard, V. W., and Wheeler, G. W.: Am. J. Dis. Child. **52**: 61, 1936.
16. Lippard, V. W., and Johnson, P.: Am. J. Dis. Child. **49**: 1411, 1935.
17. Aycock, W. L., and Kramer, S. D.: J. Exper. Med. **52**: 457, 1930.
18. Herrmann, C.: Arch. Pediat. **40**: 678, 1923; Arch. Pediat. **41**: 301, 1924.
19. Debré, R., and Joannon, P.: Bull. et mém. Soc. méd. d. hôp. de Paris **49**: 682, 1925.
20. Finkelstein, G. S.: Vrach. delo. **14**: 794, 1931. Abstract, J. A. M. A. **98**: 92, 1932.
21. Jorge, R.: Bull. Office internat. d'hyg. pub. **24**: 978, 1932.
22. De Souza, J. S.: Arch. de méd. d. enf. **35**: 633, 1932.
23. Bryce, L. B., and Burnet, F. M.: J. Path. & Bact. **35**: 183, 1932.
24. Scholtz: Hyg. Rundschau. **8**: 417, 1898.
25. Schumacher, H.: Ztschr. f. Hyg. u. Infektionskr. **37**: 323, 1901.
26. Staubli, C.: Centralbl. f. Bakt. **36**: 441, 1904.
27. Mosse and Daunie: Compt. Rend. Soc. de biol. **49**: 238, 1897.
28. Peduzzi, F.: Boll. d. Ist. sieroterap. milanese **13**: 217, 1934.
29. Timmermann, W. A.: Ztschr. f. Immunitätsforsch. u. exp. Therap. **70**: 388, 1931.
30. Neff, F. C., and Schwartz, Eugene J.: Bull. Univ. Kan. School Med. p. 10, July, 1933.
31. Cooke, J. V.: Am. Rev. Tuberc. **6**: 127, 1922.
32. Halban, J., and Landsteiner, K.: München. med. Wchnschr. **49**: 473, 1902.
33. Hirszfeld, L., and Zborowski, H.: Klin. Wchnschr. **4**: 1152, 1925; Compt. Rend. Soc. de biol. **92**: 1253, 1926; Compt. Rend. Soc. de biol. **94**: 205, 1926; Klin. Wchnschr. **5**: 741, 1926.
    Hara, M., and Wakao, R.: Jahrb. f. Kinderh. **114**: 313, 1926.
    Smith, C. H.: Am. J. Dis. Child. **36**: 54, 1928.
    Lazarewicz, M., and Zborowski, H.: Compt. Rend. Soc. de biol. **95**: 1212, 1926.
34. Halban, J.: Wien. klin. Wchnschr. **13**: 545, 1900.
    von Decastello, A., and Sturli, A.: München. med. Wchnschr. **49**: 1090, 1902.
    Martin, E.: Zentralbl. f. Bakt. **39**: 704, 1905.
    Collon, N. G.: Compt. Rend. Soc. de biol. **94**: 418, 1926; Compt. Rend. Soc. de biol. **96**: 144, 1927; Arch. Internat. de méd. expér. **3**: 237, 1927.
35. Nattan-Larrier, L., Ramon, G., and Lepine, P.: Compt. Rend. Soc. de biol. **97**: 673, 1927.
36. Nattan-Larrier, L., Ramon, G., and Lepine, P.: Compt. Rend. Soc. de biol. **98**: 1279, 1928.
37. Nattan-Larrier, L., and Richard, L.: Compt. Rend. Soc. de biol. **103**: 1084, 1930.
38. Von Oettingen, K., and Witebsky, E.: München. med. Wchnschr. **75**: 385, 1928.
39. Ratner, B.: Am. J. Dis. Child. **36**: 277, 1928.
40. Anderson, A. F., Schloss, O. M., and Myers, C.: Proc. Soc. Exper. Biol. & Med. **23**: 180, 1925.
    Schloss, O. M.: Harvey Lectures, Series XX, p. 156, 1924-25.
41. Cooke, R. A., and Vander Veer, A.: J. Immunol. **1**: 201, 1916.
42. Spain, W. C., and Cooke, R. A.: J. Immunol. **9**: 521, 1924.
43. Clarke, J. A., Donnally, H. H., and Coca, A. F.: J. Immunol. **15**: 9, 1928.
44. Bell, S. D., and Eriksson, Z.: J. Immunol. **20**: 447, 1931.
45. Ratner, B.: J. Pediat. **12**: 730, 1938.
46. Famulener: J. Infect. Dis. **10**: 332, 1912.
47. Little, R. B., and Orcutt, M. L. J.: J. Exper. Med. **35**: 161, 1922; Smith, T., and Little, R. B.: J. Exper. Med. **36**: 453, 1922.
48. Howe, P. E.: J. Biol. Chem. **49**: 115, 1921.
    Orcutt, M. L., and Howe, P. E.: J. Exper. Med. **36**: 291, 1922.
49. Lewis, J. H., and Wells, H. G.: J. A. M. A. **78**: 863, 1922.
50. Boyd, G. L.: Canad. M. A. J. **12**: 724, 1922.
51. Ratner, B., Jackson, H. C., and Gruehl, H. L.: J. Immunol. **14**: 267, 1927.
52. Ratner, B., Jackson, H. C., and Gruehl, H. L.: J. Immunol. **14**: 275, 1927.
53. Toomey, J. A.: Am. J. Dis. Child. **47**: 521, 1934.
54. Dreyfus-Sée, G.: Arch. de méd. d. enf. **33**: 16, 1930.
    Wadsworth, A., and Hoppe, E. N.: J. Exper. Med. **53**: 821, 1931.
55. Murphy, J. B., and Sturm, E.: J. Exper. Med. **60**: 293, 1934.

56. Nattan-Larrier, L., Ramon, G., and Grasset, E.: Quoted by Roux. Rev. Internat. de L'enfant 2: 1112, 1926.
57. McKhann, C. F., and Chu, F. T.: J. Infect. Dis. **52**: 268, 1933.
McKhann, C. F., Green, A. A., and Coady, H.: J. PEDIAT. **6**: 603, 1935.
McKhann, C. F.: J. A. M. A. **109**: 2034, 1937.
58. Bloomfield, A. L.: Bull. Johns Hopkins Hosp. **33**: 61, 1922.
59. Kneeland, Y., Jr.: J. Exper. Med. **51**: 617, 1930.
60. Barenberg, L. H., Greene, D., and Abramson, H.: J. A. M. A. **92**: 440, 1929.
61. Kneeland, Y., Jr., and Dawes, C. F.: J. Exper. Med. **55**: 735, 1932.
62. Sutliff, W. D., and Finland, M.: J. Exper. Med. **55**: 837, 1932.
63. Fothergill, L. D., and Wright, J.: J. Immunol. **24**: 273, 1933.
64. Davies, J. A. V.: J. Immunol. **33**: 1, 1937.
65. Baumgartner, L.: Yale J. Biol. & Med. **6**: 403, 1934.
66. Happ, W. M.: J. Exper. Med. **31**: 313, 1920.
Mitchell, J. M.: Am. J. Dis. Child. **36**: 486, 1928. Am. J. Dis. Child. **37**: 1008, 1929.
67. Friedberger, E., and Bock, G. L.: Klin. Wchnschr. **8**: 1858, 1929.
Friedberger, E., Bock, G. L., and Fürstenheim, A.: Ztschr. f. Immunitätsforsch. **64**: 294, 1929.
Thomsen, O., and Kettel, K.: Ztschr. f. Immunitätsforsch. **63**: 67, 1929.
68. von Gröer, F., and Kassowitz, K.: Ztschr. f. Immunitätsforsch. **23**: 108, 1915; **26**: 277, 1917; **28**: 327, 1919.
Zingher, A.: Am. J. Dis. Child. **25**: 392, 1923.
69. Ribadeau-Dumas, L., Loiseau, and Lacomma: Bull. et mém. Soc. méd. d. hôp. de Paris **49**: 1121, 1925.
70. Zingher, A.: J. A. M. A. **83**: 432, 1924; J. A. M. A. **84**: 806, 1925.
Cooke, J. V.: Am. J. Dis. Child. **35**: 762, 1928.
71. Aycock, W. L., and Kramer, S. D.: J. Exper. Med. **52**: 457, 1930. J. Prev. Med. **4**: 201, 1930.
72. Freund, J.: J. Immunol. **18**: 315, 1930.
73. Frankenstein, L.: Ztschr. f. Kinderh. **25**: 12, 1920.
74. Halber, E., Hirszfeld, H., and Mayzner, M.: Ztschr. f. Immunitätsforsch. **53**: 391, 1929.
75. Freund, J.: J. Immunol. **13**: 285, 1927; **17**: 465, 1929.
Valtis, J.: Compt. rend. Soc. de biol. **99**: 554, 1928.
Valtis, J., and Saenz, A.: Compt. rend. Soc. de biol. **99**: 1563, 1928.
76. Von Gröer, F., and Kassowitz, K.: Ztschr. f. Immunitätsforsch. **30**: 154, 1920.
Cooke, J.: Proc. Soc. Exper. Biol. & Med. **24**: 314, 1926.
Cooke, J., Keith, H. R., and Ermatinger, L.: Am. J. Dis. Child. **34**: 969, 1927.
Kuntz, H., and Nobel, E.: Ztschr. f. Kinderh. **42**: 372, 1926.
Kuttner, A., and Ratner, B.: Am. J. Dis. Child. **25**: 413, 1923.
Paunz, J., and Csoma, E.: Klin. Wchnschr. **7**: 498, 1928.
77. Von Gutfeld and Nassau, A.: Jahrb. f. Kinderh. **112**: 135, 1926.
78. Tschertkow, L., and Belgowskaja, E.: Ztschr. f. Immunitätsforsch. **67**: 475, 1930.
Selter, H.: Ztschr. f. Immunitätsforsch. **69**: 517, 1931.
McKenzie, G. M., and Hangar, F. M.: Proc. Soc. Exper. Biol. & Med. **21**: 442, 1924.
79. Topley, W. W. C., and Wilson, G. S.: The Principles of Bacteriology and Immunology, New York, 1929, William Wood & Co.
80. Clausen, S. W.: Physiol. Rev. **14**: 309, 1934.
81. Jungeblut, C. W., and Engle, E. T.: Am. J. Dis. Child. **43**: 523, 1932.
82. McKhann, C. F., Steeger, A., and Long, A. P.: Am. J. Dis. Child. **55**: 579, 1938.
83. Hirszfeld, L.: Klin. Wchnschr. **3**: 1180, 1924; Ergebn. d. Hyg., Bakt., Immunitätsforsch. u. exper. Therap. **8**: 367, 1926; Klin. Wchnschr. **6**: 1881 and 1929, 1927.
Halber, W., and Hirszfeld, L.: Ztschr. f. Immunitätsforsch. **48**: 34, 1926.
Hirszfeld, L., and Halber, W.: Ztschr. f. Immunitätsforsch. **53**: 419, 1927.
84. Grasset, E.: Publ. S. African Inst. M. Research No. 24, **4**: 171, 1929.

American Academy of Pediatrics

Proceedings

EIGHTH ANNUAL MEETING OF THE AMERICAN ACADEMY OF PEDIATRICS

DEL MONTE, CALIF., JUNE 9, 10, AND 11, 1938

Round Table Discussion of Clinical Immunology

Chairman: Dr. K. F. Meyer, San Francisco, Calif.

Some Fundamental Principles in Clinical Immunology

K. F. Meyer, Ph.D., M.D.*

The classical methods of controlling a communicable disease consist of procedures which prevent the transmission of the infective agent. This so-called exposition prophylaxis is directed against the existence and distribution of the disease agent and is primarily applicable to the diseases which are colloquially designated as avoidable. Sanitation of the environment, with special reference to the protection of the food and water supplies, effectively suppresses, in fact, eliminates these diseases.

In principle, these general measures are mostly ineffective in the control of the so-called civilization diseases, since contagion is eventually a function of the crowding and intimate contact of human beings, and thus unavoidable. Without a thorough knowledge of the epidemiology of the disease, it is obviously impossible to institute prophylactic measures based on isolation, disinfection, and control of carriers. Isolation as a means of suppressing measles may be effective provided the importance of notification is more universally appreciated. Physicians are lax in reporting when they know that no service is being rendered by the health department or the community.

The control of diphtheria, scarlet fever and poliomyelitis through isolation is extremely difficult since a relatively small percentage of human beings exhibit signs of the infection in form of clinical disease. In whooping cough the isolation is usually too late. The various procedures of disinfection, except concurrent disinfection, are mostly symbolic and ineffective. A search for carriers from the standpoint of a general control of civilization diseases appeared justified at a time when the so-called practical ubiquity of the disease agents was not known. Today one must be grateful for the failure to eradicate the carriers even if such a procedure would have been temporarily successful. The process of immunization by means of subclinical infections would have been strangulated, and on reintroduction of the disease, the population would have had to meet it in an utterly unprotected state. The experiences on the Island of Nauru (1910) with respect to poliomyelitis and, in fact, on the Faroe Islands (1873 to 1875) in connection with measles, offer excellent examples of what might have happened. General hygienic measures are not very promising, particularly since exposure is not preventable; a protection of the host before the onset of an infection is valuable. This so-called disposition prophylaxis is known as the immunobiologic control of a communicable disease.

*Director, Hooper Foundation for Medical Research.

The noteworthy successes which have been recorded encouraged the belief that a great many other maladies not classed with the civilization diseases may be prevented by an immunobiologic approach. It is doubtless profitable to subject the procedures to a critical inquiry. In this connection one is equally tempted to analyze the vast field of clinical serum and vaccine therapy. Thus before a few selected methods and procedures are chosen for general discussion, it may be appropriate to define the position of the immunologist in its relation to the problems involved.

Nobody will deny that in clinical and in public health work, a critical evaluation of a process of immunization is most important. The present state of affairs is in many ways untenable. A definite dogmatism or doctrinism is evident. This attitude is particularly true in those instances in which one group of workers wishes to *promote* an immunization procedure. The same position is taken when it is necessary to protect a method against an attack by others. This dogmatic concept is accompanied by an unmistakable empiricism. Theoretic considerations or experimental facts are ignored; one proceeds and accepts as conclusive only mass tests on man. The consequences of such a tendency are clearly shown in the attempted immunizations against tuberculosis and poliomyelitis.

Quite generally one is guided by the principle that the immunizations must be harmless. As an ideal, one considers a reactionless vaccination, but an immunization without manifest pathologic consequences or an immunization with a latent reaction is better. The primum non nocere predominates and overshadows the efficacy of a method. In principle, this concept is in my opinion not sound for the following simple reason: If a procedure of vaccination produces no reactions and is relatively harmless, it is reasonable to conclude that it is of little value and consequently its facultative or obligatory use is not justified. If, on the other hand, a procedure is satisfactory with respect to intensity and durability of the protection conferred, severe immunisatoric reactions must be accepted as inevitable, always provided that the risk, inherent to any effective immunization, is quantitatively and qualitatively counterbalanced by the dangers which the omission might entail.

In recent years one justifies the experimentations with an immunisatoric procedure because it is harmless, long before the value or lack of value of a certain method has been accepted by the experts as proved. As a result thousands of human beings have been injected with preparations, and no effort has been made to specify the purpose and the reason for the tests. The introduction of a method of immunization as a means to propagandize such a procedure long before the experimental evaluation of the principle has been completed is certainly not within the jurisdiction of a profession or an agency which is entrusted with the health of the people.

The purpose of all immunizations is the protection of a human or animal host: (1) against the manifest symptoms induced by the infectious process, or (2) the modification of the course of the disease, or (3) a reduction in the case fatality rates. All the known immunobiologic procedures are obviously directed towards the pathogenic effects and not against the infection per se. In fact, a great deal can be achieved provided the immunization transforms the manifest infection into a latent or abortive process.

The observations on measles show how a superimposed latent infection may effectively exert an immunisatoric effect.

Convalescent serum administered after exposure confers an immunity for three to four weeks. On the other hand, if children so treated are exposed a few days later to measles, a permanent immunity of many years' duration will result. Doubtless, the latent minimal infection transforms the ephemeral passive into an active immunity. As a rule, present-day methods are more effective in preventing the localization of an infection than in paralyzing the pathogenic manifestations, since the factors leading to the disease are unknown. Exceptions to this general conclusion are the bacterial intoxications caused by toxicogenic saprophytes, tetanus and botulism, perhaps diphtheria and certain types of dysentery.

Today some doubts have arisen as to the general concept that the test tube toxins are responsible for the total disease picture in diphtheria and, consequently, the active or passive immunization with these toxins as now practiced may not be the proper method to follow. The present-day position in this matter may be stated as follows:

(1) According to the many observations now available, it is admitted that immunity against diphtheria is primarily antitoxic; however, other factors such as bactericidal forces and primary toxin resistance participate in the defense and recovery from the disease.

(2) A human being lacking one or the other of the functions may contract the disease provided he is sufficiently exposed. In case he lacks every one of the defensive forces, he may pass through a severe disease, and should he be unable to produce them sufficiently or for a long period, the chance of repeated infections is a decided possibility.

(3) As a rule, those who possess an antitoxic immunity or other as yet unknown defensive forces never contract the disease. Furthermore, those who may be able to mobilize humoral and cellular defenses in sufficient quantity at the time of contact with the disease organism may remain unaffected.

(4) The majority of people acquire an immunity to diphtheria either by recovery or through subclinical infection. Intensity and duration of this immunity depend on (a) exogenic (antigenic) factors and (b) genotypic factors (variable ability in the individual to produce antitoxin or other defensive forces).

(5) As a rule, a lowered antitoxin content has been demonstrated at the beginning of the disease. The few exceptions (10 per cent) are attributable to the formation of antitoxin during the first few days of the illness.

(6) It is a fact that in mild diphtheria, without serum treatment during the course of the disease and following recovery, inability to demonstrate antitoxin does not preclude the possibility that the antitoxin, which is generated rather slowly, may be recognizable only after a lapse of several months. These examples merely indicate that recovery and resistance of the host to the diphtheria bacillus are not conditioned by the antitoxin alone.

Next of importance are the latent and abortive infections, which may in themselves constitute a process of immunization of the individual, but at the same time become sources of disease. Such immunizations conducted in population groups may protect the person who has been injected with the infective agent, but may injure the unprotected individual in the immediate environment. For example, the morbilloid or mitigated measles induced by serum prophylaxis is infectious, and experiences in institutions have taught that a new generation of measles within an epidemic or a new epidemic may be traced to such cases. The consequences are quite obvious. Many of the methods of immunization now in use fail to reduce the possibilities for the spread of the infection; in consequence, they will never permit a reduction of an immunization program which has been inaugurated in a certain region. What has been initiated on the present living generation must be continued for an indefinite time if it is desired to maintain the protection of the masses at a high peak. That method of immunization, which prevents the localization of a disease-producing agent and thus transforms a probable host into a nonsusceptible one, will not only protect the individual but will ultimately reach the utopian goal, the radical elimination of the infectious epidemic disease. These considerations lead to the pertinent question: What criteria must be used to evaluate a method of immunization?

Observations during the past thirty years have shown that the recovery from *certain* infectious diseases leaves a dependable and permanent protection against a subsequent reinfection of similar etiology; while in others not only no specific immunity is noticeable, but, in fact, a definite increased disposition is recorded. In the first group predominate the diseases caused by viruses; in the latter the bacterial infections. Although this distinction is not absolute, it is obvious that the efforts in the direction to produce an effective protective immunization are much more promising in the field of viruses than in the bacterial diseases. Furthermore, it is generally recognized that an infectious disease process supplies the protection to a malady of identical nature. As to whether a latent infection induces the same condition is by no means established for every disease. Abortive or latent yellow fever, measles, and Rickettsia may with considerable certainty create protection.

The importance of latent infections as factors in the individual resistance to diphtheria, scarlet fever, and other diseases of childhood is by no means clear. The theory of latent epidemization is based on statistic-epidemiologic mass observations. It is not appreciated that one rarely knows the history of specific infections of an individual who, despite innumerable chances of exposure, remains well. The absence or the presence of antitoxin in the blood is not necessarily conclusive proof that the individual has or has not passed through a latent diphtheritic or streptococcic infection. The epidemiologist has always been puzzled by one fact; the latent infections are not sufficiently widely distributed to induce a far-reaching change in the state of immunity of a large population group. What has been definitely established is briefly this: (1) The morbidity from diphtheria or scarlet fever stands in intimate relationship to age. However, no data are available to prove that this relationship is equally prevalent in the epidemic as well as nonendemic areas, and (2) even in the different age groups, the ability to contract the disease is never uniform. During the period of maximum liability, only a relatively small percentage of the exposed individuals contracts diphtheria or scarlet fever. Members of one family give usually all positive or all negative antitoxin findings. And yet diphtheria rarely selects more than one or two persons in a family (Neisser and Heymann). These and other observations make it doubtful that the latent epidemization is the sole dominant factor in creating the resistance.

Although no final explanation regarding the resistance in diphtheria and scarlet fever may be offered at this time, the procedure to immunize by inducing mild infections is theoretically sound and most useful in many infections. On the other hand, *antigen immunization* with killed organisms or their toxins leaves a great deal to be desired. Even if the injections of vaccines confer a certain degree of protection, it must be emphasized that in such diseases as typhoid, cholera, and plague in which the reports are mostly indefinite impressions and not scientifically proved facts, the duration of the protection, whether for one year or only a few months, is by no means known or definitely established.

Preliminary to any practical application of procedure of immunization, it is important to test its supposed efficacy by animal experiments which are so planned that they give complete information and prevent the physician from disappointments. In this respect, a great deal is still left to chance. The animal stock must be uniform in susceptibility. Quantitative studies must be made on large series; this is particularly true for the evaluation of the toxoids. The question has been by no means settled concerning the relationship of immunisatoric value of toxoid and its flocculating value.

Studies by Prigge in the Ehrlich Institut have shown that toxoids with an equal flocculating value possess variable antigenic properties. Thus it is imperative that the immunizing value of a toxoid preparation be compared by direct tests on guinea pigs of uniform susceptibility. The German regulations proceed in practice as follows: 125 guinea pigs are injected with standard toxoid; an equal number of animals receives an equal amount of the unknown preparation. Twenty-eight days later each animal receives an injection of test toxin. A preparation which fails to protect the same or a larger percentage of guinea pigs injected with the standard toxoid is refused general distribution. Until toxins standardized according to a like procedure are available, it is doubtless futile to argue the advantages and disadvantages of plain versus alum toxoid. Suffice it to state that alum toxoid is now produced both in Germany and Denmark with an immunizing value of not less than 30 units per 1 c.c. The average plain toxoid contains approximately 1 unit. The use of these highly potent antigens has many advantages but does not preclude the necessity of adhering as heretofore to the fractionated method of immunization.

Despite the noteworthy achievements which the animal experiments have granted the immunologist, it must be frankly admitted that the study is incomplete in many ways. It is impossible to reproduce the infectious disease with respect to portal of entry and dosage of disease agents.

When a method of immunization is ultimately tested on human beings, it is important to divide it into two acts; (1) the immunization and (2) the determination of the refractory state. The latter may be evaluated as follows: (1) by intentional infection, (2) by intentional exposure to a natural infection, (3) by permitting the prevailing epidemiologic factors to act freely without favoring the natural infection, and (4) by testing certain reactions which may indicate the altered state of immunity in the immunized (antitoxins, humoral antibodies, Schick and Dick tests, tuberculin test, etc.).

The first named procedure was used by Jenner (vaccinia-variola) and was justifiable because variola was quite prevalent. Today this mode of evaluation is probably applicable only in exceptional instances. Similarly, the second method is useful only in professional or occupational groups (laboratory workers) provided the control group is large enough and comparatively uniformly exposed.

Far more effective are the tests in which consideration is given to the interplay of disposition and exposition on the immunized; thus the influence of the immunization on the natural hazard of infections may be evaluated far more accurately than by any other method. When the disposition is maximal and the exposition is great (smallpox), dependable information may be readily obtained. On the other hand, an absence of these premises may render the information secured uncertain. A tendency has thus developed to increase the number of vaccinations in order to be able to express the effect of the immunization by statistical figures. This method has a great many inherent difficulties since the morbidity and mortality for many of the diseases involved in the mass immunizations are subject to great variations. For example, the statistics concerning typhoid vaccination during the War are greatly invalidated since they ignore the faults of the reporting system, the differences between mobile and stationary warfare, the improved condition in the care of the sick, and the inadequate differential diagnosis between typhoid and spotted fever. It is regrettable that these mistakes have not been corrected in connection with evaluation of immunizations against diphtheria and tuberculosis.

The fourth method is for all intent and purposes based on an analogy deduction. In order to be valuable, it is important that the following questions be definitely answered: (1) Are the reactions merely accompanying auxiliary phenomena or (2) are they absolute and essential conditions of the changed state of susceptibility?

In the evaluation of the Schick test, these prerequisites have not been taken into account. It is well known that occasionally Schick-negative individuals may contract diphtheria. As a test, it does not give absolute certainty but merely a high probability for a single case and indicates that an individual has an average resistance against an average infection. Furthermore, it is doubtless questionable to evaluate an immunization method by a procedure which has not been generally recognized as valid. Therefore, the Schick test can merely be used as an orientation. The antitoxin tests of the blood serum give more information concerning the immunisatoric response than the Schick test. Cases have been reported in which even one antitoxic unit failed to protect against an attack of diphtheria. Furthermore, the antitoxic serum mirror may vary in one and the same individual within a very short time. Severe fatigue or profuse perspiration may reduce or enhance the serum titer. Hamburger and, more recently, Hottinger have noted the interesting fact that children who recovered from diphtheria without the aid of therapeutic injection of antitoxin failed to produce antitoxin. The fact that recovery from diphtheria does not necessarily protect against a second or third attack is usually overlooked, although, according to Zucker's statistic, which embraces only the most susceptible age group, at least 0.9 per cent of the children contract diphtheria a second and 0.13 per cent a third time. Schick and Karasawa even saw a fourth attack.

One may in this connection raise the question: Why does the latent infection and not infrequently the active immunization with toxoids produce far more regularly and more permanently a persistent antitoxin? This important question has not been answered but deserves consideration. At one time the analysis of these observations suggested a desire to revise the theoretic foundations of the active immunization against diphtheria. How this is to be done is not clear. One has, therefore, adhered to the following thought:

The reports on the failures are numerous but in the available statistics the morbidity and the fatality rates of the nonimmunized surpass those of the immunized. The international inquest, which was conducted by the League of Nations, has shown that ten times more nonimmunized contract diphtheria than the immunized, and that the mortality is greatly reduced in some countries even to the zero point.

These critical remarks are not intended to create undue skepticism. Successful immunizations are the crowning achievements of medical research.

However, in the interest of the scientific character of the principles involved and in order to forestall eventual disappointments, it is imperative to check the numerous attempts to discredit valuable and useful methods of immunization by a criticless and planless empirical tendency to propagandize the public for an insufficiently tested procedure of protection which in the natural course of events must lead to mass immunizations and their disappointing consequences.

In order to encourage a general discussion, a few common and then a few less frequently employed methods of immunization may now be briefly presented:

(1) *Smallpox.*—All children should be vaccinated between the sixth and twelfth months of age. This should be repeated whenever the disease is epidemic or in the presence of unusual likelihood of exposure, travel, or contact with cases. The multiple pressure method: 10 to 15 strokes through the drop of virus is generally recognized as the best procedure. In recent years, aside from the well-known glycerinated, vaccinia, vaccine, several newer antigens have been recommended: the chorion-allantoic chick embryo vaccine prepared according to the method of Goodpasture and the lyophile tissue vaccine of Rivers. The latter is administered intracutaneously and is particularly useful when children with skin diseases require vaccination, and when the vaccine has to be shipped under climatic conditions which may readily destroy the potency of the vaccine. The newer preparations are bacteriologically free from micro-organisms other than the elementary bodies of vaccinia. Large comparative series intended to evaluate the antigenic values of the preparations have been carried out by several health departments. The final reports are not yet available.

The type of reactions which must be observed following vaccination, is beautifully illustrated by a chart prepared by the Baltimore Health Department.

Potent antivaccinial sera have been prepared and their use may be considered in the future. For the present, serum treatment of smallpox is in the experimental stage.

At this point, it may be profitable to reflect briefly on the immunity in virus infections. While the knowledge concerning these most intriguing agents of disease was being collected, certain observations assumed the position of facts. For example, it was believed that an active immunity could only be induced by an actual infection, that the resistance was cellular or a tissue immunity, and that the serum antibodies did not react with the virus but as part of the immunity mechanism united with the susceptible cells and protected them against invasion. The increasing number of reports on the immunizing power of heat-killed or formalin-killed virus of herpes, foot-and-mouth disease, vaccinia, psittacosis, and influenza virus cannot be questioned. There is of course the undoubted fact that some of the viruses in a killed state are poor antigens. The absence of serum antibodies in many virus infections does not justify the conclusion that the state of resistance is a true tissue immunity. There is ample evidence to show that if the passive protection against a virus is to be effective, the specific antibody must come into intimate contact with the susceptible cells; it will, therefore, disappear from the circulation or its production will rarely proceed far enough to become demonstrable in the blood stream. True tissue immunity may be operative in the so-called interference phenomenon in yellow fever. The immunity mechanism in poliomyelitis, concerning which there is quite some discussion, may possibly be classed as cellular. From the available data, one could visualize the immunity as follows: The cells of the central nervous system produce their own specific antibodies independent of those found in the circulation. But how does this antibody do its work? Perhaps there is an immunity of the neurons which is independent of the antibody; the insusceptibility is perhaps determined by the persistence of the virus. Since it is not unlikely that the infective agent of poliomyelitis on account of its small particle size is probably a heavy molecular weight protein, this explanation appears reasonable. Equally important in this connection in the question as to whether or not the insusceptibility to infection is dependent on physiologic (endocrines and vitamins) or hereditary factors.

Thus, in all probability, the immunity to animal viruses is only in rare instances of the nature of a tissue immunity. In the vast majority of cases, the antibody is the all-important factor in the immune state. Concerning the mode of action of the neutralizing antibody, it is now strongly suspected that the loose virus-antiserum union, which may be observed by various methods, prepares the virus for phagocytosis and destruction within the cells. Thus the antibody, by uniting with the virus, prevents its penetration in the cells or prepares it for intracellular destruction. But, whichever mechanism it employs, the protection afforded is always relative. Small quantities of virus survive, multiply within cells, and when set free they stimulate antibodies which in turn prevent the level to rise to a stage sufficient to cause clinical symptoms. Thus persistent infections in the immune state or the well-known latency develops. This phenomenon is not only of importance in an explanation of the durable immunity, which so many virus diseases leave behind them, but it plays a prominent role in the epidemiology and has a far-reaching bearing no the immunobiologic methods which are used for the purpose of prophylactic immunization. At this point it may not be out of place to consider the following:

(2) *Rabies Prophylactic Treatment.*—The disease is unduly prevalent, and with increasing frequency decisions have to be made concerning the advisability in recommending the specific prophylactic treatment. During the past fifty years, the original Pasteurian procedure has been modified, primarily to increase the immunity and

secondarily to reduce the complications in form of paralysis or even infection (Högye's method). The fixed virus is subjected either to heat or to the action of chemicals such as carbolic acid or ether. The so-called Semple or phenol-treated vaccine is quite generally used, and although the statistics regularly presented by McKendrick (Bull. Health Organization **6**: 17, 1937) would indicate that the killed vaccines give rise to a substantial degree of immunity when given in adequate dosage. There is definite evidence that some preparations on the market are inactive and that, as a whole, they are inferior to vaccines in which the virus is alive but attenuated. On a comparative basis, the etherized vaccines prepared according to Alivisato's method are generally considered superior to the Semple vaccine. Since the immunity mechanism in rabies is by no means understood, it is indeed difficult to evaluate the protection which may be conferred by certain preparations. It is not unlikely that the resistance of the ganglion cells to the virus is independent of the antibodies found in the circulation. For example, a veterinarian, who had been bitten on the thumb by a rabid dog, was thoroughly treated with Semple vaccine, developed neutralizing antibodies in his serum, and yet succumbed to rabies.

While there are several objections to the use of live vaccines in the prophylaxis of most diseases, the fact that the case mortality rate in rabies is so high and the patient is already infected at the time of vaccination does seem to warrant the taking of greater risks. The so-called mixed treatment consisting of etherized vaccine followed by Högye's dilution method or vice versa seems to be justifiable, particularly in deep bites with localization on the head. Those who are frequently brought in contact with the problem of antirabic treatment may profitably consult a recent monograph by Marie J. Van Stockum (New Principles of Antirabic Treatment, Hague, 1935).

(3) *Staphylococcic Infections.*—Based on experimental evidence, it is now believed that pyogenic cocci exert their harmful effect on the tissues by means of toxins, while the resistance is antitoxic in nature. Patients suffering from staphylococcic infections, furunculosis, osteomyelitis, etc., have usually a high antitoxic serum titer. Expressed in so-called international units (1 unit equals amount of specific antitoxic activity contained in 0.5 mg. of dry standard serum; antitoxic activity tested as neutralization of hemolysin, or skin necrotizing effect or death of mouse), it may vary from 1 to 15 units, while in normal persons it is always less than one (0.25 to 0.75 units per cubic centimeter). Highly potent antisera capable of neutralizing the hemolytic, skin-necrosing, lethal, and leucocidic properties have been prepared by inoculation of horses with formalin-treated and later pure toxins. The use of the serum on man is still in an experimental stage, and its usefulness is not established. From a few observations, it appears not unlikely that the antitoxic sera are not capable of neutralizing the intracellular toxins, nor do they protect the leucocytes from the destruction through leucocidins. A serum prepared by treating animals with young staphylococcic cultures contains sensitizing antibodies, which prepare the capsulated cocci for phagocytosis and subsequent leucocidin action. The antibacterial immunity in staphylococcic infections is probably not solely antitoxic.

Staphylococcal toxoid carefully prepared from known strains, which produce no enterotoxic poisons, is used in chronic staphylococcic infections with some success. There is for the present no agreement with regard to dosage and spacing of the injections. Dolman recommends eight weekly injections of 0.05 c.c. progressively increased until 0.5 c.c. is given. Ramon, on the other hand, found that three injections (0.25 c.c., 0.5 c.c., and 2 c.c.) at intervals of from two to three days yielded the highest antitoxin titer on the seventh day. From the evidence at hand, the toxoid is of considerably more value than vaccines, particularly in chronic processes (boils and chronic osteomyelitis). As a whole, the procedure is still in the testing stage and may in time be modified. However, just as in every other method of immunization, perhaps slightly more so in the staphylococcal antitoxin vaccination, the individual variations in response are quite considerable. Consequently, it is by no means surprising that in small serial observations, the disappointments may overbalance the successes. It is of interest to note that Ramon and his colleagues recommend the combination vaccination with a mixture of staphylococcal toxoid and triple typhoid paratyphoid vaccine.

(4) *Streptococcic Infections.*—Despite a vast amount of research in the field of streptococcic infection, the immunity mechanism is still shrouded in uncertainties. Immunobiologic procedures of various sorts have appeared on the scene like the ebb and flow of the tide. With the advent of sulphanilamide alone or better in combination with convalescent serum, the problem of active immunization has been pushed in the background. In fact, the recent achievements with the erythrogenic toxin as so-called scarlet fever toxoid have not received the attention they deserve. The subject should be discussed, particularly in the light of the reports by Gaylord W. Anderson of the Massachusetts Department of Public Health, who has analyzed a community immunization program involving 14,000 children in orphanages, schools, etc. They had received 0.1, 0.5, and 1 c.c. of toxoid at three weekly intervals. By comparing the attack rates of the immunized and nonimmunized groups, it was consistently noted that the rates were significantly lower among the vaccinated. It is equally noteworthy that the local and general reactions were in no way greater than those observed following diphtheria toxoid.

(5) *Tetanus.*—The tetanus antitoxin acts, not by interfering with the germination of the spores, but by neutralizing the toxin as fast as it is formed. It should be used prophylactically in cases in which there is danger of contamination of a wound with manure, soil, stable dust, etc. The initial dose of 1,500 units (800 to 1,000 units) should be repeated on the fifth day after the initial dose. In fact, third and even fourth injections may be indicated when the wound is very bad. Since the protection wears off in the course of two to three weeks, sensitization with horse serum is undesirable, and sometimes when severe serum reactions accompany the treatment, there is a tendency to reinforce the passive immunity by means of active immunization. The latter procedure is equally advisable in children, who are constantly subject to injuries which may be followed by tetanus. The French Army has pioneered in this field of active immunization. Postinfectional preventive serum therapy is now enhanced by the injection of 1 c.c. of tetanus toxoid about fifteen minutes after the administration of the serum, followed by two injections of 2 c.c. of toxoid at two weekly intervals. Such a treatment raises the antitoxin level of the patient's serum over one quarter unit per c.c., and although at least $1/200$ unit may be demonstrable nine years after the injection of the toxoid, it is advisable to repeat the treatment every time a new injury is acquired. One injection of toxoid seems to push the titer over the minimal requirements. Ramon recommends highly the systematic active immunization of children against tetanus by using the combined diphtheria-tetanus toxoid mixture. Three injections at three-week intervals in dosages of 2 c.c. are used in France. The usual contraindications, malnutrition, and skin diseases equally apply to this procedure. As a rule, the local and general reactions are observed in about 20 per cent of the vaccinated regardless of the dose. Tetanus-toxoid alum precipitated has been used by McBryde and by Goldman in this country. Two injections of 1 c.c. each at an interval of two months, followed by a third injection at the time of injury, permit the practitioner to immunize the allergic child effectively and securely against tetanus.

Whether or not antitoxin is of any value in man when given subsequently to the development of tetanus is a question that has received no definite answer. The evidence merely goes to show that in therapeutic treatment of tetanus, large and repeated doses of serum reduce the mortality. In practice, it seems advisable to administer the serum by the intravenous and intramuscular routes. Patterson, who treated twenty-six consecutive children suffering from tetanus, with only seven deaths (26 per cent mortality), used the intravenous and intramuscular routes and enormous doses of serum (120,000 to 1,970,000 units). His critics claim that he could have reduced the mortality even further had he adopted the intrathecal administration of one dose of serum (20 to 30 c.c.) by the cisterna magna route as practiced by Yodh in India. The lumbar puncture route is quite generally considered less effective and even harmful.

(6) *Typhoid Fever.*—Typhoid immunization is only recommended for universal application among those who are brought in active contact with the infection, or those who live or travel in regions where the incidence of typhoid fever is great. The heat-killed suspension of typhoid bacilli as vaccine is prepared from carefully chosen strains of potent antigenic make-up. The injection of 0.5, 1.0, and 1.0 c.c. (children 0.25, 0.5, and 0.5) may be given five to fourteen days apart, but equally satisfactory results with less severe reactions are noted when the injections are merely forty-eight hours apart. Vaccination against typhoid fever reduces the case mortality rate and the incidence: for example, in Franklin County, Tennessee, it was 7 per cent in the immunized and 14 per cent in the nonprotected groups. The duration of the immunity is sometimes quite short and it is, therefore, recommended in order to secure continuous protection. One dose should be given each year following the original course of three.

Nonspecific shock therapy with lysed vaccines prepared according to the method of Caronia and even bacteriophage therapy by the intravenous route deserve recognition.

(7) *Tuberculosis.*—It is not within the scope of this general introduction to consider the theoretic views on the immunity in tuberculosis, which have encouraged the search for a practical method of specific acquired immunity. As a whole, the attempts to immunize with dead vaccines or their analogues have been disappointing. Believing that the infection immunity in tuberculosis depends on the persistence of living bacilli, Calmette developed his B.C.G. Although tested on a very large scale, it is very difficult indeed to assess its value. With regard to its use as an immunizing agent for children, at least three questions usually have been answered:

(1) Is the B.C.G. harmless? Aside from the Lübeck catastrophe in which seventy-three out of 251 vaccinated infants died of tuberculosis, and which was almost certainly caused by contamination of the vaccine with a human strain of tubercle bacilli, in no instance could bacteriologic evidence be obtained by competent workers of an increase in virulence or change in type.

(2) Is B.C.G. effective in preventing tuberculosis among vaccinated children? The most reliable and most critically analyzed data show that the death rate is, as a rule, lowered among those children who received the vaccine.

(3) Should the B.C.G. vaccination be used as a public health measure? It is generally admitted that the chances against dying from tuberculosis during the first year of life are about 1,000 to 1. In face of such a low risk, general vaccination by an agent which confers only a moderate protection is out of the question. Finally, both the Scandinavian and American experiences suggest a more effective vaccination by parenteral instead of oral administration of B.C.G. The former has decided disadvantages in causing abscess formation which may ulcerate. Under American conditions, B.C.G. vaccination is not recommended.

(8) *Brucella Infections.*—Clinical infections with Brucella types are relatively rare in childhood, and prophylactic vaccinations are not indicated. Experiments on domesticated animals to immunize with killed vaccines have been disappointing. This is by no means surprising since the Brucella organisms are intracellular parasites, and it is not unlikely that the artificial cultivation may create antigens, which are fundamentally different from those developed during the parasitic existence (T. Smith). Only a true infection may, therefore, produce an immunity. On the other

hand, the possibility must be faced that the susceptible mesenchyme cells and their descendants become immunized during the infection. Consequently, contrary claims, notwithstanding active immunization, require the use of living organisms with the danger in causing latent infections. Therapeutically lysed vaccine administered intravenously may induce shock reactions which, at certain stages of the disease, may hasten recovery. Experience has shown that this form of treatment is valueless during the leucopenic stage, and preparation of the patient by injection of liver preparations is indicated.

(9) *Rickettsia Infection.*—In the western states, the problem of protecting children sent to Rocky Mountain fever areas on vacation has to be faced by the physicians. As a careful critic of the prophylactic vaccination, R. R. Parker has after ten years of experience concluded that the vaccine prepared from comminuted ticks preserved with 2 per cent phenol or a mixture of phenol-formalin is of definite value. Children less than 10 years of age are injected twice with 1 c.c. of the vaccine at weekly intervals. They are better protected than adults, and among them full protection against virus strains of high case fatality seems to be more frequent. It appears that persons who have received vaccines during two or more successive years possess greater resistance than those who have received vaccines only one year. In allergic children the local and general reactions may be quite marked, and intracutaneous test injections are indicated.

(10) *Plague.*—With the recognition of sylvatic plague in many recreational areas and the observations of bubonic plague in children who have handled sick rodents, discussion relative to the needs and merits of prophylactic vaccination has been repeatedly stimulated. The risk of becoming a victim of plague is so small that those familiar with the problem have advised against the use of vaccines even in the most exposed groups. The protective value of heat-killed and avirulent but living vaccines is difficult to assess. The most convincing data collected in the Dutch Indies by Otten strongly favor the use of living avirulent culture vaccines.

Sera have been used in the treatment of plague, and although the evidence that this form of treatment is beneficial is largely circumstantial, it is believed that the patient should have the benefit of this type of therapy. Dried antiplague serum prepared by the Pasteur Institute is available in San Francisco (Hooper Foundation), and will be furnished upon request. The serum should be given in large doses and early in the course of the disease. Surgical interference of the buboes should be carefully avoided.

DISCUSSION

DR. E. B. SHAW (SAN FRANCISCO).—Dr. Meyer always proves to be such a gold mine of information. My principal function on this Round Table has been to bring Dr. Meyer to Del Monte to serve as chairman of this group. I noted that whooping cough was omitted and various phases of the tuberculosis problem were not covered in his paper. There must be many questions in your minds, and the meeting is now open to general discussion.

DR. H. H. PERLMAN (PHILADELPHIA).—Did Dr. Meyer mean that it is impractical to vaccinate newborn infants against smallpox? I understand that the tendency in some clinics at the present time is to vaccinate much earlier than between the sixth and twelfth months of age.

CHAIRMAN MEYER.—It is all right to vaccinate during the first few months of life if one remembers that the degree of immunity conferred is decidedly relative. In some instances the immunity may be very slight so that if a definite exposure occurs later on, even during the last half of the first year, the child must be revaccinated. The reason for stating that the optimum time for vaccination is between the sixth and twelfth months of age is that the child is less likely to be immunologically immature at that time.

DR. A. F. ABT (CHICAGO).—Is it not true that infants in neonatal life react differently in production of humoral immunity than in later life?

CHAIRMAN MEYER.—Yes, and it is the result of many factors, such as heredity, environment, etc.

DR. R. J. DOSTAL (SANTA MONICA).—Since intradermal immunization has been successful in typhoid fever, is it satisfactory in immunizing against scarlet fever?

CHAIRMAN MEYER.—Yes, if the material used is not a formalin preparation, since the latter causes necrosis in many children. When given intradermally the vaccine is administered in ½ c.c. doses in several spots at forty-eight-hour intervals.

DR. ABT.—Do you think that streptococcic toxoid has value?

CHAIRMAN MEYER.—Yes, I do, and it may be of particular value in mass scale.

DR. ABT.—Do you think that each separate type of scarlet fever streptococcus will produce individually different toxoid?

CHAIRMAN MEYER.—No, I do not.

DR. J. W. AMESSE (DENVER).—Is the oral administration of typhoid vaccine to be recommended?

CHAIRMAN MEYER.—Yes, with reservations, if one remembers to prepare the patient before giving the vaccine. Bile should be administered first to increase absorbability. That is rarely done. However, when Dr. Shiga was visiting in San Francisco last year I asked him how he immunizes himself against dysentery, and his answer was most emphatically, "By subcutaneous injections." When large series of individuals have been given the vaccine orally some failures have occurred with later exposures. My friendly advice is "no oral administration of vaccine!"

DR. M. L. BLATT (CHICAGO).—In our prenatal clinic we are determining which mothers and which members of the immediate families are tuberculous so that within the first five days following birth alternate cases are inoculated with B.C.G. The mothers do not know of the two groups and consequently do not know that their babies have not been inoculated if they are in the control group. We are averaging 300 to 500 cases per year. All of the patients are seen monthly for a follow-up study and tuberculin tests and x-ray studies are made from time to time. Having done all this and continued the follow-up for a number of years will you be willing to accept these data when reported?

CHAIRMAN MEYER.—The most critical certainly will say "No!" Even with the best follow-up system there are many obstacles which are difficult to overcome. How long and what kind of exposure will take place? And keep in mind the uncontrollable fluctuations and changes in the social status of these patients. Then there is the danger of the control observations. Who is doing the controlling, the public health nurses, physicians, or who? Remember that the B.C.G. preparation is the easiest part. But the control of the environment is very difficult.

The question of dosage is important. How do we visualize these "massive infections" of which we speak so glibly? Most of the so-called massive infections really represent a cumulative effect of repeated minimal infections. My opinion is that massive infections rarely occur.

Specific acquired immunity to tuberculosis probably does not exist. Sensitization does not mean we are immune. If specific acquired immunity is an important factor our mortality figures would be different. The mortality from tuberculosis in newborn groups is frightfully high because the exposure occurs in the most susceptible age group. If one cuts off the source of infection immediately following the birth of these babies, even in those families with a bad history of phthisis, the children will be free of infection. A tuberculous family does not necessarily have a high incidence of susceptible offspring. Here on the Pacific Coast, however, we have found that approximately 31 per cent of all freshmen students entering the university have a positive tuberculin reaction. After residence at the university there is a 10 per cent increase each year. How far are we going to go? Remember that man has an inherited disposition to the tubercle bacillus and when exposed 100 per cent, infectious, but not tuberculous, disease will follow. The ability to react to the tuberculous infection is not synonymous with the disposition and is individually quite variable.

DR. BLATT.—This year has seen in Chicago the largest recorded epidemic of measles in recent years. Through the Cook County blood bank we have had available a large amount of bacteriologically tested blood. In the wards we administered pooled adult whole blood to every patient, 10 c.c. to infants, and 20 to 30 c.c. to children more than 1 year of age. Each patient was reinoculated on the eighth day following. Even though a new case of measles occurred about once every week among the new admissions, in spite of rigid precautions to exclude patients in the pre-eruptive stage, there have been not more than one or two cross-infections. How would you evaluate these observations?

CHAIRMAN MEYER.—I would accept that fully! Your observations provide one more solid pillar on which we are building up the house of measles prophylaxis. Remember though that other antibodies may have been transferred inasmuch as adult whole blood was used.

DR. SHAW.—What is your attitude toward immunization against whooping cough?

CHAIRMAN MEYER.—Because another round table discussion will be devoted entirely to pertussis immunization I purposely did not mention this subject in my paper. But it brings up many questions. Do we know anything but that recovery from pertussis leaves immunity? The mechanism of the immunity we do not know; the *B. pertussis* has a specific organotropism. Is the subcutaneous administration of an antigen imitating the disease process and does it immunize the host cells which are usually disordered by the bacillus? With large doses of carefully killed organisms injected subcutaneously we probably can bring about some degree of immunity of variable and limited duration.

The theory is that during the invasive stage the organism is virulent, but later it changes into a variant which produces the mucoid material causing the whoop. There have been many attempts to devise proper antigens. Sauer has given additional support to various previously reported observations of other workers regarding the effect of injections of Phase I bacilli. His work has demonstrated that large doses of killed organisms are necessary. The idea of toxoid is now being promoted. As yet not enough experience is available and will not be until another five years or so have gone by. It is difficult to evaluate what is really a pertussis infection. And remember that the contagion index of pertussis is between 70 and 80 per cent. The published data are full of errors and discrepancies, but Sauer's vaccine deserves consideration since it has given a striking degree of protection for a limited period of time in a number of serial observations.

DR. SHAW.—Does not the fact that rabies can be prevented by killed rather than by living virus, reopen the entire subject of virus immunity in other diseases such as in poliomyelitis?

CHAIRMAN MEYER.—Killed rabies virus has reduced the postvaccinal complications of paralyses. However, probably phenol reduced the amount of fixed living virus; most of the phenol-treated viruses on the market for the prevention of rabies are valueless in producing immunity. The ether-treated rabies vaccine probably is of the greatest value. Only about 35 per cent of individuals and animals bitten by a rabid animal will develop the disease if unprotected. I am sanguine about the development of an immunizing agent against poliomyelitis.

DR. J. R. LEMMON (AMARILLO, TEX.).—Should antitoxin in epidemic meningitis be given intravenously only?

CHAIRMAN MEYER.—The pathogenesis and variability of the disease is not completely understood. For this reason, some intraspinal serum of high bacteriotropic potency is probably indicated.

DR. DOSTAL.—Has enough work been done to make advisable the use of combined diphtheria and tetanus toxoid?

CHAIRMAN MEYER.—Yes. It should be given in at least two doses with a rather long time interval between injections. If injuries should occur later which ordinarily would make the use of tetanus antitoxin advisable, an injection of tetanus toxoid alone should be given. This avoids the use of horse serum and the dangers of serum reactions and gives more protection.

DR. V. E. STORK (LOS ANGELES).—Is the tetanus toxoid as effective when given with diphtheria toxoid as when given alone?

CHAIRMAN MEYER.—Apparently it is, because of the synergistic effect, the one antigen stimulating the effect of the other. But not all of the tetanus toxoid available commercially at the present time is satisfactory.

DR. W. A. MCGEE (RICHMOND, VA.).—Is it advisable to combine simultaneously two or more different immunizing procedures?

CHAIRMAN MEYER.—One toxoid preparation enhances another toxoid. There are, however, contraindications to combining simultaneously toxoid preparations with other immunizing agents, such as pertussis vaccine, but not with virus procedures, such as smallpox vaccinia vaccination.

DR. A. E. VARDEN (SAN BERNARDINO, CALIF.).—Please discuss some of the differences between alum precipitated toxoid and regular toxoid.

CHAIRMAN MEYER.—The addition of alum to toxoid reduces the absorbability so that the effect is prolonged. Also the alum apparently has the synergistic effect of which I spoke. When the alum preparations were first introduced I defended the use of plain toxoid because I preferred three doses of plain toxoid to one dose of alum precipitated toxoid. Recently, however, fine alum toxoid has been made available with 30 immunizing units per cubic centimeter. But one dose never will produce durable immunity. The first injection produces only basic immunity and further injections are necessary for a high protection. The Danes now are using one dose of alum toxoid and six months later are administering plain undiluted toxoid intranasally. After the child attains school age the intranasal toxoid may be repeated the first of every school year.

DR. FAIRFAX HALL (NEW ROCHELLE, N. Y.).—Is it true that diphtheria incidence has dropped in countries where active immunization is not done routinely as in this country?

CHAIRMAN MEYER.—Yes. That is why we should be exceedingly careful in jumping at conclusions. All we can say is that the mortality has been reduced. We may wake up some fine morning and find that a great many of these children whom we supposedly immunized against diphtheria are actually susceptible to the disease. Biologically we can only expect about 96 per cent protection. And remember that the presence of decent environmental factors is the essential thing in reducing incidence of contagious disease.

Secretaries.

EDWIN J. BARNETT, M.D., *Spokane, Wash.*
NORMAN NIXON, M.D., *Beverly Hills, Calif.*

EIGHTH ANNUAL MEETING OF REGION III OF THE AMERICAN ACADEMY OF PEDIATRICS

The eighth annual meeting of Region III of the American Academy of Pediatrics was held Oct. 27-29, 1938, in Detroit, Mich. The meeting was attended by 180 members, 175 guests, 69 wives accompanying their husbands, and 39 exhibitors—a total registration of 463.

The regional state chairmen met at luncheon on October 28. Dr. A. Graeme Mitchell is chairman of Region III; Dr. Edgar E. Martmer, associate chairman, was chairman of the committee on arrangements.

Six radio interviews broadcast from Detroit stations constituted an important innovation on the program:

The Functions of the American Academy of Pediatrics	Henry F. Helmholz
The Endocrines	A. Graeme Mitchell
The Relation of Mental Hygiene to Pediatrics	Bert I. Beverly
Preventive Pediatrics	Clifford Grulee
Immunization Procedures	John Toomey
Rheumatic Heart Disease	Hugh McCulloch

The following papers were presented:

SESSION I. THE NEONATAL PERIOD

The Significance of Intrauterine Respiration

James L. Wilson, M.D.*

A discussion is given of the status of investigations concerning intrauterine respiration. The expression "intrauterine movements of respiratory muscles" is suggested in preference to "intrauterine respiration" since as yet it is doubtful whether these movements produce a significant pulmonary tidal flow of amniotic fluid.

Cerebral Injury in the Newborn Due to Anoxia at Birth

Frederic Schreiber, M.D., Professor of Clinical Neurological Surgery, Wayne University, Detroit

Asphyxia in the newborn with depression or fatigue of the respiratory center is an important etiological factor in many cases of convulsions, spasticity, and mental retardation in children. These fixed brain lesions, which frequently first manifest themselves a few months after delivery, are secondary to anoxic degenerative cerebral changes.

---

*All authors are from Detroit except when stated otherwise.

Relation of Maternal Sedation and Anesthesia to Neonatal Asphyxia (Analysis of 5,000 Deliveries)

Warren C. C. Cole, M.D., F.A.A.P., and David C. Kimball, M.D.

Five thousand deliveries at the Woman's Hospital have been analyzed with a view of determining the relationship between sedatives and anesthetics given to the mother and asphyxia in the newborn baby. Scopolomine in any dosage does not seem to increase asphyxia. The barbiturates and similar drugs, while frequently retarding respiration, seldom cause severe asphyxia. Morphine, while seldom given within four hours of delivery, is a definite depressant. Ether or gas anesthesia as used at the Woman's Hospital is not a factor in the production of neonatal asphyxia. By far the majority of severe asphyxias are due to obstetric complications of one type or another. There is evidence that the judicious use of sedatives and anesthetics tends to reduce "birth shock" and the incidence of cerebral injury.

Certain Etiological Factors and the Pathological Lesions in Anoxia

Frank Hartman, M.D., Pathologist, Henry Ford Hospital, Detroit

Anoxia may be due to the operation of one or more of the following physiologic types: the anoxic, anemic, stagnant and histotoxic. In barbiturate poisoning we have early, nearly pure histotoxic anoxia, but later the stagnant type comes into play through the low blood pressure. In acute alcoholism there is again histotoxic anoxia plus the stagnant type, and in one case described, anoxic anoxia resulting from morphine administration and respiratory failure. In the newborn infant histotoxic anoxia results from drugging of the mother, and anoxic anoxia if the delivery is effected under nitrous oxide anesthesia. In concussion, there is stagnant anoxia due to edema and vasodilation with possible histotoxic anoxia as a direct effect of the blow. Shock with falling blood pressure may also be a factor. In fever therapy cerebral anoxia is due to a combination of histotoxic anoxia resulting from heavy sedation in the face of the high temperatures which increase the oxygen demands of cellular metabolism. Stagnant anoxia may also play a role if vascular collapse occurs.

Cerebral Hemorrhage in the Newborn (A Group Treated by Drainage)

John C. Montgomery, M.D., F.A.A.P., and Philip J. Howard, M.D., F.A.A.P.

This is an analysis of 129 cases of intracranial hemorrhage of the newborn, the final outcome of which was known. Eighty-six of these cases were treated by spinal drainage, and 43 were not. Of the 86 children treated, the outcome proved to be 31 normal children, 4 normal mentally but with greater or less neuropathologic findings, 9 idiots, and 42 deaths. A plea is made that tentatively intracranial hemorrhage of the newborn should be treated in the light of a head injury occurring at this age period, and the belief is expressed that it is justifiable to retain a hope that some benefits can be derived from treatment and that only by making such attempts can a final solution of this difficult question be acquired.

Erythroblastosis of the Newborn

Thomas B. Cooley, M.D., F.A.A.P.

There are discussed the distinction of this condition from malignant jaundice due to sepsis, the frequency and importance of the condition, the desirability of its recognition by obstetricians, the relation to anemia of newborn, and possible theories of etiology and pathogenesis.

SESSION II. NUTRITION AND METABOLISM

Relation of Growth and Skeletal Maturity to the Mineral Balances of Children

Icie G. Macy, Ph.D.

A longitudinal study extending over six continuous months showed that ten children, carefully selected as representative of average healthy American children, varied greatly in their calcium storage and accumulation in spite of a three-month prefeeding period and an adequate and fairly constant calcium intake. The range of the individual variations narrowed each successive month. The variations in calcium retention are related to previous state of nutrition, and bone development and growth.

Biological Time Patterns in Gastrointestinal Motility of Children

Lawrence Reynolds, M.D., Associate Professor of Clinical Roentgenology, Wayne University, Detroit

The individual variation in the gastrointestinal motility of children and the variation in motility produced by different types of meals is indicated by thirty-two series of roentgenograms consisting of 280 films of eight children living under standardized conditions of diet and environment. Meals of barium-and-water, -milk, -glucose, -cream, and -meat, were given upon different days and followed by means of roentgenograms taken at short intervals for several hours after ingestion. Films were also exposed at twenty-four and forty-eight-hour intervals after administration of the meals.

The biologic time patterns shown by the different series of roentgenograms are compared: for the stomach alone, for the entire gastrointestinal tract at the end of twenty-four hours, and for the entire tract after forty-eight hours.

Metabolism of Citric Acid in Infancy

A. H. Smith, Ph.D., Professor of Physiological Chemistry, Wayne University, Detroit

Thirteen infants (3 to 14 months of age) metabolized the citric acid occurring naturally in the diet to the extent of 79.5 to 96 per cent. In general, more citric acid was excreted in the urine than in the feces, the renal elimination amounting to 3.9 to 13.3 per cent of the intake.

Serum Phosphatase in Relation to Vitamin D

Donald J. Barnes, M.D., F.A.A.P.

Measurements were made of vitamin D effects upon the serum phosphatase in infants, using different vitamin D sources. The studies include attempts to establish normals for serum phosphatase during the first year of life, effects upon the serum phosphatase of different dosage levels of vitamin D in patients who show rachitic tendencies, and correlations of these with calcium and phosphorus storage.

Vitamin C Requirements of Artificially Fed Infants

Brenton M. Hamil, M.D.

Four hundred and twenty-seven (427) infants were observed for data relative to the "plane of health" through the first year of life. On a controlled dietary containing 10 mg. of ascorbic acid (200 international units) daily, evidence of mild (preclinical) scurvy according to the criteria of Park and co-workers was observed to develop in 20 cases (4.68 per cent). An analysis of these data for this factor is presented. The individual requirement is variable and is influenced by prenatal as well as postnatal factors. Scurvy is apparently a definite pathologic entity but does not become evident or retard development until the absence of the specific physiologic functions of the vitamin is manifest.

Relation of Craniotabes to Diet and Growth

Marsh Poole, M.D., F.A.A.P.

In four hundred and twenty-seven infants who were cared for in the clinic of the Children's Fund of Michigan and the Children's Hospital throughout the years 1933 to 1936, craniotabes was found in a considerable percentage. A control group of 1933-1934 received no vitamin D except that naturally contained in the diet. In this mixed group of colored and white infants 46 per cent had moderate or severe rickets, and 60 per cent showed softening of the cranial bones at some time during the year. A superior group cared for in 1935-1936 who had vegetable soup in their diet from the first clinic visit and received cod liver oil throughout, developed the same percentage of craniotabes, but there was only 5 per cent of slight rickets as shown by roentgenograms. Analysis of the records of other groups showed practically the same percentage of softening in the skulls of colored and white infants. The highest percentage of craniotabes was found among premature infants and twins. Of twenty-one babies diagnosed as having mild scurvy by x-ray, nineteen showed softening of some degree.

The majority of babies with moderate or severe craniotabes had severe or repeated respiratory infections, eczema, vomiting, parenteral diarrhea, loss of appetite, or some other disturbance which may have accounted for the inability to deposit sufficient calcium in the rapidly growing cranial bones.

Metabolic Observations on a Child With Essential Hyperlipemia

Samuel Bernstein, M.D.

A short metabolic study was made of a six-year-old boy with a marked, chronic idiopathic lipemia. The following data were determined while the boy was on a low and then on a high fat diet: nitrogen balance and distribution in the urine, lipin distribution in the blood and stool, and mineral balance. In addition, his respiratory quotient and specific dynamic response to fat and carbohydrate were studied.

Session III. Endocrine

Metabolic Effects of Growth and Thyrotropic Hormones Administered With and Without Iodine

O. H. Gaebler, M.D., and Paul Bartlett

In experiments on dogs, daily records were kept of the weight, water intake, urine volume, the excretion of total nitrogen, creatinine, and creatine, and the basal metabolism. Addition of 1 c.c. of Lugol's solution to the daily ration did not significantly alter the nitrogen storage or calorigenic effect resulting from single injections of the growth preparation. Marked storage of creatine accompanied the storage of nitrogen. Single injections of thyrotropic hormone produced just detectable calorigenic effects, but produced a marked creatinuria which was not prevented by administration of iodine, and differed in this respect from the creatinuria of human hyperthyroidism. The animals become refractive to the action of the thyrotropic hormone on creatinuria after as few as three small injections at ten-day intervals.

Relation of Diet to the Experimental Production of Goiter

G. R. Sharpless, Ph.D.

In five to seven weeks the thyroid gland is enlarged to four times normal in rats fed a diet of raw soy bean flour, yeast, butterfat, sugar, and salts. Iodine will prevent the enlargement, but the minimum requirement is greater than that for rats fed on other diets. Treating the flour by prolonged heating or extracting with solvents reduces its goiterogenic activity even though the iodine content of the diet may be reduced.

Effect of Thyroid on Nitrogen and Calcium in the Growth Period

John W. Maroney, M.D., F.A.A.P., and J. A. Johnston, M.D., F.A.A.P.

Continuous calcium and nitrogen balances with concurrent basal metabolic determinations were made on a cretin to whom thyroid was administered and an adolescent with hyperthyroidism whose gland was removed. Retention of both calcium and nitrogen was increased with the administration of thyroid. The child with hyperthyroidism showed a negative calcium balance which became positive with thyroidectomy. However, when the basal metabolic rate fell to –20 per cent following the removal of both lobes, a slightly positive calcium balance became definitely more positive with the administration of thyroid. The improvement was referable to a diminished stool loss. The negative balance in the hyperthyroid state was associated with a high urinary output. A similar anabolic effect was noted in the case of nitrogen.

A Continuous Calcium and Nitrogen Balance in a Case of Legg-Perthes' Disease Treated With Growth Hormone and Thyroid

C. L. Mitchell, M.D., and J. A. Johnston, M.D., F.A.A.P.

A continuous calcium and nitrogen balance for sixty-six days with concurrent basal metabolism determinations was obtained on a boy with Legg-Perthes' disease. The calcium balance was negative on an average intake, was not appreciably changed by growth hormone, but was made definitely positive by thyroid. The basal metabolism was low. The intercurrence of an acute throat infection rendered the balance again negative, but, following its subsidence, it became positive again with thyroid. Clinically the patient improved rapidly.

Continuous Nitrogen and Calcium Balances Throughout the Periods Just Preceding and Following the Menarche

J. A. Johnston, M.D., F.A.A.P.

Continuous nitrogen and calcium determinations before and after the menarche show a fall in the retention of these substances following the menarche. The basal metabolism throughout this period was irregular, but was relatively elevated before and depressed following the first menstrual period; the retentions of calcium and nitrogen were, accordingly, higher with the more elevated rates and lower with the depressed rates.

Session IV. Clinical Topics

Comparison of Specific and Nonspecific Serum Treatment in Scarlet Fever

Donald C. Young, M.D., Medical Director, Communicable Disease Division, Herman Kiefer Hospital, Detroit

The results of the treatment of alternate cases of moderately severe scarlet fever with scarlet fever antitoxin, scarlet fever convalescent serum, and a nonspecific horse serum are given. The trial period covered one epidemic year. Comparability of the several groups was determined by statistical methods and satisfied the requirements of random selection. No significant difference could be demonstrated in the results obtained with convalescent serum and with specific scarlet fever antitoxin, but little or no value could be demonstrated to result from nonspecific serum.

The Common Ground of Pediatrics and Orthodontics

Samuel J. Lewis, D.D.S.

Like the pediatrician, the orthodontist is dealing with an unfinished product—the child. The dentition of the child is an organ in transition and must be appraised only in accordance with the stage of development attained at the time it is observed. Orthodontic treatment, then, should be instituted when it will do the most good and be of undoubted benefit to the child.

Sulfanilamide in the Treatment of Gonorrheal Ophthalmia

Merrill Michels, M.D.

We have observed a reduction of hospitalization from 28.5 days for a control series of thirty-two patients with gonorrheal ophthalmia to 5.8 days for a series of fifteen patients similarly treated but with the addition of sulfanilamide. Sulfanilamide is warranted in the treatment of gonorrheal ophthalmia because: (1) it reduces the length of hospitalization, (2) its ease of administration, (3) the lack of complications, (4) the rapid improvement noted, and (5) general increase in comfort of patient.

The Use of Small Intestinal Decompression in the Treatment of Intestinal Obstruction

Charles G. Johnston, M.D., Professor of Surgery, Wayne University, Detroit

Intubation of the small intestine with suction drainage has been used in a sufficient number of cases of ileus of the dynamic and adynamic types to determine its advantages and disadvantages. A brief description of the method and a discussion of the results of its use are presented.

The Endogenous Reinfection Type of Tuberculosis in Childhood With Particular Reference to the Girl at Puberty

Bruce Douglas, M.D., Controller of Tuberculosis, Department of Health, Detroit, and J. A. Johnston, M.D., F.A.A.P.

A study of over 900 children over a period of ten years, many of whom were originally familial contacts to tuberculosis, indicated a larger number of re-infection type cases of tuberculosis developing than would be expected ordinarily in spite of the fact that these children were removed to foster homes free from tuberculosis. Girls developed active tuberculosis at puberty under these circumstances much more frequently than boys, suggesting that certain physiologic changes allow the already present infection to become active.

Phlyctenular Conjunctivitis: Course and Treatment

Philip J. Howard, M.D., F.A.A.P.

A series of 18 children with phlyctenular conjunctivitis was followed. The most satisfactory treatment consisted of desensitization with tuberculin after first carefully determining the threshold of reactivity by doing skin tests with serial dilutions. The most minute amount of intradermally administered old tuberculin to which the child would react was taken as the threshold, and desensitization was carried out by subcutaneous injections at five-day intervals, starting with an amount smaller than the lowest skin sensitivity dose. As desensitization progressed, the eye lesion healed.

Undulant Fever: Diagnostic and Therapeutic Measures

John Sander, M.D., F.A.A.P., Lansing, Mich.

A résumé of the signs and symptoms of juvenile brucellosis, with a critical analysis of the diagnostic and therapeutic measures currently available.

Sulfanilamide Therapy in Erysipelas

Harry T. Mernagh, M.D.

Approximately one hundred cases of erysipelas of the face, body, and extremities were treated with sulfanilamide. These are grossly compared with the results of treatment covering an experience of five years just prior to the introduction of sulfanilamide. The value of this drug in the treatment of erysipelas following such a comparison appears to be demonstrated.

Jaundice: An Epidemiological and Bacteriological Study of a Small Outbreak in Detroit

Joseph G. Molner, M.D., Director, School Health Service, Department of Health, Detroit

The study reported of 185 cases of jaundice is presented with a discussion of clinical and bacteriologic findings and an hypothesis of the transmission of the condition.

Diaphragmatic Hernia in Children

John B. Hartzell, M.D.

An analysis was made of 68 cases of diaphragmatic hernia in children under 10 years of age, treated by operation. Criteria for diagnosis, methods of treatment, and mortality statistics are presented.

SESSION V. PAPERS FROM THE DEPARTMENT OF PEDIATRICS, UNIVERSITY OF MICHIGAN

Acidosis Associated With Sulfanilamide Administration

Harry A. Towsley, M.D., and John J. Engelfried, M.D., Ann Arbor, Mich.

A study was made of the relationship of the carbon-dioxide combining power of the plasma and the blood concentration of sulfanilamide. Results showed a definite and sometimes very marked decrease in the CO_2 combining power of the plasma during the administration of the drug. For the most part a compensated acidosis was produced, and in a few an uncompensated acidosis, which is relieved by the administration of alkali.

The First Heart Beats and the Beginning of the Circulation of Blood as Shown by Micromoving Pictures of Living Embryos

Bradley M. Patten, M.D., Professor of Anatomy, University of Michigan, Ann Arbor, Mich.

The adaptation of tissue culture methods to handling entire embryos of laboratory animals in specially constructed glass chambers is beginning to be developed to a point which makes possible continued observations of developmental phenomena in living material. This paper deals with the application of such methods to the study of the initiation of cardiac contraction and the first movement of blood corpuscles in chick embryos. Microcinematography has been used as a method of recording and demonstrating these events and some of the significant changes that occur in the action of the embryonic heart during its conversion from a primitive tubular structure into the chambered organ characteristic of older embryos and adults.

Our Clinical Experience With the Treatment of Thirty Cases of Hirschsprung's Disease (Megacolon)

John L. Law, M.D., Ann Arbor, Mich.

A discussion is given of thirty cases of megacolon with reference to etiology, pathology and treatment. Highly encouraging results have followed the use of mecholin in the last several years which are comparable with those of sympathectomy.

The Role of the Pediatrician in Mental Hygiene

Paul H. Jordan, M.D., Ann Arbor, Mich.

It is now an accepted fact that most personality and behavior disorders of adults have their beginnings in unwholesome reactions to childhood experiences; therefore, the pediatrician, because of his particular field in medicine, is in a strategic position from the standpoint of mental hygiene. Emotional problems in children may arise associated with, or entirely separate from, actual physical disease and should be recognized and the proper treatment instituted at the earliest possible moment. While the pediatrician can and should handle many of the less complex disorders of children himself, in more serious cases, because of their complexity, he should seek the services of certain technical specialists, the child psychiatrist, the clinical psychologist, and the psychiatric social worker, just as he now makes use of the contributions of the roentgenologist, the otolaryngologist, and other medical specialists in the case of obscure physical disease.

A Mechanical Presentation of the Effects and Interrelationships of the Human Female Hormones of Reproduction During the Menstrual Cycle and Pregnancy

Wayne L. Whitaker, M.D., Ann Arbor, Mich.

An apparatus has been constructed in an attempt to illustrate graphically the cyclically changing amounts of various hormones of reproduction present in the body during the several stages of the menstrual cycle and pregnancy. The hormones considered are the follicle-stimulating, luteinizing, and lactogenic factors of the anterior pituitary, folliculin, and progestin from the ovary, and the pregnancy estrogen and anterior pituitary-like substances probably produced by the placenta. Cause and effect relationships between the hormones as well as endocrine influence on the reproductive organs are suggested.

Academy News

Region I of the Academy held its annual meeting on Friday, November 11, and Saturday, November 12, at Rochester, N. Y.

Region II held its annual meeting on Wednesday, November 16, at Oklahoma City, Okla. This meeting was held at the time of the Southern Medical Association.

Region IV will hold its next annual meeting on April 27, 28, 29, 1939, at Oakland, Calif. Dr. Clifford Sweet, state chairman for northern California, will be in charge of the scientific program.

At the meeting of Region III of the Academy in Detroit, the following resolution was adopted:

''Within the past month Dr. Russell Sturgis Rowland, of Detroit, has passed away. Dr. Rowland was an early member of the American Academy of Pediatrics and vitally interested in its inception and development. He was not only a notable exponent of the best in pediatrics as a practitioner but contributed importantly as well by his investigations to its scientific progress. In view of the sad loss occasioned by Dr. Rowland's death,

''BE IT RESOLVED that this body expresses its grief in his demise and extends to Mrs. Rowland and family its profound regret and sympathy.''

News and Notes

The **American Board of Pediatrics** will hold examinations during 1939 as follows:

April 26, 1939, in New York, N. Y. Appointments for this examination must be made before Dec. 26, 1938.

May 16, 1939, in St. Louis, Mo., during the meeting of the American Medical Association. Appointments for this examination must be made before Jan. 16, 1939.

November 14 and 15, 1939, in Cincinnati, Ohio, preceding the annual meeting of the American Academy of Pediatrics. Appointments for this examination must be made before July 14, 1939.

The **Pediatric Section** of the American Medical Association has had Hotel Chase assigned as headquarters for the St. Louis meeting May 15-19, 1939. It is suggested that those expecting to attend the meeting make reservations early. Rates: Single from $3.00; double from $4.00; and twin bed double from $5.00. For advance reservations address John Reinhardt, A. M. A. Housing Bureau, 910 Syndicate Trust Building, St. Louis, Mo., since all reservations must clear through this agency.

Announcement is made by Dr. A. Graeme Mitchell, director of The **Children's Hospital Research Foundation**, Cincinnati, and Dr. Glenn E. Cullen, director of laboratories, that upon authorization of the board of trustees a scientific advisory council has been appointed. This consists of:

Dr. O. T. Avery, member of the Hospital of the Rockefeller Institute for Medical Research.

Dr. Ernest Goodpasture, professor of pathology, Vanderbilt University School of Medicine.

Dr. A. Baird Hastings, professor of biological chemistry, Harvard University Medical School.

Dr. A. N. Richards, professor of pharmacology, University of Pennsylvania School of Medicine.

The second meeting of this council was held in Cincinnati on Sept. 28 and 29, 1938.

The Children's Hospital Research Foundation was created in 1929 through the generosity of Mr. William Cooper Procter. Its facilities include its own laboratory building and affiliations with the Children's Hospital of Cincinnati, the Pediatric Department and the Contagious Disease Pavilions of the Cincinnati General Hospital, the Children's Convalescent Home, the Babies' Milk Fund Association, and the Ohio Soldiers' and Sailors' Orphans' Home at Xenia, Ohio. The Children's Hospital and its Research Foundation are affiliated by agreement with the University of Cincinnati, the professor of pediatrics in the University of Cincinnati being the director of the medical service and the director of the Foundation. Approximately one hundred and fifty publications have appeared from the Research Foundation. Present plans contemplate additions to the staff and certain new lines of investigation.

Dr. Haskell Talamo, Worcester, Mass., died July 10, 1938, of subacute bacterial endocarditis. Dr. Talamo was an instructor in the Department of Pediatrics of Tufts Medical College.

Dr. Rolf R. Struthers has been appointed professor of pediatrics at McGill University and physician-in-chief at the Children's Memorial Hospital in Montreal to succeed Dr. H. B. Cushing, who becomes emeritus professor of pediatrics and honorary physician-in-chief, respectively.

Dr. C. A. Earle, of Des Plaines, Ill., died October 29.

The following have been certified by the **American Board of Pediatrics** since the last report.

Dr. I. Pat Bronstein, Chicago, Ill.
Dr. Daniel Budson, Detroit, Mich.
Dr. Vernon Richard DeYoung, Chicago, Ill.
Dr. George L. Drennan, Jacksonville, Ill.
Dr. Joseph A. Gilmartin, Pittsburgh, Pa.
Dr. Brenton M. Hamil, Detroit, Mich.
Dr. Samuel J. Hoffman, Chicago, Ill.
Dr. John L. Law, Ann Arbor, Mich.
Dr. Benjamin M. Levin, Chicago, Ill.
Dr. George Calvert Malley, Zanesville, Ohio
Dr. Charles Miles McKinlay, Lexington, Ky.
Dr. Frederick William Munro, Detroit, Mich.
Dr. Samuel J. Nichamin, Detroit, Mich.
Dr. Mila I. Pierce, Evanston, Ill.
Dr. Joseph Nathan Rappaport, Evanston, Ill.
Dr. Walter J. Siemsen, Chicago, Ill.
Dr. Ralph Spaeth, Chicago, Ill.
Dr. M. I. Vinnecour, Chicago, Ill.
Dr. Robert Breckinridge Warfield, Lexington, Ky.
Dr. Dwight Addison Weir, Mansfield, Ohio
Dr. Lawrence J. Wilhelmi, Joliet, Ill.
Dr. James L. Wilson, Detroit, Mich.

Book Reviews

Babies Are Human Beings. C. Anderson Aldrich and Mary M. Aldrich, New York, 1938, The Macmillan Company, pp. 128, Price $1.75.

This little volume by Dr. Aldrich and his wife may be regarded in a certain sense as marking a real epoch in pediatric literature. It is the first successful attempt to put modern scientific knowledge of the growth and development of the infant into an understandable form for parents. On this basis a method of approach is offered to an understanding of just what the young growing organism is doing and why he is doing it. It must not be confused with the scores of books on the care of the baby with which the market is flooded. While the authors have drawn freely on the recent work of students of development, they have contributed an invaluable selection of material based on Dr. Aldrich's experience and knowledge of what parents need.

An idea of the method of treatment of the subject may be gathered from the chapter headings: "Beginnings"; "The Baby's Dilemma"—the conflict between normal growth processes and the environment in which he finds himself; "The World Comes to the Baby"—perception through the development of the special senses; "The Baby Responds to the World"—motor development; "Babies Are Different"—the matter of individual variation; "The Baby's Way of Sleeping"; "Eating"; and "Eliminating"; "Among the Do's and Don't's"—all too brief; and "Implications for Older Children."

While written primarily for the parent, the book presents in an interesting non-technical way so much factual data unknown to many practitioners of medicine that it has a real value for the physician. The reviewer has encountered one teacher of pediatrics who has already put it on the reading list for his medical students. It is, moreover, a real pleasure to run across a book by a physician (not forgetting the coauthor) which is so well written from a purely literary standpoint. The authors are to be congratulated on having made a real contribution.

Interneships and Residencies. Report by The New York Committee on the Study of Hospital Interneships and Residencies. New York, 1938, The Commonwealth Fund, Price $2.50.

This report is an outstanding study of the complex problem of hospital internships and residencies. In recent years there has been an increasing realization that the hospital services are a part of and must be integrated with the medical education program. In fact, the internship is regarded by many educators as a part of the undergraduate training of the physician. The newly formed specialty boards to a large extent have passed the training of the "specialist" back to the hospital residencies. If the problem of preparing the physician for practice necessitates, as it apparently does, an internship, and a residency is the sine qua non for the specialist of the future, it is time the various types and kinds of house services, the methods of appointment, the character of the training received, and similar subjects be approached from the general viewpoint of education rather than the viewpoint of the demands and needs of the institution.

Although this report is based on a study of hospitals in New York City, we feel its findings apply with a few minor exceptions to the conditions existing in any large city. New York differs only in two particulars. One is that the five local medical colleges can and do furnish less than half of the annual appointments. The balance come from seventy-two American and Canadian schools in which the training is similar, and from thirty-one foreign institutions, many of which have uncertain standards. Thus the selection of the house staff constitutes more of a problem than in other cities. In the work of the New York intern the "ambulance service" forms a constantly increasing chore, disrupting the education of the house staff to an extent not found in many other cities. With these two exceptions the study in all probability reflects the situation as it exists in other large cities and hence has a general rather than a local importance.

The study was made by a joint committee of the five local medical schools and the New York Academy of Medicine, with Dr. Jean A. Curran as executive secretary. It is excellently written, and the material presented with care and understanding. Of the 182 hospitals in New York, 77 are approved by the Council on Medical Education of the American Medical Association. All of these were surveyed, and in addition 20 of the 105 nonapproved hospitals were studied as a sample for comparison. In the approved hospitals, which form the basis of the report, there were 1,760 approved positions. Of the 1,245 internships, 902 (72 per cent) are rotating. The services to which the intern is assigned on a rotating service show infinite variation. While the average is from five to seven services, in two hospitals the interns served on fourteen different services. Although the majority of rotating services are two years in length, the "block," or period of time, devoted to the important services was too short in the opinion of the committee in almost every instance. There were 545 residencies in the approved hospitals, of which 35 were pediatric.

Much of the report is necessarily statistical, but there is an excellent discussion of such topics as the relation of the internship to practice, libraries and their use, the preparation of the intern for his work, the training of the intern, health and housing, method of appointment, and the like.

The chief criticism made of the pediatric training is the short time allowed for this service in the rotating internship. The committee feels that three months of pediatric service should be included in the rotating internship. In the 43 hospitals with rotating internships of eighteen months or more, 35 have pediatric assignments of less than three months. "The relationship noted between the short assignments and the quality of work was more striking in pediatrics than on any other service." There are 35 pediatric residencies available in the New York hospitals. In 24 of these the training received was estimated as good, in 10, fair, and in 1, doubtful. Sixteen of the men holding these 35 appointments plan to enter the field as a specialty.

This report should be required reading for hospital administrators, chiefs of staff, and members of intern committees, for it is upon these groups that the fate of the house officer depends. The New York committee has rendered a valuable service to colleagues throughout the country.

B. S. V.

Erratum

In the article, "Serum Treatment of Pneumonia in Childhood," by Rosa Lee Nemir, M.D., New York, N. Y., which appeared in the August issue of the JOURNAL, line 8 on page 221 should read:

> "the swab. Occasionally good material may be found on the back of the"
>
> instead of
>
> "the Neufeld (quellung) reaction as adapted originally by Sabin[5a] for"

INDEX TO VOLUME 13

A

Aballi, Arturo J., and Kato, K., 364
Abrams, Alfred L., 513
Abramson, Harold, and Tunick, A. M., 94
Abscess, subphrenic, in children with special reference to roentgen signs of transphrenic infection, 157
Acidosis associated with sulfanilamide administration, 939
Acrodynia, nervous system in, 515
  nicotinic acid in treatment of, 891
Address, presidential, 1
Adenoidectomy, poliomyelitis, acute anterior, following tonsillectomy and, 63
Aldrich, C. Anderson, and Aldrich, M. M., 943 (B. rev.)
Aldrich, Mary M., and Aldrich, C. A., 943 (B. rev.)
Allergy, role of, in pediatric practice, panel discussion, 582
American Academy of Pediatrics, news, 301, 617, 941
    report, executive, 120
      of general meeting, 258
      of meeting of Region III, 933
      round table discussion, 143, 277, 434, 444, 605, 919
    panel discussion, 582
Anemia of newborn, round table discussion, 143
Anesthesia, relation of maternal sedation and, to neonatal asphyxia, 934
Anosmia following zinc sulfate nasal spraying, 60
Anoxia, cerebral injury in newborn due to, at birth, 933
  certain etiological factors and pathologic lesions in, 934
Anspack, William E., 157
Aorta, coarctation of (adult type), recognition of, during childhood, 303
Arena, Jay M., and Rasmussen, L. P., 352
Ascorbic acid (*see* Vitamin C)
  plasma concentration of, relation between, and diet of newborn infant, 309
Asher, Cecile, Hartmann, A. F., Perley, A. M., Basman, J., Nelson, M. V., and Morton, M., 692
Asphyxia, neonatal, relation of maternal, sedation, and anesthesia to, 934
Atelectasis, of lungs in newborn baby, resulting from lesion of nervous centers, 208

B

Babies are human beings, 943 (B. rev.)
Banana, ripe, as complementary feeding in infants, 239
Barbiturates transmitted through breast milk, 86
Barnes, Donald J., 935
Barraclough, W. Wray, Griffin, J. D. M., and Hawke, W. A., 75
Bartlett, Paul, and Gaebler, O. H., 936
Basman, Jack, Hartmann, A. F., Perley, A. M., Nelson, M. V., Asher, C., and Morton, M., 692
Behavior problems, pediatric, in infancy and early childhood, critical review, 417
Beres, David, and Schatia, V., 555
Bernstein, Samuel, 936
Bierman, Jessie M., Eliot, M. M., and Van Horn, A. L., 678
Biggs, Alfred D., and de Takats, G., 819
Biophotometer as test for vitamin A deficiency, 506
Blackfan, Kenneth D., and May, C. D., 627
Blanchard, Kenneth, and Goldberg, L. E., 381
Bleeding (*See* Hemorrhage)
Blood, carotinoids and vitamin A of, 635
  plasma, concentration of ascorbic acid in, relation between, and diet in newborn infant, 309
  vitamin C content of tonsils and; incidence of hemolytic streptococci in tonsils of children as related to, 322
Bolduan, Nils W., 357
Bone shaft, end of: Irregular extension of, in x-ray photograph in congenital syphilis, 748

Book review, Babies are human beings, 943
Interneships and residencies, 943
Tuberculosis among children and young adults, 302
Botsford, Thomas W., and Krakower, C., 185
Bromides transmitted through breast milk, 91
Brown, Alan, Tisdall, F. F., and Defries, R. D., 60
—, Tisdall, F. F., and Drake, T. G. H., 891
Bumbalo, T. S., and Jetter, W. W., 334

C

Calcium and nitrogen balance, continuous, in Legg-Perthes' disease treated with growth hormone and thyroid, 937
throughout periods just preceding and following menarche, 937
effect of thyroid in growth period, 937
Carbohydrate, use of honey as, in infant feeding, 465
Carotinoids and vitamin A of blood, 635
Celiac disease, ultimate prognosis in, 390
Central nervous system, lesions of, atelectasis of lungs in newborn baby, resulting from, 208
Cerebrum, hemorrhage in, in newborn, 934
injury to, in newborn, due to anoxia at birth, 933
Chemoprophylaxis, future of, as measure for practical control of poliomyelitis, 38
Childhood, early behavior in, some pediatric problems in infancy and, 417
endogenous reinfection of tuberculosis in, with particular reference to girl at puberty, 938
pneumonia in, serum treatment of, 219
recognition of coarctation (adult type) of aorta during, 303
Children, convulsive disorders in, histopathology of, 859
crippled, service for, accomplishments in maternal and child health, under Social Security Act, 678
gastrointestinal motility of, biological time patterns in, 935
hernia, diaphragmatic in, 939
mineral balance of, relation of growth and skeletal maturity to, 935
sulfanilamide in treatment of gonorrheal ophthalmia in, 527
Children—Cont'd
tuberculous, effect of supplementary synthetic vitamin C on urinary output of vitamin C by, 334
Christie, Amos U., 434
Circulation, blood, beginning of, first heart beats and, as shown by micromoving pictures of living embryos, 940
Citric acid, metabolism in infancy, 935
Clausen, S. W., and McCoord, A. B., 635
Cole, Warren C. C., and Kimball, D. C., 934
Comments, 454
Conjunctivitis, gonorrheal, sulfanilamide in treatment of, 938
in children, 527
phlyctenular, course and treatment of, 939
Convulsion, histopathology of, in children, 859
Cooke, Jean V., 651
Cooley, Thomas B., 143, 934
Craig, John Dorsey, 239
Craniotabes, relation of, to diet and growth, 936
Critical review, congenital syphilis, 101
heredity in disease, 555
immunity and susceptibility to disease in early infancy, 907
some pediatric problems of behavior in infancy and early childhood, 417

D

Darrow, Daniel C., 670
Davis, John A. V., 341
Debré, Robert, Marie, J., Lamy, M., and de Font-Réaulx, 208
Defries, R. D., Tisdall, F. F., and Brown, A., 60
Dehydration, deficit of sodium and chloride in, 670
Diabetes and pregnancy, 772
mellitus, round table discussion, 444
Diamond, Louis K., 143
Diaphragm, abscess of, special reference to roentgen signs of transphrenic infection, 157
Diet, relation of, to experimental production of goiter, 937
craniotabes to, and growth, 936
Diphtheria, polyneuritis from, 352
Disease, heredity in, critical review, 555
Diverticulum, Meckel's, ulceration of, relation of intestinal bleeding to heterotopic gastric mucosa, 513
Douglas, Bruce, and Johnston, J. A., 938

Drake, T. G. H., Tisdall, F. F., and Brown, A., 891
Drinker, Philip, and Roy, E. L., 71
Drugs, transmitted through breast milk, barbiturates, 86
bromides, 91
Dunham, Ethel C., and Whipple, D. V., 101
Durand, Jay I., 434

E

Eimas, Aaron, 550
Eisenberg, George, 303
Eley, R. Cannon, and Flake, C. G., 63
Eliot, Martha M., Bierman, J. M., and Van Horn, A. L., 678
Encephalitis, acute epidemic in St. Louis, 724
rheumatic (chorea minor of Sydenham), 741
Engelfried, John J., and Towsley, H. A., 939
Erythema annulare rheumaticum, 94
clinical significance of, in rheumatic states in childhood, 94
Erythroblastosis, of newborn, 934

F

Faber, Harold K., 10, 277
— and Lubin, A. J., 515
Feeding, infant, use of honey carbohydrates in, 465
Fetus, injury of, by roentgen ray during pregnancy, 894
Flake, Carlyle G., and Eley, R. C., 63
Fleming, Arthur W., and Sanford, H. N., 314
de Font-Réaulx, Debré, R., Marie, J., and Lamy, M., 208

G

Gaebler, O. H., and Bartlett, P., 936
Gastrointestinal system, motility of, biological time patterns in, 935
Gaucher's disease in early infancy, 364
Gerber, Alexander, and Stein, J. L., 547
Gesell, Arnold, 455
Goiter, experimental production of, relation of diet to, 937
Goldberg, Louis E., and Blanchard, K., 381
Gonococcus filtrate (Corbus-Ferry), treatment of gonorrheal vaginitis with, 381
Gonorrhea, vaginal, treatment of, with Corbus-Ferry gonococcus filtrate, 381
Griffin, J. D. M., Hawke, W. A., and Barraclough, W. W., 75
Growth, craniotabes, relation of, to diet and, 936
linear, vitamin D effect on, in infancy, 730
metabolic, effect of, and thyrotropic hormones administered with and without iodine, 936
period of, effect of thyroid on nitrogen and calcium in, 937
skeletal maturity and, relation of, to mineral balances of children, 935

H

Hass, Sidney V., 390
Hamil, Brenton M., 935
Hamilton, Paul M., 605
Hartman, Frank, 934
Hartmann, Alexis F., Perley, A. M., Basman, J., Nelson, M. V., Asher, C., and Morton, M., 692
Hartzell, John B., 939
Hawke, William A., 236
—, Griffin, J. D. M., and Barraclough, W. W., 75
Health, child and maternal, accomplishment in, and Crippled Children Services and, to Social Security Act, 678
systemic work in, for mother and child, 798
Heart beat, first, and beginning of circulation of blood as shown by micromoving pictures of living embryos, 940
hypertrophy, congenital idiopathic of, remarks on a case of, 760
Hemorrhage in cerebrum of newborn infant, 934
intestinal, relation of, to heterotopic gastric mucosa and relation of Meckel's diverticulum, 513
Hempelmann, T. C., 724
Heredity, in disease, 555
Hernia, diaphragmatic, in children, 939
Hirschsprung's disease (*see* Megacolon)
Honey, use of, as carbohydrate in infant feeding, 465
Hospital, orthopedic, mental hygiene in, 75
Howard, Philip J., 939
— and Montgomery, J. C., 934
Hygiene, mental, in orthopedic hospital, 75
role of pediatrician in, 940
Hyperlipemia, essential, metabolic observation in child with, 936
Hypertrophy, idiopathic congenital, of heart, 760
Hypogonadism, treatment of, in adolescent male, 847

I

Immunity and susceptibility to disease in early infancy, critical review, 907
Immunology, clinical, round table discussion, 919
Infancy, behavior in, some pediatric problems of, and early childhood, critical review, 417
early, Gaucher's disease in, 364
immunity and susceptibility to disease in, critical review, 907
effect of vitamin D on linear growth in, 730
metabolism of citric acid in, 935
pneumatosis of intestine in, 185
Infant, artificially fed, vitamin C requirements of, 935
feeding, complementary, ripe banana as, 239
newborn, anemia of, round table discussion, 143
asphyxia in, relation of maternal sedation and anesthesia to, 934
atelectasis of lungs in, resulting from lesions of nervous centers, 208
blood in, vitamin C content of, 314
cerebral hemorrhage in, 934
injury in, due to anoxia at birth, 933
diet in, relationship between plasma ascorbic acid concentration and, 309
erythroblastosis of, 934
evaluation of serologic tests for congenital syphilis with special reference to, 341
nursing care in, round table discussion, 434
rupture of liver in, 542
pancreas in, inspissation of secretion, dilatation of ducts and acini, atrophy and fibrosis of, 627
tonic neck reflex in, 455
Infantile paralysis (*see* Poliomyelitis)
Inoculation, intranasal, early lesions of poliomyelitis after, 10
Interneships and residencies, report of New York committee on study of hospital interneships and residencies, 943 (B. rev.)
Intestine, hemorrhage of, relation of, to heterotopic gastric mucosa and ulceration in Meckel's diverticulum, 513
obstruction of, use of small intestine decompression in treatment of, 938
pneumatosis of, in infancy, 185
Intestine—Cont'd
small, decompression of, in treatment of intestinal obstruction, 938
Iodine, metabolic effect of growth and thyrotropic hormones administered with and without, 936

J

Jackson, Deborah A., and Park, E. A., 748
Jaundice, epidemiologic and bacteriologic study of small outbreak in Detroit, 939
Jeans, P. C., and Stearns, G., 730
Jetter, W. W., and Bumbalo, T. S., 334
Johnson, F. Elmer, 891
Johnston, Charles G., 938
Johnston, Joseph A., 937
— and Douglas, B., 938
— and Maroney, J. W., 937
— and Mitchell, C. L., 937
Jordon, Paul H., 940
Josephs, Hugh W., 143

K

Kaiser, Albert D., and Slavi, B., 322
Kanner, Leo, 417
Kapnick, Israel, and McKhann, C. F., 907
Karelitz, Ruth F., and Karelitz, S., 195
Karelitz, Samuel, and Karelitz, R. F., 195
Kato, Katsuji, and Aballi, A. J., 364
Kimbal, David C., and Cole, W. C. C., 934
Klingman, Walter O., 805
Knott, Elizabeth M., and Schlutz, F. W., 465
Krakower, Cecil, and Botsford, T. W., 185
Krasnow, Frances, and McCall, J. O., 498

L

Lamy, Maurice, Debré, R., Marie, J., and deFont-Réaulx, 208
Law, John L., 940
LeCompte, Philip M., and Powers, G. F., 760
Legg-Perthes' disease, continuous calcium and nitrogen balances in, case of, treated with growth hormone and thyroid, 937
Leucemia, acute, experimental therapy with extract of bone marrow, 651
Lewis, Samuel J., 938
Liver, rupture of, in newborn infant, 542

Lubin, Albert J., and Faber, H. K., 515
Lungs, atelectasis of, in newborn baby, resulting from lesion of nervous centers, 208

M

Macy, Icie G., 935
Marie, Julien, Debré, R., Lamy, M., and deFont-Réaulx, 208
Maroney, John W., and Johnston, J. A., 937
Marriott, Williams McKim, dedication, 619
  bibliography, 622
Marrow, bone, extract of, experimental therapy of acute leucemia with, 651
Maturity, skeletal, relation of growth and, to mineral balance of children, 935
May, Charles D., and Blackfan, K. D., 627
McCall, John Oppie, and Krasnow, F., 498
McCoord, A. B., and Clausen, S. W., 635
McCulloch, Hugh, 741
McKhann, Charles F., and Kapnick, I., 907
Measles prophylaxis, study of, significance of conditions of exposure in, 195
Megacolon, congenital, observations on, 819
  neurogenic, treatment of, with selective drugs, 805
  treatment of, experience, clinical with, 940
Meningitis, meningococcus, treatment of, 357
Menstruation, inception of, continuous nitrogen and calcium balances throughout period just preceding and following, 937
Mernagh, Harry T., 939
Metabolism, influence of, on teeth, 498
Methyl salicylate, poisoning by, in infant, 550
Meyer, Karl F., 919
Michels, Merrill W., 527, 938
Milk, breast, drugs transmitted through, barbiturates, 86
  bromides, 91
Miller, John J., 277
Mindlin, Rowland L., 309
Mitchell, C. L., and Johnston, J. A., 937
Molner, Joseph G., 939
Montgomery, John C., and Howard, P. J., 934
Morton, Marie, Hartmann, A. F., Perley, A. M., Basman, J., Nelson, M. V., and Asher, C., 692
Myers, J. Arthur, 302
Myotonia, congenita, treated by quinine, 236

N

Narcosis, maternal, relation of, and anesthesia to neonatal asphyxia, 934
National health conference, 400
Nelson, Martha V., Hartmann, A. F., Perley, A. M., Basman, J., Asher C., and Morton, M., 692
Nemir, Rosa Lee, 219
Neuritis, multiple, diphtheritic, 352
News and notes, 301, 618, 941
Nicotinic acid, in treatment of acrodynia, 891
Nitrogen and calcium balance, continuous, in Legg-Perthes' disease treated with growth hormone and thyroid, 937
  throughout period just preceding and following menarche, 937
  effect of thyroid on, in growth period, 937
Nursing care in newborn infant, round table discussion, 434

O

Olney, Mary B., and Smyth, F. S., 772
Ophthalmia (*see* Conjunctivitis, gonorrheal)
Orthodontics, common ground of pediatrics and, 938
Oxygen therapy by open box method, 902

P

Pachman, Daniel J., 902
Pancreas, inspissation of secretion, dilatation of ducts and acini, atrophy and fibrosis of, in infants, 627
Panel discussion, role of allergy in pediatric practice, 582
Park, Edwards A., and Jackson, D. A., 748
Patten, Bradley M., 940
Peckham, C. H., 474, 484
Pediatrician, role of, in mental hygiene, 940
Pediatrics, common ground of, and orthodontics, 938
  practice of, role of allergy in, panel discussion, 582

Perley, Anne M., Hartmann, A. F., Basman, J., Nelson, M. V., Asher, C., and Morton, M., 692
Perlman, H. H., Tyson, R. M., and Shrader, E. A., 86, 91
Pneumatosis of intestines in infancy, 185
Pneumonia, serum treatment of, in children, 219
Poisoning, methyl salicylate, in infant, 550
Poliomyelitis, anterior, acute, following tonsillectomy and adenoidectomy, 63
  control, future of chemoprophylaxis as measure for, 38
  lesions, early, after intranasal inoculation, 10
  respiratory failure in, construction of emergency respirator for use in treating, 71
Poole, Marsh, 936
Powers, Grover F., and LeCompte, P. M., 760
Pregnancy, diabetes and, 772
  injury of fetus by roentgen ray during, 891
Prematurity, effect of certain obstetric factors, incidence of, and, 474
  incidence of, and effect of certain obstetric factors, 474
  mortality of, and effect of certain obstetric factors, 484
  statistical study of, incidence of and effect of certain obstetrical factors, 474, 484
Prophylaxis, chemical, future of, as measure for practical control of poliomyelitis, 38
Pylorus, stenosis, hypertrophic congenital of, 787

Q

Quinine, myotonia congenita treated by, 236

R

Rasmussen, Lester P., and Arena, J. M., 352
Ratner, Bret, 582
Reflex, tonic neck, in human infant, 455
Reproduction, human female hormones of, mechanical presentation of effects and interrelationship of, during menstrual cycle and pregnancy, 940
Respiration, failure of, construction of emergency respirator for use in infantile paralysis, 71
  intrauterine, significance of, 933
Respirator, emergency, construction of, for use in treating respiratory failure in infantile paralysis, 71
Reynolds, Lawrence, 935
Rheumatic fever, erythema annulare rheumaticum, clinical significance in, of childhood, 94
Roentgen ray, injury of fetus by, during pregnancy, 891
  sign of transphrenic infection in subphrenic abscess in children, 157
Round table discussions, anemia of newborn, 143
    clinical immunology, 919
    diabetes mellitus, 444
    nursing care in newborn infant, 434
    sulfanilamide, 605
    vaccine prophylaxis of whooping cough, 277
Roy, Edgar L., and Drinker, P., 71

S

St. Louis, encephalitis, acute epidemic in, 724
Sander, John, 939
Sanford, Heyworth N., and Fleming, A. W., 314
Scarlet fever, serum treatment of, comparison of specific and nonspecific, 938
Schatia, Viva, and Beres, D., 555
Schermerhorn, L. J., 277
Schlutz, F. W., and Knott, E. M., 465
Schreiber, Frederic, 933
Schultz, E. W., 38
Sedation (*see* Narcosis)
Serum phosphatase, in relation to vitamin D, 935
  therapy of pneumonia in childhood, 219
  treatment, comparison of specific and nonspecific, in scarlet fever. 938
Sharpless, G. R., 937
Shepardson, H. Clare, 444
Shrader, Earl A., Tyson, R. M., and Perlman, H. H., 86, 91
Silver, Harry B., 542
Singer-Brooks, Charlotte H., 277
Slavin, Betty, and Kaiser, A. D., 322
Smell, loss of, following zinc sulfate nasal spraying, 60
Smith, A. H., 935
Smyth, Francis Scott, and Olney, M. B., 772
Snelling, Charles E., 506

Social Security Act, accomplishment in maternal and child health and crippled children's service under, 678
Sodium lactate, metabolism and clinical uses of, further observations on, 692
Spine, fusion of, treatment of tuberculosis of spine by, 248
  tuberculosis of, treatment of, by spinal fusion, 248
Spray, nasal, zinc sulfate, persistent anosmia following, 60
Stearns, Genevieve, and Jeans, P. C., 730
Stein, Jacob L., and Gerber, A., 547
Steward, W. Dean, 510
Stomach mucosa, heterotopic, relation of intestinal bleeding to, and ulceration of Meckel's diverticulum, 513
Streptococci, hemolytic, incidence of, in tonsils of children as related to vitamin C content of tonsils and blood, 322
Sulfanilamide, administration of, acidosis associated with, 939
  in treatment of gonorrheal ophthalmia, 938
  in children, 527
  round table discussion of, 605
  therapy by, in erysipelas, 939
Susceptibility and immunity to disease in early infancy, critical review, 907
Swift, Walker E., 248
Syphilis, congenital, evaluation of serological tests for, 341
    irregular extensions of end of shaft in x-ray photograph, 748
    prevention and treatment, critical review, 101

T

de Takats, Geza, and Biggs, A. D., 819
Tallerman, Kenneth H., 787
Teeth, congenital absence of, 547
  influence of metabolism on, 498
Test, serologic, for congenital syphilis, evaluation of, 341
Thyroid, continuous calcium and nitrogen balance in Legg-Perthes' disease treated with growth hormone and, 937
  gland, effect of, on nitrogen and calcium, in growth period, 937
    therapy, metabolic effect of growth and, administered with and without iodine, 936
Thyrotropic hormone (*see* Thyroid gland)
Tisdall, Frederick F., Brown, A., and Defries, R. D., 60
—, Drake, T. G. H., and Brown, A., 891
Tonsils, hemolytic streptococci in, incidence of, in children, as related to vitamin C content of tonsil and blood, 322
  vitamin C content of blood and, incidence of hemolytic streptococci in tonsils, of children as related to, 322
Tonsillectomy, acute anterior poliomyelitis following, and adenoidectomy, 63
Towsley, Harry A., and Engelfried, J. J., 939
Tuberculin patch test, new, 510
Tuberculosis among children and young adults, 302 (B. rev.)
  endogenous reinfection type of, in childhood, with particular reference to girl at puberty, 938
  treatment of, of spine by spinal fusion, 248
  vitamin C in, 334
Tunick, Arthur M., and Abramson, H., 94
Tyson, Ralph M., Shrader, E. A., and Perlman, H. H., 86, 91

U

Undulant fever, diagnostic and therapeutic measures, 939
Urine, vitamin C output of, effect of supplementary synthetic vitamin C on, by tuberculous children, 334
Utheim-Toverud, Kirsten, 798

V

Vaginitis (*see* Gonorrhea)
Van Horn, A. L., Eliot, M. M., and Bierman, J. M., 678
Van Ingen, Philip, 1
Veeder, Borden, 619
Vitamin A, carotinoids and, of blood, 635
    deficiency of, biophotometer as test for, 506
  C (*see* also Ascorbic acid)
    blood content of, in newborn infant, 314
    in tonsil and blood, incidence of hemolytic streptococci in tonsils of children, 322
    in tuberculosis, 334
    requirement for artificially fed infant, 935

Vitamin C—Cont'd
synthetic, supplementary, effect of, on urinary output by tuberculosis, 334
D, effect of, on linear growth in infancy, 730
serum phosphatase in relation to, 935

W

Webster, Bruce, 847
West, Howard F., 444
Whipple, Dorothy V., and Dunham, E. C., 101
Whitaker, Wayne L., 940
Whooping cough, prophylaxis vaccine of, round table conference, 277
Wilson, James L., 933

Y

Young, Donald C., 938

Z

Zimmerman, H. M., 859
Zinc sulfate, persistent anosmia following nasal spraying, 60

5919
1-a